Simulation Champions
Fostering Courage, Caring, and Connection

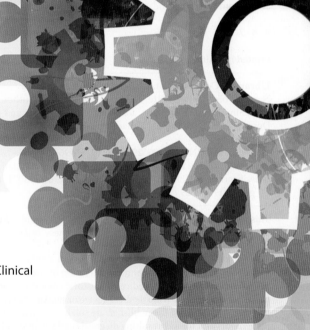

**Colette Foisy-Doll,
MSN, RN, CHSE**

Director, Clinical Simulation Centre
Professional Resource Faculty
Faculty of Nursing
MacEwan University
Edmonton, Alberta, Canada

**Kim Leighton, PhD, RN,
CHSE, CHSOS, ANEF**

Assistant Dean
Research & Simulation Faculty Development
DeVry Medical International's Institute for Research & Clinical
Strategy
Iselin, New Jersey

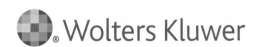
Wolters Kluwer

Philadelphia • Baltimore • New York • London
Buenos Aires • Hong Kong • Sydney • Tokyo

Executive Editor: Emily Lupash
Director of Product Development: Jennifer K. Forestieri
Senior Development Editor: Roxanne Halpine Ward
Editorial Coordinator: Jennifer DiRicco
Editorial Assistant: Hilari Bowman
Production Project Manager: Bridgett Dougherty
Design Coordinator: Teresa Mallon
Illustration Coordinator: Jennifer Clements
Manufacturing Coordinator: Karin Duffield
Prepress Vendor: SPi Global

Copyright © 2018 Wolters Kluwer

All rights reserved. This book is protected by copyright. No part of this book may be reproduced or transmitted in any form or by any means, including as photocopies or scanned-in or other electronic copies, or utilized by any information storage and retrieval system without written permission from the copyright owner, except for brief quotations embodied in critical articles and reviews. Materials appearing in this book prepared by individuals as part of their official duties as U.S. government employees are not covered by the above-mentioned copyright. To request permission, please contact Wolters Kluwer at Two Commerce Square, 2001 Market Street, Philadelphia, PA 19103, via email at permissions@lww.com, or via our website at lww.com (products and services).

9 8 7 6 5 4 3 2 1

Printed in China

Library of Congress Cataloging-in-Publication Data
Names: Foisy-Doll, Colette, author. | Leighton, Kim, author.
Title: Simulation champions : fostering courage, caring and connection / Colette Foisy-Doll, Kim Leighton.
Description: First edition. | Philadephia : Wolters Kluwer, [2018] | Includes bibliographical references and
    index.
Identifiers: LCCN 2017006629 | ISBN 9781496329776
Subjects: | MESH: Education, Nursing—methods | Simulation Training | Education, Medical—methods
Classification: LCC RT71 | NLM WY 18 | DDC 610.73071/1—dc23 LC record available at https://lccn.loc.
    gov/2017006629

This work is provided "as is," and the publisher disclaims any and all warranties, express or implied, including any warranties as to accuracy, comprehensiveness, or currency of the content of this work.

This work is no substitute for individual patient assessment based upon healthcare professionals' examination of each patient and consideration of, among other things, age, weight, gender, current or prior medical conditions, medication history, laboratory data and other factors unique to the patient. The publisher does not provide medical advice or guidance and this work is merely a reference tool. Healthcare professionals, and not the publisher, are solely responsible for the use of this work including all medical judgements and for any resulting diagnosis and treatments.

Given continuous, rapid advances in medical science and health information, independent professional verification of medical diagnoses, indications, appropriate pharmaceutical selections and dosages, and treatment options should be made and healthcare professionals should consult a variety of sources. When prescribing medication, healthcare professionals are advised to consult the product information sheet (the manufacturer's package insert) accompanying each drug to verify, among other things, conditions of use, warnings and side effects and identify any changes in dosage schedule or contraindications, particularly if the medication to be administered is new, infrequently used or has a narrow therapeutic range. To the maximum extent permitted under applicable law, no responsibility is assumed by the publisher for any injury and/or damage to persons or property, as a matter of products liability, negligence law or otherwise, or from any reference to or use by any person of this work.

LWW.com

Cover image credit: Chunyan Zhang, Simulation Technologist, MacEwan University, Edmonton, Alberta, Canada

Dedication

Our Simulation Champions book is dedicated to all the innovators, early adopters, and pioneers of simulation in nursing and our partners in healthcare. We are, because you are.

Colette and Kim

Contributors

Marguerite Abel, MSN, RN
Professor
Seminole State College
Altamonte Springs, Florida

Katie Anne Adamson Haerling, PhD, RN
Assistant Professor
University of Washington Tacoma
Tacoma, Washington

Michelle Aebersold, PhD, RN, FAAN
Clinical Associate Professor
School of Nursing
University of Michigan
Ann Arbor, Michigan

Leslie Allen, MA
NICU Parent Volunteer
Oregon Health and Science University
Hospital
Instructional Designer
GP Strategies
Portland, Oregon

Dimitri J. Anastakis, MD, MHPE, MHCM, FRCSC, FACS, FICS
Professor
Department of Surgery
Faculty of Medicine
University of Toronto
Chair, Board of Directors
SIM-one
Toronto, Ontario, Canada

Andrew Anderson
Chief Executive
Association for Simulated Practice in
Healthcare (ASPiH)
Banbury, Oxon, United Kingdom

Meghan Andrews, MD, BSc, FRCP(C)
Staff Anesthesiologist
Montfort Hospital
Lecturer
University of Ottawa
Ottawa, Ontario, Canada

L. Dawn Ansell, BN
Head, Interdisciplinary Simulation Centre
NorQuest College
Edmonton, Ontario, Canada

Teresa W. Atz, PhD, RN, CHSE
Assistant Professor
Director of Simulation
College of Nursing
Medical University of South Carolina
Charleston, South Carolina

Nasreen T. Bahreman, MSN, RN, PCNS-BC
Nurse
Johns Hopkins University
Baltimore, Maryland

Lance Baily, BA, FF1
Founder
Simghosts.org and Healthysimulation.com
Las Vegas, Nevada

Irmajean Bajnok, PhD, MScN, BScN, RN
Former Director
International Affairs and Best Practice
Guidelines Centre
Registered Nurses' Association of Ontario
Toronto, Ontario, Canada

Anthony J. Battaglia, MS, BSN, RN
President
Pocket Nurse®
Monaca, Pennsylvania

Alexis Battista, PhD
Assistant Professor
Department of Medicine
F. Edward Hérbert School of Medicine
Uniformed Services University of the
Health Sciences
Bethesda, Maryland

Eric B. Bauman, PhD, RN, FSSH
Assistant Dean
Institute for Research and Clinical
Strategy
Chair
Department of Educational Technology
and Game-Based Learning
DeVry Medical International
Iselin, New Jersey
Founder and Managing Member
Clinical Playground LLC
Madison, Wisconsin

Bryn Baxendale, MB ChB, FRCA, FAcadMedEd
Director
Trent Simulation & Clinical Skills Centre
Nottingham University Hospitals NHS
Trust
Nottingham, United Kingdom

Anne Blunden, DCUR, MCUR, RN, A
Executive Director of Nursing
King Abdullah Bin Abdullaziz University
Hospital
Riyadh, Saudi Arabia

Teresa Boese, DNP, RN
Simulation Operations Manager
American University of the Caribbean
Cupecoy, Dutch Lowlands, Sint Maarten

Catherine Bowman, MN, RN
Assistant Professor
Faculty of Nursing
MacEwan University
Edmonton, Alberta, Canada

Ruth Braga, MSN, BA, RN
Surgery Education Coordinator
School of Medicine
University of Utah
Salt Lake City, Utah

Ken Brisbin, EMT, CD
Simulation Regional Manager
Alberta Health Services
Edmonton, Alberta, Canada

Diana P.E. Callender, DM, MBBS
Chair
Department of Clinical Sciences
Director
Clinical Skills and Simulation Center
Geisinger Commonwealth School of
Medicine
Scranton, Pennsylvania

Mary Ann Cantrell, PhD, RN, CNE, FAAN
Professor of Nursing
College of Nursing
Villanova University
Villanova, Pennsylvania

Linda C. Carl, EdD, MSN, RN
Chair
American Health Information
Management Association (AHIMA)
Foundation Research Network
Education Consultant
North Charleston, South Carolina

Kathy Carver, MN, RN
Zamierowski Family Endowed Professor
Johnson County Community College
Overland Park, Kansas

Mary Cato, EdD, RN, CHSE
Assistant Professor
School of Nursing
Oregon Health and Science University
Portland, Oregon

Dustin Chan, BScN, RN
Associate Chair
Practical Nurse Program
NorQuest College
Edmonton, Alberta, Canada

Michelle Chiu, MD, FRCP(C)
Assistant Professor
Department of Anesthesiology & Pain
Medicine
Department of Innovation in Medical
Education
University of Ottawa
Ottawa, Ontario, Canada

Vimal Chopra, MD, PhD, FRCA
Section Head
Leiden University Medical Center
Leiden, The Netherlands

Timothy C. Clapper, PhD
Director of Education
Weill Cornell Medicine New York
Presbyterian Simulation Program & Center
Assistant Professor of Education in
Pediatrics
Weill Cornell Medical College
New York, New York

Sarah Clark, MSN, RN, CCRN, CHSE
Simulation Center Coordinator
Cone Health
Greensboro, North Carolina

Benjamin J. Damazo, BA
Loma Linda University School of
Medicine
Loma Linda, California

**Rebekah J. Damazo, MSN, PNP, RN,
CHSE-A**
Professor of Nursing
Rural SimCenter Director
California State University, Chico
Chico, California

**Joanne Lorraine Davies, MSc, RM,
CHSE**
Director
Simulation Department
Sidra Medical and Research Center
Doha, Qatar

Sharon I. Decker, PhD, RN, ANEF, FAAN
Associate Dean for Simulation and
Professor
School of Nursing
Covenant Health System Endowed
Chair in Simulation and Nursing
Education
Executive Director
The F. Marie Hall SimLife Center
Texas Technical University Health
Sciences Center
Lubbock, Texas

**Desiree A. Díaz, PhD, RN-BC, CNE,
CHSE-A**
Assistant Professor
University of Central Florida
Orlando, Florida

**Peter Dieckmann, PhD, Dipl. Psych.,
FSSH**
Psychodrama Director
Head of Research
Copenhagen Academy for Medical
Education and Simulation
(CAMES)
Center for Human Resources
Capital Region of Denmark
Herlev, Denmark

**Marion Donohoe, DNP, APRN,
CPNP-PC**
Assistant Professor
Loewenberg School of Nursing
University of Memphis
Memphis, Tennessee

Thomas J. Doyle, MSN, RN
President and CEO
SimOne Healthcare Consultants, LLC
Saint Petersburg, Florida

Bonnie Driggers, MS, MPA, RN
Professor Emerita
School of Nursing
Oregon Health and Science University
Portland, Oregon

Debra L. Duncan, BS, MLS
Instructional Designer/VLE Designer
Chamberlain College of Nursing
Weston, Wisconsin

Jane Duncan, EdD
Director, Learning and Development
Shock Trauma Air Rescue Society
Calgary, Alberta, Canada

Petra Duncan
Standardized Patient Educator/Trainer
University of Alberta
Edmonton, Alberta, Canada

Eliana Escudero Zúñiga, Msc.NU
Director
School of Nursing
Finis Terrae University
Providencia, Santiago, Chile

Tobias C. Everett, MBChB, EDRA, FRCA
Assistant Professor
University of Toronto
Staff Anesthesiologist
The Hospital for Sick Children
Toronto, Ontario, Canada

**Susan Gross Forneris, PhD, RN, CNE,
CHSE-A**
Excelsior Deputy Director
NLN Center for Innovation in
Simulation and Technology
National League for Nursing
Washington, District of Columbia

**Cynthia Foronda, PhD, RN, CNE, CHSE,
ANEF**
Associate Professor of Clinical
School of Nursing and Health Studies
University of Miami
Coral Gables, Florida

**Ashley Franklin, PhD, RN, CCRN, CNE,
CHSE**
Assistant Professor
Texas Christian University
Fort Worth, Texas

**Amy Fraser, MD, MSc, BScH, FRCP(C),
MHPE**
Anesthesiologist
The Ottawa Hospital
Assistant Professor
The University of Ottawa
Ottawa, Ontario, Canada

John Gillespie
Educational Solutions Account Executive
Laerdal Medical
Wappingers Falls, New York

**Sandra Goldsworthy, PhD, RN,
CCNCC(C), CMSN(C)**
Associate Professor
Faculty of Nursing
University of Calgary
Calgary, Alberta, Canada

**Teresa Gore, PhD, DNP, FNP-BC, NP-C,
CHSE-A**
Associate Professor
Director of Experiential Learning
College of Nursing
University of South Florida
Tampa, Florida

Leslie Graham, MN, RN, CNCC, CHSE
Professor
Durham College
Adjunct Professor
University of Ontario Institute of
Technology
RPN-to-BScN Coordinator
BScN Collaborative Nursing Program
Oshawa, Ontario, Canada

David J. Grant, MBCHB, MRCP, MRCPCH
Chair
Bristol Medical Simulation Centre
University Hospitals Bristol NHS
Foundation Trust
Bristol, United Kingdom

Vincent J. Grant, MD, FRCPC
Associate Professor
Departments of Pediatrics and
Emergency Medicine
Cumming School of Medicine
University of Calgary
Medical Director
KidSIM Program
Alberta Children's Hospital
Calgary, Alberta, Canada

Doris Grinspun, PhD, MSN, RN, LLD(Hon), O.ONT
Chief Executive Officer
Registered Nurses' Association of
Ontario (RNAO)
Toronto, Ontario, Canada

Paula Gubrud, EdD, RN, FAAN
Associate Professor
Special Assistant to the Dean
School of Nursing
Oregon Health and Science University
Portland, Oregon

Beth Fentress Hallmark, PhD, MSN, RN, CHSE
Director of Simulation
Gordon E. Inman College of Health
Sciences and Nursing
Belmont University
Nashville, Tennessee

Nicole Harder, PhD, RN
Assistant Professor
Faculty of Health Sciences
University of Manitoba
Winnipeg, Manitoba, Canada

Margaret Hassler, MSN, RN-BC, CHSE
Coordinator
Clarke Learning Laboratory
School of Nursing
Saint Louis University
St. Louis, Missouri

Bonnie Haupt, DNP, RN, CNL, CHSE
Clinical Nurse Leader
VA Healthcare System
West Haven, Connecticut

Damian A. Henri, RA, LEED AP
Senior Associate
Bostwick Design Partnership
Cleveland, Ohio

Helen Higham, MBChB, FRCA, SFHEA
Senior Clinical Research Fellow and
Director
OxSTaR
University of Oxford
Consultant Anaesthetist
Oxford University Hospitals NHS
Foundation Trust
Oxford, United Kingdom

Julie Hoffart, MN, BScN, RN
Coordinator
Clinical Simulation Centre
Senior Instructor
Faculty of Nursing
University of Calgary in Qatar
Doha, Qatar

Trisha Leann Horsley, PhD, RN, CHSE, CNE
Assistant Professor
Marcella Niehoff School of Nursing
Loyola University Chicago
Maywood, Illinois

James L. Huffman, MD, BSc, FRCPC
Associate Medical Director of
Education
Transport Physician
Shock Trauma Air Rescue
Society
Emergency Medicine Physician
Foothills Medical Centre
Clinical Lecturer
Cumming School of Medicine
University of Calgary
Calgary, Alberta, Canada

Caralise W. Hunt, PhD, RN
Associate Professor
Auburn University
Auburn, Alabama

Carol L. Huston, MSN, DPA, FAAN
Professor Emerita
California State University, Chico
Chico, California

Peter L.L. Jarvis, BA, MVA
Standardized Patient/Storyteller
MacEwan University
Edmonton, Alberta, Canada

Pamela R. Jeffries, PhD, RN, ANEF, FAAN
Dean and Professor
School of Nursing
The George Washington University
Washington, District of Columbia

Jayne Josephsen, EdD, RN, CHPN
Associate Professor
Boise State University
Boise, Idaho

Kirstyn M. Kameg, DNP, PMHNP-BC
Professor of Nursing
School of Nursing and Health
Sciences
PMHNP Program Coordinator
Robert Morris University
Moon Township, Pennsylvania

Fran Kamp, MS, RN, CHSE
Clinical Associate Professor
Learning Resource Center Coordinator
Georgia Baptist College of Nursing
Mercer University
Atlanta, Georgia

Suzan Kardong-Edgren, PhD, RN, CHSE, FSSH, ANEF, FAAN
Professor and Director
The RISE Center
School of Nursing and Health Sciences
Robert Morris University
Moon Township, Pennsylvania

Michelle Kelly, PhD, MN, BSc, RN
Associate Professor
School of Nursing, Midwifery and
Paramedicine
Director
Community of Practice
Curtin University
Perth, Western Australia, Australia

Karen Kennedy, MEd, BScN
Co-Owner
Eriter Creations Inc.
Stirling, Alberta, Canada

Sharla King, PhD
Director
Health Sciences Education and Research
Commons
Associate Professor
Department of Educational Psychology
University of Alberta
Edmonton, Alberta, Canada

Mike Lamacchia, EMT-P, CMTE
Vice President Operations, Alberta and
Saskatchewan
Shock Trauma Air Rescue Service
Calgary, Alberta, Canada

Sarah Lynn-Sells Lambert, MEd, BSN, RN
Distinguished Professor of Health
Simulation Facilitator
Sandhills Community College
Pinehurst, North Carolina

Timothy J. Laughlin, BA, CHSOS
Senior Simulation Specialist
Johnson County Community College
Overland Park, Kansas

Tracy Levett-Jones, PhD, MEd, RN
Professor of Nursing Education
University of Technology
Ultimo, New South Wales, Australia

Adam I. Levine, MD
Professor
Department of Anesthesiology,
Perioperative and Pain Medicine
Vice-Chair of Education
Icahn School of Medicine at Mount
Sinai
New York, New York

Karen L. Lewis, PhD
Administrative Director
Clinical Learning and Simulation Skills
Center
School of Medicine and Health Sciences
The George Washington University
Washington, District of Columbia

Lori Lioce, DNP, FNP-BC, RN, CHSE, FAANP
Clinical Associate Professor
Executive Director
Learning and Technology Resource
Center
College of Nursing
University of Alabama in Huntsville
Huntsville, Alabama

Michael Paul Lundin
Coordinator, Northern Clinical
Simulation
Northern Health Authority
Prince George, British Columbia,
Canada

Deepak Manhas, MD, FAAP, FRCP(C)
Clinical Assistant Professor
Division of Neonatology
Department of Paediatrics
Director
UBC Neonatal-Perinatal Medicine
Subspecialty Residency Training
Program
Neonatologist
BC Women's Hospital
Vancouver, British Columbia, Canada

Jennifer L. Manos, MSN, MBA, RN
Executive Director
Society for Simulation in Healthcare
Washington, District of Columbia

Bette Mariani, PhD, RN
Assistant Professor of Nursing
College of Nursing
Villanova University
Villanova, Pennsylvania

Dee McGonigle, PhD, RN, CNE, FAAN, ANEF
Director
Virtual Learning Experiences
Professor
Graduate Programs
Chamberlain College of Nursing
Dillon, South Carolina

Bernadette Mazurek Melnyk, PhD, RN, CPNP/PMHNP, FAANP, FNAP, FAAN
Vice President for Health Promotion
University Chief Wellness Officer
Dean and Professor
College of Nursing
Professor of Pediatrics and Psychiatry
College of Medicine
The Ohio State University
Columbus, Ohio

Charlene Mercer, MALAT, RRT, CHSE
Simulation Instruction Specialist
Sidra Medical and Research Center
Doha, Qatar

Robin June Miller, PhD, RN, CNE
Associate Clinical Professor
School of Nursing
University of Connecticut
Groton, Connecticut

Margaret Milner, MN, RN
Assistant Professor
MacEwan University
Edmonton, Alberta, Canada

AnneMarie Monachino, MSN, RN, CPN, CHSE
Simulation Educator
Children's Hospital of Philadelphia
Adjunct Faculty
Graduate School of Biomedical Sciences
and Professional Studies
College of Medicine
Drexel University
Philadelphia, Pennsylvania

Susan Morhart, RN (Retired)
Simulation Administrator
Northern Ontario School of Medicine
Thunder Bay, Ontario, Canada

Jason L. Morris, MD, FACP
Associate Professor
University of Alabama at
Birmingham
Birmingham, Alabama

Jonathan M. Mould, PhD
Simulation Coordinator
Joondalup Health Campus
Joondalup, Washington

Wendy M. Nehring, PhD, RN, FAAN, FAAIDD
Dean and Professor
College of Nursing
East Tennessee State University
Johnson City, Tennessee

Louis Oberndorf, MBA, BA
CEO
Oberndorf Holdings, LLC
Sarasota, Florida

Holldrid Odreman, PhD, MScN-Ed, RN
Professor of Nursing
Program Coordinator
Niagara College Canada
Welland, Ontario, Canada

Brandi Pawliuk, MN(MH), BScN, RN, CPMHN(C)
Unit Manager
Alberta Health Services Royal Alexandra
Hospital
Edmonton, Alberta, Canada

Barbara Peterson, MSN, RN
Simulation Specialist
Children's of Minnesota
St. Paul, Minnesota

Marcia A. Petrini, PhD, FAAN
Visiting Professor
Faculty of Nursing
Chiang Mai University
Muang, Chiang Mai, Thailand
Emeritus Dean
Professor
School of Nursing
Wuhan University
Wuhan, Hubei, People's Republic of
China

Oralea A. Pittman, DNP, FNP-BC, FAANP
Clinical Assistant Professor
College of Nursing
The Ohio State University
Columbus, Ohio

E. Carol Polifroni, EdD, RN, CNE, NEA-BC, ANEF
Dean and Professor
School of Nursing
University of Connecticut
Storrs, Connecticut

Summer Langston Powers, DNP, CRNP, ACNP-BC, AACC
Assistant Professor
The University of Alabama at Birmingham
Birmingham, Alabama

Susan Prion, EdD, RN, CNE
Professor
School of Nursing and Health Professions
University of San Francisco
San Francisco, California

Renee Pyburn, MS, RN, CHSE
Faculty, Masters in Nursing Program
College of Medicine and Health Sciences
University of Rwanda
Kigali, Rwanda

Rochelle Quinn, MSN, RN, CHSE
Associate Professor of Nursing
Healthcare Simulation Center
Johnson County Community College
Overland Park, Kansas

Purnima Rao, MD, BSc(Hon), FRCPC
Lecturer
University of Ottawa
Anesthesiologist
The Ottawa Hospital
Ottawa, Ontario, Canada

Scott Reeves, PhD, MSc, PGCE
Professor in Interprofessional Research
Kingston University & St. George's,
University of London
London, United Kingdom

Andrew Reid, MEdHSE, BScN, RN
Simulation Consultant
Alberta Health Services
Edmonton, Alberta, Canada

Kerry Reid-Searl, PhD, MClinEd, BhlthSc, RN, RM
Professor
Deputy Head of Program
School of Nursing, Midwifery and Social Science
CQ University Australia
Rockhampton, Queensland, Australia

Karol C. Renfroe, MSN, RN
Assistant Clinical Professor
School of Nursing
Auburn University
Auburn, Alabama

Mindy Ritter, MS, RN, CEN
Nursing Faculty
Healthcare Simulation Center
Johnson County Community College
Overland Park, Kansas

Mary Anne Rizzolo, EdD, RN, FAAN, ANEF
Consultant
Scotch Plains, New Jersey

Pamela Rock, BSc, PT
Associate Director
Health Sciences Education and Research Commons (HSERC)
University of Alberta
Edmonton, Alberta, Canada

Lisa Rohrig, BSN, RN
Director
Technology Learning Complex
College of Nursing
The Ohio State University
Columbus, Ohio

Cynthia Rubbelke, MEd, MSN(R), RN
e-Technology Coordinator
School of Nursing
Saint Louis University
St. Louis, Missouri

Sharon Saidi, MSN, RN, CNE
Adjunct Professor
Seminole State College
Altamonte Springs, Florida

Jill S. Sanko, PhD, MS, ARNP, CHSE-A
Assistant Professor
Academic and Research Director of Simulation
School of Nursing and Health Studies
University of Miami
Coral Gables, Florida

Susan A. Schory, MEd, BSN, RNC-OB
Visiting Clinical Instructor
University of Illinois, Chicago
Chicago, Illinois

Carolyn Schubert, DNP, CNE, RN-BC
Assistant Professor of Clinical Nursing
The Ohio State University
Columbus, Ohio

Ella Scott, RN, RSCN, Grad Cert PIC MA
Senior Simulation Operations Manager
Sidra Medical and Research Center
Doha, Qatar

Michael Seropian, MD, FRCPC, FSSH
Professor of Anesthesiology and Pediatrics
Oregon Health and Science University
Portland, Oregon

Barbara Sittner, PhD, APRN-CNS, RN, ANEF
Professor of Nursing
Bryan College of Health Sciences
Lincoln, Nebraska

Jayne Smitten, PhD, MEd Dipl. AdultEd., BA, RN, CHSE-A
Interim Director
Clinical Simulation Center
Chair and Professor
Baccalaureate Nursing Program
College of Health and Society
Hawai'i Pacific University, Hawai'i Loa Campus
Kaneohe, Hawaii

Andrew E. Spain, MA, NCEE, EMT-P
Director of Accreditation and Certification
Society for Simulation in Healthcare
Washington, District of Columbia

Stephanie N. Sudikoff, MD
Director of Simulation
SYN:APSE Center for Learning, Transformation, and Innovation
Yale-New Haven Health System
Associate Clinical Professor of Pediatrics
Pediatric Critical Care
Yale School of Medicine
New Haven, Connecticut

Rita Swanson, BSN, RN
Adjunct Professor
Simulation Educator
Seminole State College
Altamonte Springs, Florida

Natalie Lu Sweeney, MS, CNS, RNC-NIC
Adjunct Faculty
Dominican University of California
San Rafael, California

Sandra M. Swoboda, MS, RN, FCCM
Clinical Research Program Coordinator
Simulation Educator
Johns Hopkins University
Baltimore, Maryland

M. Elaine Tagliareni, EdD, RN, CNE, FAAN
Chief Program Officer
Director, Center for Excellence in the Care of Vulnerable Populations
National League for Nursing
Washington, District of Columbia

Antoine Tesniere, MD, PhD
Director
iLumens Simulation Department
Paris Descartes Medical School
Sorbonne Paris Cité University
Paris, France

Susan L. Thelen
Artist
Madison, South Dakota

Cynthia M. Thomas, EdD, MS, BSN, RNC
Associate Professor
Ball State University
Muncie, Indiana

Jillian Thomas, BScN, RN, CPMHN(C)
Nurse Educator
MacEwan University
Edmonton, Alberta, Canada

Maureen Tremel, MSN, ARNP, CNE, CHSE-A, ANEF
Nursing Professor
Seminole State College of Florida
Altamonte Springs, Florida

Mark Tuttle, BS, PMD
EMS/Coordinator
Suncoast Technical College
Sarasota, Florida

Philomène Uwimana, MSN, RN
Acting Director of Simulation and Clinical Skills Center
Assistant Lecturer
University of Rwanda
Kigali, Rwanda

Mohamud Verjee, MBA, MBChB, BSc(Hon), DRCOG, CCFP, FCFP
Director
Primary Care Clerkship
Associate Professor
Weill Cornell Medicine, Qatar
Doha, Qatar
Adjunct Associate Professor
University of Calgary
Calgary, Alberta, Canada

Colleen Dianne Ward, BSHEc
Co-Owner
Eriter Creations Inc.
Stirling, Alberta, Canada

Penni I. Watts, PhD, RN
Assistant Professor
Director of Clinical Simulation and Training
School of Nursing
University of Alabama at Birmingham
Birmingham, Alabama

Peter Weinstock, MD, PhD
Director and Anesthesia Chair in Pediatric Simulation
Senior Associate
Critical Care Medicine
Boston Children's Hospital
Associate Professor
Harvard Medical School
Boston, Massachusetts

Norbert Werner, MEd, ACP
Instructor
Advanced Care Paramedic Program
School of Health and Life Sciences
Northern Alberta Institute of Technology
Edmonton, Alberta, Canada

Graham Andrew Whiteside, BSc(Hons) Nur Sci, DipHE MHN, RMN, RGN
Vice President of Sales and Marketing
SIMnext, LLC
Urbana, Illinois

Nikki Wiggins, MSN, RN, CCRN
Assistant Nurse Manager
Doernbecher Neonatal Intensive Care Unit
Oregon Health and Science University
Portland, Oregon

Carol Wild, MScN, BN, RN
Assistant Professor
Grant MacEwan University
Edmonton, Alberta, Canada

Amanda R. Wilford, RGN (Hons), Dip ANC, ENB 254, ENB 998
Group Leader
CAE Healthcare International Academy
Burgess Hill, West Sussex, United Kingdom

Paul Woodcock
Virtual Learning Environment Developer
Chamberlain College of Nursing
Downers Grove, Illinois

Leanne Wyrostok, MN, BN, RN(r)
Senior Instructor Emerita
University of Calgary
Calgary, Alberta, Canada

H. Michael Young, BBS, MDiv, CHSE
Director of Healthcare Education and Business Development
Level 3 Healthcare
Stephenville, Texas

Bin Zheng, MD, PhD
Associate Professor
Endowed Research Chair in Surgical Simulation
University of Alberta
Edmonton, Alberta, Canada

Reviewers

Nancy Barker, EdD, MSN, BSN, ADN
Assistant Professor
Immaculata University
Immaculata, Pennsylvania

Alicia Book, MSN, RN
Assistant Professor
Louisiana State University at Alexandria
Alexandria, Louisiana

Carol Butler, MScN, MEd, BScN, RN
Coordinator of Clinical Learning and
Simulation
Fanshawe College
London, Ontario, Canada

Catherine Cantrell, MSN, RN, OCN, BLS
Outcomes Coordinator
Aquinas College
Grand Rapids, Michigan

Jeffrey Carmack, DNP, MSN, RN, CHSE
Instructor
University of Arkansas at Little Rock
Little Rock, Arkansas

Lorraine Chiappetta, MSN, CNE, RN
Faculty
Washtenaw Community College
Ann Arbor, Michigan

Irene Coulson, PhD, BScN, RN
Nursing Professor
MacEwan University
Edmonton, Alberta, Canada

Sally Davis, MSN, RN, CNE
Nursing Instructor
Program Chair
Western Technical College
LaCrosse, Wisconsin

Christina Devlin, MSN, RN, FCN
Faculty
Hannah E. Mullins School of Practical
Nursing
Salem, Ohio

**Marci Dial, DNP, ARNP, NP-C, MSN,
BSN, RN-BC, LNC, CHSE**
Professor
Valencia College
Orlando, Florida

Barbara Doyer, MS, BSN, RN
Lecturer, Coordinator, Skills Lab
California State University, Fullerton
Fullerton, California

Ana Fernandez, DNP, MSN
Assistant Professor
Nova Southeastern University
Cape Coral, Florida

Dawn Ferry, MSN, RN, CHSE
Professor
Widener University
Chester, Pennsylvania

Gina Fieler, MSN, RN
Simulation Facilitator/Lecturer
Northern Kentucky University
Highland Heights, Kentucky

Chris Gabourie, AEd, CMA
Paramedic Educator
Ornge Transport Medicine
Mississauga, Ontario, Canada

Kateri Gabriele, MSN, BS
Simulation Coordinator
Dayton VA Medical Center
Dayton, Ohio

**Laura Gonzalez, PhD, ARNP,
CNE, CHSE**
Clinical Assistant Professor
Simulation Coordinator
University of Central Florida
Orlando, Florida

**Kristen Mathieu Gonzalez,
MSN/Ed, RN**
Assistant Professor
Laboratory Manager
Northeastern University
Burlington, Massachusetts

Claudia Haile, MSN, RN
Associate Professor
Corning Community College
Corning, New York

Amy Hamilton, MSN, RN, CNE
Instructor
Gaston College
Dallas, North Carolina

Margaret Hassler, MSN, RN-BC, CHSE
Laboratory Coordinator
Saint Louis University
Saint Louis, Missouri

**Glenenna Haynes-Smith, DNP,
MSN, RN**
Associate Professor
St. George's University at Grenada
True Blue, Grenada

Belinda Hermosura, MS
Clinical Simulation Lab Clinical
Instructor
University of Maryland
College Park, Maryland

Pamela Hicks, MSN, RN
Skills Lab Coordinator
Simulation Specialist
Middlesex County College
Edison, New Jersey

**Elizabeth Horsley, MEd, MSMS, RN,
CHSE**
Director of Simulation Lab
The Brooklyn Hospital Center
Brooklyn, New York

Susie Hutchins, DNP
Simulation Lab Coordinator
University of San Diego
San Diego, California

Ashley Johnson, MSN, BSN
Simulation and Skills Lab Coordinator
Bethel University
Saint Paul, Minnesota

**Denise Johnson-Dawkins, DNP, MSN,
RN, CNL**
Simulation and Skills Lab Coordinator
California State University, Bakersfield
Bakersfield, California

Sharla King, PhD
Director
Health Sciences Education and Research
Commons
Associate Professor
Department of Educational Psychology
University of Alberta
Edmonton, Alberta, Canada

Tywana Lawson
Director of Nursing
Nash Community College
Rocky Mount, North Carolina

Melissa Leal, MSN, RN, CHSE
Simulation Director
Instructor
Texas Tech Health Science Center
Lubbock, Texas

Kathee Long, MSN, BSN
Lab Coordinator
Simulation Director
Wright Career College
Overland Park, Kansas

Dawn MacGibeny, EdD, MSN, RN, Certificate in Simulation
Lab and Simulation Coordinator
Our Lady Lourdes School of Nursing
Camden, New Jersey

Shirley MacNeill, MSN, RN, CNE
LNV to ADN Program Coordinator
Lamar State College
Port Arthur, Texas

Melissa Morris, MSN, RN, CHSE
Clinical Manager of HPS and Skills Lab
Nova Southeastern University
Fort Lauderdale, Florida

Robbie L. Murphy, BSN, RN
Simulation Coordinator
San Jacinto College, North
Houston, Texas

Janet Peterson, MSN, RN
Nursing Skills Lab Coordinator
Kent State University
Kent, Ohio

Sami Rahman, MEd, MSN, RN
Director of Simulation
Blinn College
Brenham, Texas

Scott Reeves, PhD, MSc, PGCE
Professor in Interprofessional Research
Kingston University & St. George's,
University of London
London, United Kingdom

Carol Reid, MS, RN
Assistant Clinical Professor
Metropolitan State University
Saint Paul, Minnesota

Pamela Roberts, MSN, RN
Nursing Laboratory Manager
Montgomery County Community
College
Montgomery County, Pennsylvania

Jacqueline Robinson, PhD(c), MBA, MSN, CCRN, ACNS-BC
Gerontology Certificate Manager
Nursing Resource Laboratory
Cleveland State University
Cleveland, Ohio

Katie Robinson, MSN, RN
Simulation Coordinator
Jacksonville State University
Jacksonville, Alabama

Cynthia Rubbelke, MEd, MSN(R), RN
e-Technology Coordinator
School of Nursing
Saint Louis University
St. Louis, Missouri

Rosemary Samia
Simulation and Clinical Lab Educator
University of Massachusetts, Boston
Boston, Massachusetts

Erica Santelmo, MSN, RN
Instructor
Rockland Community College
Suffern, New York

Elizabeth Scarano, MEd
Associate Professor
Lewis-Clark State College
Lewiston, Idaho

Jacqueline Semann, MSN, RNC-LRN, CNS
Nursing Faculty
Lake Superior College
Duluth, Minnesota

Mary Ann Shinnick, PhD, ACNP, CCNS, CCRN
Director of Simulation
School of Nursing
University of California, Los Angeles
Los Angeles, California

Becky Shuttlesworth, BSN, RN
Simulation Coordinator
San Jacinto College South
Houston, Texas

Lisa Sparacino, PhD, RN, CCRN, CNE
Assistant Professor
New York Institute of Technology
New York, New York

Tracey Stehman, EdD
Simulation Coordinator
St. Johns River State College
Jacksonville, Florida

Donnean Thrall, DNS, RN
Assistant Professor
Hackensack UMC/Mountainside
Glen Ridge, New Jersey

Elizabeth Vega, DNP, CNE
Assistant Professor
Sim Lab Educator
Concordia University—Irvine
Irvine, California

Amy Weaver, PhD, RN, CNE
Assistant Professor
Youngstown State University
Youngstown, Ohio

Teressa Wexler, EdD, MSN, RN
Assistant Professor
Simulation Coordinator
East Tennessee State University
Johnson City, Tennessee

Jean Yockey, PhD, FNP-BC, CNE
Assistant Professor
University of South Dakota
Vermillion, South Dakota

Bin Zheng, MD, PhD
Associate Professor
Endowed Research Chair in Surgical
Simulation
University of Alberta
Edmonton, Alberta, Canada

Foreword

The hardest thing is not to get people to accept new ideas; it is to get them to forget the old ones…

—John Maynard Keynes

The clinical apprenticeship method and the academic model used to teach nursing have remained unchanged for half a century, even as the underlying assumptions of those strategies were crumbling. Changing patient demographics, changing reimbursement for hospitalizations, the mass adoption of electronic health records and medication administration, and increasing calls for demonstrated competencies of health providers all created the perfect climate for the advancement of simulation in health professions education.

The pioneers of simulation in nursing were experimenting in the early 2000s. They wrote the first articles, conducted the first nursing research studies in simulation, wrote the first scenarios, experimented with debriefing techniques for nurses, and drafted policies and procedures. Arguably, one of the most important things these simulation pioneers did was become simulation champions within their own programs. As they witnessed the power of simulation, they were convinced early on that it was going to create a major shift in nursing education as we know it. But how to convince the other faculty? These authors, these simulation champions, have gathered other like-minded early adopters of simulation to write a compendium of collected wisdom to move faculty and nursing programs or hospitals forward with the successful adoption of simulation as a major part of teaching, onboarding, or competency evaluation.

Although many programs and hospitals now have well-developed simulation programs, many others are only now beginning to develop those nascent programs in earnest, with one or two simulation champions to lead the way. Luckily, today, there is no reason to reinvent the wheel! This book provides strategies and tools, garnered through personal experience and reaching out to other simulation champions, to more efficiently evaluate the readiness of the existing culture for simulation, and to develop strategies for simulation adoption, maintenance, and evaluation from a variety of perspectives. *Simulation Champions* is edited by two of our most experienced simulationist colleagues, who for more than a decade each have been immersed in simulation center design, program development, instrument development for measuring simulation outcomes, and further large-scale evaluation of simulation programs. They provide the gift of a collection that will nurture all simulation champions. Enjoy!

Suzie Kardong-Edgren, PhD, RN, CHSE, FSSH, ANEF, FAAN

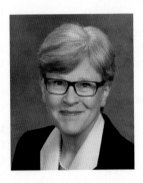

About This Book

Simulation Champions: Fostering Courage, Caring, and Connection is a book for nurses and other healthcare providers, from both academia and clinical practice, whether they are newcomers to simulation or seasoned simulationists in search of new perspectives and ideas. "Simulation Champions" are those individuals and teams that assume various roles and functions in the planning, deployment, evaluation, and advancement of simulation in healthcare worldwide. Simulation Champions are *difference makers*, working to cultivate culture change toward safer, more effective, reliable, and ethical patient- and family-centered healthcare. The title also contains three important words: *courage, caring, and connection.* We believe that these are the core values that bind us and that emanate through our collective achievements over our decades of work in simulation education.

Simulation Champions: *Courage*

This book could have been titled "The Chronicles of Courage" because it contains personal accounts of the courage it took to spearhead simulation as a disruptive innovation in our institutions and clinical practice settings at a time when only innovators could see its potential and the courage it took to stand up for much-needed change; the courage it took to push nursing education and training to places it had not gone before. But mostly, it speaks of the courage it took to become change leaders and to do the right thing by our learners and our patients and their families. We proudly offer this book as a legacy—a way of marking the contributions of many simulation pioneers throughout the world. Their collective stories provide a unique historical perspective on simulation in nursing and nursing education.

Simulation Champions: *Caring*

We are a community that cares very deeply about excellence in simulation-based learning and in healthcare education. We believe that experiential learning is inextricably tied to the learning process and that using best practices in simulation produces positive outcomes for the learners and populations we serve.

We care about finding solutions to the big problems we face in academe and clinical practice settings. Today's healthcare systems are highly complex and complicated; therefore, the solutions needed to address these problems require astute and capable leaders, followers, and managers. This book is about caring enough to make great things happen. We feature and celebrate *leadership, followership,* and *managership* for the Simulation Champion and offer current evidence for how we can acquire the essential skills we all need to move simulation forward into the 21st century.

You will notice as you read that the book is written in both the first and third person, which may seem an unusual approach. However, this writing style was intentionally used, as it provides you with a more personal connection. Our goal is to address simple to complex subjects in an easily digestible and nonintimidating fashion—as if you were learning the concepts side by side with a trusted friend, which is what we strive to be to all members of the simulation community.

Simulation Champions: *Connection*

This book is about connection and connecting people. It is our way of reaching out to join simulationists from around the world to give voice to their unique stories. Regardless of our diverse cultural backgrounds and work environments, we are working together to advance our global mandate to transform healthcare and healthcare education through the use of simulation.

We have assembled the narratives and contributions of over 150 simulation champions from all over the world and proudly feature their stories. Several sections of the book also feature the incredible contributions of our partners in allied health and medicine. We also offer chapters featuring the groundbreaking contributions of our formal communities of practice: the *International Nursing Association for Clinical Simulation and Learning* (INACSL), *the National League for Nursing* (NLN), and the *Society for Simulation in Healthcare* (SSH), as well as other simulation associations from around the world.

We enthusiastically welcome new members to our simulation community of practice, providing you with a plethora of helpful tools. We sincerely hope that you will enjoy and appreciate this collection of evidence, along with perspective sharing and storytelling, and the account of nursing's history and future in simulation.

The Text

The book contains 28 chapters that are divided into eight units. Each of the chapters offers grounding theory related to the specific content addressed, and then provides practical suggestions for application and a host of helpful tools.

The breakdown of the content is as follows:

Section 1, The Evolution of Simulation

Section 1, The Evolution of Simulation, charts the course of simulation in nursing and healthcare partners. *Chapter 1* provides a brief synopsis of the trajectory of simulation in healthcare, with an emphasis on nursing and nursing education, as well as an overview of the key drivers in the evolution of simulation in healthcare. *Chapter 2* takes a look at how early simulation leaders connected within their schools, within geographical regions, and across countries, to create steadfast networks to support pioneering simulationists. *Chapter 3* offers a historical account of the development of the International Nursing Association for Clinical Simulation and Learning (INACSL) and features current strategic directions and the many initiatives undertaken to meet their goals. *Chapter 4* delivers a historical overview of key milestones in the development of the Society for Simulation in Healthcare (SSH) and provides a summary of its many initiatives and services. *Chapter 5* features the National League for Nursing (NLN)'s work to advance simulation within nursing education and in the broader interprofessional context, while also addressing some of the challenges and opportunities arising from the use of simulation in nursing education. *Chapter 6* focuses on today's cutting edge simulation typologies, the tools we use to enact simulation delivery modalities. *Chapter 7* provides an overview of the many educational platforms used to deliver effective simulation learning events, which we termed in this book as Simulation Delivery Modalities.

Section 2, Leadership and Management in Simulation

Section 2, Leadership and Management in Simulation, addresses the essential leader, follower, and manager roles and functions that Simulation Champions enact to advance simulation from local to global. *Chapter 8* leads you through a review of key concepts for the 21st century leader. Simulation Champions are invited to reflect on new leadership paradigms and on how to use contemporary leadership approaches to leadership, followership, managership, and most of all, relationship. *Chapter 9* discusses relevant information on organizational change, culture, and climate and provides tools and perspectives to promote positive change experiences in the adoption and curricular integration of simulation in your milieu. *Chapter 10* focuses on how to go about building a simulation team where the right people, the right chemistry, the right skills, and the right attitudes make amazing things happen. *Chapter 11* walks you through the key steps to managing and operationalizing simulation programs. This chapter is loaded with resources to help you get your program off the ground! *Chapter 12* discusses key considerations for developing and managing a comprehensive simulated/standardized patient (SP) program.

Section 3, Globalization and Culture in Simulation

Section 3, Globalization and Culture in Simulation, is an exciting section that offers different views on simulation in nursing through the lenses of culture, diversity, and globalization. *Chapter 13* deals with the many competencies required of simulation champions working and collaborating in a globalized world. *Chapter 14* focuses on cultural competence, safety, and humility and why these are key competencies and considerations in simulation education. *Chapter 15* includes global perspectives on simulation and gives voice to the fascinating stories of simulation champions from Africa, Australia, Canada, China, Europe, the Middle East, Latin America, and the United States.

Section 4, The Art and Science of Simulation

Section 4, The Art and Science of Simulation, presents both the scientific and artistic dimensions required for best practices in delivering effective simulation education. *Chapter 16* guides you through a reflection on the importance of having a solid theoretical foundation for your simulation-based teaching practices. *Chapter 17* is the first chapter ever written on evidence-based practice (EBP) in simulation and explores the many ways you can integrate EBP and inquiry into your institution's simulation program. *Chapter 18* addresses the state of the science in nursing simulation research, past, present, and future and provides our readers with suggestions to help plan for and develop a research project, get it funded, and start your simulation research program. *Chapter 19* shares the tips and tricks of the artistic, theatrical side of simulation and reminds us that "Cinema should make you forget you are sitting in a theater" (Irving, 2010).

Section 5, Developing Simulation Education

Section 5, Developing Simulation Education, introduces fundamental concepts and approaches to developing, deploying, and evaluating simulation education events. *Chapter 20* will guide you from start to finish in designing simulation-based learning experiences grounded in simulation design best practice and offers words of wisdom on cost-effective ways of managing simulation design. *Chapter 21* discusses the roles of educators and technical and support personnel in simulation while keeping in mind that with significant overlap in these roles, it is not always clear "who is supposed to do what." *Chapter 22* is all about our learners: how to support them, how to create safe spaces for learning, and what proven methods decrease their stress. *Chapter 23* is a simulation idea factory, with numerous examples stemming from a broad range of nursing practice settings to provide you with interesting ideas for simulation integration in your programs.

Section 6, Simulation Across Health Disciplines

Section 6, Simulation Across Health Disciplines, invites the perspectives of nursing's frontline partners in healthcare simulation. *Chapter 24* explores the efforts of pioneers in medical simulation, the current types and uses of simulation for medical healthcare professionals, and the future of medical simulation for learner assessment and competence-based training. *Chapter 25* provides a brief introduction to the use of simulation in the context of allied health education and then uses an exemplar demonstrating the championing of simulation in various applications within an institute of technology. *Chapter 26* outlines the practical strategies and approaches that one partnership developed and implemented to ensure that learners had access to high-quality simulation-enhanced interprofessional education.

Section 7, Developing Learning Spaces

Section 7, Developing Learning Spaces, consists of *Chapter 27*, "The Simulation Champion's Ten Step Approach to Space Planning, Design, and Build," and the online Companion Workbook Series. Together, these resources offer a wealth of information for those tasked with designing and developing simulation learning spaces.

Section 8, Future Directions

Section 8, Future Directions, is comprised of the final chapter, *28*. This chapter envisions VIP-U, the Virtual Interprofessional University of the future. Let your imagination soar and think of what the healthcare school of the future and simulation-based learning will look like in 10, 15, or 20 years from today.

We are pleased to be able to include a glossary with this book. We worked toward providing a cohesive taxonomy but were challenged to find a perfect fit each term used in this book and the comprehensive resources provided by the *INACSL Standards of Best Practice: Simulation*[SM] glossary (INACSL Standards Committee, 2016) and the *Healthcare Simulation Dictionary* (Lopreiato et al., 2016). We have, therefore, provided definitions of the terms that seemed most valuable to have on hand for quick reference, and have referred the reader to these other resources when necessary. Both the INACSL Standards glossary and the Healthcare Simulation Dictionary are available online and are living documents, so the reader would be well served to consult the most current version available.

Book Design

As editors, we challenged the publisher's graphic design team to create a theme for the *Simulation Champions* book. We wanted a striking color scheme and motif to capture the essence of both the art and science of simulation-based learning. To us, this meant visually bringing to life key concepts of courage, caring, connection, teamwork, evolution, innovation, exploration, problem solving, engagement, learning, and transformation. It was a tall order and we want to thank the talented design team for meeting the task at hand and for their skillful depiction of the cogs and puzzle pieces that make up the beautiful design throughout the book.

Features of the Text

Notable in-text features include the following:

- **Key Terms.** Each chapter begins with a list of *key terms* that are defined in context (and bolded) when used for the first time in-text. Key term definitions are found in our glossary.
- **Guiding Questions.** This book is different from a student textbook, so we opted to provide readers guiding questions instead of learning objectives at the start of each chapter, allowing you to anticipate the content you should expect to learn about. Once you have finished reading the chapter, you should be able to answer the questions you were challenged to answer at the beginning.
- **Reflection Activities.** Some chapters include points for you to ponder more deeply. They may also invite you to reflect and create a plan for action.

- **Voice of Experience.** Another excellent feature of the book is the personal narratives of simulation champions presented in the *Voice of Experience* features throughout the book. Each story is unique to their lived experiences and explains a challenge encountered involving simulation, how they were able to meet the challenge, the outcomes, lessons learned, and inspirational quotes or messages from them to you.
- **Simulation on a Shoestring** offers creative ideas to save your program valuable dollars. Not all simulation programs have adequate access to funding, and simulationists are very creative people!

- **Standards of Best Practice.** Wherever chapters refer to the implementation or use of the INACSL Standards of Best Practice: Simulation^{SM}, we have earmarked them with a special icon. Look for the "Standards" symbol throughout the book for evidence of how the authors are using and implementing the Standards.

- **Online Toolkit Resources.** Whenever a helpful tool is available in our Online Toolkit, a special icon in the text will let you know! A list of all Toolkit items associated with each chapter appears at the end of the chapter.

- **Figures, tables, and boxes** colorfully highlight important content and reinforce key information.

thePoint® **Online Toolkit**

Simulation Champions: Fostering Courage, Caring, and Connection has an Online Toolkit designed with your needs in mind, available on thePoint® website. We wanted to provide our readers with practical key resources in the areas where we all seemed to struggle. To that end, the Online Toolkit contains a treasury of helpful tools and resources for you, ranging from the Simulation Manager's Booklet Series to the amazing step-by-step online workbooks that accompany The Simulation Champion's 10 Step Approach to Space Planning, Design, and Build (Chapter 27), and more! You can access the Online Toolkit via thePoint by redeeming the scratch-off code found in the inside front cover of this book.

Closing Note

We sincerely hope that you benefit from this book. Enjoy and welcome to the simulation community of practice!

Colette Foisy-Doll and Kim Leighton

Acknowledgments

Expressions of Gratitude: Colette

I love reading and telling stories, so my expressions of gratitude are tied to a meaningful personal story. My roots are firmly planted at Lac St. Cyr, a small lake community in Northern Alberta, Canada, where I spent each summer of my life and where I engaged in much of the writing and editing of this book. I learned all of life's most important lessons at the lake, including having an appreciation for and connection to life, beauty, and nature; the essential role of family and community; the value of hard work for the benefit of others; the importance of creative self-expression; the desire to understand nature; and the need to be grateful for everything this world so generously offers. The picture you see below is the view of the lake from my Pépère Foisy's old outdoor swing. The swing had been neglected and forgotten for many years, and my Papa, unable to part with it, asked that I restore it. Now back to its former glory, it resides on the front porch of my family's cottage. While rocking on the old swing, I read Kathy Malloch's and Tim Porter O'Grady's work on *Intentional Sharing of Knowledge and Wisdom* and was profoundly struck by their explicit mandate to pass on to the next generation their life-long body of work, encompassing a vast collection of intellectual property amassed over their careers in nursing. I recognized the deep sense of gratitude I hold for generational wisdom in all its forms. With the same spirit of sharing as Malloch and Porter O'Grady, I hope also to pass on the wisdom I have gained over many years of working in simulation education.

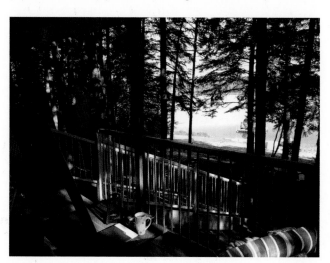

With thanks to my parents and late grandparents for the gift of their love and for the generational wisdom they imparted to me—*merci beaucoup Papa et Maman*. To my husband Greg, and my two sons, Justin and Patrick, you have been *my best teachers in life*, and I love you dearly. I am ever so grateful for my sisters: Suzanne, Christine, Michelle, and Danielle, and for my brother Paul, and my extended family and their many children. Your precious friendship and unwavering support (tempered with cautionary warnings to slow down) is what carries me through always.

Of the many who assisted me on my simulation journey, one person stands out. She was the person who first agreed to allow me to take my 3rd year students to "try out this simulator thing" at the hospital and then wrote the grant submission that brought simulation to MacEwan University. Former Dean Sharon Bookhalter, your courage, dedication, and spirit of innovation, as well as your belief in me brought us to where we are today. I also want to acknowledge all my nursing colleagues at MacEwan University for being such exemplary and creative nurse educators: you teach, inspire, and amaze me every day. Thank you!

Last but not least, I want to thank my trusted friend, my simulation mentor, and beautiful Simulation Champion, par excellence! Dr. Kim Leighton, thank you for sharing this journey with me, it has been just as amazing as you are.

Expressions of Gratitude: Kim

I'm a firm believer that everything happens for a reason and that we should always consider the "road less taken" as it will likely lead us into adventure and expose us to opportunities we didn't even know existed. When I reflect on how I reached this point in my career, two key people stand out as having made a difference in my decision as to which path to follow.

Mrs. Phylis Hollamon Berg was the President of Bryan College of Health Sciences, where I began my teaching career. On a very cold January day, Phylis asked if I would go to a conference in Tampa and tell her whether we should buy a patient simulator. I responded with an emphatic yes. Later, I asked "What's a patient simulator?" I remember calling her my first night in Tampa to tell her to write the check. Upon my return, Phylis put me in charge of integrating simulation throughout our curriculum because I was now the "expert." Knowing what a patient simulator was equated with expertise at that time! Phylis gave me the responsibility and then, a greater gift, she let me figure out how to make it all happen. It was her faith and trust in me that allowed me to experiment, to try new and different ways of teaching, and to determine how best to manage that one simulator—that eventually grew into an 11-bed simulation center.

Dr. Sheldon Stick was my doctoral advisor and supported me even when I changed my dissertation topic after writing the full proposal. He about ran out of red ink when reviewing drafts of my work! Dr. Stick was also a stickler for proper use of the English language, which has been a tremendous help to my ambition to be a better writer. He also stimulated in me a love for research. After surviving a dissertation that included 33 research questions and required approval of five IRBs, I found myself equipped to pursue a career trajectory that focused on educational research. Sheldon has continued to support me long after he retired, recently meeting me for lunch when I presented at a conference near his home and staying until he could hear my introduction as the speaker. I am indebted to him for his guidance and friendship.

My gratitude to my parents can never be overstated. They were both educators and instilled in our family the importance of education and life-long learning. They freely gave their support to my endeavors (or crazy ideas, depending on your viewpoint!) and always told me how proud they were of my accomplishments. I miss them immensely but know they continue to support me from heaven.

Lastly, my dear friend Colette. We have laughed, we have cried, we have been frustrated, and we have been joyous. What an adventure this has been. Thank you for asking me to take this journey with you. I never cease to be awed by your passion and wisdom.

Shared Gratitude

Together, we are grateful to our many colleagues in simulation, in nursing, and our partners in healthcare. These amazing healthcare professionals have taught us the true meaning of the word *interprofessional team*. We acknowledge and commend each of you for your dedication to the provision of better, safe, ethical, effective, and compassionate patient care. Lastly, we wish to thank our mentors in nursing, nursing education, and in simulation who have encouraged, empowered, and inspired us to be the best version of ourselves. You know who you are.

Colette Foisy-Doll and Kim Leighton

Contents

SECTION 1: THE EVOLUTION OF SIMULATION

SECTION 2: LEADERSHIP AND MANAGEMENT IN SIMULATION

SECTION 3: GLOBALIZATION AND CULTURE IN SIMULATION

SECTION 4: THE ART AND SCIENCE OF SIMULATION

SECTION 5: DEVELOPING SIMULATION EDUCATION

SECTION 6: SIMULATION ACROSS HEALTH DISCIPLINES

SECTION 7: DEVELOPING LEARNING SPACES

SECTION 8: FUTURE DIRECTIONS

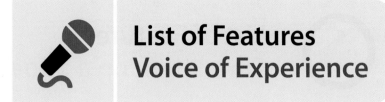

List of Features
Voice of Experience

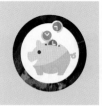

List of Features
Simulation on a Shoestring

1

Historical and Current Key Drivers for Simulation in Healthcare

Colette Foisy-Doll, Kim Leighton

 Key Terms

Simulation Champions, Innovator, Early Adopter, Simulation-Based Learning, Simulation-Based Education, Globalization, Learning Paradigms, Learning Theory, Benchmark, Guidelines, Accreditation Standards, Standards of Best Practice: Simulation, Patient Safety, Aviation, Secretive Culture, Culture of Blame, Just Culture, Systems Approach, High-Risk Industry, Person-, and Family-Centered Care, Disclosure, Error Tracking, Human Factors, SIM-IPE, Complex Adaptive Systems, Complexity

 Guiding Questions

1 Are you aware of the evolution of simulation in nursing and healthcare worldwide?

2 If you were asked to present a case for simulation integration to transform nursing education in your workplace, would you have timely and accurate information you need about the key drivers that formed the cornerstone of all simulation initiatives?

3 Should simulation be used to complement or replace traditional clinical experiences and practice hours in your nursing program?

4 Within today's global mandates for patient safety, person-centered care, team competencies, and improved patient care outcomes, what can you, as a Simulation Champion, do to transform nursing education?

5 How can the Simulation Champion work to eradicate the culture of punishment and blame in healthcare to transform our work environments to a culture of safety?

We live in amazing yet challenging times. Our world seems fraught with the dichotomy of chaos amidst seemingly endless opportunity. Likewise, today's healthcare and healthcare education contexts are replete with complexity amidst astonishing innovation. It is in this context that **Simulation Champions** emerged to confront head on the need to impact meaningful change in healthcare. Simulation Champions, in the context of this book, are all past, present, and future courageous, caring, and connected leaders, followers, and managers that drive the advancement of simulation around the world. They come from many backgrounds, disciplines, and industries. These Simulation Champions are the

● Emergent simulationists who bravely forged the road to what we now know as current practice in simulation

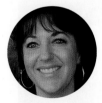

Colette Foisy-Doll,
MSN, RN, CHSE

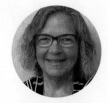

Kim Leighton,
PhD, RN, CHSE, CHSOS, ANEF

- Pioneers who first connected and collaborated to form international organizations and local communities of practice
- Educators who advocated for best practice and high standards in simulation through a commitment to excellence in teaching, transformational learning, research, and scholarship
- Healthcare professionals and clinicians from diverse disciplines working to improve as teams that provide safer, effective, ethical patient care
- **Innovators** and creators of new technologies that support simulation delivery and learning; they are the doers in the trenches who work hard day in, day out to deliver excellence in simulation
- Committed administrators of our institutions and policy makers who care to support and enact organizational and system change

Simulation Champions are *difference makers*, working to cultivate a cultural shift toward safer, more effective, and ethical person-, and family-centered healthcare.

It is said that *context is everything*, so to that end, we begin this book by providing a brief synopsis of the trajectory of simulation in healthcare, with an emphasis on nursing and nursing education. Our legacy as passionate simulationists of this generation is what we will leave to the next generation of simulationists. Together, we are the collective creators of tomorrow's reality, the ones who initiate change, and are, therefore, in a better position to manage the change that is ultimately inevitable. Both the choices we have made over the past 10 to 15 years and those we make in the years ahead will impact the evolution of simulation pedagogy, simulation programs, simulation modalities and typologies, and the future of healthcare itself in very significant ways. Therefore, it is vital for us to take pause, reflect on the past and present, and then look to the future. In doing so, we will discuss simulation in healthcare and explore its development and advancement in light of key global, international, and national historical and current drivers that continue to influence and shape its trajectory. Key drivers in the evolution of simulation in healthcare in recent decades are the demand for **patient safety** and quality improvement, marked advancements in technology, and the call for transformation in nursing and healthcare education.

In this chapter, we provide a brief overview of the history of simulation in healthcare and nursing education. We examine a broad overview of current educational realities and calls for radical transformation in nursing education and healthcare programs, a key driver for simulation. Additionally, we offer an account of the key lessons learned from other high-risk industries, such as aviation, nuclear power, and engineering, and an overview of key drivers for organizational change in healthcare. These include human factors, patient safety, person-, and family-centered care, interprofessional competency development, workforce transformation, shifting scopes of practice, and systems-based approaches. Lastly, we review current benchmarks and emerging **standards and guidelines** for simulation and the need for accountability and risk management in simulation.

History of Simulation in Healthcare

For as long as humans have played, there has been simulation. As far back as 3,000 years ago, the Chinese army used a war game called "Wei-Hai" as a means of simulating war strategies where black and white tokens were moved around a game board, reminiscent of modern chess. In 300 B.C., Herophilus, the ancient Greek father of anatomy, employed simulation as a means of modeling the human body. In the 18th century, jousting afforded knights valuable experience in the development of battlefield skills (Bradley, 2006).

The dawn of the information age dates back to the 1970s with the revolution in computer technology, networking, and information systems. It is within this context that early healthcare simulation took root and evolved to its current level of sophistication. In recent decades, **high-risk industries** have progressively introduced more technologically advanced forms of simulation. For example, dating back to the 1930s, the armed forces used simulation for training. The nuclear power industry has developed highly sophisticated nuclear power plant operations simulators for development and testing of nuclear systems to avert the devastation of nuclear reactor meltdowns. Moreover, simulation throughout aviation history has served as means of testing flight craft, as well as for educational and training purposes. Today, in the **aviation** industry, terms such as *aviation training* or *flight simulator* have become commonplace (Fig. 1.1). Moreover, flight aviation simulation principles have had a direct impact on simulation in healthcare, for example, the emergence of *Crew Resource Management* (CRM) that "promotes the development of superior non-technical skills such as communication, teamwork, situational awareness, and leadership" (McMaster University, 2013, para. 1). It was later adapted

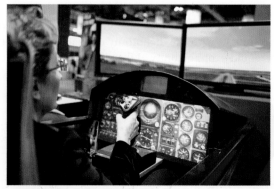

Figure 1.1 Flight simulator. (Editorial credit: pcruciatti / Shutterstock, Inc.).

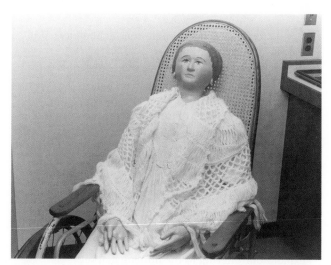

Figure 1.2 The Creation of Mrs. Chase in 1911 Marked the Advent of Human Simulators. (Used from The Hamilton Archives, Hartford Hospital, with permission.)

to become *Anesthesiology Crisis Resource Management* (ACRM), regularly used today as CRM training in healthcare (Blum et al., 2004; Bornais, Foisy-Doll, & Wyrostok, 2014; Bradley, 2006). The aviation industry continues to lead and innovate using simulation, especially in the areas of *Crew Resource Management* and safety through the study of human factors to mitigate harmful and sometimes disastrous outcomes. Today, when passengers board an airplane, they know with certainty that the crew has trained using simulation. Why then, are such standards not applied to healthcare?

In nursing, the use of simulation dates back to the early 1900s, a time when oranges served as the tool of choice for practicing injections. Later, in 1911, marked the advent of human simulator use with the creation of *Mrs. Chase* (Herrmann, 1981, 2008) (Fig. 1.2), a static, low-fidelity, non-interactive mannequin that offered little realism but provided an opportunity for nursing students to practice patient care. The modern era of simulation was initiated in the 60s, bringing with it the more interactive *Sim One* human simulator, Asmund Laerdal's *Resusci Anne* cardiopulmonary resuscitation trainer (Fig. 1.3), and *Harvey*, equipped with

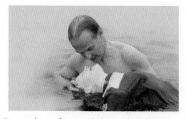

Figure 1.3 Founder of Laerdal Medical, Asmund Laerdal, with Resusci Anne in 1969. (From *The Story of Resusci Anne and the beginnings of Modern CPR*. Retrieved from http://www.laerdal.com/gb/doc/2738/The-Story-of-Resusci-Anne-and-the-beginnings-of-Modern-CPR. Photo courtesy of Laerdal Medical. All rights reserved.

more sophistication such as movement and audible sounds. In the decades that followed the introduction of Mrs. Chase in nursing education there was a lack of urgency to adopt mannequins as teaching tools, and the subsequent uptake of static simulators was slow. At the time, the vast majority of psychomotor skills practice in nursing education took place in the clinical setting on patients at the bedside. This practice was part of the contemporaneous apprenticeship model of the day (Bradley, 2006). In addition to a lack of urgency to change traditional practices, static mannequins were also limited in availability, lacked portability, were costly, and had design and maintenance challenges (Bornais et al., 2014).

It was not until the 1960s that Denson and Abrahamson, both anesthesiologists from the University of Southern California, developed the first fully interactive full-body computer-controlled mannequin simulator. The simulator, named Sim One, proved useful in anesthesia for training induction and endotracheal intubation. This prototype operated via a large computerized mainframe attached to the mannequin via tethered electrical and gas cords. The narrow scope of functionality that Sim One offered, coupled with its large price tag, eventually led to a lack of adoption in medical education. The 1980s saw the dawn of more sophisticated and less expensive computer hardware and software systems, and a resulting increase in development of simulation systems used in aviation, military training, nuclear power generation, and space flights.

In 1985, Dr. David Gaba, a professor of anesthesiology at Stanford University, and a small team of faculty and students set out to build a simulator for training purposes, adopting a "just do it" Nike approach. Fueled by his background in biomedical engineering and a passion for aviation, the design and development of simulators was a great fit for Gaba (Rosen, 2013a). In 1987, the C.A.S.E. 1.2 Simulator (Comprehensive Anesthesia Simulation Environments) was born. The simulator's crude design featured an off-the-rack static mannequin head, neck, and thorax and such supplies as plastic tubing and bags for lungs (Rosen, 2013a). Crude or not, it was impressive that this partially retrofitted mannequin with its' technological supports offered the first physiological and pharmacological modeled states. The C.A.S.E. 1.2 first went into production through a Canadian aviation simulation company, CAE-LINK. In the years that followed, more than one company took ownership and the name evolved to include both The Eagle Patient Simulator and, later, the Med-Eagle Patient Simulator. The Eagle Patient Simulator was the first to offer eyes that opened and closed, pupillary constriction and dilatation, heart and breath sounds, changeable airway anatomy, palpable carotid and radial pulses, and a thumb twitch to mimic nerve stimulation (Gaba, Howard, Fish, Smith, & Sowb, 2001; Smith & Gaba, 2001). The Eagle was used for anesthesiology training and the care of critically ill patients (Stanford University, 2015). By the 1990s, anesthesia simulation development expanded to include the HPS—Human Patient Simulator (HPS), another physiologically driven simulator created by Medical Education Technologies Inc. (METI). The HPS mannequin proved useful in the implementation of anesthesiology training, characterized by dynamic, intense, uncertain environments where problems were ill-structured and ill-defined (Gaba et al. 2001). Later, with the influence of simulation for Crew Resource Management in aviation, medicine also integrated simulator training to create and practice systematic emergency procedures and practice technical and nontechnical skills for challenging situations. Later, simulator use spread to other medical specialties like critical care, obstetrics, emergency medicine, and internal medicine (Lateef, 2010). However, at that time, use still lagged in nursing education due, in large part, to the cost of the simulators.

Read about how Lou Oberndorf, then President and CEO of Medical Education Technologies, Inc., leveraged his company's resources to pioneer and advance simulation technologies in nursing education.

1-1 Voice of Experience
METI History: How We Introduced METI High-Fidelity Simulators into Nursing Education

● ●

Louis Oberndorf, MBA, BA

● ●

The Challenge

In 1996, I started METI by selling one of the first commercial human patient simulators to medical schools. From the moment I witnessed the simulator in action, I recognized its potential to transform healthcare learning. The simulator had a clear purpose for anesthesia. Yet one of our key strategic challenges as a business was to expand its use beyond anesthesia. What piqued my interest early on was its potential to revolutionize nursing education.

Meeting the Challenge

The academic medical community and even a few of the inventors were skeptical. Whenever I presented the METI Human Patient Simulator, the HPS, as a learning tool for nursing, I would hear the same three questions. Why do nurses need high-fidelity simulation? Can they handle the technology? Will they be able to afford it?

Despite the obstacles, we made a strong commitment to focus on nursing education. At the same time, Betty Castor, who was Florida's Secretary of Education, was eager to introduce this new technology into Florida's community colleges. With support from Governor Jeb Bush, they made a brave decision to purchase two of the first simulators for Tallahassee Community College and Santa Fe College. We partnered with them to deliver the pilot program. Later, the state provided matching funds for the purchase of four simulators in community colleges each year. Their financial support paved the way for us to expand our offering to the nursing market.

From the beginning, we understood that the models of training for medicine and nursing are significantly different but also the same. We knew we would have to customize our technology for nursing education. We reached out to nurse educators, and we partnered with nursing faculty to write a curriculum for nursing that integrated the use of simulation technology. We committed our support to professional nursing organization such as NLN and AACN and INACSL.

Outcome

One of the highlights of those collaborations was the creation of the Program for Nursing Curriculum Integration, known as the PNCI. With Texas Woman's University as the lead, we partnered with a faculty and institutions to completely revamp the undergraduate nursing curriculum and build a 4-year curriculum around the use of simulation.

We developed a library of Simulated Clinical Experiences (SCEs), a storehouse of learning scenarios. It also provided flexibility, so educators could pick and choose how and when to incorporate simulation. I think the arrival of PNCI will be remembered as one of the hallmarks in advancing nursing education.

Once we committed to nursing education, we integrated it into every R&D project for new patient simulators—PediaSim, BabySim, iStan, and METIman. Each new simulator had at its core a foundation of experience from the perspective of nursing.

During that early period of skepticism, what kept me going was the reaction of the nursing students and their wonderment at the technology. The power of simulation, not only for building competency but also for instilling confidence, was a constant source of motivation for me.

Twenty years later, simulation today is the gold standard for nursing education, and it has followed nursing into hospital-based simulation practice and continuing education. The innovators and **early adopters** within nursing are now leading the major professional organizations.

Most Valuable Lesson Learned

When we entered the uncharted territory of delivering new technology into the nursing classroom, my mantra was this: if it's valuable for physician education, simulation is absolutely essential for nursing education and all of healthcare. The lesson learned is not to listen to anyone who would try to create a pyramid or a hierarchy of learning in healthcare education.

Our foray into nursing education allowed us to evolve from a simulation company to an education company and to realize the full potential of simulation to transform learning for all of healthcare.

Early in the 21st century, the price point for patient simulators drastically fell as computer technology changed. During that time, computers moved from requiring large mainframes for computing to using the compact, personal computer. These smaller components made simulator redesign possible, producing more portable, less expensive options such as the Emergency Care Simulator (METI) and SimMan (Laerdal). All of a sudden, simulators became viable alternatives that nursing budgets could manage. In the mid-2000s, simulation curriculum design also took hold, filling a critical niche for experiential learning in nursing programs. As the use of simulation began to take root, both educators and administrators recognized that scenario development was a layered, time-consuming process. Off-the-shelf products such as the Program for Nursing Curriculum Integration (METI) and the NLN Simulation Scenarios (Laerdal) were designed to enable faculty to integrate simulation into their curriculum more quickly. Despite these advances and the ready availability of simulators, we are still seeing simulators sitting in boxes, purchased, yet unused. There are many reasons for this— all of which this book is designed to help overcome.

The past decade has given rise to significant advancements in simulation with the introduction of highly sophisticated, increasingly user-friendly, computer-driven *human patient simulators* that offer higher levels of fidelity (realism), increased interaction, and ease of use. Now, there are diverse simulators that cover gender, skin tone, and age spectrums (See Figure 1.4). Simultaneously, a paradigm shift was taking place with a marked shift to improved patient safety and total quality improvement in the delivery of patient care. As a result, there

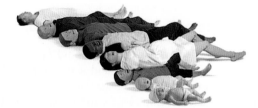

Figure 1.4 Laerdal Family of Simulators. Photo courtesy of Laerdal Medical. All rights reserved.

is now widespread acknowledgment that development of undergraduate competencies can no longer come at the expense of patient safety. The *"see one, do one, teach one"* apprenticeship approach that had students trained at the point of care on live patients was no longer acceptable. It became possible to employ a *no risk to the patient* approach using **simulation-based learning** (SBL) to bridge the gap between theory, lab skills practice, and clinical practice (Gates, Parr, & Hugen, 2012; Jeffries, 2007b). Contemporary educational methodologies shifted to place a stronger emphasis on *active learning in curricula* using a host of simulation modalities (the educational platforms used to deliver simulation) and simulation typologies (the tools used to enact the modalities) (INACSL Standards Committee, 2016. Simulation Design). Read how Dr. Adam Levine became the recipient of the first patient simulator sold and how the support he received from his organization's leadership helped to grow their simulation program.

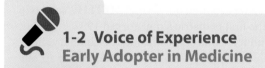

1-2 Voice of Experience
Early Adopter in Medicine

Adam I. Levine, MD

The Challenge

My experience getting "THE" very first simulator is really no different than someone today getting "THEIR" very first simulator in terms of challenges. At a cost of $175,000, we officially took receipt and installed the very first Loral Human Patient Simulator during April 1994. Though the first simulator was remarkably sophisticated, it only recognized seven intravenous agents, ran on DOS software, and was not easily programmed.

(Continued)

1-2 Voice of Experience (*Continued*)

We had 3 months to prepare and create scenarios for the new residents and a research study; we needed every moment of that time to create the curriculum and develop cases with the existing technology. The lessons learned proved invaluable as the simulation technology improved and scenario building and programming became possible.

Meeting the Challenge

As a new attending physician with interest in education, I was honored to be involved in the new simulation initiative at Mount Sinai. I quickly realized the critical importance of mentorship, departmental leadership support, and the presence of a productive, effective team was going to be key to the success of our program. We assembled a faculty team and met frequently as we developed an entirely new method of teaching. We designed the new simulation-based curriculum, focusing on the importance of scenario building and debriefing.

Outcome

We achieved several milestones during the early years:

- Installed the first simulator in an existing operating room—a true first "in situ" simulator.
- Became one of the first multisimulator centers when we acquired our second METI HPS and one of the first pediatric simulators in 1997.
- Conducted one of the first interdisciplinary simulations in 1997. We moved our simulator to our level 1 trauma center so we could create simulations for a NOVA special on head trauma. We gathered attending physicians and trainees from several specialties, respiratory therapists, and ER nurses to trial simulations for a day, followed by actual filming the following day. It's ironic to think that we were only planning for a TV spot and what we actually did was deliberate multidisciplinary team training.

Most Valuable Lessons Learned

Don't be afraid to dive in, experiment, and learn through creative trial and error. Much of how I conduct simulation today was formulated during my very early experiences with this wonderful new teaching tool.

We learned a lot about simulation, **simulation-based education** (SBE), formative assessment, and debriefing as a whole. We were fascinated by the process of introducing simulation to a broader audience and were convinced that this technology was hugely advantageous to medical educators and would naturally become part of all training programs. Recognizing the power of mistakes, errors, and failure was born from our early experiences and has set the tone of our simulation scenarios and our research efforts to this day.

Inspiration for Simulation Champions

"The best way to meet any challenge can be summed up in one sentence 'don't go it alone', and starting one of the world's first simulator programs is no different."

Excerpts from Levine, A. I., DeMaria, S., Schwartz, A., & Sim, A. (2013). *The comprehensive textbook of healthcare simulation* (Chapter 2, pp. 33–39). New York, NY: Springer Science and Business Media.

Simulation in healthcare has reached far beyond its North American roots to countries all around the world. A recent market research report titled *Global Medical Simulation Market Outlook: 2013–2020* reports simulation industry growth projections of compound annual growth rate (CAGR) of 14.8% from 2015 to 2020. The report lists factors that have impeded growth as being "principally, the high cost of simulators, and reluctance to adopt new training methods" (p. 4). The major global simulation market continues to be North America, where a steady growth is anticipated during the forecast period, followed by Europe and Asia Pacific (namely, India and China) (Meticulous Research, 2015). Growth in the latter is tied to increasing economic development, an increased awareness the need for patient safety and the growing focus on the global simulation players in these markets. Furthermore, they predict an explosive expansion in the global virtual patient simulation. The reports states that "Markets in healthcare simulation will reach $508.7 million by the year 2019 at a CAGR of 21.1% over the period of 2014 to 2019 ¼ where in 2014, academic settings accounted for a 58.6% increase in the use of virtual simulation" (para. 3).

The report cites major players in the industry as dominated by "Laerdal and CAE (formally METI, Inc.), followed by Simbionix USA Corporation. Other contributors to the industry are Simulaids, Inc.; Gaumard Scientific; Kyoto Kagaku Co., Ltd; Limbs and Things, Ltd.; Education Management Solutions; Adam, Rouilly Limited; Altay Scientifics; S.P.A.; IngMar Medical; Moog, Inc.; Surgical Science Sweden AB; KaVo Dental GmbH; Medical Simulation Corporation; Simulab Corporation; Yuan Technology Limited; and Mentice AB" (Meticulous Research, 2015, p. 5). There are ever more companies emerging. In the past decade, healthcare simulation stakeholder groups have also expanded to include academic healthcare programs; hospitals and clinics; professional societies; government organizations, such as the military; research and consulting firms; simulation vendors and training providers; medical device companies; insurers; and regulatory and credentialing bodies.

Simulation Modalities and Typologies

Today, simulation is recognized as a valid and effective pedagogical approach for the teaching and learning of healthcare competencies, including critical thinking, psychomotor skills, and interprofessional competencies (Bornais et al., 2014). In the past decade, there has been a veritable explosion in the integration of SBL. Along with it came purpose-built simulation learning spaces and a wide array of simulation modalities and typologies. In nursing, Nehring and Lashley (2010) described the *continuum of simulation* consisting of seven elements: "partial and complex task trainers, role-play, games, computer-assisted instruction, standardized patients, virtual reality and haptic systems, integrated simulators (low through high-fidelity)" (p. 8). Simulation modalities and typologies for learning in healthcare have continued to evolve over the years, and their definitions have gone through a variety of interpretations and iterations within disciplines. Most recently, publication of the Healthcare Simulation Dictionary (Lopreiato, Downing, Gammon, Lioce, Sittner, et al., 2016) aims to provide a universal taxonomy for simulation in healthcare. The International Nursing Association for Clinical Simulation and Learning (INACSL) Simulation Design standard defines a simulation modality as "the platform for the experience" (INACSL Standards Committee, 2016, p. S7). The following are examples of simulation education modalities:

- *Simulated clinical immersion*
  - Also referred to as simulated clinical events (SCE) (INACSL^SM or full-scale or full-mission simulation [Seropian, Brown, Gavilanes, & Driggers, 2004b])
- *Computer-based, screen-based simulation or computer-assisted*
  - *Virtual reality*, 3D *augmented virtual reality*, gaming, holographic simulation
- *Mobile simulation*
- *In situ simulation*
- *TeleSim* or *broadcast simulation*
- *Boot camp simulation*
- *Classroom simulation*
- *Procedural simulation (e.g., training for specific technical skill sets)*
- *Domestic simulation* (simulations that unfold in a home care setting)
- *Expert modeling*
- *Deliberate practice*
- *Hybrid simulation* (the blending of two or more simulation modalities to deliver simulation (INACSL Standards Committee, 2016, Simulation glossary, p. S7)

To achieve a given simulation modality, we use a variety of means or tools classified by type, known as simulation typologies. Many approaches to classifying simulation typologies have emerged over the years. In the context of this book, we adopted the INACSL description of a simulation typology as the means by which a given simulation modality is enacted (Design Standard). For a detailed discussion on the evolution of modalities and typologies, see Chapter 6.

Common simulation typologies include:

- *standardized patients and simulated patients (SP)*, patient volunteers, and embedded SPs/actors—sometimes referred to as a confederate or embedded simulated person
- *mannequins, ranging from static or low-fidelity to mid and high-fidelity full-body integrated computerized simulators* (model or instructor driven)
- *partial task trainers* (discrete body parts, e.g., hip injection trainers)
- *hybrid simulators (combine physical models with computers* [Kneebone, 2003]*), or some combination of simulators;*
- *case studies and human or animal tissue* (i.e., cadavers or organs), simulated cadavers, plastinates, and, in the virtual world, avatars, haptic systems and devices, virtual workbenches or integrated (i.e., endoscopy trainers), and holograms (Kneebone, 2003; INACSL Standards Committee (2016, December), Simulation glossary; Maran & Glavin, 2003)

Simulation has also been labeled according to levels of fidelity (low, mid, and high) where the degrees of realism and interactivity impact the student experience (Waldner & Olson, 2007).

Simulation use has become the new normal, being employed in clinical education and training throughout undergraduate, graduate, and postlicensure environments. High-fidelity simulation-based learning was cited as far back as 2006 as "one of the most important issues in nursing education today" (Bremner, Aduddell, Bennett, & VanGeest, 2006). As technological capabilities evolve, so too will the continued advancement of simulation pedagogy and programs. Roger Kneebone's words still ring true today, "any simulator device can only ever be as good as the educational programme in which it is embedded and many simulators are purchased every year and then underutilized due to lack of educational goals to underpin their use" (2003, p. 27). The simple truth is that using high-tech equipment will never be synonymous with high-quality learning. Excellence in SBL, therefore, involves the application of instructional design principles to create realistic, experiential, socially and physically contextual, immersive, and adult-centered learning experiences for formative assessment and/or evaluation, summative evaluation, and, under controlled conditions, high-stakes evaluation embedded within curricula.

Simulation Defined

Over the past decade, many definitions of simulation and SBL have evolved. Recent attempts to standardize definitions and terminology are producing a more cohesive taxonomy, but varying definitions prevail and it is worth looking them over.

The INACSL Simulation Glossary defines simulation as "An educational strategy in which a particular set of conditions are created or replicated to resemble authentic situations that are possible in real life. Simulation can incorporate one or more modalities to promote, improve, or validate a participant's performance" INACSL Standards Committee. (2016, Simulation Glossary, p. S44).

The *National League for Nursing* defines simulation as

An attempt to mimic essential aspects of a clinical situation with the goal of understanding and managing the situation better when it occurs in actual clinical practice. A technique that uses a situation or environment created to allow persons to experience a representation of a real event for the purpose of practice, learning, evaluation, testing, or to gain an understanding of systems or human actions. (Reprinted with permission from the National League of Nursing. Retrieved on March 21, 2017 from the Simulation Innovation Resource Center [SIRC] Glossary at http://sirc.nln.org/mod/glossary/view.php?id=183)

The *Society for Simulation in Healthcare* (SSH) defines healthcare simulation as "the imitation or representation of one act, or system by another. Healthcare simulations can be said to have four main purposes—education, assessment, research, and health system integration in facilitating patient safety". SSH also purports that

"each of these purposes may be met by some combination of role play, low and high tech tools, and a variety of settings from table-top sessions to a realistic full-mission environment. Simulations may also add to our understanding of human behavior in the true–to–life settings in which professionals operate. The link that ties together all these activities is the act of imitating or representing some situation or process from the simple to the very complex. Healthcare simulation is a range of activities that share a broad, similar purpose—to improve the safety, effectiveness, and efficiency of healthcare services" (SSH, 2016a. Quote retrieved from http://www.ssih.org/About-Simulation on January 17, 2017.)

Dr. David Gaba (2004), a well-known pioneer of medical simulation, defines simulation as "… technique, not a technology, to replace or amplify real experiences with guided experiences, often immersive in nature, that evoke or replicate substantial aspects of the real world in a fully interactive fashion" (p. i2). When conducted under specific conditions, Gaba also notes that simulation creates an ideal educational environment because learning activities can be made to be immersive, predictable, consistent, standardized, safe, and reproducible.

Bland, Topping, and Wood (2011) conducted a conceptual analysis and examination of empirical referents related to simulation. The resulting definition of simulation in undergraduate nursing education is as follows: "Simulation is a dynamic process involving the creation of a hypothetical opportunity that incorporates an authentic representation of reality, facilitates active student engagement and integrates the complexities of practical and theoretical learning with opportunity for repetition, feedback, evaluation and reflection" (p. 668). *Simulation-based learning* (SBL) is also described as a

Revolutionary pedagogy: an art and science that is challenging traditional teaching and learning approaches and, in doing so, is transforming the face of nursing [and healthcare] education. It is a powerful experiential learning process that involves patient actors, computer-based virtual platforms, the use of human patient simulators, and task training devices. Additionally, simulation is characterized by the emergence of associated teaching and learning methods grounded in reflective learning processes for the student [and the teacher]. (Bornais et al., 2014)

These emerging learning models also spawn the need for educators with the conceptual knowledge and technical ability to enact transformational, discovery-driven, collaborative learning.

Simulation offers an innovative alternative to the classroom and to traditional clinical settings as it can be adapted and integrated to complement existing nursing curricula. As much as it holds great promise, offering effective simulation also brings with it significant challenges (Hetzel Campbell & Daley, 2008). Among the many difficulties for educators is the ability to design teaching and learning for the most technosavvy generation of nursing students in history. Today's learners spring from a digital culture: a culture that demands engagement, fast processing, rapid communication, and high-quality learning and innovation (CNA, 2012a; Hetzel Campbell, Pagano, O'Shea, Connery, & Caron, 2013; Prensky, 2001, 2005a, 2007). Educators must keep pace by being visionary and open minded if they are going to be able to meet these new learners where they are, and embrace the richness they have to offer. Millenials may not, for example, understand the "need to enter lengthy, hand-written descriptions of an acute wound into a file when they could snap a photograph and enter assessment data using a smartphone … then share it instantly or drop it into a digital record" (CNA, 2012a, p. 35). Actually, today's educators face shaping a new learning-scape for a generation of *entrepreneurial learners* (Seely-Brown, 2012). These learners are constantly looking around them for new ways and new resources to learn new things. Learning in the network age provides each of us with unprecedented and immense volumes of information to assimilate. Knowledge is no longer static. Knowledge is continuously undergoing metamorphosis as it is being reshaped by a world of digital connectors (Seely-Brown, 2012).

Today's educators are confronting the need to balance long-standing academic traditions that still offer relevant and meaningful learning with the need to embrace and engage the strengths of technosavvy millennial learners

(Prensky, 2013b; 2015). In the above example, it makes perfect sense that the nurse use image capture technologies to optimize the visual accuracy of wound tracking, facilitate communication, and provide timely documentation. If we want to keep up with the digital revolution, it just simply isn't the time to say, "I don't get Twitter®" or "What's the point in blogging?" or "That simulator is just a chunk of plastic." Rather, as Watson says, "it is the time to embrace new technologies, social media, and a myriad of platforms through which contact can be maintained and influence exerted" (2014, p. 23). Prensky (2013b) encourages today's educators to embrace students' technological abilities as a way to foster new capacities in them by actually having them learn through doing. He recommends designing effective curricula that are proactive about integrating learners as capable, positive contributors to their communities, their country, and their world. Simulation environments and associated technological tools can serve as powerful "mind extenders" that allow students to reach places they could not have in past educational contexts.

In doing so, educators must also be mindful of how their effective or ineffective use of technology can impact nursing education outcomes. We are called to consider the ethical use of technology in simulation, giving careful thought to its use, for example, engaging in ethical practices in both the use and storage of video recordings to protect learners and uphold learning.

In recent years, educators have voiced a perceived shift away from philosophy-based curricula to a focus on teaching and learning with technology as its core (Day-Black & Watties-Daniels, 2006; Parker & Myrick, 2009). Therefore, there is a heightened need for nurse educators to keep nursing values, theories, and principles at the heart of nursing curricula employing technology as a powerful extender of learning. Patients come to us as trusted healthcare providers, "not for what it is that we do, but for what they get from us" (O'Grady, 2014, p. 15). What patients expect, and have a right to, is exceptional value and expert care. It is no longer simply enough to say that nurses add value by simply doing; we must know and understand the value that a professional nurse brings to those in our care. Likewise, the same goes for those leading pedagogical innovation and curricular transformation in nursing education. Educators must be held accountable for bringing value to the programs and the learning environments we create. As we embark on the expanded use of simulation, we need to focus on well-designed learning that demonstrates impact, outcomes, and value. In other words, simply doing more simulation does not in and of itself bring value to learners in nursing programs; rather, doing more of what is proven best practice in simulation brings value to our learners. In order to take on this task and do it well, educators must keep the past in mind, while looking to the horizon to see well beyond the status quo. It takes a significant commitment to excellence and effort, for example, to keep the simulation as "real" as possible and to develop key dimensions of fidelity and enhance authentic lived experiences for the learner (Hetzel-Campbell & Daley, 2013).

Educators and those in charge of educational institutions must be courageous and take evidence-informed and evidence-based risks to create revolutionary and transformational growth in nursing education. We are paradoxically in the midst of, and on the cusp of tremendous transformation in nursing education.

Simulation Theory and Theory to Support Simulation

The simulation revolution has brought with it the need for educators to foster relevant, meaningful learning to prepare better graduates that are equipped for the healthcare environments of today. As such, simulation is now a well-established learner-centered pedagogy rooted in diverse learning theories.

As we were writing this chapter, there was excitement mounting about the first-ever simulation theory: The NLN/Jeffries Simulation (Jeffries, 2015a). Jeffries Simulation Theory is rooted in constructivist educational philosophy from which both experiential and adult learning theories are derived (Jeffries, 2014; Waxman, 2010). Constructivism is not as much scientific or educational theory as it is an epistemology (the study of how humans acquire knowledge) and a philosophical life view on how humans learn and make meaning of their experiences (Ultanir, 2012). Constructivist philosophy stems from the seminal works of Dewey (1938), Piaget (1953), Bruner (1961), Vygotsky (1978), and other theorists that viewed learning as "temporary, developmental, socially, and culturally mediated" (Brooks & Brooks, 1993, p. vii). Read how Dr. Pamela Jeffries identified the need for a framework for simulation educators to use as they develop, implement, and evaluate simulation education.

1-3 Voice of Experience
Early Adopter in Nursing

Pamela R. Jeffries, PhD, RN, ANEF, FAAN

The Challenge

When I first became involved in simulation pedagogy, I explored the literature, journals, and texts looking for a "cookbook" type of approach based on theoretical underpinnings telling me how to create,

(Continued)

1-3 Voice of Experience (*Continued*)

implement, and evaluate the use of clinical simulations in my teaching. Over a decade and a half ago, there were no "cookbooks or recipes" and the literature was sparse on these topics. Authors provided little information on how simulation was designed, implemented, and integrated as a part of clinical education. Initial simulation work was undertaken by eight different project coordinators selected by the NLN with me as the project director.

Meeting the Challenge

As any researcher should do, I explored the literature, which was sparse a decade ago. Even when simulation was mentioned, there was no clarity on how the simulation was designed, implemented, or used, whether it was a teaching–learning intervention, or used as a mechanism for assessment/evaluation.

After the NLN/Simulation Research project concluded, the research team, project coordinators, and I wrote our "cookbook," "*Clinical Simulations in Nursing Education: From Conceptualization to Evaluation*" (2007), to help the next wave of educators and researchers. Three learning theories and their constructs were explored and used to explain simulations from creation to implementation and then evaluation of using this new type of pedagogy.

Outcome

The second edition of our book was published in 2012, followed by a contemporary book, *Advanced Clinical Simulations: The Concepts, Trends, and Opportunities* (2013), and most recently, the NLN monograph titled *The NLN Jeffries Clinical Simulation Theory (2015)*. The *NLN Jeffries Simulation Framework* has been declared a midrange theory based on work by many nursing researchers led by nursing theory development expert, Dr. Beth Rogers. In addition, numerous research studies have been conducted using the NLN Jeffries Simulation framework, not only in nursing education but across disciplines.

Most Valuable Lessons Learned

It is importance to have a framework or model to help introduce a new innovation, model, or pedagogical approach to educators and researchers. Creating a theory-based framework helps researchers to test components of the framework, allowing for more deliberate, rigorous research on the model. The model helps to guide not only research but also

implementation and integration of simulations in a nursing curriculum.

The other lesson I learned was how to work with a national organization. When working with a large organization, such as the NLN, it is necessary to communicate, communicate, communicate to ensure they understand your intent, trajectory, and expectations. I also had to understand that the work I did wasn't just a reflection on my professional self but also on the organization. Clear communication, discussion of activities, and intent of disseminating the work elsewhere all need to be communicated since the work is collegial and collaborative. Working with a national organization helps move one's research forward in a much greater way than when individually disseminated. This has been a wonderful, collegial, collaborative relationship!

Inspiration for Simulation Champions

"Color outside the lines."
                                        —John Jacob Zwiegelaar
"If you can dream it, you can do it!"
                                        —Walt Disney
"I would rather attempt something great and fail, than to attempt nothing and succeed."
                                        —Robert H. Schuller
"Opportunities don't happen, you create them!"
                                        —Chris Grosser

Constructivist learning involves the active, cyclical, somewhat messy building process by which meaning and understanding and, therefore, knowledge is built. Knowledge construction requires that a person first filter new experiences internally, then probe, explore, and weigh them against existing beliefs and prior knowledge. Once these experiences have been passed through a person's internal sifter, new insights and meanings emerge. Because of the subjective, internal nature of personal knowledge, its development is unique to each of us and remains a moving target that is fluid, dynamic, and ever changing. This fact accounts for why groups of people can experience the same event, yet emerge with entirely different perspectives and interpretations. Over the years, our students have appreciated the image in Figure 1.5 we've titled "How Teams See Elephants" to demonstrate that even though facilitators and learners may all be seeing the same elephant, each will formulate different assumptions based on their unique vantage point and prior experiences with elephants. As a result, team members will formulate a broad range of perspectives while engaged in the same learning situation.

Although constructivism is the most commonly cited educational approach today, educational practices and

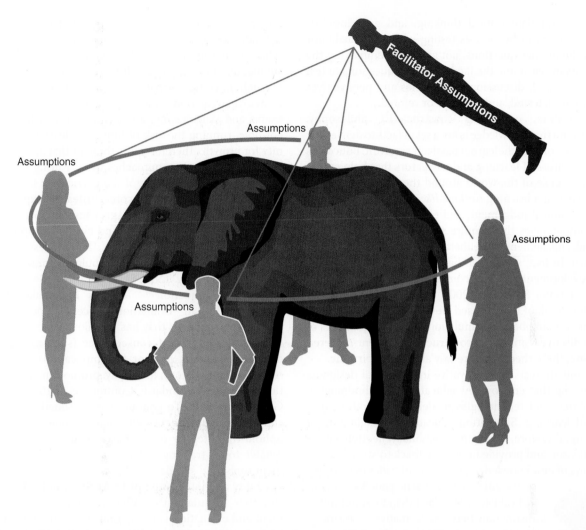

Figure 1.5 "How Teams See Elephants" Demonstrates How Learners All See the Same Elephant but Have Very Different Perspectives and Vantage Points. (C. Foisy-Doll, personal tool.)

theory change with shifts in communication and technology and the influences of **globalization** and the knowledge economy (Brown, 2005). Shifts in education and **learning paradigms** over past decades can be characterized as the movement from reproductive (rote memorization) to productive learning, from behaviorism to constructivism, from teacher-centered to learner-centered, from teaching to the facilitation of learning, from context-based to outcomes-based, and from content-based evaluation to outcomes-based assessment (Brown, 2005). In today's global- and technology-rich learning environments, constructivism has given way to social constructivism (evident in online social platforms); knowledge production has given rise to knowledge navigation; linguistic intelligence has expanded to include gamification and play through human connection in virtual worlds; and facilitation, coaching, and mentoring have replaced the sage on the stage (Brown, 2005; Kerchner, 2011). These significant shifts are impacting the core of long-standing beliefs and assumptions in teaching and learning, forcing us to reexamine and change the "way we have always done things in education." SBL encourages

knowledge construction through the use of active, experiential learning in high-context, immersive, lifelike situations that offer learners real-world problem-solving. Knowledge is created when learners get out of their seats and onto their feet and bring together mind, heart, and hands to work through true-to-life dilemmas.

Reflection is a core activity in simulation where learners think about and process theirs and others' lived experiences to construct new meaning and understanding in debriefing sessions (Rudolph, Raemer, & Simon, 2014; Rudolph, Simon, Rivard, Dufresne, & Raemer, 2007). Safe learning spaces, or *safe containers*, as coined by Rudolph et al. (2014), are environments "where learners face professionally meaningful challenges and are held to high standards in a way that engages them but does not intimidate or humiliate them" (p. 339). Paul and Elder's (1997) seminal work on critical thinking denotes the need for Socratic questioning: a method that is based on the teachings and practices of Socrates, the famous Greek philosopher. Socratic questioning is characterized by facilitator-initiated inquiry and discussion between members of a group/team to find answers, stimulate critical thinking, and gain insights. It is grounded in hypothesis testing where the facilitator offers the learner questions, not answers—employing the elements of reasoning the facilitator asks questions to test ideas and spark discussion. Possibilities and perspectives are explored, tested, and accepted or refuted.

Educators, embracing constructivist philosophy, understand that knowledge is not a set of facts to delivery or give away, nor does the learner passively receive it. Educators are facilitators of learning and navigators that help others to make sense of the world around them. These are vital supports when learning to *think like a nurse*. Critical reasoning, clinical judgement, and clinical decision-making are competencies that require significant time, exposure to, and engagement in deliberate practice and reflection to learn. In fact, simulation has proven to be effective in the development of these competencies (Lasater, 2007a, 2007b; Lasater & Nielsen, 2009; Tanner, 2006). We can't help but think of how pleased Dewey, Piaget, Bruner, and Vygotsky would be with simulationists. As the pioneers of active discovery and social constructivist student-centered learning, these theorists were way ahead of their time.

Simulationists are innovative instructional designers of learning that employ new educational methodologies, modalities, and technologies to deliver impactful experiential learning. Simulation educators as facilitators of learning, therefore, must guide personal reflection, coach and mentor, and provide honest feedback to stimulate the building of new knowledge, skills, and attitudes in learners.

The 2013 INACSL Participant Assessment and Evaluation Standard (Sando et al.) noted a distinction between formative assessment, and summative and high stakes evaluation. Based on a review of current educational literature the new standards focus exclusively on evaluating simulation outcomes using formative, summative, and high-stakes evaluation. Oermann (2017) describes clear differences between the terms assessment and evaluation, noting that the terms are related, but not synonymous. She describes assessment as the "process of obtaining information to use for making educational decisions" (p. 2), and evaluation as the "process of making a judgement as to value and worth based on the information" (p. 2). Formative assessment is considered process-oriented and involves ongoing monitoring of how learning is unfolding with giving feedback for improved performance (Oermann, 2017). In simulation, formative assessment, and subsequent evaluation extends to include debriefing and reflection. Formative evaluation focuses on outcomes related to formative assessment strategies used in teaching and learning with the aim of enhancing learning (or the overall formation of the learner) (Oermman). Summative evaluation is product-oriented and involves gauging what has been learned in totality. Summative evaluation infers judgement about the quality and totality of what has been learned at a terminal point in time (i.e., course end). In the past, summative evaluations in nursing

included written examinations or skills testing as terminal indicators of knowledge or skill attainment. Instead of reliance on summative evaluation strategies, learning in simulation nurtures and cultivates student development through ongoing formative assessment, culminating in formative evaluation. Traditional testing methods, such as exams and skills testing, are seen as too constrictive and episodic, running the risk of limiting a learner's opportunity for growth. Therefore, it is thought that applying conventional summative approaches to measuring knowledge might lead to a narrowing of the curriculum by reducing simulation learning to test scores, instead of expanding it.

In recent years, there is growing support to move beyond formative assessment and evaluation approaches to include high-stakes testing. This process is under debate within the simulation practice community. INACSL Standard of Best Practice: Simulation[SM] defines high-stakes testing as an "evaluation process associated with a simulation activity that has a major academic, educational, or employment consequence (such as a grading decision, including pass or fail implications; a decision regarding competency, merit pay, promotion, or certification)" (INACSL Standards Committee, 2016, Simulation Glossary, p. S41). To conduct such evaluations, specific conditions must be present that include measures to uphold the integrity of the participant, use of valid and reliable tools, training of faculty on the use of measurement tools, and standardized processes such as interrater reliability and integration of **INACSL Standards of Best Practice: Simulation**[SM]. Whatever approach to assessment and evaluation is used, "only when the nurse is able to make the connection between the information [content] and clinical experience [context], will a nurse reach the level of competence" (Galloway, 2009, para. 6).

Diverse **learning theories** are employed in simulation, for example, Knowles *Adult Learning Theory* (1990), Kolb's *Experiential Learning Cycle* (1984), Schön (1983, 1987) and Argyris and Schön's (1978) *Double Loop Learning and Reflection*, Lave and Wenger's (1991) *Situated Cognition*, Benner's (1984) *Novice to Expert*, and National League for Nursing/Jeffries *Simulation Theory* (Jeffries, 2007b, 2015b; Kardong-Edgren, Dieckmann, & Phero, 2015). Other relevant theory includes Zones of Proximal Development (Vygotsky, 1978), Cognitive Load Theory (Sweller, Ayres, & Kalyuga, 2011), Deliberate Practice Theory (Ericsson, Ericcson, Charness, Feltovich, & Hoffman, 2006), Stress Inoculation Theory and Training (Meichenbaum & Deffenbacher, 1988), and a rich body of literature from human factors, organizational training, and cognitive psychology on social development and cognition and skill decay (Kardong-Edgren et al., 2015; Weaver, Newman-Toker, & Rosen, 2012). Aligning these theories helps us to understand that simulation learning is deeply rooted in deliberate, repetitive active experimentation and reflection that is situated within authentic sociocultural processes and practices.

Therefore, SBL ideally plays out within true-to-life sociocultural contexts where experienced facilitators can guide learning. Learners are prompted to think about their own and others' thoughts and actions while exploring the consequences of those actions in context. Using an iterative reflective process, learners along with their facilitator cocreate new patterns of thinking and transform ways of being (INACSL Standards Committee, 2016, Facilitation Standard; Debriefing Standard; Hetzel-Campbell & Daley, 2013). Further discussion on learning theory is found in Chapter 16.

Whereas classroom and clinical learning offers value in education, simulation learning also adds unique value by delivering timely, relevant experiences for learners (Harder, 2015). Simulation provides a means of bridging theory and clinical while allowing deliberate and repeated clinical skills practice. Over 20 years ago, Polifroni, Packard, Shah, and MacAvoy (1995) noted that students spent 44% of their time on clinical units not engaged in patient care activities. The authors reported that 75% of clinical time was spent unsupervised with the other 25% taking place in the presence of a clinical instructor or registered nurse. Moreover, students reported losing valuable learning time trying to operate in unfamiliar settings, voicing a fear of harming acutely ill patients due to lack of knowledge and experience. Studies also showed that students report a lack of supervised one-on-one time with clinical educators (Hartigan-Rogers, Cobbett, Amirault, & Muise-Davis, 2007; Hickey, 2010). It is disturbing that despite these findings, current models of clinical instruction have remained relatively unchanged.

Faculty have also voiced concerns regarding the limited time they have to devote to nursing competency development in areas of clinical decision-making, clinical reasoning, and clinical judgement. They also reported that 70% of their time was task focused and trapped on the psychomotor skills supervision treadmill (Henderson, Cooke, Creedy, & Walker, 2012; Ironside & McNelis, 2010). In the end, this leaves only 10% of educator time to devote to clinical teaching (Norman, Buerhaus, Donelan, McCloskey, & Dittus, 2005). We fail to see how this clinical education model meets the needs of future nursing education.

Clinical placements are difficult to secure and do not ensure consistent or quality experiences (Henneman & Cunningham, 2005; Oldenburg, Maney, & Plonczynski, 2013). Acuity levels are high, with patients suffering from multiple comorbidities, often surpassing the ability of the novice learner to provide knowledgeable and safe care. Often, students are further limited by access restrictions to the electronic health record (EHR) and in the administration of certain medications. In clinical settings, they also reported that 14% of their time was spent receiving inconsistent information from multiple healthcare providers where gaps in staff instruction or knowledge play out (Polifroni et al., 1995). To further confound the situation, skill decay occurs with a lack of opportunity for repetitive skills practice (Jeffries, 2012a). Yet, the apprenticeship clinical training

model in nursing remains alive and well. The Carnegie Foundation for Teaching, the National Council of State Boards of Nursing (NCSBN), and the Joint Commission in the United States have issued reports concluding that nurses entering the workforce are not prepared for practice challenges. It is clear that the current educational model has failed students, faculty, and patients (Jeffries, 2007b). When compared to conventional clinical practica, simulation offers educators and learners the opportunity for increased meaningful interaction and clinical learning that is just as if not more effective (Alinier, Hunt, Gordon, & Harwood, 2006; Bland et al., 2011; Brewer, 2011; Fountain & Alfred, 2009; Harder, 2009; Hayden, Smiley, Alexander, Kardong-Edgren, & Jeffries, 2014; Jeffries, 2007b; Meyer, Connors, Hou, & Gajewski, 2011; Oldenburg et al., 2013).

We have come a long way since Pamela Jeffries and Mary Anne Rizzolo spearheaded the NLN/Laerdal Project (2006a) and the subsequent seminal report that shaped the progression and rapid advancement of simulation in nursing education. There is now consensus in the simulation practice community and current research to support that simulation offers incredible potential for quality learning. Thankfully, we are beyond questioning simulation as a bona fide teaching and learning technique. However, at the same time, there is consensus about the need for increased rigor in simulation research so that we maximize and optimize its use in nursing and healthcare education. In-depth inquiry into simulation teaching and learning needs to extend beyond participant self-perception and satisfaction studies. As we move forward, simulation researchers must conduct quality studies grounded in theoretical frameworks and current evidence, and use valid and reliable instruments to measure downstream outcomes. Moreover, Issenberg, Ringsted, Ostergaard, & Dieckmann (2011) encourage educational research in three categories using Kirkpatrick's four levels of evaluation: Instructional Design, Translational (T1-T2-T3) Research, and Outcomes Studies. There is a consensus that future simulation research needs to ramp up its focus on rigor (Boyd & Salameh, 2006; Hayden et al., 2014; Issenberg et al., 2011; Jeffries, 2012a; Kardong-Edgren et al., 2015; McGaghie, Draycott, Dunn, Lopez, & Stefanidis, 2011). Fey (2016) reported that the INACSL research committee conducted a survey of the membership to ascertain membership body research priorities. Research priorities feature:

a) translational research; b) evaluation methods; c) validity and reliability of instruments; d) ratio of clinical time to simulation time; e) pre-briefing and briefing; f) use of theory in simulation measurement of higher order thinking (e.g., clinical reasoning); g) faculty development; h) facilitator competence communication. (p. 845)

Benchmarks and Emerging Standards

Benchmarking in healthcare and simulation refers to "a process of seeking out and implementing best practices at best cost … the fundamental principle of benchmarking consists of identifying a point of comparison called the **benchmark**, against which all else can be compared" (Ettorchi-Tardy, Levif, & Michel, 2012, p. e102). The key benefit to benchmarking comes with its integration into comprehensive policy development and continuous quality improvement processes (CQI). In simulation, benchmarks are emerging for education, technology, human resource development and qualifications, and practice. The NCSBN has published the *National Simulation Guidelines for Prelicensure Nursing Programs* Alexander, Durham, Hooper, Jeffries, Goldman, Kardong-Edgren et al., (2015). The SSH has published has recently updated the Society for Simulation in Healthcare **Accreditation Standards** (2016). Simulation programs as well as credentialing programs for simulation educators and technicians. INACSL has disseminated the *Standards of Best Practice: Simulation* since 2011. In prior years, such standards did not exist, whereas today, these evolving standards play a vital role as benchmarks for simulation program development, development, educational best practice, and staff development in simulation.

There is a growing awareness of the need to examine value propositions in simulation. The Global Network for Simulation in Healthcare (GNSH, 2015) recently conducted a survey to collect data with the intent to create consensus guidelines for establishing the value of simulation for key stakeholders. Global stakeholder groups that are involved include, but are not limited to, the financial sector, governmental regulators, educational bodies, politicians, patient advocacy groups, healthcare and college executives, and policy makers.

Education for the 21st Century: A Transglobal Call for Transformation

Calls for the transformation of healthcare education are now heralded worldwide appealing to educators and policymakers from all sectors to be *difference makers* through active engagement in shaping education on a global scale. Today, there is unprecedented urgency for designers of education and stakeholders groups from around the world to reexamine and transform our teaching and learning practices and to do so ethically and efficiently within the context of shifting global realities. Indeed, this is no small charge. "The challenge now is to transform education systems into something better suited to the REAL needs of the 21st century. At the heart of this transformation, there has to be a radically different view of human intelligence and creativity" (Robinson, 2011, p. 14).

Globalization and its evolution present us with both unique opportunities and gnarly challenges. The emergence of globalization has brought sociopolitical–economic–ecological trends that are complex and multifaceted, and as such, educators are tasked with thoughtful consideration to create new educational models for the 21st century. Key trends associated with globalization include the following:

1. Growing inequities between the low-, mid-, and high-incomes countries, as in those who have benefitted from globalization and those who have not
2. Low employment growth for graduates in shrinking global job markets
3. Positive and negative effects of migration, mobility, and cultural diversity
4. Growing demands for personal voice at local, national, and transnational levels
5. Radical transformation related to the digital revolution
6. Shifting patterns of educational governance
7. Privatization of knowledge
8. Emphasis on corporate social responsibility
9. Demands to develop global citizens
10. Calls for sustainability in educational practices; and alarmingly
11. The deprofessionalization of teachers, such as the contracting of unqualified teachers for postsecondary education in countries that do not have the means to pay for quality education (UNESCO, 2013, pp. 10–15)

Recently, the *United Nations Education Scientific and Cultural Organization*, UNESCO (2013), published its revisioning report, setting forth a plan for reexamining the fundamental principles upon which approaches to education play out in the context of globalization—and new world realities. The proposal calls for a renewal of principles built on previously published UNESCO documents: the Faure report (1972), *Learning to Be*, and the Delors Report (1996), *Learning: The treasure within*, that featured the now infamous four pillars of learning:

1. *Learning to live together*, expanding our knowledge of each other
2. *Learning to know*, knowledge as part of culture
3. *Learning to do*, competency acquisition, especially in teams
4. *Learning to be*, developing independence in judgement toward realizing our collective destiny (p. 9)

A UNESCO senior expert group is tasked with creating a more contemporary framework for education within today's complex, uncertain, and rapidly changing environments. Recently, their work reintroduced a global debate aimed at, "reexamining the implications of multifaceted social transformation on education, and how in a global context, knowledge skills, and values are created, reproduced, transmitted, validated, appropriated, and used" (2013, p. 3). Currently, there is a strong commitment to refresh previously defined concepts to incorporate a more balanced approach of diverse perspectives. The following concepts and terms have been earmarked for revision with a need to be more inclusive and universally acceptable:

Development versus other worldviews and conceptualizations; Equity versus equality; Respect for diversity versus cultural relativism; Procedural democracy versus democracy based on human rights that are inclusive; Education versus learning; Formal versus non-formal or informal education; Lifelong Learning; Information Society; Knowledge Society; Learning Society versus Education Society; Skills versus competencies, and; Short-term; mid-term; and longer-term perspectives.

Understanding and incorporating these concepts in formal and informal educational endeavors are crucial; they serve as beacons for all educators working to develop sustainable, ethical, and responsible education on a global platform. Paulo Freire (1972), in his book, *The Pedagogy of the Oppressed*, reminds us that in doing so, "One cannot expect positive results from an educational or political action program that fails to respect the particular view of the world held by the people. Such a program constitutes cultural invasion, good intentions notwithstanding" (p. 95).

Other global initiatives that have impacted not only education but also healthcare include the Sustainable Millennium Development Goals (SDGs) (http://www.undp.org/content/undp/en/home/sustainable-development-goals.html), Millennium Development Goals (MDGs), Education for All (EFA), the Decade of Education for Sustainable Development (DESD), the United Nation's Literacy Decade (UNLD), and the more recently launched Global Education First Initiative (GEFI) (UNESCO, 2013, p. 9; United Nations, 2015). Based on preliminary work, the group's mandate is to be *Rethinking Education in a Changing World.* This group endeavors to develop a more "coherent international framework for educational development in the 21st century" (UNESCO, 2013, p. 9). Educators and policymakers are employing collaborative approaches to chart a course for future generations and a more global, human-centered vision of education. To that end, we are challenged with developing new and diverse global educational model(s), articulating renewed guiding philosophies and strategic directions, and redefining our hopes and aspirations while maneuvering social, political, and economic influences.

Globalization trends are also affecting healthcare education. Teaching and learning and the delivery of healthcare unfold on a world stage. Learner and educator mobility is enhanced by technological connectivity and ease of travel. Today, educators share their expertise around the world as international borders become increasingly blurred and transglobal teaching and learning are fast becoming the new reality. For example, there is a global dispersion of **simulation-based education** (SBE) as simulationists with expertise in program development, curriculum design, instructional methods and assessment, operations management, and physical space design work across international borders.

In 2006, the World Health Organization (WHO) projected a shortage of 4.3 million healthcare providers (HCP) worldwide. There are increasing numbers of newly educated HCPs from low-income nations leaving their native countries for work in high-income countries causing a *brain drain effect.* This continuous movement for learning across international borders presents unique circumstances where education delivery models must now consider how to prepare HCPs for other contexts and health delivery systems. We no longer have the traditional *local student with local teacher* learning configuration. Dominant configurations now reflect *local student with the international teacher,* or *international student with local teacher.* These configurations necessitate creative and innovative educational delivery models, such as the use of computer-based learning using virtual simulation (WHO, 2011b). Implicit in the development of new delivery models is the need for educators and policy makers to enact collectively shared goals for education. Now, we must also plan for equitable dissemination of knowledge, skills, and wealth across the globe while honoring diversity. Approaching each other with a stance of cultural humility and curiosity helps us to understand personal biases when interacting with cultures that differ from our own. Ultimately, we are all members of a global collective of difference makers that must work together to create short-, mid-, and long-range planning toward building the new global knowledge society.

Calls for Radical Transformation in Nursing Education around Our Globe

Can you hear the call for transformation beckoning nurses around the globe? The World Health Organization (WHO), in its 2009 report titled *Global Standards for the Initial Education of Professional Nurses and Midwives,* estimated that the global nursing workforce comprises approximately 35 million nurses. Even with those large numbers, making up the shortfall of nurses through training will require injections of funding ranging from 1.6 to 2 million USD per country per year. Given the great disparities between countries in areas such as social determinants of health, economic status, effects of globalization, free trade, migration, and telecommunications, many countries will, unfortunately, remain with significant shortfalls. This lack of funding will leave millions of needy individuals around the world without access to much needed professional healthcare services International Council of Nurses (ICN, 2014a, 2014b). It is fascinating to note that of the known 35 million nurses worldwide, very few are involved in policy development or high-level strategic decision-making. According to the WHO (2013), the need for global standards in nursing education has arisen because of "the increasing complexities in healthcare provision, the increasing number of health professionals at different levels, and the need to assure more equitable access to healthcare" (p. 8). The Independent Commission on Education of Health Professionals for the 21st Century (2010) identified that simply producing more health professionals would be insufficient; rather, what we need is to educate competent, context-relevant qualified healthcare professionals who can both thrive and respond to a given populations' evolving needs. Moreover, the WHO (2013) published a document titled *Transforming and Scaling up Health Professionals' Education and Training*. This report issues a plea to the designers of healthcare education to create "the sustainable expansion and reform of health professionals' education and training to increase the quantity, quality, and relevance of health professionals, and in so doing strengthen the country's health systems and improve population health outcomes" (p. 11). The guidelines fall into five domains: (1) education and training institutions, (2) accreditation and regulation, (3) financing and sustainability, (4) monitoring and evaluating, and (5) governance and planning. Additionally, the WHO report stipulates the dire need for competent educators and trainers who understand and effectively employ educational methods and tools and have access to needed resources.

Among the many guidelines, item 5 speaks to curriculum development using simulation:

Simulation methods (Recommendation 5): Health professionals' education and training institutions should use simulation methods (high fidelity methods in settings with appropriate resources and lower fidelity methods in resource-limited settings) of contextually appropriate fidelity levels in the education of health professionals. The quality of the evidence supporting these recommendations is moderate, and the strength of the recommendation is strong. (WHO, 2013, p. 14)

Dr. Judith Shamian, current president of the ICN, voices with fervor, "the urgency for nurses to effectively reverse the worldwide erosion of nursing and its impact on health and public policy" (Nagle, 2014a, para. 5). She urges with a passion that nurses must participate in the global development and global transformation of healthcare. Shamian challenges us to take our vast amounts of underutilized "knowledge, information, experience, expertise and research ... and to have a serious look at how we prepare our nurses for leadership roles" (para. 5). Additionally, she asks that we consider expanding our nursing education programs to include subjects such as political science, public health, economics, and epidemiology, to name but a few. Shamian believes that unless nurses take their place at decision-making tables, either as elected officials or sitting alongside them, *we risk losing out and taking a back seat while the visibility of nursing becomes nonexistent.*

Nurses, therefore, need to commit to redesigning education to meet the current and future demands arising from complex issues in healthcare that are playing out in global, national, and local contexts. Educational programs must deploy graduate nurses with the leadership competencies required of front line healthcare leaders. Today's nurse leaders must fight for equity and access to healthcare, strengthen health systems, develop effective interprofessional teams, and manage health services to better resource our health systems. Regardless of geographical location and context, nurses, educators, regulators, professional organizations, unions, management, leaders, and policy makers must unite and act in the call for the advancement of nursing and nursing education, including simulation.

It is clear that simulationists from both clinical practice and academe are well positioned to insert leadership competency development into curricula and then bring learning to life through well-designed and well-deployed simulation. The immense challenge we face is to ensure that learners acquire the core competencies required of new graduates while also educating those same nurses to thrive as capable transformational leaders, followers, and managers. The nurse leader of the future must be adept as a patient advocate, change leader, and change manager in primary care, public health, long-term and continuing care, home care, community care, and global health (MacMillan, 2014).

The use of simulation is ever-expanding. Simulation-based performance assessments and evaluations are increasingly commonplace for certification and licensure. Moreover, as the practice of replacing real clinical time with simulation grows, "evidence to support its application needs to be gathered to identify a theoretical basis" for the educational choices we make (Jeffries, 2012a, p. 53). Mounting evidence clearly dictates that simulation offers a viable alternative to clinically based learning (Alinier et al., 2006; Cant & Cooper, 2010; Cook et al., 2011; Meyer et al., 2011; Schlairet & Pollock, 2010). Evidence supports that up to 50% up to 50% of clinical practical can be effectively replaced by simulation that is grounded in best practice (Hayden et al., 2014). Therefore, what we need to learn more about is when, how, and how much simulation is needed (Jeffries, 2012a). To that end, it is also time to re-examine our clinical teaching practices to ensure that learners are gleaning maximum return on the time they spend in clinical practice, whether that learning occurs using simulation or within actual clinical practice settings.

New research is needed to explore such questions as, "Where and how do learners attain maximum gain from experiential learning toward the attainment of required competencies?" or "What degree of immersion in actual clinical settings yields sufficient opportunities for effective socialization and professional acculturation of learners?" In the future, new knowledge is vital to designing relevant, responsive, and evidence-informed/evidence-based educational programs. Currently, for example, due to the focused and intensive nature of SBL, many schools assign double or triple clinical credit hours for time spent in simulation (e.g., 1 hour in simulation being the equivalent of 2 hours in clinical). Currently, global standards for clinical replacement credit hours do not currently exist, and as we see a progressive increase in the use of simulation, it is imperative to examine the value of the time spent in clinical as compared to simulation. Educators must ask, "What is learned? When, how, where, and why?" It will be important to ascertain which core knowledge, skills, and attitudes are best attained through experiential learning in simulation, as opposed to the *hit and miss* approach currently playing out in clinical practica. Ultimately, quality evidence is needed to create a nexus between the worlds of simulated and traditional clinical learning.

In North America over the past 50 years, nursing science and nursing education have advanced through periods of profound change. Predominant influences throughout these periods include dynamic shifts in sociopolitical and economic forces, the advent of technology-mediated approaches to teaching and learning, and dynamic alterations in healthcare delivery and the healthcare needs of an aging population. Concurrently, we have also experienced changes in healthcare practices, that includes moving high-acuity patients from acute care to community settings; the need for safer healthcare delivery by interprofessional teams of clinicians; increasing patient activism; and the ever-expanding scopes of practices across and within disciplines.

These shifts and subsequent demands have contributed to the need for new sets of competencies in nursing graduates in all levels of education. In response to these contextual realities over the years, numerous iterations of nursing curricula and pedagogical approaches have been implemented. One powerful example is today's technology-mediated, theory-based, simulation pedagogy. When implemented using best practices in simulation and education, this methodology provides rich experiential learning to help bridge the gap between theory and professional practice settings. *The Future of Nursing: The Focus on Nursing Education* (IOM, 2011) reports that simulation offers a way to transform nursing through new models for clinical practice. Therefore, a well-recognized need for immediate change has resulted in innumerable calls from nurses and stakeholders around the globe, all expressing the dire need for sweeping and pervasive change to meet current and future challenges in healthcare.

A Nursing Call to Action, published by the Canadian Nurses Association (CNA, 2012a), calls for "collaboration among professional associations, educators, scientists, unions, and employers to reach consensus on the scientific knowledge, education, competencies, and skills sets demanded of effective 21st century registered nurses" (p. 37). Key collaborators working across disciplines and sectors must engage to serve as catalysts that will build a new healthcare education system and science. Needed

changes will also require funding models and support structures that give the right to registered nurses to make autonomous patient care decisions within broader scopes of practice and a more patient- and family-centered healthcare system (CNA, 2012a). One example of such collaboration is *Hacking Health* (http://hackinghealth.ca/), a global initiative that brings together technology creators and healthcare professionals to find realistic, human-centric solutions to tough healthcare problems (Hacking Health, n.d.).

What is needed is a paradigm shift that moves us out of our silos and toward a renewal of our shared values of collaboration, caring, and competence. For this to transpire, we need to see more intersectoral and cross-industry work to discover innovative technology-mediated solutions. In Canada, much has happened since the release of the Baker and Norton report (2004). The Canadian Patient Safety Institute (CPSI, 2016a) has ramped up patient safety programs and competency training across the country where recent findings indicate improvements in healthcare outcomes and a beginning shift in healthcare culture (Baker et al., 2004; CPSI, 2016a; Frank & Brien, 2008).

In the United States, many nurse leaders and national nursing organizations have led the charge in the call for the transformation of nursing education. In 2010, the American Association of Colleges of Nursing (AACN) released the *Tri-Council for Nursing Issues New Consensus Policy Statement*, stating that

Healthcare reform initiatives call for a nursing workforce that integrates evidence-based clinical knowledge and research with effective communication and leadership skills [that] require increased education at all levels…. Without a more educated nursing workforce, the nation's health will be further at risk. (2010, p. 1).

The Quality and Safety Education for Nurses initiative (QSEN, 2014) in the United States has called for "curricula that would assure that future nursing graduates had competencies in patient-centered care, teamwork and collaboration, evidence-based practice, quality improvement, and informatics" (para. 1 to 2).

Influenced by the recommendations of the seminal Flexner report of 1910, Benner, Sutphen, Leonard, and Day (2010) appeal to nurse educators with a plea for radical transformation in nursing education. Their vision is one where nursing education is grounded in a commitment to skills and moral/ethical practice for the greater public good. The authors state that "human welfare ultimately depends upon the cultivation of values, such as, care and responsibility, that cannot be produced by self-interest alone" (Benner & Sullivan, as cited in Benner et al., 2010, p. 9). That said, nursing in North America faces many challenges. For example, employment shortages for healthcare professionals in the United States alone are reported at an estimated 5.6 million vacancies between 2010 and 2020 (Rieteg & Squires, 2015). Workplace dissatisfaction and burnout remain prevalent for nurses working in complex and sometimes chaotic healthcare environments. Confounding high levels of stress in nursing is the constant need for change. Workplace transformation has brought with it shifts in scopes of practice and subsequent turf wars that play out in the workplace within nursing disciplines, as well as between healthcare disciplines. Moreover, the ability for healthcare systems to pay for skilled, competent nurses is met with shrinking fiscal resources.

Globally, other nations are heralding a similar call to action. This book gives voice to a cross section of simulationists carrying out their mission to transform education all around the world. Simulationists, working in other countries, share with us their personal narratives so that we might connect and engage in collective problem-solving and solutions-seeking for the benefit of all. It is through this type of exchange that we will build a strong global village of simulationists. To that end, in June of 2012 the INACSL Board of Directors created a new board position titled, *Vice President of International Collaboratives.*

By the time this book goes to print, the incumbent will already be at work to create synergies that have been lacking on the global platform. There is a great deal to be learned from and with each other.

The European Federation of Nurses Associations (EFN) strongly advocates for the development of a highly qualified and competent nurse workforce. In the United Kingdom, the Willis Commission published *Quality with Compassion: The Future of Nursing Education,* stating that, graduate nurses "have played and will continue to play a key role in driving up standards", with patient-centered care as "the golden thread" that runs through all nursing education. (Royal College of Nursing, 2012, p. 6)

In Australia, "key pressures within undergraduate nurse education … include competition for scarce clinical placements and increasing enrollment numbers" (Health Workforce Australia, 2013). Nurse educators in New Zealand are working to ensure that healthcare providers meet and maintain high standards for competent and safe practice (New Zealand Ministry of Health, 2015).

In Africa, nurses face unique challenges such as working to reverse the effects of Colonialism that affected nursing and nursing education as much as it affected African society as a whole. The development of professional nursing in Africa unfolds in varying ways. "A vast difference, for example, can be seen when comparing South Africa, which was the first country in the world to start state registration of nurses, to Mozambique and Niger, which have no nursing councils at all" (Klopper & Uys, 2013, p. xxiv. Used with permission ©The Honor Society of Nursing, Sigma Theta Tau.) Even so, within these tremendous challenges are many triumphs for nursing education in Africa, especially where collaboration within and outside the country has led to the progressive advancement of the discipline. Hester C.

Klopper, past president of Sigma Theta Tau International (STTI), and coauthor Leanna R. Uys extend a request to all by inviting us "to join forces with us to leave a legacy of improved nursing and nursing education systems for generations to come; let's work together!" (2013, p. xxvix).

In 2009, the Chinese Nurses Association in China celebrated its 100-year anniversary as nursing education in China forges ahead to meet future challenges for improving healthcare education in a demanding complex healthcare system with the future goal of university-level degree education. The Commission on the Education of Health Professionals for the 21st Century in China stipulates the need to develop a broader range of new competencies for nursing graduates. Of note are disease prevention, health promotion, core ordination, evidenced-based practice, quality care, and patient safety (Gao, Chan, & Cheng, 2011; Hou et al., 2014). Learners need additional experience in the community, long-term care and home settings, and schools. Nursing is working to provide more opportunities for upward mobility in education from basic training programs to universities through attempts to standardize prelicensure nursing education by promoting stronger international links to build alliances for best practices that are key to the global development of nursing education and practice in China (Gao et al., 2011). In similar fashion, nursing education in other Asian countries has moved toward a baccalaureate for entry-level nursing practice or from a 3-year curriculum to a 4-year curriculum in programs that are government accredited or approved. These countries include Hong Kong, Japan, Korea, Macau, and Thailand (ICN, 2014a, 2014b, pp. 1–5).

Numerous national nursing associations in Latin America have called for innovative educational models for all levels of nursing to prepare the region for the next century. They aim to enhance teaching and service programs to develop capacity in educator and learners, to increase learning in interdisciplinary teams, and to create a learning focus on primary health while working to remove institutional, economic, and language as obstacles to education access. Canever, Prado, Backes, and Gomes (2012) identify three main obstacles and challenges to expanding access to nursing education in Latin America. The first is the lasting effects of a disease-focused medicalized curricula. Second is the commodification and subsequent privatization of college education, and lastly, the financial and personal cost of procuring an education where there is a lack of federal support and dollars for investment in science and technology.

The time for talking has passed, and the time to act is now. The road ahead is not an easy one, nothing of value ever is. In nursing education, we currently face tremendous pressures in chaotic environments. The list includes funding shortages, mounting social pressures, the ongoing shortage of nurse educators, and mounting demands for new nurses. In fact, such demands contributed to the creation of multiple modes of entry to practice and varying types and levels of credentialing for nurses in the United States

(Benner et al., 2010). Despite these challenges, nurses, out of all the healthcare professions, deliver the most frontline care to patients in our hospitals and communities. Therefore, nurses as leaders and advocates of quality care are also well positioned to effect positive and lasting change in the development of new health delivery frameworks and processes. Educators and employers involved in deploying and employing nurses of the 21st century are tasked with both the initial and ongoing development of nurses of excellence (CNA, 2012a). This can be accomplished by setting new standards for the delivery of high-quality education, grounded in evidence-based standards for design, implementation, and evaluation as indicated in the best practice standards for simulation (INACSL Standards Committee, 2016, INACSL Standards of Best Practice: Simulation).

 We need nurses capable of advancing the profession within a team-based healthcare environment to provide value in the delivery of ethical, effective, safe, and compassionate nursing care. Nurses of the 21st century must possess new competencies that align with what is needed to thrive in complex and rapidly changing environments. Nurses, therefore, must have the ability to engage as effective leaders, followers, and managers within and outside of their discipline.

Future nurses must be adept in their roles as providers of person-, and family-centered care, team members, case managers, coordinators of care, project managers, patient advocates, and change agents, but our curricula have struggled to keep up with these realities. Dr. Shamian reminds us to

Embrace leadership, influence and impact … within and outside healthcare … to be courageous and take on positions in non-traditional healthcare organizations; find employment in government, and community and social agencies; run for office and expand your horizons; continue your education; apply for international jobs … to be a player on the world stage … and finally, to seize the day—the world is waiting! (Nagle, 2014b, para. 13)

The simulation practice community, in tandem with other healthcare organizations, educators, scientists, researchers, clinicians, and policymakers, has been at the forefront of transforming healthcare education in many parts of the world. Simulation-based team learning efforts are on the front line, breaking down silos and turfism to create evidence-based pedagogical practices that include interprofessional, team-focused curricula; however, we have a long way to go. Simulationists worldwide are urged to heed the call for educational transformation through the use of innovative and evidence-based simulation. Together, we can anticipate, predict, and guide the adaptation of simulation for nursing and healthcare. We are the simulation educators, researchers, and leaders that are shaping the future of nursing for our world.

High-Risk Industry—Aviation, Engineering, and Nuclear Power Safety

About 30 years ago, the aviation industry set its sights on improving the industry's poor safety track record (Plane Crash Information, 2015). Figure 1.6 depicts the trajectory in the number of fatal accidents between 1950 and 2014. It was evident that by 1970 that the aviation industry would need sweeping and widespread change. Also, "prior to 1970, there were no standards for flight simulation devices and accreditation was based on individual country regulatory authorities, providing vastly different performance criteria" (2016, p. 5). What ensued over the next decade and in the years that followed was large-scale organizational change that comprised the integration of systemic transformation in every facet of the aviation industry. The outcomes of this sweeping change were remarkable. Aviation accidents in 1950 averaged one death for every 2 million flights, and by 2014, that number had plummeted to one death for every 11 million flights (Plane Crash Information, 2015). The aviation industry having successfully maneuvered the road to systems change, therefore, provides the healthcare industry with valuable lessons for organizational and systems change.

In the year 2000, the Institute of Medicine (IOM) (Kohn, Corrigan, & Donaldson, 2000) in the United States published its seminal report informing the American public that an estimated 44,000 to 98,000 iatrogenic deaths occurred in US hospitals annually. According to Dr. Lucien Leape, that estimate was low. Based on several published studies of the time, he estimated that closer to 180,000 US citizens died annually, or the equivalent of three jumbo jetliner crashes every second day (1994). Moreover, an additional 1 million patients or more were harmed by sentinel events annually. If one compares healthcare statistics to the death rates in the aviation industry during the worst performing years, healthcare statistics are far worse (see Fig. 1.4). Kalra compared the risks associated with healthcare and other industries and found that bungee jumping and healthcare topped the list for highest risk for deaths (Fig. 1.7).

Some challenged the high figures cited by Leape (1994) and the IOM report (Kohn et al., 2000). These objections were later deemed unsubstantiated (Sox & Woloshin, 2000). Kalra (2011) cites the following studies that have clearly upheld the IOM's claims:

- Schimmel (1964) reported that of 1,252 admissions in a university hospital, 20% experienced adverse outcomes with an 8% fatality rate stemming from medication and diagnostic procedures
- Steel et al. (1981) reported that of 815 admissions in a university hospital, 36% experienced adverse events with a 2% fatality rate from medication and diagnostic procedures

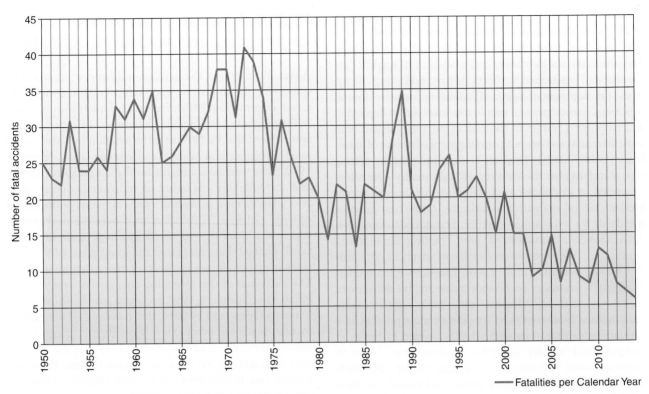

Figure 1.6 The Trajectory in the Number of Fatal Accidents in Airliners with Greater Than 19 Passengers between 1950 and 2014. (Source: Plane Crash Information. (2015). *Statistics.* Retrieved from http://www.planecrashinfo.com/cause.htm.)

- Brennan et al. (1991) studied 30,121 records from New York hospitals and found 3.7% experienced adverse events with a 13.6% fatality rate from medication and surgical procedures
- Wilson et al. (1995) found that of 14,000 admissions in New South Wales and South Australia, 16.6% experienced

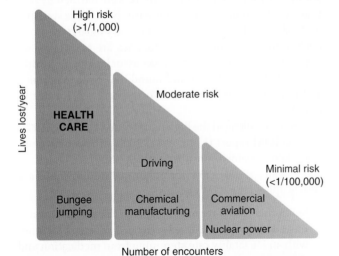

Figure 1.7 Comparison of Risk in Healthcare and Other Industries. (From Kalra, J. (2011). *Medical errors and patient safety: Strategies to reduce and disclose medical errors and improve patient safety.* New York, NY: Deutsche Nationalbibliothek.)

adverse events with a 4.9% fatality rate from medication and surgical procedures
- Vincent et al. (2001) found that of 1,014 records from two hospitals in the London area, 10.8% experienced medical complications, and 8% experienced complications from surgical procedures
- Forster et al. (2004) reported that of 620 patients from Canadian teaching hospital, 12.7%/4.8% respectively suffered medication/operative complications
- Baker et al. (2004) studied records from 25 hospitals and 3,745 hospital charts to find that between 9,000 and 24,000 adverse events occurred in Canada each year (p. 5).

The truth is that even if we allow for a large margin of error in the numbers, the healthcare community is well past the point of denying that huge problems exist. It was no longer about the precision of numbers reported decades ago; it is about commitment to processes and human practices that do far less harm to our patients! Recent evidence from a study out of John Hopkins University cites medical error as the third leading cause of death in the United States, right behind cancer and heart disease as the number one killer (Makary & Daniel, 2016). According to the National Center for Health Statistics, medical error is accountable for 251,454 deaths per year, or to put it into context, that is 689 deaths in the United States each day.

It may seem that comparing healthcare to other industries is a flawed approach because healthcare is very complex, inherently risky, and prone to failure in different ways than other sectors. It begs the question, "Why haven't we been able to apply lessons learned from aviation with the same rate of success over the past 10–15 years in healthcare?"

John J. Nance is a native Texan of the United States of America, decorated Veteran Air Force and commercial pilot, a publically recognized authority on flight education safety, and author of the book *Why Hospitals Should Fly* (2008). Nance offers readers a fictional depiction of patient care at St. Michael's Hospital. Although the characters and the hospital are fictional, the problems associated with offering patient care in high-risk hospital environments are very real. So to, are the solutions he proposes that align with recommendations of the now infamous IOM report *To Err is Human* (Kohn et al., 2000). St. Michael's hospital goes through an incredible transformation that reflects the IOM vision for healthcare as safe, patient-centered, efficient, effective, timely, and equitable. Through this poignant story, Nance delivers a powerful appeal to healthcare providers worldwide to turn the tide on the cataclysmic loss of life that has taken place over the last century in healthcare environments. He leaves us wondering why it has taken us so long to get there. Nance pleads that like aviation, healthcare needs deep, pervasive, and sustainable organizational culture change.

Organizational Culture in Aviation Had to Change

The airline industry set out to embed within their organizations the principles, practices, and values inherent in a **safety culture** using lessons from high-consequence, **high-risk industries**. From the beginning, the aviation industry employed a rigid, top-down management approach with individually based safety systems that held individuals, not groups, accountable for outcomes. There was a clear, defined hierarchy that positioned the senior pilot or captain, as having full authority over the crew. As a result, pilots were revered as highly skilled individuals and were not questioned. During that period, pilot training and promotion was solely based on individual competency attainment and the ability to maintain an error-free track record. The approach to training pilots did not include any training in teamwork or leadership. Before organizational change, pilots rarely consulted others, and anyone who dared to question pilots was quickly silenced (Skiles, NSC conference presentation, 2012).

Organizational changes in the airline industry used proactive approaches instead of the reactive approaches of the past. Instead of waiting for terrible events to occur, they would use an integrated **systems approach** to predicting potential threats to avoid disasters. A complete integrated systems transformation transpired over the next decade

involving both bottom-up and top-down change. Indeed, Skiles noted that the most remarkable shift occurred when everyone on the crew was held responsible for everything that happened, whether good or bad (2012). This remarkable philosophical and operational paradigm shift led to the development of entirely new processes that catapulted communication and team competency training to the forefront of organizational culture. Gone were the days when ego was a barrier to safe practices. The new focus was on flattened hierarchy and team development by creating opportunities for the crew get to know each other as human beings and friends. One of the ways to mitigate perceived power distances was to have everyone dress in casual clothes during training sessions rather than being in full uniform. The word *crew* came to mean that *everyone* had to speak up and challenge every mistake or potential mistake. Effective communication, mutual respect, and a clear understanding of each crewmember's critical role replaced autocracy. Integrated systems like preflight checklists and cross-checks for pilots and copilots now required two sets of eyes, two brains, and the introduction of the third party in cases of disagreement. A captain's authority was now rooted in team trust, not fear. One decade after the airline industry implemented changes, the culture that pervaded it for so many decades was no longer even traceable (Skiles, 2012).

Patankar and Sabin (2010, as cited in Patankar, Brown, Sabin, & Bigda-Peyton, 2012) depict the cultural change that occurred in aviation in the *Safety Culture Pyramid Model* (Fig. 1.8). This model depicts how a safety culture lives within a dynamically balanced, adaptable state inside organizations. Unfolding within organizations is a continuous interplay of inculcated values, leadership strategies, and attitudes that together promote sustainable safety practices.

A secretive culture thrives when trust at all levels of the organization is low and when mistakes or latent failures are known but remain hidden or not verbalized. In secretive organizations, evaluation of events relies exclusively on data from operational reports and punishment for mistakes follows swiftly (Patankar et al., 2012). Similarly, in healthcare, many issues go unreported for fear of reprisal or of shame and ridicule. A **culture of blame** is also present in highly reactive, low-trust organizations. Within a culture of blame, individuals are punished for mistakes or negative events (Patankar et al., 2012). For changes to occur, the progression toward a *reporting culture* means that employees must be understood as trusted key informants that provide vital information to fuel individual and systemic change.

In a **just culture**, the level of trust throughout the organization is very high. Employees are encouraged, even rewarded as key informants whose voices serve to reinforce the development of risk-conscious safety behaviors. To sustain the shift to a just culture, organizations need

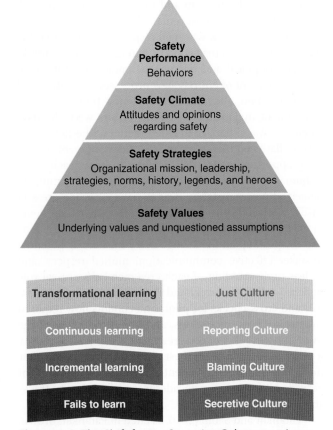

Figure 1.8 The Shift from a Secretive Culture to a Just Culture. (Based on ideas found in Patankar, M. S., Brown, J. P., Sabin, E. J., & Bigda-Peyton, T. G. (2012). *Safety culture: Building and sustaining a cultural change in aviation and healthcare*. Aldershot, UK: Ashgate Publishing.)

both a bottom-up, top-down, commitment to continuous assessment, intervention, and evaluation of critical success factors. Critical success factors in just culture include behavior, climate, strategies, and underlying values. As Captain Skiles revealed, the aviation industry decided to exchange the ability to reprimand and punish an individual for the capacity to gain greater knowledge about the organization. The airline industry accepts the fact that human beings are fallible for personal and human factor–related reasons. Today, instead of punishment or litigation, procedural solutions are used to mitigate error as patterns emerge in the data (Skiles, 2012).

Aviation Accounted for Human Factors

Mistakes are rarely the result of one individual's actions. As human beings, our very nature is to learn from our mistakes. We are all subject to moments of inattention, poor judgement, a lack of focus, oversight, misinterpretation, fatigue, forgetfulness, distraction, and a myriad of other factors that confound our ability for peak performance. So,

if we cannot change the human condition, we need to shift our focus to changing the conditions under which people work (Reason, 1990). **Human factors** in healthcare is a discipline that aims to do just that: to uncover and address elements that manifest as mismatches between people, the tools they use, and the environments in which they work.

Apply Lessons Learned to Complex Adaptive Systems in Healthcare

Human factors, also known as human factors engineering or ergonomics, are a human-centered and task-centered systems-based design process that studies interactions between humans and other elements of a system. Human factors draws on the theory, principles, data, and methods of other disciplines, such as nuclear and aerospace engineering, and even mainstream consumer product development to enhance overall human well-being and performance (International Ergonomics Association, 2000, in Patient Safety Education Program©). The human factors approach in healthcare views employees as humans that are working within a larger system while also being part of a whole system. It is interesting to note that in human factors, both humanists (those who study and work in human science fields) and mechanists (those who work in computer and technology industries) must interact and engage in designing together. It takes an intentional bridging of the gap that exists between these two disciplines to create an effective human-centered design. In order to achieve effective design "technologies must be a good fit with: a) human physical abilities; b) human cognitive abilities; c) communication facilitation; and d) particular political and organizational characteristics, such as, laws or organization culture" (PSEP—Canada, Module 2, pp. 7–9).

A common misconception is that because human factors engineering is touted to be human-centered, it is thought to focus on changing human beings and their behavior. This is completely false. Rather, overarching goals in human factors in healthcare are focused on improving (1) patient safety, (2) efficiency, (3) technology adoption, and (4) user experience and to (5) reduce the resources required for user training, so the focus is on improvement in systems and technology.

One simple example of a human factors initiative in aviation is the Pilot's Quick Reference Handbook that Captain Skiles reached for in the Hudson River emergency. The handbook is printed in big bolded font to accommodate vision changes in aging pilots or a cockpit that is smoke-filled. Another more complex example would be digitized dashboard equipment that sends verification messages to pilots when programming altitude, asking them if they are certain of their actions. These types of prompts are also common in human-centered healthcare systems design to mitigate error. Some of the benefits of having technology, tools, and systems that are designed to be readily usable by humans are as follows:

1. Increased productivity.
2. Reduced errors through effective design that incorporates "forced functions" that direct a user to question and verify equipment function or prevent the use of certain functions under certain circumstances.
3. Reduced training and support by providing a mechanism to reinforce learning.
4. A well-designed and usable system that can reinforce learning, thus reducing training time and in-person teaching sessions.
5. Improved acceptance as easy, effective design makes the user interface experience pleasant.
6. Improved user acceptance is often an indirect outcome from the design of a usable system.
7. Enhanced reputation for product sales through positive user comments (Maguire, 2001).

Systems-Based Approaches to Change in Healthcare

High-performing organizations in high-consequence industries such as aviation, healthcare, nuclear, and chemicals **are recognized for having** resilience as their core. Patankar et al. (2012) define resilience in high-consequence industries as the ability for people in organizations, functioning either in teams or as individuals, to engage in self-regulatory practices in complex situations to change behaviors and ultimately achieve success. Through a learned process of vigilance and the ability to recognize misaligned safety practices, the individual and/or team proactively engages in corrective action to return balance to the system. Therefore, a deeply embedded culture of safety will result in an unwavering commitment from people in the organization to prevent harm, as well as the ability to recover from accidents when they do occur. Once employees are committed to this approach, their commitment becomes the moral force that drives the proactive and autocorrective behaviors that build a strong safety culture and a safe industry for consumers. On the other hand, when resilience is absent or weak, vulnerabilities and cracks appear quickly and systems crumble as employees hide or blame others for fear of reprisal and the ability to defend against threats is undermined.

A *nonreprisal policy and philosophy* was adopted by the aviation industry with the guiding principle that if an error by one person is a mistake, an error by five people is an organization hazard that requires an organizational solution. As long as the individual crewmembers operated within their legal scope of practice and did not engage in risk-taking behavior that was unsafe, employees would not be held accountable for outcomes, either good or bad. The caveat is that the nonreprisal policy no longer applies when someone other than the employee reports the near miss or error. In such circumstances, the nonreporting employee is no longer covered under the risk-free reporting clause.

According to Patankar et al. (2012), two other hallmarks of resilient organizations are risk-taking and risk management to optimize performance. *Risk-taking* occurs when common sense dictates trying out new approaches and strategies, even if they are incongruent with current policy. This approach is only effective when such decisions are made collectively and are grounded in overarching safety principles and values. *Risk management*, on the other hand, is the ability not only to effectively navigate a storm but also to project and plan for the most significant risks and then work to reduce those risks. *Integrated risk management* (IRM) is used in healthcare and provides a framework for "understanding and prioritizing different types of risks that arise from across and within an organization, such as, the effectiveness and accountability of governance, organizational performance, levels of reliability and resiliency, and alignment with accreditation and regulatory (government) expectations" (Healthcare Insurance Reciprocal of Canada, 2014a, pp. 1–4). When risk management processes are not effectively carried out in high-consequence industries, effects will range from poor performance to catastrophic failures, such as death or harm to patients and families, harm or distress to individuals or teams, or even a threat to the continued existence of the organization (Caldwell, 2012).

Applying Aviation Approaches to Reduce Medical Error

Healthcare literature refers to medical error in different ways: adverse events, sentinel events, errors of omission, errors of planning, error of execution, etc. (Kalra, 2011). Although there are slight variations in their meaning, ultimately, the end result of all types of error can be patient death or significant or disabling harm (Kohn et al., 2000). Since the release of the IOMs preliminary *To Err is Human* report in 1999, adverse events and subsequent harm to patients are widely accepted as a crisis in healthcare that comes at high cost to patients, significant others, families, communities, nations, and our world.

Historically, data on error and error outcomes in healthcare were generated from either retrospective review and analysis of charts or institutional error reporting results. This type of data relies exclusively on the extent to which a healthcare provider chooses to report an adverse event. Historically, patients and families had few, if any formal mechanisms to report error in hospitals; error, if reported, was usually brought to the attention of hospital staff/management or to professional regulatory bodies where disciplinary measures could be taken. Note that it is important to make the distinction between **disclosure** of error and reporting of error in that a person can engage in the act of disclosure to a patient or other HCP but could choose to not formally report the error. In the end, the choice to disclose or report an adverse event resides with the individual, and that choice is always impacted by personal and professional beliefs, assumptions, moral and ethical principles, as well as the perceived degree of negative outcome for the patient (Kalra, 2011). The pervading healthcare culture of blame and shame, still present in most healthcare contexts, also impacts the extent to which reporting occurs. Perception, then, is everything, and when confronted by issues of personal culpability and blame within the prevailing organizational culture, decisions about whether or not to report can be confusing.

Airlines used human factors theory as the basis for full disclosure and as such have systems that require reporting of all errors and near misses, regardless of outcomes. The reason for use of **error tracking** is that, "it is vastly more important to identify the hazards and threats to safety, than to identify and punish an individual for a mistake" (Skiles, 2012). With error tracking, organizations exchange the ability to reprimand an individual for greater knowledge of the system problems that lead to error and individual and system failure. The evidence is clear. If healthcare systems unilaterally adopted both individual-, and systems-based approaches to adverse event reporting as part of a wholesale culture change management process, as in aviation, patients and families would indeed be benefactors.

Adopting these approaches in healthcare will require us to develop and implement system-wide self-reporting mechanisms using deidentified reporting systems (report does not identify the person reporting—individual remains unknown) that can easily be accessed and completed in a timely manner. Error tracking systems contain direct data links to deidentified data, allowing error and near miss reports to be uploaded, tracked, and analyzed. From there, all facets of the organization can work to generate new procedures and training programs designed to combat threat and error and trap them before they become adverse events. Lastly, self-reporting and data gathering must be supplemented by deidentified observational safety audits where individuals are planted as observers to record team performance and document live events as they unfold in the trenches, without reporting individual identifiers. To that end, organizations must continue to strive toward creating systems that use proactive versus reactive approaches to create resilient safety systems, the hallmark of learning organizations.

Organizations, and the healthcare providers working within them, must also develop effective error disclosure practices for sharing adverse events with patients and families. As well, organizations must explore means for full restitution for any harm incurred. This is a huge challenge, especially when operating within a highly litigious society, where legal action has become a viable option for victims and family members of adverse events. Time and again, there is strong evidence that when full disclosure of adverse events and the circumstances surrounding them is accompanied by a sincere apology as well as efforts for full restitution, the victims and/or their families can move forward in their grief and loss, not as adversaries but as partners in changing the culture of healthcare. The Patient and Family Story section of the Canadian Patient Safety Institute website provides an example of how patients and families, along with healthcare providers and safety agencies, are banding together to create policy and practice changes from exceptionally devastating circumstances (CPSI, 2012). The patient and family must be central to our purpose, mission, and vision for safer healthcare. Now, just imagine the power of an *error disclosure simulation.*

Healthcare systems, professional regulatory bodies, government, administrators, and all employees in healthcare must understand and accept that an error happens, even with the best of the best. If we are ever to shift the tide from a culture of individual blame and shame in healthcare, we must be willing to accept and embrace that errors are the result of multifaceted and complex systems that are populated by human beings: well-intentioned individuals that despite having high standards for knowledge, skills, and attitudes are nonetheless fallible and prone to human factors–related occurrences.

Healthcare environments must develop effective teams, where those teams, in essence, fuel the safety organization by generating the data needed to learn and create procedural, team-oriented solutions. This process in aviation, known as Barrier to Error Management, results in the creation of tools like team emergency procedure, Quick Reference Handbooks, Standard Operations Protocol, or start-up and crosscheck checklists that have become industry standards with which all teams become intimately familiar through team training.

To realize the full benefits of a systems-based approach in healthcare, we must commit to integrating system-wide, nonpunitive team development methods, coupled with individual-based performance management that serve to hold professionals accountable for their professional practice. This dual system attends to both individual and team functions (see Fig. 1.9). Individual performance management is required for those who step outside their professional scopes of practice or who engage in unethical or illegal practices, such as criminal activity, intentional falsification, substance abuse, or use of controlled substances. Although healthcare and aviation are not the same, failing to apply aviation's safety science principles will be detrimental to patient safety and improved healthcare outcomes. ***We need an organizational culture shift that***

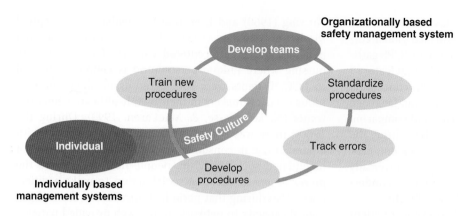

Figure 1.9 Individually Based and Organizationally Based Management Systems. (Based on ideas from Skiles, J. (2012, May). Was it really a miracle on the Hudson? Aviation meets healthcare safety [Plenary session]. National Patient Safety Foundation 2012 Meeting.)

views high-risk environments as the source of informing our practices to minimize risk. What is needed is a large-scale and lasting culture change that moves us away from lingering practices that punish individuals for error, to systems that learn from, and respond to full-disclosure environments and error-tracking (Fairbanks, 2012).

How Is Healthcare Change Advancing?

Meaning-filled change, calls for meaning-filled action. Healthcare workers and the public, as well as, government and government agencies, were all shocked by the IOM report (2000), To Err is Human. Since its release nearly twenty years later, billions and billions of dollars have been earmarked to fund patient safety and total quality initiatives. It is now 2017, and the healthcare scorecard is showing improvement, especially with targeted initiatives, such as a decrease in hospital-acquired infections, and other targeted safety programs such as TeamSTEPPS in the United States (AHRQ, 2011) and Safer Healthcare Now interventions through the Canadian Patient Safety Institute (CPSI, 2016a). When we compare the results in healthcare against those in aviation over time, change in healthcare is lagging (Classen et al., 2011; Fairbanks, 2012; Landrigan et al., 2010; Levinson, 2010). There is a consensus that at the 10-year mark, we should be doing better.

In recent years, there have been amazing stories shared by healthcare professionals from all disciplinary backgrounds, who openly shared the effects of perfectionism and elitism on team performance and patient outcomes. One common thread in these narratives is the acknowledgment that we are all products of professions in which we were socialized for perfectionism and competition (Anderson, 2015). The pervading message in education must change from being perfect to understanding that "We are not Gods!" We are human beings and even when we are on top of our game, we can and do make serious mistakes. Together, we have the potential to be less fallible.

What Are We Doing in Healthcare?

Crossing the Quality Chasm, the second IOM report (2001), recommended six key dimensions, in no particular order of priority, to support the delivery of healthcare in the 21st century that are expressed as the acronym, STEEEP. Policymakers, purchasers, regulators, health professionals, healthcare trustees and management, and consumers are called to develop and implement the following:

- **Safety**—Avoid injury to patients from the care that is intended to help them.
- **Timeliness**—Reduce waits and harmful delays.
- **Effectiveness**—Provide services based on scientific knowledge to all who could benefit and refrain from providing services to those not likely to benefit (avoiding overuse and underuse, respectively).
- **Efficiency**—Avoid waste.
- **Equitability**—Provide care that does not vary in quality because of personal characteristics such as gender, ethnicity, geographical location, and socioeconomic status.
- **Patient-centeredness**—Provide care that is respectful of and responsive to individual patient preferences, needs, and values (IOM, 2001, pp. 39–40).

Below, we flush out in more detail these dimensions and related concepts by examining (1) focus on patient safety, (2) focus on person-, and family-centered care, (3) interprofessional education and developing healthcare teams, (4) using systems approaches to make better decisions, and (5) using systems approaches to mitigate harm from medical error.

Focus on Patient Safety

As previously mentioned in this chapter, patient safety is a key, if not the most important driver in healthcare education using simulation. Today, we have a plethora of tools at our disposal for teaching patient safety to enact positive change in healthcare outcomes. The International Classification for Patient Safety (ICPS), spearheaded by the WHO, developed a standardized classification of key patient safety concepts, intended to enhance global collaborative learning, sharing, and patient safety. ICPS gathered a group of experts from across the globe that featured 48 preferred concepts and an accompanying conceptual framework. It is hoped that the use of common language and resources will promote global sharing and comparing of safety incidents and reports, ultimately benefitting the collective whole. If terms like patient safety incident, near miss, harm, and reportable circumstance are universally adopted and employed, we are better positioned to understand their impact on a global level (WHO, 2015b).

The WHO (2011b) has also published an entire patient safety curriculum for use by all healthcare disciplines. This resource is a treasure for educators in search of core content, tools, and resources for course development. Similar products have been developed around the world in different countries to educate the public and healthcare providers in safety concepts while other programs offer training in patient safety. Some of these programs include the Canadian Patient Safety Institute (CPSI); Patient Safety Education Program (PSEP), 2016b; National Patient Safety Foundation (NPSF); and the Certification Board for Professionals in Patient Safety (2015).

As educators, we are charged with infusing patient safety concepts into student learning experiences. Healthcare curricula across the board must include the core concepts of patient safety outcomes. These include, but are not limited to, (1) historical trajectory of patient safety; (2) the language of patient safety and person- and family-centered care; (3) the culture of blame and shame; (4) transparency and accountability in delivering safe effective care; (5) disclosure and reconciliation in adverse events; (6) flattening of power structures to create well-functioning teams; (7) leadership and followership; (8) communication; (9) systems thinking and healthcare as industry; (10) healthcare delivery systems engineering; (11) high-reliability organizations and lessons learned from aviation, engineering, and nuclear; (12) human factors and technology; (13) risk management and total quality improvement, and (14) knowledge of tools and resources for healthcare providers (PSEP, 2016b; WHO, 2011b). The INACSL **Simulation-enhanced interprofessional education** (Sim-IPE) standard states that:

Simulation-enhanced interprofessional education (Sim-IPE) enables participants from different professions to engage in a simulation-based experience to achieve shared or linked objectives and outcomes" (INACSL Standards Committee, 2016, p. S34).

Focus on Person- and Family-Centered Care

Person-centered care (PCC) is a term coined over 50 years ago by nurse theorists, beginning with Faye Abdellah's work on the grand theory Patient-Centered Approaches to Nursing (1960) and Ernestine Wiedenbach's Conceptual Model of Nursing (1964). These theorists promoted patient-, and family-centered care (PCC) in maternity nursing where unique personhood is viewed as central to PCC. Patients were considered as qualified, autonomous decision-makers in their own healthcare needs and wants (Nickel, Gesse, & MacLaren, 1992). During the 1960s, there was a substantial rise in consumerism with a parallel rise in consumer voice. Through this period of heightened social activism, people now understood the *power of one* in effecting social action to make a difference. Also during that period, an increase in the technological capacity to network on the web provided patients and their families a platform to share personal stories online. In fact, patients and family members have shared horrific accounts of the harm and death that was experienced while receiving healthcare. Today, public outcry coupled with the rise of the PCC movement in healthcare is seeing patients and their loved ones as key partners in social and system change. Patients and their families now have a strong presence in online platforms, they deliver presentations at healthcare conferences, and within many organizations they have a seat at the table in healthcare boardrooms. Another result of the PCC revolution is that hospitals are beginning to develop formal processes to ensure error disclosure and are also adopting reconciliatory processes that ensure victim compensation for loss of life and injury. Here are two excellent examples of patient story websites (http://www.patientstories.org.uk/) and (http://www.patientsafetyinstitute.ca/en/toolsResources/Member-Videos-and-Stories/Pages/default.aspx).

Currently, provider- and system-centered approaches still dominate in healthcare: the emphasis continues to reside with provider evaluation and treatment of disease where the patient is expected to comply with those care regimes and families are generally not part of the patient–provider relationship. Emanuel, Taylor, Hain, Combes, Hatlie, Karsh et al. (2011) state that, "the main characteristics of 20th century healthcare may be summarized as physician autonomy, usually in the context of solo practice … where physician competence was determined by a physician's knowledge" (p. 3). PCC, on the other hand, deems the patient in charge of his/her own unique health regime: evaluating and choosing from treatment options through shared decision-making, through collaborating with family members at their discretion, and through self-determination of outcomes and associated treatment choices. Studies have clearly demonstrated the benefits, including a financial upside to enacting PCC (Stewart et al., 2000).

Additionally, as part of the IOM's charge to improve the quality of healthcare in America, healthcare professionals were called to re-examine healthcare in its totality. Part of that total re-examination involved health professionals having to look inward at themselves and the ideologies and principles that underpinned professional practice. In the years that followed IOM's report, Don

Berwick, an American physician, spearheaded a discourse that went viral on the need for providing patient-centered care. Berwick proposed a radical, unfamiliar, and disruptive shift from old ideas that had to change to allow for new consumer-centered healthcare practices (Berwick, 2009). Berwick stated, "I think it wrong for the profession of medicine—or any other healthcare profession, for that matter—to reserve to itself the authority to judge the quality of its work" (p. w559). A decade later, the significant shift that would see dialogue between healthcare providers and their patients' change from profession-centered to truly patient-centered is progressing, but we are not yet there.

In 2006, the International Alliance of Patients' Organizations (IAPO), in its *Declaration on Patient-Centered Healthcare*, states that the "essence of patient-centered healthcare is that the healthcare system is designed and delivered to address the healthcare needs and preferences of patients so that healthcare is appropriate and cost-effective" (p. 1). Within the declaration, five principles of care are identified: respect, choice and empowerment, patient involvement in health policy, access and support, and information (p. 1).

So how does one enact patient-centeredness? Berwick (2009) suggests three helpful tenets: "1) The needs of the patient come first, period; 2) Nothing about me without me; and 3) Every patient is the only patient" (p. w560). Deeply entrenched ways of being and values do not change easily or quickly; therefore, it is important that the shift to patient-centeredness occur at all levels of healthcare. To attain PCC in healthcare, we must engage all stakeholder groups: learners in educational programs, clinicians in practice, educators in academe, administrators at all levels, politicians making policy and funding decisions, and most importantly, patients and their families.

Within simulation-based learning events, many of these concepts play out with learners for the first time. Within simulated learning events, we have ideal conditions under which we can allow learners to test out new ways of being patient-centered; through our words, actions, attitudes toward patients and families, and policy formulation, we help students to learn the art of patient-centered ethical care. Educators are encouraged to

Reverse the academic notion that we must suppress our emotions in order to become [clinicians].... We will not teach future professionals emotional distancing as a strategy for personal survival. We will teach them instead how to stay close to emotions that can generate energy for institutional change... (Berwick, 2009, p. w560) ... we need a new professional who can confront, challenge, and help change the workplace. (Palmer, 2007, p. 10)

So what of the critics? Those purporting that the patient does not have the ability, knowledge, or skill to manage their own healthcare decisions? Palmer (2007) reminds us that throughout history, those whom the powerful have deemed to be *powerless* have in fact moved mountains. Think, for example, of the power exercised in the black struggle for liberation in apartheid. The power of the human soul, or human light (as per Palmer), has repeatedly demonstrated that positive social change emanates from an inner belief and the will to make it so. Future healthcare practitioners must understand that patient-centeredness is synonymous with professional competence. Today's learners are the leaders and change agents of tomorrow and will need to be emotionally and intellectually adept. They must possess the parallel competencies of leadership and emotional intelligence while advocating for others and themselves through the ability to translate their feelings into knowledge and skill.

This vision is not a pipe dream; it is unfolding around us and becoming reality. Kaiser Permanente KP HealthConnect (2016), for example, has opened access to personal electronic healthcare records to empower patients and encourage them to be more engaged in their own healthcare. They have also created secure patient–healthcare provider email capabilities to promote effective messaging, especially for diabetes and hypertension care. What they found was that in improving connectivity, healthcare outcomes also improved (Kaiser Permanente, 2016). Key healthcare documents all around the world now include patient-centered care as a keystone of excellence in the provision of healthcare. It is now up to each one of us to determine the pace at which this vision becomes reality.

Develop Interprofessional Competencies and Improved Team Outcomes

Historically, healthcare education has occurred in silos with little emphasis on learning the professional roles and scopes of practice in healthcare disciplines (Accreditation of Programs in Health Professional Education (AIPHE), 2016; Dillon, Noble, & Kaplan, 2009; Orchard, Curran, & Kabene, 2005). Over the past decade, there has been a marked global shift in postsecondary and postlicensure programs toward the education of healthcare professionals to include interprofessional competencies. Interprofessional competencies are defined as the complex integration of knowledge, values, skills, and judgements integrated into collaborative practice (Canadian Interprofessional Health Collaborative (CIHC), 2010). A Joint Commission task force on sentinel events led by the National Patient Safety Institute (2008) reported miscommunication and communication failure in teams as a core cause of sentinel events in healthcare. There is an urgent need for the rapid ramping up of our focus on the integration of patient safety and healthcare team competencies in undergraduate and workplace education programs (Hammick, Freeth, Koppel, Reeves, & Barr, 2007; Reeves, Lewin, Espin, & Zwarenstein, 2010; WHO, 2010a; Zwarenstein & Reeves, 2006).

Disappointingly, there is evidence supporting the notion that baccalaureate programs in nursing are not adequately preparing students for proficiency in interprofessional communication (CIHC, 2010; Frank & Brien 2008; Utley-Smith, 2004). Moreover, new graduate nurses self-identified a lack of confidence and competence in professional communication (Duchscher, 2008, 2009; Kelly & Ahern, 2007). IPE recommendations support the use of simulation-based training as a powerful strategy for teaching these competencies in healthcare programs (AIPHE, 2007; American Institutes for Research, 2011; Decker et al., 2015; Dillon et al., 2009; Reeves et al., 2010; Thomas, Bertram, & Johnson, 2009). Educators employing simulation pedagogy are able to create effective learning opportunities for students to interact, practice, and reflect on communication skills in teams. Furthermore, using a Sim-IPE approach allows students to use skill practice, repetition, and reflection with their peers while gaining proficiency in team communication competencies (INACSL Standards Committee, 2016, Sim-IPE). Communication is clearly defined as a competency and graduate outcome of baccalaureate in nursing undergraduate programs (AACN, 2008b, 2011; CNA, 2009a; Duchscher, 2008, 2009; Thomas et al., 2009; Utley-Smith, 2004).

Note: Chapter 26 focuses on IPE and addresses in more detail the need for global expansion of IPE in all healthcare contexts.

Using Systems Approaches to Making Better Decisions in Healthcare

Complexity in healthcare is a term that has become ubiquitous, but what does it really mean? In this section, we will look at tools that can help us understand the **complex adaptive systems** we work in.

The *Cynefin Framework* (Fig. 1.10) is a sense-making tool to help us understand levels of complexity in situations and offers varied approaches to solving simple, complex, complicated, and chaotic issues (Cognitive Edge, 2015) Cynefin (pronounced *kun-ev-in*), is Welsh for "a place of multiple belongings" (Cognitive Edge, 2015).

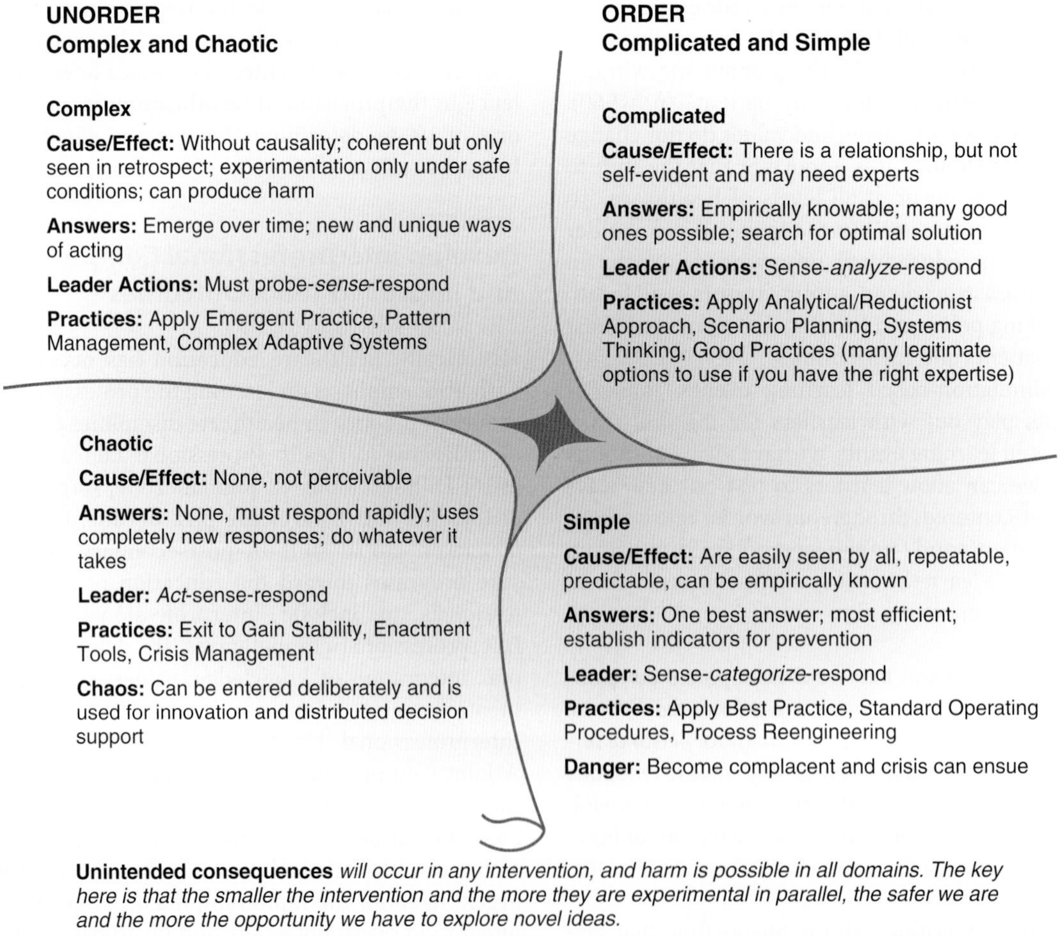

UNORDER
Complex and Chaotic

Complex

Cause/Effect: Without causality; coherent but only seen in retrospect; experimentation only under safe conditions; can produce harm

Answers: Emerge over time; new and unique ways of acting

Leader Actions: Must probe-*sense*-respond

Practices: Apply Emergent Practice, Pattern Management, Complex Adaptive Systems

Chaotic

Cause/Effect: None, not perceivable

Answers: None, must respond rapidly; uses completely new responses; do whatever it takes

Leader: *Act*-sense-respond

Practices: Exit to Gain Stability, Enactment Tools, Crisis Management

Chaos: Can be entered deliberately and is used for innovation and distributed decision support

ORDER
Complicated and Simple

Complicated

Cause/Effect: There is a relationship, but not self-evident and may need experts

Answers: Empirically knowable; many good ones possible; search for optimal solution

Leader Actions: Sense-*analyze*-respond

Practices: Apply Analytical/Reductionist Approach, Scenario Planning, Systems Thinking, Good Practices (many legitimate options to use if you have the right expertise)

Simple

Cause/Effect: Are easily seen by all, repeatable, predictable, can be empirically known

Answers: One best answer; most efficient; establish indicators for prevention

Leader: Sense-*categorize*-respond

Practices: Apply Best Practice, Standard Operating Procedures, Process Reengineering

Danger: Become complacent and crisis can ensue

Unintended consequences *will occur in any intervention, and harm is possible in all domains. The key here is that the smaller the intervention and the more they are experimental in parallel, the safer we are and the more the opportunity we have to explore novel ideas.*

Figure 1.10 Four Quadrants of Complex Adaptive Systems. (Framework from Cognitive Edge. (2016). *Introduction Cynefin framework*. Retrieved from http://cognitive-edge.com/videos/cynefin-framework-introduction/. Adapted for simulation education with permission.)

Complexity in healthcare is no different; it is a space where thousands upon thousands of influences play out in unpredictable, fast-paced environments, where issues are not easily understood, and decisions are not easily made. Snowden (2015) explains the Cynefin Framework as an emergent, analytic model that uses data to retrospectively recognize causal relationships between systems to inform future processes. It is, therefore, not a "plug and play" prescriptive model that spews out process before data are available. A decision-maker can look back at a given situation to analyze whether the decisions he or she made or intends to make are well aligned with the level of complexity. Different problems require different courses of action and it is through probing our failures, as well as successes, that best responses are unearthed. It is true in healthcare that we have focused on developing system robustness by attempting to prevent failure, when our efforts would be better exerted in promoting resilience, where "we accept that failure is inevitable and focus instead on early discovery and fast recovery from failure" (Cognitive Edge, 2016). We need to embrace our increasingly complicated, complex, and sometimes chaotic environments to better learn from them how to fashion a resilient system.

According to Snowden (2015), the best spaces to reside within the framework are either within the central space of *indecision* or in the complicated or complex domains. This is because those domains require the use of continuous approaches to solution finding, whereas in simple situations, there is always the danger of stagnancy or complacency that can lead to harmful outcomes. *Ordered* domains are divided into complicated and simple domains, and *unordered* into complex and chaotic. Within each of the domains are varying descriptions of causal relationships, answers, leader actions, and practices.

Using Systems Approaches Instead of People Approaches to Mitigate Error in Healthcare

In 1990, James Reason first published the Model of Human Error Causation, in which he purported that highly engineered systems have fail-safe mechanisms that serve to protect from hazards. Ideally, fail-safes engage, but some do fail, and when they do, the results can be catastrophic. The slices of Swiss cheese in the model (Fig. 1.11) represent those layers of defense that are designed to protect and holes in the cheese represent gaps or failure to protect. Holes in defenses occur for two reasons: active failures and latent conditions. Active failures are a result of peoples' actions and comprise "slips, lapses, fumbles, mistakes, and procedural violations" (p. 769). Reason refers to latent conditions as inevitable "resident pathogens" within the system that arise from decisions made by designers, builders, procedure writers, and top-level management that either can create conditions provoking

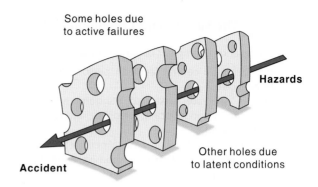

Figure 1.11 Depiction of James Reason's Swiss Cheese Model. (Adapted from Reason, J. T. (1990). *Human error*. Cambridge, UK: Cambridge University Press, with permission.)

error potential, such as "time pressure, understaffing, inadequate equipment, fatigue, or inexperience... or can create long-lasting holes or weaknesses in the defenses, such as untrustworthy alarms and indicators, unworkable procedures, design, and construction deficiencies" (p. 769). These conditions lie dormant until they are triggered, and when they line up perfectly, the perfect storm is created, making way for adverse events. Usually, when one layer fails, other defenses are present, stopping the untoward event from occurring, but when multiple layers of holes in defenses line up, the unintended error results. Lessons learned from the Swiss Cheese Model in healthcare are that we must proactively determine the presence of latent conditions and retrospectively learn from all active failures if we are to see meaningful change.

"We cannot change the human condition, but we can change the conditions under which humans work" as a premise for change in how we view and understand medical error" (Reason, 2000, p. 769).

Summary: How Can Simulation Improve Healthcare Systems and Outcomes?

Simulation grounded in best practice and embedded within new learning paradigms is a powerful means of promoting the acquisition of requisite knowledge, skills, and attitudes for healthcare professionals in today's complex healthcare contexts. Together, we are called to transform nursing and healthcare education by mobilizing our collective efforts as difference makers working to turn the tide toward safer person-, and family-centered healthcare. This chapter is a callout to each of us in

---

Box 1-1   **The Simulations Champion's Mission**

As Simulation Champions of the new millennium, we will:

1. Unite behind a central focus on person-, and family-centered care.
2. Work as *difference makers* to transform nursing and healthcare education locally, regionally, and throughout the in the world.
3. Seek to understand global and local perspectives on education to effect change that is responsive, equitable, and relevant using simulation.
4. Advocate for change as transformational and transcendent leaders, good followers, and competent managers of simulation at local, national, and international levels.
5. Partner and work with organizations, groups, and teams at all levels to collaborate on simulation initiatives.
6. Commit to being change leaders by modeling effective change in professional practice and our workplaces.
7. Work to inculcate essential humanistic values in all simulation teaching and learning: enacting compassion, respect for humankind, integrity and ethical practice, commitment to excellence, and equity and justice in healthcare and education.
8. Reach out to collaborate outside our discipline specific silos to work with other healthcare professionals, clinicians, and Simulation Champions from diverse disciplines to provide safer, effective, ethical patient care.
9. Work to change healthcare systems through enacting cultural change in daily teaching practices, for example, enact safe conditions for error and near miss and adverse event reporting in simulation and clinical contexts.
10. Adopt a mindset of risk mitigation and total quality improvement in program development, keeping what works and learning from what doesn't.
11. Commit to excellence in program development and curricular integration of simulation-based learning.
12. Design learning inclusive of the core concepts of patient safety, person-/family-centered care, just culture, systems thinking, and complexity.
13. Collaborate with other educators and healthcare practitioners to engage in and create team training through IPE.

14. Innovate, innovate, and innovate.
15. Promote the delivery of high-quality simulation delivery through a commitment to:
    a. Adopt, uphold, and imbibe standards and use them to set and attain simulation program benchmarks, such as adopting the INACSL Standards of Best Practice: Simulation (2016) or the SSH Accreditation Standards (2016).
    b. Engage in rigorous, evidence-based, and informed teaching and learning practices in simulation to support the attainment of requisite graduate outcomes and professional practice expectations.
    c. Conduct quality research to build disciplinary knowledge and evidence.
    d. Adopt a stance that learners are highly motivated and desire to engage in simulation learning to be their best and, therefore, require well-defined objectives, challenges that offer appropriate levels of difficulty, and opportunities for focused, repetitive, and deliberate practice of well-defined skills.
    e. Create psychologically safe learning spaces in small groups that foster conditions for deep reflection and transformational learning, through modeling and becoming adept master facilitators.
    f. Design learning that is realistic, with strong fidelity to best support the replication of realistic clinical practice environments and encounters.
    g. Create conditions that promote self-regulated, adaptive learning founded on strengths-based, supportive, and genuine feedback aimed at individual and team performance excellence.
    h. Promote the best use of technology to support learning, while ensuring the efficient and effective use of technology in simulation.
16. Celebrate the successes of learners, colleagues, and simulation teams—everyday.
17. Be true to the main edict of simulation-based education by learning from our mistakes!

---

whatever capacity we are serving, to transform organizations and systems to improve healthcare outcomes. We close this chapter by offering you The Simulation Champions Creed (Box 1-1).

We dedicate this creed to all Simulation Champions everywhere: each of them *difference makers*, working to transform healthcare systems through a united commitment to improve patient safety, engage in effective interprofessional collaboration, and to enacting person-, and family centered care. Let's make the most of the amazing opportunities we have to transform our world through simulation.

2

Coming Together: The Evolution of Communities of Simulation Champions

Kim Leighton

 Key Terms

Leadership, Networking, Organization, Collaboration

 Guiding Questions

1. Where can you go for help when you are told that you are responsible for integrating simulation throughout your school's curriculum?

2. What organizations are available for simulationists and what do they offer to their members?

3. I'm interested in networking and connecting a regional group of simulationists in order to support each other. How do I go about that?

Introduction

Imagine being asked to convince the entire faculty at your school that using patient simulation is necessary. Imagine that you are given two semesters to get every course to have at least one simulation experience for their students. Now, and this is the most challenging of all, imagine that you don't know anyone to ask how to do this. You heard that a community college 4 hours away has a simulator like yours, and of course, the vendor can teach you how to use the equipment, but where else can you turn?

Scenarios like this were common in the early 21st century, less than just 15 years ago. There were no books about simulation, no associations, no journals, and no shared scenarios. There was, however, literature on the topic in other industries, such as aviation, nuclear power, and, for healthcare, in anesthesia training. Many early simulation

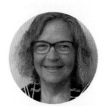

**Kim Leighton,
PhD, RN, CHSE, CHSOS, ANEF**

enthusiasts dove into that literature, gleaning some pieces of the puzzle that they could begin to apply to nursing and other healthcare professional education. But the progress was slow. Not all faculty members were enthused about learning a new teaching strategy, especially one that was technology based and labor intensive. The thought of using simulation in lieu of some existing clinical experiences led to heavy debate. And leaders were hesitant to spend money—a lot of money—on an untried method that had no documented outcomes in nursing education.

Fast forward to today. Look how simulation resources have grown! This chapter is designed to provide you with an understanding of how early leaders connected within their own schools, within geographical regions, and across countries, to create steadfast networks to support pioneering simulationists. Learn about the challenges of the time, the gaps that confronted those educators in their work, and the solutions that their entrepreneurial spirits developed. Not only will you better understand the growth of simulation but you will also benefit from understanding the decisions that were made and how they have impacted the work that you do today. Someday, new simulationists will be looking back to learn about what you did and why. In this quickly growing area of education, the history is short, but important to consider as we now make our own decisions about how to move forward. From small groups to large networks, educators have come together to build strong communities that commit to furthering the efforts of simulation as a teaching strategy.

Inside the Organization

Creating momentum within one's educational environment can be very challenging. While the simulation enthusiast is often an innovator, they are challenged to convince others that their plan for teaching with simulation should be embraced. Rogers (2003), creator of the Diffusion of Innovation Theory, defines innovators as a small group (the lower 2.5% of a normally distributed bell curve) that show the highest proclivity to understand and adopt an innovative idea, technique, or piece of equipment—in this case the idea of teaching utilizing simulation technology. Diffusion of Innovation Theory is presented elsewhere in this book (see Chapter 16), but suffice it to say that innovators did not typically have an easy job.

Finding the first follower is as important as being the lead in moving technology and other ideas forward. Nurturing followers and building critical mass are necessary to get enough people to buy into the idea of simulation. Organizational change and **leadership**, followership, and managership are presented in greater detail in Chapter 8, so instead, let's look at some of the ways that simulation was moved forward within individual institutions.

The top-down, autocratic approach is fraught with potential problems, such as putting one person in charge of simulation and simply telling the faculty that they will be expected to use simulation in their courses. While this clearly identifies the leader, it strips the potential followers of engagement and decision making related to how they will deliver their course content. Mandating how faculty are expected to teach will often result in backlash based on the premise that academic faculty and institutional educators should have academic freedom and professional autonomy in their teaching practices (AAUP, 2015). Another challenge with mandating that all faculty use simulation is that all faculty are not yet qualified with the skill set necessary to teach with simulation. Early practices were to move skills lab personnel into the simulation role—or to add it to their current workload. While this seemed to make sense, over time we have come to realize that patient simulation education is very different from psychomotor skills-based training, which is a subset of simulation. In addition to demanding that unqualified people teach in simulation, educators who had no interest or desire were also forced into the role. Imagine being asked to teach in a way that you don't understand, have no interest in learning, and don't value. To be the best at what we do, it must come from the heart. Even worse, imagine being that teacher's student. In many cases, it is best to leave behind the laggards, those who may never move past resisting change (Rogers, 2003) and focus energy

and resources toward those willing to learn. Workload can then be redistributed accordingly.

Another method that has worked for many schools is to develop a committee that is responsible for simulation use in the program. The composition and role of this committee will vary depending on the faculty governance structure and organizational model of the **organization**. In some schools, a less formal committee meets monthly or quarterly to support the role of simulation, plan training, identify equipment needs, and respond to other concerns such as space, workload policies, clinical replacement questions, and the like. This type of committee may have decision-making power or may have a more advisory role. In other schools, the curriculum committee envelops simulation. This is a strong place for this work to reside, as the program objectives, curriculum threads, and course objectives should help to guide simulation integration. However, an assessment committee should also lay claim to simulation in its role of determining if educational outcomes are met across the curriculum. It is easy to see how it can become a complicated matter to determine where simulation best fits. Each school needs to examine its organizational structure to determine where responsibility best lies or if a shared model works better. Reporting structure for the committee should be a solid line to a leadership position that has decision-making authority and a budget to support the identified needs related to equipment and faculty development.

Read about the experiences of Dr. Beth Hallmark as she moved the simulation program forward at Belmont University. She shares both the challenges and successes, as well as a caution about monitoring your commitments to prevent burnout.

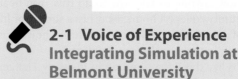

2-1 Voice of Experience
Integrating Simulation at Belmont University

Beth Fentress Hallmark, PhD, MSN, RN, CHSE

The Challenge

I do not think our center is different from many small academic centers; we received funding from local foundations that enabled us to build a phenomenal space. When we moved into our space in May of 2006, simulation was just beginning to "come on the scene" in nursing schools. We had over 20 mannequins, no one knew how to use them and classes beginning in the fall with the expectation of integrating the new tools into our courses.

Meeting the Challenge:

The program director asked me if I was interested in being the "Lab Director" and I literally laughed, because I did not see the value in using "plastic dummies" to teach. I subsequently began doing some reading and research and found that simulation seemed to fit with my love for technology. We were also involved with a community grant that included educating faculty in simulation pedagogy and I was given the lead at Belmont to move this forward. The challenges were numerous; developing a program that was new and was not supported in the evidence became almost impossible. I quickly realized I was in over my head and brought in consultants and experts to help me articulate how they had integrated simulation in their programs. In addition, the community grant allowed us to have an annual simulation conference at Belmont and I was mentored by some amazing nurse educators.

Outcome

In the summer of 2010, we formed simulation groups to adopt an evaluation rubric and debriefing method; these two decisions were pivotal to the faculty beginning to take some ownership of simulation. In 2012, we were able to hire a postdoctoral fellow who also became an important voice for simulation within our program. Together we submitted the SSH accreditation application and were successful in our application for provisional accreditation.

Lessons Learned

I have sought out experts in the field to help me understand the pedagogy around simulation; I volunteered Belmont to be a pilot site for studies, and I read as much research as I could find. I have learned many lessons as I have volunteered to speak and worked with vendors, publishers, technology companies, and other independent groups; the knowledge I have is valuable and I am much more careful about simply volunteering to help them develop their products. I am not in this profession for the money, but I did exhaust myself both physically and emotionally by giving to so many people. I do think that healthcare providers and particularly nurses are vulnerable to this. One additional challenge was lack of

infrastructure within the simulation program. I ran the program single-handedly for over 7 years; currently, our program is supported by two additional staff positions. I accomplished this by taking my dean to see programs across the region, demonstrating to her the value of simulation. Having an advocate within your administration is key. I will be forever grateful for the opportunities that simulation has given me; I have grown both professionally and personally during my journey. The journey is not over, as we are in the midst of a curriculum revision, and simulation will have a much more prominent place in our program. We have developed an experiential learning model and will have a true simulation team in place.

Inspiration for Simulation Champions

This is an exciting time in simulation for us and for health education in general.

Reaching Out

While many schools have adopted a committee structure of some type to support simulation activities, others, particularly smaller and independent nursing programs, may only have one person responsible for simulation: knowing how to use the equipment, creating scenarios, running scenarios with students, and evaluating them. There may not be anyone else on campus that has similar responsibilities or interest in learning more. This is a very lonely position to be in. There is no one to commiserate with when simulation experiences don't go well; after all, if you complain, then you may be losing a potential ally in the quest to integrate simulation. It is important, especially when you are a committee of one, to project a positive image of simulation, even when you might be struggling. While there are now journals and books from which to glean ideas, there is significant value in discussion with other people who speak the same simulation language and understand the challenges involved in this type of teaching. When there is no one within, then it is time to reach out to others.

Many new simulation educators begin their education in simulation by visiting other simulation labs and centers to "see how they do it." This is an effective way to learn what has worked—and not worked—for other educators, then take the information and adapt it to your own environment. Most schools and organizations are happy to show you their labs and the work that they do; just call ahead and schedule a time to meet. While you are there, also pay special attention to the equipment, props, and supplies that are available for simulation. You will likely be amazed that almost every single item that is available in the traditional clinical environment is also available for simulation. These tools that are used to increase the fidelity, or realism, of the simulation experience range from expensive equipment to "home-grown" solutions. I have seen a ventilator created from a washing machine box, while another school rents a ventilator from a durable medical equipment company for the days it is needed. These are examples of cost-effective ways of avoiding the capital purchase of a ventilator. Throughout this book, you will find these ideas in the Simulation on a Shoestring feature. Additional ideas can be found on the Simulation Innovation Resource Center (SIRC) site in the Home-Grown Simulation Solutions section, an initiative of the International Nursing Association for Clinical Simulation and Learning (INACSL) and the National League for Nursing (NLN). Simulation employs a lot of very creative people.

The major simulation organizations have LISTSERVs and LinkedIn pages for their members to use to communicate about a wide variety of topics that include staffing models, determining return on investment, how to best use video, and scenario ideas. Archives have been created for examples of position descriptions and low-cost solutions for common problems. These provide an easy method for contacting others for assistance with routine everyday problems as well as challenging questions for which the literature has not yet provided answers. Many members list their contact information in the membership directories. For those who do not, it is easy to search "[first and last name] simulation nursing" or a similar combination to find out where the person works. Then, go to their college's website, and use the faculty/staff directory to find the contact information. This is also an easy way to seek out presentation materials from a conference session that you were unable to attend. Most simulation educators are happy to share their work—after all, that is the purpose of presenting at a conference! One thing that has amazed me is the generosity of our simulation practice community, likely born of our initial isolation in the workplace.

Major simulation organizations also have communities of common interest, called Special Interest Groups (SIGs), Sections, or Affinity Groups. These groups have different compositions, sizes, and roles. These subsets of the greater organizations often meet face-to-face at annual conferences as well as monthly or quarterly in between. Meeting minutes may be archived, and continuing education opportunities, often with associated continuing education credit, are provided. Examples of these groups include nursing, critical care, pediatrics, simulation operations, serious games, and numerous others.

Growing Regionally

One of the first regional groups to develop for simulation educators occurred in the Midwest in 2003—the same day that a simulator first appeared on network television.

Watching a simulated patient experience of a cocaine overdose, while inept medical students provided care, supported the reasons that this group believed in the power of simulation education. That group of people included a nurse educator and technician from Prairie View A&M University in Houston, Texas, a nurse educator from Johnson County Community College in Overland Park, KS, a nurse educator and technician from Bryan School of Nursing (now Bryan College of Health Sciences in Lincoln, NE), and a nurse representative from Medical Education Technologies, Inc. (now known as CAE Healthcare). The day was spent sharing successes and challenges, problem-solving and troubleshooting, and brainstorming where to head next as we tried to move simulation forward in our schools.

Since that first meeting many years ago, the Midwestern Regional Users Group grew to encompass the entire Midwest; followed by other regions of the country creating their own User Groups. These regional meetings continue across the country and some have evolved into larger conferences that attract attendees from across the country. Additional user groups have formed in Canada, the United Kingdom, and in other countries. While some are informal, others have developed mission statements to direct their work, and a small number have progressed to the point of creating consortia or simulation collaboratives.

Simulation Collaboratives

Bonnie Driggers, MS, MPA, RN

Paula Gubrud, EdD, RN, FAAN

Michael Seropian, MD, FRCPC, FSSH

Collaboration around simulation is not new; it is, however, becoming more formalized as simulation becomes increasingly accepted in both the academic and practice settings. Collaboration involves "two or more entities work[ing] together towards a common goal" (Frey,

Lohmeier, Lee, & Tollefson, 2006). Other common names for collaboratives are "alliance" and "consortium." Merriam-Webster's dictionary defines an *Alliance* as "an association to further common interests of the members," a *Collaborative* as an association "to work jointly with others or together especially in an intellectual endeavor," and a *Consortium* as "an agreement, combination, or group (as of companies) formed to undertake an enterprise beyond the resources of any one member." The common goal is coming together to educate healthcare students and practitioners using simulation modalities to improve patient outcomes in the long term. Models of collaboration vary depending upon the mission and goals of the entities participating, their simulation needs and access to resources, financial situation, and politics and previous relationships. Many collaboratives have developed out of opportunity, rather than from a need-based planning process with a deliberate plan outlining the educational, patient safety, and/or research purpose of the entity. Without a specific mission, vision, or business and sustainability plan, collaboratives struggle. For this reason, it is important to develop collaborations that meet the needs of the partners within the resources available to them.

The Impetus for Collaboration

The impetus for developing collaborations are primarily related to access to resources, both human and capital. Simulation-based education (SBE) is an expensive undertaking, often beyond the resources of any one entity. When resources are combined and shared, the collaborators gain by enhancing the quality of simulation, creating operational efficiencies, and leveraging limited resources. Collaboratives may develop to address a problem or need, such as workforce shortages or lack of clinical experiences; address an opportunity that arises out of receipt of grant funds; or as a grass-roots effort to address the above problems. Simulation programs are often started by innovative faculty members with clinical, educational, and research skills and expertise but without the business, management, technical, and facility design skills necessary for sustainable success (Jeffries & Battin, 2011). Collaboration with others allows organizations to maximize resources, leverage strengths, streamline processes, avoid duplication of efforts, share resources, test theories, and develop best practices (Maxworthy & Waxman, 2014) (Table 2.1).

Not All Collaboratives Are Alike

It is important to note that not all collaborations are alike; they vary by mission, size, geography, discipline, specialty, funding source, and formality in structure

Table 2.1	Benefits of Collaboration
Networking	Share best practices
Facilitate research	Shared grant development
Shared fundraising	Access to job descriptions, policies and procedures, scenarios
Assistance with equipment specifications, procurement, troubleshooting	Standardize facilitator competency through locally offered education and apprentice opportunities
Access to expertise and consultation	Access to interdisciplinary training and educational opportunities
Inspire innovation	Bargaining power for pricing and discounts
Creation of common products (templates, models)	Sharing curricula

and governance. Examples of collaboratives are listed in Table 2.2.

Some collaborations are designed for a single discipline or specialty, while others have arisen from the need to provide interdisciplinary experiences. Some are specific only to simulation and others include simulation as part of a broader purpose such as the Oregon Consortium for Nursing Education (OCNE), a partnership of Oregon Schools of Nursing with shared curricula, including simulation. Many collaboratives were founded in response to future workforce shortages, primarily in nursing. As a result, grants came from workforce development funds and foundations like the Robert Wood Johnson Foundation, the Northwest Heath Foundations, and other funders that support more than simulation initiatives. A variety of structures exist for collaboratives and are listed in Table 2.3.

The First Simulation Collaborative

The first simulation collaborative noted in the literature is the Oregon Simulation Alliance (OSA) established in 2003. "The core objective of the Oregon Simulation Alliance was to address the demand for quality simulation by making expertise accessible and by developing a system that was sustainable and robust" (Seropian, Driggers, Taylor, Gubrud-Howe, & Brady, 2006, p. 56). This was accomplished through program development consultation and education, small equipment grants, simulation specialist training and faculty development apprenticeship opportunities, and intentional **networking** and local coalition building activities. Key to the success of the OSA

Table 2.2	Examples of Collaboratives	
Coverage	**Example**	**Website**
State	California Simulation Alliance (CSA)	https://www.californiasimulationalliance.org
	Tennessee Simulation Alliance	http://tnsim.org
Regional	Bay Area Simulation Collaborative (BASC)	http://www.bayareanrc.org/BayAreaSimulationCollaborative.aspx
	Victorian Simulation Alliance (AU)	http://www.vicsim.org.au
National	Veterans Health Affairs SimLEARN	http://www.simlearn.va.gov
International	International Network for Simulation-based Pediatric Innovation, Research, and Education (INSPIRE)	http://inspiresim.com
	International Simulation Alliance	http://internationalsimulationalliance.com
Research based	INSPIRE	http://inspiresim.com
Practice based	Kaiser Permanente National Healthcare Simulation Collaborative	http://kp.simmedical.com
Academic	Oregon Consortium for Nursing Education (OCNE)	www.ocne.org
	Chicago Simulation Consortium (CSC)	http://128.248.91.60/chicagosim

was encouraging local coalitions that were multidisciplinary and multisector in nature.

Like many other statewide simulation collaboratives, the OSA was primarily grant funded at first. The OSA made the case to potential funders (Oregon Workforce Investment Board, Northwest Health Foundation, Federal Department of Labor, and others) that simulation could positively impact workforce shortages by using simulation to create more efficient and effective clinical experiences and by decreasing the strain on clinical sites caused by increased enrollment. The OSA and many other collaboratives initially offered free services to advance the goals of the collaborative and then began to struggle for sustainable funding sources without major foundation funding. Some have transitioned to subscription or member fee organizations that raise revenue through fees for course offerings, vendor advertising and sponsorship, product development and sales, and community grants and philanthropy. Depending on the size of the collaborative, and its mission, vision, and funding model, the collaborative may operate only with volunteers, or have a paid executive and staff, a shared executive with another state, or may contract with others for services to provide to collaborative members.

Developing a Simulation Collaborative

Key to the development of a simulation collaborative is identifying a shared need and bringing potential collaborators together to share information, gather data, and begin the conversation about working collaboratively. Experience tells us that inclusivity is important in the initial phases of developing a collaboration, as it is harder to bring in additional parties after the mission, vision, goals and objectives, and governance are established. Consider inviting not only those who are engaged in simulation-based learning but also those who might be if they had the resources or would be likely to do so in the future: schools of medicine, nursing, and allied health; hospitals and health systems; emergency medical services; police and fire; STEM (science, technology, engineering, and mathematics) programs; and previous partners in other related endeavors. The consensus model of community engagement suggests a phased approach, beginning with:

1. Informing others about the problem or need and the opportunities,
2. Consulting with them regarding options to solve the problem or address the need,

Table 2.3	Structure of Collaboratives	
Free-standing, for Profit	**Nonprofit, Embedded into Partner Site**	
Joint venture limited liability company (LLC)	Memorandum of understanding (MOU)	
Fee for service	Nonprofit 501c3, exempt from federal income tax	
Subscription or membership fee	Partner funding, equal or based on utilization	

Box 2-1	**Understanding Collaboration**
Variants of Collaboration	**True Collaboration**
✓ Networking ✓ Coordination ✓ Cooperation ✓ Coalition	✓ Members belong to "one" system ✓ Frequent communication characterized by trust ✓ Consensus decision making

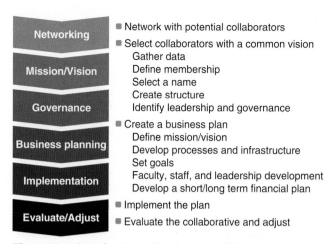

Figure 2.1 Developing a Simulation Collaborative (Courtesy of Oregon Consortium for Nursing Education [OCNE])

3. Involving them in planning and collaborating around solutions, and
4. Empowering the collaborators with "the skills, information, authority and resources they need to make a decision" (Powell, Gilliss, Hewitt, & Flint, 2010, p. 59).

Once the need for collaboration is identified and a desire to collaborate is established, then members with a common vision are recruited. Defining the level of collaboration desired is a very important next step in the development of collaboration (Box 2-1). Many collaborations start as loosely defined networks and become more formalized and integrated as the need is more clearly defined and funding is secured.

Frey, Lohmeier, Lee, and Tollefson (2006) created the Levels of Collaboration Scale, a tool designed to measure the degree of collaboration for evaluating grants. We have found the Scale and model useful to help newly forming collaboratives define the level of collaboration desired.

The levels of the Scale differ by purpose, structure, decision making, type and frequency of communication, and leadership (Table 2.4). The complete Scale is located in the Online Toolkit.

Once the desired level of collaboration is defined, the partners can then determine the structure and governance of the collaboration and give the arrangement a name. Steps in the development of a simulation collaborative are outlined in Figure 2.1. Depending upon the level of collaboration, the next logical step is to create a business plan for the collaborative that clearly delineates the mission, vision, goals and objectives, organizational description, financing plan, market/risk analysis, organizational structure, and governance. Once this is complete, a written commitment is recommended. This could be in the form of a memorandum of understanding (MOU) for less formal collaborations or a formalized contract for legal entities or joint ventures. The next step is implementation of the business plan and commitment followed by regular strategic review and adjustments to the plan as necessary.

Table 2.4	**Levels of Collaboration Scale**				
	Five Levels of Collaboration and Their Characteristics				
	Networking 1	**Cooperation** 2	**Coordination** 3	**Coalition** 4	**Collaboration** 5
Relationship Characteristics	- Aware of organization - Loosely defined roles - Little communication - All decisions are made independently	- Provide information to each other - Somewhat defined roles - Formal communication - All decisions are made independently	- Share information and resources - Defined roles - Frequent communication - Some shared decision-making	- Share ideas - Share resources - Frequent and prioritized communication - All members have a vote in decision-making	- Members belong to one system - Frequent communication is characterized by mutual trust - Consensus is reached on all decisions

From Frey, B. B., Lohmeier, J. H., Lee, S. W., & Tollefson, N. (2006). Measuring collaboration among grant partners. *American Journal of Evaluation, 27*(3), 383–392, with permission.

Keys to Successful Development of Collaborations

Leadership with simulation and business expertise are key to the success of the collaborative. It is important that leaders be able to take time from their own institutional priorities to support the shared vision of the collaborative. The collaborative partners should "own" the collaborative, rather than any one institution or individual. Deliberate planning is ongoing, from initial planning through developing the business plan and implementing the strategic plan to achieve long-term sustainability. The collaborative must be willing to change and evolve as simulation grows and other avenues to meet the original needs become available. It's important to long-term success to be clear on what the collaborative is and what it is not. For example, if the collaborative's activities are managed by volunteers, then the services that it provides, and activities that it undertakes, must be congruent with the human and financial resources that are available. Nurturing relationships through communication and shared work will be key to long-term success. This is true at the simulation educator, technician, collaborative governance, and staff levels. Most importantly, the institutional leadership must continue to support the participation of their institutions in terms of time and money.

Creating Organizations

Internal committees, regional groups, and collaborations fulfilled the needs of many early simulation enthusiasts; however, the need for formal organization at a larger scale was evident. Two large simulation-specific organizations were formed: the INACSL and the Society for Simulation in Healthcare (SSH). The impetus for development, history of evolution and growth, and key contributions and initiatives for each organization are described in further detail in Chapters 3 and 4, respectively. The National League for Nursing (NLN), an organization that promotes excellence in nursing education, has also made a substantial commitment to the advancement of simulation in an effort to advance global health. The work of this organization is discussed in greater detail in Chapter 5. In addition to these large organizations, several others have developed to fill the needs of more specialized audiences and will be discussed in the sections to follow: the Association of Standardized Patient Educators (ASPE), the Association for Simulated Practice in Healthcare (ASPiH), the International Pediatric Simulation Society (IPSS), the Society in Europe for Simulation Applied to Medicine (SESAM), and the Global Network for Simulation in Healthcare (GNSH). Additional organizations have formed in countries around the world, and many have affiliated with existing organizations to leverage resources. A list of simulation organizations and their websites are included in Table 2.5.

Association for Simulated Practice in Healthcare: Development of a National Organization in the United Kingdom

Andrew Anderson

Bryn Baxendale, MB ChB, FRCA, FAcadMedEd

Helen Higham, MBChB, FRCA, SFHEA

In the United Kingdom (UK) the National Association for Medical Simulation (NAMS) was a network of early adopters of medical simulation that grew organically between 1999 and 2008. In parallel to NAMS, nurse educators interested in simulation developed the Clinical Skills Network (CSN). This exacerbated a disconnect between medical and nursing training programs in the adoption of simulation-based methodologies and restricted opportunities for promoting and implementing interprofessional learning and team training. The requirement for interested practitioners to join both organizations provided a barrier to the development of active collaboration among academic and professional communities. In 2009, the leadership of each organization agreed to merge into a single learned body called the Association for Simulated Practice in Healthcare (ASPiH).

ASPiH serves the UK and Ireland healthcare sectors by supporting an active and diverse community of simulation practitioners from different professional, specialty, and academic backgrounds. Acting as a critical communication and networking portal between members and the wider healthcare community, ASPiH has expanded its membership and influence to become the leading UK organization in driving improvement and implementation of SBE to improve quality of healthcare and patient safety. ASPiH has strengthened relationships with those leading the wider domains of Technology Enhanced Learning (TEL) and innovation in education and practice. ASPiH has established a significant presence and strong reputation in the healthcare education sector as well as in patient safety improvement in the UK and around the world (Fig. 2.2).

Table 2.5	Simulation Organizations
Organization	**Website**
Australian Society for Simulation in Healthcare (ASSH)	http://www.simulationaustralasia.com
Brazilian Association for Simulation in Healthcare (ABRASSIM)	http://www.abrassim.org.br
Latin American Association of Clinical Simulation (ALASIC)	https://www.alasic.org
The Association of Standardized Patient Educators (ASPE)	http://www.aspeducators.org/
Association for Simulated Practice in Healthcare (ASPiH)	http://www.aspih.org.uk
Canadian Network for Simulation in Healthcare (CNSH)	http://www.cnsh.ca
Dutch Society for Simulation in Healthcare (DSSH)	http://www.dssh.nl/en/
French Association for Simulation in Healthcare (AFSARMU)	http://www.afsarmu.fr
International Nursing Association for Clinical Simulation and Learning (INACSL)	http://www.inacsl.org/
International Pediatric Simulation Society (IPSS)	http://ipssglobal.org
Italian Society for Simulation in Healthcare (ISSiH)	http://www.issih.it
Japan Society for Instructional Systems in Healthcare (JSISH)	http://www.asas.or.jp/jsish/index.html
Korean Society for Simulation in Healthcare (KoSSH)	http://kossh.or.kr/english/
New Zealand Association for Simulation in Healthcare (NZASH)	http://nzash.co.nz
Polish Society of Medical Simulation (PSMS)	No website; contact: czekajlom@gmail.com
Russian Society for Simulation Education in Medicine (ROSOMED)	http://rosomed.ru/en/
Sociedad Chilena de Simulacion Clinica y Seguridad del Paciente (SOCHISM)	http://www.sochisim.cl
Sociedade Portuguesa de Simulação Aplicada às Ciências da Saúde (PSMS)	http://www.spsim.pt
Spanish Society for Simulation in Healthcare (SESSEP)	http://www.sessep.eu
Pediatric Simulation Training and Research Society of India (PEDISTARS)	http://www.pedistarsindia.com
Society in Europe for Simulation Applied to Medicine (SESAM)	http://www.sesam-web.org
Society for Simulation in Healthcare (SSH)	http://www.ssih.org

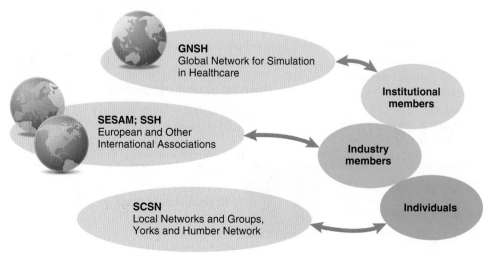

Figure 2.2 ASPiH Network.

ASPiH's members are from healthcare practice and leadership, higher education and workforce development, and patient safety backgrounds. This includes academics and researchers, learning technologists, workforce development or education managers, administrators, and healthcare staff and students. This community bridges undergraduate (preregistration) and postgraduate (postregistration) education and training and ongoing professional development for all of the health and social care workforce.

Mission, Vision, and Purpose of the Organization

ASPiH began as a community of enthusiasts wishing to exchange activities and experiences as the adoption of simulated practice increased in healthcare. Its subsequent successful growth and maturity has seen the Association formalize its structure into a not-for-profit company with limited liability that includes a part-time Chief Executive Officer role. This period has also seen the organization establish greater clarity about its purpose and future, describing an overarching mission to enable wider sharing of knowledge, expertise, and educational innovation related to simulated practice across the healthcare professions. This is supported by clear aims that include providing an effective communication network and exemplars of best practice, linking simulated practice with improved patient safety and quality of care, developing resources, supporting scholarly development and member recognition, and providing expertise, advice, and information about healthcare simulation.

Value for Members and Future Plans

The enduring value to ASPiH members has been the creation and enhancement of opportunities for networking and to encourage sharing experiences among members. This has been underpinned by a financial model that focuses on revenue from membership (corporate, institutional, and individual) and an annual scientific conference, which has become the major scientific meeting for healthcare simulated practice in the UK and now attracts over 500 delegates plus support from industry. This conference also provides a significant opportunity for members to engage with representatives from key national commissioning and policy forming bodies in relation to healthcare workforce development and patient safety.

A number of recent initiatives in pursuit of growth and maturity of the Association have been identified, namely:

- Pursuing purposeful and transparent collaboration among key stakeholders and networks nationally
- Articulating and refining standards of practice and quality indicators of excellence that can be adopted nationally and help guide high-quality commissioning (funding) practices

- Leading the creation of new opportunities for peer-reviewed publication in order to promote high-quality simulation-based research across the UK and contribute more effectively to the evidence base supporting the use of simulation in healthcare.

In the past 10 years, regional simulation networks developed based on local funding support and vision. Other simulation opportunities were available through membership in medical specialty professional groups. However, there are still barriers to sharing resources and to multiprofessional collaboration. A key longer-term goal for ASPiH is to develop a more comprehensive, cohesive, and collaborative national network that can benefit from the collective experiences of existing regional or specialty networks, but without being disruptive to their own sustainability. ASPiH engages with international networks and societies to share ideas and develop relationships that will benefit the ASPiH membership. This is intended to help promote excellence in simulation practice, strengthen the development of a scientifically rigorous evidence base, and support leadership development in healthcare education and practice.

One important project that will help coordinate different groups and networks is development of more explicit standards for SBE with an underpinning of a quality indicator framework. The aim of this collaborative UK-wide work program is to offer valuable benefits to providers, commissioners, and professional bodies when seeking to ensure high-quality SBE across different sectors and networks.

In relation to improving the research evidence for SBE and TEL, ASPiH has partnered with the British Medical Journal (BMJ) and launched an online, peer-reviewed journal: BMJ Simulation and Technology Enhanced Learning (www.bmjstel.com). This will increase the capacity for publication of high-quality research and will help build a research-oriented community that can benefit from activities and resources made available or coordinated by ASPiH related to research design.

In summary, ASPiH is widely recognized as a model for national association and society development. The organization seems set to expand significantly in the coming years, as the use of SBE and TEL becomes a key platform for improving patient safety and performance improvement.

Association of Standardized Patient Educators: Building a Community of Standardized Patient Educators

Karen L. Lewis, PhD

Founding members agree that the impetus for establishing the Association of Standardized/Simulated Patient Educators (ASPE) reached its peak in 1999 when the Association of American Medical Colleges decided to no longer sponsor SIG sessions. Although there were six national meetings dedicated to the use of standardized patients (SPs) during the 1990s, these meetings often included a wider audience of faculty and researchers. The Standardized Patient Educator (SPE) SIG was the only regular forum available for educator skill development and support. With the forum lost and new programs popping up around the country, SPE who had worked to legitimize the inclusion of SPs in medical education were naturally concerned.

The development of the national medical licensing exams in both Canada and the United States added fuel to the fire. Working on the board exams gave educators the opportunity to practice their craft, work collaboratively, and vet and produce scholarly applications. The dialogue begun during this work helped shape the thinking about forming an association and what it could do for its members: provide informed practice on how to run a program, demonstrate effective SP training techniques, expand case development, and assess and demonstrate the quality of the methodology.

The time was ripe for ensuring that the SPE was a recognized profession. In February 2000, The University of Texas Medical Branch, Galveston, sponsored a meeting focused on professional development for SPEs. During this conference, there was discussion about the possibility of starting an association: a place to go for skill and professional development, a place that legitimized their work, and a place where they could say, "I belong." Not wanting to lose the momentum created in Galveston, Mary Ann Cantrell, ASPE founding president, invited a group of SPEs to Arkansas for a brainstorming weekend. With the help of a lawyer and sample bylaws from other associations, the ASPE was created. Once incorporation was complete, the next step was to build the membership, starting with the first annual ASPE Conference in Ottawa in 2001, a 1-day event held the day before the Ottawa Conference on Medical Education. The theme, significantly, was "Advancing the Practice." It drew 150 members and provided the impetus and money for the 3-day conference in Virginia Beach the following year and every year thereafter.

Today, ASPE is an international organization of 600 educators from 24 different countries who are dedicated to transforming professional performance through the power of human interaction. Its mission is to:

- Promote best practices in the application of SP methodology for education, assessment, and research
- Foster the dissemination of research and scholarship in the field of SP methodology
- Advance the professional knowledge and skills of its members

The annual conference provides an outstanding forum for carrying out this mission, but ASPE provides other opportunities for professional development year round. ASPE award grants annually to help members further their scholarship, holds webinars throughout the year, and keeps members abreast of the latest trends with the ASPE e-News. The website's Virtual Learning Center houses video recordings, articles, tool kits, how-to guides, cases, and archived webinars and newsletters. ASPE recognizes those educators who have done outstanding work in the organization with the prestigious ASPE Outstanding Educator Award and honors those who do significant work in the field with the Howard Barrows Invited Presenter Award. For those new to the field, ASPE offers a mentoring program that pairs new educators with more experienced ones at the annual conference and throughout the year. Another form of mentoring takes place for members who participate in the Scholars Certificate Program, where an experienced SPE works with the participant to prepare a scholarly project for presentation.

There is much on the horizon for ASPE and its members. On the international front, educational leaders from countries all over the world are approaching ASPE for help in starting SP Programs and creating regional ASPE chapters. On the educational front, advances in simulation technology are expanding the content of SP scenarios, enabling educators to teach learners with the help of SPs as well as whole patient and task-specific simulators and devices that can simulate physical findings. Innovations in virtual reality and gaming have the potential to expand even further what educators can do clinically with SP scenarios, while at the same time retain at the forefront what is most important about the methodology: the real human being that is the basis for its existence. Educator thinking has also evolved into fields beyond the medical patient. The same pool of people called standardized/simulated patients are beginning to perform the roles of healthcare professionals, pharmacist and veterinary clients, lawyers, law enforcement personnel, teachers, and students. On the association front, ASPE members have always been collaborative and will seek opportunities to work with simulation associations and societies committed to advancing simulation practice.

ASPE was created because of a need to connect people with common education goals and methods, and no matter what innovations and trends emerge in the coming years, that need and the goal to promote best practices and emerging trends and scholarship in the field of human simulation will remain central to its vision. All who share this vision are welcome to join ASPE in building a stronger simulation community. Resources available in the toolkit include a list of books and articles related to SP education and a scenario development template in MedEd Portal format.

Championing the Art and Science of Pediatric Simulation: The Birth of the International Pediatric Simulation Society

Stephanie N. Sudikoff, MD

David J. Grant,
MBCHB, MRCP, MRCPCH

Ella Scott, RN, RSCN, Grad Cert PIC MA

Peter Weinstock, MD, PhD

The seed for a dedicated pediatric simulation society was planted at the Second International Pediatric Simulation Symposia and Workshops (IPSSW) meeting in Florence, Italy, in 2009. A small group of individuals embarked on a fact-finding mission to explore the feasibility of establishing a pediatric simulation society with a plan to report back to the international audience at IPSSW the following year. Given the unique nature of the pediatric patient and family unit, this group identified the need to establish a community focused exclusively on pediatric simulation, which provides an alternative to trainee "practice" on children, minimizing risk and maximizing safety. As a result, the simulated environment is now considered an essential component to educating all pediatric healthcare disciplines. Although SIGS provided one forum, the international pediatric community was not satisfied with being "shoe-horned" into existing adult-oriented societies. A dedicated pediatric organization could not only represent the global population of pediatric simulation enthusiasts committed to advocating for this special population but also could serve as a catalyst for a larger, and more interprofessional movement.

After presentation of these facts, the nearly 300 international, interprofessional attendees at IPSSW 2010 voted unanimously to establish the IPSS; it was officially signed into existence on April 8, 2011. At that time, the primary focus was to ensure at least an annual opportunity to bring the international pediatric simulation community together. This was achieved through our IPSSW meetings, held in strategic venues, specifically chosen to stimulate local development of pediatric simulation, as we "walked around the world."

Mission, Vision, and Values

The International Pediatric Simulation Society (IPSS) is dedicated to pediatric, perinatal, and associated healthcare providers and organizations utilizing SBE to improve care and safety for children (Table 2.6).

IPSS plays a vital role in the evolution of pediatric simulation by facilitating interaction among these providers and integration across both geographic and professional domains. IPSS leadership considers the notion of "community" to be paramount to achieve our future goals. These goals include:

1. Optimizing pediatric simulation resources to ensure the establishment of affordable and appropriate technology for all types of environments. This is a vital element to ensure global application in both high and low resource settings.
2. Eliminating the artificial divide between high-quality service delivery and education by identifying new ways to integrate simulation into our healthcare systems.
3. Applying simulation as a vehicle to innovate and develop new technologies and methods to enhance healthcare outcomes.

Table 2.6	Mission Statements of IPSS
Mission Statement	To inspire, grow, and lead the global pediatric simulation community
Vision Statement	Optimal healthcare for children and families through simulation
Core Goals	Reflect and empower the global pediatric and perinatal simulation community Develop and sustain a dynamic community of practice for pediatric and perinatal simulation-based innovations, education, research, and advocacy Support effective, safe, and efficient individual, team and system improvements Promote innovation for implementation and dissemination of pediatric simulation networks With a unique focus on pediatric and perinatal healthcare, complement and enhance efforts of other organizations Champion solutions for resource limited environments

4. Promoting the use of simulation-based methodologies to investigate key areas in healthcare most likely to effect positive patient outcomes.

5. Inspiring and leading the global pediatric and perinatal healthcare community by advancing our field to improve global child health.

In addition to establishing relationships with key global stakeholders, IPSS strategic goals and plans are all designed to provide vital support for, facilitate communication and interaction among, and promote growth and diversity of our global membership, both within and beyond the healthcare domain. Now, 5 years out from our formal incorporation, we are currently focused on creating a stable financial and administrative infrastructure that can support growth and enhance connectivity.

The Society in Europe for Simulation Applied to Medicine

**Peter Dieckmann,
PhD, Dipl. Psych., FSSH**

Vimal Chopra, MD, PhD, FRCA

Antoine Tesniere, MD, PhD

Our Mission is to encourage and support the use of simulation in healthcare for the purpose of training and research (www. sesam-web.org)

Copenhagen, Denmark, 1994—Three simulation pioneers meet in a bar at the end of long meeting day. Vimal Chopra from the Netherlands, Arne Rettedal from Norway, and Per Føge Jensen from Denmark not only meet in this bar, but have one more thing in common: They all are involved in building patient simulators, and they decide that it is time to create a society that can facilitate the meeting of like-minded enthusiasts. They filled napkin after napkin to find the right name. A small pile of papers later, the Society in Europe for Simulation Applied to Medicine was born as the first international society in the world dealing with simulation in healthcare: SESAM. The society

thus began as a network of producers of simulators and yet they made important decisions to keep its focus open and oriented toward the future. Although the society was based in Europe, it was and still is an international player and open to simulation enthusiasts from all over the world. The founders also saw that it is the use of the simulators—the resulting simulations—that are the core tool to reach the goal of simulation. The word Medicine, in the name, might seem a limitation nowadays, but the society very quickly involved professionals from all fields and disciplines working with health-related simulations—even though mostly the acute care disciplines responded to the call for participation.

For some years, the main activities of SESAM were to create a network of people working with simulation—both users and developers. Those people met during the Annual Meetings of the Society, which rotated through many European cities. Slowly, yet steadily, the size of the meetings grew, as did membership in the society. The SESAM web-page (www.sesam-web.org) provides an overview of important steps in the history of the society, including a list of the past and current presidents.

The SESAM annual meetings provide a mix of scientific presentations, work in progress sessions, and hands-on workshops. With a size of approximately 600 participants—many of them "frequent flyers"—those meetings provided ample opportunity for exchange of ideas and networking. In recent years, SESAM's organizational backbone was improved, and several activities and initiatives beyond the annual meetings were established, the most important likely being the establishment of an open-access journal: Advances in Simulation (AIS—www. adavancesinsimulation.com). In the Literature Highlights, content experts make recommendations to interested people about material to study about a respective topic. Other initiatives include the creation of smaller meetings—the SESAM-supported working meetings that can have an educational or developmental focus.

SESAM's role in the community has long been the role as a "hub" in connecting people and groups. This was evident in 2009, when the first European-Latin-American Meeting for simulation in healthcare was held in Coimbra, Portugal, in collaboration between SESAM and the Asociación Latinoamericana de Simulación Clinica (ALASIC—www.alasic.org). This meeting and subsequent meetings held in Brazil (2011) and Costa Rica (2013) were a contribution toward the Latin-American simulation meetings now established (Chile, 2015). Pursuing this open initiative, SESAM also reached out to different parts of the world, opening new perspectives of collaboration for training and research with simulation, and organized joint meetings in the Middle East (SESAM—Middle East Northern Africa meeting in Dubai) in 2014. SESAM is proud of its role in facilitating exchanges with the very active simulation scene in different regions, connecting people and organizations, to create not only great facilities but more importantly, great concepts.

There are many benefits for members, as SESAM is committed in offering many important features, such as the opportunity to engage and participate in a network of like-minded and enthusiastic people, facilitated access to the new journal *Advances in Simulation*, the potential to organize SESAM-sponsored working meetings around their field of interest, or easy exchanges on simulation through SESAM's Center database. The idea of moving the simulation community forward is a strong driver behind the motivation of SESAM members.

Many projects are envisioned for SESAM to develop in the future. Among those, one goal is to increase interaction with specialty societies and to grow an influential network to interact more strongly with the European authorities to help build a sustainable foundation for simulation. In Denmark, the first country in the world to establish simulation as a mandatory part in the specialist education for anesthesiology, there is a long history of experience to help the society in these efforts. Work within European and other countries help to build this expertise further.

Global Network for Simulation in Healthcare

Kim Leighton, PhD, RN, CHSE, CHSOS, ANEF

During a conversation at the International Meeting on Simulation in Healthcare (IMSH) conference, a thought was shared that it would be interesting to have a meeting and invite the president of every simulation organization around the world to attend. By the end of that conference, a date had been chosen, a location secured, and planning commenced toward developing an agenda. The initial planning committee included leadership from INACSL, SSH, SESAM, ASSH, and the London Deanery.

The first meeting of what would be named the Global Network for Simulation in Healthcare was held in August 2010 in London. Twenty-seven people, representing 16 organizations focused on simulation in healthcare, attended this leadership summit. This first meeting was a fact-finding mission to learn more about the work of each organization, build relationships, and determine how to move forward. The goal was to empower the organizations to work together as simulation continues to expand around the globe. The group achieved consensus to form the GNSH and agreed upon a mission statement: "A global network of organizations, committed to enhancing patient safety and quality of healthcare by promoting the appropriate use of simulation through collaboration, advocacy and support" (GNSH, 2015). Working groups were formed for the areas of governance, communication, and organizing.

The following year, 30 attendees from 19 organizations attended, with the main focus on the goal of identifying international simulation needs relevant to GNSH. A concordat was produced to consolidate strategic goals and to engage all potential partners. The group continues to meet annually, with the following objectives:

1. To promote the appropriate use of simulation in healthcare to improve patient care and safety, clinical service, training, research and education,
2. That the network will act as a source of expertise
3. That the network will act as a global resource
4. Through shared advocacy, to support and promote the use of simulation in healthcare,
5. Terms of reference and ways of collaborative working (GNSH, 2015).

By 2014, the GNSH had grown to 24 member organizations from around the world with the purpose "to connect all sectors of the healthcare simulation community and to enhance value through shared vision, resources, and tools" (GNSH, 2015). The group is now inclusive of both commercial and noncommercial representatives that come together to "advance patient care, efficiency, and efficacy through healthcare simulation." The work of the GNSH for the current session is to develop consensus guidelines to establish the value of simulation for different stakeholders. Key stakeholders include financial, governmental regulators, educational bodies, politicians, patient advocacy groups, healthcare and college executives, and policy makers.

Summary

In just over a decade, simulation has grown from work often conducted in isolation, where educators were challenged to "learn on the fly," using trial and error to identify teaching strategies that might help their students to learn, all while using very expensive equipment with little internal or external support. Thankfully, many of these innovators and early adopters were tenacious and built support within their own facilities, then reached out to others in their area, until that reach ultimately spanned the globe.

This chapter has shared the beginnings of our simulation communities—what prompted people to reach out and then to organize. Creating nonprofit organizations is not easy, yet these pioneers understood that if the use of simulation as a teaching pedagogy was to expand, then a unified approach would be needed. Interestingly, it was pointed out that sometimes "too many" different groups can in itself become a barrier to networking and unification. At this time, large regional groups that oftentimes cover an entire continent or country are the most common organizations for simulationists to seek resources from. Other, larger organizations with a worldwide membership have also partnered with other organizations (both large and small) to combine resources for both novice and experienced simulation educators. If this is any indication, we can only imagine the growth that will occur over the next decade as we continue our quest to determine how to best impact learning for our students and ultimately, improve patient care.

3

INACSL: International Nursing Association for Clinical Simulation and Learning

Teresa Gore, Teresa Boese

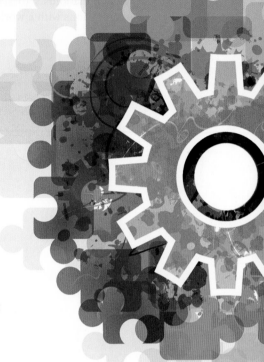

 Key Terms

Simulation, Standards of Best Practice, Learning Resource Center, Association Management Company, Mission, Vision, Impact Factor, Fellowship

 Guiding Questions

1 How were the *INACSL Standards of Best Practice: Simulation* developed and why are they important in evidence-based simulation?

2 What are the educational and leadership opportunities provided by INACSL?

3 Why is collaboration among simulation organizations/groups important to the simulation community?

Introduction

The International Nursing Association for Clinical Simulation and Learning (INACSL) is nursing's portal for educators using **simulation** as a strategy for experiential learning of safe, competent patient care. Its beginning can be traced back to the 1970s with the inception of **Learning Resource Centers** (LRCs). At that time, practice and audiovisual laboratories in colleges of nursing were commonly consolidated together to create an LRC. As computers were developed, and universities needed to reach beyond their brick and mortar, technology and distance

education also came under the auspices of the LRC. This unique, niche community of nurse educators realized there was a strong need to develop opportunities for networking and the exchange of ideas. Drs. Charlene Clark, Kathleen Mikan, Kay Hodson-Carlton, and Joanne Crow were leaders in their respective nursing LRCs. As forward-thinking leaders in the community, they understood the power of sharing their successes and challenges with others in the community. They organized the first conference for nursing educators dedicated to issues of psychomotor skill education and learning resources. Over the course of the next 20 years, the Learning Resource Center conference was held biennially at various locations across the United States.

In the mid-1990s, the University of Texas Health Science Center at San Antonio's School of Nursing began a new continuing education conference focused on nursing education and psychomotor skills. This conference was held in San Antonio during years the LRC conference was idle. Both conferences drew many of the same participants, which enabled nursing faculty to form permanent connections that continued beyond the conferences. Throughout the years, the idea of establishing an official organization to serve this growing community had been discussed, but the time did not seem right until the 2000 LRC conference.

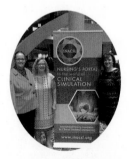

Teresa Gore, PhD, DNP, FNP-BC, NP-C, CHSE-A

Teresa Boese, DNP, RN

During this conference, a session was dedicated to determining interest in the establishment of a specialty organization that would bring together educators with nursing learning laboratory expertise. At the same time, nursing faculty administrators, faculty, and staff focused on educating students in the practice laboratory setting saw their roles start to shift and expand with the use of advanced technology, such as high-fidelity mannequins.

These educators formed the INACSL. The original INACSL founders saw a need for a formalized network to meet the needs of the directors, managers, and coordinators responsible for this part of the curriculum in their institutions and to recognize the distinct contributions they made to nursing education.

A group of volunteers (Table 3.1), endorsed by participants at the Fourth National Conference on Nursing Skills Laboratories, served as the initial members of the Board of Directors for the organization. This group, led by Dr. Debra Spunt and Dr. Teri Boese, drafted a **mission** and **vision** based on a survey identifying core issues facing those active in nursing laboratory settings. There was a strong sense that an organization would provide mutual support and ongoing communication among people in this community of practice beyond the yearly opportunity at conferences to share best practices. The original mission was "to promote and provide the development and advancement of clinical simulation and learning resource centers." The vision statement listed 17 objectives focused on communication, lab management, and scholarship activities that INACSL was committed to and supported. In addition, the group developed the groundwork for INACSL's infrastructure by crafting bylaws, leading to the incorporation of the organization in 2003. The original Board of Directors served until 2005, when the first elections were held.

Table 3.1	Founding Board of Directors	
President	Teri Boese	Dr. Debra Spunt
Vice President for Communication	Dr. Janis Childs	
Vice President for Program	Dr. Linda Haynes	
Vice President for Finance	Reba Moyer-Childress	
Membership Chair	Margaret Meccariello	
Nomination Chair	Chris Lafferty	
Member-at-Large	Eva Vigo	
Advisor	Dr. Charlene Clark	Dr. Kay Hodson-Carlton

Organization Development

The INACSL Board of Directors has continued to grow and refine, similar to the growth and refinement of simulation. In 2010, to help the organization's continued growth, INACSL hired an administrative assistant to manage the secretarial type of work and allow the board of directors more time to grow the organization. At that time, the membership in INACSL exceeded 1,000 members.

As an all-volunteer board and executive committee experiencing exceptional growth, the INACSL Board of Directors hired a professional **association management company** (AMC) to help sustain that growth. This allowed INACSL to have an Executive Director. Hiring of the AMC led to the next pivotal moment in the organization's growth and development. With the help of the AMC, the INACSL Board of Directors could now transition from a working board to a more visionary board. The AMC allows the board to concentrate on growth and opportunities to provide better services to the members by being the point of contact, answering members' questions, maintaining necessary paperwork, and meeting the day-to-day needs of the organization. Board members could then focus on strategically seeking opportunities for advancing the science of simulation and the organization.

INACSL has experienced great leadership since the beginning of the organization by individuals dedicated to simulation that donated their time and talents. The Presidents of INACSL have been Dr. Debra Spunt, Dr. Teri Boese, Dr. Karen Tarnow, Dr. Jana Berryman, Dr. Kim Leighton, Dr. Valerie Howard, Dr. Carol Durham, and Dr. Teresa Gore. Each brought talents and unique skill sets that helped the organization to move forward through the exceptional work ethic of a diverse board of directors. Each member of the Board of Directors has contributed to the foundation and/or growth of INACSL through their strengths and dedication to advancing simulation.

Strategic Planning

INACSL's leadership has consistently been cognizant of their stewardship responsibility to members of the organization. The leadership formalized strategic planning to support the mission and goals of the organization. The strategic plan identified four areas of focus, which remain constant today: (1) increase professional recognition and advancement of INACSL, (2) advance the science of simulation and learning environments, (3) enhance membership, and (4) strengthen organizational structure of board of directors. In addition, the mission and vision of the organization was revised to reflect the changing needs of simulation and the community of practice for 2010:

- **Mission:** "The mission for the International Nursing Association for Clinical Simulation and Learning is to promote research and disseminate evidence-based practice standards for clinical simulation methodologies and learning environments."
- **Vision:** "INACSL is Nursing's portal to the world of clinical simulation pedagogy and learning environments."

The strategic plan has been refined with specific goals, but the outcomes remained the same. In 2015, the INACSL Board of Directors examined the current state of INACSL and the community of simulation. The board believed that the mission and vision had been accomplished for promoting research and disseminating evidence-based practice standards for clinical simulation methodologies and learning environments as Nursing's portal. The board decided to focus on all of healthcare simulation and how simulation can impact patient safety. The new Mission and Vision is as follows:

- Mission: "Global leader in transforming practice to improve patient safety through excellence in healthcare simulation."
- Vision: "Advancing the science of healthcare simulation."

In 2016, the organization revisited their strategic and operational plan to better meet the needs of the INACSL membership and the simulation community. The new strategic plan is to (1) provide innovative education and networking, (2) create and disseminate healthcare simulation research, (3) build future leaders, (4) set the standards for healthcare simulation, and (5) advance healthcare simulation globally. A plan for operationalizing the strategic plan was also developed to meet the community of simulation and INACSL membership needs.

Member Recognition: Awards, Grants, and Scholarships

As INACSL continued to grow, the organization began to recognize outstanding work among the membership. Recognition for our members is accomplished through awards, grants, and scholarship.

Awards

Awards were developed and presented for the first time in 2004. Since that time, members in three areas of expertise have been acknowledged annually: research, excellence in the academic setting, and service to the organization. The awards are as follows:

- *Excellence in Research Award:* Member or group of members that has completed quality research in the field of nursing simulation.

- *Excellence in Academia Award:* Member that demonstrates a sustained record of excellence in simulation teaching and learning in academic settings.
- *Excellence in Service Award:* Member or company that has given their time, talent, or resources to better INACSL.

In 2015, additional excellence awards were developed to include the following:

- *INACSL Best Practice Innovator Excellence Award:* Member of INACSL who goes above and beyond the ordinary, to demonstrate extraordinary commitment and the use of innovative approaches to the development, promotion, dissemination, and/or utilization of the *INACSL Standards of Best Practice: Simulation.*
- *Spirit of Simulation Leadership Excellence Award:* Member of INACSL that is a visionary and inspiring nurse leader in the INACSL simulation practice community who exemplifies the characteristics of a transformational leader.
- *Front Line Simulation Champion Excellence Award:* Member of INACSL who goes above and beyond the ordinary, to demonstrate an extraordinary commitment to the development, promotion, dissemination, and/or utilization of the *INACSL Standards of Best Practice: Simulation.*

Grants

The Debra Spunt Research Mini-Grant Award was established in 2007 to honor the memory of Dr. Spunt who was one of the founding organizers of INACSL and a leader in simulation. This $500 mini-grant was awarded to members whose research continued the advancement of the science of simulation, which was Dr. Spunt's passion at the time of her death. The grant award is now $1,000 due to donations from Laerdal in support of advancing the science of simulation. In 2016, a $10,000 contribution was made by Chamberlain College of Nursing/DeVry Medical International's Institute for Research and Clinical Strategy to support the work of experienced researchers and promote multisite studies. Since 2007, eleven research grants have been awarded to scholars studying simulation. As a result, research has been conducted in areas of simulation as a teaching method, its impact on the learning process, faculty development, debriefing, evaluation, and clinical judgement.

The research committee conducted a needs assessment to identify gaps in the literature in need of further research. The gaps and emphasis of research should focus on translational research, evaluation methods, validity and reliability of instruments, ratio of clinical time to simulation time, prebriefing and briefing, use of theory in simulation, measurement of higher-order thinking, faculty development, facilitator competency, and communication (Fey, 2016). In order to meet the needs and bridge the gaps, INACSL is seeking more funding from corporate sponsors to fund higher-level research to meet the identified gaps in the literature (Fey, 2016).

Scholarships

In addition to the research grant, a scholarship was developed as a result of the generous donation from Pocket Nurse. This award provides assistance to members attending the INACSL conference for the first time. The Anthony Battaglia Scholarship award covers recipients' registration fee. This scholarship provides an opportunity for up to 10 participants each year to attend the INACSL conference.

Journal

The first issue of the organization's journal *Clinical Simulation in Nursing Education* (now known as *Clinical Simulation in Nursing*) was published in June 2005. Launched with the vision of editor Dr. Linda Haynes, and followed by Dr. Suzie Kardong-Edgren, *Clinical Simulation in Nursing* provides INACSL with an opportunity to share the organization's ongoing commitment and contribution to the science of healthcare simulation. The journal publishes research, literature reviews, lessons learned, and other articles about the development of simulations, programs, alliances, and interprofessional education.

A major benefit of *Clinical Simulation in Nursing* is that it is an electronic journal. This allows all members access to all previous articles, while eliminating costs of printing. The journal has increased the number of publications from six times a year to monthly. This increases the access and availability of new information.

Another major accomplishment occurred in July 2016 when an **impact factor** (IF) of 1.36 was assigned to *Clinical Simulation in Nursing*. The IF is retroactive for the last 3 years. The importance of an IF is the resulting increase in status of the journal, which will attract additional authors who publish only in journals recognized in this way, potentially increasing the submissions of scholarly research that will advance simulation. This provides our members with more information to advance the science of simulation. For some academicians seeking promotion and tenure, an IF is required for the articles to be submitted for consideration in that process.

Conferences

Never forgetting the original events that brought people in our community of practice together, conferences remain an important part of INACSL. In 2008, the two separate nursing laboratory and resource center conferences were merged and renamed the Annual International Nursing Simulation/Learning Resource Center Conference, which is held in June each year.

As INACSL's membership and leadership grew, INACSL began coordinating its own conference. Over time, the main focus of the conference transitioned to simulation and not just nursing lab coordination. In 2015, the name of the conference was changed to the INACSL Conference followed by the year of the conference. With the increase in simulation use in various programs and settings, the number of attendees continued to grow. With the increased acceptance of simulation as a teaching strategy, more rigorous research was produced, and the conference more prominently featured research. The conference meets the needs of the novice simulationist who attends to gain knowledge about simulation as well as the advanced practitioner who seeks research opportunities and outcomes.

INACSL Standards of Best Practice: Simulation

In 2009, INACSL recognized the profound need for guidance in the simulation community of practice and spearheaded work on standards of best practice for healthcare simulation. The INACSL published the first standards for simulation: The *INACSL Standards of Best Practice: Simulation* (INACSL BOD, 2011a), as follows:

- Standard I—Terminology
- Standard II—Professional Integrity of Participant
- Standard III—Participant Objectives
- Standard IV—Facilitation Methods
- Standard V—Simulation Facilitator
- Standard VI—The Debriefing Process
- Standard VII—Evaluation of Expected Outcome

The standards were written, reviewed, vetted, and published in a period of 2 years by the Board of Directors. The board then established a Standards Committee to refine the publication. The Standards Committee continues to refine and revise the publication as the field of clinical simulation develops.

In 2013, the Standards Committee revised the *INACSL Standards of Best Practice: Simulation* and constructed guidelines for each standard, creating the second edition of the Standards (INACSL, 2013). The guidelines were added to provide a more in-depth explanation of the standards based on emerging evidence. These Standards remain freely accessible on the *Clinical Simulation in Nursing* website www.nursingsimulation.org. INACSL created a Standards Advisory Board for reviewing the Standards and providing feedback to the Standards Committee. This advisory board is composed of subject matter experts in the field of simulation and included representatives from academia, practice, interprofessional, international, and major simulation organizations.

During this time period, the National Council of State Boards of Nursing (NCSBN) published the results of their National Simulation Study (Hayden, Smiley, Alexander, Kardong-Edgren, & Jeffries, 2014). This longitudinal, multisite, controlled, experimental study concluded that simulation could be a substitute for traditional clinical for prelicensure students for up to 50% of clinical time when high-quality simulations were used, a high level of planned debriefing based on an educational theory was implemented, facilitators were trained, and the *INACSL Standards of Best Practice: Simulation* were incorporated into the simulation program. These results and the inclusion of the Standards helped launch INACSL and the Standards to a larger audience.

Two new INACSL Standards of Best Practice were developed in 2015: Simulation Enhanced Interprofessional Education (Sim-IPE) (Decker et al., 2015) and Simulation Design (Lioce et al., 2015). As nursing strives to meet the Institute of Medicine (IOM) recommendations, the Standards were also vetted and reviewed by 14 organizations for adoption into other healthcare professions outside of nursing and internationally. Based on the feedback from these organizations, the Standards Committee has restructured the simulation standards. The revised *INACSL Standards of Best Practice: Simulation* (INACSL Standards Committee, 2016) are included in their entirety in this book with the permission of the INACSL leadership.

The newly revised Standards include the following:

- Debriefing
- Facilitation
- Outcomes and Objectives
- Participant Evaluation
- Professional Integrity
- Sim-IPE (Interprofessional Education)
- Simulation Design

One additional Standard is under development for Simulation Operations. The Terminology Standard has become a Glossary (appendix) in the new version. The 2016 Standards will be operationalized within Chapter 20, "Curriculum Development in Simulation Nursing Programs."

Collaborations

In order to support the various needs of the simulation community, strengths of various organizations can produce a better product to advance the science of simulation than any single organization. Collaboration with other organizations continues to be a priority for INACSL.

Society for Simulation in Healthcare

INACSL and Society for Simulation in Healthcare (SSH) began to work collaboratively in 2009 to improve simulation practice by affiliating with each other. This affiliation was important to provide an interdisciplinary approach to simulation. This affiliation provides members with discounts to join the other organization and provides educational sessions at each other's annual conference. This partnership continues to grow and expand with collaboration on publications and endorsement of the Standards, certification, and accreditation. SSH developed the certification for simulation educators and operations specialist, while INACSL developed the Standards.

The newest collaborative effort, regional workshops, has been developed to better meet the needs of the individuals working on the front line of simulation. These workshops are designed to meet educational needs in relation to the Standards, Guidelines, fellowships, certification, and accreditation.

National League for Nursing

The INACSL collaborated with the National League for Nursing (NLN) on the examination of the NLN Jeffries Simulation Framework constructs. This state-of-the-science project undertook extensive literature review to examine the research surrounding each construct, with resulting recommendations to strengthen the framework.

The INACSL and NLN developed the HomeGrown Solutions Program. The HomeGrown Solutions concept was initiated by Margaret "Meg" Meccariello to recognize individuals that developed low-cost solutions to simulation needs. Due to Meg's dedication to INACSL and simulation, one session at the annual conference is recognized as the Meg Meccariello Session during Hot Topics for Low-Cost Solutions presentations. In November 2015, the INACSL membership mourned the loss of Meg who will always be remembered for her hard work and dedication to INACSL, her role as conference administrator, and pioneering low-cost solutions for simulation. INACSL will continue her legacy of the HomeGrown Solutions for low-cost alternatives in simulation.

As part of NLN's Vision Series, *Debriefing across the Curriculum* (NLN, 2015a) was published as a collaborative effort with INACSL. This white paper states that debriefing is a major part of simulation; however, debriefing should be used in other areas of nursing education, not just simulation. Instead of postconference sessions after clinical, debriefing should be used to help students link the clinical experience with didactic material and to further develop clinical reasoning.

Laerdal Medical

Laerdal Medical has been a longtime supporter of simulation and nursing. One of the first projects directly impacting INACSL was the NLN/Laerdal National Simulation Research Team project. INACSL provided a platform for dissemination of this important early simulation research as part of both postconference sessions and keynote addresses.

Laerdal has also provided funding for various INACSL activities and projects, most notably the Debra Spunt Research Grant and funding for the examination of the NLN Jeffries Simulation Framework (Jeffries, 2016).

American Association of Colleges of Nursing

To increase awareness of the *INACSL Standards of Best Practice: Simulation*, INACSL collaborated with the American Association of Colleges of Nursing (AACN) to provide three free annual webinars regarding the use of simulation and the Standards since 2011. AACN provides recorded sessions to their members along with a link that is posted on the INACSL website for our members. This provides simulation information to a larger group of nursing educators.

National Council of State Boards of Nursing

INACSL collaborated with the NCSBN and other organizations for the development of the NCSBN National Simulation Guidelines (Alexander et al., 2015). These guidelines were published to provide guidance to institutional leadership, faculty, and those conducting simulation and to provide each state board of nursing a framework for simulation use and policy development. This is the first time that INACSL participated in policy development for simulation.

INACSL Chapter Europe

As INACSL's membership and the community of practice grew, the importance of building relationships across simulation organizations and international borders became increasingly important. The INACSL leadership worked diligently to strengthen these relationships and represent INACSL's voice at the international table to discuss issues common to all healthcare simulation educators. The inaugural INACSL Chapter Europe was chartered in 2012. This chapter was especially important to the organization to meet the growing needs of healthcare simulation educators worldwide. It is necessary to involve other cultures, aspects, and perspectives to meet our organizational goal to be international. INACSL Chapter Europe's focus is to strengthen and expand the collective for evidence-based clinical simulation and clinical skills using all modalities for the education of nurses and postgraduate nurses in all fields. INACSL Chapter Europe aims to become one of the leading voices in simulation-based healthcare education in Europe.

CAE Healthcare

INACSL collaborated with CAE Healthcare on the printing of the Standards in 2011 and cosponsored the printed publication in 2013 with Elsevier Simulations. The sponsored educational grants and funding allowed the printed version to be mailed to each member of INACSL. This helped INACSL to meet their goal of developing and disseminating evidence-based practice standards.

Another joint venture between CAE Healthcare and INACSL was the development of the Hayden Vanguard Lectureship Series. Mrs. Jennifer Hayden was the primary researcher responsible for the NCSBN National Simulation Study. She passed away in 2014. To honor her contributions to simulation, INACSL developed the Hayden Vanguard Lectureship in 2015, which is sponsored by CAE Healthcare. The recipient of the lectureship is selected by a committee for his/her contribution and/or innovation that contributes to simulation. The first recipient of this award was Amy Cowperthwait, whose contributions to simulation include the design and development of SimUCare products, which are wearable overlay devices for standardized patients or students to add realism to hybrid simulation. In 2015, INACSL and CAE Healthcare cosponsored the INACSL-CAE Healthcare Simulation **Fellowship**.

Fellowships

INACSL-CAE Healthcare Simulation Fellowship

The INACSL-CAE Healthcare Simulation Fellowship was developed and based on the *INACSL Standards of Best Practice: Simulation* and the Essentials of Simulation by CAE. This immersive fellowship is offered approximately four times a year in the United States and worldwide as formal education on the incorporation of the standards into simulation practices. It provides an immersion into each of the Standards, scenario building using the Standards, facilitation, debriefing, and evaluation. The fellowship is vendor neutral and focuses on the pedagogy of simulation. This fellowship supports a community of practice with mentoring and resources necessary to build a successful program for simulation scholars. A majority of the first cohort fellows focused on basic and intermediate simulation faculty development as their final simulation project. Another cohort focused on assessment, research, and publication. The mentorship portion of the fellowship is designed to meet the specific needs of the participants.

Research Fellowship

In 2016, a Research Fellowship for novice simulation researchers was developed. This fellowship is competitive and restricted to approximately six participants a year. The goal of the Research Fellowship is to advance the science of simulation by improving the rigor of simulation research. All scholars work in teams and will produce a grant proposal for submission to Sigma Theta Tau International, NLN, INACSL Debra Spunt Grant, SSH, or a foundation agency. The major focus is developing files and resources necessary for quality simulation research.

Future of INACSL

The future of INACSL is to advance the science of simulation using evidence-based education and practices, rather than tradition for our 21st century learner. An outgrowth of the narrative pedagogy, which is the basis of higher-level debriefing used in simulation, is becoming more common in university-wide classroom and curriculum. The narrative pedagogy of debriefing is being adopted by non–healthcare disciplines.

The INACSL Standards are a major contribution of the simulation world. The Standards are freely accessible, so people have access to best practices as they evolve. We will continue to develop, refine, and disseminate the Standards. The use of best practice for simulation is reaching the tipping point for critical mass worldwide. INACSL will be a leader in this process. As nurses, we will always be the largest group of end users of simulation due to the number of nurses compared to other disciplines.

Another area to grow simulation is in graduate education. With the information provided about the NCSBN National Simulation Study for best results with prelicensure nursing students, the education of graduate students using simulation requires examination. INACSL would like to collaborate with other simulation organizations, nursing education, advanced nursing practice organizations, and the practice world to evaluate the use and efficacy of simulation in preparation of our graduate school nurses.

As the variety of simulation users continues to expand, methods, programs and technology will also continue to evolve. Education is one topic that spans across all these areas. INACSL is positioned to be the leader in simulation education to meet the future needs of the simulation community.

Summary

The International Nursing Association for Clinical Simulation and Learning is the organization that supports nursing's simulation community of practice. INACSL specializes in developing and disseminating the best practices in healthcare simulation. The mission of the original leaders, "to promote and provide the development and advancement of clinical simulation and learning resource centers," has been met and surpassed. INACSL's current vision and mission will serve to guide the organization into the future as the science of simulation develops.

4

Society for Simulation in Healthcare

Jennifer L. Manos, Andrew E. Spain

Key Terms

Simulation, Accreditation, Certification, SimOps, Research, Strategic Plan

Guiding Questions

1 What is the purpose of the Society for Simulation in Healthcare (SSH)?

2 What contributions has SSH made to the healthcare simulation community?

3 What two programs developed standards for simulation programs and simulation educators?

History

The Society for Simulation in Healthcare (SSH) is a 501c(3), nonprofit, member-based organization that facilitates and supports educators, researchers, administrators, and technicians in the field of healthcare simulation. It is a volunteer organization that is continually adapting to meet the needs of this changing profession. SSH is the world's largest professional organization representing multiple disciplines in healthcare and multiple simulation methodologies utilized in the field of healthcare simulation. SSH's interdisciplinary and multispecialty demographics are represented throughout its membership, programs, and leadership. The mission of SSH is to be a leading interprofessional society that advances the application of simulation in healthcare through global engagement (Society for Simulation in Healthcare, 2016a).

SSH has evolved, grown, and changed since its inception based on the needs of its members and the changing landscape of simulation in healthcare. The history of the organization can be traced back to 1995 when simulation was first being adopted in anesthesiology. The University of Rochester sponsored a symposium entitled *First Conference on Simulators in Anesthesiology Education* in May of 1995 at Rochester, New York (Raemer, 2008). Over the next several years, interest and use of simulation in healthcare continued to grow. This could be seen by the growing number of abstract submissions and panel presentations at the Annual Meeting of the Society for Technology in Anesthesia (STA). In 2000, STA decided to host a simulation-specific meeting, and in January 2001, the first International Meeting on Medical Simulation (IMMS) was held in Scottsdale, Arizona (Raemer, 2008). As attendance at the meeting grew and interest in healthcare simulation increased across multiple disciplines and specialties, a decision was made to begin a separate society. In 2004, the first meeting of the Board of Overseers was held for the Society for Medical Simulation (SMS). The first elected board was William Dunn, MD; David Feinstein, MD; David Gaba, MD; James Gordon, MD; Bernadette Henrichs, PhD; Bosseau Murray, MD; Dan Raemer, PhD; Elizabeth Sinz, MD; and Jeffrey Taekman, MD (Raemer, 2008). The organization was incorporated in California

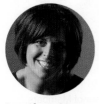

Jennifer L. Manos, MSN, MBA, RN

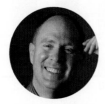

Andrew E. Spain, MA, NCEE, EMT-P

in 2004, and in 2006, it changed its name to the Society for Simulation in Healthcare to represent the broadening scope of membership, and consequently the annual meeting became the International Meeting on Simulation in Healthcare (IMSH).

Society membership has grown exponentially since 2004. SSH membership includes physicians, nurses, allied health and paramedical personnel, researchers, educators, technicians, and developers from around the globe. SSH fosters the application and advancement of a variety of simulation-based modalities. The multidisciplinary and multispecialty focus of the organization has contributed to its growth from approximately 200 members to more than 3,400, as of November 2015 (Fig. 4.1).

Healthcare Simulation Impact and Contributions

SSH is committed to being an organization that advances the application of simulation in healthcare. The organization holds the dissemination of simulation education, practice, and research in the utmost regard. In the dynamic field of healthcare simulation, the organization strives to provide a sense of community among its members and also allow for growth and development within the profession itself. SSH has developed a number of programs to contribute to the field of simulation in healthcare while being committed to making an impact on the profession now and into the future.

Journal

Simulation in Healthcare is the official publication of the Society for Simulation in Healthcare and is published by Lippincott Williams & Wilkins, a division of the publishing house, Wolters Kluwer. It is a multidisciplinary

publication including all areas of application and research in healthcare simulation. The first editor-in-chief, David M. Gaba, MD, was appointed in 2005. Dr. Gaba provided over 10 years of service to the development of the journal, and through his dedication and the dedication of the associate editors, *SIH* has become the preeminent peer-reviewed publication for healthcare simulation research. In late 2016, Dr. Mark Scerbo was appointed editor-in-chief upon Dr. Gaba's retirement. The inaugural issue, *SIH* Volume 1, Number 1, was published January 2006. Milestones throughout the history of the journal include (1) acceptance for indexing in MEDLINE in 2008, (2) increased publications to six times per year in 2010, and (3) in 2011, assigned its first impact factor.

The journal, indexed in Medicus/MEDLINE and the Science Citation Index, is relevant to a broad range of clinical and biomedical specialties and publishes original basic, clinical, and translational research on a variety of topics related to simulation in healthcare (Society for Simulation in Healthcare, 2016b). In addition to being the official publication of SSH, *Simulation in Healthcare* is also the recognized journal for many other simulation-based professional organizations. The journal is available in print and electronic formats via the web and iPad app to SSH members. A complete listing of organizations that recognize *SIH* as the/an official journal can be found at http://www.ssih.org/News/Journal. The electronic subscription to the Journal is included with SSH membership and members living in North America also receive the printed journal by mail.

International Meeting on Simulation in Healthcare

The International Meeting on Simulation in Healthcare (IMSH) is the world's largest multidisciplinary, multispecialty conference dedicated to healthcare simulation. It is a

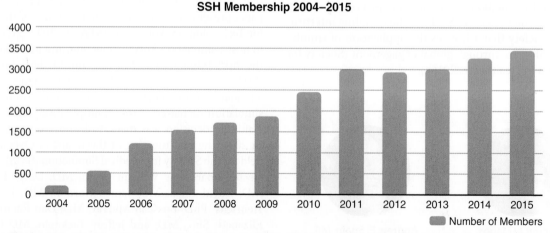

Figure 4.1 SSH Membership Growth Through 2015. (Data courtesy of the Society for Simulation in Healthcare.)

IMSH Attendance 2003–2016

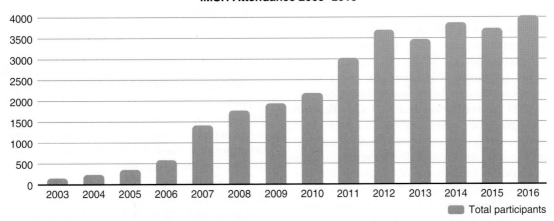

Figure 4.2 IMSH Attendance Growth Through 2016. (Data courtesy of the Society for Simulation Healthcare.)

unique opportunity to network with healthcare simulation professionals from around the world, learn and experience innovative ways healthcare simulation is being incorporated into education, gain insight into the latest trends and research, and influence the national discussion and evolution of healthcare simulation. IMSH just celebrated its 16th annual meeting, and it has experienced exponential growth and development in this short time (Fig. 4.2).

The first meeting, the International Meeting on Medical Simulation, was held in 2001 in Scottsdale, Arizona. In 2006, the name of the meeting was changed to IMSH to incorporate the multidisciplinary/multispecialty focus of the organization. Since 2001, the conference has grown from just over 100 attendees to over 3,400 individuals representing educators, clinicians, researchers, operations specialists, administrators, students, and industry. Today, the conference features world renowned faculty and keynote speakers, preconference and immersive courses taught by leaders in the field, over 300 educational sessions, and poster presentations including research abstracts, program innovation, technology innovation, and student categories. In addition, IMSH provides showcases highlighting innovations in healthcare simulation, which include the Annual Serious Games & Virtual Environments Arcade and the Annual Spectrum of Innovation Showcase. IMSH is also proud to have a prominent and expansive exhibit hall with over 100 industry partners and exhibitors.

Over the past 16 years, IMSH has evolved content to support continued professional development of the attendees and the healthcare simulation community. SSH, through IMSH, is committed to providing learning opportunities for novice, intermediate, and advanced learners by offering the latest developments in cutting edge innovation. In addition, the organization is committed to providing education that advances leadership skills to allow for continued growth of the community and the organization.

Regional Meetings

As SSH has grown and developed so have the needs of its members. Regional meetings provide the opportunity to meet a specific need related to geographic location, simulation specialty or role, or both. In addition, regional meetings offer attendees the opportunity to expand their simulation knowledge, engage in networking opportunities, and leverage their experience in a local setting that allows for increased accessibility.

The Asia Pacific Meeting on Simulation in Healthcare (APMSH) provides an exciting and unique experience for a diverse population of stakeholders striving to promote excellence in patient care through innovation and collaboration in this region. The first meeting was held in 2011 in Hong Kong and the second held in Shanghai, China, in 2013. Both meetings included over 400 participants from throughout the Asia-Pacific region. APMSH provides a spectrum of education that spans from introductory to advanced topics through a variety of engaging sessions including interactive workshops, expert panels, roundtable discussions, and expert keynote presentations. The development of an international regional meeting is directly supportive of SSH's mission. It provides learners from all over the world an opportunity to engage in collaboration to further promote and develop healthcare simulation.

SSH **SimOps** was developed to provide education and training to operations specialists in a unique hands-on environment. This regional conference is aimed at providing the learners with a comprehensive menu of basic to advanced levels of integration of simulation technology and information to further develop technological and supportive advances within a simulation program. The first SimOps Regional meeting was held in 2014 in Pittsburgh, PA, at the Peter M. Winter Institute for Simulation, Education, and Research (WISER). The goal of this program is to partner with simulation programs from across the country to provide an immersive experience to the attendee.

Accreditation and Certification

Many of the initiatives of SSH involve complex projects that are quite extensive and work intensive for development and ongoing delivery. While this type and scope of work is not unique to SSH, there are two projects that deserve recognition as being under this category of complexity: SSH **Accreditation** and SSH **Certification**. These two programs are often confused for each other. Accreditation is for programs (institutions or entities), and certification is for individuals. The term program was deliberately chosen to be inclusive of all entities that perform simulation activities. Not all simulation activities occur in fixed buildings (centers). This can create confusion with programs in the sense of educational programs (e.g., courses).

These projects were initially approved for development by the SSH Board of Directors in 2007 when the Committee on Certification, Accreditation, and Technology & Standards (CATS) was formed. Much of the catalyst for the creation of this committee was the fact that healthcare simulation had evolved as so many things do—with tremendous energy, ideas, and goals. However, it was also recognized that this had created some notion of divergence in practice; healthcare simulation risked being fundamentally different in how it was delivered. These committees were tasked with identifying ways to prevent this problem.

For Accreditation and Certification, it was recognized that the way to continue to harness the energy and ideation in healthcare simulation, while simultaneously creating some standardization, was through adhering to some key principles:

- Developing frameworks in which healthcare simulation activities are delivered
- Focusing on outcomes as well as processes
- Ensuring nonprescriptive ideas and concepts
- Inclusivity of the various components identified in healthcare simulation, including, but not limited to:
  o Modality (e.g., virtual reality, standardized/simulated patients, mannequins)
  o Types of simulation activities (e.g., research, education, assessment)
  o Setting (e.g., academic, hospital based, mobile)
  o Cultural (e.g., ethnicity, language, beliefs)
  o Clinical (e.g., professions, methods)
  o Experience (e.g., new learners, experienced healthcare providers)
  o Regulatory (e.g., laws, regulations)
  o Purposes (e.g., patient safety, improved outcomes, competency verification)

The goal was to create a voluntary evaluation process for programs and individuals that, by adhering to these principles, recognizes performance to a set of standards.

Focus on the end point rather than the specific path, supports creativity, flexibility, and evolving practices.

Accreditation

Program accreditation involves the external evaluation of a program by independent reviewers for the purposes of ensuring quality to a published set of standards (Prus & Strein, 2011). Previously, the focus in accreditation was on the structures, resources, and processes in place to effectively perform the functions being accredited. However, the last few years have seen a shift to a much more outcomes-oriented focus for accreditation (Prus & Strein, 2011). SSH Accreditation is no exception to this in that programs applying for full accreditation must be able to demonstrate at least 2 years of outcomes data. However, the structures, resources, and processes are not ignored. Accredited programs must demonstrate how they achieve quality outcomes that meet the standards through having sufficient facilities, structures, and resources, as well as consistent and continually evolving processes.

The Accreditation Committee determined this evaluation to be more comprehensive and yet also flexible. No specific mandates were given in the standards for what must be present, but rather what concept must be met and demonstrated. For instance, there are no requirements on what physical space or financial resources must be present beyond that the program must state what is necessary to support what simulation activity is performed. This creates the freedom of flexibility while still maintaining the requirement to meet the quality of the standard.

After great deliberation, the committee developed standards for five functional areas in healthcare simulation, commonly referred to as the Core-ART/S model:

- Core—the criteria regarding fundamentals that must be in place for each program (e.g., governance, finances, staff qualifications)
- Assessment—the criteria regarding simulation activities where formal assessment (either formative or summative) is performed (e.g., for objective structured clinical examinations [OSCE], psychometric expertise)
- Research—the criteria regarding research activities where healthcare simulation is utilized in the research activities (e.g., ethics, research design, investigator qualifications)
- Teaching/Education—the criteria related to the use of simulation to teach, train, and educate individuals (e.g., educational design methodology, instructor qualifications)
- Systems Integration—the criteria related to the use of simulation to investigate and improve patient care activities in a healthcare setting (e.g., hospital), often focused on patient safety efforts (e.g., feedback loops, continuous improvement activities)

All programs are required to become accredited in the Core standards. Programs then must become accredited in at least one of Assessment, Research, and/or Teaching/Education. If desired, a program can also apply for accreditation in Systems Integration but must be accredited in at least one of the previous three areas to be eligible for accreditation in Systems Integration.

The first accreditations were awarded in January of 2011 at IMSH in New Orleans. Those first seven programs were the first of many to come over the next few years. Since these first accreditations were awarded, a new program has also been added in 2013 for those programs that do not yet have the 2 years of outcomes data. Many programs, due to regulatory requirements, must be accredited prior to performing any healthcare simulations. Other programs desire to begin the accreditation path and begin capturing outcomes. Provisional Accreditation was created to meet this need. Since the programs cannot demonstrate the outcomes, the evaluation process is focused more on the intended outcomes, evaluating what is or will be in place as stated by the applying program.

As of January 2016, there are 65 programs from 7 countries that have successfully become accredited, and 10 programs from 3 countries that have successfully become provisionally accredited. Nine of the fully accredited programs have achieved the distinction of being accredited in all four areas beyond the Core area.

Certification

"Professional accountability requires a self-regulating profession to set and maintain credible, useful standards for its members. Voluntary certification and recertification—evaluation by peers—serves the responsibility of the profession to establish and enforce its own standards" (Benson, 1991, p. 238). Based on feedback as well as on results of a 2010 survey ($n = 1,221$) done by SSH, the healthcare simulation community stated they felt there was a need for a set of standard behaviors and guidelines that could frame the practice of simulation. Additionally, 88.3% shared that much of their learning had occurred "on the job," that is to say informally and as learned through actual practice, rather than through formal education. This indicated to the Committee that certification offered a way to frame the desired behaviors. Bolstered by the 71% of respondents who also indicated that certification was desirable, the Certification Committee set about the development of certifications to serve the community.

It became readily apparent that the work required to develop the certifications was significant. Table 4.1 represents key milestones of work in the development of the Certified Healthcare Simulation Educator, Certified Healthcare Simulation Educator-Advanced, and the Certified Healthcare Simulation Operations Specialist certifications (CHSE, CHSE-A, and CHSOS).

Table 4.1	Key Milestones in Certification Program Development
Date	**Milestone**
2008	Certification Subcommittee of CATS officially formed
May 2010	Statement of Principles of Certification adopted
September 2010	CHSE and CHSE-A to be developed based on needs survey; CHSE to be exam based, CHSE-A to be portfolio based
January 2011	Request for Proposal (RFP) issued to obtain vendor to develop exam-based CHSE
June 2011	Schroeder Measurement Technologies Inc. (SMT) selected as vendor
August 2011	CHSE/CHSE-A Practice Analysis performed (completed in October)
November 2011	CHSE item writing and form development underway
June 2012	CHSE launched in pilot mode
December 2012	Pilot ends, first CHSEs awarded; open to all applicants
January 2013	CHSOS development approved by Board of Directors
May 2013	CHSOS Practice Analysis performed (completed in November)
August 2013	CHSE-A launched in pilot mode
December 2013	CHSOS item writing and form development underway
January 2013	Pilot ends, CHSE-As awarded
April 2013	CHSE-A review completed, open to all applicants
May 2014	CHSOS pilot launched
October 2014	CHSE practice exam launched
January 2015	Pilot ends, first CHSOSs awarded; open to all applicants
January 2016	CHSOS practice exam launched

All of the work that is represented in the timeline has been to certification industry norms and standards. Key elements of these certifications are described as follows.

Overview of Certifications

CHSE and CHSOS were developed for the 2-year competent level healthcare simulationist. A 2-year competent individual has been identified as someone who has had enough experience and education over a period of time to incorporate lessons learned into their practice and can be considered to be functional with minimal direction within the expected policies, procedures, mission/vision, and functions of the simulation program. The CHSE is for individuals focused on the educational development principles and processes in simulation, whereas the CHSOS is more for individuals who are focused on the operational and delivery principles and processes, especially those that are grounded in computer and technological fields. The two groups of individuals served by these certifications are believed to represent the largest portions of the teams often in place to develop and deliver healthcare simulation activities.

The CHSE-A certification is an additional level that can be achieved by individuals who have achieved CHSE, have more experience and education, and have moved into a higher level of leadership as demonstrated through a portfolio. The portfolio serves as a platform for the applicant to demonstrate their performance of the same fundamental knowledge of the CHSE certification, but at a much higher level that indicates their expanded and extended skills and leadership.

Statement of Principles

The Certification Committee adopted a set of principles that guided the development and delivery of the certifications. Through adopting these principles, the Committee believed this would best serve the healthcare simulation community and support the integrity of the certifications.

- Certification is a voluntary process.
- Certification will be seen as a service to SSH members and our communities of interest.
- Certification will confirm the knowledge, skills, and attitudes essential to individuals in the field of simulation.
- Certification, in order to maximize efficiency and impact, should be a cooperative effort between simulation and professional organizations.
- Certification will be time limited and renewable.

Practice Analysis

The foundation of a standards-based certification program is the establishment of the link between the requisite knowledge for competent practitioners to perform their jobs and what content appears on the examination. The CHSE and CHSOS examination development began with a practice analysis (also referred to as a role delineation study or RDS), which provided the critical foundation for developing a psychometrically sound and legally defensible certifying examination. The RDS ensures that the examination content is valid and determines the critical knowledge competencies required of practitioners within the field. A RDS provides a detailed description of the

content knowledge that practitioners within a specified field need to competently perform their job roles, and the information gathered is used at all stages of examination development.

Adherence to Industry Standards and Best Practice

The SSH CHSE and CHSOS examinations are professionally developed and adhere to industry standards such as those promulgated by the American National Standards Institute (ANSI), National Commission for Certifying Agencies (NCCA), Accreditation Board for Specialty Nursing Certification (ABSNC), the Joint Technical Standards of the American Psychological Association (APA), American Educational Research Association (AERA), and the National Council on Measurement in Education (NCME). By following these standards, as well as best practices within the certification and testing industries, the CHSE and CHSOS examinations provide an exemplary model for the certification of healthcare simulationists. Continuous adherence to these standards and best practices provides stakeholders the assurance that the CHSE and CHSOS examinations are valid and reliable measures of practitioner's knowledge of essential competencies to practice within the field.

Status of the Certification Programs

As of February 1, 2016, 720 individuals from 22 countries had successfully passed the CHSE exam and become certified (since June 2012). From this group, 18 individuals from 3 countries have taken the next step and become a CHSE-A. The newest certification, CHSOS, has seen 73 individuals from 6 countries successfully pass the exam and achieve this certification.

Support and Recognition Initiatives

SSH gives back to the greater healthcare simulation community by recognizing the need for mentorship and scholarship. It is important for the community to foster new initiatives for the future of simulation while also recognizing the contributions of leaders who have paved the way for healthcare simulation today. SSH is privileged to be able to provide for the development of current and future leaders and is committed to serve as a collaborative venue for the international simulation community to positively affect quality and safety in healthcare.

Beverlee Anderson Scholarship

At the International Meeting on Simulation in Healthcare (IMSH) in 2008, the SSH showed its gratitude and appreciation for its first Executive Director, Beverlee Anderson, who retired on July 1, 2008. Beverlee's vision and promotion of simulation helped the Society achieve significant milestones. Beverlee was recognized for her efforts at the January 12, 2008, Board of Directors meeting as well as the membership business meeting in San Diego. It was with great honor that the Board of Directors announced the establishment of the Beverlee Anderson Education Scholarship Fund (BAESF) to continue her mission to provide support to attend IMSH and other SSH-sponsored educational activities.

After the untimely death of Beverlee in September of 2009, the SSH Board set up a memorial fund to build on the already established Scholarship fund. Members are invited to contribute to the fund. Application is tied directly to Beverlee's interest and past commitment of providing "scholarships" to those she identified as having a need for support in order to attend IMSH. SSH currently provides two scholarships per year and is hoping to provide more in the future. The Society is honored to be able to provide this opportunity to the simulation community.

Research Grant

In 2012, the SSH Board of Directors approved the development of a research grant to support novice investigators in the field of healthcare simulation research. The first award was granted in 2013. The Society continues to provide this award annually with the goal of increasing funds for future research development.

The SSH Research Grant provides up to two $5,000 grants to support promising pilot studies. The main objective is to support novice investigators with less than 5 years of simulation-based research experience in performing health-related, simulation-based pilot studies. SSH seeks studies that are both novel and have strong potential for a positive impact on healthcare delivery processes and outcomes through, for example, education, assessment, usability testing, or system integration.

Pioneer in Simulation

The Pioneer in Simulation Award was initiated in 2014 by the SSH Board of Directors to recognize those who have played a pivotal role in the development of healthcare simulation. The first Annual Pioneer in Simulation award was presented to Dr. Stephen Abramson at IMSH in 2014 for the development of the first computer-controlled mannequin simulator; SimOne. In 2015, Dr. Michael Gordon was bestowed the honor for his contributions in life-saving cardiovascular training through the development of Harvey, the Cardiopulmonary Patient Simulator. Lou Oberndorf received the award in 2016 for industrialization of the Human Patient Simulator and other significant contributions to the healthcare simulation industry.

Key Contributor(s) and Teams

With having a large membership, it is almost impossible to pull together the list of all individuals who have contributed to SSH—its founding, growth, evolution, and all the activities therein. The time, input, work, and passion of the literally thousands of individuals who have contributed to SSH is extensive, and all should be thanked.

SSH Presidents

The contributions of a select group of individuals, the presidents—past, present, and future—must be recognized as having been essential to taking SSH to where it is now and what it will become in the future (Table 4.2)

2016 Board of Directors

The SSH Board of Directors works with the president to make key decisions and shape the direction of SSH. As the largest interprofessional simulation society, SSH strives to ensure diversity of representation on the Board in order to capture the range of perspectives and input that makes up all of healthcare simulation. The membership of the 2016 Board of Directors is composed of representatives from medicine, education, nursing, research, industry, business, and hails from several countries.

Commissions, Committees, Sections, Special Interest Groups, Affinity Groups

There are many teams and groups that are working toward meeting the directives and directions from the Board and also continue to move SSH and healthcare simulation forward. The Commissions and Committees are the working groups assigned in the bylaws to carry out the business of SSH. These groups are made of volunteers who work to complete the tasks and duties assigned.

The Sections, Special Interest Groups, and Affinity Groups are composed of individuals with shared interests. One key distinction between these and the Commissions and Committees is that these groups originated at the request of the SSH members—not the Board of Directors. Essentially, members who identified in some common way—simulation expertise, clinical background, or other grouping—petition the board to be recognized as such. Upon approval, this creates an Affinity Group (AG). The AG can become a Special Interest Group (SIG) after maintaining membership and activity for a period of time then can move onto Section status after further time and activity. Sections hold a special place in that they are more involved in the decision making and input for SSH for activities such as conferences.

Table 4.2	SSH Presidents	
Dates	**Name**	**Affiliation**
2004–2006	Dan Raemer, PhD	Center for Medical Simulation (CMS)
2007	Elisabeth (Lisa) Sinz, MD, FCCM	Penn State Milton Hershey Medical Center
2008	William (Bill) Dunn, MD	Mayo Clinic
2009	Michael DeVita, MD	Harlem Hospital Center
2010	Mary Patterson, MEd, MD	Children's National Medical Center
2011	Michael Seropian, MD, FRCPC	Oregon Health and Science University
2012	Mary E (Beth) Mancini, PhD, RN, NE-BC, FAHA, ANEF, FAAN	The University of Texas at Arlington
2013	Paul Phrampus, MD	University of Pittsburgh—WISER
2014	Pamela R Jeffries, PhD, RN, FAAN, ANEF	George Washington University School of Nursing
2015	Pamela Andreatta, EdD, PhD, CHSE	University of Central Florida
2016	Chad Epps, MD	University of Alabama at Birmingham
2017	Christine Park, MD	Northwestern Center for Clinical Simulation, Northwestern University

Future Direction

The future of SSH is guided by its approved strategic plan. The SSH **Strategic Plan** outlines the goals and objectives of the organization through 2020. The plan was developed after obtaining SSH member input and with careful deliberation to accommodate the growing numbers and diversity of membership (Society for Simulation in Healthcare, 2016b). The current strategic plan was unanimously approved by the SSH Board of Directors in 2015. The plan establishes a framework for growth that is nimble enough to facilitate member engagement, leadership, and professional development opportunities through multiple, coordinated objectives. The principle elements of the plan include identity, sustainability, value, and leadership with goals and objectives associated to each element.

Get Involved

SSH invites anyone involved in healthcare simulation to join the organization and experience the benefits the organization has to offer. Join over 3,000 colleagues as the international voice advocating healthcare simulation in education, practice, and research. SSH membership provides opportunities to network with peers, share ideas, learn about best practices, and discover new research. As an SSH member, one can access resources to stay current with advances in simulation practice, develop and promote standards of simulation-based education and research, connect with peers via shared interest groups, and participate in interprofessional collaboration. To learn more about what SSH has to offer, visit www.ssih.org.

5

National League for Nursing and Simulation Innovation Resource Center

Susan Gross Forneris, M. Elaine Tagliareni, Pamela R. Jeffries, Mary Anne Rizzolo

 Key Terms

Theory Development, High Stakes Assessment, Debriefing, NLN/Jeffries Simulation Theory, Leadership Development, Vision Statement

 Guiding Questions

1 How has the NLN promoted simulation pedagogy and leadership since 2003?
2 Describe the evolution of the NLN Jeffries Simulation Theory.
3 How might your school operationalize the recommendations in the NLN vision statements?

Introduction

The integral relationship between practice and education is a core truth for the National League for Nursing (NLN). The NLN maintains that advances to promote this relationship must underpin how the nursing profession deliberates and strategizes and how the NLN implements and evaluates its mission, to promote excellence in nursing education to build a strong and diverse workforce to advance the health of the nation and the global community. The NLN implements its mission guided by four dynamic and integrated core values that permeate the organization and are reflected in its work: Caring, Integrity, Diversity and Excellence. For more than a decade, the NLN has promoted simulation as a teaching methodology to prepare nurses for practice across the continuum of care in today's complex healthcare environment.

The NLN's work to advance simulation within nursing education and in the broader interprofessional context and to lead simulation innovation is evidence of the NLN's commitment to its mission and core values. That legacy, reinforced by the League's mission and core values, furnishes a strong foundation to address the challenges and opportunities arising from the use of simulation in nursing education.

Historical Overview

The Early Years

The NLN's leadership in simulation design and faculty development began in 2000, at the dawn of the new millennium.

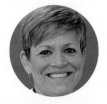

Susan Gross Forneris,
PhD, RN, CNE, CHSE-A

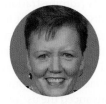

M. Elaine Tagliareni,
EdD, RN, CNE, FAAN

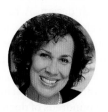

Pamela R. Jeffries,
PhD, RN, ANEF, FAAN

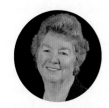

Mary Anne Rizzolo,
EdD, RN, FAAN, ANEF

Medical Education Technologies Inc. (METI),[1] a company that was founded in 1996 by Mr. Lou Obendorf, contacted the NLN about administering a program that would provide funding for simulation research projects that focused on the use of METI's Human Patient Simulator (HPS) in nursing education. The 3-year agreement provided funding for four awards of $10,000 each year. Applicants were required to already own a METI HPS mannequin for use in their nursing education program. Grant recipients made presentations about their work at METI's annual Human Patient Simulation Network (HPSN) conference each year and several awardees also presented during a session sponsored by METI at the NLN Summit.

Initial Testing of Simulation Models

In 2003, Laerdal Medical approached the NLN about funding a simulation project that would develop and test models of simulation that nursing faculty could implement to promote student learning. Rosie Patterson, currently Vice President for Business Development at Laerdal, and Dr. Terry Valiga, NLN Chief Program Officer and Dr. Mary Anne Rizzolo, Senior Director of Professional Development at the time, outlined initial plans for a national multisite project. The NLN issued a competitive nationwide call for a project director and schools that wished to be considered as project sites. After many applications were received for the project director position, Dr. Pamela Jeffries was the unanimous choice. There were over 170 applications for the school project sites, with only eight schools being selected in the process, representing diversity of geographic locations and type of program. The schools and project coordinators are outlined in Box 5-1.

The project was launched in June 2003 with a kickoff meeting at the Laerdal Headquarters in Gatesville, Texas, to clarify goals and responsibilities, explore a theoretical framework for the research design, and explain the process for implementing the research over the 3 years of the project. The project director, NLN staff, and project coordinators collaborated on conducting a literature review and found that while there were many anecdotal articles, there was little evidence-based literature to guide the development and use of simulations.

Following the June meeting, the project director developed the framework to design, implement, and evaluate the use of simulations in nursing education (Jeffries, 2005) and completed the four-phase research design. A review of existing measurement tools revealed that none were adequate for the purposes of this study, so new research instruments had to be developed and tested: the Simulation Design Scale, the Educational Practices Questionnaire, and the Student Satisfaction and Self Confidence in Learning. These instruments have been used by hundreds of doctoral

---

[1]Note: CAE Healthcare acquired METI in 2011.

Box 5-1	Project Sites and Coordinators

Case Western Reserve University
Frances Payne Bolton School of Nursing
Cleveland, Ohio
Project Coordinators: Melissa Horn, Marcella Hovancsek

Community College of Southern Nevada
Las Vegas, Nevada
Project Coordinators: Nina Carter, Ruth Politi

Texas Tech University Health Sciences Center, School of Nursing
Lubbock, Texas
Project Coordinator: Sharon Decker

Tulsa Community College
Tulsa, Oklahoma
Project Coordinator: Cheryl Feken

University of Maryland School of Nursing
Baltimore, Maryland
Project Coordinator: Debra Spunt (deceased)

University of Southern Maine
Portland, Maine
Project Coordinator: Janis Childs

University of Virginia
Charlottesville, Virginia
Project Coordinator: Reba Childress

The Washington Hospital School of Nursing
Washington, Pennsylvania
Project Coordinator: Kristen Rogers

students and researchers since their development and are currently available on the NLN Simulation Innovation Resource Center (SIRC) website (http://sirc.nln.org/).

By the end of year 3 of the project, Dr. Jeffries, Dr. Rizzolo, and the project coordinators had delivered more than 60 presentations, published 17 articles and book chapters, and published a book on simulation, titled "*Simulation in Nursing Education: From Conceptualization to Evaluation*" (Jeffries, 2007a). Their dissemination efforts extended to Singapore, China, South America, Japan, Africa, Thailand, Egypt, Vietnam, Korea, Australia, Israel, Russia, Jordan, Canada, Iceland, United Kingdom, Ireland, Scotland, Norway, and Italy. Dr. Jeffries and Dr. Deborah Spunt, Director of the Simulation Center at the University of Maryland, were invited to participate on a national task force created by the Division of Nursing (U.S. Department of Health and Human Services, Health Resources and Services Administration) to study the feasibility of funding a faculty development initiative to prepare nurse educators for the use of technology and simulated learning. The result was nine federally funded collaborative projects, each with over 1 million dollars in funding over 5 years, which provided faculty development to hundreds of nurse educators and advanced the use of technology, including simulation, in schools of nursing throughout the nation. The project director and project coordinators also received many honors and awards, and they sought and received funding amounting to almost 2 million dollars to expand and support their simulation equipment, the laboratory environment, and new research efforts. This 3 year national project marked the first significant research on the use of simulations in nursing education. It contributed significantly to the body of knowledge about simulation and the science of nursing education (Jeffries & Rizzolo, 2007). It launched a movement toward the use of simulation as an essential teaching strategy. It also forged a relationship between the NLN and Laerdal Medical that has grown and thrived and continues to this day with collaboration on a variety of simulation projects.

Development of the NLN Simulation Innovation Research Center

Following the original research project, the NLN continued to promote the use of simulation through various faculty development initiatives. Perhaps the most significant and comprehensive faculty development effort by the NLN to date is the Simulation Innovation Resource Center (SIRC), a website was developed with Laerdal funding to meet an important and timely need for faculty development.

In 2007, a call was issued to recruit simulation experts who were willing to participate in the development of the SIRC. The NLN received 159 applications, nine were selected from the United States, and they were joined by eight nurse educators from Australia, Canada, Chile, China, Japan, Norway, and Scotland.

The SIRC (http://sirc.nln.org) was created to provide core educational programs and resources for faculty. The main educational resources are 15 interactive web-based modules designed to prepare nurse educators to design, implement, and evaluate the use of simulations in nursing education that can be purchased by individuals or schools. A number of free resources can also be found on the website including a glossary, annotated bibliography, list of simulation centers around the world, links to vendors who sell products related to simulation, a discussion board, and a number of other free resources such as templates and reports of simulation projects. Research conducted in 2014 (Fey, 2014) reported that 28.7% of 307 faculty members who responded to her survey cited the SIRC as the source of their training on debriefing, demonstrating the need, impact, and success of this early faculty development resource for faculty.

Advancing the Science

From Simulation Framework to Theory

As noted above, Dr. Jeffries designed the original simulation framework to guide the NLN/Laerdal simulation research study in 2003. The first image, which was called the "Simulation Model," was modified in 2005

and published by the NLN to describe the framework and each of its components: student, teacher, educational practices, design characteristics, and outcomes (Jeffries, 2005). Over the course of time, the framework was revised, and a third variation was published (Jeffries, 2007a); the constructs remained relatively consistent. A historical overview of the three iterations of the Nursing Education Simulation Framework (Rizzolo, Durham, Ravert & Jeffries, 2016) provides a thorough description of the modifications; the framework provided a solid foundation for research by simulation scholars to investigate the powerful learning opportunities with simulation as a teaching methodology.

By 2010, there was recognition within the simulation nursing community that a review of the framework, in light of studies conducted using the framework as a theoretical foundation, was the next step in building the science of simulation in nursing education. In the summer of 2011, the International Nursing Association for Clinical Simulation and Learning (INACSL), in consultation with Dr. Pamela Jeffries, convened nursing simulation educators and researchers to examine the application of the Nursing Education Simulation Framework. The NLN provided partial funding through the NLN's research grants program. Volunteer simulation experts formed five teams to investigate one of the five framework constructs: student, teacher, educational practices, simulation design characteristics, and outcomes. Each construct team was asked to examine the literature in light of the following questions:

1. How is the concept defined in the literature to date?
2. What is the state of the science (what evidence is available) surrounding the assigned framework constructs to date?
3. What are the major knowledge gaps and research opportunities in these areas?
4. What are the important future directions for research surrounding the concepts in the framework? (Ravert & McAfooes, 2014, p. 335)

Significant findings that emerged include:

- The term facilitator was more consistently used in the literature than teacher (Jones, Reese & Shelton, 2014).
- The word participant, rather than student (Durham, Cato, & Lasater, 2014), more adequately described the many roles required during simulation scenario implementation.
- The term simulation design characteristics was a guiding principle, but little evidence was found to support the construct (Groom, Henderson, & Sittner, 2014).
- Debriefing and feedback were used interchangeably in the literature (Hallmark, Thomas, & Gantt, 2014).
- Components of the framework listed for outcomes were widely used, but outcomes related to teamwork and roles and responsibilities were lacking (O'Donnell, Decker, Howard, Levett-Jones, & Miller, 2014).

The next iteration of the framework (Jeffries & Clochesy, 2012), now termed the NLN Jeffries Simulation Framework, included revised terminology for the constructs of student and teacher that were changed to participant and facilitator.

Following this initial work, the NLN, with partial funding from Laerdal, in collaboration with INACSL, convened a think tank to continue this important analytical work. The NLN asked an internationally known expert in **theory development**, Beth Rogers, PhD, RN, FAAN, to join the think tank. Her charge was to evaluate the potential for moving the NLN/Jeffries Simulation Framework from a framework to a theory. While the discussion reaffirmed the importance of the NLN/Jeffries Simulation Framework and the appropriateness of its components and content (Rizzolo et al., 2016), Dr. Rodgers determined the need for a comprehensive literature review with high-quality evidence tables, focused on completed rigorous research, in order to clarify the constructs in the framework and the relationships among the various components. Additionally, the intent was to identify gaps in the literature in order to clarify directions for further research (Rizzolo et al., 2016).

In 2014, the NLN contracted with Dr. Katie Adamson to complete a systematic review of the literature related to the use of the NLN Jeffries Simulation Framework (Adamson, 2015; Adamson & Rodgers, 2016) in order to render the specificity needed to advance development of

the framework to a theory. The review illuminated what is currently known about best simulation practices, what research exists to support these practices, and priorities for future research. The resulting **NLN/Jeffries Simulation Theory**, (Jeffries, 2016), Figure 5.1, provided evidence to develop the theory to a predictive level such that it provides clear guidance to those who use simulation in teaching–learning situations. Recommendations were developed based on the assumption that the theory would be regarded as a guide not only for implementation of simulation in a variety of contexts but as a solid foundation for future testing of simulation experiences and techniques.

Constructs for the NLN Jeffries Simulation Theory were modified from previous iterations of the framework, resulting in some changes to the conceptual illustration (Jeffries, Rodgers & Adamson, 2016):

- Context: Simulation is used in a variety of contexts, which include diverse disciplines, purposes, and environmental supports. An important starting point in designing and evaluating simulation, this construct also includes, for example, whether the intent is formative or summative.
- Background: This construct includes the goal(s) of the simulation and specific expectations or benchmarks that influence the design of the simulation, including such factors as how the simulation activity is situated

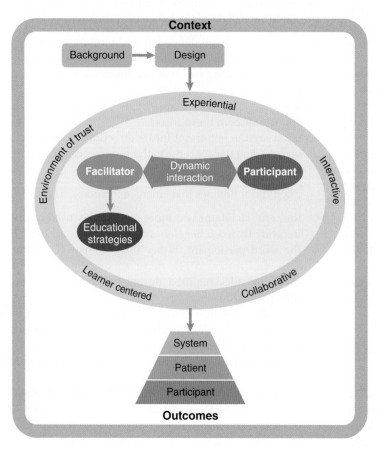

Figure 5.1 NLN/Jeffries Simulation Theory. (Copyright © 2015 by the National League for Nursing. Used with permission.)

within the larger curriculum, the expectations or benchmarks established for the simulation, and more specifically, the learning objectives for the simulation activity.

- Design: This construct, which solidly emerged from the systematic literature review, was expanded to highlight the specific learning objectives, which are directly related to the activities and complexity of the scenario. Essential to design are also decisions about equipment, predetermined facilitator and participant dialogue and interventions, as well as role responsibilities. This construct is complex and multifaceted.

- *Simulation Experience*, in the theory illustration, is characterized by an environment that is experiential, interactive, collaborative, and learner-centered, recognizing that the participant and the facilitator share responsibility for the learner environment, in the context of sound educational practices.

- Outcomes of the simulation, in the revised illustration, are separated into three areas: Participant, patient (or care recipient), and system. "The illustration depicts outcomes in a triangular format based on the hierarchy of outcomes with participant, patient, and system outcomes as defined and extracted from the body of literature found on simulation outcomes" (Jeffries et al., 2016, p. 41). The literature review revealed that most past and current studies focus on participant outcomes; there is a need to expand to health outcomes of patients and caregivers and more system-based measures, for example, cost-effectiveness and changes in practice.

NLN High-Stakes Simulation Project

The NLN's Project to explore the use of simulation for high-stakes assessment (Rizzolo, Kardong-Edgren, Oermann & Jeffries, 2015) was designed to lay the groundwork for use of simulation for high-stakes assessment in prelicensure RN programs. Phase 1 began by gathering experts in the use of simulation in nursing and medical education, outcomes assessment, and clinical judgement for a 2-day think tank meeting. These experts identified end-of-program outcomes that are amenable to assessment through simulation, outlined scenarios that could be designed for that purpose, and provided recommendations for their implementation.

In Phase 2, a team of experts, led by Dr. Pamela Jeffries, developed four simulation scenarios along with three parallel forms for each scenario. They were pilot tested at schools of nursing across the country and then revised. While the simulation experts were designing the scenarios, a second team, led by Dr. Marilyn Oermann and Dr. Suzan Kardong-Edgren, constructed the research plan, selected the tools for scoring the scenarios, and designed the training for the evaluators.

During Phase 3, revised scenarios were field tested at schools of nursing across the country that were geographically diverse and represented different types of RN prelicensure programs. The schools video recorded student performance of the scenarios. Raters, selected via a competitive application, were trained on use of the Creighton Competency Evaluation Instrument (CCEI) tool and then they normed and scored the video performances. Statistical analysis revealed inconsistencies in application of norming criteria. The final evaluation phase employed the simulation authors to establish the criteria for scoring the CCEI and then the same raters independently viewed and scored the student video performances at two separate points in time. Statistical analyses were completed to determine interrater and test/retest reliability. The project report (Rizzolo et al., 2015) details recommendations regarding the use of simulation for high-stakes evaluation in nursing education and areas for future research related to this practice.

The significance of this project cannot be underestimated. In Spring of 2014, 605 people responded to a survey about the use of high-stakes assessments in preparation for a report that was presented at a Town Hall meeting at the INACSL conference. Forty-two percent of the respondents said they were using high-fidelity simulations to evaluate their students and 28% were using objective structured clinical examinations (OSCEs). However, few had determined the reliability and validity of their scenarios (Rutherford-Hemming, Kardong-Edgren, Gore, Ravert, & Rizzolo, 2014). The findings from this project have already raised awareness and generated new studies that can refine and improve this process.

Faculty Development Initiatives

The NLN has offered faculty development programs on simulation throughout the United States and internationally, beginning in 2007 when Basic Simulation Workshops were offered across the country. Content on simulation has been incorporated into Summit sessions and other signature NLN conferences since that time and webinars on a variety of simulation topics have taken place each year.

The NLN is acutely aware that the current advances in the delivery of care in today's changing healthcare system are informing necessary changes in nursing curricula. Nursing education is challenged to coach and mentor students to make important connections between what they have learned and how they will practice nursing. Students do not learn from just textbooks and lectures but from their ability to discuss and apply their own experiences and ideas. Learning is contextual; therefore, teaching should focus on the best strategies to achieve learning outcomes. The NLN has focused current faculty development strategies on the belief that simulation as a teaching strategy moves students from knowing *what* to knowing *how* and knowing *why*, as well as determining what is meaningful and relevant within the context of practice. The use of simulation and theory-based **debriefing** strategies incorporates opportunities to use knowledge within context. Reflection and dialogue are important components engaging the student to observe, reflect, and dialogue with experts to identify variations in practice that lead to effective approaches in care. To that end, simulation provides a venue for nurse educators to assist students by modeling both professional nursing behaviors and the thinking underpinning the behavior. This section explores the role the NLN is currently playing to foster leadership and faculty practice in simulation excellence.

Fostering Leadership in Simulation Excellence

The NLN continues to build on these initiatives through innovative programming. The **Leadership Development** Program for Simulation Educators began in 2010 under the direction of Drs. Pamela Jeffries and Mary Anne Rizzolo. Each year, simulation educators apply for admission into this competitive program. Evidence of the need for such a program was clear when 142 applications were received in its inaugural year. More than 100 simulation leaders have participated in the program to enhance their leadership skills to advance simulation education initiatives both nationally and internationally. Participants from Australia, Singapore, South Africa, and Canada have provided valuable insights into how simulation is developing outside of the United States.

The accomplishments of our Sim Leaders have been phenomenal. They have conducted research, presented their work at national and international conferences, and published dozens of articles that have advanced the science of simulation. They have taken leadership positions in their own institutions, provided faculty development, and engaged in strategic planning for their simulation centers and for the integration of simulation throughout the nursing curriculum and more broadly for interprofessional education. The NLN has engaged many of them to author scenarios, present workshops and in other projects. Sim Leaders have also provided service and leadership to the Society for Simulation in Healthcare (SSH) and INACSL. Some of our participants have initiated regional and statewide consortium groups. Many have received awards for their work and have obtained funding for simulation projects. One developed a new start-up company with products that provide increased authenticity in simulation experiences and another was appointed to lead a 5-year, multimillion dollar initiative to provide faculty development in simulation in her state. We continue to be delighted whenever our Sim Leaders tell us about their rewarding experiences, large and small.

The Simulation Leader program is part of the Leadership Institute within the NLN Center for Transformational Leadership. Simulation educators admitted to the program participate in year-long leadership mentoring that includes executive coaching, team building, and scholarship initiatives that build on the growing body of evidence in nursing education focused on simulation.

Advancing Care Excellence for Seniors

In 2007 the NLN, in collaboration with the Community College of Philadelphia and funded by the Independence Foundation, the John A. Hartford Foundation, Laerdal Medical, and, since 2012, the Hearst Foundations, began developing the Advancing Care Excellence for Seniors (ACE.S) project and the ACE.S framework to improve the care of older adults (Tagliareni, Cline, Mengel, McLaughlin, & King, 2012). ACE.S was the first national effort to prepare students in all prelicensure nursing programs to deliver high-quality care to older adults in a variety of settings by providing unfolding cases utilizing simulation scenarios embedded within each case, teaching tools, and other resources to help prelicensure nursing faculty offer geriatric content to their students.

A key component of ACE.S is that nursing students understand how older adults and their families interact with multiple health professionals along a continuum of care and how they make decisions about care before, during, and following life transitions. Coordinating care during significant life transitions is fundamental to ensuring competent, individualized, and humanistic care for older adults and their caregivers. Recognizing that adding new content to an already full and intense prelicensure nursing curriculum is challenging, ACE.S was designed to work without adding additional content. Instead, ACE.S provides modifiable, unfolding cases and simulation scenarios along with classroom-ready teaching tools, strategies, and opportunities for interactive learning, in the classroom, skills laboratory, simulation lab, and through direct patient care experiences in a wide variety of environments, including hospitals, rehabilitation centers, long-term care facilities, and community settings. The resources are free and available on the NLN website (nln.org).

In 2009, at the start of the ACE.S grant, four nursing faculty were chosen through a selective process to create and develop the original four unfolding cases for ACE.S, under the direction of Dr. Mary Anne Rizzolo and Dr. Pamela Jeffries. The unfolding cases were developed to fully incorporate the emerging ACE.S Framework (http://www.nln.org/professional-development-programs/teaching-resources/aging) and to represent a diverse population of seniors. The resulting cases were piloted and distributed on the website for all faculty to download and use in the classroom, in the simulation lab, and for clinical education. Since that time, the ACE.S cases: Sherman "Red" Yoder, Millie Larson, Henry and Ertha Williams and Julie Morales and Lucy Grey, have become known to prelicensure students in over 800 nursing programs nationally. As they begin, the journey to understand about and advocate for older adults, these cases lay a foundation for individualizing person-centered care for seniors and their caregivers. In 2013, the ACE.S site was expanded to provide unfolding cases and related teaching strategies for veterans to meet their special physiological and mental health needs (ACE.V). In addition, with funding from the MetLife Foundation, three cases focused on patients with Alzheimer disease and their caregivers (ACE.Z) were added to the ACE.S library in 2014 and are available on the NLN website. Cases are written to be modified to address the needs of diverse curricula, different teaching methods, and individual style.

Each case includes the following:

- A first-person monologue that introduces the individual or couple and the complex problems to be addressed.
- Simulation scenarios with links to appropriate evidence-based assessment tools.
- A final assignment that asks students to finish the story.
- An instructor toolkit with suggestions on how to use the various components of the unfolding cases and incorporate them into the curriculum.

Data from NLN analytics indicate that the ACE.S unfolding cases are widely used to enhance gerontology content in a wide variety of schools of nursing; in 2015, for example, over 40,000 hits were recorded on the ACE.S website.

Scenario Development Across Platforms

Recognizing the need for well-designed and developed scenarios, the NLN began developing scenarios that were available for purchase on SimStore beginning in 2007. Simulations that address fundamentals, medical-surgical nursing, obstetric and pediatric nursing have relieved faculty of the time consuming burden of developing and pilot testing. In 2012, the NLN, in collaborative with Laerdal and Wolters Kluwer, recognized the need to advance simulation to screen-based scenarios. Using the NLN scenarios as a foundation, and then creating new scenarios in specific topic areas, the partnership resulted in the creation of a virtual simulation product, vSim for Nursing (NLN, 2015a). Currently, vSim scenarios are available for the following content areas: medical-surgical, pediatrics, obstetrics, gerontology, pharmacology, and fundamentals.

In 2014, the NLN conducted a pilot study of faculty use of the vSim scenarios within a wide variety of schools of nursing. The results are available in an implementation guide on the NLN website. Two key findings relate to the

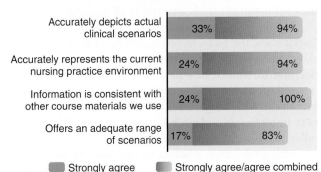

Content Quality:
Percent that strongly agree and agree with statements about vSim

Accurately depicts actual clinical scenarios — 33% | 94%

Accurately represents the current nursing practice environment — 24% | 94%

Information is consistent with other course materials we use — 24% | 100%

Offers an adequate range of scenarios — 17% | 83%

■ Strongly agree   ■ Strongly agree/agree combined

Figure 5.2 vSim for Nursing Content Quality: Participants in a Pilot Study Identified that vSim Content Accurately Depicted Actual Clinical Scenarios with a Good Range of Content. (From *vSim for Nursing Implementation Guide for Faculty.* Wolters Kluwer and National League for Nursing, 2014. Available online at: http://www.laerdal.com/us/vSimGuide.)

quality of vSim content (Fig. 5.2) and the achievement of student learning outcomes. Pilot faculty concluded that vSim content accurately depicted actual clinical scenarios with a good range of content and 67% of faculty identified vSim as a strategy to enhance prioritization and reasoning skills.

NLN Vision Statements to Guide Faculty Innovation

In 2015, the NLN published two vision statements: *Teaching with Simulation* (NLN, 2015b) and *Debriefing Across the Curriculum* (NLN, 2015c), which fully support the NCSBN landmark study exploring the role and outcomes of simulation in prelicensure clinical nursing education in the United States (Hayden, Smiley, Alexander, Kardong-Edgren & Jeffries, 2014). The NLN has consistently challenged nurse educators to learn about and implement teaching methodologies that prepare novice nurses to practice in a participatory and information-driven consumer environment. The **vision statements** were designed to uphold that commitment, to encourage new paradigm thinking about the role of the teacher: facilitator of knowledge cocreation.

A key message in the first vision statement, *Teaching with Simulation*, emphasized that context is an essential component of the transformational learning experience that occurs for all nursing students in simulation. Learning in simulation allows for situated cognition—or learning in context—a concept at the forefront of contemporary educational reform. As teachers and learners move away from content-laden curricula to curricula that emphasize experiential learning, it is critical that nurse educators have the requisite knowledge and skills to use simulation to its full potential. Experience followed by learner self-reflection provides diverse perspectives on caring for patients across the continuum of care and is core to all methods.

In the vision statement, *Debriefing Across the Curriculum*, the NLN, in collaboration with the INACSL, stated that integrating debriefing across the curriculum—not just in simulation—has the potential to transform nursing education. This approach to learning holds great promise in educating nurses to be the reflective practitioners necessary in today's healthcare system. Developing reflective practitioners requires a thoughtful approach to nursing education wherein faculty and learners question and reorder how they think, act, and understand. Reflection is at the core of debriefing and is therefore central to being critical, that is, the ability to examine information to see the whole of reality (Freire, 2000). It is a process of assessing what is relevant and determining the reasons for our actions. Debriefing provides educators with an evidence-based means to cocreate this paradigm.

Both vision statements included recommendations for faculty; selected recommendations include:

- Purposefully integrate simulation into the curriculum with clear connections toward achievement of student learning outcomes.

  - Incorporate simulation standards, including INACSL Standards of Best Practice (INACSL Standards Committee, 2016) in the design, implementation, and evaluation of simulation-based experiences.
- Engage in faculty development in simulation pedagogy and theory.
- Pursue continuing education to develop expertise in the use of debriefing techniques in the classroom, clinical postconference, and patient care settings.
- Use evidence-based resources consistently to ensure evaluation of and competence in debriefing.
- Seek simulation leadership development opportunities.

Building Innovative Workshops to Advance Simulation

The newest faculty development collaborative initiative between the NLN and Laerdal is Simulation Education Solutions for Nursing (SESN). The goal of this program, to help nursing programs better use simulation to prepare students for practice, is achieved through: a *comprehensive assessment* of current practice; *implementation* of recommendations custom-tailored to address the teaching, program infrastructure, curriculum, debriefing methods, and clinical environment; and regularly occurring *pulse checks* to keep the program on track. A set of faculty development workshops have been developed that will be available to schools who participate in the

complete SESN program: (1) Foundations in Simulation Pedagogy; (2) Curriculum Integration; (3) Debriefing of Simulation. Additionally, the NLN has embarked on an initiative to bring like workshops to select regions across the United States.

The NLN Center for Innovation in Simulation and Technology

In 2013, the NLN embarked on its historic move to Washington, DC. As part of the redesign during the transition, the NLN created centers of transformative teaching excellence. The NLN Center for Innovation in Simulation and Technology was developed to formalize the NLN's simulation work and to engage in resource development and collaborative partnerships to advance the faculty role with simulation and emerging technology. In 2015 Susan Forneris PhD, RN, CNE, CHSE-A was appointed to lead the center as its Deputy Director with funding from Excelsior College. Dr. Forneris is working to provide professional development resources for faculty to:

- Incorporate standards of practice in simulation pedagogy and theory-based debriefing.
- Integrate simulation into nursing curricula.
- Enhance faculty expertise in the use of theory based debriefing in simulation.
- Evaluate simulation experiences and debriefing using valid and reliable instruments.

The center continues to collaborate with key stakeholders (e.g., INACSL, SSH, NCSBN, Laerdal, Wolters Kluwer) to develop and disseminate best practices in the use of simulation in teaching and learning and integrating debriefing into learning activities throughout the curriculum. Working with other NLN centers, specifically the NLN Chamberlain College of Nursing Center for the Advancement of the Science of Nursing Education, Dr. Forneris is actively engaged in developing simulation research scholars, increasing support of multisite research studies in simulation pedagogy, and securing support grants and scholarships to fund nursing education research in the use of theory-based debriefing and student learning.

Additionally, the center works in collaboration with other centers at the NLN. The Leadership Development Program for Simulation Educators is housed in the NLN Leadership Institute, a cornerstone of the NLN Center for Transformational Leadership. In collaboration with the NLN Center for Diversity and Global Initiatives, Dr. Forneris serves as a resource for the global community; she has traveled extensively in China and Korea to bring simulation best practices to faculty actively engaged with simulation. Dr. Jeffries and Dr. Rizzolo also bring the NLN message and on-going work to South America, Europe, and the Far-East.

Summary

The NLN mission is clear, to promote excellence in nursing education to build a strong and diverse nursing workforce to advance the health of the nation and the global community. With its unique ability for broad outreach and dissemination to the entire nurse educator community, the NLN has been pleased to take a leadership role in promoting simulation as an innovative and effective pedagogy. We were pleased to participate on the expert panel convened by the National Council of State Boards of Nursing to develop national simulation guidelines for prelicensure programs (Alexander et al., 2015) and will continue collaborative partnerships through ongoing initiatives that foster leadership in simulation innovation and provide faculty development in quality simulation research and teaching practices. The NLN supports nurse educators and practicing nurses as they reframe the student–teacher relationship to cocreate meaningful learning experiences through simulation. Consistent with this commitment, the NLN fully acknowledges the vital role that nurse educators play in preparing our nation's diverse nursing workforce to enhance patient care outcomes.

6

The Evolution of Cutting Edge Technology: Today's Simulation Typologies

Kim Leighton

Key Terms

Anatomical Models, Avatars, Embedded Actors, Fidelity, Haptics, High-fidelity Simulator, High-fidelity Simulation, Holograms, Hybrid Simulation, Low-fidelity Simulators, Mannequin/Manikin, Mid-fidelity Simulators, Patient Volunteers, Plastinates, Procedural Simulation, Simulated Patient, Simulated Person, Simulator, Standardized Patient, Static Mannequin, Task Trainer, Typology, Virtual Patient, Virtual Reality, Wearable Technology

Guiding Questions

1   What is included when we talk about using "simulation" and how does the educator decide what type is the right one to use when designing a simulated learning experience?

2   What are the benefits and challenges associated with simulation typologies most commonly used today?

3   How does the way we define different types of simulation impact our ability to study and compare research outcomes?

Introduction

When many educators hear the term simulation, they immediately picture a **simulator**, such as a full-body life-size **mannequin**. However, there are several entities that fall under the **typology** of simulation. Merriam-Webster (2015) defines typology as classification based on types or categories. One might think that it would be very straightforward to categorize simulation; however, a review of Table 6.1 will give you a historical perspective of the ways in which simulation typologies have changed over time.

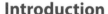

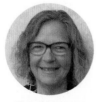

Kim Leighton, PhD, RN, CHSE, CHSOS, ANEF

Mueller (1997) categorized types of simulation by what the activity focused on—a patient or disease process, a procedure or piece of equipment, a healthcare provider, or an expert practitioner while further identifying whether the simulation was active, passive, or interactive. Seven years later, Beaubien and Baker (2004) defined three levels of simulation—a case study or role play exercise, partial task trainers (which included standardized patients [SPs]), and full mission simulations within the realm of team training. Alinier (2007) increased the number of levels by adding screen-based simulators as early versions of computer software became available. These were low on the list due to the lack of interactivity and realism at the time. He also further separated full-body simulators into intermediate and high **fidelity**, depending on the programmability of the computer and whether the physiology of the simulator was model driven and interactive. Decker, Sportsman, Puetz, and Billings (2008) included peer-to-peer learning, **virtual reality**, and **haptic** systems in their typology. Finally, Nehring (2010) also delineate seven typologies. Of most interest is the inclusion of **low-fidelity simulators** in the integrated simulator category; however, she then identifies

Table 6.1	Historical Typologies	
Author	**Typology**	**Example**
Mueller (1997); 4P's	P1: patient, disease process P2: procedure, test, equipment P3: physician or paraprofessional P4: professor or expert practitioner Active (a), passive (p), or interactive (i) element	P1 = **anatomical models** (resuscitation, wounds); a, p, i P2 = mannequin with computer program P3 = mannequin with software to simulate patient, equipment looks real but has no real function P4 = represents all elements of clinical interaction; theoretical, "dream machine"
Beaubien & Baker (2004); 3 Levels	Case study/role play (CS/RP) Part **task trainer** (PTT) Full mission simulation (FMS)	CS/RP: Paper and pencil, discussion PTT: standardized patients, simulated machines FMS: simulated mission, scripted, rotate through roles
Alinier (2007); 6 Levels	Level 0: written simulations Level 1: 3D models Level 2: screen-based simulators Level 3: standardized patients Level 4: intermediate fidelity patient simulators Level 5: interactive patient simulators or computer model–driven simulation	0 = pen and paper 1 = basic mannequin, model, part task trainer 2 = software, videos, DVD, virtual reality, surgical simulators 3 = trained actors, role play 4 = computer controlled, programmable, full body 5 = computer controlled, model driven, interactive
Decker et al. (2008); 7 Typologies	Partial task trainers (PTT) Peer-to-peer learning (PP) Screen-based computer simulation (SB) Virtual reality (VR) Haptic systems (HS) Standardized patients (SP) Full-scale simulation (FSS)	PTT: procedural models PP: peer collaboration SB: computer programs VR: computer with sensory stimuli via PTT HS: simulator with real-world plus virtual reality SP: individuals trained to portray patients using case studies, role play FSS: programmable computerized full-body simulator with realistic physiologic responses
Nehring (2010); 7 Components	Partial/complex task trainers (PTT) Role-play (RP) Games (G) Computer-assisted instruction (CAI) Standardized patients (SP) Virtual reality/haptic systems (VR/HS) Integrated simulators (low through high fidelity) (IS)	PTT: anatomic model RP: assigned roles, group G: more structured than role play CAI: interactive, multiuser, multiformat SP: person instructed in how to act VR/HS: computer based with tactile stimulation IS: part or full body

that these mannequins are really task trainers. It is easy to see how the advancement of computers and technology created frequent change to the terminology associated with simulation typology.

This frequently changing typology has created a problem. Huang, Rice, Spain, and Palaganas (2015) provide an excellent discussion of what has led to the lack of standardized definitions, the resulting challenges, and the plan toward standardization. Because of the lack of clear and consistent definitions, researchers and authors are left to provide their own definitions for each study or article written. This creates havoc for the person conducting a literature review in an attempt to further define their own research and is a barrier for those conducting systematic reviews of the literature. A variety of terms must be used in order to attempt to capture the available literature. As a result, this slows simulationists in their quest to express "projects, research, assessments, techniques, and data" (p. xxii). This further makes it difficult to compare outcomes and create guidelines for best practice. In the

end, this also impedes the industry's ability to be recognized as a specialty and to access funding.

Many authors have identified the need for consistency in definitions related to simulation (Alinier, 2007; Edler & Fanning, 2007; Huang et al., 2015; Issenberg, McGaghie, Petrusa, Lee Gordon, & Scalese, 2005; Sinz, 2007). As you can see by the dates of these citations, this is not a new problem. I recall attending a business meeting in 2006 at the first conference on simulation sponsored by the Society for Simulation in Healthcare (SSH): the International Meeting on Medical Simulation (IMMS). Almost the entire business meeting was spent deciding whether **mannequin or manikin** should be the preferred way of denoting that piece of equipment when writing about simulation. In 2006, a Simulation Summit was held in Chicago with representation of 33 organizations considered stakeholders of simulation. Efforts were made toward a common definition of simulation, and the need for common terminology was one of the themes identified as a "first-tier" priority (Sinz, 2007).

In 2011, the International Nursing Association for Clinical Simulation and Learning (INACSL) released the first *Standards of Best Practice: Simulation^{SM}*. Standard I: Terminology, updated in 2013, was designed to "promote consistency and understanding in education, practice, research, and publication" (INACSL, 2013a, p. S4). However, the terms included are only those used in the Standards document and are not all-inclusive. These definitions provide a foundation for nursing educators and researchers to use in their written and oral communications about simulation. To further the work of definitions, in 2012, the SSH formed the Simulation Terminology and Concepts committee. This committee released the *Healthcare Simulation Dictionary*, a compilation of definitions of 127 terms, in June, 2016. The *Dictionary* is designed to promote communication and clarity in simulation discussions (SSH, 2016e). The Terminology Standard, now a Glossary, located in Clinical Simulation in Nursing at http://www.nursingsimulation.org/issue/S1876-1399(16)X0014-X. The SSH Dictionary is located at http://www.ssih.org/Dictionary.

One of the biggest challenges with defining the typology of simulation is the common attempt to classify according to fidelity or realism. Fidelity is the "degree to which a simulated experience approaches reality" (INACSL Standards Committee, 2016, p. S42). It is often thought that the higher the fidelity, the better the learning experience, or that simulators with the most advanced capabilities are of higher fidelity than other simulation methods. However, many now understand that it is not so much the simulator, but what you do with it that creates the fidelity of the experience. Static mannequins and anatomical models can be used in such a way as to create high-fidelity experiences with the right amount of creativity. Conversely, highly complex mannequins have also been used in ways that are very low fidelity. In fact, Hamstra, Brydges, Hatala, Zendejas, and Cook (2014) suggest that the term fidelity no longer be used when discussion simulators as several studies have shown that fidelity does not correlate with educational effectiveness.

The remainder of this chapter will focus on several simulation typologies, or the means by which we enact a given simulation modality (the educational platform used to deliver a simulation event). Simulation modalities are covered in depth in Chapter 7 and include simulated clinical immersion, computer-based simulation, **procedural simulation**, and augmented 3D virtual reality, to list a few. With the exception of the mannequin discussion, the concept of fidelity will be avoided. It is not possible to fully classify simulation according to fidelity. Recall those who listed SPs low on their typologies of simulation fidelity? Many now state that they are the highest fidelity simulation of all. But, what if the SP doesn't portray their illness or disease process accurately? Is it still a high-fidelity experience? The issue of fidelity and its significance when creating high-fidelity experiences will be further explored in Chapters 19 and 20.

This chapter will explore various typologies, which are grouped into three categories: living people (SPs, simulated patients, simulated persons, patient volunteers [PVs], and embedded SPs/actors), nonliving simulated tools (mannequins/simulators, task trainers, simulated cadavers, human and animal tissue, and **plastinates**), and virtual tools (**holograms, wearable technology, avatars**, and virtual patients). Simulationists will share their experiences with enhancing available typology by improving fidelity with equipment, real human bodies, and use of volunteers. These overviews will help the reader to develop foundational knowledge of various typologies that they might want to incorporate into their programs.

Living People

Standardized Patients

Petra Duncan

Pamela Rock, BSc, PT

From the time of inception in the 1960s by Dr. Harold Barrows and with the addition of Dr. Paula Stillman's work in the 1970s (Rideout, 2001), the use of SPs in medical and other health professional education programs has undergone phenomenal growth. Standardized patients, defined as a person who has been "carefully coached to simulate an actual patient so accurately that the simulation cannot be detected by a skilled clinician" (Barrows, 1987, p. 17), are common in healthcare education today. INACSL Standards of Best Practice Simulation: Simulation Glossary defines the **standardized patient** as "a person trained to consistently portray a patient or other individual in a scripted scenario for the purposes of instruction, practice, or evaluation" (INACSL Standards Committee, 2016, p. S44). "In performing a simulation, the SP represents the gestalt of the patient being simulated; not just the history, but the body language, the physical findings and the emotional and personality characteristics as well" (Barrows, 1987, p. 17).

According to the Association of Standardized Patient Educators (ASPE, 2015), SPs are trained to:

- Portray specific patient conditions
- Repeat portrayal in a realistic and standardized way
- Interact with more learners than a real patient would

- Focus on the learner
- Further the education of healthcare students and professionals
- Give feedback and evaluate learner performance

Advantages of Using Standardized Patients

SPs provide learners with a safe and controlled method in which to practice and learn psychomotor skills as well as higher-order thinking skills, such as clinical judgement, critical thinking, decision making, problem solving, prioritization, and communication (Kameg, Szpak, Cline, & Mcdermott, 2014). SPs and other simulation modalities have been shown to reduce learner anxiety, particularly when learning how to care for those with mental illness (Lehr & Kaplan, 2013). Using mannequin-based simulation for mental health has not been successful due to their inability to provide nonverbal cues to learners (Doolen, Giddings, Johnson, de Nathan, & Badia, 2014). When using SPs, no real person risks injury, is hurt by unintentional words, or dies, and there are no upset or angry patients and family members, unless scripted for learning purposes. SPs provide verbal or written feedback from the patient perspective, also allowing opportunities for learners to repeat scenarios for mastery. Debriefing sessions that include the SP allow the learner to self-reflect on their learning while receiving constructive support to create new learning to later transfer to practice.

Integrating Use of Standardized Patients

SPs have been used for decades in medical schools; however, nursing educators only recently began more widespread adoption of this teaching modality. The challenge of providing realistic, meaningful clinical experiences is one factor that has led to increased use (Anderson, Holmes, LeFlore, Nelson, & Jenkins, 2010). Most commonly, SPs are trained to represent a patient; however, they can also be trained to take the role of a healthcare professional, a family member, or can interface with another simulation modality, such as a task trainer or mannequin (**hybrid simulation**). A well-trained and experienced SP is able to depict a wide array of scenarios and situations.

Planning and design of a SP program is covered elsewhere in this text (Chapter 12); however, many authors have published examples of how SPs can be integrated into various courses throughout the nursing program. Anderson et al. (2010) outline how SPs are used in the four levels of an undergraduate baccalaureate program, as well as in graduate level courses. SPs take on the role of various patients, parents, and grandparents. Multiple encounters with SPs are offered in every clinical course throughout the program, and the authors provide the expected outcomes and scenario details. Examples are also provided for advanced physical assessment and for psychiatric, family, and pediatric nurse practitioner students. SPs have also been used to teach specific areas of content such as leadership skills (Sharpnack,

Goliat, & Rogers, 2011), autism (McIntosh, Thomas, Allen, & Edwards, 2015), end-of-life care (Fink, Linnard-Palmer, Ganley, Catolico, & Phillips, 2014), and fall safety (Beischel, Hart, Turkelson, & Churchill, 2013) among others.

SPs are used in high stakes licensing examinations for nurse practitioners to evaluate history taking, interview, and physical assessment skills. These types of examinations are known as objective structured clinical examinations (OSCE). This type of examination is also used at the undergraduate level, both for summative and formative evaluation. A 2014 survey prior to the INACSL conference revealed that 28% of responding schools were using OSCEs for high-stakes assessment. During a town hall meeting, at that conference, discussion indicated that quality control of the practices used to develop these OSCEs was lacking (Rizzolo, Kardong-Edgren, Oermann, & Jeffries, 2015).

Challenges for Use of Standardized Patients

Locating appropriate persons to train as SPs can be a challenge, particularly when a SP program does not exist or when the program is located in a rural area. Husson and Zulkosky (2014) share how they identified potential SPs by contacting the alumni association, all graduates of the college, and then all of the college's employees. Other programs arrange for payment of their SPs, a decision that has budgetary implications. A process also needs to be identified that includes agreement or contract forms, liability waivers, information about the volunteers, method for training, and internal communication for the courses using SPs (Husson & Zulkosky, 2014). Time for creation of validated scenarios and training of the SPs must be taken into consideration when developing a SP program as this hidden time factor can be extensive and impact the workload of involved faculty. These costs may be mitigated somewhat by using resources associated with a consortium; however, this too comes at a price (Jeffries et al., 2013; Schram & Mudd, 2015). These and other considerations, such as space and supply management, are found in Chapter 12.

Simulated Patients and Simulated Persons

Kim Leighton, PhD, RN, CHSE, CHSOS, ANEF

In the past several years, SP terminology has received greater scrutiny in comparison with the term **simulated patient**. While many use the terms interchangeably, others define them differently creating challenges for researchers and simulation facilitators. Churchouse and McCafferty (2012) outline the evolution of definitions for standardized and simulated patients and compare them for differences.

The key differences are that the SP is not an actor and presents his or her own healthcare history to each simulation in the same way, while the simulated patient is acting in a role and portrays the history and information that they are directed to. Churchouse et al. state that these distinctions drive preparation for these roles.

Reviewing literature related to simulated patients uncovers a review of pediatric simulated patients (Gamble, Bearman, & Nestel, 2016) defined as well people trained to portray patients in a realistic way. Nuzat, Salem, Al Shehri, and Al Hamdan (2014) also define simulated patients as those who are coached to portray specific signs and symptoms. Other authors cross-reference simulated patients as "also known as" patient actors or SPs (Weller, Nestel, Marshall, Brooks, & Conn, 2012). The INACSL Standards Glossary lists "Standardized Patient (also known as Simulated Patient)" (INACSL Standards Committee, 2016) while Palaganas, Maxworthy, Epps, and Mancini (2015) list "Simulated Patient (also known as Embedded **Simulated Person**)". The Healthcare Simulation Dictionary (Lopreiato et al., 2016) defines the simulated patient similarly to Churchouse and McCafferty (2012), however, add an additional definition for the simulated person. This person can be a simulated patient, family member, or healthcare provider within the simulation—and may also be known as the SP, family, or healthcare provider.

Based on the origin of the literature, it appears that the term SP is most commonly used in North America, while the term simulated patient has gained footing in Australia, the Middle East, and beyond. Benefits and challenges to using simulated patients and simulated persons are the same as those faced by SPs—recruitment, training, and performance. It is reasonable to believe that training outcomes for SP programs can guide development of simulated patient training programs. It would be wise for the simulationists to consider the literature for SPs, simulated patients, and simulated persons when planning to use these roles in the simulation-based learning experience.

Embedded Standardized Participants as Learner Engagers, Often Overlooked, but Vitally Important Champions of Simulation

Jill S. Sanko, PhD, MS, ARNP, CHSE-A

Alexis Battista, PhD

When planning, evaluating, and running simulation encounters, embedded standardized participants (ESPs) (sometimes called confederates, actors, **embedded actors**, embedded simulated person, scenario guide) are often overlooked (Sanko, Shekhter, Kyle, & Birnbach, 2015). However, ESPs' impact on learner engagement needs to be fully understood and considered. This section will discuss the role of the ESP, summarize their role as learner engagers and scenario enhancers, and discuss training and preparation needs.

The SP, a "cousin" of ESPs, has a longer history in healthcare education, and therefore is better understood in terms of what they offer to simulation-based educational encounters. SPs have been in use in healthcare education for over five decades (Barrows & Abrahamason, 1964) and are most often associated with summative assessments of medical students. However, their use across healthcare education has broadened (Owens & Gliva-McCovey, 2015) as simulation-based education has grown. Trained SPs realistically depict patients, replete with the ability to record data on learners' performances. SPs must portray a high level of realism, standardization, and reliability, in addition to being able to provide feedback and evaluation of learners. As such, their training is often in depth, and their roles tightly and carefully scripted to ensure they accurately present the "gestalt" of a patient and their illness.

By comparison, ESPs are less described; thus, they are less carefully considered, trained, or standardized. This creates opportunities for their role to have negative implications on learning and engagement. ESPs are most often found playing the role of a health or social care professional or the relative of the patient (Nestel, Mobley, Hunt, & Eppich, 2014). During scenario-based simulations, students often engage ESPs in diverse social interactions, including diagnostic questioning, education and counseling, or providing social and emotional support (Battista & Sheridan, 2014). Thus, ESPs' interactions with the learners, SPs, mannequins, and other ESPs during scenario-based simulations become important drivers of the scenario itself.

Nestel et al. (2014) consider ESPs as educators who are "hidden in plain sight," because they are immersed in the scenario as an agent of education. For example, participants who struggle with the use of equipment during a scenario (e.g., IV pump) may become discouraged, give up quickly, or be easily distracted (Battista & Sheridan, 2014). ESPs who are charged with the responsibility of judging when to provide guidance during simulations can help students persist to overcome deficits in their knowledge, while continuing to support the narrative of the scenario (Battista & Antonis, 2015). A well-trained ESP has the ability to draw learners into a scenario, deepening their engagement, and improving the educational impact (Nestel & Bearman, 2014a). Conversely, ESPs who fail to enact their role in a way that supports the goals of the scenario run the risk of misleading students, potentially altering the sequence of their participation, or making it difficult for them to suspend disbelief (Sanko et al., 2015).

ESPs must be properly trained to deliver high-quality, valid, and consistent education as part of the larger team of educators providing simulation-based education (Nestel et al., 2014; Sanko, Shekhter, Kyle, Di Benedetto & Birnbach, 2013). Their roles must be carefully outlined, complete with specific and guided scripting for verbal interactions, and timing of prompting if this is part of their role. Their "costume" (dress) must be consistent with the role that they are playing. Casting decisions should take into account if those being considered for a role will be able to realistically portray their role, while also being comfortable with improvising, should learners take the scenario in an unexpected direction. They must be able to elicit a range of appropriate emotions that correspond to the action taking place in the scenario. ESPs must have a high level of knowledge around who the learners are, what the objectives of the scenario/encounter are, and how much assistance they should give to the learners (Sanko et al., 2015). Finally, they must also be evaluated routinely and given feedback so that they can sharpen their skills and hone their craft.

Simulation-based learning environments are complex and dynamic, where the elements used to create complexity (e.g., ESPs, SPs) increase the possibility that students may be negatively influenced. For some students, this can result in their failing to fully engage the scenario, which can have an impact on what is learned. Therefore, all educators, especially ESPs, must be prepared to engage learners through sound practices. These practices should include those mentioned earlier (being well prepared, dressed appropriately, and tightly scripted), as well as being trained to quickly notice disengaged learners so that corrective actions can be taken to re-engage them. Special consideration should also be given if ESPs will be expected to observe and assess learners' engagement and performance. Taking note of times where learners were solidly engaged as well as where engagement was lost in association with the timing of interactions or actions of the ESP can serve as a way for EPS to learn how to mimic or correct actions to maintain engagement throughout a scenario. A review of recorded videos looking at interactions can be used to train ESPs what to look for. Common ESP caused situations that lead to loss of engagement include talking to the "voice in the sky," failing to play the role/character realistically, depicting emotions that are inconsistent with the gravity of the situation being played out, and not staying in role/character.

The next section will discuss a novel undergraduate nursing program that trains students from various departments to perform as PVs. Learn how this differs from the traditional SP role and how such a program may be feasible in your school.

Students as Trained Patient Volunteers for Healthcare Simulation

Natalie Lu Sweeney, MS, CNS, RNC-NIC

Simulation programs of all types and maturity strive to maximize resources and minimize cost to sustain a robust offering of simulation experiences. Hundreds of students cycle through pediatric simulation experiences each year in our undergraduate nursing program. Over a period of 3 years, a training program was developed for PVs for our nursing simulation program. A proposal was developed to streamline and integrate the existing Standardized Patient/**Patient Volunteer** (SP/PV) educational training program in our undergraduate nursing simulation program.

There are two main goals:

1. Maximize successful attainment of student learning objectives by using students to play quality, controlled roles as PVs in scenarios for formative simulations. Use of peer-to-peer teaching/learning pedagogy greatly enhanced student reports of satisfaction and offers a potential resume building item.
2. Minimize lost productive learning time and operational costs (e.g., faculty, manager time, lab resources, technical support) due to inadvertent, unplanned, or inappropriate actions by untrained, ad hoc student or faculty playing roles resulting in salvaging sessions and/or aborted simulations.

Historically, a 5-hour in-person PV training was developed and offered once or twice a semester to our nursing students. To date, we have used several trained PV alumna, as well as current students, in about 100 scenarios over the last 5 years. Our current streamlined approach involves 4 hours of hybrid training including completion of 2 hours of online learning modules focusing on foundational simulation concepts, case development, providing verbal and written feedback, and learning a variety of SP/PV cases. The modules were coupled with a 2-hour workshop culminating with face-to-face implementation and evaluation of skills acquired. The training uses components of the longer best practice-based training workshop developed by nursing faculty with expertise in simulation and a professional SP/PV trainer.

The participants in the PV training are drawn from the Dominican student body, particularly Health and Natural Sciences and Fine Arts/Drama students. Participants may or may not concurrently be student workers in the nursing labs. Up to 10 trainees participate per session. Following completion of the training, students play at least two PV trainer-facilitated roles in scheduled scenarios. More sessions may be required if determined by PV faculty. A certificate is issued after the completion of the facilitated roles that can be included on a resume, and the PV is then added to the SP/PV pool. The potential to hire trained experienced PVs occurs at the discretion of the Simulation Manager/Director.

Once PVs are trained, pediatric and other simulation faculty recruit and coordinate scheduling with the Simulation Program Manager/Director. Assessment labs, simulation labs, and a debriefing room are available after approved by simulation leadership. Our program uses the Sweeney-Clark Simulation Performance Rubric© to evaluate PV-integrated scenarios. This provides data to reveal learner strengths and to support revisions of unique educational offerings to address patterns of weakness in skills or knowledge gaps.

Program Planning:

- Annual training program revision to create or refresh online activities and documents from existing workshop agenda items.
- Extend invitation to nursing student groups on campus to participate in training as well as Drama Club and other targeted groups.

- With approval of Simulation Program lead, reserve minimum of 3 hours of funding per semester for the SP trainer to assist with the face-to-face PV training.
- The goal is to offer the PV training once a semester with Simulation Program Manager/Director consultation and approval.
- Some cost reduction may be possible, but the goal is to break even while increasing availability of pediatric PVs.

There are many considerations related to return on investment when implementing a training program involving students. Although they are trained for a volunteer position, there are other costs to consider. There are many pros as well, some not attached to tangible dollars, but important nonetheless (Table 6.2). Some general expectations can be drawn from our cost analysis, but each program will have a unique break-even, revenue loss or gain.

Multiple points of feedback will be gathered on initial and ongoing program operations as well as PV performance:

- Online evaluation of learning via posttest and in-person assessment during the workshop
- Satisfaction surveys by participants after workshop (one for each phase: online, in-person, and first two facilitated role plays)
- Satisfaction survey after participating as a PV
- Feedback from Simulation Manager/Director re: operations successes/failures

Table 6.2	Pros and Cons of Training Program Implementation
Pros	**Cons**
Builds ongoing pool of trained amateur actors to play roles of children, specifically pediatric adolescent roles	Time needed and scheduling dates that trainees will actually attend
Cost savings of $20/h ($80/session) when using VP instead of SP	Fiscal ROI is not appreciated until first two scenario roles played.
Opportunity exists for OT/Psych and other interdepartmental scenario participation	Limited to students 18 years and older in young adolescent roles as using or employing minors in simulation is often a prohibitively difficult legal process
Offers resume building	Time/labor constraints with other operational activities
Pathway to keep in contact with DUC nursing alumna	Locating, vetting, and paying for an experienced, effective SP/PV trainer
Good marketing press for use in the community and alumna returning to use new state-of-the-art simulation facility	Initial investment in time and resources; funding may not be in budget or supported with other fundraising efforts.
Enhances attraction to attend DUC by prospective students	
Ongoing cost reduction potential if PV volunteers as alumna after graduation	
Interest by others in healthcare simulation and education community about the program	

Nonliving Simulated Tools

Mannequin-Based Simulation

Kim Leighton, PhD, RN, CHSE, CHSOS, ANEF

Simulators, a term often used interchangeably with mannequins (manikins), come in adult, pediatric, infant, and neonatal sizes, as well as with the ability to birth babies. The term simulator is typically reserved for a mannequin that is computer controlled, while mannequin is used more commonly for models that are not. These non–computer-controlled mannequins are referred to as static mannequins because they do not respond to the learner's verbal or physical interaction. Mannequin-based simulation has been described as low-, medium-, and high fidelity; however, as with simulation terminology in general, there is no set agreement on where each simulator or mannequin falls into the fidelity scale. Early definitions of simulator fidelity corresponded to the cost of the simulator. As the cost increased, so did the assumption of fidelity. Manufacturers of simulators also entered the discussion, with each new model purporting to be of higher fidelity than the competitor's model.

The INACSL Standards of Best Practice: Simulation Glossary (INACSL Standards Committee, 2016) define the levels of mannequin fidelity as:

- Low: static mannequins
- Moderate or midlevel: more technologically sophisticated, more realistic than a **static mannequin** (e.g., with breath sounds, pulses, or other features) (Fig. 6.1)
- High: computerized patient simulators, high interactivity and realism

These definitions are fairly subjective, leaving the reader to wonder where their particular model might fall on the continuum. Nehring (2010) provide further criteria:

- Low: "usually provide for simple, gross movements without joint movement and are best used for the instruction of psychomotor skills" (p. 15)
- Moderate: "allow the student to listen for breath and heart sounds and to feel for some pulses, but lack the ability to show chest movements when breathing or eyes that blink or pupils that dilate" (p. 15)
- High: "computerized full-body mannequin that is able to provide real-time physiological and pharmacological parameters of persons of both genders, varying ages, and with different health conditions" (Nehring, Ellis, & Lashley, 2001, p. 195) (Fig. 6.2).

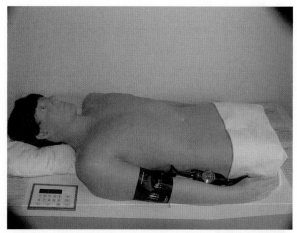

Figure 6.1 Mid-fidelity Simulator With Heart and Lung Sounds. (From Gregory D., Raymond-Seniuk C., Patrick L., Stephen T. C. (Eds.) (2014). *Fundamentals: Perspectives on the Art and Science of Canadian Nursing.* Wolters Kluwer Health.)

The most important consideration when determining the fidelity of the simulator needed is the learning objectives of the planned activity. It is the educator's responsibility to use resources that are appropriate, yet cost-effective. To use an expensive **high-fidelity simulator** to teach wound care is inappropriate when a lower-fidelity, less expensive model is available. Conversely, it is more difficult to teach a student to respond to the gas exchange complications that occur during general anesthesia by using a low-fidelity mannequin. Read the Voice of Experience feature to learn how simulationists created their own mannequin features to meet the multidisciplinary needs of their team.

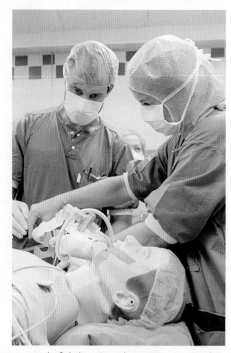

Figure 6.2 High-fidelity Simulator Mimics Real Patient Findings. (Photo courtesy of Laerdal Medical. All rights reserved.)

6-1 Voice of Experience
Cardiac Charlie

Andrew Reid, MEdHSE, BScN, RN

Ken Brisbin, EMT, CD

The Cardiac Charlie project grew from the need to give cardiac surgery residents and ICU staff the opportunity to integrate open-chest CPR and internal defibrillation into simulations of post-op cardiac arrest. The Provincial Simulation Program of Alberta Health Services worked with educators from the Mazankowski Alberta Heart Institute and the University of Alberta Faculty of Medicine to create the curriculum and a mannequin system to support learning of the surgical tasks (Fig. 6.3).

We laid out a scenario plan involving nurses, physicians, respiratory therapists, and perfusionists—every clinical profession in the chain from the bedside to the bypass pump. To create a simulated reality to engage participants from so many

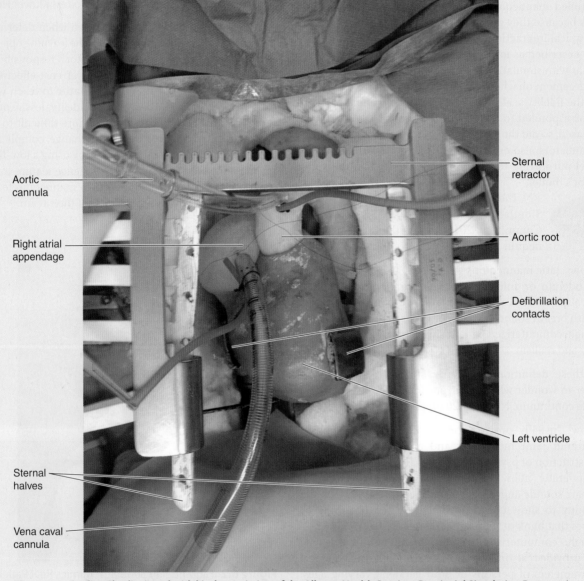

Figure 6.3 Cardiac Charlie. (Used with kind permission of the Alberta Health Services Provincial Simulation Program.)

professions, we realized that we'd need confederates from every profession as well. With input from educators in every participant discipline, we settled on the mannequin system's requirements:

- The chest will accept full force CPR.
- The sternal halves will be wired together using standard sternal wire with the usual surgical technique. The wires will be cut and the sternum retracted using unmodified instruments and standard procedures.
- The heart model will be compressible, using the correct technique of internal cardiac massage.
- Electrical contacts on the heart will allow full-energy defibrillation using unmodified internal paddles.
- The surgeon will cannulate the aorta and right atrium models using unmodified cannulas and standard technique. Once connected to the perfusion circuit, the model will accept perfusion flow up to 5 L/min.

We were fortunate that we were about to replace one of our older mannequins, a METI HPS (CAE, Montreal, QC) from which we removed all the thoracic contents below the trachea. We built the rib cage and sternum of steel and then cut the sternum along the midline to simulate the fresh post-op state. Holes drilled in each sternal half accommodated the sternal wires; we bolted the whole assembly into the mannequin's chest.

The aorta and vena cava models posed a real challenge. Surgeons from our educator group found DragonSkin20 silicone rubber (Smooth-On Plastics, Macungie, PA) to offer the best combination of tactile feedback, watertight sealing, and stitch-holding strength. We built casting molds for the great vessel models by hand using Sculpey polymer clay (KJP Crafts, Nepean, ON) and orthopedic plaster. Once poured and cured, we secured the vessels to half-inch vinyl tubing using barbed connectors. While each use of the mannequin requires casting a fresh pair of great vessels, and a fresh chest skin, the heart with its electrical contacts and the rib cage are completely reusable.

Given the loss of mannequin function entailed by removal of chest components, we always insert several discipline-specific confederates within scenarios with Charlie as the patient; generally, we invite educators from the disciplines involved to play the confederate roles.

We approach every exercise with Cardiac Charlie as an opportunity to improve him and to expand the range of curricular options he can support for our educator clients.

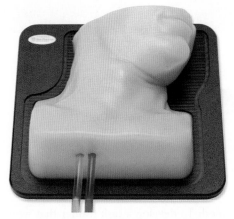

Figure 6.4 Simple Procedural Simulator. (©2017 Image Courtesy of CAE Healthcare.)

Partial Task Trainers

Perhaps the types of simulation most familiar to nursing educators are task trainers and partial task trainers, also known as procedural simulators (Fig. 6.4) and anatomical models of individual body parts. Most skills/simulation laboratories use a variety of these simulators to teach students how to perform skills. These skills include giving injections, inserting urinary catheters, and inserting intravenous catheters, among many others. The simulators or task trainers used to teach these skills range from simple to complex and may or may not represent the actual part of the body where the skill takes place. For example, many faculty have used hotdogs to train students in the skill of administering intradermal medications. Other, more sophisticated, models have higher fidelity and respond to interventions via haptic devices that document the location of touch or degree of pressure (Fig. 6.5). An example

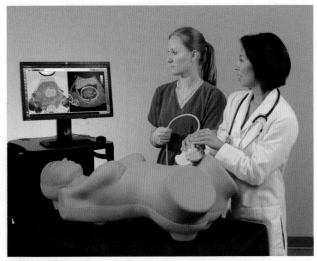

Figure 6.5 Sophisticated Procedural Simulator. (©2017 Image Courtesy of CAE Healthcare.)

Female Urinary Catheterization Task Trainer

**Colette Foisy-Doll,
MSN, RN, CHSE**

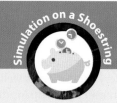

1. **The Need:** To develop a task trainer that would allow students to practice urinary catheterization off campus, that was portable, lightweight, and effective.
2. **The Shoestring Innovation:** a portable, low-cost simulator was designed to allow independent skill practice for nursing students outside of the skills labs.
3. **Supplies Required:**
   a. One disposable absorbent pad, approximately 1 ft × 1 ft (blue pad)
   b. One recycled catheterization plastic tray or other container such as styrofoam bowl
   c. One large elastic band
   d. One anatomical image of female perineum (paper)
   e. Lamination device or transparent MACtac vinyl sticky paper
   f. Scissors or pen
   g. One stapler
4. **Step-by-step instructions and use of solution (Fig. 6.6):**
   a. Lay the absorbent pad flat, noting center.
   b. Place image of perineum in the center of the blue pad and laminate both top and bottom. This allows students to use cleaning solution and affixes the image well.
   c. Approximately 2 inches from center, fold a segment toward the middle to form the labia. Tack the fold with a piece of tape to hold. Repeat on other side,

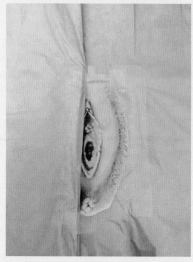

Figure 6.6 Urethral Catheterization Task Trainer.

and then tack the folds in place just above and below the image with several staples.

   d. Poke a hole through the urinary meatal opening and the container with a pen or scissors, ensuring the opening is large enough to allow the catheter to pass through.
   e. Take the folded absorbent pad and affix over the bottom of the container with an elastic band to secure (must not be too loose or too tight).
   f. The task trainer is ready to use by positioning it on a pillow to give it the correct insertion angle. It has also proven useful for students to apply the task trainer to each other for realism in positioning and to develop empathy or an understanding of client vulnerability in this position. To preserve the integrity of the learner, it is suggested that a folded towel cover the subject's perineum before laying the simulator in place (Fig. 6.7A–C).

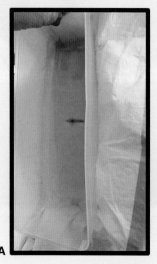 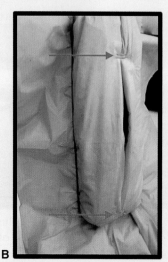 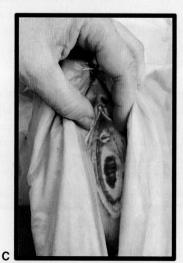

A   B   C

Figure 6.7 A–C. Development of a urethral catheterization task trainer.

is a pelvic examination simulator that documents where the student touches on the internal exam as well as the amount of pressure applied—all of which cannot be determined by a facilitator who is observing the learner.

Examples of procedural simulation activities are found extensively in the literature. Ramponi and Ross (2015) taught several skills to doctoral students prior to an international clinic experience. Some skills were taught using commercial task trainers, while abscess incision and drainage was creatively designed by injecting yogurt under chicken leg skin. While animal skin and hotdogs have been used to teach suture skills, the authors opted for an inexpensive wound closure pad that provided a more realistic feel and allowed students to take the materials home for further practice. Operating room skills, more commonly learned by physicians, are practiced on partial task trainers that exist in the physical and virtual world. For example, laparoscopic surgery skills are learned by holding surgical tools in one's hands while watching how they are manipulated in the virtual world via a computer screen.

Obtaining the necessary simulators, mannequins, and task trainers for your lab can become costly. Read how one simulationist created a female urinary catheterization task trainer in the Simulation on a Shoestring feature.

Tissue, Cadavers, and Plastinates

Many of us do not fondly remember our time in school spent dissecting various types of small animals, reptiles, or body parts. Visiting the cadaver lab to observe bodies in various stages of dissection gave us an idea of what the inside of the human body looked like, in the hope that it would help us to better understand anatomy and physiology of the living person. Science educators continue to use these methods, but additional options are now available, particularly as animal scientists work to decrease experimentation on live animals. Many of these products have a higher price point than their predecessors; however, they can be reused by numerous students and reportedly have long life.

Cadaveric and animal tissue simulation is most commonly used in medical education and surgical training for procedures such as vein cannulation and laparoscopic techniques (Sirimanna & Aggarwal, 2013) and falls outside the scope of this text. Substitutions for these methods have become available recently. One product creates synthetic tissue that simulates arterial and venous vasculature, nervous system, muscles, bones, organs, and skin. The model can pump blood and has ventilator capabilities (SynDaver™ Labs, 2016), creating live tissue replacement (Fig. 6.8). By the time this book is published, there may be similar products on the market.

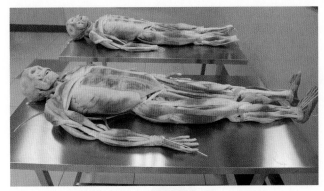

Figure 6.8 Synthetic Human Body. (Courtesy of SynDaver™ Labs.)

Plastinates are another alternative found in approximately 400 medical and nursing schools around the world (Von Hagens Plastination, 2016). Deceased human bodies are dissected in a variety of ways such as removal of all tissue other than the circulatory system, longitudinally in half, or in a specific pose such as shooting a basketball with the muscles, tendons, and ligaments exposed (Fig. 6.9). The dissected bodies undergo a lengthy process called plastination that preserves the body in its current position and hardens it so that it can be touched or observed in its motion. Individual organs, bones, and tissues can also undergo plastination so that numerous students can handle the material

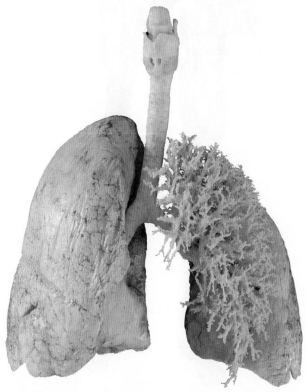

Figure 6.9 Plastinated Respiratory System. (Courtesy of Gobener Plastinate GmbH/con Hagens Plastination–Real Anatomy for Teaching.)

without it deteriorating (The Human Body Exhibit, 2016) (Fig. 6.10). Graham Whiteside shares his knowledge of the types of plastinates and how they are used for healthcare education in the following Voice of Experience.

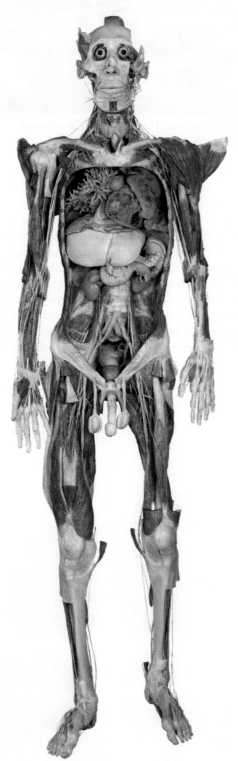

Figure 6.10 Whole Body Plastinate. (Courtesy of Gobener Plastinate GmbH/con Hagens Plastination–Real Anatomy for Teaching.)

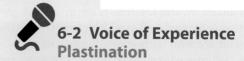

6-2 Voice of Experience
Plastination

Graham Andrew Whiteside, BSc(Hons) Nur Sci, DipHE MHN, RMN, RGN

My first exposure to plastination was in 2002, when Prof. Gunther von Hagens demonstrated his dissection skills and plastination techniques during a live television broadcast in the UK. The program, just like his successful Body World's and Animals Inside Out Exhibitions, was primarily aimed at health education.

Plastination commonly produces two types of specimens. Individual specimens are used to compare healthy and diseased organs, that is, a healthy lung with that of a smoker, to emphasize the importance of a healthy lifestyle. Whole-body plastinates can be posed to illustrate the position of our organs and what we are: naturally fragile in a mechanized world. The exhibits help visitors to become aware of the naturalness of their bodies and to recognize the anatomical beauty inside of them.

Plastination is a method to permanently preserve prosections or slices of cadavers in a safe, strong, dry polymer that is odorless, nontoxic, durable, flexible, authentic, shrinkless, and permanent. These models are increasingly being used in medical, nursing, and allied health programs as they have none of the drawbacks of traditional anatomy classes that use formaldehyde-preserved specimens, such as:

- Difficulty in obtaining and preserving quality specimens for all healthcare programs and ensuring predictable teaching opportunities in a cost-effective manner
- Difficulty in identifying anatomical structures as cadaveric specimens lose color, the correct anatomical alignment, and relationships during preservation
- Odorous, toxic chemicals with a risk of fume inhalation and specimens requiring careful handling, elaborate ventilation, and cold storage equipment

Additionally, anatomy programs exclusively using living anatomy, imaging, and/or virtual learning packages without dissection have received mixed feedback in relation to student satisfaction and the potential inadequacy of the student's anatomical knowledge (Baker, Slott, Terracio, & Cunningham, 2013).

These issues led Prof. von Hagens to develop anatomical specimens that provide superior learning and teaching opportunities (Table 6.3). The anatomical knowledge gained is crucial to simulation-based education related to the performance and interpretation of physical examinations, invasive procedures, ultrasound, and other radiological techniques. It is critical that a healthcare practitioner understands the organ structures they are aiming at or passing by as they examine, diagnose, and treat their patients.

Once medical professionals study human biology and pathology through plastinated specimens, they invariably view traditional specimens as relics of medical history. The use of plastinated specimens has been linked to an increase in student satisfaction, an increase in students' long-term retention of anatomical knowledge evidenced by an improvement in high stakes test scores, and a more efficient use of anatomy department resources (Baker et al., 2013).

I have witnessed the "Aha!" moments from many students and professionals when I have demonstrated plastinated specimens. They encourage a considered encounter with human biology and anatomy that drives student engagement and dramatically enhances their healthcare simulation education.

Table 6.3	The Broad Range of Plastinated Specimens
Type of Plastinate	**Description**
Silicone plastinates	Meticulously dissected whole-body, regional, or systemic anatomy specimens highlight even the smallest details and ensure anatomical accuracy.
Sheet plastinates	Real tissue specimens encased in organic glass illustrate fine anatomical structures and can be studied down to the finest tissues, at the microscopic level.
Anatomy glass	High-resolution acrylic glass prints of original body slices that can be examined under a submacroscopical scope. The anatomical structures have positioning errors corrected before printing and can be used on light tables or overhead projectors for comparison to radiological images.
Blood vessel configurations	Perfect castings of the inner blood vessels, created through a process that involves the injection, curing, and removal of real tissue. They show the smallest filigree blood vessels and beautifully illustrate the complex network of blood vessels within organs.
Skeletons and skulls	Produced with a level of detail and durability that cannot be replicated using plastic models

Virtual Tools

Virtual reality as defined by Owens and Taekman (2013) is "a term that applies to computer-simulated environments that can replicate physical presence in places in the real world, as well as in imaginary worlds" (p. 233). Augmented reality "supplements the real world such that actual objects existing in the real world appear to coexist with virtual objects" (Bauman, 2012, p. 249). As mentioned earlier, procedural simulation can take place in the physical environment or virtual environment, often a combination of the two. In nursing education, one common example is a physical model in which the learner inserts an intravenous cannula according to procedure. The model feels and responds like real skin and the learner can palpate the "vein." The haptic devices inside the model provide feedback to the computer about pressure, needle angle, and insertion of the cannula. The **virtual patient** on the computer screen responds accordingly, such as bleeding if the needle goes through the vein. This type of simulation allows for learners to face challenging intravenous cannula insertion, while allowing educators to standardize psychomotor skill development in the same manner for all students. When hybrid models are used, the experience is limited to the physical area where the models are housed, but still allows for repetition of the experience.

Virtual patients can be created to meet learning objectives for any type of patient condition, allowing expansion of opportunity that does not exist in the traditional clinical environment. Using virtual reality, and other types of simulation, gives educators full control over the types of patients their learners will care for. In cases where the entire virtual experience takes place online, the learner can access the patient repeatedly and outside of classroom hours. To care for the virtual patient, the learner may adopt the appearance of an avatar—a character that exemplifies a combination of their on-screen identity (such as a nurse) with their real-world identity (middle-age female) (Bauman & Ralston-Berg, 2015); however, some learners—and educators—create a new persona for themselves when learning in the virtual environment.

Wearable technology, such as optical head-mounted displays (glasses), allows the leaner to participate in a virtual or augmented world. The learner experiences varying degrees of immersion into the learning experience. The learner may be standing in a regular classroom, but when they apply the glasses, they see another environment entirely, such as a patient room that has a bed with a patient, intravenous pumps, art on the wall, oxygen outlets, and anything else the designer includes. They may hear the pump beeping, an overhead page, or someone arguing in the hallway. They may see the electrocardiogram tracing moving across the cardiac monitor or the pulse oximetry number changing every few minutes. The learner is immersed in the environment and communication is through regular voice. It is important to note that augmented reality can be achieved through a variety of technologies including desktop computers and handheld devices (Wu, Lee, Change, & Liang, 2013). This technology is not new and has been used in the gaming environment for a number of years. Over time, applications to education have been realized.

Holograms are no longer only a part of Star Trek lore, but are being used in healthcare education to help teach anatomy, patient safety, and a wide variety of other topics. Holograms were invented back in the 1940s and, with ongoing development, have evolved into digital format that allows them to be visualized without glasses (Hackett, 2013). Holograms are images that appear three-dimensional and change position as the learner moves them (Bassendowski, 2013), moves around them, or even moves inside them (e.g., walking into a holographic heart chamber). Providing learners with three-dimensional images facilitates understanding of human anatomy and physiology in a way that is more efficient than learning with pictures and diagrams found in books (Walker, 2013).

A variety of other applications of wearable technology are in development, allowing users to access a computer in glasses that function just as a laptop does, giving access to electronic mail, applications, and conferencing. One application allows the wearer to access a patient's electronic health record and record notes as they examine their patient. Applications, such as this, remain in development due to privacy and data access concerns. However, there have been several examples of surgeons wearing this technology to broadcast surgery online so that students could observe remotely. Other surgeons have used this method to allow a consulting surgeon, who may be on the other side of the world, to observe and provide input during surgery.

Think of the opportunities this type of technology brings to simulation. We can use augmented reality to place learners in environments and situations they might not otherwise have the chance to participate in and to provide care for virtual patients with conditions or circumstances they might not encounter in traditional clinical environments. We can also broadcast simulation to remote learners, giving them the caregiver's vantage point, as opposed to the view from a camera in the room. Walking through holographic chambers of the heart gives new meaning to the term active learning! Technology changes rapidly and ideas will evolve that will impact how we teach our students with various simulation typologies.

Summary

This chapter has provided an overview of just some of the different typologies of simulation and the rationale for how those categories have changed over time. It will be interesting to see how these change in later editions of this book. Technological capabilities are not going to slow down so we should continue to expect changes in the equipment that we have available to teach our students. We will also see current simulators evolve, while at the same time, virtual worlds of learning will become better defined. Wearable technology and holographic images are new now, but by the time this book hits the shelves, how will we be using this technology? Or, will even more opportunities be available? The world of simulation is for the nimble who can keep up with the changes. Meanwhile, we need to carefully consider the words of wisdom that implore us to provide clear, meaningful definitions that will help guide our research into outcomes.

7

Simulation Program Delivery Models

Kim Leighton

Key Terms

Modality, Computer-Based Simulation, Simulated Clinical Immersion, Boot Camp, Procedural Simulation, Expert Modeling, Hybrid Simulation, Games, Virtual Learning Environments, In Situ, Mobile Simulation, Telesimulation, Classroom Simulation, Just-In-Time Training

Guiding Questions

1 Now that I've learned about the various types of simulation, how can I use one or more of them in my teaching environment?

2 What are best practices for different simulation delivery models?

3 How can I overcome some of the inherent challenges of different delivery models for simulation-based education?

Introduction

In the previous chapter, we discussed the various typologies of simulation including the categories of living people, nonliving simulated tools, and virtual tools. In this chapter, we will consider how each of these types of simulation can be used. Delivery models, or modalities, are "the platform for the experience" (INACSL Standards Committee, 2016, Simulation Design, pg. S7). When determining how to best create a simulation experience for summative or formative evaluation, a **modality** should be chosen that best supports the learning objectives, participants, and resources that are available.

Many people think of a simulation lab when they are first asked to become involved in simulation. That lab could be envisioned as a one-room space or a large, multiroom

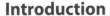

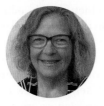

Kim Leighton, PhD, RN, CHSE, CHSOS, ANEF

center. In many locations, the lab is part of an existing skills lab space.

In the early days of mannequin-based simulation, we were confined to one location due to the various cords and connections that were needed to make the simulators run. Many of today's mannequins are tetherless, requiring only a Bluetooth connection to run. This allows mannequins to be moved so that simulation can be provided in almost any environment. Further, expansion of the typologies of simulation allow for education to be conducted in smaller physical spaces and even in virtual environments. This gives simulationists greater freedom in designing the right experience to meet the desired outcomes.

This chapter will consider three categories of simulation modalities: experience-driven, virtual, and location. The intent of this chapter is to cover common modalities, and it may not be inclusive of all simulation modalities presently available. Modalities that consider the experience include **computer-based simulation, simulated clinical immersion, boot camps, procedural simulation, expert modeling**, and **hybrid simulation**. Virtual modalities include **games** and **virtual learning environments**. Modalities that consider location will include **in situ, mobile simulation, telesimulation** (broadcast), **classroom**, and **just-in-time training (JITT)**.

Modalities That Consider the Learning Experience

Computer-Based Simulation

Many simulation activities are conducted via computer programs. These programs are designed to meet a variety of learning objectives, including knowledge gain, skill acquisition, and immersive patient care and range from simple to complex (Huang, Rice, Spain, & Palaganas, 2015; Weller, Nestel, Marshall, Brooks, & Conn, 2012). Some simulations are designed to help the learner grasp facts, while others allow the students to apply what they have learned and see the outcomes of their actions, or failure to act. Higher-order thinking skills are also tested as learners solve problems and engage in decision-making activities (Koenig, Iseli, Wainess, & Lee, 2013). A wide variety of learning activities can be designed by educators, who also may have access to vendor-developed scenarios.

Advantages of computer-based simulation include portability as the simulation programs can often be accessed via the Internet from any computer. Alternatively, some programs must be downloaded to an individual computer for access. These simulation programs are less expensive than simulation typologies that involve mannequins and supporting equipment such as audiovisual capabilities and other peripherals such as a medication administration cart, ventilator, or electronic health record. Computer-based simulations can be repeatedly accessed by learners, who complete the activities for either summative or formative evaluation. Some programs are designed so that the learner completes a different scenario each time the program is accessed, while others allow for repetition. Evaluations designed within the computer program are not prone to the objective nature of evaluations conducted by people; therefore, there may be less bias introduced to the learning process.

A variety of programs exist and, for our purposes, will be categorized by anatomy/physiology, pharmacological or physiological modeling, and patient cases. The type and variety of programs increases exponentially as vendors attempt to fill the practice gaps identified by educators and clinicians. Computer-based simulations that are designed for anatomy and physiology tend to be created for knowledge acquisition. Joints might be viewed from a variety of angles or while in various degrees of flexion or extension; layers can be divided to see what is underneath as in viewing a surgical incision that cuts through layers of skin, muscle, and subcutaneous fat; organs can be viewed from the interior such as the chambers of the heart; or physiology can be demonstrated through showing how oxygen flows through the airway and into the lungs, with or without restriction. Many of these types of activities could be completed using real people; however, by integrating computer-based simulation, opportunities are expanded so that learning is not restricted to place and patient availability.

Pharmacological and physiological modeling are common programs, though they often are designed for medical students and practitioners, including nurse anesthetists. Typical programs show the effect a medication or intervention has on the physiological parameters of the patient. For example, the learner enters a dose for an anesthetic agent based on his or her evaluation of a patient. The computer program is mathematically modeled to respond to that dose based on the patient's weight, BMI, physical condition, comorbidities, and other programmed parameters. The learner then sees how the dose chosen will affect the patient, providing them with feedback to determine if the dosage was correct, too high, or too low. Similar simulations can show physiological response to blood loss, volume infusion, or hypoxia, sharing resultant blood pressure, heart rate, pulse oximetry, arterial blood gases, cardiac output, and various other parameters (Fig. 7.1).

Patient cases, in this environment, are further on the continuum toward immersive simulation, which is discussed more fully in the next section. Numerous simulations of this type exist for a variety of types of patients (neonatal, obstetric, trauma), conditions (cardiac, respiratory), interventions (blood gases, ultrasound, electrocardiogram, invasive procedures), and events (bioterrorism, conscious sedation, advanced cardiac life support [ACLS]). Patient cases may be designed for a singular purpose, such as to determine whether the learner can intervene with a specific intervention, or may encompass everything from introduction to the patient, taking of history, conducting physical exam, communicating findings to the healthcare provider, prioritizing interventions, evaluating outcomes, and documenting activities. Some of these programs are designed to follow a novice to advanced trajectory, increasing in difficulty as the learner demonstrates proficiency.

It is beyond the scope of this discussion to help educators create computer-based simulation, but there are criteria that should be considered when evaluating adoption of healthcare simulation programs: "1) goals of the simulation, 2) learning objectives, cognitive demands, and assessment, 3) affordances of the simulation, 4) the instructional strategies used, and 5) motivation considerations for users" (Koenig et al., 2013, p. 47). It is important that the computer-based simulation have goals and learning objectives that align with the planned curricular integration and that knowledge, skills, and attitude promoted by the product match educator expectations. Related to fidelity, do the anticipated actions of the learner match with real-world actions? If the learner chooses an action incorrectly, does the simulation respond accordingly? The criteria for choosing computer-based simulation programs are closely aligned with the expectations of how all simulation experiences are designed, regardless of modality. Simulations that are computer based should

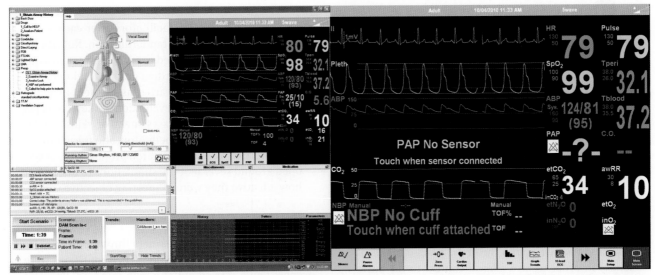

Figure 7.1 Physiological Display Monitor. (From Orbaugh, S. L., & Gigeleisen, P. E. (2012). *Atlas of airway management: Techniques and tools* (2nd ed.). Philadelphia, PA: Lippincott Williams & Wilkins.)

also adhere to the best practices outlined by McGaghie, Issenberg, Petrusa, and Scalese (2010) in their meta-analysis of simulation research and the INACSL Standard of Best Practice for Simulation: Simulation Design (INACSL Standards Committee, 2016). These are further discussed in Chapter 20 Curriculum Development in Simulation Nursing Programs. Motivation for engagement by the learner takes on a bit different context as there is not generally a facilitator present to guide this activity, requiring motivation to come from within the activity in the form of intuitive design, such as including an interactive vital sign display that changes based on learner interventions (Koenig et al., 2013).

Simulated Clinical Immersion

Simulationists strive to create learning environments that fully engage the participants so that they perform as they would in real-world situations. To fully immerse the learner in the experience, educators develop scenarios that encourage them to suspend disbelief and make real-time decisions (Huang et al., 2015). The effort to create this immersive environment should address various human senses such as tactile, auditory, and visual (Wucherer, Stefan, Weidert, Fallavollita, & Navab, 2013). Unfortunately, many published manuscripts about immersive simulation projects or research fail to describe how the immersive environment was created.

There is considerable debate among simulation experts as to how much fidelity is enough to promote learning, and this is addressed in other chapters. This healthy discussion is important to have as resources, including time, money, and equipment, are limited and, therefore, should be put toward experiences that lead to the best learning outcomes.

Some believe that for learning to occur, full immersion into the environment is required (Wucherer et al., 2013); however, the choice of resources should also be tied to the desired educational outcomes (Talbot, 2013).

Creating an immersive experience helps learners to make the connection between classroom learning and application of that material when caring for real patients. Immersive experiences can be created using any of the simulation typologies but most often are associated with mannequins, standardized patients, and virtual reality. The focus of this modality is the environment and how to make it as realistic as possible thereby allowing learners to participate in an experience that replicates their work environment (Stefaniak & Turkelson, 2014).

The most realistic option may be to place the experience within the true practice environment (Mowry & Crump, 2013) such as a mental health unit that includes an admissions office, patient rooms, seclusion rooms, and therapeutic communication rooms. This type of in situ simulation is described in more detail later in this chapter. However, these environments can also realistically be created within dedicated simulation space, which would allow learning to occur without disrupting the routine of the practice environment and associated patient care activities. Immersion has also been equated with time (Onello & Regan, 2013), suggesting that scenarios must be longer than usual in order to be immersive. Increasing time does allow for the scenario to play out—students can obtain diagnostic test results in real time or evaluate the patient post-intervention at increased time intervals, for example. Appropriate simulation design can create these situations in shorter time periods as well. Read Diana Callender's Voice of Experience to learn how one college manages scheduling and faculty development to successfully deliver 3,000 hours of simulation experiences every 4 months.

7-1 Voice of Experience
Large-Volume Simulation Integration

Diana P.E. Callender, DM, MBBS

The Challenge

At Ross University School of Medicine, we integrated simulation activities into the first 2 years of medical school in order to give clinical context to the basic science courses and enhance clinical thinking among learners. The challenge was scheduling and delivering two high-quality simulation activities to approximately 1,500 students in four different semesters, three times a year. Approximately 12 clinicians from different disciplines and levels of expertise facilitated these activities. In two activities, clinicians were paired with nonclinical facilitators. As learners had summative assessments, which included performance on these activities in their clinical skills assessments, we needed to ensure that quality activities were delivered in a consistent manner.

Meeting the Challenge

We analyzed how we would have to schedule learners so we could have approximately 300 to 350 students complete a simulation within a week so the material could be integrated with classroom activities. We had to determine how to deliver approximately 3,000 hours of simulation every 4 months, plus assess learners on their mastery of at least one activity each semester. We realized that we needed a rigorous faculty development process to ensure that all facilitators understood the objectives and facilitated and debriefed in a consistent manner so that all students had comparable experiences. Because of the narrow window for the delivery of each simulation, we needed backup simulators in case one malfunctioned. We also had facilitators stand by in case a faculty member was ill or unable to participate. We developed a rigorous quality improvement process around curriculum delivery and the assessment of both learners and the quality of facilitation. Faculty development included facilitator training and refresher sessions every 4 months, reviewing scenarios/activities with facilitators before each

activity, and debriefing facilitators after each activity, using video clips for standardization. Rubrics for assessments were reviewed every semester and sample tapes used to standardize grading and decrease intergrader variability. Learner assessment included pre- and posttests and evaluation of key concepts on written exams and assessment of skills taught. Surveys of learners and facilitators about each simulation were also done. A research proposal was developed around several of the simulations to document how effective they were in meeting objectives.

Outcome

We were able to put all learners through the simulations with minimal disruption. The simulations were consistently carried out at a high standard. Pre- and posttests showed significant increases in learner knowledge after simulation and written tests showed increased mastery of some concepts, with the greatest gains being in the lower third of the class. Evaluations of simulation activities were positive. The procedures and processes implemented in this program were central to our being accredited by the Society for Simulation in Healthcare for teaching and research.

Most Valuable Lessons Learned

A rigorous quality improvement process is central to the sustained success of a program.

Overall, the point of immersion is to create an environment realistic enough for learners to engage with their simulated patient to the level that they would engage with a real patient in various healthcare environments. Three general categories of fidelity must be considered when developing an immersive simulation: physical, conceptual, and psychological/emotional/experiential (INACSL Standards Committee, 2016, Scenario Design; Rudolph, McIntosh, Simon, & Raemer, 2015a). Physical aspects include the patient (standardized, simulator, virtual), environment, and equipment, including props. Any additional personnel, such as a confederate, must be realistic in appearance and purpose. Environmental fidelity includes the methods used to address the senses, such as visual, tactile, auditory, and olfactory aspects of the patient being cared for. Conceptual fidelity ensures that the scenario makes sense and is logical in its content and flow. Vital signs, lab results, patient responses, cues, etc. should all be realistic for the patient being cared for. Psychological fidelity (emotional/experiential fidelity) is enhanced when the scenario includes methods that will impact the emotional response of the learner, such as time pressures, stress, changing priorities, or emotional family members.

While immersive simulation may be considered the standard for engaging students, the level of fidelity must be weighed in light of the desired learning outcomes: available space, equipment, and supplies, and personnel. Additionally, the simulationists should consider the correlation of the scenario design with learning theories. For example, when attempting to impact psychological fidelity, it is common for educators to include too many distractors, thereby increasing the cognitive load for the learner. Examples of ways to enhance fidelity in all areas are included in Chapter 19, Leading Artistry in Simulation: Moulage.

Developing Psychomotor Skills Using a "Boot Camp" Approach to Training

Michelle Aebersold, PhD, RN, FAAN

The development of psychomotor skills is a necessary component of nursing education, but despite our best efforts, students are still often unprepared to perform even the most basic skills when at the clinical site. Many programs teach skills only once during a fundamentals course, expecting students to retain the ability to perform the skill, despite the fact that skills often begin to decay soon after being learned (O'Donnell et al., 2011). Ericsson's (2004)

work on deliberate practice shows that skills must be practiced repetitively. Learners must also receive feedback to guide improvement. One model to support the deliberate practice of skills and incorporate formative feedback and assessment is a boot camp approach. The boot camp approach is similar to the military approach to basic training where new recruits are put through a series of training tasks designed to improve their skills in several areas. This approach has been used by surgical residency programs to train new residents on surgical skills through the use of surgical task trainers and simulators and also in the areas of team training (Malekzadeh et al, 2011; Nishisaki et al., 2009).

The boot camp approach to skills training can be used at any level of nursing education, including prelicensure education, graduate education, and continuing education for practicing nurses. This approach is competency based and generally provides formative feedback, as well as a method to help learners prepare for a summative or high-stakes test or evaluation. The content and delivery schedule can be adapted to the learners' needs. The experiences are generally short bursts of training done over several days or a few weeks. Boot camps can be timed to develop skills as students enter a clinical rotation, such as learning newborn bathing, injections, breast care, and postpartum checks prior to an obstetrics course. Boot camps can be designed to prepare students for end of the term skills checkoffs. Another option is to have a boot camp the week before classes start to help students refresh skills they have not been able to practice over the summer to reduce anxiety as they return to class. Boot camps are a good way to learn new skills and practice skills that have not been used regularly. Table 7.1 outlines sample skills and equipment for a medical–surgical boot camp.

Table 7.1	Sample Boot Camp Skills Stations for Medical–Surgical Prelicensure Students	
Station	**Skill**	**Equipment**
#1	Tracheostomy care	Nasogastric tube and tracheostomy care trainer Tracheostomy tube/tube holder Tracheostomy care supplies
#2	Central line dressing change	Central line task trainer Central line for setup Central line dressing trays
#3	Program infusion pump to deliver intravenous piggyback medication (IVPB)	Intravenous (IV) infusion pump IV tubing Prepared IVPB medications
#4	Insert peripheral IV catheter	IV training arm IV insertion supplies Simulated blood
#5	Initiate code and defibrillate a patient	Automatic external defibrillator (AED) trainer Midfidelity mannequin

Each student rotates through each station in 1-h time blocks. Times can vary depending on student to instructor ratios. Each student must have a chance to practice the skills.

Designing Your Boot Camp

The first step in designing a boot camp is to determine the needs of the learners. This can be done by conducting a needs assessment, reviewing skills needed for upcoming clinical rotations, or reviewing the literature to determine which skills are important for your students to develop. Once you have decided which skills to focus on, then determine how to set up the learning stations to teach those skills. For example, if learners need to practice sterile technique, will you have them insert an indwelling urinary catheter or do an intermittent straight catheterization? Consider which skill they are more likely to perform in the clinical setting. A task trainer is appropriate to use for this activity since the focus is on psychomotor skill development (Fig. 7.2). If learners are practicing advanced airway skills, with a focus on learning to intubate a difficult airway, a task trainer for that purpose is most appropriate. The boot camp is all about psychomotor skill development, not demonstrating higher-order thinking skills, communication, or prioritization—behaviors that might be better suited for mannequin-based simulation (Malekzadeh et al., 2011).

Once you have identified the skills to focus on, gather the associated equipment and supplies needed, ensuring you have an adequate supply for the number of learners. The important next step is to determine how to set up the space and schedule. A small learner to instructor ratio is important, as is adequate space for the instructor to observe the practicing learners. Boot camp training is an observed and supervised training. Based on Ericsson's (2008) deliberate practice model, the instructor should provide immediate feedback, allowing the learner to reflect and correct their technique. Scheduling learners to complete the boot camp can take several forms depending on the number of learners, faculty, and space availability.

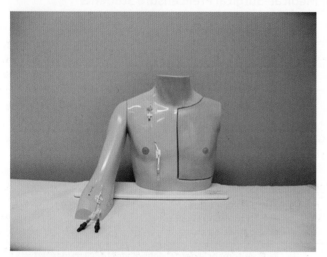

Figure 7.2 Intravenous Boot Camp. (From Gregory D., Raymond-Seniuk, C., Patrick, L., and Stephen, T. (2015). Fundamentals: Perspectives on the Art and Science of Canadian Nursing. Philadelphia: Wolters Kluwer Health. Photo courtesy of David P. Bornais.)

Learners might rotate through multiple stations in one day or come to one or two sessions a day over the course of a week or more. It is possible to use higher-level students to assist with the stations; however, the students must be adequately trained ahead of time and teach the skills in the same manner as you. Consistency is crucial to success.

To prepare for a successful skills boot camp, it is critical that each skill has a well-designed rubric. The rubrics should identify the essential steps for each skill as well as the rationale for the steps, when appropriate. These rubrics should be shared with the learners ahead of time so they can review and prepare, along with any other essential materials to help them prepare such as videos, reading materials on how to perform the skills, evidence-based practice articles, or agency policies important to the skills. Rubrics also help to ensure each instructor teaches the skills the same way.

In summary, the key elements of boot camp–style training include the following:

- Generally done as formative assessment where learners are focused on practicing a skill with the goal of moving toward competency.
- Small learner-to-instructor ratio.
- Focus is on psychomotor skill development.
- Use skill stations set up with task trainers or equipment such as intravenous infusion pumps.
- There is a well-defined rubric for each skill.
- Learners are provided information to prepare ahead of time.
- Boot camps occur over a short period of time.

Procedural Simulation

Kim Leighton, PhD, RN, CHSE, CHSOS, ANEF

Perhaps the types of simulation most familiar to nursing educators are task trainers and partial task trainers, also known as procedural simulators. Most skills/simulation laboratories use a variety of these simulators to teach students how to perform skills. These skills include giving injections, inserting urinary catheters, and inserting intravenous catheters, among many others (Fig. 7.3). The simulators or task trainers used to teach these skills range from simple to complex and may or may not represent the actual part of the body where the skill takes place. For example, many faculty have used hotdogs to train students in the skill of administering intradermal medications. Other, more sophisticated, models have higher fidelity and respond to interventions via haptic devices that document the location of touch or degree of pressure. An example is a pelvic examination

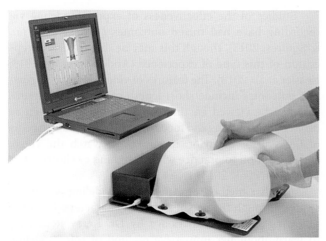

Figure 7.3 Pelvic Exam Task Trainer. (Image courtesy of Carla M Pugh, MD, PhD, Susan M Behrends, MD, Professor of Surgical Education, University of Wisconsin)

simulator that documents where the student touches on the internal exam as well as the amount of pressure applied—all of which cannot be determined by a facilitator.

A major benefit of task trainers is that they are generally low cost and can be used repetitively over long periods of time without significant maintenance or replacement costs. The low cost also allows for multiple purchases of each trainer (Weller et al., 2012). As a result, faculty should be able to provide the learner with multiple opportunities to practice their skills. Psychomotor skills, such as aseptic technique, may not be transferred from the skills laboratory to the clinical environment due to lack of repetition, as well as other factors such as product design (Gonzalez & Sole, 2014). Mastery learning may be achieved by using a deliberate practice model that promotes repetition of skills practice (Carson et al., 2015; Cohen et al., 2013; Ericsson, 2004; McGaghie, Issenberg, Barsuk, & Wayne, 2014) and also decreases instructor-to-student ratio (Carson et al., 2015). However, there is still little research in nursing education about skill acquisition and simulation (Ross, 2012).

Examples of procedural simulation activities are found extensively in the literature. Ramponi and Ross (2015) taught several skills to doctoral students prior to an international clinic experience. Some skills were taught using commercial task trainers, while abscess incision and drainage was creatively designed by injecting yogurt under chicken leg skin. While animal skin and hotdogs have been used to teach suture skills, the authors opted for an inexpensive wound closure pad that provided a more realistic feel and allowed students to take the materials home for further practice. Operating room skills, more commonly learned by physicians, are practiced on partial task trainers that exist in the physical and virtual world. For example, laparoscopic surgery skills are learned by holding surgical tools in one's hands while watching how they are manipulated in the virtual world via a computer screen.

There are a large number of partial- and full-task trainers available for nursing educators to teach psychomotor

skills; however, some choose to teach these skills using high-fidelity simulators. The educator should weigh the value of having students perform repetitious skills on models that were not designed for that purpose. The task trainers have been designed to be rugged and hold up to repeated use. The mannequin simulators were not designed for this purpose, though they all allow a variety of skills to be performed on them. In general, educators should consider having students perform repetitious practice on task trainers while having them perform skills on the simulators if called for in the scenario design and to meet learning objectives. For example, the simulators have the capability to have an intravenous (IV) line started on them; however, it is not like starting an IV on a real person. If the learning objective is to start an IV using sterile technique, then a task trainer should be chosen for the activity. If the learning objective is for the student to start IV fluids in response to hypotension in their patient, then the simulationist may want to consider creating a patient story in which an IV is already in place so that the focus (and associated time) is not spent starting an IV on a model not designed for that purpose. One school always leaves a saline lock in the simulator so that IV access is available for learner interventions.

Procedural simulation has been a large part of nursing education for many years; however, as outlined above, transfer of these skills to practice is still a challenge. A careful review of mastery learning (Ericsson, 2004) shows that a significant number of practice hours must take place before learners are proficient in their skills. Not only is it the number of hours, but it is the quality of the practice hours. Practicing a technique 10,000 hours will not result in mastery if the educator does not correct bad technique. Despite the ease at which most task trainers are used, it remains vital that an educator oversee the practice.

Expert Modeling

Expert modeling is a method supported by Bandura (1977b), who theorized that skills could be learned or enhanced by observing someone modeling the behavior to be learned. One of the factors that lead someone to adopt an observed behavior is the consequences of the model's actions. For example, if an expert role model provides appropriate patient care in a scenario and the patient improves, the impetus for modeling that behavior is greater than if care led to a poor outcome for the patient. While observing the expert perform, learners create their own mental image that they can refer to when called upon later to demonstrate the same behaviors or skills.

Expert role modeling can be done in person or by video recording. One method of expert role modeling uses the instructor or clinical expert to demonstrate responses and interventions expected during a scenario while the learners observe. The expert model explains the skill, behavior, and knowledge that are applied during the simulated experience (LeFlore & Anderson, 2009). This is typically followed by the group of observers then completing the same scenario. One of the challenges of this type of simulation is that perfection must be demonstrated by the person(s) modeling the behaviors or there is a risk that the observer will mimic incorrect actions that they observed. Other challenges with role modeling occur when more than one person is the model. It is very difficult to make sure that all models show how to manage a behavior or skill in the exact same way. Again using the skills lab as an example, at the start of each semester, all faculty agree to teach the various skills the same way, using the checklists in the textbook as the guide. But, at the end of the semester, students commonly complain that each teacher showed them a different way to accomplish the skill and wonder who is right. Novice students are concrete thinkers and have not yet developed the abstract thinking that allows them to see that there is more than one correct way to change a sterile dressing.

Many of us are familiar with videotapes used for skills lab preparation. Skills lab instructors often require their students to review the recordings prior to coming to the skills lab so that they have a reference mental image to use when practicing. It is thought that watching the videos in combination with required readings from the text will help to improve performance when the learners practice their skills. However, many instructors have also been frustrated by these same videos because they often feature inaccurate techniques or do not teach the skill the way that we want it to be taught. As someone who used to review skills videos, I can report that inaccuracies such as failure to wash hands, failure to put on gloves prior to touching body fluids, and errors related to other common procedures were frequently observed. An excellent example of how to develop an expert role-modeling video is described by Aronson, Glynn, and Squires (2013). They developed a practice video that shows an expert nurse providing competent care to a patient who is deteriorating. The video was scripted and rehearsed numerous times to ensure it depicted expert care. In addition, the team members independently rated the nurse's performance to ensure validity of the video. The video was designed for students to watch prior to engaging in a simulation.

Anderson, LeFlore, and Anderson (2013) offer an overview of advantages for using videotape instead of in-person role modeling. Although initially it is time-consuming and costly (in terms of faculty time) to create the video, it can be reused, saving time and cost in the long run. The recording can also be viewed outside of class time, freeing this time to focus on application of what is learned in the recording. Students can watch the recording as many times as they wish without impacting faculty time and visual cues in the video may prompt recall of information.

Studies of the effectiveness of expert modeling via recording have had mixed outcomes (Aronson, Glynn, & Squires, 2013), though this may be due to lack of repetition of this type of experience (Anderson et al., 2013; Kessler et al., 2013). The features of videos leading to positive outcomes include short length of under 25 minutes that can be viewed anytime, anywhere, and as often as desired; instructions and focus on most important aspects of the skill or behavior; incentives to watch the video; and the option to practice while watching or shortly after (Anderson et al., 2013).

Another method of expert role modeling is demonstrated through the use of Mask Ed characters. Read the following Voice of Experience by Dr. Kerry Reid-Searl to learn about her immersive method of role modeling within simulation.

7-2 Voice of Experience
Mask Ed (KRS Simulation): Transforming the Educator—Addressing All Elements of Human Care

Kerry Reid-Searl, PhD, MClinEd, BhlthSc, RN, RM

The Challenge

For decades, nursing educators and students have adopted role-play to simulate the patient or nurse role in the classroom. There are numerous advantages with the educator adopting the patient role: knowing content that needs to be covered, understanding the role from experience, and often no rehearsed scripts are required. The disadvantage, however, is that when an educator plays the role of the patient, it is difficult for students to become totally immersed when the educator remains visually present. The power imbalance existing between student and educator cannot be ignored. In an effort to overcome this, the idea of totally hiding the educator's face was considered as the best option.

Meeting the Challenge

In 2008, I conceived the idea of wearing silicone props. The silicone body parts initially included lifelike masks, arms, and hands sought from United States companies. I then designed body torsos including catheterizable genitalia. Soon, the impact on students would be realized. The props were so real that students became suspended in disbelief and forgot that the educator was hidden behind the props. The impact of this technique led me to advance the technique by designing a teaching framework to inform what I was doing and ultimately inform others.

The technique was named Mask Ed (KRS Simulation). Mask Ed represents masking of the educator and the education process and involves the educator donning realistic silicone props. The educator adopts mannerisms and assumes the personality and history of a character relevant to the learning experience. The character emerges as the platform for teaching and coaching. The hidden educator directs the learning process informed by his or her knowledge and expertise. The KRS component of Mask Ed (KRS Simulation) stands for knowledgeable, realistic, and spontaneous simulation.

- Knowledgeable: Educator has a deep understanding of the content being imparted; understanding of different learning styles in order to develop strategies within the simulation experience that engage the learners.
- Realistic: Simulation experience mimics a real situation, based on the educator's experience and deep understanding of their discipline and the simulation experience.
- Spontaneous: Reaction of the character is unprompted. However, the character is directed by the educator who is in turn influenced by the learner response. Because scripts are not set, the reactions can be immediate in response to learners.

Outcome

The outcome has been learner engagement, student satisfaction, positive student evaluations, exciting teaching opportunities, numerous and extensive teaching awards, invitations to speak across the world, and the design of a teaching approach that would be fine-tuned into workshops and now being implemented into health-related programs across the world.

The challenge has been listening to critics who do not understand the process. Without an understanding of Mask Ed, there are risks. These include not adhering to the pedagogy and thinking this is just about donning silicone props. When the pedagogy is not followed, then learning situations can be compromised. The technique requires preparation, an understanding of the learning objectives, and careful debriefs. Additionally, there are risks in terms of ethics and placing students in difficult situations. The characters in this technique need to be carefully crafted; they must be warm, friendly, vulnerable, and always wise and knowledgeable. The teacher/coach must be transferred through the character. If this does not occur, then the essence of Mask Ed is lost and the character becomes a standardized patient.

Most Valuable Lessons Learned

Never give up on an idea that you believe can make a difference for others.

Inspiration for Simulation Champions

Dare to think differently. Be brave to let your ideas come to fruition. Ignore the dream thieves in your life.

Hybrid Simulation

Hybrid simulation is defined as "the integration of multiple modalities of simulation (e.g., simulators and standardized patients) to achieve learning objectives in a simulation; a simulation that combines constructive, live, and/or virtual simulation, typically in a distributed environment" (SSH Accreditation, 2014b). In other words, sometimes just one type of simulation isn't enough! The decision on whether to use more than one type of simulation and what options to choose should be based on the learning objectives of the simulation experience. There are many ways to combine simulators; examples are shown in Table 7.2.

Early on, simulationists worked diligently to try to integrate mannequin-based simulation throughout the nursing school curriculum. Often, that was the mandate given to us by our college leaders. In many courses, scenarios were easily created to complement the didactic and clinical-based portion of the courses; however, there was one course in particular where we struggled—mental health. As those who have taught mental health know, there are many nonverbal cues and emotions that a nurse will look for when working with mentally ill patients. How does one identify those cues when the patient is a plastic mannequin, devoid of emotion? Try as we might, mannequin-based simulation just was not the answer! We started to add to our scenarios by including a faculty

Table 7.2	Examples of Hybrid Simulation Experiences	
Scenario	**Objectives**	**Modality Used**
Patient requires intravenous fluids (IVF).	Start IV infusion; manage deteriorating condition.	Place IV arm in bed next to patient simulator.
Patient undergoing laparoscopic surgery develops hypovolemic shock	Psychomotor skill development for laparoscopic surgery. Manage large fluid volume replacement.	Use surgical trainer for skill attainment; move to high-fidelity simulator for management of complications.
Patient death and family notification	Notify family, in person, that patient has died.	Static mannequin with standardized patient as family member
Patient complains of lower abdominal pain	Communicate with patient while conducting pelvic exam.	Pelvic exam model next to standardized patient
Disaster drill	Manage multiple casualties	Simulators, static mannequins, and standardized patients

member playing the role of a family member or by having a "charge nurse" enter the room to provide cues to the students: "Mrs. Jones, I see that your hands are shaky and you keep looking over in the corner of the room. Can you tell me what you see?" or "Mom, I see tears in your eyes...." By adding these roles to the simulated clinical experience, we had unknowingly created hybrid simulation experiences. We also now know that using a mannequin for all simulation is not the most cost-effective or efficient way to meet learning outcomes. We can use the variety of simulation modalities now available to choose the best teaching strategy. One creative use of hybrid simulation resulted in PartoPants™, a modified pair of surgical scrubs worn by a simulated patient and used to demonstrate delivery of a baby (Fig. 7.4).

There are many examples in the literature of ways to create hybrid simulation. At an Utstein-style meeting designed to set a simulation research agenda, those present agreed that there is "ample evidence that single modality simulation leads to long-term retention of certain

skills"; however, the same cannot be said for hybrid simulation modalities (Issenberg, Ringsted, Ostergaard, & Dieckmann, 2011, p. 157).

Virtual Modalities

Games and Virtual Learning Environments

Eric B. Bauman, PhD, RN, FSSH

Over the last 5 years, multimedia and digital educational content have experienced a significant increase in the level of sophistication in nursing and other types of clinical education. These modalities are no longer a novelty and are becoming a standard educational practice for nursing education at all levels. This section serves as an introduction to game-based learning, contemporary screen-based simulation, and importance of mobile or application-based learning. Best practices for game-based learning, application development, and integrating such technology into curricula for nursing and clinical education are shared.

Defining Games, Applications, and Virtual Worlds

Games are goal-oriented and rule-based events that engage players through consequence. The consequences provide a system of rewards for achievement and often provide a negative repercussion for actions that do not subscribe to the goals or rules of the game (Deterding, Dixon, Khaled, & Nacke, 2011).

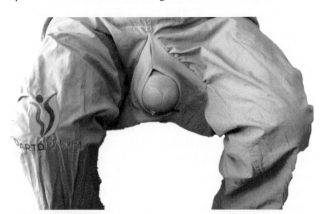

Figure 7.4 PartoPants™. (Reprinted from Pronto International, with permission. http://prontointernational. org/partopantstm-birith-simulator.)

Applications are software designed for mobile devices, such as smartphones and tablets, to support existing curricula goals and objectives. If applications are well designed and mobile, they are capable of becoming powerful cognitive aids to support future practice and continuing professional development (Jeffries, Bauman, & Shaefer, 2014).

Virtual worlds (also referred to as virtual reality environments) are digital environments that exist synchronously, meaning players inhabit a digital space in real time. Virtual worlds are capable of hosting multiple people or players, represented as avatars, facilitated by networked computers (Bauman, 2012; Bell, 2008).

Game-based platforms provide a narrative and a system of rewards to encourage players to accomplish specific tasks and objectives. Game-based platforms use virtual environments to stage the game (Bauman, 2010, 2012). Not all virtual environments are game-based. For example, the popular virtual reality environment Second Life is a virtual world, providing a stage; however, it lacks essential elements of a game. Read how Dee McGonigle began using Second Life as a virtual teaching environment in her Voice of Experience.

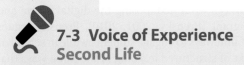

7-3 Voice of Experience
Second Life

Dee McGonigle, PhD, RN, CNE, FAAN, ANEF

The Challenge

When we were first trying to get our arms around distance education, we moved from mailed text, to emailing, to listservs, to web-based interactions such as web pages, wikis, and blogs. Then, Second Life (SL) appeared on the scene in 2003 and changed the landscape of distance education forever. There were five challenges that we identified:

1. Learning how to incorporate this virtual world into our coursework and other educational offerings while still completing normal faculty workload
2. Determining if students would have the computing strength necessary to use this program

3. Assessing the learning curve for students prior to developing educational episodes
4. Providing support for the students
5. Evaluating the educational episodes in this new delivery modality

Meeting the Challenge

Since this was a new frontier, SL was difficult to get started. Most educators either had not heard about it or had not explored it. One of the best ways to learn about anything is to consult the experts, which I did in order to learn more about this new virtual world. We soon realized that most students would not be able to access SL easily. Since we did not want to frustrate them with technology issues, we needed another way for them to experience this new educational arena. We discussed our alternatives: (1) in-class demo, (2) computer lab experience, or (3) create a video for them. After some debate, we decided to begin with an observation; the students could watch a video instead of having to enter the world on their own (Fig. 7.5).

Outcome

We integrated one video module into the course management system. The experience was very low level and lacked interactivity in world; however, it exposed the students to this new educational medium. We provided detailed information on the time and cost to develop what they observed. The students enjoyed the experience and gained insight into another technology since none of them had even heard of SL prior to that learning episode.

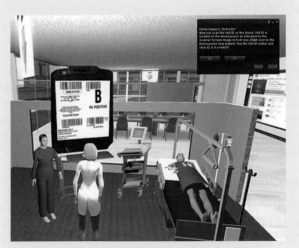

Figure 7.5 Second Life Virtual Environment.

(Continued)

7-3 Voice of Experience (*Continued*)

Most Valuable Lessons Learned

The learning curve for programming while developing an educational module is steep. It is best to have a developer who can do the heavy lifting of programming while the educator focuses on the learning activities.

Inspiration for Simulation Champions

"Learning by doing, peer-to-peer teaching, and computer simulation are all part of the same equation."
—Nicholas Negroponte

Best Practices

Game-based learning and educational games should engage and motivate students through experiences occurring within the game while mapping back to course objectives. Students must understand how playing an educational game supports academic achievement and how playing the game will help them reach their goals. Educational games ought to provide a number of opportunities to learners:

- To explore situated phenomena
- To provide possibilities for testing hypotheses within the curriculum and profession that the learner hopes to join
- To provide activities and experience in ways that are not practical or possible using traditional educational modalities (Kiili, 2005)

Educational game and application designers should develop experiences that engage learners and that are relevant and situated to the curriculum (Bauman, 2007; Kiili, 2005; Squire, 2006), replicating real-world environments and activities. Well-engineered or created digital spaces promote the suspension of disbelief to produce sufficient authenticity or environmental fidelity to allow for deep meaning making (Bauman, 2007, 2010, 2012).

The goal of an educational game is to prepare players for the real world. A successful educational game will move players from the digital environment to the real world as quickly and efficiently as possible by supporting and reinforcing didactic content and preparing students for additional experiential learning activities such as traditional mannequin-based simulation and supervised clinical rotations.

Evaluation

Digital games are capable of collecting vast amounts of data to evaluate skill acquisition and knowledge transfer. Standard evaluation tools built into game-based learning platforms are capable of collecting quiz scores, measuring time-in-state, how long a player spent on any particular part of a game, or how long it took a player to play through a level of a game or the game in its entirety. In addition, it is possible to record the total number of times and total time a player has spent playing a game or application. Game designers can create scoring matrixes, which allow for multiple attempts to encourage knowledge acquisition and demonstration. In this way, evaluation becomes both summative and formative.

Vetting and Fit

Our role as faculty is first and foremost to evaluate games and applications for appropriateness and accuracy. We must also look at the triad of cost, time, and complexity when we select games and applications to support nursing and health sciences curricula. For example, if a game works well, is easy to use, and requires little infrastructure for support, but costs a million dollars to license and implement on your campus, it may not be adopted because the cost is prohibitive. If a game is affordable, contextually accurate, but clunky, such that faculty struggle to deploy it and students find it difficult to play from a user interface perspective, it likely will not meet your program's objectives (Bauman & Ralston-Berg, 2014).

Conclusion

Many teachers interested in the digital revolution are familiar with Prensky's work juxtaposing the digital native and digital immigrant (Prensky, 2001, 2010). Prensky argues that we must find ways to engage students while in school or in the context of structured learning in the same ways that they are engaged in their social, personal, and recreational lives. The traditional classroom and traditional academia simply do not approach engagement with the type of active play that exists and is possible through a digitally connected environment. Embracing the 21st century digital experience offers choices that drive engagement and promote learner agency (Prensky, 2005b). We have an obligation to teach and guide students in ways that prepare them for the type of practice that they will work in. We must strive to serve students', employers', and patients' interests.

Space Modalities

In Situ Simulation

Kim Leighton, PhD, RN, CHSE, CHSOS, ANEF

In situ simulation typically involves team-based training and occurs in a real patient care environment (Clapper,

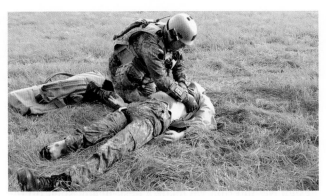

Figure 7.6 Military In Situ. (Photo courtesy of Laerdal Medical. All rights reserved.)

2013a; Patterson, Geis, Falcone, LeMaster, & Wears, 2012). Most commonly, we think of inpatient hospital units; however, in situ education has occurred in clinic rooms, stairwells, on mountains, and on battlefields (Fig. 7.6). In situ simulation can help uncover potential causes of error not evident in well-controlled simulation laboratory environments because it occurs where patients, visitors, and staff may be present during learning, equipment may be poorly located or maintained, and communication and team work may be interrupted by real-time patient care activity. This section discusses advantages and challenges and suggests best practices for in situ simulation.

Advantages and Challenges

In situ simulation provides opportunities for those without access to a simulation lab setting because of costs, location, or space. The advantages tend to create the challenges. Team members remain in their work environment, limiting time away from patient care. However, that convenience can be challenged by competing demands generated by the patient care. When a patient deteriorates shortly before the educator's arrival, learner focus must remain on the patient's needs but is disruptive and interferes with meeting practitioner learning needs. Resolving this remains one of the greatest challenges to in situ training.

Training in situ offers the advantage of learning in a familiar environment, using equipment and supplies that the learner typically uses. This does not mean that learners are confident or competent using the equipment or that it is located in a readily accessible place. Read the Simulation on a Shoestring feature to learn how one simulationist created the SimHide, an equipment transport unit that doubles as a control station but is designed to blend in with the environment. Latent threats to patient safety are uncovered, interventions implemented, and improvements realized (Barbeito et al., 2015; Patterson et al., 2008). In situ training is used even prior to opening new units or facilities to help determine patient care flow. One hospital reported they

had not realized the time it took to transport critically ill patients from one department to another.

While advantageous to train in the clinical environment, serious risk to patients was highlighted when 40 patients received intravenous fluids using a product intended only for simulation use, falling ill as a result (Szabo, 2015). The product, labeled for simulation use, is only sold to academic institutions; however, it found its way to the clinical environment—in seven different states. Simulationists frequently deactivate potentially dangerous equipment such as defibrillators. Open, unused, and now unsterile kits and outdated supplies are donated (e.g., central line) to simulation labs. It is high-risk practice that may result in supplies and equipment designated for simulation use accidentally being used for real patient care.

An interesting phenomenon that occurs in situ but not in the simulation laboratory is the potential for real patients, families, and visitors to observe training. Some are concerned that observers may believe training takes time away from the provider attending to their needs or may observe mistakes and believe that the care provider regularly errs. Others argue that the observer may be reassured that their caregiver receives ongoing training and efforts at care improvement are evident (Patterson et al., 2008).

There are several aspects of in situ training that may increase costs. Transporting equipment poses risk of damage (Clapper, 2013a). A significant cost can be accrued by employee-related activities. For example, when a simulationist is working entirely within the confines of a sim lab, supplies are handy, the rooms that require setup are close, and learners come to the simulationists. When training in situ, supplies and simulators must be gathered and packaged for transport; the simulationist is not available for other work within the lab. This may be considered unproductive time in some labs, depending on calculation of usage hours (Clapper, 2013a) and the lab's mission.

However, from the learner perspective, they are not taken away from their working environment so continue to be productive up to and immediately following training. The educational opportunity is brought to them, eliminating time to transport themselves to the lab and, in many cases, avoiding payment of overtime as they do not need to attend training during time off (Patterson, Blike, & Nadkarni, 2008). The cost-efficiency of in situ training is dependent upon the relationship of the lab and the in situ location. Various methods to control costs can be undertaken, such as sharing costs of equipment purchases among departments. The management of budget needs for in situ training is beyond this section's scope.

Best Practices

The process of identifying learning needs, developing objectives, scenario design, debriefing, and evaluation

Creating SimHide

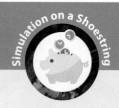

Tobias C. Everett, MBChB, EDRA, FRCA

The Challenge

We run in situ interprofessional team training programs and transported equipment on a wheeled garage shelving unit, which doubled as a display stand for the vital signs monitor. The garage shelves were, needless to say, incongruous in the clinical environment! In addition, the sim technician seated behind the shelves was a distraction for learners. During in situ simulation exercises, the learners should interact with the mannequin but ideally, the computer operator and associated paraphernalia should not physically intrude. We needed a solution that could house, transport, and hide all the gear (and a computer operator) but not be conspicuous in the real clinical areas where we were running simulations.

Innovative Solutions

I've improvised solutions before (e.g., multiple GoPro cameras as a mobile a/v solution) but projects work out better when you involve someone who is properly trained! I had an idea of how to solve this challenge but would need help from our biomedical engineers. They would think of factors to do with structural integrity, load bearing, maneuverability, etc. We identified furniture large enough (once "gutted") to accommodate all the simulation equipment, universal to all clinical care areas, and amenable to "gutting." A tall, double-fronted medical supply cart fit the bill, and we salvaged a damaged one. From the front, the unit would still have to look like clinical supply shelves, but from the back it had to be hollow. Taking the shelves out of the unit was easy, but then, we had to create sham shelf-fronts that gave the impression of well-stocked shelves but in reality had no depth. We sawed off the front of the shelves, and glued in a divider behind so that they were only an inch deep. With enough expired medical disposables

wedged in the fake shelves, the disguise was complete. To allow the computer operator to view the action, we made a plexiglass viewing window onto which we stuck reflective film to create an effective one-way glass. To design the interior, we made a desk-height shelf on the same side as the viewing window so that the operator could use the laptop seated on a stool while still being able to see out of the viewing window. We added flat shelves to accommodate the various components of simulation and audiovisual equipment. Cable holes allowed us to feed the data and power cables from one compartment to the next. We mounted cameras discretely, either nestled among the medical supplies on the shelves or stuck on the frame exterior. Live video feed from these cameras to a separate laptop inside the SimHide meant that the operator had added perspectives beyond what's visible through the window. We mounted a hospital-grade power bar on the SimHide so that on location we only need to plug into a single electrical outlet. We reinforced the base of the unit so that we could house the mannequin's compressor and not require a nearby medical air outlet. There is sufficient space to easily transport the baby or child-size mannequin. Figures 7.7 and 7.8 show the front and rear sides of SimHide, respectively. We would have to revisit the design if it was to transport an adult-sized mannequin. We are planning to add a cargo net across the back of

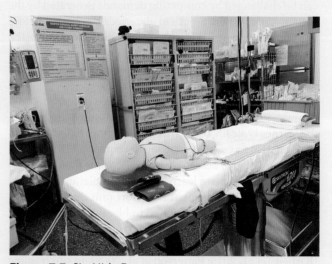

Figure 7.7 SimHide Front.

Creating SimHide (*Continued*)

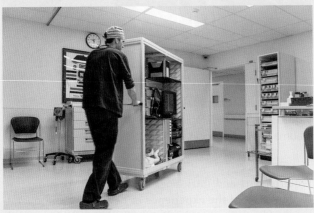

the unit for use during transport to prevent items falling out if we take a sharp corner too quickly! We visit all corners of the hospital with SimHide—everywhere we do in situ interprofessional team training. It fit on all the elevators. It is quite a large unit so we've found space at a premium in some of the tighter areas. Aside from this, there have been no drawbacks to introducing SimHide except rolling it out has induced immediate requests for another one!

Figure 7.8 SimHide Back.

is covered in Chapter 20. Best practices related to the logistics of preparation and implementation are suggested:

- Determine cost/benefit ratio.
- Evaluate if adequate physical space for equipment and learner movement.
- Determine how to safely transport equipment. Is there secure storage at a repetitively used site?
- Schedule time to pack and transport equipment. If transfer by private vehicle, ensure personal insurance coverage for potential damage or loss.
- Verify learners are scheduled to be present as planned.
- Obtain contact information for key personnel (e.g., distribution department to obtain additional supplies).
- Boldly label equipment and supplies "for simulation use only."
- Develop checklist similar to that of a "sponge count" to ensure supplies not left behind.
- Collaborate with leadership to determine response to training interruptions. Will training be postponed, paused, rescheduled?
- Schedule too much, rather than too little time. Ensure time for adequate debriefing.
- Notify patients, families, and visitors of training activities and expectations.
- Determine how in situ training will be reflected in simulation program metrics.

- Provide regular debriefing sessions for facilitators and simulation personnel to identify strengths and areas for improvement.

There are many considerations, particularly if training is to take place outside of the organizational system in which the simulation lab resides. Clapper (2013a) provides additional insight into the level of detail needed, as well as offers a checklist to help organize the experience.

Conclusion

In situ simulation education provides important opportunities for healthcare providers without access to simulation labs or equipment by bringing the training to them. Learning in the environment in which one practices has identified latent hazards to patient safety (Barbeito et al., 2015), built interdisciplinary teamwork and confidence (Klipfel et al., 2015), transfer of outcomes such as task speed and task completion rates to clinical practice (Steinemann et al., 2011), and result in improved recognition and management of deteriorating patients (Theilen, Leonard, & Jones, 2013). A systematic review (Rosen, Hunt, Pronovost, Federowicz, & Weaver, 2012) found positive learning and performance outcomes; however, there was inconsistency with simulation design and implementation. It is important for simulationists to adhere to best practices in simulation design and delivery for in situ simulation in order to mitigate the challenges that occur when teaching and learning in real clinical environments.

Mobile Simulation-Based Medical Education

Mike Lamacchia, EMT-P, CMTE

James L. Huffman, MD, BSc, FRCPC

Jane Duncan, EdD

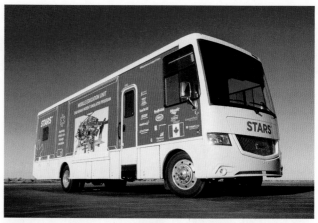

Figure 7.9 Mobile Simulation Laboratory. (Courtesy of Shock Trauma Air Rescue Society [STARS]. Photo by Dave Stobbe.)

Introduction and Background

Healthcare training, regardless of geographical proximity, poses very real challenges in terms of time, equity, resource availability, and expertise. This problem is further exacerbated by the significant percentage of healthcare providers working in remote or rural areas who have limited or no access to urban simulation centers or to in situ simulation. To promote equity and quality training of healthcare professionals, various alternative delivery models have been utilized, including mobile simulation, distributed simulation, and virtual simulation. This section will look specifically at mobile simulation, referred to here as mobile simulation-based medical education or mobile SBME.

For the purposes of this section, mobile SBME is defined as an SBME program, not necessarily tied to a specific curriculum, which is delivered by facilitators who travel to the participants' location to deliver SBME (Fig. 7.9). These facilitators bring equipment (mannequins, mobile simulation laboratory, etc.) and their expertise in operating the hardware and software as well as leading and debriefing the simulation session. The participants are generally in a nonacademic center (often rural) and usually don't have ready access to other opportunities for SBME.

Mobile SBME helps address issues of equity, resource availability, and expertise while presenting interesting opportunities and challenges. While increasing access for teams and individuals who may not otherwise get the opportunity to participate in SBME, it also adds complexities in logistics and funding to those that already exist for nonmobile simulation programs.

This section will explore some of the specific requirements and intricacies of mobile SBME programs. Examples from the experience of developing and operating the Shock Trauma Air Rescue Society (STARS) mobile SBME program in Western Canada will be used to illustrate some of these concepts.

Logistics, Funding, and Staffing for Mobile Simulation

Mobile SBME programs have specific demands for logistics, funding, and personnel that differ from programs in purpose-built simulation laboratories, large tertiary or academic hospitals. Some mobile programs use large motor homes designed to include control rooms, debriefing spaces, and mock patient care areas stocked with equipment used to represent anything from the back of a helicopter to a makeshift ICU room. Other programs simply provide equipment (mannequins, task trainers, etc.) and rely on local resources such as a resuscitation bay or a meeting room for space. Advancements in mannequin technology made it easier to run scenarios in a destination site's own facility (in situ simulation) and provide an opportunity to look at issues such as space design, human factors, and functional use of space (Miller, Riley, Davis, & Hansen, 2008; Mullan, Wuestner, Kerr, Christopher, & Patel, 2013). Using an existing simulation laboratory creates a more controlled environment, increases efficiency by eliminating a great deal of setup and takedown time, and decreases chance of equipment malfunction because it is moved less frequently. Figures 7.10 and 7.11 show examples of how STARS has configured simulation space.

From a funding perspective, a hurdle for mobile SBME programs is maintaining ongoing operational funding distinct from the costs of start-up and hardware. Mobile programs require budgets for gas, lodging, meals away,

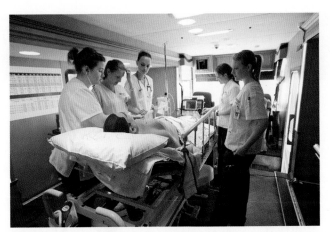

Figure 7.10 Space Design for Running Scenarios. (Courtesy of Shock Trauma Air Rescue Society [STARS]. Photo by Dave Stobbe.)

travel time for staff, maintenance of simulation equipment and vehicles used for transportation, and unanticipated equipment failure at a destination site. Obtaining funding for specific capital purchases (new mannequin, ventilator) is generally easier than obtaining ongoing funding to run the program. Some funding sources for STARS have included private and corporate donors, provincial programs designed to support rural healthcare providers, and service organizations.

When staffing mobile simulation programs, we found it helpful to include a multiprofessional facilitation team, for example, having a nurse available to help debrief nurses or a physician when the team includes physicians. This has helped increase buy-in from the participants. Anecdotally, running and delivering a mobile simulation program may lead to increased staff turnover compared

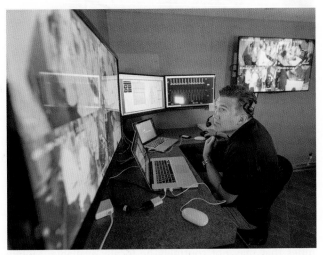

Figure 7.11 Space Design for Control and Monitoring of Scenarios. (Courtesy of Shock Trauma Air Rescue Society [STARS]. Photo by Dave Stobbe.)

to nonmobile programs. This may be related to time away from home, family, and support networks, a sense of disconnectedness from other team members, the potentially repetitive work, and long hours facilitating preceded and followed by long hours traveling. As a result, good support and a sustainability plan are essential for maintaining a program over time.

Finally, due to time, capital, and physical resource requirements, it is essential to have commitment from participants well in advance of the trip. When recruiting participants and planning sessions, consider approaching multiple disciplines (physicians, nurses, respiratory therapists, nursing assistants, etc.). Doing so increases the conceptual fidelity of the scenarios and the likelihood of adequate numbers of participants (Rudolph, Simon, & Raemer, 2007). Consider running multiple sessions, possibly over several days, to allow multiple groups or teams to participate within one road trip.

Education Delivery

Differences in participant emotion, stress, and cognitive load during mobile SBME compared with nonmobile SBME have not been studied; however, it has been the experience of the STARS mobile simulation leadership group that participants at rural sites have higher negative emotion, stress, and cognitive load than participants who have more access to simulation education. This may be due to lack of familiarity with the modality, but there may be some aspect of feeling as if "the experts are coming to judge me." Modifications can be made to mitigate some of these factors and enhance learning.

Ensure cases align with the participants' learning needs, objectives, and resources. Select cases that could be realistically encountered and that utilize available resources. For example, planning a case that requires the local presence of a neurosurgeon despite the fact that there would rarely be such a resource available in that community decreases the applicability of the case. In situ educators are often challenged by lack of audiovisual capabilities in the clinical environment. Learn about an inexpensive mobile recording option in the Simulation on a Shoestring feature.

Participants are often healthcare providers with limited local resources who generally have less routine experience with the types of cases being simulated. With that in mind, and also considering research on the impact of emotion and stress on learning, provide several lifelines, such as contact with a mock-receiving physician in a tertiary care center or access to various web resources, within the cases to assist learners who may be struggling. Also, Fraser et al. (2014) suggest that when participants have high cognitive load and negative emotions, it is likely better to avoid unexpected death of the mannequin,

Portable Debriefing

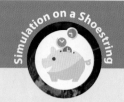

Michael Paul Lundin

The Challenge

Our Clinical Simulation Program had three sites requiring a recording system for debriefing. After some contemplation of the $25 to $40K systems on the market, I decided to focus on finding a more affordable user-friendly solution. The software in existing systems posed a barrier for instructors to use. Another challenge was having only one technician supporting the three sites, so remote tech support was a desired feature. I decided to use something that everyone is familiar with and is relatively inexpensive—an iPad.

Innovative Solutions

Using an iPad combined with an IV pole and connection cables provide each site with a low-cost solution. The components include: iPad, iPad locking number bracket, pole mount locking adjustable mount, IV pole, VGA cable with 3.5-mm audio, iPad adaptor to VGA and 3.5 mm as that is our current debriefing room input, VGA gender bender for connecting to existing cabling, 3.5 coupler for connecting to existing cabling, and FaceTime accounts on all iPads. The connections and setup are illustrated in Figure 7.12. This has been very well received and used by instructors since implementation. They especially like the ease of use with one-touch recording, quality of recordings, and connection to the AV system. The recordings are deleted at the end of each session in front of the learner group. Another key benefit is that we can provide live remote tech support to each site through FaceTime. This is especially handy to walk instructors through troubleshooting steps for the simulator operation or support cabling.

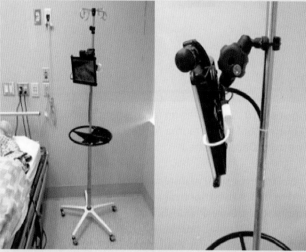

Front view of setup   Side view showing iPad adaptor
                                    to VGA/3.5

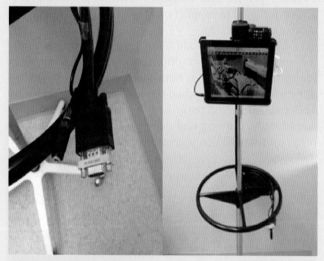

VGA Cable with adaptors for   Front view showing Bracket and
connection   lock release

Figure 7.12 iPad Mobile Recording.

unless managing death is a specific objective for the learning experience. Another suggestion for maximizing participant learning, particularly with those less experienced with the material and the modality, is to choose minimally complex tasks/cases and offer participants an opportunity to run a case for the facilitators.

Conclusion

Mobile SBME programs provide unique opportunities for rural healthcare practitioners to access learning opportunities that may not routinely be locally available. Mobile programs come with challenges in logistics, funding, staffing, and program development. As evidenced by STARS' experience in mobile SBME programs, these challenges can be mitigated in service of the community's learning needs.

Telesimulation (Broadcast)

Deepak Manhas, MD, FAAP, FRCP(C)

Telehealth uses secure videoconferencing technology to exchange health information across geographic barriers (Ried, 1996). Telesimulation uses these telehealth links and other methods of two-way interactive video (e.g., Skype) to provide simulation experiences to those restricted by those geographic barriers. Healthcare providers at the participating site use their equipment to run a scenario that can be observed by others. Experts in the medical field and in simulation are able to develop appropriate clinical scenarios, provide them to educators in other locations to implement, and observe the simulated scenario at a distance via the telehealth link. The experts are then able to provide feedback with debriefing following the encounter.

In Situ Telesimulation

Using this method, healthcare providers working in rural, geographically restricted, or resource-poor healthcare centers can practice in situ simulation while eliminating the cost of travel for participants and instructors. The participants benefit from having expert instructors providing them feedback. However, this modality does require the participating site to have the appropriate simulation equipment.

An example of a simulation scenario designed for this type of situation is the use of the Neonatal Resuscitation Program (NRP) algorithm for a newly born infant who is limp and apneic. If the learning objective is to apply the NRP for an infant in distress, a neonatal mannequin would be ideal and the scenario should take place in a delivery room. Additional equipment that would be beneficial includes a radiant warmer and neonatal supplies in order to establish an airway and circulation. Ideally, the expert instructor could control the mannequin remotely in order to adjust vital signs and clinical findings in a manner that is consistent with the steps the participants are performing during the resuscitation. If the instructor cannot control the simulation equipment remotely, changes in vital signs may need to be provided via the telehealth link, or an additional technology support staff may need to make adjustments to the simulation mannequin under the guidance of the instructor. Not all healthcare facilities have access to simulation equipment but may benefit from involvement in these scenarios in an effort to improve patient outcomes.

In the previous example, a healthcare facility may not have a neonatal mannequin. However, perhaps a pediatric mannequin may suffice if the participants are able to suspend disbelief sufficiently. Alternatively, a doll (essentially an extremely low-fidelity mannequin) may be used. In this case, the expert instructor may have to verbally provide the participants with the vital signs and clinical examination findings or perhaps on a screen shared via the telehealth link that displays a cardiorespiratory monitor. Use of lower-fidelity equipment and supplies would limit the ability of the participants to perform procedural skills such as establishing an alternate airway (with a laryngeal mask airway or endotracheal tube).

Expert Modeling Telesimulation

Occasionally, the learners are not yet ready to participate in a hand-on simulation, or due to limitation in resources, participation may not be possible. In this case, the use of expert modeling may be useful. In this approach, the learner is able to gain insight into the expert's thought process while he or she is dealing with an authentic problem. The learner is able to establish a scaffold for the process or problem in question and strive to achieve the same result as the expert. Modeling through a demonstration is an effective learning strategy for procedural skills (Anderson & Warren, 2011). In the apprenticeship model, this is the basis of the old medical maxim, "see one, do one, teach one." Though now the need for deliberate and repetitive practice for mastery learning is appreciated, the concept of expert modeling is still crucial.

Returning to the previous example of neonatal resuscitation, healthcare providers in outreach areas may benefit tremendously by actively observing a live demonstration of a neonatal resuscitation by experts in the field via a telehealth link. Though these healthcare providers don't have a hands-on experience in this scenario, they are able to observe the flow of the resuscitation, experience the thought process of the expert leading the scenario, and observe the technical aspects of any procedural skills. Scenarios can also be designed that provide opportunities for observers to direct the next steps of care as they observe the patient management from a distance, allowing development of critical thinking, clinical judgement, communication, teamwork, and prioritization skills. Furthermore, those observing can also actively engage in the debriefing session following the scenario.

Limitation of Telesimulation

These examples demonstrate some potential limitations of telesimulation and some potential methods to circumvent these barriers. Unfortunately, some centers have experienced increased technological difficulties using the telehealth technologies as well as the simulated technologies. One common difficulty involves insufficient bandwidth with the telehealth technologies that results in significant audio or visual delays leading to disruption of flow and frustration with participants on both sides of the telehealth link. Trying to participate in telesimulation with a low bandwidth is like watching a movie that keeps skipping or the audio is not proceeding at the same rate as the visual pictures. As bandwidths in hospitals continue to improve, this may no longer be as significant an issue. Some centers have had recurring issues being able to connect via the telehealth bridge and sometimes give up on the entire endeavor because of this. Having accessible IT support can help immensely in this regard. Technical support staff may also be able to assist with the setup of simulation equipment in the community hospital. Developing a good relationship with the technical support staff is key for telesimulation to be efficient and effective.

Using Simulation in the Classroom

Margaret Milner, MN, RN

Simulation in the classroom provides a unique opportunity for students to explore theoretical concepts at the point of learning. Creating intersections in the learning environment where theoretical knowledge is realized through practice assists students to find meaning in clinical encounters, realize personal strengths, and identify opportunities for continued growth. Classroom simulation is increasing as educators search for innovative and effective ways to engage students in meaningful learning activities. To achieve classroom simulation, educators use a variety of simulation typologies such as mannequins, standardized patients, actors or role-players, avatars, holograms, VR gear and head display mounting, or other tools such as case studies. Classroom simulation can be combined with other modalities such as screen-based virtual reality (VR) or broadcast simulation (Fig. 7.13).

Theoretical Underpinnings

Simulated learning experiences (SLE) in the classroom provide educators with a unique opportunity to engage students in transformational learning for the purpose of bringing awareness to emotional reactions and responses to enacted situations. Transformational learning theory (TLT), first described by Mezirow (1991), refers to adult learning processes where shifts in beliefs and identity occur because of the integration of new information into

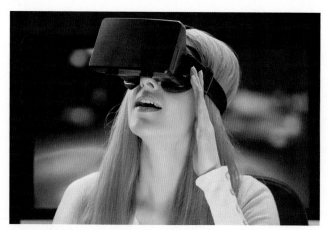

Figure 7.13 Virtual Reality Goggles. (Courtesy of Shutterstock.com.)

pre-existing schema (Taylor, 2009). TLT closely approximates with situated cognition but expands learning beyond the cognitive realm, where openings for a shift in the learner's "state of being in the world" are realized, including their sense of agency and relatedness (Lange, 2004).

Current Evidence to Support Classroom Simulation

Few studies have examined the use of simulation in the classroom. Students who participated in an unfolding scenario using a high-fidelity simulator projected onto a video screen reported increased confidence in their clinical reasoning skills (Norman, Thompson, & Missildine, 2013). Evaluation of exam scores following a learning experience using simulation videos and debriefing versus traditional didactic instruction and case studies found no significant difference in final exam scores (Zulkosky, 2012). Hooper, Shaw, and Zamzam (2015) also found no differences in pre/post scores after conducting classroom simulation that included participants and observers who watched the scenario via video streaming in another room. The authors describe methods that classroom educators can use to provide opportunities to engage large numbers of learners when either time or space is not available in the laboratory setting. Additionally, Pollard and Wild (2014) discuss the use of role-play to teach leadership competence with an emphasis on situational awareness and effective team communication. By interspersing simulation exercises throughout the semester, students had opportunities to enhance teamwork, leadership, and followership roles. Debriefing and critical reflection encouraged double and triple-loop learning while exposing students to transactional, transformative, and transcendent leadership styles.

Computer-Based and Virtual Classroom Strategies

Technological development has led to reasonably priced, high-quality virtual reality (VR) simulation applications.

These screen-based applications are primarily for individual learning and assessment but can be easily adapted for use in classroom simulation. Computerized classroom simulation can facilitate student immersion into virtually any clinical practice world to unleash imagination, provide exposure to "real" patients and families, and allow for active experimentation. Patient simulation software and VR in the classroom allows students to participate in a realistic scenario where they can apply their newly acquired skills and knowledge. Simulation software can be projected on the screen, and as scenarios progress, students can anticipate, predict, and explain physiological changes while prioritizing the nursing interventions that should occur as a result. Two-way interactive video can be used to connect participants in the sim lab with observers in the classroom. Additional examples of how to use simulation in the classroom can be found in Leighton (2016). Read the Simulation on a Shoestring feature to learn how one simulationist created a mobile headwall to take into the classroom and other areas outside the clinical environment to increase fidelity of the environment. Examples of some products available to enhance classroom simulation are included in Table 7.3. Game-based learning in the virtual world

Table 7.3	Examples of Classroom Virtual Reality Tools
VSim	https://youtu.be/UiLFUKpMSAk
Second Life	http://secondlife.com/
MUVE Market	https://youtu.be/FWUpXar6sh8
Shadow Health	https://youtu.be/A3g0Gcw8Op8
Cyberanatomy	https://youtu.be/4vsP93OqlN8
SimX	https://youtu.be/5E0Hg4k9Ems
Anatomage	https://youtu.be/Q7SHE_s8-P8
Google Glasses	https://youtu.be/4EvNxWhskf8
Meta 2 Vision	https://www.metavision.com
Oculus Rift	https://www.oculus.com/en-us

offers expanded options for classroom-based simulation (Bauman, 2012). A case exemplar outlining use of video and small group activities to create a simulation activity is in Box 7-1.

Box 7-1   Classroom Simulation Case Exemplar

A video was created for senior undergraduate nursing students that focused on conflict management while transitioning to the role of the registered nurse. In the video, two recent graduates of the program and two faculty members engaged in role-play to portray incivility toward a new graduate by a senior nurse. Students prepared for the class by reading an article on advocacy and inquiry as a communication strategy to elicit frames when providing feedback (Rudolph, Simon, Dufresne, & Raemer, 2006), in addition to an article on cognitive rehearsal, a strategy used to assist new graduates to deal effectively with horizontal violence in the workplace (Griffin, 2004). The class started with a prebriefing that included a discussion of the readings and setting the stage for the scene in the video. The facilitator discussed the simulation objectives, drawing attention to the fictional contract and psychological safety for enactment of the scenario (INACSL Standards Committee, 2016, Facilitation). Students then viewed the video as a large group. Immediately following the viewing, individual students spent time journaling about their immediate response to the vignette. They then broke into small groups that they had been working in during the semester—an additional safety factor. Students took on the role of the various individuals from the video and re-enacted the scenario, taking turns practicing cognitive rehearsal techniques with the senior nurse. In their small groups, students

were then given time to debrief themselves using a Plus Delta Gamma framework (Anderson & Decker, 2013), drawing attention to what went well and what they would change if they could enact the scenario again while reflecting on the effectiveness of the cognitive rehearsal techniques and their experience practicing with advocacy and inquiry. The facilitator conducted a large group debrief, focused on advocacy and inquiry as a method for giving feedback and uncovering frames (INACSL Standards Committee, 2016, Debriefing). Emphasis in the debriefing was directed toward creating meaning rather than the rightness or wrongness of particular approaches or interventions. Toward the end of the class, a second video was shown where the same actors engaged in reconciliation, modeling advocacy, and inquiry. Students then had time to respond to the second video as a large group, reflecting on their capacity for moral courage to advocate for themselves and others in future practice situations. Anecdotal feedback provided in student written reflections following the classroom simulation was, for the most part, positive. Some students indicated that they felt uncomfortable playing the role of the new graduate or the senior nurse in the scenario and preferred to observe rather than engage in the small group role-plays. It should be noted that in the briefing, students were given permission to observe rather than actively role-play to ensure a sense of psychological safety.

Mobile Headwall

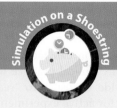

Barbara Peterson, MSN, RN

The Challenge

As a simulation specialist, I provide mobile customized training experiences for internal and external customers. Some simulation sessions require staging in nonclinical areas where there is no access to a medical headwall with oxygen flow and suction. As an educator, I had concerns about building proper muscle memory and was disappointed when I received negative feedback about the lack of clinical realism in my simulations. Commercial products I researched lacked important features, could not be customized, and did not collapse enough for car transport.

Innovative Solutions

My vision for a mobile headwall was shared with our biomedical engineers who had a reputation for innovation. They had built a facade that increased clinical realism in our mobile simulation bus. Their clinical and product knowledge, combined with my ability to find a silent air compressor and quiet suction unit to place behind the headwall, resulted in a customized mobile headwall that simulates oxygen flow, suction, and additional requested features. I now have a product that I can take apart, load into a car (with other simulation equipment), rebuild, and roll into an area for a realistic simulation.

This mobile headwall has been very effective in creating a sense of realism in the numerous nonclinical spaces at sites I travel to (Figs. 7.14 and 7.15). Based on need, a second headwall was built with a few modifications. The only drawback to the headwall is noise from the suction machine despite its designation as "quiet." The headwall does have a storage footprint of about H6′ × W30″ × D16.5″.

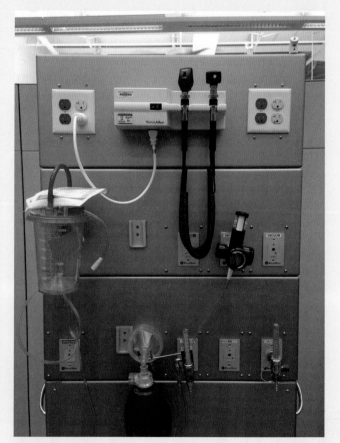

Figure 7.14 Front of Portable Headwall.

Figure 7.15 Back of Portable Headwall.

Challenges and Opportunities in Classroom Simulation

Ensuring appropriately educated facilitators conduct in-class simulation is critical. Enacting interactive pedagogy in the classroom is a serious endeavor and educators should follow the INACSL Standards of Best Practice:

Simulation^{SM}, regardless of the location or type of SLE. Rudolph, Raemer, and Simon (2014) identify practices to ensure student psychological safety when conducting simulation in the classroom, including structured and intentional prebriefing of students (i.e., reviewing objectives, addressing confidentiality, identification of roles, and clearly laying out expectations), "establishing a fictional contract, and conveying respect and interest in the learner's perspective" (p. 341).

In-class simulations create unique challenges for educators and students alike, stemming in large part from the uncontrolled nature of the classroom environment. A primary goal when conducting in-class simulations is to be flexible and responsive to the needs of the learners and portray willingness to change the planned sequence of events if warranted. One teacher working with a larger group of students is not able to make detailed observations of individual students so it is important to consider the tone of the classroom during activities. For this reason, the timing and group size of in-class SLEs are important considerations. Establishing trust and conveying genuine interest in student perspective helps ensure success. Debriefing at intervals throughout the simulation event may address emerging issues as they arise. Evaluation of student performance should be done with caution unless an adequate number of evaluators are available. Encouraging students to write a short self-reflection can be an effective way to assist them with finding meaning inside the simulation encounter and provide the facilitator with feedback to adapt in-class simulations in the future.

In summary, simulation in the classroom can foster meaningful student engagement in the learning environment. Thoughtful consideration in development of SLEs, paying attention to pedagogy, best practice standards, and creating psychological safety are important antecedents for success.

Just-In-Time Training

AnneMarie Monachino, MSN, RN, CPN, CHSE

Introduction/Background

Just-in-time education refers to training that is conducted directly prior to a potential intervention (Huang et al., 2015). Oftentimes, nurses are asked to perform complex procedures, and if that nurse has not performed the skill on a regular basis, he or she may lack confidence in their ability. This real-time refresher training may increase a clinician's self-confidence and decrease the risk of harm to a patient (Monachino & Tuttle, 2015). This concept of just-in-time education can be integrated fairly easily into simulation programs. Simulation provides a unique educational strategy to promote the development of psychomotor, critical thinking, teamwork and communication skills, as well as preparing clinicians to work in interprofessional teams (IOM, 2011). As a nurse and an educator who employs simulation as a teaching methodology, I see simulation as a combination of art and science. The art of simulation is how the educator chooses from a diverse spectrum of simulation typologies and modalities based upon the learning objectives, the intended audience, and the timeframe for the education while incorporating his or her understanding of the educational principles (science) behind simulation.

As per the INACSL Standards of Best Practice: Simulation, an educational activity should be guided

by specific learning objectives (INACSL Standards Committee, 2016, Scenario Design). The objectives of this section are to discuss the benefits and challenges of using just-in-time simulation-based training as an educational strategy; identify opportunities for using just-in-time simulation, including skills refresher training, impromptu team training, preparing for low-frequency/high-risk situations, and exploring latent safety risks; and discuss methods to incorporate just-in-time simulation-based training with limited resources.

Benefits and Challenges

In the healthcare setting, just-in-time simulation-based training occurs right before the learner needs to perform the intervention in a clinical situation. Some of the benefits to this type of training are that it provides the learner, who has already achieved some level of competency in the skill or behavior, an opportunity to refresh or practice a skill that he or she may not have performed recently. It can be done in the clinical setting with minimal interruption to clinical responsibilities, and it provides real time education and feedback. This type of simulation can be challenging in that an educator may not be available to conduct the training or the equipment or space may not be easily obtained (Monachino & Tuttle, 2015).

Opportunities for Just-In-Time Training (JITT)

As a simulation educator, you may encounter opportunities to develop just-in-time programs. This type of training works well for psychomotor-based skills such as CPR, urinary catheter insertion, tracheal intubation, lumbar puncture, and IV insertion, to name a few. This education requires an appropriate simulator (i.e., partial task trainer, full-body mannequin), the necessary equipment or supplies, a procedure or checklist, and an educator or content expert to provide feedback. For more details as to how to implement JITT, see the Step-by-Step Plan for Just-in-Time Training found in the online toolkit (Monachino & Tuttle, 2015).

For those of you who do not have the luxury of having an educator or a content expert readily available, it is possible to still provide this training. Create your own video of the skill being properly performed or access an online video of the skill (make sure it matches your institution's procedure). Include directions on how to access the video in your just-in-time skill training documents. Although the learner will not get feedback, he or she can practice while watching the expert perform the task. This rehearsal will refresh their knowledge and increase muscle memory of the psychomotor skill.

In addition to skills training, the just-in-time concept can be applied to affective learning objectives (communication/teamwork) and higher-level cognitive (synthesis/analysis) or critical thinking objectives. One may consider this type of training for interprofessional teams, especially those who are called upon to participate in a low-frequency/high-risk event such as a multiple birth delivery that requires many hands-on deck, a complicated surgical procedure such as the separation of conjoined twins or a bilateral hand transplant, or a precipitous delivery that requires a maternal team to respond to the mother and a neonatal team to resuscitate the newborn. In my institution, we have executed interprofessional just-in-time simulations for events such as these. In each case, the objectives addressed not only the steps of the surgical and medical procedure but effective communication techniques, resource management, situational awareness, and role definition. An added bonus was that the in situ simulation exposed potential safety issues that could be addressed prior to the actual patient care event.

Imagine being a new member of a Rapid Response or Code Team. While an expert in the field of critical care nursing, you are new to working on this team of physicians, respiratory therapists, and perhaps a pharmacist, a social worker, and a security officer. The Interprofessional Education Collaborative Expert Panel (IPECEP) found that effective communication and teamwork is essential to maximizing patient outcomes and improving patient safety (IPECEP, 2011). While many recognize the importance of training teams, it is not easy to accomplish and requires engagement and support from key stakeholders and leaders. Involving members from the various professions in the planning of the just-in-time simulation program will enhance your potential for a successful outcome.

Delivering excellent care to our patients is something we as nurses and other healthcare clinicians strive to do. As a simulation educator, you may not be directly providing care, but you have so much influence on those who do. By using simulation as a teaching tool, especially just-in-time simulation training, you are providing contextual guidance, feedback, and experiential learning opportunities, which contribute to the development of competent providers who deliver safe, quality care.

Conclusion

This chapter has covered numerous modalities for using various simulation typologies, with the goal of expanding your thoughts as to how best to use simulation to meet the needs of your learners and the objectives you've developed for the simulation-based learning experience. The chapter provided background into the methods, advantages, and challenges to the modalities and provided suggestions for best practice when implementing these engaging ways to use simulation in often nontraditional ways. A variety of experts shared their experiences creating and implementing simulation experiences within a modality, while others shared their inexpensive solutions to help overcome the challenges. Be wary of getting caught in the thinking that only simulators can be used for simulation education—and that it can only occur in the simulation lab. You can make simulation happen anywhere!

8 Simulation Champions as Leaders, Followers, and Managers: Advocating, Dreaming, Influencing, Challenging, and Executing!

Carol Wild, Colette Foisy-Doll

"When you are just EXISTING, life happens to you… and you manage; When you are truly LIVING, you happen to life… and you lead."—Steve Maraboli, Unapologetically You: Reflections on Life and the Human Experience

Key Terms

Leadership, Management, Followership, Transactional, Transformational, Transcendent, Relationships, Values Based, Complexity Science, Moral Courage, Change, Models, New Science of Leadership, Reflexivity

Guiding Questions

1 How can Simulation Champions leverage leadership, followership, and managership theory to excel in their leader, manager, and follower roles?

2 Have you spent time reflecting on your leadership style and how it might impact team performance and simulation program outcomes?

3 How can the modern Simulation Champion move beyond the pioneering all-in-one leader/manager approaches of yesteryear to embrace new facets of leader/manager roles?

Introduction

Leaders, followers, and managers: much has been written how to become them, what not to do; why one is better than the other; how we can blame them, how corrupt they are; why they are essential, indeed why we cannot live without them; and how we admire and want to be like them. Leadership, followership, and managership have been evident in written work starting primarily in the 20th century and have illuminated our thinking and understanding of the importance of being people focused. Contemporary leadership approaches have shifted their focus to relationship. Relation-based leadership focuses on relationships within the structures, processes, and outcomes—in change, transformation, communication, and teams—and the efficacy of organizations, groups, and communities. This focus has provided new direction for leadership in the 21st century. Together, these concepts have challenged the thinking and being of persons in groups, teams, collectives, and organizations thus influencing local, regional, and global perspectives.

This chapter is for Simulation Champions, a.k.a., the simulation advocates, supporters, and dreamers that have taken on the managership of simulation and want to be introduced to the importance of followership and the significance of transformational leadership for system change.

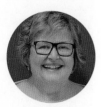

Carol Wild,
MScN, BN, RN

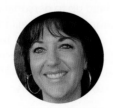

Colette Foisy-Doll,
MSN, RN, CHSE

Today, there are many innovative and inspiring Simulation Champions in healthcare. At the forefront are nurses and nurse educators, and we have noted that many of them have not had the experience of formal training in leadership, followership, and managership. Therefore, the main goal of this chapter is to stimulate you to reflect and act on new leadership paradigms for Simulation Champions of the 21st century. Using a social lens, we provide a brief historical summary of leadership and followership development. Also, some grounding in the historical significance of management, leadership, and followership theory is presented but comprehensive dialogue and debate of leadership theory are left to experts and scholars in the field.

In this chapter, we honor the contributions from the following leadership theorists and authors: Burns, Bass, Kellerman, Kelly, Chaleff, Bennis, Kouzes and Posner, Goleman, Senge, Wheatley, and Porter O'Grady. As the reader, you are asked to reflect on personal knowledge throughout the chapter. This chapter is also about empowering you to use and apply knowledge from this century toward a needed paradigm shift in leadership for the 21st century. To facilitate this process, we review concepts critical to the developing leader, manager, and follower within each Simulation Champion and each simulation team member. Effort has been made to link to the INACSL Standards of Best Practice: Simulation^SM (2016), and each reader is encouraged to be familiar with the standards as they engage in discourse with our topics.

"We all know much more than what we do. When it comes to leadership, knowledge isn't power. Only applied knowledge is power."—**Jim Clemmer (p. 10, Growing the Distance)**

Historical Significance of Leader and Leadership Theory

Our belief is that leader, follower, and manager are each different but uniquely related. Different competencies and characteristics define each of these roles, transpiring across multiple continuums. Consequently, leadership, followership, management, and managership involve processes and theories simultaneously designed to assist Simulation Champions in the development of their role. The champion will need knowledge of each role and each theory to optimize effectiveness and efficiency as they develop their unique being.

The Origins of the Constructs Leader and Leadership

"Leadership probably has a long evolutionary history. It may have emerged as a solution to specific group coordination challenges—group movement, intragroup conflict, and intergroup competition are prime candidates. Arguably, individual fitness would be enhanced by living in groups with effective leadership"—**Van Vugt, Hogan, and Kaiser (2008, p. 184)**.

Reflection Activity 8-1
Personal Leadership Development Activity and Journal

If you have begun to read this chapter, you are obviously on a leadership journey or at least intrigued with the notion of it or find yourself thrust into it. Welcome! Leadership is about *development from the inside out*. Simulation Champions don't become great leaders, managers, and followers because of a conferred title or assigned task. They take the time to learn about these roles and engage in a continuous improvement process of *becoming*.

PERSONAL DEVELOPMENT: *Reflection activity* boxes are inserted periodically to ask you to take a development moment. You can find a leadership journal in the online Toolkit (Toolkit 8-1) that you can personalize, giving you a place to write your thoughts, inspirations, and plans for change! This process is about working with your ingrained mental models or internal pictures: bringing them forth to be held up to personal scrutiny. It is about revealing your understanding of personal assumptions and beliefs and how they impact your awareness and your actions. You will also be asked to reflect at the end of the chapter on all the information you have gathered to enhance the leader and follower that resides inside of you. The intent is that the chapter will inform, suggest, provoke, and extend. It is all about increasing personal consciousness or reflexivity.

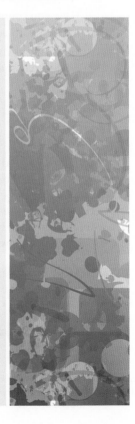

Social groups where cooperation and internal accord were necessary for survival could well be the basis for the evolutionary development of the constructs of leader and leadership (Van Vugt et al., 2008). These authors describe the cognitive processes required to support leadership as the perceived need for coordination; proactive planning; collective courses of action including "specialized decision rules"; initiating selected courses of action; and maintaining group cohesion through "communication, perspective taking, and conflict management" (p. 184). Furthermore, the authors suggest that cognitive processes utilizing intelligences, temperaments, empathy, social identity, and language were critical to leadership function development. Thus, the notion of leader and leadership emerged resulting from *social processes* (followership too, but this will be discussed later). These processes occurred purposefully in collectives, offering us an interesting evolutionary historical perspective of leadership. The word leadership came into common usage at the beginning of the 20th century where early notions are truly based on the role of a leader. Still today, we tend to group the words leader and leadership together. Four nominal stages of leadership practice in human societies are hypothesized and described in the research by Van Vugt et al. (2008). Each of these stages from their perspectives is described below and continues to have global relevance.

Stage 1

Prehuman leadership involved leader–follower structures for coordinating group movement, such as seen in insects, schools of fish, migrating birds, and nonhuman primates. The leader is any individual or alpha in a situational or dominance hierarchy where the leader–follower relations are democratic and/or despotic (autocratic/or dictatorial) (pp. 186–187). It makes logical sense to suggest that leadership and followership are purposeful behaviors in nature and so are similar or natural to human groups and team functioning.

Stage 2

Band and tribal leadership involved seminomadic hunter-gatherers with no formalized leadership role but where the leader as the "big man or head man" had egalitarian and consensual leader–follower relations. These types of leader–follower relationships utilized standards such as "fairness, integrity, competence, good judgement, generosity, humility, and concern for others" (pp. 187–188). It is interesting that these continue to be criteria for measuring 21st century leadership today.

Stage 3

Chiefs, kings, and warlords developed within communities some 13,000 years ago when agricultural and dependable food sources allowed groups to settle and populations to grow. The growth of communities heralded the potential for the growth of intra- and intergroup conflict that resulted in power being used to defend resources, keep and hoard resources, and create dynasties of hereditary leadership. Leaders became powerful due to the legitimization of their roles from the followers. Preindustrialized societies had warlords and soldier classes as norms. The leadership structure was formal and centralized, and the relations between leaders and followers were hierarchical and unilateral (p. 188). Further to these, the command and control hierarchy that we associate with the military did much to advance our knowledge of leadership.

Today, we also see similar warlord societies whenever centralized governments in countries do not function on a democratic equalitarian basis and where political unrest and abuses toward humanity are common occurrences. We can also reflect on the *Great Man theory* of leadership founded on these kings, chiefs, and warlords, and we have been inspired by the autobiographical works and glorious tales of these persons: all great leaders whom have accomplished dreams and overcome challenges. Is it really that they possessed innate abilities as great "men" or "women," or did their life path and choices guide them to become great leaders? Sometimes, we focus so much on, and exalt about, the extraordinary person that the attainment of personal leadership does not seem plausible. Remnants of those early leadership beliefs still echo in statements like, "Who am I to think I can be a great leader?" or "Do I have what it takes to be a great leader?" Simulation Champions today need to understand that extraordinary things can be and are done by ordinary people (Kouzes & Posner, 2007, 2014) who have a dream and do not stop until that dream is accomplished.

Stage 4

State and business leadership covers the time period from the Industrial Revolution, some 260 years ago (Van Vugt et al., 2008). Communities became nations and countries; and large businesses developed, all requiring and having implications for the development of management theories and leadership. Leadership structure became centralized and democratic with individuals as leaders whom were heads of state, managers, and executives with both hierarchal and participatory leader–follower relations. Hierarchal relations existed where the leaders and managers were more responsive and accountable to upper level superiors than to subordinates (pp. 188–192). Herein lays the challenge for the Simulation Champion of today where new generations of workers are changing the landscape of organizations and relationships. Today, transformational leaders encourage followers to see themselves as group members with collective commitment and vision in participatory and partnering relations.

What of Managers, Management, and Managership During This Stage?

In any historical review of the development of leadership, there needs to be discussion about management. The "state and business" perspective originally identified the roles of manager and leader as synonymous. The 1940s, both before and after World War II, saw leadership and management primarily concerned with how to get subordinates to do what was wanted and, in some cases, how to do it (Kellerman, 2008, p. 15). Leadership today has moved away from the command and control model of hierarchical and bureaucratic organizations (p. 15) but not without, even today, some general confusion about the similarities and differences between management and leadership. For example, are leadership and managership roles separate and clearly defined in your current simulation role, or are they presumed to be one?

Zaleznik (1977) wrote a seminal article about the differences between managers and leaders suggesting that "leaders and managers are basically different types of people; the conditions favorable to the growth of one may be inimical to the other" (p. 67). Whereas "leadership inevitably requires using power to influence the thoughts and actions of other people," managerial leadership may not (p. 67). "While ensuring the competence, control, and the balance of power relations among groups with potential for rivalry, managerial leadership unfortunately does not necessarily ensure imagination, creativity, or ethical behavior in guiding the destinies of corporate enterprises" (p. 67). Contemporary views continue to identify the difference between the two as "leaders doing the right thing and managers doing things right" (Bennis & Goldsmith, 2010, p. 31). The Simulation Champion will focus on building capacity as both. At the time, Zaleznik (1977) suggested that myths about who a leader is needed to be challenged, identifying that "managers and leaders differ in motivation, personal history, and in how they think and act." Furthermore, a manager is a problem solver focusing on win–win or win–lose scenarios, while a leader works from a high-risk situation to develop choices and fresh approaches to chronic problems or new issues, engendering strong feelings of identity, indifference, love, or hate (pp. 70–74). Managers were seen as relating to persons based on the roles people were in, while leaders relate in more "intuitive and empathic ways" (p. 73). "There is a call, at the beginning of this tumultuous twenty-first century, for a new brand of leaders who are distinct from what we think of as traditional managers" (Bennis & Goldsmith, 2010, p. 30). Knowing the distinction between managers and leaders becomes vital to understanding the difference between efficiency and effectiveness and progressing to understanding the importance of efficacy and relationship and value-based leadership for today. The leader/manager distinction also has implications when designing Simulation Center position descriptions and organizational structure. As you read through

this section, think about how this could play out in your milieu.

Traditionally, management has been defined as inclusive of five primary functions: controlling, staffing, directing, organizing, and planning. Sometimes, a sixth, leading, is included. Today, managership is a seldom used but is a legitimate term to refer to administration or the overall coordination done by a manager or administrator. It is a term utilized in references to the acceptance of the managership of civic responsibilities, as in town or city or county administrators. Managers, on the other hand, have designated roles within managership as in frontline manager or middle manager or upper administrator.

Leadership within an organization uses similar designations indicating a level of managerial responsibilities and accountabilities with terms such as clinical leader, executive director or leader, and chief executive officer (CEO). Hierarchies and bureaucracies have deliberate intentions in designating roles and titles to denote function, relationships, and lines of accountability and responsibility. Leadership may or may not be attached to these frontline roles in an organization but is sometimes indicated as part of an executive role or upper administrative role in future or strategic planning. Increasingly, the importance of distributed leadership in organizations is recognized in successful and competitive organizations.

Traditional systems of past management models are at their core, dedicated to mediocrity and to forcing people to work harder and harder rather than appreciate the spirit and collective intelligence of teams, partnership, and collaborations (Senge, 2006). Cummings et al. (2010) conducted a systematic review of studies between 1985 and 2009 and found that transformational and relational or people-focused leadership is needed to enhance employee satisfaction, recruitment, retention, and healthy work environments within healthcare settings for nursing staff and ultimately quality care of healthcare consumers. Organizations and individuals, therefore, need to focus on relationship and distributed, people-focused leadership competency development. Ask yourself if this is the case in your environment?

Organizations must have both leaders and managers, and controlling managerial structures and systems must give way to more democratic structures and systems where leaders identify goals and rally support; and managers accomplish concrete goals (Bennis & Goldsmith, 2010, p. 32). "Managing [optimally] works at a certain level of discourse in organizations where processes are predictable. Leading goes beyond that" (Kowch, 2013, p. 30).

Peter Senge published the first edition of his book *The Fifth Discipline* in 1990 about managerial systems and the learning organization. Its premise was that a competitive advantage would only be achieved by the organization that learned the fastest. Senge's 2006 revised edition features stories of how applying these learning principles resulted in transformation of management systems and organizations. Learning disabilities and five integrated "learning disciplines" integral to a management system are illustrated. Bottom line: lifelong learning occurred at all levels of an organization, and the fifth discipline, systems thinking and complexity science, is the cornerstone that underlies all of the disciplines (Senge, 2006, p. 69).

Can a Manager and a Leader Be the Same Person or in the Same Role?

Progression of thoughts and knowledge on the subject indicate that truly understanding the *transactional* nature of leadership as described in a manager role and combining it with *transformational* leadership principles, or balancing leadership and managership, is the critical act of doing and being in these roles.

It has been the authors' experience that the pioneering Simulation Champion was the all-in-one leader/manager, whereas the evolution of simulation has brought with it new opportunities for leader/manager role delineation. This is why our leadership journey in this chapter will now take you in that direction. The various aspects of each of these roles must be respected and valued in partnerships and collaborations, as much as in individual endeavors, to accomplish either synergy or holism. Our goal as champion of change and project initiator requires skill sets and competencies as well as clear collective collaborative partnerships to function in these tumultuous turbulent times. Managership without leadership and the leader's ability to inspire change feels much like hitting your head against a brick wall in attempts to get people to move; leadership without managership and the manager's ability to see a project through will result in inefficiencies, lack of organization, and an inability to operationalize a vision.

How Was Leadership Developed Within State and Business Perspectives?

One of the more widely quoted statements about leadership is that: "Leadership is one of the most observed and least understood phenomena on earth" (Burns, 1978, p. 2). There are multitudes of descriptions and definitions of leadership. Specific theoretical perspectives for classifying leader characteristics and behaviors (Hibberd, et al., 2006) have been identified and described through general developmental classifications.

Personality Trait Theories

It was considered that *leaders* were born not made and could be identified by characteristics such as height, weight, intelligence, and energy level. Socially elite and monarchies were identified as born leaders having innate characteristics of a leader (Hibberd et al., 2006, p. 374). *Great Man leadership theory* as one of the earliest notions about leaders derives from the notions discussed earlier in this chapter– chiefs, warlords, and kings– but sometimes is identified separately from trait theories. Great Man identifies that leaders are persons born into the right family and possessing inherited traits that made them a natural leader (Grossman & Valiga, 2013, p. 2). Does the Queen of Canada fit within this model or do we see the changes in the monarchy as more transformational or transcendent today?

Have you heard someone described as a *born leader*? This is probably one of the greatest myths about leadership and leaders. What do you think this means? Is being a leader about a given person's advantage, behaviors, or characteristics, or is it more about our emotional reactions to a charismatic person? Some people may seem to have natural leadership abilities. However, we do know today that leaders are developed and they are not born from a privileged gene pool! Personal traits can enhance leadership but do not alone make a leader. Further discussion about charisma will become part of the early notions about transformational leadership theory.

Behavioral Theories

In the 1940s, studies at two American universities identified two dimensions of leadership behavior. *Consideration* involved concern about the welfare and job satisfaction of employees (employee orientation) and *initiating structure* for the organization and definition of work tasks for employees (production orientation). These behavioral leadership theorists identified that context or situation was critical to leader effectiveness. A continuum of leadership behaviors or decision-making styles from *laissez faire* (hands-off approach) through *democratic* (participatory) and *autocratic* (top-down) was identified as influencing group performance and satisfaction in a classic 1939 study (Lewin, Lippitt, & White as cited in Hibberd et al., 2006, p. 376).

Behaviorists in the 1960s described leadership on a continuum ranging from autocratic to democratic and in relationship to varying degrees of task versus relationship orientation (Tannenbaum, Weschler, & Massarik as cited in Hibberd et al., 2006, p. 376). Participatory leadership was really about decision making and the degree to which followers or subordinates participated with their leader or manager in the process. Participation varied from providing opinions, to influencing, to actual decision making. Behaviorists concluded that the leader, the followers, and the situation all determined the style selected. Personal values, confidence, comfort, tolerance of ambiguity, independence, security needed, perceived urgency of the problem, and organizational culture and effectiveness in group decision making were all factors within leaders, followers, and organizations that influenced the selection of a given style within leadership (Hibberd et al., 2006, pp. 374, 376).

Contingency Theory

In the late 1960s, Fiedler considered leadership styles as relatively inflexible and that effective leadership was dependent on a fit with the situation. Fiedler identified leader–member relations as critical to leadership, and the power to influence members through *formal authority* was based on three factors: the degree of mutual trust, respect, and admiration; the structure or rigidity of tasks; and position of power or perceived authority of the leader. Fiedler developed a measurement tool for leadership style based on a task or relationship orientation (Hibberd et al., 2006, pp. 376–378). Fiedler's *Least Preferred Co-worker* *Scale* (LPC; Toolkit 8-2) identified a low LPC score as a person with a task orientation and a high LPC score as a person with a relationship orientation. When taking the scale, one is asked to think of their past work experiences and identify the most difficult ever to work with person and then rate that person using a group of statements. This approach is based on the assumption that under severe stress, our natural predisposition toward a set leadership style will be made obvious and is contingent upon our preference for task versus people.

The 1980s saw the work of P. Hersey and K. Blanchard in the development of a *Tridimensional Leader Effectiveness Model* where leadership style is determined by both task and relationship behaviors. Others described leadership behaviorally as the leader was influencing the group. Their work progressed to the development of *The Situational Leadership Model* (A registered trademark of the *Center for Leadership Studies Inc.*, Escondido, CA, USA). This model emphasizes the amount of socioemotional support, the amount of guidance and direction provided by the leader, and the readiness or maturity of the follower for task performance. Four leadership styles are identified as telling, selling, participating, and delegating. The leader makes a judgement about the readiness of followers and a style is then selected for effective leadership (Hibberd et al., 2006, pp. 378–380). Iterations of this model are widely used in organizations and in leadership development enterprises today. A quick Google search reveals that *Situational Leadership Model II* is current today after more than 30 years of use and development.

Transactional and Transforming Leadership: Changing the Way Leadership Was Viewed

Initiating structure and related considerations had been the foundational notions of the leadership theories well into the 1970s (Hibberd et al., 2006, p. 382). Using a

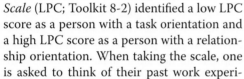

Reflection Activity 8-2
Personal Leadership Development LPC Survey

Take the LPC assessment in the online Toolkit. What do the results of your score reveal about your basic leadership orientation? Are you classified as more task or relationship oriented? Do you agree? Why or why not? Have you always considered yourself as having a certain leadership style or style preference? Are you made uncomfortable with the inference of a preferred style? What do you assume contributes to these feelings and emotions?

Write a narrative about your behaviors in a group at a time when you have experienced or observed extreme conflict within the group's members (perhaps your simulation team). How did you set out to resolve the situation? Were you more focused on getting the job done or on individual members' needs? This narrative should feature your preferred orientation. Did it match with the LPC results? Reflective practice asks that we be open to the full truth about ourselves while considering a new truth about ourselves.

DID YOU KNOW: What we know from a polarity viewpoint is that both orientations exist simultaneously and that we may have a preference for one but can access and develop the other and balance both perspectives! Team functioning can be enhanced with understanding team members' preferences for certain styles. Have an open discussion with your simulation team.

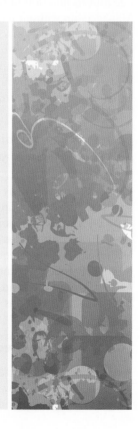

new approach, Burns (1978) identified the concepts of transactional and transforming leadership based on his observations in the military (he was a combat historian), political office, educator/professor; and studies in psychology, philosophy, sociology, economics, and political science (Bailey & Axelrod, 2001). *Transactional leadership* is based on an exchange between the leader and the followers similar to that used by the traditional manager engaged in the course of day-to-day operational details where negotiating and bargaining within relationships deliver needed transactions (Hibberd et al., 2006, p. 382). Contingent reinforcement is involved in transactional leadership where followers are motivated by rewards in exchange for services rendered (Bass, 1995, p. 466).

Transforming leadership occurred when leaders and followers engaged with one another in such a way that both experience higher levels of motivation and morality (pp. 19–20) where in fact transformation may occur. Transforming leaders attract and develop followers into leaders (Bass, 1995, p. 467). Transforming leaders were seen to elevate the concerns of followers higher on Maslow's hierarchy to a need for achievement and self-actualization (p. 467).

Burns (1978) suggested that transforming leadership could not easily be established in bureaucratic or hierarchical organizations (p. 298) and distinguished between the terms moral and ethical. Ethical leadership was viewed as being about professional standards and acting as a role model; and moral leadership was concerned with the "highest values of a country" (Bailey & Axelrod, 2001, pp. 115–116) that we interpret today as social and distributive justice, civil rights, equality, and equity. Burns (as cited in Bailey & Axelrod, 2001, p. 118) suggests a liberal arts education and qualities of compassion, knowledge, and strong values for development of moral leadership. Today, we recognize that transforming, or as it is later termed transformational leadership, is a critical element in our healthcare safety agenda, empowerment, evidence-based practice, and work environments; thus, organizations need to establish transformational leadership practices in administrative and frontline leadership roles and positions (Cummings et al., 2010; Everett & Sitterding, 2011; Kramer, Schmalenberg, & Maquire, 2010; Samner et al. 2010; Wong & Cummings, 2009).

Burns (1978) defined leadership as "the reciprocal process of mobilizing, by persons with certain motives and values, various economic, political, and other resources, in a context of competition and conflict, in order to realize goals independently or mutually held by both leaders and followers" (p. 425). In an interview set in this century, James McGregor Burns felt his definition should still stand as reflective of 21st century leadership and acknowledged that the work of Bernard Bass and his associates were the most exciting developments in leadership theory (Bailey & Axelrod 2001, p. 115).

Transformational Leadership: The True Start of Relationship-Based Leadership

"The secret of leadership is simple: Do what you believe in. Paint a picture of the future. Go there. People will follow."—**Seth Godin, Tribes: We Need You to Lead Us**

Bernard Bass (1995) identified with the work of J.M. Burns and in 1980 began his research and development of what Burns had described as transforming leadership into what we now understand to be the theory of transformational leadership. Bass (1995) further distinguished leadership between a transactional and transformational foci, and his research identified *four transformational factors*: idealized influence, individualized consideration, intellectual stimulation, and inspirational motivation.

- **Idealized Influence**: Focused on envisioning, setting standards, and role modeling. Originally, Burns identified this factor as charismatic, but Bass initially felt that charisma and consequently transformation leadership were in fact amoral. Further research and discourse, including discussions about the absence of morality in such charismatic leaders as Adolf Hitler and Jim Jones, changed Bass' approach to emphasize the morality of transactional and transforming leaderships as Burns had originally envisioned them. The change in factor description from charismatic to idealized influence more closely aligned this morality as a critical factor (Bass & Steidlmeier, 1999, p. 187). It also resulted in development of the concepts of authentic and pseudo transformational leadership styles critical to the development of 21st century leadership understanding.

- **Individualized Consideration**: Focused on development and concern for each follower as an individual utilizing coaching, mentoring, and learning opportunities. Ensuring that followers have attainable goals is critical in this factor (Bass & Steidlmeier, 1999, p. 189). A focus on followers and followership theories is developed later in this chapter and identify the importance of the leader–follower relationship. Leadership theory and development and beginning followership theory have largely been leader centric, and development of current constructs should take a closer look at being follower centric and as such would describe additional insights about leadership (Carsten et al., 2010; Epitropaki et al., 2013; Sy, 2010).

- **Intellectual Stimulation**: Involved logic and critical inquiry and reflexivity. "*A sine qua non* of intellectual stimulation is arousing consciousness and awareness in followers of what is right, good and important, which new direction must be taken and why" (Bass, 1995, p. 29). The openness created provides a transcendent and spiritual dimension that promotes a questioning of assumptions to develop inquiry skills and creativity

(Bass & Steidlmeier, 1999, p. 188). This of course is the key to innovation.

- **Inspirational Motivation**: "Provides followers with challenges and meaning for engaging in shared goals and undertakings" (Bass & Steidlmeier, 1999, p. 188). Bass (1998) identified that the inspiring leader behavior builds confidence and enthusiasm through managing meaning and impressions, molding follower expectations, envisioning, and intellectually stimulating followers (p. 22). The ability to inspire passion and to find our own passion is what motivates and generates energy in leader–follower and follower–follower relationships.

Factors were found across cultures though some variance existed: charisma or idealized influence was found to be the largest component in transformational leadership. Bass (1995) further identified that transformational leaders could be participative or directive, authoritarian, or democratic in decision making. He identified that the transformational leader needed mature moral development and that the best leaders were both transactional and transformational. It is generally in defining moments that leaders are identified as transformational (Bass & Steidlmeier, 1999, p. 184). Bass and Burns built on earlier work and changed the direction of leadership theory. Many subsequent theories and models all reflect notions about task and relationship and transformational factors.

As you read through this section, consider your leadership experiences in simulation-based learning. Have you or others demonstrated transactional, transformational, or even transcendent leadership? Which of the four factors described by Bass do you deem most impactful and how have they played out in your organization or team?

Wong and Cummings (2009) identify authenticity and *authentic leadership* as the root or core construct of positive forms or strength-based leadership approaches. Authenticity has been suggested as critical in building trust and healthier work environments. The authors define authentic behavior as "acting in accord with one's values and needs rather than to please others, receive rewards, or avoid punishments" (p. 525). Kaiser and Overfield (2010) identify *flexible leadership*, the ability to respond effectively in diverse situations (p. 106), as vital to organizational adaptability and performance. This is defined within a complexity framework and considers the abilities to assess and execute actions in response to opposing but complementary factors in management. Dolan and Garcia (2002) identify *agility* for organizational effectiveness in describing *Management by Values* (MBV) as a leadership tool and the necessity of decentralized and flattened hierarchies to meet the challenges of a global community in leadership. The terms competencies and traits are often used in discussing the important attributes of leaders and managers in leadership. Specific models can help in understanding the attributes and competencies needed.

Leadership Models: So…What of Leadership Attributes Anyway?

Using a Model From Bennis and Goldsmith as an Illustration

Leadership is a multidimensional concept, particularly in the 21st century when uncertainty, chaos, and change are the constants. Bennis and Goldsmith (2010) provide a long description of leaders as being "people of principles," "both reflective and action oriented, imaginative, and practical." Leaders are persons that "generate and sustain trust," "relish diversity," and maintain qualities that are compassionate and "encourage transparency and eschew the use of fear." They are humble and lifelong learners and teachers; and "they prepare the ground of acceptance for what has not yet been imagined" (p. x). The discussion of characteristics of a leader in the preface of their book is an impressive and seemingly overwhelming list of attributes! Oddly, we have come to understand leadership as more than a list of characteristics yet we still describe leadership in this way!

What better guides the developing Simulation Champion than a list of leader attributes is to understand the *competencies* needed to meet the challenges of our century? Bennis and Goldsmith (2010) identified that competence, ambition, and integrity must be in balance for constructive, and what they term *audacious leadership* (p. 29). Are you an audacious Simulation Champion? Bennis and Goldsmith (2010) identified six clear and powerful competencies shared across "brave and brilliant leaders": mastering the context, knowing you, creating a vision, communicating with meaning, building trust through integrity, and realizing intention through actions.

Mastering the Context

To master is about understanding the big picture and the impact and influences that both internal and external factors contribute (p. 50). External refers to the larger context in which we live and work and understanding the big-picture issues such as demographic changes, modern technologies, and social, economic, and political unrest. The internal context described by these authors encompasses values, political and faith beliefs, theoretical frameworks, and intellectual standards and commitments inclusive of ethical stands (pp. 49–58). As a Simulation Champion, do you compel yourself to gain an understanding of the big picture, or are your efforts focused on more transactional day-to-day functions in a skills laboratory? Have you thought about how your ability to do so either enhances or inhibits your leadership?

Knowing You

Bennis and Goldsmith (2010) describe this as referring to lifelong learning, engaging in reflective practice and humbly soliciting feedback. It is about searching for self-knowledge and risking self-evaluation and understanding intention and mindfulness; it is about enlightenment. This is the "authentic examined self" (Anna Quindlen as cited in Bennis and Goldsmith, 2010, p. 1), and genuine leadership can only be developed by "self-examination, introspection, and honest soul-searching" and being self-conscious, taking risks, and including collaborative partnerships (pp. 3–6). Are you a lifelong learner who engages in intentional reflective practice and humbly solicits feedback with an earnest desire to change and improve?

Creating a Vision

A compelling evolving vision inspires passion and mobilizes followers to collective and collaborative action. "Leaders are the most results-oriented individuals in the world" (p. 101). A vision is a living document and as followers and leader engage so does the vision grow and change to encompass all images of the future within the collaboration and partnership. The vision must be lived (p. 121). Do you have a vision for simulation in your organization? Can you articulate a clear, concise, and moving vision for simulation?

*"You have to be burning with an idea, or a problem, or a wrong that you want to right. If you're not passionate enough from the start, you'll never stick it out."—**Steve Jobs***

Communicating With Meaning

It is through actively listening to followers and developing empathy that clear and transparent messaging by a leader is achieved. This shared meaning then results in joint endeavors, as opposed to top-down directives. Leadership rhetoric, or the language we use with the intent to influence others, reflects our values and reveals what we think, feel, and want, ultimately affecting the enthusiasm and endorsement of the message. *A leader is always conscious of this.* The content of a message is not more important than the interests, needs, wants, and priorities of the listeners. Choose the media you will need to carry the message in the best way (pp. 123–130). How are you communicating messages to followers? Do you prefer to use technology (i.e., email) or are you more apt to wait and address others in person? Are you adept at tapping into the most desirous needs, wants, and dreams of healthcare educators or clinical practitioner followers?

Resolution of conflict, whether it is by confrontation, conflict resolution strategies, or reconciliation (our favorite) for chronic long-standing conflicts, is a communication

competency that needs to be developed, exercised, and wisely modeled. This means modeling by using emotional intelligence, appreciative inquiry, advocacy inquiry, and other reflective strategies within leaders, followers, groups, and organizations. Goleman (2006) acknowledges the importance of self-awareness, self-discipline, and empathy in the development of emotional intelligence (EI). Understanding personal and other emotions is part of the development of cognitive and affective empathy described as "outsight" (Kouzes & Posner, 2014) in a leader. Communication is the most important competency in leadership.

Do you truly understand that your influence in getting the right message across is hugely impacted by emotions and feelings of both leader and follower? EI is first developed on an individual basis so that the skills can be transferred to leading teams, but EI does not develop in a bubble. Each of us exists and develops within an interconnected environment comprised of social, ecological, and political systems, that is, family, community, organizations, associations, and global networks. Therefore, our unique leadership rhetoric and the way we have come to understand how to facilitate inquiry and discourse are influential in and of itself. Goleman (2006) has created a model critical for leadership development and functioning effectively in groups and teams. Indeed, reflection, as an educational strategy in self-awareness, can help prepare "emotionally capable" leaders (Horton-Deutsch & Sherwood, 2008). Have you ever taken an EI inventory? Are you aware of the various dimensions of EI and how your level of EI affects your ability to effectively lead, follow, and manage?

Building Trust Through Integrity

*"Integrity is doing the right thing, even when no one is watching."—**C. S. Lewis***

Integrity is built through consistent ethical actions that "walk the talk" and maintain constancy in both difficult and easy times. Use of the four Cs of *competency* (skill, attitude, knowledge), *congruity* (integrity), *constancy* (consistency), and *caring* (consideration and empathy) is seen in emerging leaders as they develop trust with followers (Bennis & Goldsmith, 2010, p. 40, pp. 148–152). Trusted leaders capably contribute to their organization's effectiveness through vision, empathy, consistency, and integrity (pp. 153–178). Transparency from leaders is needed for trust and integrity to flourish. Bennis, Goleman, O'Toole, and Biederman (2008) develop the notion of transparency as vital to creating a culture of candor within and between organizations. Knowledge of organizational culture is developed within another chapter of this book and, as the context setting the stage for leadership, is a primary factor in the changing faces of leadership and followership today.

Integrate these chapters in your development of your simulation role.

Healthcare identifies culture in the safety agenda and development of a culture of transparency and quality initiatives (Samner et al., 2010). In your leadership role, are you intentional about transparency? Have your actions sometimes lead to distrust or misunderstanding? Do you share vital information and entrust followers as accountable and responsible contributors? Is safety and quality improvement a priority?

Realizing Intention Through Actions

To quote a famous proverb, "the road to hell is paved with good intentions." Leaders must recognize reliance on followers and be intentional to "act with" in achieving goals and desired results. Leaders must translate commitments into goals and goals into actions or all is for not. In formulating actions, leaders are strategic, make good judgements, and focus on engaging people, by being proactive and responsive. The ability to exercise astute judgement, especially during difficult times, is at the core of one's leadership nucleus, directly affecting outcomes and how they are achieved (Bennis & Goldsmith, 2010, p. 182). Being strategic about involving stakeholders and utilizing a project management approach can effectively turn goals into actions and provides clear directions for change and innovations (Skelton-Green, Simpson, & Scott, 2007). Change and the use of a project management approach are often the strategic tool of leadership and organizations for implementing innovations and change. Some organizations even have strategic project departments. In your role as Simulation Champion, do you empower others to action, or do you prefer to do things yourself? Do you find yourself making great plans and consistently falling short of executing them? How effective are you at turning goals into actions for others? The importance of action is reflected in an historical quote from the designer of modern nursing:

"I think one's feelings waste themselves in words; they ought all to be distilled into actions which bring results"—***Florence Nightingale (1844)***

Using a Model From Kouzes and Posner as an Illustration of Transformational Leadership for the 21st Century

To understand what leadership is and is not, is to "liberate the leader in each and every one of us" (Kouzes & Posner 2007, p. 341). So what is it really? How do we bring clarity to this concept? Kouzes and Posner (2007, 2014) have completed over 35 years (since 1983) of leadership research into actual behaviors, described by people when they assert that they are at their personal best as leaders, or defining moments people describe as their "leadership best" when they have "mobilized others to get extraordinary things done." They have postulated five key behaviors or exemplary practices of leadership engaged in by leaders in organizations: modeling the way, inspiring a shared vision, challenging the process, enabling others to act, and encouraging the heart.

Kouzes and Posner (2007, 2014) identify that leadership is a set of competencies that can be learned, acquired, and engaged in by anyone. The *Leadership Practices Inventory*, initially developed by them in 1988, is a proprietary tool that can enhance the development of leaders through reflective assessment by individuals and the receipt of feedback on current behaviors and actions based on the reported practices within the inventory. The *Leadership Practices Inventory* (LPI) is regarded as one of the most widely used and effective leadership development instruments.

Leadership is about a powerful combination of our being, our credibility, and our doing (Kouzes & Posner, 2007, p. 338). Credibility, in this mix, is viewed as the basis of leadership by Kouzes and Posner (2014) and additionally defined by Grossman and Valiga (2013) as:

Reflection Activity 8-3
Personal Leadership Development

Write a story in your personal journal describing a time when you feel that you were at your leadership best. What happened and what did you do and say that made the difference? Log the answers to questions that arose in the preceding text. When you considered Kouzes and Posner's five practices did you see those behaviors in your actions?

DID YOU KNOW: Narratives are a powerful tool for reflection that can add to our critical consciousness!

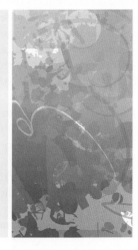

Honesty + competence + inspiration + vision = CREDIBILITY

For the 21st century, perseverance, resilience, and humility (Wheatley, 2010; 2011) should be added to the credibility formula and in fact may preempt a leader's visionary ability in these turbulent times!

Honesty + competence + inspiration + perseverance + resilience + humility = CREDIBILITY

Kouzes and Posner (2007, 2014) identify and describe *ten commitments* associated with the five practices of an exemplary leader. While reading, imagine yourself as Simulation Champion and how you currently enact or plan to enact these practices.

Modeling the Way

Modeling the way comprises the commitments, *clarify values* and *set the example.* This practice is about you as a leader being a good example by actively living out what you expect of others. Leaders need to give voice to their own beliefs and values while representing the common principles and ideals of the organization. When leaders are directly involved and are seen to act in accordance with their values and the organization's principles and ideals, respect of and for the leader is engendered. Can you identify the values and principles your actions give voice to? Do others tell you that your actions model the way to excellence in simulation?

Inspiring a Shared Vision

Inspiring a shared vision includes the commitments, *envision the future* and *enlist others.* Enthusiasm and passion must be displayed in relating the dream or vision and in developing it for and with others. In order to engage others in a vision, the leader needs to understand the needs and interests of their constituents, and constituents and followers need to believe the leadership does understand them and "have their best interests at heart." "Leaders cannot command commitment, only inspire it" (2007, p. 17). Have you inspired vision for simulation that speaks to and tugs at follower heartstrings for better outcomes in education?

Challenging the Process

Challenging the process includes the commitments, *search for opportunities* and *experiment and take risks.* Personal best stories from leaders were used in developing this model, and all involved a challenge or change from *the*

status quo and mediocrity. Terms used synonymously in describing this changing are pioneer, innovation, growth, improvement, initiative, and the unknown. Sound familiar? Simulation Champions are all of those things! To be effective, today's leaders must understand the dynamics of change and the levels of risk tolerance of their constituents and the organization. Leaders need to know that they can promote a sense of safety in the process of change by making smaller incremental changes to decrease risk and gain commitment. "Try, Fail, Learn. This is the leader's mantra." Leaders know the importance of learning from both failures and successes and modeling and encouraging that with others (2007, p. 20).

Do you beat yourself or others up when mistakes are made? Are you able to go with the flow in your response to failure or do you dwell on the failure instead of learning the valuable lesson? This is a mental skill that must be developed as for many of us; failure is deeply engrained as a negative for which we are to be held personally accountable. Learning how to reframe failure and embrace it as a valued informant is a necessary skill in challenging the process. This is also enhanced in debriefing as a Simulation Champion.

*"Sounds so obvious, but it's true that leadership occurs in moments of challenge, not during moments of ease"—**Robin Sharma***

Enabling Others to Act

Enabling others to act includes commitments to *foster collaboration* and *strengthen others or build trust.* This practice is about developing and engaging as a team. This is when individual accountability and group confidence and competence develop into trusting strong relationships. This is when accomplishments are seen as team accomplishments not as leader accomplishments. There is no me in we! The sense of teamwork involves all stakeholders, and each individual has a sense of empowerment, discretion, and ownership in the change. Authentic leadership is based on mutual trust and respect.

Encouraging the Heart

Encouraging the heart includes commitments *recognize contributions* and *celebrate the values and victories.* Genuine acts of caring, compassion, love, and appreciation create strong work relationships. A single "thank you" is extremely powerful! A strong sense of collective identity and community spirit is developed within a culture of appreciation and celebration for group, individual, and organizational accomplishments and successes.

These five practices and their accompanying commitments are foundational to our development of our doing and being as a transformational leader and as a leader of change. "Success in leading will be wholly dependent

Reflection Activity 8-4
Personal Leadership Development (LPI)

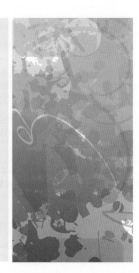

Want to assess your perception of your exemplary practices? Google *Leadership Practices Inventory* or go to https://www.lpionline.com/lpi_individual.html. Complete **the Leadership Practices Inventory (LPI)** as an online activity. (Note: To complete the survey, there is a nominal cost, but you can take the inventory multiple times.) A review and summary report is returned to you electronically and will reflect your strengths and suggest activities to strengthen your practices. This can be foundational to your leadership development. It is to your advantage to be completely honest in taking the inventory. This is not a test and all you have to gain by being transparent is to better understand yourself. Celebrate and honor your strengths!

upon the capacity to build and sustain those human relationships that enable people to get extraordinary things done on a regular basis" (Kouzes and Posner, 2007, p. 25). Understanding the five practices and commitments can be accomplished in the obvious way by reading and reflecting, but try the novel way suggested in the Personal Development: Reflective Moment in Activity 8-4 found above.

Leadership Models: So…What Is the Definition of Leader and Leadership?

Defining leadership and leader is in part a values-based exercise. Four of our favorite definitions that reflect a preference for transformational concepts are shared here. It is hard to compose single statements to truly reflect the concepts critical for both terms.

1. Essential to leadership is a process of involving people, gaining their commitment, and energizing them to participate in the tasks related to achieving mutual goals (Hibberd et al., 2006, p. 370).
2. Leaders and followers form an action circle around a common purpose, with decent values, based on a courageous relationship with mutual respect and honesty (Chaleff, 2009, pp. 2–13).
3. The leader's role is not to make sure that people know exactly what to do and when to do it. Instead, leaders need to ensure that there is strong and evolving clarity about who the organization is (Wheatley, 2006, p. 131).
4. In a learning organization, leaders are designers, teachers, and stewards. People who are truly leading seem rarely to think of themselves in that way (Senge, 2006, pp. 321 and 340).

Whatever definition or description chosen, it should reflect that leadership is a process of "engendering positive turbulence" characterized by ongoing creativity and innovation (Grossman & Valiga, 2013, p. 3) and a process of gaining commitment and involvement of persons through igniting their passion for a mutual vision and mission (Grossman & Valiga, 2013; Hibberd et al., 2006, p. 370; Kouzes & Posner, 2014).

What we have come to understand is that leadership and being a leader are hard work. It does not come naturally but it is possible through relational inquiry and an ethical lens (Bergum & Dossetor, 2005; Doane & Varcoe, 2015) that credibility is enacted. "Leadership can happen anywhere, at any time" (Kouzes & Posner 2007, p. 8). A leader inspires and influences others to achieve a collective best in an endeavor. A leader comes from the collective or creates a collective or community of others. Others within a collective are the followers. There is a dynamic and intimate relationship among leaders and followers based on mutual respect and trust, relational ethics, courage and risk, mindfulness, and intentionality. A leader is humble without hubris. The term, leaders, is deliberately plural, and leaders engage in leadership as an individual or a collective and in partnership with their followers. "From a relational inquiry perspective, every moment of nursing action involves leadership" (Doane & Varcoe, 2015, p. 430).

Leadership starts within a person and is exemplified by how we are with and for people. Leadership is reflected in how decisions are made and in how and what actions are taken. The leader is held accountable by the follower, and indeed today, the follower may be far more important than the leader. To make it even more complex, it happens within an organization and society and on a global basis. This leader being is a complex construct!

"We're here for a reason. I believe a bit of the reason is to throw little torches out to lead people through the dark."
—Whoopi Goldberg

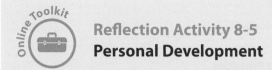

Reflection Activity 8-5
Personal Development

"You change your life, by changing your heart."—Max Lucado from Grace for the Moment

Take a moment to define the primary terms—champion, leader, follower, and manager—with your ideas and words. Flag your page.

Refer back and reflect on this page as you plan change and as you continue in this chapter and book and in your leadership lifelong journey.

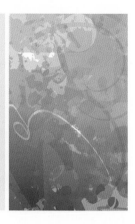

Utilizing Models: So Really! How Do We Learn to Be a Leader?

What is known is that everyone can learn to be a leader because leadership is no longer seen as an inborn characteristic or attached to a specific role or a position of authority. Note that we suggest that someone can learn to be a leader, we do not profess that we can be taught to be a leader; but one can utilize and provide knowledge and ways of enhancing and nurturing leadership competencies. Therefore, a model can only provide structure, rigor, and consistency for learning and discussion. You are left with the lion's share of the work.

Leadership development has been and continues to be a multimillion dollar industry. It has been a focus in organizational and talent development and a designated goal in educational institutions for all of this century to date and most of the last. The real challenge is in relating the success of leadership endeavors to organizational and individual goals. The political, healthcare, business, and faith-based cultures and climates have all experienced the downside of poor leadership and management as seen in scandals, bankruptcies, violations of the public trust, and unethical business and management practices. So why is there such a crisis in leadership and followership today despite all of the educational endeavors and learning? What exactly are the measurements of success and excellence in practice?

Success and excellence are about habits of quality in everything that is done, every time it is done, over and above what is expected of us, and of others (Grossman & Valiga, 2013, pp. 203–211). Is there a golden panacea for the crisis of leadership excellence? Bennis et al. (2008) challenge our thinking on the roots of today's leadership crisis and the importance of transparency and candor. The authors' observations create understanding about the changes needed in the 21st century and the importance of speaking and knowing the truth for both leaders and followers.

*"He that thinketh he leadeth and hath no one following him is only taking a walk."—**John C. Maxwell Goleman**

Goleman, Boyatzis and McGee (2002) write about "maximizing the half-life of learning" (p. 244) or developing a learning process, rather than using single topical programs, for continuous learning or sustainability or "stickiness." These authors are writing about resonant leadership skill, or emotional intelligence, and propose that the best leadership programs are self-directed processes that use multifaceted approaches focusing on individual, team, and organizational learning needs. Their examples include programs with links to culture, seminars about the process of change, emotional intelligence competencies, purposeful intentional learning goal setting, and relationship-based learning experiences such as with teams and executive coaching (p. 244).

Within the nursing profession, the *Registered Nurses' Association of Ontario* (RNAO) published the second edition of their Best Practice Guidelines (BPG) in July 2013 for the development and sustaining of nursing leadership as part of the *Healthy Work Environments Best Practice Guidelines* project (Fig. 8.1). It is important to note that leadership in nursing is encouraged at point-of-care (POC) positions, which are nonmanagerial, based on a strong belief that every nurse is and must be a leader. Furthermore, in the same document, specific competencies and knowledge are recommended for leadership by 2020 (CNA, 2009b).

Harris (2013) challenges us to consider if we are changing in nursing as quickly as we could and as quickly as we need to. Integration of BPG would be a great start to the development of leadership skills and competencies within an organization. On an individual level, development of intellectual knowledge about leadership development can be implemented as personal strategies. We can be challenged on how we teach leadership as well; knowing that leadership is learned through lived experience, we need to continue to design curricula that integrate the learning of leadership, managership, and followership competencies through the use of simulation and reflective pedagogies.

Simulation research in nursing education has increasingly been published in the last 5 years, and a sampling includes the importance of simulation in the development

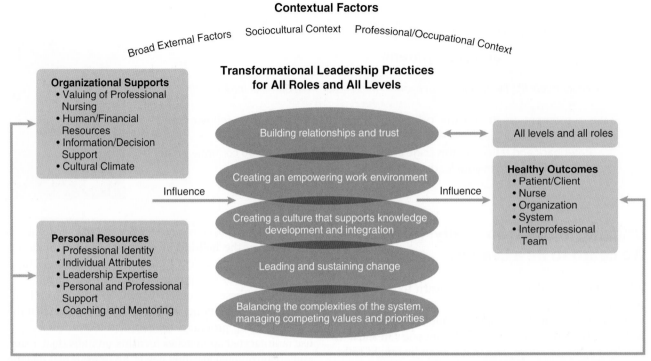

Figure 8.1 RNAO Conceptual Model for Developing and Sustaining Transformational Leadership Practices. (Redrawn from Registered Nurses' Association of Ontario (2013). Developing and Sustaining Nursing Leadership, 2nd ed. Toronto, ON: Registered Nurses' Association of Ontario. This work is funded by the Ontario Ministry of Health and Long-Term Care.)

of confidence (Zulkosky, 2012), the degree of student satisfaction with low-fidelity versus high-fidelity learning (Tosterud, Hedlin, & Hall-Lord, 2013), the learning and application of clinical judgement (Kelly, Hager, & Gallagher, 2014), low-fidelity classroom activities for leadership education (Pollard & Wild, 2014), and the case-based learning and simulation to develop assessment skills in undergraduate students (Raurell-Toredà et al., 2015). An integrated review on the place of web-based simulation in nursing education (Cant & Cooper, 2014) and meta-analysis of the effects of high fidelity and patient simulation in nursing education (Lee & Oh, 2015; Shin, Park, & Kim, 2015) showcase progression in our development of nursing simulation evidence. Additional publications indicate the potential benefits of senior-level student teachers (Dumas, Hollerbach, Stuart, & Duffy, 2015) and the use of simulation pedagogy for professional development of nursing clinical educators (Hunt, Curtis, & Gore, 2015).

Morrow (2015) completed a literature review focused on baccalaureate nursing curricula in prelicensure programs from 2008 to 2013. Her gap analysis indicated a lack of strategies to develop leadership competencies at the organizational level. This would involve quality improvement, research, and policy development areas. Professional associations and scholars both in the United States and in Canada have identified repeatedly in the last 10 years the need for imbedding leadership competencies in prelicensure programs if we are going to meet the challenges of

the 21st century (Benner, Sutphen, Leonard, & Day, 2010; CNA, 2009b, 2012b; Duncan, 2014; Institute of Medicine, 2010b; Kilty, 2005; Robert Wood Johnson Foundation, 2010). This is about a need for resocializing through an educational process about both leadership and followership. Simulation can play a critical role in this area.

Grossman and Valiga (2013) emphasize development of leadership throughout one's career in general ways. To develop as a leader, it is believed that one must "serv [e] in leadership roles" emphasizing the importance of acting on and applying knowledge and that one must develop leadership as lifelong learning by utilizing strategies that continually refine, renew, and enhance competencies (p. 178). Specific approaches to develop "leadership mindsets" are professional involvement in organizations, formal courses, conferences, workshops, newsletters, blogs, videos, and websites and participation in role-plays, games, and simulation (p. 180). The leadership student or learner must utilize and engage in reflective strategies such as debriefing, journaling, coaching, and mentoring to enhance inquiry and learning. In fact, identifying and engaging with a mentor or coach in an ongoing relationship can be beneficial in any learning endeavor.

 This type of learning endeavor through coaching and mentoring is reflected in the INACSL Facilitation Standard (INACSL Standards Committee, 2016). The need to individualize learning needs and approaches through collaboration with learners while coaching and mentoring to facilitate learning and translation of evidence into practice is what both good simulation and good leadership development are about.

Approaches such as sensitivity training, conscious and deliberate role modeling, participation in institutes and fellowships, and on-the-job training are all effective approaches designed to engage with the leader and follower in all of us (pp. 178–183). Simpson, Skelton-Green, and Scott (2011) relate over 15 years of successes at nursing's only leadership institute in Canada, the *Dorothy Wylie Nursing Leadership Institute* (DMW-NLI), with project management and change workshops and organizational change projects and research endeavors. The *National League for Nursing* (2015e) in the United States offers several options for leadership formation in nursing with the Leadership Development Program for Simulation Educators being particularly applicable to leadership development for the Simulation Champion.

Marshall (2011) identifies that a transformational leader "reads widely and is informed, interested and engaged in issues of healthcare, science, the arts, history, biography, current events and popular culture" (p. 263). Senge (2006) defines a learning organization as "an organization that is continually expanding its capacity to create the future" (p. 14). Learning is central to leadership, management, and followership as is collective learning within an organization. Within simulation, there is no reason to wait for a leader to emerge. Take the risk; learn together; take on the challenge of innovation, change, and implementation of standards. Everyone on your simulation team can be a leader. Change needs you!

Followership

What about the other part of the relationship? What is the historical development to date of the follower? When you were young, were you told to be a leader not a follower? Told to take charge and show what you are worth; be a leader, right? Have we grown up feeling that followership is an "F word" and truly not an envied role to take? Researchers suggest that individuals have preconceived or implicit notions about being followers, sometimes based on socialization or a transactional or transformational perspective, and these notions shape our interactions with others (Sy, 2010). Can we say that there is an underappreciated importance of followership and those implicit viewpoints and beliefs affect leader–follower interpersonal outcomes? Many authors agree (Chaleff, 2009; Epitropaki et al., 2013; Hurwitz & Hurwitz, 2015; Kellerman, 2008, 2014; Kelly, 2008; Riggio, Chaleff, & Lipman-Blumen, 2008; Sy, 2010). If teams are the learning units of organizations and individuals on teams think, interact, and learn from one another (Senge, 2006, p. 10), then followers are

the critical team players within an organization. Just think of the amazing potential simulation holds to shape learners' valuing and understanding of the important roles that followers play in today's healthcare realms.

"Not the cry, but the flight of a wild duck, leads the flock to fly and follow."—**Chinese Proverb**

Van Vugt et al. (2008) suggest that the psychology of followership is far more interesting than that of leadership particularly since most people are followers. Not unlike leadership, followership most likely emerged in response to a need to resolve problems through a collective effort to enhance individual and group survival (p. 189). People probably spend more hours in their lifetime being a follower than being a leader. Kellerman (2008) describes the historical "romance of leadership" during which it was believed that leaders dictated the course of human history and followers were invisible, and so the all importance of leaders became firmly entrenched in our perceptions (p. 10), when in fact without the follower, the leader can accomplish nothing. The paradox of leader and follower has been well rehearsed and acclaimed; and a prototype of both, as seen in classifications, greatly influences relationships.

In 1899 Elbert Hubbard published a classic essay in the *Philistine Magazine* entitled "*A Message to Garcia.*" The essay was a reflective article on the importance of the man who took a military communiqué to the leader of the insurgents in Cuba during the *Spanish American War*. It was an opinion that the real hero was the *person who took the message* that allowed the leader to be victorious. The follower was the hero who had initiative to get the job done. It was he who figured out how to accomplish a seemingly impossible task. He was committed to the request asked of him. Such is the follower: committed, steadfast, and true to the cause. The essay resonated with readers and became so influential that over forty million copies of the essay were printed in multiple languages, and it was regarded as having the largest circulation of any literary venture during the lifetime of the author (Hubbard, 1899). This may indeed be one of the first written influential records of the importance of the follower in an organization.

Robert Kelly (2006) began his study of followers and followership in the late 1970s when little research and scholarship considered followers, and if it did, it was leader centric (p. 5). Kelly wrote a groundbreaking article in 1988 about followers (p. 5) and the first book for followers, as opposed to leaders, in 1995 (Kellerman 2008, p. 79). Kelly identified five basic styles of followership based on independence in critical thinking and organizational engagement: the sheep, the yes people, the alienated, the pragmatics, and the star performers (Kelly, 2006, p. 9). Kelly (2006) describes the courageous conscience needed by followers to be the "primary defenders against toxic leaders or dysfunctional organizations [and the responsibility that followers] have to keep leaders and peers ethically and legally in check" (p. 14). Additional leadership scholars have theorized about followers.

Kellerman (2008) wrote about a typology of five types of followers based on level of engagement. They ranged in engagement from *isolates* being totally withdrawn, feeling and doing absolutely nothing, to *bystander*, *participant*, *activist*, and *diehard* as totally engaged, passionately committed, and deeply involved and committed to support or opposition of the leader (p. 84). Kellerman encourages followers to be bold subordinates and acknowledges the difficulties followers encounter when "leading up" or "leading from below," both aspects of being a good follower (p. 249). Kelly (2006) describes the 25 years (35 now!) he has spent developing the field of followership with his colleagues and the importance of this field, though it is in its infancy, in making "powerful contributions to society and to the individuals who make up society" (p. 15).

Evolution of the Follower

Kellerman (2014) continues to write about the evolution of relations between leaders and followers and how it has evolved throughout human history. "Beginning with the Enlightenment, marked by the American and French revolutions and continuing into the 19th and 20th centuries, there has been an expansion of democratization in both theory and practice" (p. x). Society is characterized by less respect for authority, while power and authority have devolved from the top down. "For their part, followers, ordinary people, have an expanded sense of entitlement—demanding more, giving less and demonstrating a far lower level of tolerance, not to speak of admiration, for people in positions of authority now than they did even as recently as 30, 40 years ago". Furthermore, this author identifies two phenomena of the 20th and 21st centuries that have further fuelled this shift and exacerbated leadership problems: "the changes in culture—and...in technology." Information is available both in amount and in quick time through social media and the web. The author uses regulatory environments as an example of the context that has made leading more complex and infinitely harder. Kellerman writes that it is not the people whom lead, but rather the public and the context, that makes leading and following in the 21st century so complex and difficult (pp. 18–19).

Hurwitz and Hurwitz (2015) write about followership as the "other half of leadership." Their research and work are based on their personal narratives and over 10 years of working with organizations to develop a culture that values and utilizes both leadership and followership in developing strong collaborative generative partnerships. They describe these learnings as helping people to thrive in organizations.

Followership Characteristics Across the Generations

Carsten et al. (2010) describe the current social construction of the follower as being leader centric and suggests an alternate approach to follower centrism would help us to better understanding of both followership and leadership. Dixon, Mercado, and Knowles (2013) report on two studies that consider follower behaviors and commitment levels of the three generations of workers across technical and nontechnical work groups. Dixon et al. (2013) found within one group of technology workers that there were similar behaviors across generations: in four out of five follower behaviors, baby boomers had similarities to both generations X and Y, and Gen Xers and Gen Yers held affective commitment in common.

The discussion of commitment and follower behaviors suggested that we take a closer look at the generations of workers currently in the organization and what follower and commitment behaviors of each generation would enhance the understanding of the dynamics within a work group or a team. Consider also the effect of students and adding a fourth generation, millennials, into a work or learning setting! Generational differences among follower behaviors need to be clearly understood for effective team development and as a strategy for the Simulation Champion could well be a vehicle for effective high performance team development.

The issue of diversity across generations is not exclusively explained through the five followership characteristics (Chaleff, 2009), as just like leadership, followership can be learned. Generational differences may relate to understanding or developing "outsight" (Kouzes & Posner, 2014) or cognitive empathy about team members' positions or learning needs. Chaleff (2009) identifies that a follower leads from behind and works diligently for the success of the organization and the leader. The courageous follower serves the organization and the central purpose. According to Chaleff (2009), the challenge for the follower is to develop a trusting genuine honest relationship with the leader where speaking the truth when appropriate is appreciated, and confrontation is done without malice or self-serving motives (p. 23). Within this model, five courageous followership behaviors are identified plus four styles of followership based on support given to the leader and the degree of challenge of the leader that a follower is willing to risk (p. 40). In the most recent edition, Chaleff (2009) identifies the *importance of leaders listening to followers* and followers having the courage to speak honestly to the hierarchy (p. 8). Chaleff (2009) offers a personal and reflective view of the workings of an organization and management of work by leaders and followers and is worth a read for any person employed in an organization and wishing to understand follower obligations and responsibilities in

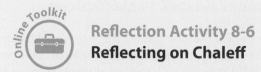

Reflection Activity 8-6
Reflecting on Chaleff

CONSIDER: How do you relate to a current authority figure? Can you speak the truth to the hierarchy without reprisal? What do you challenge? Policy, leader behavior, or both? Do you challenge when an organizational goal is in jeopardy? Are you supportive in the ways that you challenge? Do you listen and value followers?

DID YOU KNOW: The way we have been socialized to authority influences our beliefs and assumptions about leaders and followers? Have you considered that it may be time to challenge this? How were you socialized to authority? How does that history influence your leadership/followership behaviors?

Take, for example, the devil's advocate. This follower often functions from a position of low support and high challenge to the leader. The devil's advocate will also often be marginalized and growth for the devil's advocate follower must include increasing their actual and visible support for the leader's initiatives. How do you react to this type of follower? Do you shut them down? Or give them voice and value their contributions?

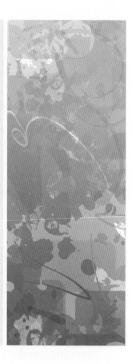

relationship to their leader and how to partner effectively with that leader.

Sy (2010) suggests from his research that action-oriented *implicit followership theory* (IFT) could well be viewed as a "two-factor structure": followership prototype (industry, enthusiasm, and good citizen) and followership antiprototype (conformity, insubordination, and incompetence). The task in the 21st century becomes one of focusing on the positive prototypes in developing individuals within a learning organization culture, but acknowledging how our personal biases across diversities can influence our view about how prototypical behavior is expressed. Epitropaki et al. (2013) challenge further organizational thinking and suggest and emphasize the "real-world" applicability of IFT and implicit leadership theories (ILT) as sociocognitive processes with implications for leader–follower relationships, job attitudes, affect, and performances. If we are successful in establishing a new paradigm, both leaders and followers will need congruent and positive implicit models of both roles. Research and scholarship in followership and leadership are needed for the 21st century. In what ways can the Simulation Champion accelerate shifting to this new paradigm within organizations?

Constructs for Leadership and Followership

In developing leadership competencies and clarifying the concepts inherent in theories for the 21st century, certain constructs stand out and are illustrated in the next segment. This is not an all-inclusive list. Just like change and leadership, our knowledge continues to change as we interact with persons, organizations, and new innovations. Clarity in presenting these concepts for the Simulation Champion is attained through a lens that includes multiple disciplines but a focus in nursing is utilized.

"I like nonsense; it wakes up the brain cells. Fantasy is a necessary ingredient in living."—**Dr. Seuss**

Complexity Science and Complex Adaptive Systems

"Transformational leaders of the future will see the world with a new vision, break old rules, discover or create new rules, and thrive in the paradoxes of complexity" (Marshall, 2011, p. 21). Nursing has identified the importance of Complexity Science, Chaos Theory, and Complex Adaptive Systems (CAS) in understanding systems thinking, organizations, and leadership. "The concept of complexity science is meant to challenge the status quo...and affords the leader the opportunity to create order out of chaos" (Chadwick, 2010, p. 157). Complexity as a construct is recommended in the development of curricula and is present in models for analysis, nursing leadership, and research (Chadwick, 2010; James, 2010; Lett, 2001; RNAO, 2013). Nursing has utilized principles of complexity to change practice and influence healthcare delivery and as members of *Learning Organizations* to understand and deal with the complexity of problems, safety systems, and the change process as CASs. Nursing has also had a rich tradition in utilizing systems thinking and quantum physics in nursing theories for the past 50 years (Holden, 2005, p. 656).

As you read through the list provided, consider your personal thoughts on complexity science thinking and how their adoption can impact the systems you work within. Characteristics that can facilitate our understanding of the natural order of things from a complexity science perspective are to understand that:

1. *Simple rules are needed* to create flexibility and fluidity that is required to adjust to turbulences and external change (eCunha & Rego, 2010, p. 91).
2. *Improvisation* is needed as a mechanism of anticipation and prediction (p. 92).
3. *Swarm intelligence* or collective intelligence is seen in groups or teams as robust decision making and action tasking (p. 92).
4. *Nonlinearity is present,* creating uncertainty and unpredictability versus a definite cause–effect relationship (Dolan, Garcai, & Auerbach, 2003, p. 25).
5. *Fractals* exist as single patterns repeated in different scales to make up a complex whole (p. 25). Fractals are geometrical figures or images that can describe repeating, random, or chaotic phenomena in sections that are repeated and, in doing so, get smaller—conduct an Internet image search to have a look at them. Imagine your simulation center, your organization, and our healthcare system represented as fractals!
6. *Chaos, and indeed the edge of chaos,* is not avoided but rather used to self-organize through innovation and creativity (p. 25).
7. *Fuzzy logic* relates to the relationship between elements and sets of elements as a matter of more or less, rather than as yes or no, white or black (p. 25).
8. *Paradox and tension* are about the ability to get comfortable with uncomfortable environments and seen as the norm (Chadwick, 2010, p. 162).
9. *Cooperation and competition* need to be balanced or integrated together for collaboration (p. 163).
10. *Creative destruction* refers to a needed process of dismantling rigidity (p. 163).
11. *Equilibrium* is not a goal of a CAS as there is continual change and response to energy (Holden, 2005, p. 654). Equilibrium would end the CAS.
12. *Adaption or emergence* is the major consequence. Emergence is a holistic phenomenon that manifests from within the whole (p. 654).
13. *Self-organization* is how emergence occurs. "It results from each individual doing their own thing independently" (Paley, 2007, p. 235).
14. *Chunking* results in simple networks forming from CASs as they link and connect to one another (Burns, 2001, p. 477).
15. *Embeddedness* exists as CASs are embedded or nested into another and form larger systems that need to be understood as a single entity within others (Chaffee & McNeill, 2007, p. 234).

Complicated Versus Complex Systems

Characteristics of complex systems aid us in critical inquiry and understanding group and organizational behavior. Kowch (2013) provides an important distinction for us in considering complicated (mechanical and functional) and complex (learning or organizing). In complicated organizations, we add parts or structural functions to fill gaps, to fix unexpected outcomes; whereas in *complex* systems, these changes emerge as part of a networked, relational organization structure. It is increasingly important in leadership and management to understand the differences between simple, complicated, complex, and chaotic systems. When dealing with systems, it is essential to use systematic approaches to solutions finding: formulaic approaches are key to defining the source(s) or a problem and creating a strategic plan to solve the problem in simple systems and some complicated. Complicated systems are not simple and solving issues within them will often require additional coordination and inputs from others with expertise.

For example, pulling together a simulation schedule means being able to meet the demands of multiple users with finite resources: you must consider mannequin or standardized patient bookings and requirements, time frames, supply requirements, technology use, room functions, and personnel requirements. A simulation schedule can in fact be considered a complicated system that can be accomplished using systematic project management approaches. In contrast, using formulaic approaches will not solve complex systems issues. Whereas the complicated systems have a high degree of certainty and predictability in outcomes, complex systems are *unpredictable.* They are not, therefore, easily understood using step-by-step processes and rules, procedures, and project management. Rather, they demand that you understand relationships that thrive on self-organizing, evolving, and deep connection.

Consider now, an intensive end-of-life simulation event using 15 standardized patients (SP) (10 of them brand new to this role), 140 learners, and 14 faculty members with varying levels of experience. The reality is that a rulebook cannot be consistently applied to the host of issues that will arise; SP success with one event does not guarantee success with another; faculty expertise can help, but in and of itself does not ensure success; and finally, every learning encounter is unique, and relationships and interactions that unfold within them will not play out in a predictable way. So as you see, problems arising from complicated and complex systems manifest differently and require different cognitive and psychosocial processes to resolve.

Snowdon and Boone (2007) wrote a seminal article in 2007 that has been republished illustrating the complexity of decision making by leaders and managers. They have developed a proprietary model or framework called the *Cynefin* framework for decision making in contextually relevant ways. The value of this framework is in teaching leaders how to identify context and how to behaviorally respond to match the context. Leadership and management in the complex knowledge age of the 21st century need to be approached as a humanistic and moral endeavor rather than a scientific one (Kowch, 2013, p. 31). Quantum characteristics such as nonlinear structures, a focus on relatedness, center-out decision making, interdependence of all things, and value-driven actions (Porter-O'Grady & Malloch, 2003, pp. 20–22) will dominate in CAS in the years to come.

Reflection, Reflexivity, and the Reflective Learner

"Reflection is a learning journey of becoming a reflective practitioner…through our everyday experiences towards realizing one's vision of desirable practice as lived reality."—**Johns (2013, p. 1)**

For us, becoming reflective practitioners is about developing leadership of self and developing skills for critical inquiry and decision making. Personal reflection can make your learning time more constructive and fruitful. It allows time for contemplation, mindfulness, and consequently the time to sort and refine ideas and decisions by challenging personal beliefs and deeply held assumptions (Marshall, 2011, p. 29). Reflective practice is about becoming aware of our assumptions, how these assumptions govern our practice, how these assumptions must shift to embrace change, how our resistance to assumptions shifts, and finally that changing assumptions support creating a better state of affairs. Without doubt, much of what passes as reflection is "surface" work that does not address the deeper structures that govern the way the world is. This is not to say that surface work is not important. We just need to commit to dig a little deeper each time (Johns, 2013, p. xv).

Reflection is always purposeful and reflects a being as "who I am" rather than a doing or "what I do" (p. 2). The being is at its pinnacle in *mindfulness* or "seeing things for what they really are without distortion" (p. 3). This mindfulness is at the core of transformational thinking in followers and leaders. Curiosity and commitment are prerequisites of reflection, and contradiction is the creative tension that is worked through in reflection, often intuitively, but with voice (pp. 2–12). Multiple reflective models exist in the literature and offer a developmental approach for reflective practice critical to a professional clinician and nurse. Reflective practice is a method of quality improvement and control, ensuring that quality is the professional responsibility for which every practitioner is held accountable (p. 209). Transformational leaders work with the reality of risk, daring to find their creative edge at the edge of chaos. Reflection, in a sense, is the application of chaos theory, nurturing relationships and connectedness. Group-guided reflection is a tool that can work to empower and create team effectiveness and allow self-organization and emergence (pp. 193–196). "Self-reflective

practice is the missing link for understanding and developing authentic leadership, particularly as it relates to the quality of self-awareness" (Raffo, 2014, p. 191).

Reflective practice pedagogy, whether in academic or clinical settings, provides important opportunities for nurses to explore their professional and individual commitment to quality and safety in their emerging practice (Sherwood & Horton-Deutsch, 2012, p. 37).

Reflection is a critical tool for simulation in debriefing and in reflection beyond the simulation (pp. 149–168). Here lies a great link for the leader and follower and champion of simulation with development and learning from reflection in leadership development. Celebrate this linkage and strength and role of reflexivity.

"The creation of learning environments that utilize reflective practice is offered as an effective grounded method…to help organizations continually learn and improve to meet the rapid change [and]…[in] creating resilient practitioners who [when] utilizing reflective practice will be the cornerstone of the [healthcare] future" (K. Kerfoot in Forward of Sherwood & Horton-Deutsch, 2015, p. xl).

Reflective practice is about leadership of self, others, and organizations and is a professional imperative. It is about learning and mindfulness, all skills required in simulation and Simulation Champions. The linkage is clear!

 Simulation Champions, who either teach or conduct prebriefing and debriefing in simulation, should aim toward promoting reflective thinking. "Reflection is the conscious consideration of the meaning and implication of an action, which includes the assimilation of knowledge, skills, and attitudes with pre-existing knowledge. Reflection can lead to new interpretations by the participants; cognitive reframing is essential to learning" (INACSL Standards Committee, 2016, Debriefing, p. S21).

The Ethics of Leadership and Followership

Six moral virtues have emerged as consensual across cultures and time: *wisdom and knowledge,* characterized by creativity, curiosity, open-mindedness, love of learning, perspective; *courage,* characterized by bravery, persistence, integrity, vitality; *humanity,* characterized by love, kindness, social intelligence; *temperance,* characterized by forgiveness and mercy, humility or modesty, prudence, self-regulation; *justice,* characterized by citizenship, fairness, leadership; *and transcendence,* characterized by an appreciation of beauty and excellence, gratitude, hope, humor, spirituality (Peterson & Seligman as cited in Crossan & Matzutis, 2008).

Courage, as a basic virtue in early nursing, has been identified as missing or uncelebrated in nursing today and is needed for our foundation in caring and compassion (Hawkins & Morse, 2014). Nursing has recognized virtues that have played a role in our historical development and identity but also relational ethics (ethical action within relationships) as foundational to our practice. This also links closely with current leadership and followership perspectives.

Relational ethics comprise four ongoing processes of mutual respect, engagement, embodiment, and environment (Bergum & Dossetor, 2005). It is so important for us to recognize that commitment to fostering *ethical space in relationship* may be the only way to ethically approach diversities of values, beliefs, cultures, knowledge, and gender: mutual respect is the glue that ethically holds relationships together (p. xxix) and is about how we "are with" not "for" others (p. 97). Clarity and choices arise from this relational space.

The ethical space needed for relational practice allows for clear recognition of mutual respect and the professionalism needed to ensure excellence in simulation (INACSL Standards Committee, 2016, Professional Integrity). The diversities respected in this ethical space extend to safe learning environments whether it is for leadership development or required in each simulated event.

Within nursing, we also look to the work of Doane and Varcoe (2015) in understanding the *relational inquiry* that is required in practice with self, others, families, communities, and organizations and in leadership. Relational inquiry further clarifies the role of the relational space and the relational ethics required in practice but most importantly defines the inquiry or the taking on of action with that relational consciousness.

Being is our personal knowing (Johns, 2013) in relationships and how we enact an *ethical and moral being* in all that we do. Ethical Fitness is a personal social awareness and engagement characterized by caring and compassion, honesty, responsibility, respect, fairness, and courage (Kidder, 2005, pp. 50–55). Like any fitness element, ethics and morality require deliberate and constant practice. Moral courage is "the true gauge of our maturity and civilization" (Kidder, 2005) and reflects "a commitment to moral *principles*, an awareness of the *danger* involved in supporting those principles and a willing *endurance* of that danger" (p. 7).

Character matters. "True leaders take responsibility for failures and openly and actively acknowledge mistakes" (Bennis & Goldsmith, 2010, p. 76). Authentic transformational leadership must rest on a moral foundation of legitimate values and in behaviors that are authentic. Deception and manipulation are part of pseudotransformational leadership, a space where true transformational leadership does not reside (Bass & Steidlmeier, 1999, p. 186). It is immoral when information is withheld, when bribes and manipulation are utilized, when authority is abused, and even when nepotism is practiced within an organization (Bass & Steidlmeier, 1999, p. 192). Simulation leaders and followers are called to uphold the values required for authentic transformational leadership with colleagues, as much as with learners. Bass and Steidlmeier (1999) identify that leadership is best served by a moral compass that reads true (p. 193). Three pillars of ethical leadership are identified:

1. "The moral character of the leader;
2. The ethical legitimacy of the values embedded in the leader's vision, articulation, and program which followers either embrace or reject; and

Reflection Activity 8-7
Personal to Group Values Assessment

WHO ARE YOU? Values define us as a person. What are your top values? Consider doing this as you develop your group of champions to build simulation. This may be the "stickiness" of high performance teams. Answer the questions. I am _____. We are _____. If you are further along in your inner leader development consider the values suggested by Kidder (2005) as needed for moral courage: compassion, respect, fairness, responsibility, and honesty. Knowing that (principles + endurance + danger = moral courage), how courageous are you? Where do you stand on moral agency (your personal ability to act from knowing what is right or wrong)? Do you waver? Are you certain? If unsure, what do you do to risk movement? Have you tried and failed? Are you open about personal failure?

DID YOU KNOW! THINK ABOUT THIS: Some consider beliefs as having been based on or formed by past experiences, while values are needed to inform future actions. Articulate your values in your journal and tie them to actions you will take. Consider the belief that was tied to the value and how the two relate. How do beliefs and values differ to you? Why are they important in your role as Simulation Champion? Do not get stalled by beliefs and assumptions!

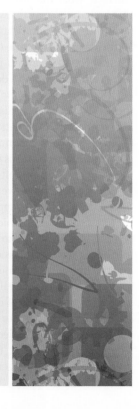

3. The morality of the processes of social ethical choice and action that leaders and followers engage in and collectively pursue" (p. 182)

Strong leader *value positions* are needed in *humility,* acknowledging others over self; *respect,* unconditional regard and consideration for others and self; *honesty,* speaking the truth; *service,* citizenship and a belief in caring for others; *competency,* excellence in skills/tasks and relationships; and *perseverance,* to continue determinedly, intentionally, and mindfully.

Change

Transformational leadership is by definition about change. Leaders, followers, and managers initiate change and sustain momentum through understanding the creative process. Senge (2006) recommends the use of organizational tools and principles that actualize openness, reflection, deep conversations, personal mastery, shared vision, and understanding the broader system. The use of advocacy inquiry is featured as one approach to facilitation that leaders can use and is discussed in more detail in another chapter. Scharmer (as cited in Senge, 2006) identifies three thresholds a leader must pass "in leading profound change: opening the head, opening the heart, and opening the will." Skelton-Green, Simpson, and Scott (2007) at the Dorothy Wylie Nursing Leadership Institute (DMW-NLI) in Toronto, ON, Canada, developed a comprehensive methodology for change initiatives based on change theory and project management (see Fig. 8.2). The richness of this model is that it incorporates the three typical project foci to leading change within an organization: *people-driven approaches, project management, and strategic planning* (pp. 3–4) and principles of transformational leadership. The model also uses two key underpinnings:

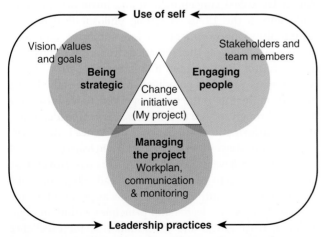

Figure 8.2 DMW-NLI Leading Change Framework. (Redrawn from Skelton-Green, J., Simpson, B., & Scott, J. (2007). An integrated approach to change leadership. *Canadian Journal of Nursing Leadership, 20*(3), 1-15.)

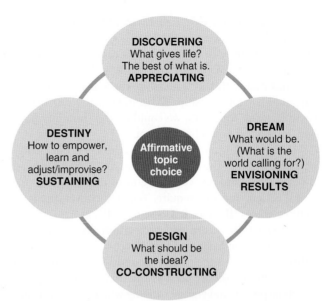

Figure 8.3 Appreciative 4D Cycle. (Redrawn from Cooperrider, D. L., & Whitney, D. (2005). *Appreciative inquiry: A positive revolution in change.* San Francisco, California: Berrett-Koehler Publishers, Inc.)

- Kouzes and Posner's Exemplary Leadership Practices (2007, 2014)
- Use of Self: Personal integrity, Goleman's Emotional Intelligence Model and Lifelong Learning (Skelton-Green et al., 2007, p. 5)

Change theories and approaches can be integrated into the model and assist in the change process and structure. Appreciative inquiry (AI) can be utilized as both an approach and a strategy for transformational organizational change (Moody, Horton-Deutsch, & Pesut, 2007, p. 319). As a change management process, AI accesses organizational human potential, increasing engagement, and *focuses on the positive* of what is working well (Cooperrider and Whitney, 2005). AI is also used as a debriefing model for simulation activities and scenarios. The visioning and dreaming stage is critical as in transformational leadership, but discovering what is currently the best begins a 4D cycle of appreciation (Fig. 8.3).

Bad, Ineffective, and Toxic Leadership

What happens when competence and ambition and integrity are not in balance? To suggest that leadership is only a positive concept is neglectful of the true situation. Bennis and Goldsmith (2010) identify a *three-legged stool* on which true leadership sits. If competence, integrity, and ambition are out of balance, negative outcomes occur (p. 29). Today, we see a crisis in leadership ranging from immoral to unethical to violations of the public trust. What happens to organizations and to people exposed to bad leadership? Who has the responsibility to "keep leaders in check"? Kellerman (2008; 2014) would indicate that followers could have a clear responsibility and accountability to leaders and to organizations to be the check and balance for the integrity of leadership. She identifies that with bad leadership, there is bad follower-ship and toxic followership. We would like to think that as exemplary star followers, we could be the "humility handler" for leaders and other followers.

Understanding about how to live ethically in our changing world is about "the emerging understanding of the need to respect relational space as an ethical responsibility" for ethical action, and this requires ongoing conversations of multiple voices (Bergum & Dossetor, 2005, p. 221). Varied voices need to be heard and respectfully contradicted as "no one voice can truly represent all others" (p. 221). These authors have based their research and work on the belief that we cannot objectify persons and that we need to know the whole person and engage with the whole person. So, are ineffective and toxic leaders lacking in ethical responsibility? YES. Can we change them? Perhaps, probably no, but we can voice concerns and change the circumstances for self, others, and organizations and hope that as a person they focus on development of self and engage in introspection. As a Simulation Champion, you can be alert to toxicity within your group and in the context of change within your organization. Marshall (2011) makes an important distinction for us when she writes: "be vigilant in your own experience. Neither your career nor your life is long enough to spend any of your finite time working with a bad leader. When you recognize that you are in a bad situation ... where there is no hope, no dealing with a person who is irrational and unable to take a healthy leadership perspective, where the person is truly doing harm... honestly evaluate the situation" (p. 202).

Lipman-Blumen (2005) and Pelletier (2011), both internationally recognized as experts in this area, describe a complex toxicity associated with leadership. One that is demoralizing and destructive and not easily rectified. Suggestions from both authors provide guidelines: understand the dynamics of toxicity, speak the truth but in a safe environment, document, provide information to the leader, challenge only when safety is uncompromised, use supporters, and, if necessary, work to oust the leader or leave the organization if change is not possible. Pelletier (2011) also created a useful typology to assist in understanding the categorization of behaviors and the rhetoric associated with bad, ineffective, and toxic leadership.

Being a "whistle-blower" takes moral courage and happens when values trump fears (Kidder, 2005, p. 80). Moral courage is needed to confront the bad or toxic leader or follower. Ethical decision making at these times is often a decision about right versus wrong, but sometimes, the more difficult decision is right versus right and this calls for moral courage (p. 86). A dysfunctional culture in which bad leadership and bad followership occurs requires moral courage to surmount the communication barriers (p. 179).

"Moral courage has a defining role when organizational cultures are in disrepair...yet we must strive to create organizations [and cultures] where moral courage is not needed" (p. 179). Thus, it is the paradox of complexity. Principle-based or values-based leadership is required in organizations if they and people are to thrive and survive.

Additional Leadership Perspectives

Learning about leadership is a journey of considering as many and as varied a viewpoint as is written by our experts, our scholars, and our researchers. The journey of self-discovery of leadership is an ongoing lifelong journey, and the quest for understanding should incorporate reading as many leadership texts as possible from as many disciplines as possible. The future of leadership and indeed followership and management will be the result of discourse, inquiry, reflection, and application of the new sciences and a new worldview of how organizations can best thrive. Leadership for tomorrow will be directed at the importance of relationship and people-focused orientations. This is what we have come to understand.

The process of deconstructing our old frameworks and ways of doing business is always in process. We need to inform ourselves and evolve our competencies and skills, being open to experience the joy of learning. Some additional viewpoints on learning about leadership are shared and recommended for your further perusal. Do not limit your experience to these comments but engage more deeply in the scholars' perspectives in your own way and time. Seek a balanced perspective and look outside the discipline of nursing to other disciplines and their historical and contemporary gurus. Your learning potential is limitless.

Servant Leadership

Robert Greenleaf conceptualized and introduced servant leadership in the 1970s. A strong philosophical base in community, empowerment, shared authority, and relational power suggests the "servant as leader" as a construct for the future (Bass as cited in Sendjaya & Sarros, 2002). At its core is a marked paradigm shift that sees the leader move from the top of the leader pyramid, to lead from the bottom through service to followers. Servant leadership is about transformation, and the chief difference is that a servant leader or steward serves first and then leads (Greenleaf as cited in Sendjaya & Sarros, 2002). This has proven true in the development of transcendent leadership concepts. Research by these authors suggests that as persons become grounded in servant leadership principles within an organization, trust grows and the foundation for excellence is developed (p. 62). Current role models of this type of leadership are seen in altruistic Nobel Peace Prize winners Mother Teresa and most recently Malala Yousafzai.

Primal Leadership

Primal leadership (Goleman, Boyatzis, & McKee, 2002) came about as a result of work in emotional intelligence (EI) realizing that emotions matter for leaders in management (p. 245). Emotional intelligence offers the essential competencies for resonant leadership, a form of leadership that uses skills in emotional and social intelligence to foster positive relationships and fostering healthy spaces for themselves and others to thrive and attain common goals. These are competencies that can be developed and strengthened in individuals and teams and distributed throughout an organization. These authors argue that the fundamental task of leaders is "to prime good feelings in those they lead" and that the deep reverberating resonance that is created is a reservoir of positivity that "frees the best in people" (p. viii). They further emphasize that the emotional task of the leader is *primal*, both in originality and in importance; and "the driving of emotions in the right direction" ensures that success, performance, and power are derived for the individual, team, and organization. The authors indicate a shared belief in the power and empowerment of distributed leadership in organizations but acknowledge that the leader has maximal power to sway everyone's emotions for better or for worse. Positively, it is resonant; negatively, it is dissonant. Cummings et al. (2010) classify or categorize leadership styles as resonate or dissonant and indicate the positive effects in organizational culture with resonate or people or relationship-focused leadership styles. This emphasizes the importance of not just focusing on *what leaders do* but on *how they do it*.

Quantum Leadership

The authors approach the topic of leadership through the issues of the fast rate of change and changes in the responsibilities of providers and consumers of healthcare services. Porter-O'Grady and Malloch (2003) integrate systems theory, complexity theory, and quantum theory to illustrate the structure components of the new framework of this century as we move from the *Industrial Age* to the *Technology Age (or Information Age)*. The authors identify that leaders must anticipate the path of change, see it as a journey, and act as agents or strategists of change. Quantum theory describes changes or transformations not as an event or a thing but as a dynamic, such as the Internet and fiber optics, portability and accessibility of information, intentional and mindful personalization's of relationships, and miniaturization that allows less costly mobility, connectedness, and innovations (pp. 1–23). Leaders will change from a focus on "What have you done? [To] What difference did it make?" (p. 21) since sustainability stems from the

point of service in an organization. Quantum leadership is responsive to the *Technology Age* and incorporates a strong complexity science approach to developing a new paradigm for leadership as organizations restructure in this new century.

New Science of Leadership

Margaret Wheatley (2006) advocates that we ground our thinking in the "science of our times" and uses three sciences: quantum physics, self-organizing systems, and chaos theory to suggest a new worldview. It is within this worldview that we come to understand the importance of relationship in a new paradigm for management and leadership and a greater understanding of the importance of followership (p. 14). The author clearly identifies that the promise of a new paradigm brings renewed hope for the resolution of seemingly insolvable problems (p. xiv). The emphasis in the new science is that our world coevolves as we interact in it and with it and with others; and the *focus is on holism*, not on parts: a system is understood as a whole and *attention is given to relationships within those networks* (p. 10). Sometimes, the solutions come by learning to understand the complementary nature of different phenomena and knowing the right questions to ask!

"The participatory nature of reality … focuses attention on relationships…Nothing exists independent of its relationships" (p. 163). Wheatley (2006) suggests that the contemporary leadership problems are a result of being human: that we struggle to learn to work with diversity, uniqueness, and teams; that we are terrified of emotions of conflict, loss, and love; and that overall, we do not know how to work together (p. 164). This becomes a challenge for the new leadership, as persons in Western cultures have not been socialized to these new worldview values of collaboration, synergy, holism, and connectedness. We are called to evolve beyond the individualistic, competition-based, and mechanistic views of the 19th and 20th centuries.

Transcendent Leadership

*"Average leaders raise the bar on themselves; good leaders raise the bar for others; great leaders inspire others to raise their own bar"—**Orrin Woodward, LIFE***

Sometimes referred to as visionary leadership, enlightened leadership, or responsible and accountable leadership; transcendent leadership was initially introduced in 2006 and 2007 as a global imperative. Transcendent leadership is grounded in servant and transformational leadership and shared governance to establish the trust needed for global sustainability (Gardiner, 2009). This situates leadership as service to humanity and society and is achieved through relational values-based inquiry. Crossan and Mazutis (2008) describe an integrative framework for leadership through transcendence and the necessity of multiple levels of leadership: levels of self, others, organization, and society. Transcendent, in the sense that the leader transcends levels through a quality of going above and beyond, within and between levels (p. 132). A transcendent leader is better positioned to leading in complex, turbulent, and highly transparent environments (p. 133), and an emphasis on the importance of leadership of self in strategic decision making is emphasized. Leadership of self includes self-awareness and self-regulation through reflection and introspection. Leadership of others is an integration of leadership of self with authentic and transformational behaviors directed toward other centric leadership development. Leadership of self and organizations is accomplished by integrating self with strategy and flexible management structures and adapting creatively to the internal and external environments and constant change. Through consistence with corporate social responsibility and transparency, transcendence results with the organizational level changing to include the social level (p. 137).

New Paradigm Needed: A Call to Action for a New Paradigm of Leadership, Management, and Followership!

"Go to the people. Learn from them. Live with them. Start with what they know. Build with what they have. The best of leaders when the job is done, when the task is accomplished, the people will say we have done it ourselves"—**Lao Tzu**

What About Leadership in the New Paradigm?

"Another new paradigm is needed—one that provides a context for leaders to understand their responsibility to lead the transformation of economic, social and political conditions. This new paradigm of leadership must be based on ethical values and a commitment to be fully integrated and evolved human beings" **(Bennis & Goldsmith, 2010, p. 73)**.

Values-based leadership is critical for the new paradigm. Leaders "must be able not only to see into the darkness of the future but to live comfortably inside the potential that risky, unsettled space between the present and the future. And because leaders cannot pull people into a future only they have conceived of, they must bring everyone to the table to shape the future through collective dialogue and concerted action" (Porter-O'Grady & Malloch, 2003, p. ix).

"There go the people. I must follow them for I am their leader"
—**Alexandre Ledru-Rollin**

The applications of quantum theory, complexity science, and chaos theory in understanding how organizations are formed, reformed, and structured have altered the landscape of leadership forever (Porter-O'Grady, & Malloch, 2003, p. 41). Senge (2006) uses a three-legged stool metaphor (another one!) to symbolically represent the core learning capabilities of teams: *aspiration*, personal mastery and shared vision; *reflective conversations*, mental models and dialogue; and *understanding complexity*, systems thinking. Senge (2006) further describes a belief that "people are socialized in ways of thinking and acting that are embedded in their most formative institutional experiences" and that the prevailing system of management will not be changed unless our system of education changes or is transformed. That is unless the three-legged stool is intact and the core learning capabilities are realized (p. xiii). Senge (2006) advocates an alternative system of management based on *love* (not fear), *curiosity* (not insistence on right), and *learning* (rather than controlling). Diverse thinking paradigms and use of "out-of-the-box" thinking are required in our new paradigm for leadership. An uncommon sense approach to arriving at new knowledge in complex situations has been developed from Tao leadership philosophy and illustrates this innovative and creative thinking needed by leaders for the 21st century (Fu & Bergeon, 2012).

What about followership in this new paradigm? Hurwitz and Hurwitz (2015) identify two trends that characterize work in the 21st century: "the increased use of teams as the primary way to get things done; and the amount of interpersonal change in the workplace" (p. 3). Complexity requires multiple players and their cognitive abilities and contributions in multiple teams to accomplish the tasks and work of organizations. We become members of multiple teams and at the same time experience changes in work settings, bosses, organizational restructuring, and colleagues such that we have a "near-constant state of building and re-building relationships" (p. 5). The authors further suggest that this constant change in relationships is the "most disruptive and difficult type of change because it affects our sense of self." These authors have developed a model called *The Generative Partnership Model* (GP Model) to emphasize the importance of the understanding, acknowledging, and optimizing of the roles of both followers and leaders among members of team as true respectful partners. This is a model for the 21st organization that recognizes complexity and the importance of relationship. The model "opens up leadership to everyone while normalizing followership" (p. 10). This is about culture building and resocialization through education in organizations. "All the leadership skill in the world is meaningless (or, at least, less meaningful) if there isn't a complementary followership skill. The two are a matched set" (p. 38).

Reflection Activity 8-8
Personal Development Summary

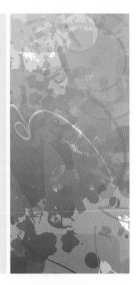

"Get to the truth: You are meant to play big with your life." Robin Sharma from *The Greatness Guide Book 2*.

CONSIDER: All that you have provided in your journaling and what it now reveals about you. Leadership and followership are in all of us; know that a great leader will draw them out. Review the LPI results or take it now. Plan to make a change right now and continue your leadership development. What are your mental models of leadership and followership now? What has influenced you?

You are a champion and a hero! Work to keep your simulation leadership development is on track for success.

Well into the 21st century, nursing must be prepared to achieve "greater equity in whose voices is heard" (Storch, Starzomski, & Rodney, 2013, p. 529). Furthermore, these authors suggest that nurses are well positioned "to take leadership roles...and shape the changes that need to occur in the future" (p. 531). An ethical lens must become embedded in healthcare in all decisions and actions and "continuous reflection and political action are required to ensure that nursing messages receive prominence in healthcare reform" (p. 532). Nurses and nursing must assume a leadership role based in moral agency to influence local, regional, societal, and global change.

So here, we are at our end and your beginning! Leadership, followership, and managership for the 21st century needs to be people and relationship focused, team focused, based on supportive managerial structures, and operationalized through a collaborative partnership of mutual trust and respect and courage; values and principle based in self, team, organizational, and global systems. It must be energized through ethical transformation and transcendence. In a world that is becoming increasingly complex "whether through interconnected global economies, technologies that transcend communication, cultural boundaries, and traditional practices, or the speed at which problems need to be solved individually or collectively, the 2050 leader must be able to work effectively and draw upon a multitude of leadership skill-sets on demand" (Jackson, 2015, p. 242). The vision we hold for the 21st century is one of caring and compassion for the environment and the beings that care for it. Indeed, it is the embodiment of leadership knowing and "the positive growth and profound personal change" in individuals that "will restore us one leader at a time to a collective ethic of service" (Burgess, 2013, pp. 19–20). Reframing the understanding of leadership and followership will take a strong commitment to resocialization and transformed education. The challenge, however, starts with the self and works from there. The world is changing and us with it. It may be our biggest challenge ever and we are confident that together, we have the capacity and courage to change to a new and better humanistic worldview. As Simulation Champions, we are charged to lead and follow by forging positive change through exemplary courage, caring, and connection!

Summary

Where are you at in your journey? Are you still in it? We sure hope so! This chapter discussion has identified and illuminated specific beliefs and assumptions about leadership and followership. We believe that:

1. Leadership and followership are socially constructed.
2. Manager, follower, and leader are different but each is created and based in relational practice and inquiry. The same holds true for Simulation Champions.
3. Learning about leadership starts with the person and develops "inside out" using reflective pedagogies to reach critical consciousness, intentionality, and mindfulness. Reflective pedagogies are inherent in and essential to effective simulation practice.
4. Leadership is about leadership of self, groups, and organizations.
5. Followership is an underappreciated and increasingly important construct.
6. The system complexity of the 21st century requires new management structures and systems defined by transformational and transcendent leadership.
7. A new paradigm of collaborative partnerships in leadership and followership is needed for the 21st century characterized by moral courage and ethical practices.
8. *A call for action* in leadership and followership development is needed. This requires a resocialization and education that starts with self and modeled outward.

9. Leadership and simulation are related in knowledge, reflective pedagogy, and relational inquiry.

10. The Simulation Champion must heed the *call to action* to develop multiple sets of integrated competencies within the "Simulation Champion being" follower, leader, and manager for excellence in healthcare education in the 21st century.

Toolkit Resources

Toolkit 8-1: My Leadership Journal
Toolkit 8-2: Fiedler's *Least Preferred Co-worker Scale* (LPC)

Colette Foisy-Doll, Carol Wild

Key Terms

Organizational Culture, Organizational Climate, Change Leadership, Change Management, Transformational Change, Executive Sponsorship, Perseverance, SWOT, SOAR

Guiding Questions

1. How has your organization's culture impacted the uptake of simulation? How would you describe your organizational culture and its impact on your simulation integration journey so far?

2. Are change leadership and management models regularly used in your organization? If not, how could you employ these models to advance simulation in your institution?

3. Do you have a Simulation Champion executive sponsor(s) in your organization?

4. Have efforts to integrate simulation been met with resistance, obstacles, and failure? Do you know how to lead and manage change to overcome those barriers?

Introduction

How do we make a difference or harness the energy in people and organizations? It helps to understand that "organizations are living, open systems capable of self-renewal" (Wheatley, 2006, p. 77). Wheatley's timeless work on change leadership tells us that leaders need to open ourselves to change by giving up the need for equilibrium and balance. Instead, be open to embracing imbalance as the new normal (2006; 2012). Equilibrium and stability are characteristics of closed systems that are no longer capable of system change. Therefore, our goal in leading change in organizations is to reside squarely in the space of *nonequilibrium*. It is in the

space that we can capitalize on the messy "off–kilter" experiences that are the seeds of growth (Wheatley, 2012). It is about understanding the complexity and connectivity of systems in the world around us and thus the relationships between people, organizations, and their environments (2005; 2012). Understanding complexity in organizations gives a way to harness the energy within our complex adaptive systems for growth and change. In fact, we are capable of so much more when we choose curiosity over certainty (Snowden, 2015).

Given what we now know about change, it is clear that leading complex systems in our 21st century requires specialized knowledge, skills, and attitudes that can be fostered within each of us to maneuver the murky waters of change. Simulation is an extremely complex endeavor that requires thoughtful attention to organizational culture, climate, and knowing how change happens in your milieu. Taplay, Jack, Baxter, Eva, and Martin (2014) rightly state, "There is more to integrating simulation into nursing curriculum than faculty buy-in" (p. 2).

In this chapter, we offer you relevant information on organizational change, culture, and climate and a host of tools and perspectives to promote positive change experiences

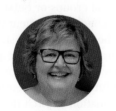

Colette Foisy-Doll,
MSN, RN, CHSE

Carol Wild,
MScN, BN, RN

in the adoption and curricular integration of simulation in your organization. Remember, people are your most valuable resource on this journey, period. We wish you success as you persevere within your organizations to make our learning world a better place. Let the changes begin!

Persevering in the 21st Century

Human beings have always had to **persevere** as a matter of survival. What is most needed of leaders and followers in organizations in these times of complexity and chaos is perseverance. Margaret Wheatley (2010) describes *perseverance* as a day-to-day decision to not give up. It is about committing to see things as they are, as they could be, and working with focused intention to make them *what they should be*. On the change journey in our complex environments, we can lose our way, become overwhelmed, feel betrayed or exhausted, and lose heart in our efforts. Does that sound like a familiar experience in your simulation change efforts? To survive the day-to-day struggles inherent in complex change, we must nurture the best in each other, celebrate even the smallest of successes, and hold on tight during the most difficult times. New ideas, inspirations, and energy are all around you; so do welcome them in.

As leaders and followers working in organizations, we are called to stretch ourselves to do things believed impossible, like fighting to change our unwieldy healthcare systems. Often in the quagmire of complexity, we can feel alone and are left wondering if one person can make a meaningful impact. We do believe that one person can and does change the world; it happens around us every day. In his classic work on change, Malcolm Gladwell tells us that the *power of one* or *very few* usually form the impetus for reaching a tipping point to accelerate change (2002). That being said, if we actually want to transform our complex systems in education and healthcare, we will need to abandon our exclusive reliance on the leader-as-hero (Wheatley, 2011). Change may start with one or very few, but it never ends with one. We need each other to succeed: high-functioning teams are grounded in a leader's willingness to build leadership capacity in others.

Change Leadership and Change Management

Change leaders and managers of today must accept that change is an ongoing *event*; it is situational and *external* to us and involves something stopping while something new is starting (Bridges, 2009). The emotion experienced during change, on the other hand, is psychological; it is lived *internally* and is often felt as loss, chaos, and confusion, and for some, it is freeing, renewing, and energizing (Bridges, 2009). What is needed to survive the dynamic change machine is excellence in *change leadership*. Change leadership for the 21st century focuses on a vision for people, relationships, and teams; it is aimed at building collaborative and transformational partnerships that are fortified by mutual trust, respect, and courage and supported by strong organizational structures and management practices.

Think for a moment of the many *difference makers* of this world and ponder their extraordinary abilities. Which change leaders would be on your list? Ours include Nelson Mandela, Malala Yousafzai, Steve Jobs, Bill Gates, Mother Teresa, Rick Hanson, Terry Fox, Deepak Choprah, Eckhart Tolle, Winston Churchill, John F. Kennedy, Martin Luther King, Oprah Winfrey, or perhaps Florence Nightingale? The list goes on. These individuals were all motivated by an urgency for change in the world and had the courage, compassion, conviction, as well as the ability to persevere, regardless of circumstance. They embraced good in the world around them and worked to make change possible.

Change leadership is a necessary solution for sustainable change that change management alone fails to accomplish. Effective organizational change requires that leaders have the *big picture view* of an organization and the ability to articulate a clear vision for the future and the urgent reasons for change. These persons are skilled motivators that inspire and empower others to take on even the most difficult change, adept connectors who foster key relationships internally and externally, with individuals and groups to mobilize necessary resources. Change leaders have the passion to put fuel on the fire, keeping change momentum on track (Kotter International, 2015a).

Change management, on the other hand, is the continuous process of aligning an organization with its marketplace and processes—and aims to do so more responsively and efficiently than its competitors. The change manager is the *doer* in the equation, the one that puts into action the change leader's great vision. Organizations across the world are using change management processes and tools to keep change leaders and stakeholders abreast of key changes and most importantly, to balance the budget. Change managers tend to be associated with discrete and containable change that can either be carried out by internal groups or outsourced to consultants specializing in change management (Kotter International, 2015a). You will be asked about sustainability of current practices and future plans. John Gillespie tells us how important it is to collect data in the form of hard facts and figures on past and future. Your executive sponsor will need this type of information to pitch the integration of simulation, so take John's advice and start collecting now!

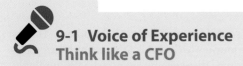

9-1 Voice of Experience
Think like a CFO

John Gillespie

The Challenge

As the former Corporate Director of Simulation Operations at Galen College of Nursing, prior to my arrival, one of the challenges that we worked through was that the college had purchased equipment that was not tied to any real objectives. After getting a better understanding of the organizational goals, we determined that we needed more equipment at a higher fidelity to meet our course objectives.

Meeting the Challenge

To be able to secure all of the equipment that we needed, I had to request the funds outside of the normal budget process directly from our CFO (Chief Financial Officer). While I made a convincing argument, he asked two data-driven questions that I couldn't answer beyond antidotal responses. His questions were:

- How can you document that you are effectively using the equipment that you have today?
- Could you please show me the integration plan that you are going to use to insure that this additional equipment will be used?

Both are great questions that I had not anticipated him asking. He was thinking like an accountant. I was behaving like an educator. The two methods would have eventually achieved the same results with the equipment being used, but it was not strong enough to allow me to compete for the funds that I needed.

Outcome

The answer came with tracking our usage on all of the equipment across all of the campuses. Additionally, we needed to document how often we were limited by not having the equipment that we had requested. Using data to capture our limitations, we were able to demonstrate "holes" in our curriculum. Additionally, through this data collection, we were able to better

identify areas that we were highly efficient as well as areas that clearly we were having challenges in. From this initial data collection starting point of how many learners were being supported in which courses, we grew to using data to measure many things. We were able to use our data to not only measure efficiencies but also quality of customer satisfaction and quality of faculty preparedness.

Most Valuable Lesson Learned

The lesson learned was that our simulation program was destined to stay in the same place that it had been if we had not started collecting. However, we not only had to collect the data but also use it to drive our needs in a competitive financial market. We had to use our data to position our needs higher than other areas in the school that were also seeking funding for other projects. With this data, we were able to show a clear need that would benefit the organization as a whole.

It is not enough to just collect the data. You also have to use the data. Goals for data collection must be in place before designing your data collection tool and should tie into organizational goals. Remember, the data that you collect are only as good as the tool that you create to collect it. If you can do this to show value back to the organization with consistency and regularly, you will likely be granted your requests more often than if you had not done any data collection at all.

Inspiration for Simulation Champions

"To do a common thing, uncommonly well brings success"
—Henry J. Heinz

Organizations do need skilled change managers and all that they bring; however, in the absence of effective leadership, even the most talented, efficient, well-intentioned managers can founder. Both are needed, and sometimes both the change leader and the manager are one in the same. We have had to learn to be both!

We have been in the educational and healthcare field for long enough to see change leadership and management mistakes recur, over and over again. They include (1) creating a lot of hype through floods of emails and messaging that somehow never gets off the ground, (2) lacking a system approach to implementing change, (3) the absence of succession planning so programs fold, (4) leaders who silo themselves in their offices and do not connect with individuals and teams on the ground, (5) absence of, or weak strategy that is not linked to organizational goals,

(6) directives given by leadership with no follow-up, and (7) development of great strategy, but no implementation plan, timelines, and goal setting. We have also been witness to great successes and feature two such exemplars in this chapter. The many organizational successes we have experienced over the years have all included great leadership. These leaders also demonstrated strong followership and managership when it best suited organizational goals.

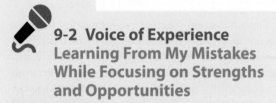

9-2 Voice of Experience
Learning From My Mistakes While Focusing on Strengths and Opportunities

Colette Foisy-Doll, MSN, RN, CHSE

The Challenge

In the 1990s, when simulation was first introduced in healthcare education and clinical practice settings, innovators and early adopters recognized the potential for meaningful learning; I was among those that were excited and inspired. However, like the vast majority of my simulationist peers, we took on simulation leadership roles for which there was no preparation and somehow muddled our way through. Over the past 15+ years, I have had the privilege of working with dozens of teams to implement simulation-based learning programs and design learning spaces. What became evident to me was that most, if not all organizations (including my own), failed to effectively plan for the organizational culture change that is required for successful simulation-based learning program integration. In the beginning, most (if not all) simulation initiatives started with a simulator purchase—followed by a "now what?" moment. Ours sat in a box for one year because we didn't have a locked storage area. I have personally seen "simulator graveyards" with unpacked and unutilized simulators ranging from tens of thousands to millions of dollars in value.

Meeting the Challenge

As my knowledge of simulation grew and I came to understand better what successful implementation entailed, so did my passion to help others. That is where the journey to the book *Simulation Champions* began for me, through my own struggles and successes and by responding to "calls for help" from others. I began to write a simulation user manual that just kept growing and growing in size over the years.

Outcome

In the early years, I partnered with a simulation enthusiast and friend, Susan Morhart. Together, Susan and I teamed up as simulation consultants, and many years later, Damian Henri—a simulation architect joined us to offer conference workshops. Together, we enhanced the "how to manual" titled *Simulation Champions* a resource to help organizations jump-start their programs. Feedback from the manual was overwhelmingly positive and colleagues urged us to publish. Over many years, that manual evolved into the book you are reading today.

Most Valuable Lessons Learned

In retrospect, I feel very fortunate that most of the requisite conditions for effective organizational culture change were present in my organization. I also worked with generous leaders who believed in me and were willing to mentor me. As a Simulation Champion, we need a balance of personal and professional skills to effectively lead and manage change because simulation is ever changing. Build on your existing strengths to become a better clinician, educator, director, politician, communicator, organizer, decision-maker, team member, follower, marketer, analyzer, system thinker, business thinker, and change leader and manager. These, in fact, are many of the executive skill sets required of Simulation Champions today.

Lead where you are. Have *courage* to follow your heart. Know when to lead, when to manage, and when to follow. Build on yours and others' strengths. Know that weaknesses fall by the wayside when you focus on doing your best. Trust in goodness, and forgive mistakes quickly—both yours and others'. *Connect* with others to build capacity. *Care* about being your best and about empowering others to do the same!

Inspiration for Simulation Champions

"Have courage to think differently, courage to invent, to travel the unexplored path, courage to discover the impossible and to conquer the problems and succeed."
—A. P. J. Abdul Kalam

Culture and Climate in Organizations: Seeing the Forest Through the Trees

"Each organization has a distinctive culture, a combination of the impact of its founders, history, successes, crises and current leadership. Organizations also have routines and rituals, the 'way we do things'— ***Kotter, 1996, p. 14***

Culture-, and climate-related concepts - effective leaders will possess knowledge of both within their organization.

Culture, Subculture, and Climate

Culture is "deep, broad, and stable: slow to change, but for many leaders is difficult to define" (Schein, 2009, p. 51). Schein, a world-renowned scholar and researcher in organizational change, describes **organizational culture** as "both a *here and now* dynamic phenomenon… a coercive background structure that influences us in multiple ways… it is constantly enacted and reenacted, created by our interactions with others and shaped by our own behavior" (p. 3). How would you describe your organizational culture? Culture in organizations is difficult to pin down. It lurks in hidden places like in the "mindsets and frames [of employees]…and are powerful in their impact but invisible, and to a considerable degree unconscious" (2010, p. 14).

Subcultures reside in smaller subgroups within the larger culture where they develop their own unique cultures. Think of the subcultures you interact with every day in your workplace. For example, universities have departments such as faculties and programs, research departments, admissions, campus life, library, human resources, etc. Subcultures not only thrive, but wield a great deal of power in organizations. Interestingly, subcultures are most often influenced by those with informal power, so knowing your people is crucial. Even for the best of leaders, understanding and shaping culture is an exercise in mental gymnastics!

On the other hand, **organizational climate,** sometimes referred to as corporate climate, is different than culture. Climate refers to the feeling or social atmosphere within a group (Schein, 2010; Schneider & Barbera, 2014). Think about the climate in your simulation centre or organization. How would you describe what it feels like to work there? Put simply, culture speaks to "how we do things around here" while climate speaks to "how it feels to do things around here." A positive work culture and climate are defining indicators of high-performing teams. If you don't feel overall positivity about your work culture and climate, chances are good that other employees think and feel the same way. Positivity in organizations is contagious and doesn't happen by accident. It takes skilled leadership and ongoing commitment to build a strong culture and positive climate.

Organizational Structure for Simulation Success

Kotter (2014) tells us how, using the Accelerate (XLR8) system, organizations in today's dynamic environments can become more agile, increase employee satisfaction, and get better results (p. 12). In today's environments, change often fails because of bureaucratic structures and processes that are too cumbersome and slow to be effective. To create effective, reliable, and efficient structures with the increased agility, speed, and efficiency required for simulation, organizations need to transform archaic bureaucracies. What is needed is a new structure with a new set of processes and procedures to achieve better organizational results. Simulation champions must be empowered by organizational structures to be "change agents who can get more done faster" (p. 14). For example, one institution spoke of taking 3 years of bureaucratic red tape to purchase one simulator! At that rate, by the time the simulator arrives, its shelf life is nearly over. In our fast-paced environments, there is simply no way for organizational leadership teams to do all they have to without sharing leadership and divesting authority to make things happen.

The XLR8 system features a "network-like structure that operates *in concert* with the traditional bureaucratic hierarchy" to create a "dual operating system" (Kotter, p. 12). Figure 9.1 depicts how a simulation team/program can be positioned off-the-grid, operating as a semiconnected entity that strategically networks with internal and external stakeholders. By pulling itself off the bureaucratic grid, the Simulation Program can be granted a certain level of functional autonomy such as having the ability to budget and purchase equipment independently, to have its own steering committee, or to develop strategic partnerships apart from the organization. In this way, the simulation team/Program also has the freedom to capitalize on opportunities in the larger simulation world while having the ability to enact rapid and responsive change to challenges. Explore how your Simulation Program fit in this dual system.

Executive Sponsorship for Simulation Adoption

As an advocate and leader of simulation adoption and curricular integration, you have the difficult mission of infusing energy and change into structures and processes. In doing so, you must promote movement, balance, and forward momentum in organizational culture. Failure to do so will result in disequilibrium, dissension, and disengagement so do not ever try to do this alone. Top-down, bottom-up, and side-to-side

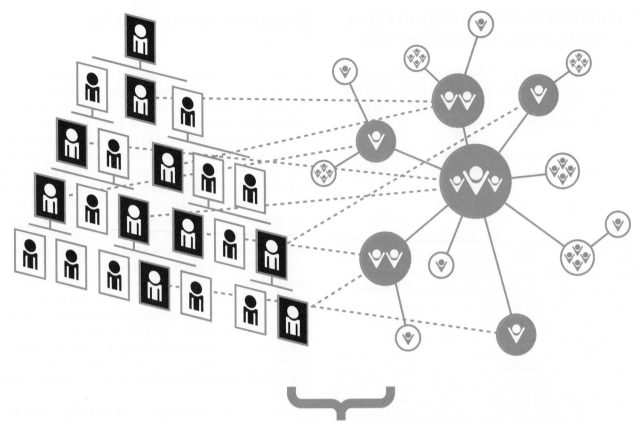

Figure 9.1 XLR8 Dual Operating System. (From Kotter, J. P. (2014). *XLR8: Accelerate*. Boston, MA: Harvard Business School Press.)

forces are at play in organizations, and it is key that you understand all of them and the forces that interplay between them. How does a simulation champion then advocate for and influence change for the successful adoption of simulation? One of the essential elements of successful change is most certainly linked to **executive sponsorship**.

Your executive sponsor(s) is an individual or team of individuals that possess a solid understanding of simulation-based education and that work to make things happen. These individuals will go to bat for you at board meetings, influence agendas at top levels, secure funding, engage other institutions, and have your back by supporting the simulation project at every opportunity. Whether you are the Chief Executive Officer, Dean/Associate Dean, or the manager of a small nursing lab, you NEED executive sponsorship. John Kotter, another organizational change guru, would call a group of such individuals your guiding coalition (2015). Prosci Solutions, Inc. (2016) reports that in over 20 years of research, executive sponsorship has consistently been cited the "greatest contributor to success when managing change and project teams" (page 4). Consistently, since the late 90s, Prosci's benchmark studies have listed ineffective change sponsorship from senior leaders as the number one obstacle to successful change.

Sadly, most employees rated nearly 50% of their executive sponsors as poor to fair and believe that their leaders do not understand the important role they play in leading change. The connection between the executive sponsor and change success is clear. Kruse and Louis found the single most important aspect of leading a change process is for the leader to maintain a *culture of positivity* and a *spirit of inclusivity and collegiality* (2009). This task is not easy, requiring leaders to be emotionally intelligent, people-centered, and value-driven amidst uncertainty and fear. Executive sponsors play a pivotal role in creating psychological safety in the change process. Therefore, those leading the change effort are wise to draw upon the existing strengths of individuals and teams when developing processes, structures, and environments to support employees through change.

In simulation endeavors, the executive sponsor must work to create a compelling, positive vision and then be able to clearly communicate it. Role modeling positive behaviors and attitudes are essential. It is crucial in times of change to provide education and training and to involve employees in planning and implementing efforts throughout the change process. In other words, give teams a chance to own the change to create buy-in. This could not be truer with simulation integration initiatives.

Keep in mind, however, that the change leader must also provide resources and time for dedicated personnel to facilitate the change. All too often the resources needed to make change happen do not accompany the command, "just get the job done." A simulation champion can quickly find themselves in over their head at the deep end of the pool.

Organizations can and do become stagnant. The world is a fast-changing place and organizations need leaders who are lifelong learners, committed to ongoing excellence. Organizations must leverage the strengths, motivations, and abilities of their senior executives and support them in building up their individual leadership competencies. Executive formation to create a high-performance organization includes such initiatives as targeted 360-degree feedback, leadership retreats, action-learning projects carried out with mentors, or to provide focused leadership programs (Zenger, Sandholtz, & Folkman, 2014). Executive leadership skills are not competencies we are born with—they must be learned!

Model for Organizational Change and the Adoption of Simulation

Although there is little research on the organizational influences that shape the adoption of simulation, one recent grounded theory study by Taplay et al. (2014) set out to learn just that. The team conducted semistructured interviews (*n* = 43) across 13 nursing programs in Ontario, Canada. Findings revealed that the leading factor in nursing programs that demonstrated the highest simulation adoption rate was *shared leadership*. Those high uptake cases consisted of a nurse administrator working collaboratively with a dedicated simulation champion(s). This study further underscores the importance of your executive sponsor! Without them, you will find yourself trying to implement a massive undertaking alone and in doing so, risk taking on too much, feeling under supported, and burning out.

Taplay et al. developed a conceptual model titled, OESSN model (Organizational Elements that Shape

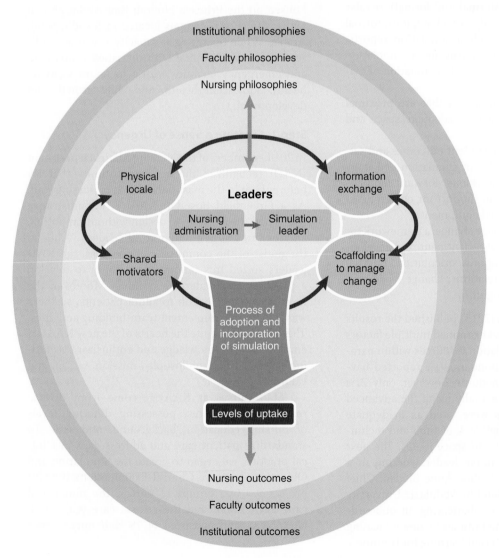

Figure 9.2 The Organizational Elements That Shape Simulation in Nursing. (Used from Taplay, K., Jack, S. M., Baxter, P., Eva, K., & Martin, L. (2014). Organizational culture shapes the adoption and incorporation of simulation into nursing curricula: A grounded theory study. *Nursing Research and Practice, 2014*, 1–12. doi:10.1155/2014/197591, with permission.)

Simulation in Nursing; Fig. 9.2). The OESSN model is made up of a series of concentric circles, each representing different levels and elements at which organizational influences impact simulation adoption and curricular integration. The three outer circles depict the guiding philosophies of the institution, of the faculty (i.e., Faculty of Health), and nursing philosophy of the nursing program. Within the inner circles are the five key elements of culture most strongly correlated with high uptake organizations (those that quickly and effectively adopted simulation): (1) nursing leaders; (2) information exchange; (3) physical locale; (4) shared motivators; (5) scaffolding to manage change. As you see, central to the entire model, is the nurse leader—your executive sponsor working in tandem with you. See the list below to evaluate how your organization measures up according to the OESSN model. Which of the following key elements for success are part of your organizational culture?

- Explicit knowledge and use of guiding philosophies such as mission, vision, and value statements are tied specifically to simulation.
- Information exchanges (informal and formal): regular communiqués from leadership and champions, formal meetings and minutes including simulation reports, sharing evaluation data for improvement, simulation journals, committee reports, and dissemination of evidence and learning.
- Physical locale: visible sim spaces that are proximal to teaching and learning spaces; adequate space and resources.
- Shared motivators: positive student outcomes and satisfaction, funding, knowledge of simulation pedagogy and equipment, assigned workload, forward momentum, training and education, support for conferences/courses, and well-maintained equipment.
- Scaffolding as a way to manage change: a framework for curricular integration, talent recruitment, and development strategy, job descriptions, orientation, internal and external stakeholder relations; change leadership and management; and recognition.

Recently, McKenna et al. (2015) published the results of a cross-sectional survey that examined multiple factors in the use and access to simulation resources within paramedic programs. Of 389 responders, 91% reported having access to advanced mannequins; however, only 71% of those programs reported actually using the advanced simulators. Reasons for this were cited as inadequate training, inadequate personnel, lack of time and technical resources, as well as, turf and space issues. The next section tells the story of a nurse leader working in a Greenfield hospital in Saudi Arabia. Anne Bluden, Chief Nurse Officer at King Abdullah bin Abdulaziz University Hospital (KAAUH), is busy implementing an onboarding program for foreign-trained nurses by first educating them, then using simulation-based learning for training.

9-3 Voice of Experience
Using Simulation To Shape Culture: Onboarding Critical and Non-Critical Care Teams in a Greenfield Hospital in Riyadh, Saudi Arabia

Anne Blunden, DCUR, MCUR, RN, A

The Challenge: Leading Large-scale Change for a New Hospital

King Abdullah bin Abdulaziz University Hospital (KAAUH) is a new 300-bed teaching hospital housed on the Princess Nourah Bint Abdulrahman University (PNU) campus located in Riyadh, Saudi Arabia. When operating at capacity, it will be a full-service general hospital with outpatient, inpatient, and emergency facilities with a focus on women's health, adolescent health, and child growth and development.

Step 1: Creating a Sense of Urgency

In 2014, members of the Nursing Affairs Department (NAD) recognized the *huge* opportunity that lay before them in the mass onboarding of nursing staff. As a Greenfield hospital, KAAUH administrative teams had the freedom to design without limitation, and then to test new and innovative ideas. While in the midst of the commissioning process, the NAD leaders seized this unique opportunity to develop a platform to standardize training. Moreover, the hospital had not begun to admit patients, so there was also time to implement team-building activities. These served to ignite the hearts of the new KAAUH employees with knowledge and enthusiasm regarding organizational philosophy, mission, vision, and values.

Staff nurses at KAAUH come from diverse regions and cultures, possessing differing levels of nursing education, background, and skill. To standardize patient care and address gaps in clinical practice, we began to create the Simulation and Objective Structure Clinical Examinations (OSCE) project for two groups of nurses: the noncritical care (NCC) staff and the critical care (CC) staff. New NCC staff consisted of 78 staff nurses from

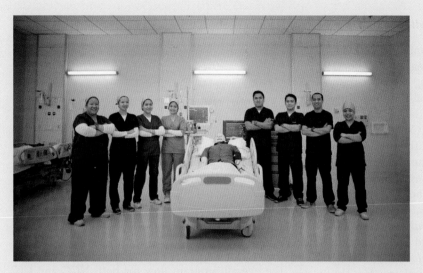

Figure 9.3 Noncritical Care Simulation/OSCE Team.

OPD, MW, SW, PW, WHW, the Nursery, and L&D. The second target group comprised a smaller group of more experienced nurses recruited to work in the ICU, NICU, PICU, OR, ED as well as the Clinical Resource Nurses who undertake clinical teaching and evaluating of Staff Nurses in the hospital.

Step 2: Building a Guiding Coalition

After establishing a clear vision and mission, the committee divided into two teams and set out to plan the onboarding and training programs for NCC and CC nurses (Figs. 9.3 and 9.4). It was vital to success that we form a steering committee with representation from all key stakeholder groups. Designated committee roles included the following: program facilitators (nurse managers), site preparation and competency check-off

(CRNs), lecture and skills demonstration (interdisciplinary), and evaluators (directors of nursing and executive director of nursing). Obtaining formal commitments from each of the concerned departments played a huge part in the success of the program. From the earliest stages of planning, weekly team meetings kept the development of the OSCE Program for noncritical and critical areas on track. Weekly task delegation and accountability to the project by all members of the committee facilitated a successful fast-track rollout.

Step 3: Form a Strategic Vision and Initiatives

With the vision and mission in mind, the CC project module was developed based on the American Association of Critical-Care Nurses (AACN) and the

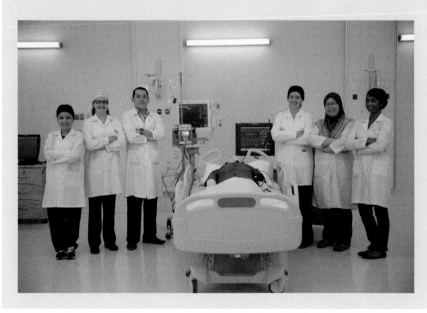

Figure 9.4 Critical Care Simulation/OSCE Team.

(Continued)

9-3 Voice of Experience (*Continued*)

AACNs Essential Critical Care Orientation (ECCO) program (http://www.aacn.org/wd/elearning/content/ecco/eccohome.pcms?menu=elearning). This program focuses on the development of critical-thinking skills for CC nurses - a skill that is essential in preparing a skillful provider of patient care (Commission on Collegiate Nursing Education, 2013). The program, as indicated above, is patterned after the OSCE framework that allows for flexibility in assessment of both theory and practice competencies. The classic Miller (1990) OSCE framework (see Fig. 9.5) depicts that *knows* and *knows how areas are best evaluated by* traditional written exams, assignments, and projects, while the pinnacle of the triangle, that is, *does* can only be evaluated within the real world of clinical practice. The OSCE sits just beneath that pinnacle, at the *shows how* level where participants' "hands on" performance is evaluated using a more objective and standardized process. Therefore, simulation-based learning was adopted as the educational methodology of choice to help prepare teams for the OSCEs.

Step 4: Enlist a Volunteer Army

An interdisciplinary planning team led the instructional design process by first conducting a thorough needs assessment and literature review. Consideration to institutional alignment meant the inclusion of innovation and cultural sensitivity. Quickly, teams from each of the clinical focus areas rolled up their sleeves and got to work building a three-phased project grounded in current research, best practices, and innovative teaching practices. Teams designed an escalating

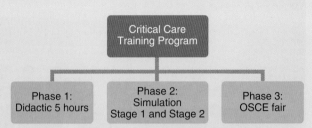

Figure 9.6 Configuration of KAAUH Simulation/OSCE Onboarding and Training Program.

structure, from basic to complex and from general to specialized level of skills, based on patient acuity and hospital requirements.

The overall program flow for both NCC and CC groups consisted of the same teaching methodologies with content being leveled accordingly. The three stratified phases were as follows (see Fig. 9.6):

- **Phase 1: Didactic and written examinations**: 5 hours covering core nursing care concepts.
- **Phase 2: Hands-on simulation:** in this phase, facilitators (experienced in simulation-based learning) employed interactive teaching methods using high-fidelity manikins, where teams engaged in collaborative learning. These sessions were highly experiential to support ongoing formative knowledge, attitude, and skill development.
- **Phase 3: The OSCE fair:** this phase took place closer to the time of the hospital operating since it was imperative that staff nurses have their skills refreshed and evaluated before and during the first few days of the Hospital's operation. The focus

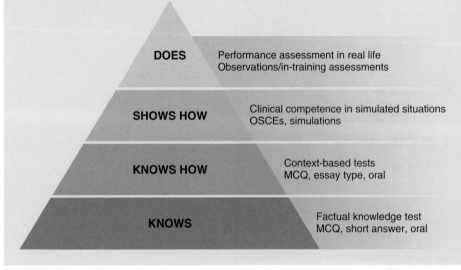

Figure 9.5 Miller's Pyramid of Medical Competence. (Source: Miller, G. E. (1990). The assessment of clinical skills/competence/performance. *Academic Medicine, 65,* s63–s67.)

for NCC and CC groups varied according to expected competencies for each area. OSCE scenarios were designed to assess team performance and as such, roll out in teams. For example, content in each NCC OSCE scenario included three generic competencies (i.e., pain assessment, hand hygiene, and safe medication administration) and two (2) unit-specific competencies (i.e., visual acuity and vaccination for OPD; predialysis teaching and care of catheter site for RDU; 12-lead ECG and NGT insertion MW; etc.).

- **Preparation and event:** before the commencement of the OSCE, teams of nurses were given an orientation to the OSCE method of evaluating clinical skills so as to allay anxiety and to prepare them for this experience. Each participating team had ten (10) minutes to perform all the required competencies and procedures at each station and rotated through multiple OSCE stations.

- **Feedback and debriefing:** simulation-based learning activities involved the use of group debriefing, whereas OSCE events employed immediate feedback sessions at the end of each station. Nurses unable to satisfy the minimum criteria for passing were scheduled for repeat OSCE experiences in 2 months' time.

Step 5: Enable Action by Removing Barriers

Simulation is a new approach for most employees at KAAUH, so it was important to take the time to educate the nurses about simulation-based learning and its intended purpose. This strategy was particularly important to allay fears of any repercussions related to poor performance. Simulation served as only one of many different assessment strategies used to empower individuals and teams. We also sought out an expert simulationist for advice about best practices in simulation instructional design.

Step 6: Generate Short-Term Wins

It was important to us that KAAUH Staff Nurses and Development Teams experience success. We tracked our progress weekly on bulletin boards and walls, making it visible to everyone. At each stage of development and delivery, we were intentional about creating opportunities to celebrate. "Wins are the molecules of results" (Kotter International, 2015c) and they are crucial to keeping momentum in the midst of rolling out of new initiatives. To keep spirits up, teams need to see and feel and be recognized for success!

Step 7: Sustain Acceleration

Evaluation is key to effective change processes. We approached each phase as an opportunity to enact total quality improvement increments. Both successes and failures informed change for the future. Three program assessment perspectives included the learner, OSCE evaluator, and steering committee program evaluations. NCC participant responses revealed very positive comments about the entire experience. Participants appreciated ample preparation time (didactic and simulation), relevancy of content, excellence in facilitation and instruction, increased culture of collaboration and teamwork, increase critical thinking and clinical judgement ability, increased time management, and an engaged mutual learning environment. Suggestions for improvement from participants included the need to incorporate more independent nursing interventions and the need for increased consistency in learning opportunities for all participants. Evaluation of the course by facilitators cited the need for enhancements in clarity regarding the evaluator role.

Evaluation of the CC program yielded a need to escalate the level of education for Critical Care Nursing Staff. Participants and facilitators cited the need for more simulation sessions to learn about the ventilated patient, advanced hemodynamic monitoring, handling a deteriorating patient, precode patients, management and assessment of PAIN, and sedations and muscle relaxation management in critical care areas. Also, to ensure skills retention, a follow-up OSCE fair took place in the high-fidelity simulation laboratory 2 months after completion of the above program.

Step 8: Institute Change

Given the large-scale success of the initial project role out, the Simulation OSCE Project will continue to be implemented. Ongoing balance between change leadership and management strategies is required to sustain momentum. We envision that as facilitator expertise in simulation grows and participant comfort with this learning process increases, so too will opportunities for the expanded use of simulation. We are also committing resources to develop our local talent pool of simulation experts. Furthermore, KAAUH staff has access to an exceptionally well-equipped simulation facility at PNU. We intend to mobilize our resources to maximize the use of simulation for the benefit of our nursing staff, patients, and their families.

Assessing Organizational Readiness for Change: SCORS and SCORS Handbook

"More than 70% of all major transformation efforts fail. Why? Because organizations do not take a consistent, holistic approach to changing themselves, nor do they engage their workforces effectively" —**John Kotter, from Kotter International**

When combined, culture and climate are powerful indicators of an organization's readiness for change. If you are a parent, you might recall your readiness level for parenthood. You might have spent months preparing (or not) for the impending life change, but once the baby arrived, so had the change and there was no going back. Whether or not you felt ready, the change was upon you. The time and energy you put into preparing, however, were important and served as an incubation period to better equip you for a successful transition to parenthood. In simulation, we did not have simulation "prenatal classes" and many did not foresee the complex care needs of the new simulator. Change leaders and managers at the time lacked the necessary knowledge and experience to effectively plan for the arrival of this disruptive little package. It was usually the simulation champion and a few eager innovators and early adopters that greeted the new simulator upon arrival, only to discover that this baby had tremendous needs. And so it was that the inevitable lack of sleep set in, as did the worries, crankiness, diaper rashes, and persistent fatigue. Of course, this parody is in jest, but the similarities run deep, and failure to plan for simulation as organizational culture change has caused a great deal of angst in many organizations.

In failing to plan, we plan to fail. Black and Gregersen (2014) liken organizational change to making a New Year's resolution, citing a reported 80% failure rate in studying over 10,000 executives, while other studies have reported 50% (p. 3). Either way, this is a very high rate of failure. He also states the current dynamics of change impact failure rates: the rate of change (fast and faster), the unpredictability of change (dynamic environments that are much less predictable), and the magnitude of change (today's changes are big) (pp. 9–11). Kotter cites reasons as ill preparedness and lack of planning, taking too long to act, being laggards in adopting an innovation, and having organizations that are too siloed to collaborate (Kotter International, 2015c).

This is why Colette Foisy-Doll and Kim Leighton have worked to create a tool for those new to simulation wanting a positive start or for those who find themselves stuck and lacking momentum to move forward. The *Simulation Culture Organizational Readiness Survey* (SCORS) and the *SCORS Companion Guidebook* (Foisy-Doll & Leighton, 2015a, 2015b) (Toolkit 9-1) are an adaptation from *The Organizational Culture Readiness for Evidence-based Practice Survey* created by Ellen Fineolt-Overholt and Bernadette Melnyk (2015c).

In 2014, the National Council of State Boards of Nursing (NCSBN) published its seminal study and findings on the conditions under which quality simulation can serve as a substitute for traditional clinical experiences (Hayden, Smiley, Alexander, Kardong-Edgren, & Jeffries, 2014). The findings supported that under specific conditions, simulation could comprise up to 50% of traditional clinical hours. Armed with the results of the NCSBN study (2014), a team of experienced nursing simulationists then developed the National Simulation Guidelines for Prelicensure Nursing Programs—listed in Box 9-1 (Alexander et al., 2015). The guidelines feature information and practical checklists for faculty and programs administrators known to contribute to the success of simulation in nursing programs. Moreover, since 2011, the INACSL Standards of Best Practice: Simulation^{SM}, 2016, continues to publish updated and expanded versions. To follow a comprehensive change management process means to begin with an environmental assessment and a determination of one's readiness for change. Box 9-2 features the Garcia & Guisado, (2013) evidence-based summary of the top success factors for simulation integration success.

Together, the SCORS tool and companion guidebook walk you through key elements of change readiness for simulation-based education including the extent to which your organization (1) has defined the need for change; (2) is ready for culture change; (3) is prepared for the time, personnel, and resources required to change; and (4) the extent to which there is a plan for sustainable education development to embed the new culture. We recommend that you carry out the assessment with a team of individuals, giving a broader purview of the questions asked. The SCORS Tool and Companion Guidebook (Foisy-Doll & Leighton, 2015a, 2015b) are housed in the. Your team will be guided through a series of questions and reflections to spur on the thinking and planning required for successful simulation-based education. Completing the tool will identify critical areas of need and serve as a basis for strategic planning.

Creating a Culture of Obstacle Transformation

An organization's ability to identify, manage, and remove barriers positively correlates with its success. Lean organizations successfully adopt ways to extricate the things that hold them back, as should educational and healthcare institutions. Many methods can be used to remove obstacles. For example, you can use the *direct approach*, by doing it yourself, as in the case of terminating an ineffective employee. Alternately, by *command and control* where you give the responsibility for obstacle removal to

Box 9-1	**NCSBN Combined Program and Faculty Preparation Checklist**

- There is a commitment on the part of the school for the simulation program that includes the following:
  - Letter of support from administrators indicating long-term program and fiscal support
  - Budgetary plan for sustainability and ongoing faculty training
  - Written short-term and long-term objectives for integrating simulation into the undergraduate curriculum, including ongoing evaluation of the program
- The school has created a framework that provides adequate resources (fiscal, human, and material) to support the simulation.
- The program has appropriate facilities for conducting simulation.
- The program has educational and technological resources and equipment to meet the intended objectives.
- Lead faculty and simulation lab personnel are qualified to conduct simulation.
- Faculty are prepared to lead simulations.
- Policies and procedures are in place to ensure quality-consistent simulation experiences for the students.
- The simulation program has an adequate number of dedicated trained simulation faculty members to support the learners in simulation-based experiences.
- The program has job descriptions for simulation faculty members/facilitators.
- The program has a plan for orienting simulation faculty members to their roles.

- The program uses a needs assessment to determine what scenarios to use.
- The simulation program provides subject–matter expertise for each scenario debriefing.
- The program and faculty members incorporate the INACSL Standards of Best Practice: Simulation.
- The program has appropriate designated physical space for education, storage, and debriefing.
- The faculty members have a process for identifying what equipment or relevant technologies are needed for meeting program objectives.
- The program has adequate equipment and supplies to create a realistic patient care environment.
- The faculty use evaluative feedback for quality improvement of the simulation program.
- The administration has a long-range plan for anticipated use of simulation in the forthcoming years (Alexander et al., pp. 40–41).

"Crossing the river of change requires that you leave the same familiar predictable self-connected to the same thoughts, same choices, same behaviors, and same feelings—and step into a void of the unknown…entering this river is stepping toward a new unpredictable, unfamiliar self. The unknown is the only place where you can create—you cannot create anything from the known"—Dr. Joe Dispenza from You Are the Placebo

---

another who possesses special skills, as in asking human resources to carry out employee termination. Also *indirectly*, by using your influence to sway others that can

Box 9-2	**Critical Success Factors for Simulation Success (Garcia & Guisado, 2013)**

1. *Orientation toward healthcare* [education] requirements/ standards
2. *Integration into the curriculum*
3. Available resources
4. *Design of the training activity* [SBE standards upheld]
5. *Fidelity in Simulation* [reality is important]
6. Team-based learning be a [learning organization]
7. *Feedback* [debriefing skills]
8. Deliberate practices [evidence-based approaches to SBE]
9. *Roles and training* of the instructor
10. Skills acquisition and retention [for learners, educators, and staff]
11. *Translation to practice* [facilitate knowledge and skill transfer from SBE]
12. *Measurement of results [what gets measured, can improve]*
13. *Organizational and educational content [aligned]*

be slow and frustrating, as in asking a peer or colleague to work more collaboratively with an ineffective employee. Lastly, by *supporting* or *coaching* using a team approach, like implementing capacity-building exercises for individuals and team members (Amory, 2011).

What happens when YOU are the obstacle? Pride and a lack of humility are enormous barriers in leadership. Black and Gregersen (2014) tell us that this is all too often the case. Pride manifests as leaders that are closed minded and not open to others' ideas. Humility is the opposite of pride. Leaders who focus on others take real joy in seeing them succeed. Mistakes leaders can make include disengagement, complacency, creating false urgency, lopsided lecanadership that focuses too much on managing, and creating boundaries instead of gateways (Kotter International, 2015c). So simulation champions, take care of the basics: be trustworthy, dependable, on time, and honest. Use deliberate practices like reflection and 360-degree feedback to critically inform and improve your leadership style. Keep your composure during change and be flexible and adaptable whenever you can: change can be scary, and not everyone will buy into the vision right away. After you succeed, don't let yourself be blinded by that success: continue to strive for better. Avoid placing yourself in the center of the universe and focus instead on and empowering others

(Black & Gregersen, 2014). See obstacles as opportunities. Root out negativity by adopting a mindset that obstacles are to be transformed into catalysts for growth.

Change Leadership Process: Kotter's 8 Steps to Accelerate Change in 2015

Many leadership models provide proven change leadership processes, but Kotter's 8-Step approach is simple, doable, and practical, even for those that are new to change leadership. Using Kotter's 8 Steps as a blueprint for leading change (2015), simulation champions can follow a proven blueprint for leading the adoption of simulation (Fig. 9.7 and Table 9.1). Don't be afraid to get messy in the process. Pull out the whiteboards, the poster papers, the computers, and go for it. Although the steps are sequential, in reality, they play out very dynamically and in a nonlinear fashion.

"Change leaders…are less adverse to getting "messy" and taking risks, influencing and inspiring behaviors that lead to large-scale transformation." —**Gregg Lestage from Inspire. Kotter International Newsletter, (2015, January)**

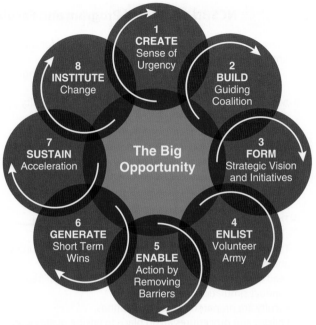

Figure 9.7 Kotter's 8 Steps for Accelerating Change. (Used from Kotter, J. P. (2014). *XLR8: Accelerate*. Boston, MA: Harvard Business School Press, with permission.)

Table 9.1	Kotter's 8 Steps to Accelerate Change in 2015	
Step	**Description**	**Result**
Step 1: Create a Sense of Urgency	Your top leaders must describe an opportunity that will appeals to individuals' heads and hearts and use this statement to raise a large, urgent army of experts.	You have a breadth of focused readiness across the workforce that is unprecedented in your organization.
Step 2: Build a Guiding Coalition	A volunteer army needs a coalition of effective people—coming from its own ranks—to guide it, coordinate it, and communicate its activities.	The linchpin of your entire transformation is in place: an accountable, diverse group bound by opportunity, strategy, and actions.
Step 3: Form a Strategic Vision and Initiatives	A vision must be bold, concise, authentic, and evoke a clear future state. Initiatives must have defined goals and link directly to the strategy designed to create that future state.	You have a single vision of the future with a credibility and authority that comes from being crafted by a diverse set of employees and validated by senior leaders.
Step 4: Enlist a Volunteer Army	Large-scale change can only occur when very significant numbers of employees amass under a common opportunity and drive in the same direction.	You have a stable body of employees excited and able to take action on critically important initiatives linked to your business strategy.
Step 5: Enable Action by Removing Barriers	By removing barriers to inefficient processes or hierarchies, leaders provide the freedom necessary for employees to work across boundaries and create real impact.	You have tangible evidence of employee innovations stemming from collapsed skills and new ways of working together.
Step 6: Generate Short-Term Wins	Wins are the molecules of results. They must be collected, categorized, and commemorated—early and often—to track progress and energize your volunteers to drive change.	A body of wins data that tells the story of your transformation in validated, quantifiable, and qualifiable terms.
Step 7: Sustain Acceleration	Change leaders must adapt quickly in order to maintain their speed. Whether it's a new way of finding talent or removing misaligned processes, they must determine what can be done—every day—to stay the course toward the vision.	You have confirmation of organizational fitness and standing that enable the reinvigoration of your mission and help you and your employees stay the course of change over time.
Step 8: Institute Change	To ensure new behaviors are repeated over the long term, it's important that you define and communicate the connections between these behaviors and the organization's success.	You have collective recognition that your organization has a new way of working with speed, agility, and innovation that directly contributes to strategically important business results.

© 2015 Kotter International. Used from Kotter, J. P. (2014). *XLR8: Accelerate*. Boston, MA: Harvard Business School Press, with permission.

Step 1: Creating a Sense of Urgency: Helping Others Feel a Gut-Level Determination to Move and Win

It is vital that your top leaders effectively create and establish a sense of urgency to garner others' cooperation (Kotter, 2008; Kotter International, 2015a). To do so, describe the big opportunity that will "ignite the hearts and minds of your people" (p. 12). Set out to identify, articulate, and communicate it!

Define the Big Opportunity, Identify, and Articulate Why you Have to Change: Your leadership must clearly articulate what is at stake should you succeed or fail. Consider things such as the need for improved graduate outcomes in the face of increasing patient acuity, increasing patient safety, a heightened consumer demand for safer care, compliance with federal/national agency/government regulations, institutional mandates, best practices in education, frameworks/theories/models, etc.

Step 2: Pull Together the Guiding Team: Getting the People with the Power to Make Change Happen

Kotter International (2015c) urges us to build a guiding coalition by strategically enlisting a volunteer army: a team devoted to helping others *see and feel* the need for change who will work to get the plan rolling. Coalition members will be key stakeholders who represent a mix of known formal and informal leaders, middle managers, and change agents from different levels of your program/institution. You must ensure that each team member brings authority, credibility, and specialized knowledge of internal and external environments, key connections, leadership and/or managerial skills, and a shared sense of urgency to change. Most importantly, you need a capable, knowledgeable, reliable, and credible leader with an inspirational, motivating, and clear vision to lead the coalition to successful implementation.

According to Kotter International (2015c), the responsibilities of your guiding coalition include:

- Developing the right vision and key networks to manage innovative change
- Communicate exactly what you HAVE to do to garner buy-in from 50% greater than members of the organization

Step 3: Form a Strategic Vision and Initiatives: Targeted and Coordinated Activities that Effectively Make Change Happen

Your team should be clear on the big idea that inspires them and set out to create a plan to make it happen. For this to happen, everyone must be on the same page. Get clarity around the change vision. Three functions are common to every single organization on the planet: what they do, how they do it, and why they do it (Simon Sinek Inc., 2015). Simon Sinek encourages us to share his simple idea with as many people as possible, so we are sharing it with you: The Golden Circle (Fig. 9.8). Using this simple tool can help your organization to discover and articulate its purpose. Take a moment to think about the three spheres using the simple guiding questions in the diagram.

To create a targeted and coordinated strategic plan and ensure timely action, consider using a SWOT or SOAR strategic planning activity.

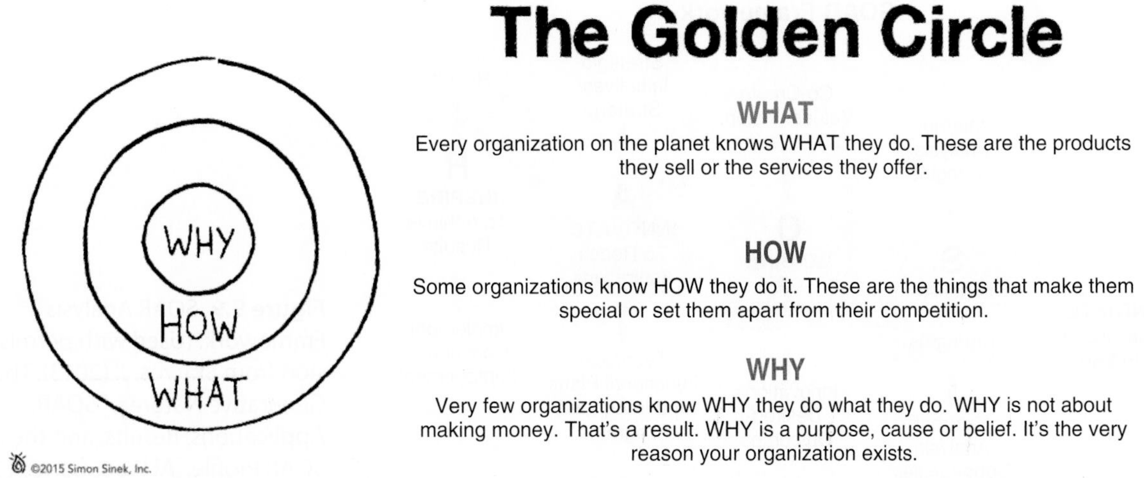

The Golden Circle

WHAT
Every organization on the planet knows WHAT they do. These are the products they sell or the services they offer.

HOW
Some organizations know HOW they do it. These are the things that make them special or set them apart from their competition.

WHY
Very few organizations know WHY they do what they do. WHY is not about making money. That's a result. WHY is a purpose, cause or belief. It's the very reason your organization exists.

©2015 Simon Sinek, Inc.

Figure 9.8   The Golden Circle. (Excerpted from "Share the Golden Circle: Presenter Slides & Notes" [©2015 Simon Sinek, Inc.] http://www.startwithwhy.com/Tools. Used with permission.)

SOAR Analysis for Uncovering Potential and Strategy

SOAR is a formulaic and strategic planning framework used by all stakeholders to explore an organization's Strengths, Opportunities, Aspirations, and Results (Fig. 9.9). This framework is grounded in Appreciative Inquiry and, therefore, focuses on exploring untapped organizational potential rather than focusing on that which holds it back. It is a fundamentally different process from the **SWOT Analysis** that sees the organization as attacked by environmental threats and internal weaknesses. Rather, the **SOAR** (Stavros, 2013; Stavros & Hinrichs, 2007) unfolds in an open process that fosters creativity, hopefulness, and courage to unleash potential and encourages full stakeholder engagement in the process (see Fig. 9.8). People engage in system-based discussion grounded in possibility thinking and conversation, instead of talking about what's wrong and needs fixing. For a sample SOAR table and questions, see the online Toolkit 9-3. Participants meticulously explore today's strengths, so that tomorrow's dream can rise from them. In the SOAR exercise, the minds of all the participants are imbued with open, creative, and the positive energy unhindered by negative impediments that stem from views of disempowerment.

SWOT Analysis for Assessment and Strategy

SWOT Analysis is a structured framework that uses a strategic approach to identifying organizational strengths, weaknesses, opportunities, and threats (both internal and external). Once completed, responses are analyzed and clustered into themes, serving as a springboard to strategically address each of the areas. SWOT Analysis focuses on awareness of internal and external forces and how they might impact the organization's future. It can improve decision making and preparedness and serves as a starting point in strategic directions and planning processes. The SWOT chart in the Toolkit depicts a fictional Simulation Centre SWOT analysis (Toolkit 9-3). A helpful worksheet is available for download at (http://www.mindtools.com/pages/article/newTMC_05.htm)

Step 4: Enlist a Volunteer Army: Engage Your People with Heart

To effect change on a large scale, you cannot do it alone. Enlist those around you in emotionally engaging ways employing approaches that allow them to see, hear, or touch the change. Find the doers and those who are interested, and then enlist the willing. It is important for the simulation champion to use clear, honest, and consistent messaging using all available strategies and modes of communication to recruit others. It is imperative to be consistent with your vision and your image when rolling out all communication activities such as face-to-face meetings, using powerful slogans and images, startling statistics on posters, emails, and the use of large display monitors and memoranda (Kotter, 1996).

What are the means you have available to enlist others? A personal invitation is usually best. Also, use PPT, Town Hall meetings, newsletters, special announcements, video footage on video monitor displays, images such as posters to build excitement and visibility for change, email, and social media. Consider conference attendance, bringing in vendors, visiting other simulation centers, etc. to create a clear vision of what can be and generate excitement. Once people are excited about what can be, they are much more likely to buy-in.

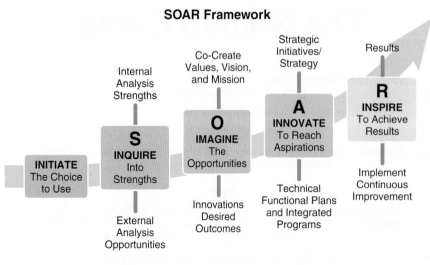

Figure 9.9 SOAR Analysis Framework. (Used with permission from Stavros, J. (2013). The Generative Nature of SOAR: Applications, Results, and the New SOAR Profile. AI Practitioner 15 (3), p. 8. To learn more, visit http://www.soar-strategy.com.)

"Changing behavior is less a matter of giving people analysis to influence their thoughts than helping them to see a truth to influence their feelings. The flow of see-feel-change is more powerful that that of analysis-think-change."—***John Kotter, 2002***

Step 5: Enable Action by Removing Barriers: Unleashing People to Do Their Best Work

When employees can *see* and *feel* a change during the entire process, an opportunity for **transformational change** is realized in organizations as much as in their people (Kotter & Cohen, 2002). However, change is never straightforward or streamlined. Many times there are *structural organizational barriers* to change, including, layers of bureaucracy that impede and squelch timely change efforts. Which barriers do you anticipate in your institution? Silos, complacency, overworked people, lack of influencers and executive sponsors, time pressures, or lack of money? They are all real barriers, and you must plan for them. Under these conditions, it is vital to empower others. Doing so might involve restructuring internal processes like creating new positions with the authority and power to make change happen or to create incentives that uphold SBL endeavors.

The guiding coalition must be open to employee reactions and ideas in the process of simulation adoption. Sometimes, it is people, not structure or process, that stand in your way. Consider a naysaying manager or administrator or that powerfully negative colleague in your milieu. Note that that person often wields a significant amount of informal power. Plan ahead and think about what you will do to empower these people as change agents? In our experience, the best option is to engage those who have reservations or anxiety about simulation by offering them opportunities to see it in action, and then to proceed with incremental engagement. Have conversations about their concerns that are grounded in honest, open dialogue. No matter how exciting the change, leaders must anticipate and plan for a sense of loss.

When Resistance Becomes Organizational Demise

In Jim Clemmer's brilliant book, The Moose on the Table (a Canadian parody for the *elephant in the room*), he describes the makings of *organizational demise* as cynicism and devaluing of core values. Seemingly small issues can spiral out of control resulting in declining engagement, shirking of responsibilities, rising absenteeism, and a decrease in productivity or missed deadlines. When left unattended, the result is low morale, low trust, negative perceptions of people in power, turf wars, lower employee health complaining of constant exhaustion and overburden, and ultimately can result in the loss of good people (2007). If you hear waves of discontentment chants like

"I am only here so I can pay my bills......I would rather be poking my eyeballs out than be here today... if that simulator breaks down one more time... I am going to lose it"... and the likes, levels of cynicism are high, and your leadership and the organization is at significant risk (Jim Clemmer, personal communication, The Clemmer Group Blog, 2015).

Effective leaders of organizational change possess skills that foster adaptation; embrace equilibrium; generate more leadership, not less; and result in nurturing of self and others. Undergirding all of these behaviors is transparency and honesty to build trust.

Step 6: Generate Short-Term Wins: Creating Visible, Unambiguous Success as Soon as Possible

"Clear improvements in performance make it difficult for people to block the needed change…Short-term wins have a way of building momentum that turns neutral people into supporters, and reluctant supporters into active helpers."—***Kotter, 2012***

Simulation champions must aim to identify relevant short-term, readily achievable goals that the team can celebrate with genuine, heart-felt pride. For example, new equipment installations early in a construction project can be celebrated by inviting staff to learn about the new equipment, attend an in-service, or stop by for cake and coffee. Planning these wins helps keep people motivated and uplifted, marks milestones, builds confidence in the project, and lessens the eroding effects of cynicism (Kotter, 1996; Mortenson, 2005). Get busy planning your celebrations because over time, small wins add up to big results. We recall with fondness the baby shower we held for the arrival of Noelle and Baby Hal: cake, coffee, cards, balloons, and donated second-hand baby gifts—the works!

Step 7: Sustain Acceleration: Don't Give Up, Consolidate Gains, Make More Change

*Simulation champion*s must use their credibility to change all systems, structures and policies that don't work during the change process. You must do what it takes. Perhaps that means to advocate for hiring new talent or to promote and develop existing employees. Most importantly, you must regularly reinvigorate the process, even adding new change agents as needs arise. We started with one position in our Simulation Program and today we are advertising to fill our sixth and seventh full-time positions. To encourage ongoing change efforts, *simulation champions* must continuously foster the development of other simulation champions: those brave, willing souls who emerge from all levels of the organization. Snap them up and work with the willing! You can quickly burn out by spinning your wheels to convert resistant individuals. Ensure that you also empower students as change agents and champions. This strategy will facilitate the ground swell you need for cultural change that grows simultaneously from the bottom-up and the top-down within the organization. Developing your *simulation champions* as change agents and leaders is the key to success.

Difficult organizational and cultural issues will arise, so take action promptly. Do not let them linger or they will weigh you down. Take care of yourself. Fatigue or burnout can set in as workload requirements of the project become increasingly heavy for you and the staff. If the leader and coalition members are cratering, the project's demise will not be far behind. Plan events to refresh and reenergize the project team.

Step 8: Institute Change: Anchor Change in the Culture to Sustain It

"Changes—whether consistent or inconsistent with the old culture—are difficult to ingrain." —***John Kotter from Kotter International, 2015***

To produce sustained, large-scale change requires significant behavioral and cultural change. It is realistic to expect that a new simulation program will take several years to roll out. During this phase, or earlier, your guiding coalition will need to formalize its presence within the organization, likely through permanent or temporary committee structure such as a steering or advisory committee. For long-term, lasting cultural change in teaching and learning practices to be realized, vigilance and perseverance on the part of simulation champion is vital. Additionally, continuous improvement and progress should be precisely mapped and measured throughout the entire process with the overall goal of achieving sustainable change. One of the biggest sources of failed change at this stage is declaring victory too soon and easing off on efforts. Your efforts will not multiply alone and sustained change will require your constant attention and monitoring.

There is ample evidence that following Kotter's 8-Step Accelerated blueprint for leading change can empower *simulation champions* to help others SEE the big opportunity, FEEL the need to change, and take the necessary bold steps toward sustained CHANGE. The following Voice of Experience features a simulation organization that used the 8 steps to effect positive change. I know you will be inspired by the Sim-one Story.

Box 9-3	SIM-one's Vision, Mission, and Values

Our Vision

The Global Leader in Healthcare Simulation

Our Mission

As a provincial initiative, Our mission is to connect and serve a large and complex healthcare simulation enterprise by:
- Advancing simulated clinical learning in the healthcare professions
- Advising and advocating for simulation in health profession education
- Further expanding interprofessional education aligned with interprofessional care, through the use of simulation
- Laying the foundations for further innovation and commercialization of simulation-related intellectual property
- Maximizing the value and return on investment of current and future provincial capital investments

Our Values

Civility, Best practices, Collaboration, Transparency, Creative disruption

---

9-4 Voice of Experience
Change Leadership to Create a Simulation Network

Dimitri J. Anastakis, MD, MHPE, MHCM, FRCSC, FACS, FICS

The Challenge

SIM-one is a simulation network that was founded in Ontario, Canada, and is a not-for-profit corporation that connects the province's simulation community (http://www.sim-one.ca). We serve over 75 simulation centers from across all healthcare disciplines and sectors (i.e., University, College, Hospital, and Emergency Medical Services). Our community includes approximately 1,400 health profession educators and staff and over 80 dedicated simulation researchers. Our vision is to further position the organization as a global leader in healthcare simulation (Box 9-3).

SIM-one's role and structure have changed over time. We evolved from an organization called NESCTL (Network of Excellence in Simulation for Clinical Teaching and Learning) that was established in 2007. NESCTL was never a legal entity but was a network under the shared leadership of its three founding organizations. A governance committee was established and made up of founding members. NESCTL received 3 years of start-up funding from the Ministry of Health and Long-Term Care (MOHLTC) to build a provincial simulation network.

Two years into the project, NESCTL was not progressing in the intended direction nor at the pace needed to fulfill its deliverables to the MOHLTC. There were a number of challenges facing the network at this point in its history. Firstly, NESCTL lacked a strategic vision. Secondly, the skills and attributes of NESCTL's governance committee members did not match the needs of the organization at this point in its evolution. Thirdly, NESCTL's management team struggled with financial and operational issues.

Meeting the Challenge

In 2009, with new leadership, a new management team and a restructured governance committee were able to become SIM-one. Using Kotter's 8-step change framework facilitated our ability to build SIM-one and successfully bring about system-wide change. I am pleased to share with you some of our experiences and the accomplishments we achieved using Kotter's framework during our early and formative years.

Step 1: Creating a Sense of Urgency

In 2009, the network had just over 1 year to fulfill its commitments to the MOHLTC. A sense of urgency was clear to both the governance committee and management team that change was crucial. In fact, this reality provided the catalyst needed to restructure the governance committee and secure unanimous agreement on a new strategic vision for the organization.

We then identified several big opportunities that would appeal to our stakeholders and help them to understand the value of having a network. These opportunities included (1) the need for better ways of reporting on the return on investments in health professions simulation equipment, (2) the need for faculty development across all sectors, and (3) the need to contain the cost of healthcare simulation. We leveraged each of these big opportunities to create a widespread sense of urgency and raise support the concept of a simulation network.

Step 2: Building a Guiding Coalition

Our first guiding coalition was our restructured governance committee that was made up of diverse and influential opinion leaders. They played an important role early in our history by helping build critical relationships and by anticipating and removing obstacles. Following incorporation, SIM-one installed a skills-based Board of Directors that provides strategic and fiduciary oversight.

Step 3: Form a Strategic Vision and Initiatives

Early in SIM-one's history, we redefined our vision and communicated that vision to all our stakeholders (Box 9-3). Several key initiatives followed including launching SIM-one's education courses and two symposia, the SIM-one's Simulation Exposition and the SIM Marketplace a virtual platform to buy, sell, rent, and share healthcare simulation products.

Step 4: Enlist a Volunteer Army

Communicating SIM-one's vision to all our stakeholders was critical to enhancing awareness and establishing engagement. The communication team leveraged all available communication channels to engage our simulation community. Initially, our communication performance indicators focused on community engagement (Fig. 9.10). The level of sophistication of our communications has evolved to mirror the evolution of SIM-one's products and services. We now communicate with increasingly global and diverse customer segments.

Early on, we built a coalition or "volunteer army" of education, research, and leadership champions. We then established a large and diverse cohort of graduates from our education stream. Also, we provided research funding to simulation researchers. By our 3rd year, SIM-one had trained over fifty simulation leaders in a Meta-Leadership Program (Harvard Kennedy School, 2013). These meta-leaders now lead within and across organizations. This growing network of simulation educators, researchers, and leaders continue to enable SIM-one's vision and mission.

Step 5: Enable Action by Removing Barriers

Removing barriers and empowering a team of bright and committed individuals is an important enabler of system-wide change. We have a team of talented self-starters who have initiated and built many great things. For example, our Director of Education and his team have pulled down traditional barriers to collaboration and created a large group of faculty from across the province and from all healthcare

(Continued)

9-4 Voice of Experience (*Continued*)

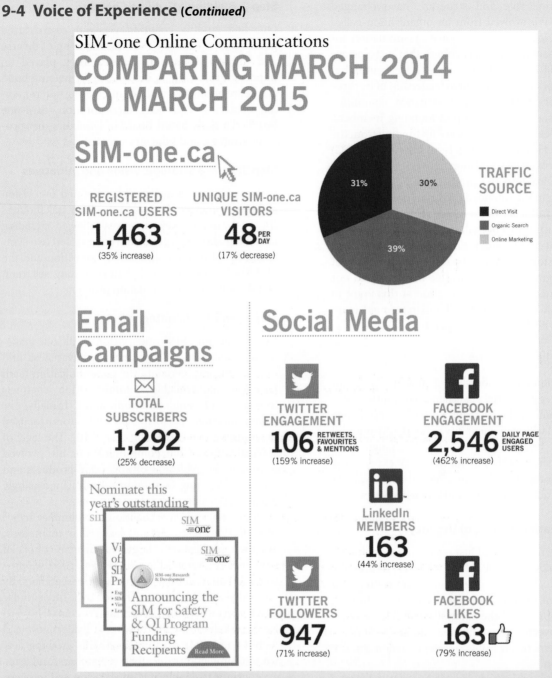

Figure 9.10 SIM-one Communications Metrics. SIM-one reports on website, email campaign, and social media metrics regularly. There has been a consistent annual increase in volumes across all metrics. The decrease in 2014/15 in email subscribers was due to the implementation of the Canadian Anti Spam Legislation that required us to obtain consent of all our email addresses. (Courtesy of SIM-one Communications.)

disciplines. Together, this group has created an impressive list of simulation-related courses and symposia (http://www.sim-one.ca/courses/course-listing).

Our largest initiative involved conducting a province-wide inventory of all simulation equipment. The SIM-one Provincial Equipment Coordination Service (SPECS) is an Ontario-wide simulation equipment coordination service that has the capacity for expanded use

within a larger network. The SPECS team has inventoried every simulation center in the province (Fig. 9.11). Today, we have a comprehensive snapshot of Ontario's current capital equipment. SPECS provides the basis for the strategic management of Ontario's investments in simulation equipment. In doing so, SPECS promotes sustainability, enabling cost-efficient access to simulated learning and—ultimately—better patient care and patient safety.

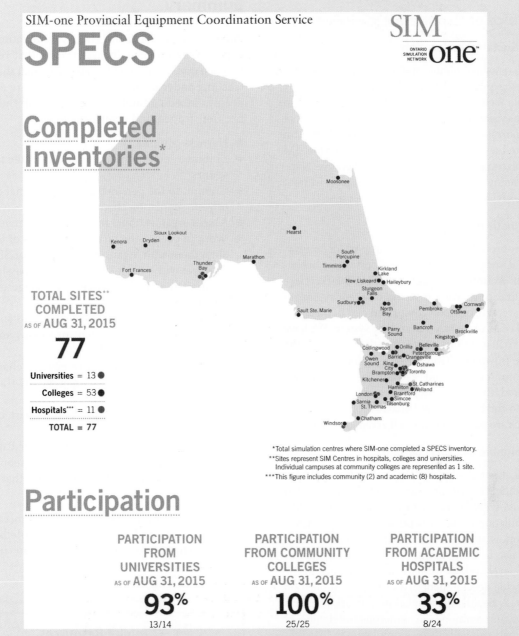

Figure 9.11 SIM-one Provincial Equipment Coordination Service (SPECS). SIM-one Provincial Equipment Coordination Service has inventoried 77 simulation centers to date. Emphasis on hospital-based simulation centers is the current focus for the SPECS team. (Courtesy of SIM-one Communications.)

Step 6: Generate Short-Term Wins

Early in our history, we renamed and rebranded ourselves as SIM-one—Ontario Simulation Network. This was an important turning point for us as we leveraged this rebranding opportunity to communicate our new vision. Another important win was our incorporation into a not-for-profit corporation. This, along with the election of our first skills-based Board of Directors, sent a powerful message to our community—that we are here to stay, and together we will position SIM-one as a global leader in healthcare simulation.

Our signature event, the SIM-one Simulation Exposition, was another important short-term victory. The SIM-one Expo is now Canada's largest interprofessional simulation exposition drawing in over 350 participants and almost every simulation manufacturer from around the world. The annual Expo affirms SIM-one's ongoing role as a connector of all things simulation.

(Continued)

9-4 Voice of Experience (*Continued*)

Step 7: Sustain Acceleration

We have remained nimble and responsive to opportunity. We have hired, promoted, and developed many incredible faculty and staff who have contributed to SIM-one's vision and created products and services that are of enormous value to our community. This team has created several spin-off products including the SIM Marketplace and SIM-one Buying Collaborative. None of these innovations would have been possible without SIM-one's talented, dedicated, and driven staff.

Step 8: Institute Change

We have brought about several important innovations that show a strong connection to new behaviors. For example, through the SIM Marketplace for the first time, we are seeing different organizations share, sell, or trade equipment and in doing so, reduced costs to themselves and the system. We have also seen institutions come together through the SIM-one Buying Collaborative to explore the power of group purchasing and warranty negotiation. We anticipated that both these innovations will contribute to further shifts in behaviors on how capital resources are purchased and utilized in our province.

Most Valuable Lessons Learned

Bringing about change at a regional or national level across different sectors can be challenging. That being said, creating a sustainable and valued healthcare simulation network is possible. Kotter's change framework is an important tool that simulation leaders can use to bring about change at a regional or national level and, as we have shown, applies to the system-wide development of a healthcare simulation network. A healthcare simulation network connects and serves its community in numerous and significant ways. A network will advance simulation in the clinical setting, it will help drive quality improvement and patient safety, and it will help solve common financial issues faced by all simulation centers. SIM-one continues to evolve and now serves a growing pan-Canadian simulation community. We continue reinvent ourselves so as to better position all our members across Canada as leaders in healthcare simulation.

Inspiration for Simulation Champions

"A higher rate of urgency does not imply ever-present panic, anxiety, or fear. It means a state in which complacency is virtually absent"
J. P. Kotter - from Kotter International

Summary

Organizational change for effective simulation integration is part of an ongoing change process that requires more than a paradigm shift; it demands a primal shift to the new teaching and learning culture in healthcare education. To deeply embed cultural change for SBE in the entire organization, leaders and managers must:

- Harness complexity
- Embrace emerging simulation leaders as change agents
- Commit to the personal and professional development of your simulation champions
- Assess organizational readiness for change
- Work to change the tacit assumptions of followers and align them with organizational goals for SBE
- Connect with people's emotions and passions
- Commit required resources for change ensuring sustainable practices
- Implement efficient, agile, flexible, and speedy change leadership and management processes and structures using proven frameworks
- Clearly communicate a strategy for change through transparency, trust, engagement, and shared leadership
- Promote knowledge translation as part of a learning organization for SBE
- Measure and monitor progress; foster capacity building, enthusiasm, and commitment in people
- Create a culture of celebration that recognizes excellence

This sums up the right stuff of organizational leaders, followers, and managers for implementing sustainable change for SBE. We wish you an incredible journey!

Toolkit Resources

Toolkit 9-1: *Simulation Culture Organizational Readiness Survey* (SCORS) and the *SCORS Companion Guidebook* (2015). To download a copy, use this link or go to the Toolkit (https://sites.google.com/site/scorsfile/)

Toolkit 9-2: SOAR Strengths-based Strategy Sample Questions

Toolkit 9-3: SWOT Analysis Example from Hypothetical Simulation Centre

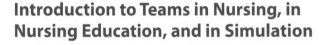

10 Leading and Developing Effective Simulation Teams

Colette Foisy-Doll, Carol Wild

 Key Terms

Groups, Teams, High-Performing Team, Simulation Delivery Team, Self-Managed Team, Distributed/Dispersed/Virtual Team, Bounded Team, Unbounded Team, Safe Container, Moral Courage, Ethical Workspace, Conflict Resolution, Reconciliation, Outrospection, Introspection, Emotional Intelligence, Intrinsic and Extrinsic Motivation, Team Assessment, Drama Triangle

 Guiding Questions

1 Is your simulation team really a team, or do you function more like a group?

2 How do simulation teams become high-performing teams? What makes a high-performing team so special?

3 How can simulation leaders empower and sustain a high-performing team of simulation champions?

4 How would you evaluate your overall simulation team's performance? Would you say you have attained status as a simulation champion team?

Introduction to Teams in Nursing, in Nursing Education, and in Simulation

Have you ever had the experience of working with an amazing team? How about an incredible simulation team? A team where the right people come together with the right chemistry, the right skills, and the right attitudes to make magical things happen? Yes, those teams, the seemingly elusive ones! If you have had the privilege of this experience, you will know that it is remarkable and inspiring to work with that team every day. We are privileged to have worked on such teams and can honestly say that those expe-

riences are remembered as peak moments in our careers and in our lives outside of the workplace. Truth be told, it is only natural to want to be on a great team; togetherness is a part of our human survival instinct! Evolutionists have studied how humans emerged and evolved in groups to build new cultures and societies ensuring their survival (or demise), productivity, and reproduction as a species (Richerson & Christiansen, 2013).

However, those exhilarating experiences are not the norm, and teamwork is challenging and at times, downright awful. Teams can experience dysfunction, disruption, and even destructive conflict. Daft (2014) found in recent surveys that "80% of employees report working in some kind of team, but that only 14% of employees rated their teaming efforts as highly effective, just over 50% reported somewhat effective, and 15% considered their efforts not effective at all" (p. 596). Dyer, Dyer and Dyer (2013) report that large numbers of employees indicate never having worked on a high-performing-team. Despite this fact, teams do have the potential to do great things and accomplish more together than apart. For the past several years, prospective employers cite teamwork as a core competency for new hires (CEB Blog, 2014).

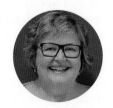

Colette Foisy-Doll,
MSN, RN, CHSE

Carol Wild,
MScN, BN, RN

Teams have become ubiquitous in work and life, with the success of organizations, and in this case simulation programs, relying heavily on the productivity of high-performing teams, sometimes referred to as high-functioning teams. However, today's healthcare team performance reports show the need for interprofessional team improvement (INACSL Standards Committee, 2016, Sim-IPE; AHRQ, 2014a; WHO, 2010a, 2011b, 2013; CNA, 2011a; CIHC, 2010; AIPHE, 2007; Reeves et al., 2007; Hammick et al., 2007). Also adding complexity to team composition and function is the demand for increased patient safety and patient- and family-centered care (Berwick, 2009; Frank et al., 2008; Baker et al., 2004). This new mandate means that healthcare teams must include patients and their loved ones as equally valued members of the healthcare team.

In nursing education, whether learners engage in online collaborative learning, live simulation, classroom role-play, psychomotor skills practice in skills laboratories, or work in healthcare settings, teamwork is implicit. As such, there is a need for learners and those who teach them to develop teamwork competencies. Students are often assigned to group work in nursing courses with the added stress of having that work graded. Yet, Dyer et al. (2013) state that educators lack understanding of high-performance teams and lack the ability to help students attain that level of performance. When learners are left to figure out teamwork, frequently there are group issues, disagreements, and inequities to the point where learners experience distaste for teamwork that stays with them well into nursing practice. Also, in both academe and clinical practice, the terms *academic incivility* and *bullying* are all too familiar, being reported with regularity as part of the team experience (Adams, 2015; Clark, 2013). In response, there is a growing demand in healthcare and educational settings to graduate professionals who possess technical, interpersonal, and communication competencies in addition to team leadership, followership, and managership abilities (AACN, 2006, 2008b, 2011; Benner, Sutphen, Leonard, & Day, 2010; CIHC, 2010; CNA, 2001, 2005, 2008, 2009a, 2011b; NLN, 2005; WHO, 2010a, 2011a, 2013, 2015d).

Simulation learning can support competency attainment of vital nursing knowledge, as well as team-building skills (Jeffries, 2007b). When grounded in simulation-enhanced interprofessional education (INACSL Standards Committee, 2016, sim-IPE), simulation learning can facilitate significant team learning. Today's learners, however, must be socialized to and acquire teamwork competencies to optimize team success. Learning about teams and teamwork in simulation is especially important, as learners are in the beginning stages of socialization to healthcare team function, process, and structure. An experienced facilitator who is knowledgeable in team development serves as a driving force in the acquisition of team competencies (INACSL, 2016).

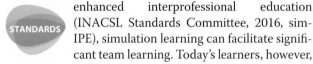

Within simulation centers, both leaders and followers aim to foster the development of high-performing simulation teams. **Simulation delivery teams** consist of diverse employees with specific skills and knowledge sets. As far back as 1985, the National Research Council report on Human Factors Aspects of Simulation stated the need for specially trained personnel for simulation centers and programs (Jones, Hennessey, & Deutsch, 1985). Rapidly expanding use of simulation-based learning and related technology has resulted in greater differentiation and increased diversity in the types of personnel we see staffing simulation programs. It is vital to positive outcomes that simulation teams have the goal of becoming a high-performing team. Simulation Champions working on such teams are necessary for positive outcomes.

As we saw in previous chapters, many factors shape healthcare teams today. They include complex, shifting, and challenging work environments; increased stress and demands of the job; rapid innovation and technological change; the need to demonstrate interprofessional competencies; and stronger patient voices demanding safer care and total quality improvement. In this chapter, we review the basics of team theory and what makes groups different from teams; the evolution of, type, and size of teams; the composition of simulation teams; and a description of simulation team member roles and functions, and lastly, we provide you with the Simulation Champions High-performance Simulation Team Discussion Tool to facilitate exploring your team's context, competencies, composition, and to change practices as an aspiring high-performance team.

Evolution of the Team Concept

"For as long as we've been around as humans, as wandering bands of nomads or cave dwellers, we have sat together and shared experiences… when the world became fearsome, we came together. When the world called us to explore its edges, we journeyed together. Whatever we did, we did it together" —**Meg Wheatley, 2009—Turning to One Another**

In the early industrial era, leadership and management theory viewed organizations as entities that had authority over employees; teams, as we know them today, did not exist. The big bosses of the day stifled creativity and innovation by taking an *autocratic* and mechanistic approach to productivity and worker functioning. Workers were subservient to managers and, generally, followed orders to increase company productivity. Years later in the 1960s, theoretical advancements supported a more humanistic view of organizations and the people working within them. Under the new psychology, teams working within institutions were considered part of *human systems* that contributed to employee self-actualization and the achievement of personal potential (Dyer et al., 2013). In the years that followed came the emergence of T-groups, team dynamics, and team skill development. According to Dyer et al., a T-group comprises a group of individuals that aim to improve team performance: they provide each other with "open and honest" feedback about their behavior, require "open and honest" responses, and encourage group members to accept responsibility for their behavior. *Group dynamics* also evolved from this era as a defined area of study that examines human behavior in teams and their interactions within them (Dyer et. al., Introduction). Likewise, team skills emerged through the acknowledgment that teams could perform well and do great things as units composed of hardworking, committed individuals. In the decades that followed T-group emergence, a notable shift to team skills development occurred, including team learning about collaboration, problem-solving, and conflict management.

In contrast, today's **high-performing teams** (HPTs) are central to organization goal attainment. Team training has become a mainstay to favorable outcomes in organizations throughout the world (Dyer et al., 2013). Whereas groups of people can pull together to get the job done, HPTs differ in that while they get the job done, they also develop a unique team identity and way of being, marked by mutuality, trust, and friendship. HPTs cocreate positive work climates through enacting empathy, outsight, and encouragement with others on the team. To that end, these teams demonstrate high degrees of emotional intelligence (EI) and have each other's backs when someone on the team is lagging. We contend that this is the stuff that makes up great simulation delivery teams and will cover more on HPTs later in the chapter.

How Groups Develop Into Teams

"Remember, all teams are groups… but not all groups are teams! Teamwork is working together, even when apart."
—*From Teams and Work Groups, 2005*

In the early 1940s, Kurt Lewin began to study groups and group dynamics in an attempt to uncover the deep layers of human interaction in groups (Lewin, 1944). Groups and group dynamics have since been further broken down into teams and team dynamics, with groups as distinct from teams.

Groups are defined by Bendaly and Bendaly (2012) as "a collection of "individuals who happen to be taking up the same space but each going in his or her own direction and working relatively independently of one another with little collaboration" (p. 14). For example, consider the current move away from multidisciplinary healthcare delivery models to team-based patient and family-centered models. Using Figure 10.1, follow the pathway that charts a patient's journey through an acute care hospitalization (from left to right). Note that each color on the graph denotes individual healthcare disciplines. Notice that the patient and care provider encounters are, for the most part, discrete one-on-one events. You will also notice that few healthcare disciplines intersect with each other during the patient's stay. Teamwork is virtually absent from this image. What you see, instead, is healthcare providers working independent of each other with few opportunities to connect. Remember that to connect and to collaborate are not the same thing. *Interprofessional collaboration* (IPC) requires teamness and working together

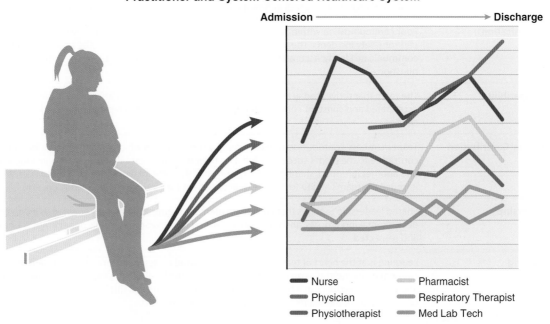

Multidisciplinary
Practitioner and System-Centered Healthcare System

Admission ⟶ Discharge

Nurse
Physician
Physiotherapist
Pharmacist
Respiratory Therapist
Med Lab Tech

Figure 10.1 Depicting The Lack Of Intersectionality Using A Practitioner-, Systems-Centered Multidisciplinary Disconnected Approach To Patient Care. This Model Does Not Support Meaningful, Regular, Team Connection And The Patient Is Not On the Team.

toward a "shared purpose, critical reflection, innovation, and leadership" (Sims, Hewitt, & Harris, 2015, p. 209). In this healthcare–centric model, the patient is not considered a member of the team and therefore does not have the formal authority to contribute to the team. Care providers focus on their individual roles to individually solve immediate concerns with no long-term patient-centered shared team vision or goal (Bendaly & Bendaly, 2012; Reeves, Zwarenstein, & Goldman, 2009). Once acute care services are completed, the patient exits the multidisciplinary health delivery system and community care may or may not be a part of the plan. If we ever hope to turn the tide in healthcare, we need to develop interprofessional HPTs with the patient and his or her significant others at the center of the team. Chatalalsingh and Reeves (2014) describe how healthcare teams could develop and empower team-learning leaders to enable day-to-day team learning.

Team Versus High-Performing Team

A *team* is very different from a *group*. Teams can, but do not automatically evolve from groups and, as such, demonstrate varying levels of teamness (Bendaly & Bendaly, 2012). Groups can remain as groups, and often this is perfectly

desirable and functional. Daft (2014) describes a team as "a unit of two or more people who interact and coordinate their work to accomplish a common goal to which they are committed and themselves mutually accountable" (p. 597). However, teams can evolve to become HPTs that exemplify greatness and accomplish amazing things. HPTs have unique attributes that are so palpable, you can sense the difference the minute you are in their presence. HPTs are marked by strong team cohesion, open communication, and flexibility to change. These teams heavily invest in cocreating a healthy team climate. They experience synergistic potential through increased levels of interdependence, shared leadership, and a unified commitment to goals. High-performing team (HPT) members openly share their talents and gifts to build capacity in others. These are the teams that never stop learning from and with each other (Bendaly & Bendaly, 2012). Through extensive team studies, Bendaly and Bendaly (2012) developed what is coined The Seven Elements of High Performing Teams (Table 10.1). Each of the seven elements described in the table is interdependent, where fluctuations in one will affect the strengthening or weakening of other elements. For example, for a team to optimally engage in *shared leadership*, a *healthy climate* must first exist. Secondly, people must be honest and open about their leadership

Table 10.1	The Seven Elements of High-Performing Teams
Healthy Climate	Healthy climate refers to how members feel about the way the team functions, including their level of comfort with team norms of behavior. If the climate is not positive, honesty and openness are lacking and team members may not fully trust and respect one another.
Cohesiveness	Cohesiveness refers to the degree to which the team pulls together in the same direction. Cohesiveness requires agreement and *commitment to what the team is in place to achieve* (mandate, goals, and objectives), as well as *how* it will achieve them (values, priorities, and procedures).
Open Communication	Poor communication within healthcare organizations is cited as a major contributing factor in patient safety incidents. The degree of open communication is reflected by a team's ability to communicate clearly, accurately, and respectfully, with the freedom to express opinions and to ask questions.
Change Compatibility	The team that thrives today must be able to maintain high performance in an environment of accelerated and constant change. Change compatibility requires receptivity and adaptability to change.
Team Members' Contribution	Team members' contribution is determined by the degree to which team members individually contribute to the team's success by fulfilling their team responsibilities. Examples include keeping one another informed, sharing the load, and actively participating by looking for opportunities to improve the team's ability to provide quality patient care by sharing ideas and concerns.
Shared Leadership	Shared leadership requires that each team member is appropriately self-directed, is involved in the decision-making process, and is an equal member of the team in that his or her input is both valued and respected.
Shared Learning	Learning is at the heart of team culture and is focused on team performance and patient safety. This element measures the degree to which the team actively reflects on experiences, shares knowledge, and provides feedback in a blame-free, "what can we learn from this" manner, so that learning becomes part of the team's regular day-to-day practice.

Used from Bendaly, L., & Bendaly, N. (2012). *Improving Healthcare Team Performance*. Hoboken, NJ: John Wiley and Sons, with permission.

and followership strengths and weaknesses. Both elements must be present to cultivate trust.

Bendaly and Bendaly (2012) express teams versus groups using the following mathematical equations: HPTs (*2 + 2 = 5 or more*), whereas Groups (*2 + 2 = 3 or* less). For a team to achieve optimal levels of innovation and creativity, all members must feel free to contribute diverse strengths, skills, experience, and perspectives. HPT members are committed to achieving and maintaining high-functioning skills through the use of continuous improvement processes to acquire and evaluate requisite team skills (Bendaly & Bendaly, 2012). Table 10.2 lists team performance indicators

in the center column, flanked by features that distinguish groups from teams on the left and right.

Determinants of High-Performing Teams

Dyer et al. (2013) list the *four Cs of team performance* as (1) the context of the team, (2) the composition of the team, (3) the competencies of the team, and (4) the change management skills of the team. Each determinant is further broken down to detail the conditions that increase team success. Interestingly, it is the context and the composition of the team that set the stage for team development.

Table 10.2	**Distinguishing Characteristics of Groups Versus Teams**	
Groups ➤		**Teams**
• Lacking or lessened potential for synergy	***Synergy**	• Amplified synergistic potential
• Little or no collaboration	***Collaboration**	• Continuous, cooperative, interactive
• Designated group leader in control	**Leadership**	• Shares or rotates leadership roles
• Independent work; leader delegates clearly articulated and holds group members accountable	***Interdependence**	• Interdependent and team members accountable for self; shared decision-making
• Goals are identical for all group members, absence of shared goals	***Goals and commonalities**	• Shared team-specific vision and purpose
• Individual products • Low quality and does not strongly impact organizational performance	**Output**	• Collective products • Higher quality with high impact on organizational performance
• One-way communication to the group, brief	**Meetings**	• Open dialogue and problem-solving sessions
• Lacking or absent	***Elements of successful teams**	• All seven elements present (Bendaly & Bendaly, 2012)
• Team skills development absent	***Team skills**	• Integration of team development processes
• Not bound • Not motivated to stay • Less concerned with team welfare	**Cohesion**	• Bounded, mutuality, trust, and friendship • Motivated to stay • Concerned with team welfare
• Measured by indirect impact on organization	**Effectiveness indicators**	• Measures team collective work and outcomes
• Members report low sense of valuing and belonging • Low team morale • Less motivated to give their personal best • Quick to sense leader negativity and hostility	**Satisfaction**	• Increased self-worth, dignity, and motivation to contribute • High morale • Attracted to the team • Share similar personal attitudes and values • Stronger ties to leaders evident
• Lack of contact with others • Little or no excitement • No social interaction • No team identity	**Social facilitation**	• Greater camaraderie and friendship • Form team identity • Release of tremendous energy and excitement • Social setting boosts performance
• Slow to respond • Slower to produce • Lesser quality • Lacks communication or communication comes from leader only	**Speed and efficiency**	• Integrated, agile, smooth-functioning teams with increased speed, efficiency, and accuracy • Problem-solving is timely, coordinated, and communicated

Information from (*) denotes Degree of Teamness. Bendaly, L., & Bendaly, N. (2012). *Improving healthcare team performance: The 7 requirements for excellence in patient care* [Books24x7 version]. Retrieved from http://common.books24x7.com.ezproxy.macewan.ca/toc.aspx?bookid=51171; Daft, R. L. (2014). *Management* (11th ed.). Mason, OH: South Western Cengage Learning.

- *Context* is the organizational environment within which teams work. Context affects team productivity and satisfaction in positive or negative ways, serving as a catalyst or a barrier.
- *The composition* of teams involves selecting the right members with the requisite skills, motivation, and attitudes to get the job done well. Teams require thought and attention to positioning new members so that they add value to the existing blend of talent and ability. Team composition involves team member selection by (1) establishing competency-based team selection criteria, (2) creating processes to build team capacity; (3) releasing members that underperform, (4) sharing management of the team, and (5) paying attention that group size is not too large or too small (Dyer et al., 2013).
- *Team competencies* include relational and interpersonal communication skills; making effective team contributions, being reliable, being trustworthy, and working to build trust; being open to mutually beneficial conflict resolution strategies for the benefit of the team; and encouraging risk taking and innovation. The goals and metrics by which teams achieve these competencies must be transparent. HPTs determine their metrics and self-regulate team performance.

Dyer et al. also feature *change leadership and management* as an HPT competency. Teams must have the ability to adapt and be flexible; to exercise good judgement in evaluating own and others' strengths and weaknesses; to self-identify the need for changing behaviors; and, to engage in continuous evaluation of context, team composition, and team competencies to achieve desired goals (Dyer et al., 2013).

Becoming a High-Performance Team Member

Becoming a high-performance team takes commitment to the processes of individual and team development. The following section outlines key factors to consider as you examine your own team performance.

Developing Empathy and Outsight

Kouzes and Posner (2012) stated that leaders are really no more intelligent, creative, insightful, or imaginative than followers; what they do have that distinguishes them from followers is *outsight*: the ability to look outside yourself and your experiences using **outrospection**. Insight, conversely, is an ability to see yourself and your experiences using **introspection**. Making the mental shift from looking within, to looking without, especially during challenges, is the mark of an emotionally connected, relational leader. As HPTs engage in shared leadership, outsight and insight are requisite abilities. Debriefing in simulation, for example, involves modeling structured outrospection and introspection to gain insight and outsight, and develop foresight.

Know What Motivates You: Intrinsic versus Extrinsic Motivation

Maslow's journey to self-actualization cultivated a shared understanding that right after our human need for food, water, sleep, and security, comes our need for love and belonging (1943). He noted, for example, that self-actualization must be preceded by the development of self-esteem through recognition, feedback, growth, and opportunity. In later years, Maslow's thinking evolved to include a *self-transcendence* dimension where "the self can only find its actualization in giving itself to some higher goal outside oneself, in altruism and spirituality" (Koltko-Rivera, 2006; Maslow, 1943). It is especially true that praise from the people you admire and value most is even more meaningful. As modern workspaces and teams continue to evolve and improve, so do motivational dynamics within organizations. Knowing what makes us and others tick can go a long way to increasing satisfaction in teams.

Would you say that you are *intrinsically* or *extrinsically* motivated? To better understand your preference, think about what brings you the most joy and pleasure in work and life. **Intrinsic motivations** arise from within and comprise experiences that are inherently pleasurable like self-accomplishment and pride in a job well done. **Extrinsic motivations** are those where the source of pleasure and energy stems from outside, such as deriving energy and pleasure from being in the company of others. There is no right or wrong way of being; there only is what is. Understanding what motivates you and those you work with is the foundation for empathy and helps contribute to greater understandings of team members to inform actions. For example, when I know that someone appreciates hearing that he or she has done an excellent job, I will go out of my way to tell them that, even if giving praise is not something that comes naturally to me.

Intrinsic and Extrinsic Rewards in Teams

There is evidence in the literature that *recognition and acknowledgment* of individual or team behaviors not only increase an organization's profile but create a whole host of overlooked benefits (Harrison, n.d.; PBrun & Dugas, 2008; Salie & Schlechter, 2012). Interestingly, employee motivations have shifted over the past few decades now showing a stronger desire for intrinsic rewards with less emphasis placed on extrinsic rewards. In the past, material rewards were preferred, such as performance bonuses, whereas today people prefer intrinsic rewards, such as meaningful work, personal discretion to make decisions about work, and working in highly-engaged teams that create and innovate. The new generation of employees also prefer intrinsic rewards in that they respond best to work that is meaningful and that allows them to learn cutting-edge skills to find their own ways of accomplishing tasks (Thomas, 2009).

Prensky (2014) tells us that our teaching and leadership practices need to align better with the fact that the new workforce generation can and do want to accomplish great things. "They are, increasingly, individually and as a group, hugely capable and powerful—and linked to each other in ways which never existed before" (p. 3–4)... moreover, by that very nature, are compelled to make a difference on a global scale. Knowing what motivates you and the people you work with certainly puts you in a better position to fuel team motivation. If you want to empower a young new employee, give them an altruistic-centered BIG goal. They want to make a difference!

In our fast-paced work environments, we seldom take the time anymore to celebrate. However, carving out small moments to encourage and motivate the team does not require huge efforts. The pay-off for the team, in particular for those who are intrinsically motivated, is to experience the joy of giving to others. These small gestures can go a long way to building team cohesion and enhance overall functioning. Take time to encourage and support each other in ways that are meaningful. We invite you to praise the people you work with daily by creating moments of personalized praise and gratitude (see Table 10.3).

| Table 10.3 | Team Rewards |

Intrinsic Rewards	Extrinsic Rewards
Promote a sense of meaningfulness: Carve out opportunities for meaningful work such as taking on new or expanded roles and self-management.	Anonymously leave someone a small gift card or a sticky note, or leave them a coffee mug with a personalized message handwritten on the paper cup.
Ask each team member to share his or her personal vision for team dreams.	Publicly announce when individual and team goals are attained. Use a team metric to quantify improvements and post colorful info-graphics.
Promote a sense of choice and high engagement: Allow team members to decide how best to feel fulfilled in their role based on passions.	Post a visible *employee recognition accomplishments board* and be faithful to celebrating the people around you for their valued contributions.
Create spaces that give people the freedom to care deeply engaging in initiatives they care most about.	Publish projects and special initiative outcomes in newsletters, blogs, newspapers, annual stakeholder reports, etc.
Promote valuing of ideas: Start a suggestion program and make a point of featuring the ideas you implement. Trust each other and be respectful in all encounters.	Find electronic ways to publicize great ideas and good deeds, such as participate in blogs or the INASCL *Linked In* platform, thanking those who have made a difference to you.
Promote collaborative teams: Support the need for flexibility at work to promote a sense of freedom, trust each other to follow through.	Arrange a special lunch with the Dean to celebrate big milestones and mark the occasion with a gift.
Promote a sense of competence: Allow employees to generate processes for performance evaluations and goal attainment tracking to self-assess progress.	Host open, public celebrations to recognize team members' accomplishments such as Ph.D./Masters degrees, or other academic achievements such as CHSE, CHSE-A, or CHSOS designations, and publish the event in your institutional newsletter.
Support the employee advancement as identified by the employee to develop new competencies or recognize existing ones, i.e., CHSE or CHSE-A designation attainment.	Award *Appreciation Certificates* for a job well done.
Promote a sense of progress: Create opportunities for employees to innovate, create, problem-solve, and lead.	Nominate an employee for external or internal awards.
Promote pride and a sense of accomplishment and ask team members to share with each other one personal success they were most proud of.	Name an in-house award or physical space after a long-standing contributor on your team, i.e., Dr. James Jane Award or Dr. Jane James Simulation Library.
Schedule regular one-on-one discussions with team members and invite them to dialogue about whatever is most important to them.	Keep a team progress board of achievements up to date and visible in your simulation center.
Promote a sense of valuing: Greeting your team members by name, with a smile wherever you encounter them.	Think about awarding those who are behind the scenes, i.e., the "Behind the Scenes Special Person" award.
Promote a sense of pride: Write an *unsolicited* letter of commendation for the person highlighting their contributions.	Acknowledge and celebrate birthdays and special days of team members to promote valuing.
Foster a sense of confidence: Allow employees to increase their participation and scope of practice as they feel they are ready.	Inscribe a personal note on your favorite book as a gift of encouragement to someone who loves reading.

Simulation team rewards created by Foisy-Doll, C. (2016), Author.

Are You an Introvert, Extrovert, or Ambivert?

Introvert, extrovert, and ambivert are terms coined by C. G. Jung that "explain different attitudes people use to direct their energy" (Myers Briggs Foundation (MBF), 2015, para. 1). *Extroverts* feel at home in the world deriving energy from active engagement with individuals or groups, places, and activities. *Introverts*, on the other hand, prefer spending less time with others deriving their energy from internal experiences, such as intellectual activities, manipulating ideas, wondering through memories, creating mental models, and pondering emotions (Myers Briggs Foundation (MBF), 2015). All human beings manifest some combination of introversion and extroversion, where *ambiversion* is used to describe landing somewhere in the middle of the two. The Myers Briggs—MBTI Type Questionnaire is a tool that makes accessible Jung's theory of personality types. The tool classifies personality types into four distinct categories: (1) extroversion or introversion, (2) sensing or intuition, (3) thinking or feeling, and (4) judging or perceiving (Myers-Briggs Foundation). You can take the MBTI assessment online where trained professionals will analyze your results and provide personalized interpretation. The follow-up can take place over a phone call or completed exclusively online. Self-knowledge of your personality typing can help you to gain insight into yourself and how and why you choose to interact the way you do in teams.

Emotional Intelligence

*"People with high EI know that angry people can be dangerous, that happiness means that someone wants to join with others and that some sad people may prefer to be alone" —**Mayer, 2009, para, 3***

Emotional intelligence (EI) *is* a relatively recent concept first introduced by Peter Salovey and John Mayer in 1990. They challenged the efficiency of intelligence quotient (IQ) and personality tests as the only legitimate measures of intelligence. The basic premise was that one's IQ is far too limiting in its ability to characterize intelligence. Later, Goleman (1995) in his book, *Emotional Intelligence*, further popularized the construct. Goleman proposed that implicit in EI are *personal competencies*, such as self-awareness, accurate self-assessment, and self-control, and *social skills*, such as conflict management, empathy, and leadership. He further divided EI into five domains: (1) knowing your emotions, (2) managing your emotions, (3) motivating yourself, (4) recognizing and understanding other's emotions, and (5) managing relationships and the emotions of others. Science in this field has advanced to the point where EI is now thought to be a better predictor of one's success than IQ (intelligence quotient). EI gives individuals an edge over others by enhancing their ability to innovate, work in teams, build trust, motivate others, and increase overall organizational performance and productivity. Moreover, an increased level of EI is strongly correlated with job satisfaction, productivity, and job performance (Zenger, Folkman, & Edinger, 2010).

EI also speaks to one's "capacity to reason about emotions and emotional information, and of emotions to enhance thought" (Mayer, 2009, para 2; Goleman, 1998). In organizations, those with a high level of EI possess a strong awareness of others' and their emotions; they harness those emotions while working on group tasks such as problem-solving; and self-regulate emotions while contributing to the

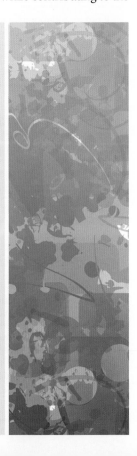

Reflection Activity 10-1
Team Situations and Emotional Intelligence

What would the emotionally intelligent simulation team member do in these circumstances? Partner with a simulation colleague to compare notes on your responses.

- **Scenario 1:** Your simulation colleague is often late for work and gives little notice when late. Your colleague text messages to say he or she is "running late today." So you are left doing double time again. What should the emotionally intelligent team member do?
- **Scenario 2:** As the simulation team director, you have worked very hard on a project for the past few weeks, completed it successfully, and received very positive feedback. You are feeling quite pleased with the team's accomplishments. The next day, you receive an email from your supervisor. The tone is angry and punitive. The supervisor berates you for your seeming lack of professionalism and for putting too much pressure on others in the completion of the project. You are stunned as your supervisor made harsh, judgemental statements that you feel are unfounded. What would the emotionally intelligent leader do?
- **Scenario 3:** Your simulation team is in the middle of an intense day of simulations. As a simulation educator, you are overseeing many students and Simulated Patients (SP) over the course of the day. As you are listening to one encounter, you notice that the SP begins to counsel the students based on their lived experience. The conversation is off-script and starts to make you feel very uncomfortable. What would the emotionally intelligent simulation educator do?

emotional well-being of others. EI offers us a much broader spectrum with which to understand and assess people's behaviors, management styles, attitudes, interpersonal skills, and potential (Goleman, 1995). People with high EI are vital in teams because they have the ability to act quickly and accurately in a variety of emotion-centered situations. They also have the ability to sway others' emotions and thinking. Would your team members say you have high, or low EI?

How can you determine your EI? There are a host of EI measurement tests you can take, many of which have been empirically evaluated while others have not. Here is a list of those tests deemed valid and reliable by the Consortium for Research on Emotional Intelligence Organizations (2015) where active links to each are located: BarOn Emotional Quotient Inventory, Emotional & Social Competence Inventory, Emotional & Social Competence Inventory—U, Genos Emotional Intelligence Inventory, Group Emotional Competency Inventory, Mayer-Salovey-Caruso EI Test (MSCEIT) , Schutte Self Report EI Test, Trait Emotional Intelligence Questionnaire (TEIQue), Work Group Emotional Intelligence Profile, and Wong's Emotional Intelligence Scale (Consortium for Research on Emotional Intelligence Organizations, 2015). Note that there are costs associated with taking these tests.

Relationality and Relational Ethics

"Before I built a wall I'd ask to know; what I was walling in or out, And to whom I was likely to give offence." —**Robert Frost (1914), Mending Wall**

Each one of us is a vulnerable human being. We come together in workplaces and carry our personal baggage, our worries, our pressing family concerns, our health issues, as well as our hopes, talents, dreams, and aspirations. We are not just complicated, we are complex and dare we say, at times even chaotic creatures. When layered upon that same complexity in others, teams become a seemingly endless web of paradoxes: an entanglement of both vulnerabilities and potential.

In healthcare teams, these relationships are further confounded by power differentials, both real and perceived that exist between team members. The same can be true for leaders and followers in teams where one person may have an increased sphere of influence and control over others. In healthcare, this applies especially to the relationship between the patient and provider where the patient enters the relationship under very vulnerable circumstances with complex emotional and intensive treatment needs. In a study of nursing relationships over 10 years ago, Austin et al. reported that "professionals seemed unaware of their power and privilege and how their projected authority is perceived" (p. 79). With the increasing awareness of the need for safer patient care, we would expect the opposite. However, cultural change is slow, and power distance in healthcare teams is very much present.

"Boundaries emphasize the limits of what the participants should or should not do to preserve the ethical sanctity of a relationship" (p. 81). Boundaries serve to demarcate clearly our zones of comfort from zones of discomfort in relationships. Boundaries are also considered as precursors to violations, where the crossing of a boundary is considered denigration of ethical and relational sanctity, the breaking of a bond of trust that results in harm to the other person (p. 82). In HPTs, we value relationships and enact relational ethics by recognizing and defining clear boundaries and honoring, respecting, and maintaining the sacred nature of those boundaries.

Doing Your Best to Stay Off the Drama Triangle

In relational dysfunction, games unfold within our interactions at work and in our personal life. We can use that discord either as a catalyst for change or as a means of perpetuating dysfunction in our life. Rooted in Transactional Analysis Psychology and Family Script Theory, Dr. Stephen B. Karpman (2011, 2014) uses the *Drama Triangle* to depict complex human interactions and entanglements that unfold in conflict situations (see Fig. 10.2). To put it simply, the drama triangle represents the "all-to-familiar three-sided way we sabotage relationships" (2014, p. 15). Life's games between people play out within drama triangles in commonplace settings such as in "dysfunctional families,…in the courtroom, bedroom, and the classroom" (Karpman Drama Triangle.com, 2015, para. 1). Coaches and therapists, self-help groups and individuals all over the world use this simple, yet very effective tool to unlock and mobilize those of us who find ourselves stuck on the web of this stressful triangle.

The original drama triangle has undergone several transformations to now include dozens of different applications; some of them highly complex (i.e., the compassion triangle, the insight triangle, the outer and inner personality triangles, and so on). In his new book, *A Game Free Life*, Karpman (2014) flushes out how we can be pulled into the "drama triangle" as one of three characters: the persecutor, the rescuer, or the victim. The ensuing triangulation can escalate to grave destabilization and emotional exhaustion,

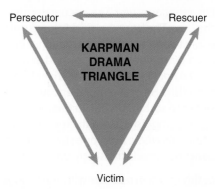

Figure 10.2 The Karpman Drama Triangle. (Used from Karpman, S. B. (2014). *A game free life*. San Francisco, CA: Drama Triangle Publications, with permission.)

in fact perpetuating the cycle of dysfunction and worsening the situation. An individual's initial participation as the persecutor, rescuer, or victim on the triangle happens for a variety of conscious or subconscious reasons. Ultimately, participants believe they are justified in being there and are usually gaining some form of psychological satisfaction, that being, a self-esteem boost, a desire to be seen as a hero, an inclination toward drama and excitement, etc. Drama triangles need at least two participants to subsist, but most often a third person is added to the mix, thereby, completing the triangle.

The victim is the person who feels victimized, and therefore, acts like a victim. They perceive themselves as oppressed, helpless, hopeless, powerless, and shamed. They express an inability to make decisions, solve problems, take pleasure in life, or achieve insight—their actions epitomize the "poor me" syndrome. As long as the triangle is intact, the victim is given permission to remain stuck on there as the victim. The victim never needs or wants to leave the triangle as long as there is fuel to stay. If allowed, the victim will covet the victim's place on the triangle in perpetuity.

After all, he or she is getting lots of attention as a victim (Johnson, n.d.; Karpman, 2014; Orriss, 2004). We have all played the victim role at one time or another.

The persecutor is the person in the drama triangle that could be described as controlling, blaming, critical, oppressive, angry, authoritative, rigid and superior, or self-righteous. The *persecutor* adopts the "it's all your fault" attitude and dishes it out in buckets (Johnson, n.d.; Karpman, 2014). It has been our experience that persecutors especially like to tackle a victim behind closed doors.

The rescuer is the person that always needs to fix things. After all, if a friend is in trouble, you should help, right? The *rescuer* adopts the classic enabler role and feels guilty if he/she fails to rescue the other. Nurses are prime targets for this role as our altruistic tendencies lead us to want to rescue others. Rescuing, however, "has negative effects: it keeps the *victim* dependent and gives the *victim* permission to fail. It also keeps the *rescuer* stuck in focusing energy on someone else's problems, not solving his/her own (Karpman, 2014). The *"rescuer's* attitude is one of 'Let me help you'" (Johnson, n.d., para. 15).

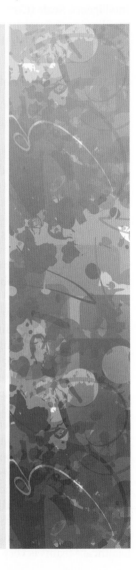

Reflection Activity 10-2
The Drama Triangle—In Work Situations

- *Enter the victim:* The victim arrives at work and finds that the boss is once again ignoring them. Upon arrival, the victim says hello to her boss and does not receive a reply. She is upset and feeling the open flesh wound of repeated rejection as this has happened many times in recent weeks. She wonders if she has fallen out of favor or has done something wrong. However, deep inside, she knows that she has done nothing to deserve this kind of treatment (at this point, you will note that the victim does not accept responsibility for his or her feelings and that the victim conveniently perceives the boss as a persecutor, even though this may be far from reality).

- *Enter the rescuer:* A work colleague and confidant enters. The victim is upset and quickly reveals the details of the encounter to the rescuer, knowing that the rescuer will support the victim in his or her interpretation of the cold, unfeeling boss. The conversation goes on a long while and escalates into a full-blown victim and rescue session where the rescuer attempts to problem-solve for the victim. Depending on the actions of the rescuer, the intensity of the conflict can escalate or subside.

- *Enter the persecutor:* The rescuer decides that it is in everyone's best interests to talk to the boss. The boss can quickly jump onto the triangle, joining as a persecutor, only to escalate and worsen the situation. Conversely, the situation can quickly be de-escalated by the boss' reactions and actions. For example, the boss makes a conscious choice *not to jump* onto the triangle by adopting a neutral stance and not buy into the "crisis." He or she might encourage the persecutor to speak one-on-one with the victim to sort things out. In this case, the situation is resolved, the victim's fuel for the fire is extinguished, and the rescuer's efforts to rescue are not supported. Alternately, situations where everyone stays active on the triangle eventually escalate, all participants become increasingly polarized, and complete dysfunction ensues.

Does this situation resonate with you? Can you see how you or others get snared onto the triangle? What skills do you need to develop to release yourself from the drama triangle?

In the preceding example of how a drama triangle might unfold, ask yourself where you might typically be positioned? When are you a victim, persecutor, or rescuer?

Staying off of the triangle begins with *introspective and outrospective self-reflection* to gain an intimate knowledge of self and others. Once you train yourself to recognize the triangle, you can get off of it quickly-or avoid it altogether!

Resilience in Teams

"At their very core, high-performing simulation teams are made up of well-intentioned, caring and complex human beings who recognize that it is through commitment, mutual accountability, and a strong belief in each other that together, they can make amazing things happen!"
—C. Foisy-Doll

Resilience can be described as the ability to "dance with life, to flex, adapt, and create as life keeps surprising us" (Wheatley, 2011, p. 126). Resilience has existed for as long as there has been life; all living systems have had to learn how to persevere to survive, but this ability does not develop in isolation. Older descriptions of resilience compartmentalized it as a personal skill that we develop on our own. Today, resilience is viewed within the greater context of the *interdependence* and *interconnectedness* of all living systems and beings. "Like any of life's strengths, resilience grows in relationships and community" (Wheatley, 2011, p. 126). In self-reliant HPTs, resiliency abounds. These teams know that they can hold onto each other. They know that they have all that they need to succeed there in their midst. There is an awareness, a shared trust that whatever they need, the world and the people around them will provide.

Teams who demonstrate resiliency are less dependent on external leadership sources. Resilient teams rely more on leadership emerging from within the team. This is because exertion of control over another is often met with abandonment or despair on the other person's part. Dependency in teams, therefore, can be the unintended consequence of a leader's helpfulness, thereby diminishing resilience (Wheatley, 2011). So, don't always jump in to rescue others or be so helpful that you disempower them. These rescuers are often referred to as micromanagers with the underlying premise that micromanaging others stems from distrust in others' abilities. When leaders are overly controlling, they can stifle others' strengths, creativity, gifts and personal resources, in fact disallowing them from coming to the surface. The team then is no longer a team but a group of doers, simply following orders. Indeed, what ensues is a lack of individual and team resilience.

Contributing to Team Efficiency: Team Composition Matters

Daft (2010) explains that "for a team to be successful over the long run, it must be structured so as to both maintain

> ### Box 10-1 Task Specialist Functions
>
> - **Initiate ideas:** Allow team members to propose new solutions to team problems.
> - **Give opinions:** Allow all team members to share opinions and to give candid, objective feedback on others' suggestions.
> - **Seek information:** Ask for task-relevant facts.
> - **Summarize:** Ask team members to take turns summarizing discussions to promote active listening and summarize various ideas to solve the problem at hand; pull everyone's ideas together to form a team summary perspective.
> - **Energize:** Ask team members to do or say something stimulating to move the team into action when interest drops (i.e., take a health break, or take turns doing a team activity).

its members' social well-being and accomplish its task [behaviors that promote team resilience]" (p. 513). In essence, teams need both efficiency and resiliency to survive. Successful teams have their needs met through two internal team roles: the *task specialist* and the *socioemotional specialist* (see Boxes 10-1 and 10-2). Task specialists focus efforts on keeping the team on task and on time by initiating ideas, giving opinions, seeking information, summarizing, and energizing, whereas socioemotional specialists focus on team spirit and emotional needs of team members and creating a positive, safe social environment (p. 513).

Task specialists tend to focus almost exclusively on team productivity, whereas socioemotional team players tend to be underproductive by focusing on social aspects of teams. Effective teams have people in both task specialist and socioemotional roles. A high-functioning team will do best over the long term because it will both be personally satisfying for team members as well as create a sense of

> ### Box 10-2 Socioemotional Functions
>
> - **Encouragement:** Establish team norms that promote warmth in workplaces and receptivity to others' ideas; praise and encourage others to draw forth their contributions.
> - **Harmonize:** Each member can play a part in reconciling team conflicts by facilitating disagreeing parties to reach a resolution.
> - **Reduce tension:** Tell jokes or in other ways draw off emotions when group atmosphere is tense.
> - **Follow:** Remember that followership is a key role in teams; everyone must respect when it is time to follow and go along with the team; that is, agree to other team members' ideas.
> - **Compromise:** Will shift own opinions to maintain team harmony.

accomplishment from team task accomplishment. Teams with mostly socioemotional roles can be satisfying, but they also can be unproductive—spending too much time socializing. At the other extreme, a team made up primarily of task specialists will tend to have a particular concern for task accomplishment—do, do, and then do some more. This team will be effective for a short period but will not be satisfying for members over the long run. Effective teams have people in both task specialist and socioemotional roles (Daft, 2010). A well-balanced team will do best over the long term because it provides a balance of personal satisfaction and team accomplishment. What does the blend of task versus social orientation look like on your simulation team?

"What we need to do is learn to work in the system, by which I mean that everybody, every team, every platform, every division, every component is there not for individual competitive profit or recognition, but for contribution to the system as a whole on a win-win basis" —***W. Edwards Deming***

Who Is on the Sim Team?

Simulation delivery teams are made up of innovators and committed hard working individuals with diverse knowledge and skills sets. Job titles and role descriptions in simulation programs will vary from place to place and by organizational size, structure, and titling practices. Depending on the size of your program, these positions and the number of employees will vary considerably. Sometimes, there is only one person responsible for simulation, although we acknowledge this is an undesirable and unsustainable practice. Whatever the size or scope of your simulation program or endeavor, all would be wise to follow the NCSBN Simulation Guidelines for Prelicensure Nursing Programs. These guidelines stipulate the need for simulation delivery teams with dedicated lead faculty and sim lab personnel that are qualified to conduct simulation and are supported in their ongoing professional development. Educators must be prepared to lead simulations, and adhere to clear policies and processes that support excellence in simulation (Alexander et al., 2015). Simulation team composition for might include:

- **Executive Sponsor:** This person is a senior administrator within your organization serving as Dean, CEO, CFO, or maybe even the Provost, Vice President, or President. They are accountable to a governing body and as such, are well positioned as key Simulation Champions. Having a positive and close working relationship with this person is vital to the health and success of your simulation team and other internal stakeholder groups, such as, faculty and staff. These leaders communicate organizational vision and mission, set the tone for corporate culture, and work closely with all stakeholder groups. More importantly, they are held accountable at the highest levels of the organization for successful simulation adoption and integration.

- **Steering, Advisory or Guiding Coalition Committee/ Team:** A team composed of high-level stakeholders who provide guidance on critical issues, marketing strategies, resource allocation, and overall program goals, policies and outcomes. Some groups serve as permanent committees that are assigned decision-making authority, while others serve in an advisory capacity.

- **Simulation Program Director:** According to Society for Simulation in Healthcare (SSH) (2016e), the Simulation Director/Program Director provides strategic leadership, business development, governance, executive, and management of the center. The primary focus of a Simulation Director/Program Director is to lead the strategic direction of the simulation program to align with the goals of the organization with a focus on corporate and business leadership. This person typically oversees simulation integration at institutional, administrative, and curricular levels across programs and works closely with internal and external stakeholder groups and the Executive Sponsor(s).

- **Simulation Program Operations Manager or Administrator:** The Simulation Center Manager (Administrator)/ Operations Manager (Administrator)/or Director of Operations is responsible for the day-to-day operations of the center and will often report to and support the Director. This person oversees the general operations and functioning of the center. They manage operational services including having input into the budget, equipment, and supplies procurement; scheduling of courses and staff; supervision of simulation educators, coordinators, and technicians; and supervision of any administrative personnel and promotion of the center (ASSH, 2012).

- **Simulation Program Business Manager** (if applicable to your milieu): This person is responsible for the business end of things in your Simulation Program and is especially important in business model approaches that must generate revenue to subsist. They can work to generate bookings, develop promotional marketing strategies, foster positive public relations, and engage in business-related research including operations analysis, statistics, and economic reports. If present, they can oversee finances, accounting, budgeting, and purchasing. It is advantageous if the person is adept at technology and business information software to support excellence in business practices.

- **Simulation Program Research Officer:** This team member is a person who conducts and implements a research strategy and then conducts and implements a research program/plan within a particular clinical specialty. The researcher plans and conducts experiments or exploration to increase the body of scientific knowledge on simulation-related topics. They may also aim to develop or improve existing processes in simulation or provide a new body of evidence for different aspects of simulation (SSH, 2012a).

- **Simulation Program Educational Lead/Coordinator:** The Simulation Education Lead (sometimes referred to as Coordinator) is responsible for implementing and sustaining best practices for simulation education programs that are consistent with the vision and mission of the Health Service or University (SSH, 2012a). In some cases, this person may be the same person as the Director. Today, this role has evolved to warrant the hiring of a qualified simulation education expert (i.e., Certified Simulation Healthcare Educator—CHSE or CHSE-Advanced through SSH, 2016e). The education lead contributes to the development of simulation educational programs and related curricula for students and educators. They might oversee simulation teaching and learning strategies to design, plan, execute, and assess or evaluate student and faculty learning as well as the evaluation of simulation program outcomes. The educational coordinator may also assume administrative tasks related to course delivery, workshop offerings, and other events, as well as participate in simulation setup and takedown of scenarios and the operation of simulators.
- **Simulation Program Instructor/Educator:** The Simulation Instructor/Educator's primary responsibility is instructional. Therefore, they enact simulation and assess learner performance on a daily basis. Some programs hire an entire team of instructors/educators that exclusively work as members of the simulation delivery team. The role may also encompass certain aspects of curriculum design, development, implementation, and evaluation of scenarios and courses (ASSH, 2012). This role could also involve technical operations and/or instruction as well as include faculty development related to simulation frameworks, implementation of best practices, and faculty roles.
- **Simulated/Standardized Patient Coordinator/Trainer:** This person is trained to work with Simulated/Standardized Patients (SPs) (in some cases, across the life span). The role they play in SP programs varies to include involvement in certain aspects of simulation development (i.e., scheduling, script writing, SP training and coaching, SP human resources management). If you are starting from scratch, we highly recommend that you seek out learning opportunities from the many training programs that offer SP educator training programs. A quick Internet search yielded twelve different programs. The larger the program, the more role differentiation will be needed, in addition to the need for adding more staff.
- **Simulation Operators:** These are people that could be specifically hired to man the control rooms and orchestrate the entire back end of simulation events (computer operations, patient voice, recording, software

management, etc.). This position could also be a cross-over position for other staff, such as a simulation technician if they are the operators of the control stations. It is strongly advisable that these people, especially those filling the role of patient's voice, have a healthcare background to maximize realism.

- **Simulation Technician(s)/Technologist(s)—Sim Tech/ Simulation Operations Specialists (Sim Ops)/or Simulation Operations Specialist (SOS)/ or Certified Simulation in Healthcare Operations Specialists (CHSOS):** The *Simulation Operations Specialist* (SOS) "possesses advanced knowledge and understanding of the many facets of day-to-day operations within a simulation lab (Gantt & Young, 2016b, p. 3). The SOSs key areas of responsibility are in planning, organizing, project management, and provide specialized technical support services solutions and maintenance for quality assurance and improvement. They come with varied backgrounds including health education, engineering, and instructional and educational technology requiring a blend of all of these talents. Gantt and Young refer in jest to the SOS role as "Just Call Me Gumby" (p. 3) speaking to how stretched these individuals are on any given day. The simulation technician can also play a role in educating and supporting staff and instructors in the use of simulation, audiovisual, and other information communication technology. From time to time, the simulation technician is also responsible for managing technology requirements of special projects (ASSH, 2012; SSH, 2016e). A person in this capacity can have an expanded role to engage in collaborative work with simulation educators on scenario development and delivery. They have varied backgrounds ranging from instructional media and design to graphic design, instructional or informational technology (IT), and audiovisual, or other computer-based professional competencies (Gantt & Young, 2016b).
- **Simulation IT/AV Specialist:** Depending on the size and scope of your center, you may access existing staff from your internal IT/AV department. If you are a smaller school, consider a shared position between your program and other departments as you may not require full-time assistance. It is essential that these persons be involved from the outset and themselves become simulation technology specialists. Whether you choose to install an integrated AV/IT recording and center management system, it is wise to engage your institution's Technology Department.

NOTE: The roles of computer operator, simulation technician, and IT/AV specialist are sometimes combined, to provide a multilayered skill set that can span the functions in each job. If you can find and individual with a healthcare and education background and a talent for technology, you have a rich resource on your team. This person can liaise with faculty to design scenarios, prepare the mannequin, stage the environment, operate the computer, vocalize the patient and manipulate the technology (Gantt & Young, 2016b).

- **Support Staff:** This person offers support for the program and other personnel. These individuals are responsible for the administrative support needed to run your facility. They may be positioned at the entrance to greet and manage the flow of customers/students/faculty or be involved in a wide assortment of duties related to computer processing, organizing, materials management, and scheduling. In the simulation facility, these individuals may be referred to as lab assistants and assume many roles in simulation from setup and takedown to moulage and designing props.
- **Custodial Staff:** This person or group of people are responsible for maintaining a clean, safe environment in the sim center. Institutional custodial staff usually covers this, but special cleaning requirements may be necessary such as dusting off of all audiovisual equipment. You will need to define who is responsible for cleaning and maintaining simulators in your organization.

Simulation Delivery Team Types

Teams are classified into types depending on form and function. Many organizations rely on cross-functional (CF) approaches to increase efficiency and productivity. Typically, CF teams are composed of individuals possessing different functions or coming from different departments. Typically, they stem from within a given organization but can come from outside. Given the fact that members are selected for their expertise, teams are also extended the freedom to make critical decisions related to their knowledge sets. They can be temporary or permanent in nature. CF teams are known to work as highly interdependent units where collaboration contributes to cohesion within the team and also within the organization (Daft, 2014).

Simulation teams rely heavily on cross-functionality. One example of a temporary CF team is to assemble team members from inside and outside the organization when building a simulation center. The CF team engages key people from, information technology, audiovisual, facilities management, human resources, academic faculty, and administrative departments and externals in design–build, city planning, and other stakeholder groups. All participating members contribute to the end product and disband at the end of the project. A permanent CF team would be the simulation delivery team itself composed of key individuals that are hired for different skills sets, that is, technology, simulation education, operations, research, materials management, moulage, etc. Each person brings unique expertise to the team that benefits the whole. These simulation delivery teams engage in CF team training to optimize outcomes and build team capacity. A CF approach is particularly useful in smaller teams where members identify functions or tasks that can be carried out by others on the team. For example, all employees (including Lab Assistants) can be trained to start up and shut down equipment. On a busy day, the team can draw on the cross-functionality of its members to execute multiple or competing demands. The more capacity you build in each team member, the stronger the team functionality. A CF simulation chart is provided for you in the online toolkit titled "Levels of Cross-Functionality in Simulation Teams" (Toolkit 10-1).

Self-Managed Teams

Do you think of yourself as an independent thinker and doer? **Self-managed teams** are groups of between 5 to 20 individuals that ideally do not require a manager. As multiskilled highly motivated individuals, they take responsibility for decision-making, expending dollars, adding new members, monitoring performance, problem-solving, adapting to change, and working toward goal attainment as they deem appropriate (Daft, 2014). In Simulation Programs, it is not unusual for team members to take it upon themselves to learn new skills allowing them to cross-cover or rotate job functions with others on the team. The most effective teams according to Laszlo, Laszlo, and Johnsen (2009) are "self-managed teams whose members have a great deal of autonomy, are valued for their skills and intelligence, feel challenged in their work, and feel that they are free to contribute to team goals in ways they see fit" (p. 32). Often, simulation teams adopt the characteristics of self-managed teams as they effectively work out program delivery details among themselves.

Distributed, Dispersed, or Virtual Teams

Distributed, dispersed, or virtual teams are just that. Each of these terms refers to teams that are not in the same geographical location, do not need to engage in real time, nor do they need to coact simultaneously. These types of teams are emerging strongly in the 21st century, and, as such, there are requisite competencies for members and their leaders. Some simulation delivery teams operate across programs, across campuses, or between organizations and, for some, across borders.

Effective use of *technology is key to building relationships in these teams and is crucial for effective virtual teamwork*. When assembling a distributed team, it is important for leaders to engage people who possess the right mix of technical, interpersonal, and communication skills to work effectively in a virtual environment. Establishing trusting relationships takes longer than with face-to-face teams, although online social networking, photo sharing, and such can enhance connection and virtual team success. "Researchers found that round-the-clock virtual workspaces, where team members can access the latest versions of files, keep track of deadlines and timelines, monitor one another's progress, and carry on discussions between formal meetings, got top marks" (Daft, 2010, p. 510). There are a plethora of online spaces available now for this type of teamwork. They include Wikis, Blogs, copy and Cloud-based File Sharing, Desktop Videoconferencing with multiple participants, screen sharing, online meeting software, etc.

 See the online toolkit for an example of a *collaborative online team communication tool* built in Google Sheets (Toolkit 10-2). (Note: You will need a Google account if you wish to adopt this form). In this example, you see how the instrument is used by a simulation team to plan for one semester. The beauty of this platform is that all members can populate the form, and then share the responsibility for team outcomes. All members can view it live (so all updates/edits are accessible), and side conversations using comments inside the spreadsheet can be sent as notifications linked to email; color coding and the ability to add comments make this a very useful tool. You can also insert URL links to key team documents. The Google Sheet will also populate Google Calendars to save your team valuable time. Many products now have the capacity to interface, offering dual or triple functionality (i.e., Facebook, Twitter, Linked In, calendars, scheduling software, etc.). It can serve a single site or connect distributed teams. Welcome to the whiteboard of the 21st century! Whiteboards, however, serve an important function for teams because they allow for larger surface views that are lacking in computer projections.

Team roles can play out in a variety of different ways in distributed teams, where evidence suggests higher success rates in e-teams that have clear and directive leadership. Daft (2014) notes that e-leaders fulfill many vital functions by establishing a socially safe environment for team interaction. In a safe team space, members are more apt to "express concerns, admit mistakes, share ideas, acknowledge fears, or ask for help" (Daft, 2010, p. 511). This open ambiance contributes to shared leadership, enhanced interactivity, team trust, role clarity, establishing of group norms, and clear communication toward a common goal.

Bounded and Unbounded Teams

Organizational healthcare teams are sometimes classified as bounded or unbounded. **Bounded teams** are composed of individuals in stable positions working independently with clearly defined rules and established boundaries, having well-defined tasks and a clear and solid presence within an organization. Simulation delivery teams would be an example of a bound team and have the benefit of

building long-standing relationships. **Unbounded teams**, on the other hand, are characterized by the fluidity of boundaries and members, such as with shift workers in healthcare teams. Student groups in simulation can be considered unbounded teams. Because of their fluid membership, they are more prone to a lack of cohesion, miscommunication, and error. These teams must develop clear and transparent systems and processes to promote effective functioning as they often face solving complex unpredictable issues (Hackman, 2011). The nature of unbounded teams underscores the need for thorough student preparation and prebriefing before a simulation experience. It is important for educators and all simulationists to recognize the impact of degrees of "boundedness" on learners in teams.

Optimal Team Size and Composition

The optimal size for top performance in quality improvement healthcare teams is reported to be between five and eight persons, although there may be variations depending on the function and task at hand (AHRQ, 2013). Auerbach et al. (2012) studied the effects of teamwork and communication on patient care outcomes on over 10,000 patients, concluding that optimal team size was between five and seven persons. However, size does not exclusively determine optimal team functioning. For effective communication to occur, select each team member for their expertise, diverse skill sets, the unique perspectives they hold, as well as their willingness and ability to work with others. Without these characteristics, even teams that are said to be an optimal size can perform quite poorly (Hackman, 2011).

Leading Teams

Leading and managing teams is currently an employment expectation for nurses, so consequently, nurses assume varied leadership and managerial roles and positions throughout the healthcare system. Accepting managership as part of leadership is the task of a leader, and accepting leadership as a part of managership is the task of a manager. Today, leaders and managers need to develop both leadership and management competencies. A wise simulation leader/manager will understand that competent leadership and management create the momentum needed for the emergence of HPTs. Excellence is deliberate. It doesn't just happen!

To that end, today's nurse leaders need specific formation and skill development in team leadership and managership, and the teaching of team competencies. Unfortunately, this is often not the case, and leaders are left to handle tough situations without the benefit of formal training (Dyer et al., 2013). We are fortunate in the simulation practice community to have opportunities for leadership development through the National League for Nursing Simulation Leadership Academy (http://www.nln.org/professional-development-programs/leadership-programs/leadership-development-program-for-simulation-educators) and the International Association for Clinical Simulation and Learning Fellowship programs (http://www.inacsl.org/i4a/pages/index.cfm?pageid=3476), in addition to other professional association and local or regional offerings.

Kotter (2002) and Kotter International (2015b) suggest that great leaders are essential to effective change leadership, providing a clear vision for followers. The leader makes the goals transparent to the followers by making them *touchable, feelable, and seeable* (Kotter, 2002). Leaders and managers who effectively elicit positive emotional responses in people are also more likely to obtain their commitment, acceptance, and an embracing of change. When simulation teams succeed, both followers and leaders are changed through a transformational process that brings about new behaviors, thoughts, and beliefs. The transformation, in fact, involves moving from being a group to becoming a team. In a recent study that surveyed over 100,000 company employees, Zenger Folkman cite the top nine leadership behaviors that boost employee performance as (1) high levels of enthusiasm and energy to inspire and motivate, (2) orientation and drive toward results, (3) a definite sense of purpose and direction with clear strategy, (4) promoting a collaborative *esprit de corps* team synergy; (5) walking the talk; (6) trusted to deliver consistent expertise and skill, (7) pushing others to develop new skills, (8) balancing results orientation with the needs of employees, and (9) courage to address issues and handle conflict while holding employees accountable.

*"Emotions are the 'switch' that connect the leader with the group…and are extremely contagious." —**Zenger, Folkman & Edinger, 2010***

Leading Teams: Forming, Storming, Norming, Performing, and Adjourning

Once groups gather, they can begin the process of developing teamness following a five-step sequential process: forming, storming, norming, performing, and adjourning (Tuckman, 1965; Tuckman & Jensen, 1977). Even though decades old, Tuckman's Stages of Small Group Development still hold true. Figure 10.3 depicts the five phases, corresponding levels of certainty/uncertainty, and group progression to team status. Creating opportunities for group members to socialize and get to know each other is the beginning process of team development.

As a leader, different approaches are required at each stage of the process. There are critical team leader behaviors that correspond to each of the phases (Fig. 10.4). These strategies will assist leaders in each stage of small group development. Simulation leaders can facilitate and expedite the process of transitioning groups into teams.

As the simulation champion leading a group in the *forming stage*, you will need to play a dominant role because someone needs to take responsibility for getting the group off to a good start and get organized. You are transactional in your approach, providing hands-on assistance at this point and educating the group. Group tasks when in the forming stage are driven by a desire for acceptance by others and include the following actions:

- Meeting and greeting
- Sizing each other up
- Establishing rules, roles, and goals
- Gathering information and assigning roles
- Discussing and establishing group norms
- Building communication systems
- Avoiding conflict
- Sizing each other up with uncertainty and some distrust

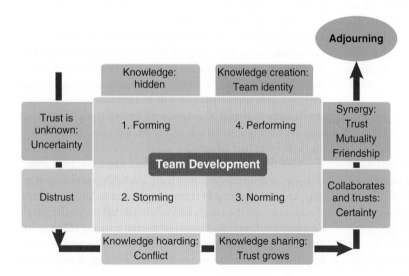

Figure 10.3 Tuckman and Jensen's Stages of Small Group Development. (Adapted from Tuckman, B.W. & Jensen, M.A. (1977, Dec). Stages of small-group development revisited. *Group Organization Management, 2*(4).)

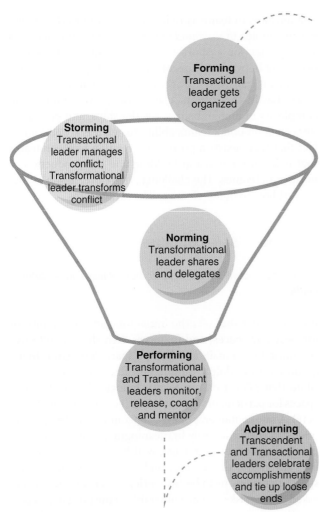

Figure 10.4 Leadership Approaches to Help Groups to Become Teams.

- Depending on one person to lead and get them organized.
- Team identity at this point has not yet formed. (Tuckman & Jensen, 1977)

In the second stage, *storming*, the leader is challenged to keep group harmony and focus amidst growing concerns. Both transactional and transformational leadership approaches should now concentrate on managing differing opinions and conflict. Facilitating the transformation of conflict is a key leader function during this stage. Keep your cool and adopt team processes to resolve conflicts. Remember to use transparent communication approaches, such as those we describe later in the chapter. Group tasks in storming focus on moving the project ahead. The group in the storming phase experiences the following:

- Resistance, opposition, and differences of opinion
- Conflict around team personalities and working styles

- Withdrawal from the group can happen at this stage, usually pressured to stay
- Mostly positive conflict resolution; however, it is possible that the team may dissolve
- Emergence of new norms from conflict resolution efforts
- Lack of team identity (Tuckman & Jensen, 1977)

In the *norming phase*, the leader pulls back and delegates the lion's share of the work, shifting focus to transformational approaches to leading team development and performance or outcomes enhancement. This is an excellent opportunity to formalize shared leadership in teams. The group in the norming phase is enjoying well-functioning processes and starts to become a team. Team identity emerges, and members congeal as the group:

- Develops a strong sense of cohesion, interdependence, and flexibility
- Develops strong relationships and camaraderie
- Enacts norms with fluidity
- Shares feelings openly; gives and receives feedback freely and respectfully
- Builds on each other's strengths
- Starts to experience team successes
- Shared responsibility is present
- Continues to test and tweak communication systems (Tuckman & Jensen, 1977)

In the fourth stage, *performing*, the team is rolling along merrily. Resist the temptation to pull back altogether, and instead use a check-in approach and assist as the team requires your direction. Allow the transcendent leader in you to encourage personal and team transformation beyond the scope of the project. Group tasks in the performing stage are characterized by:

- Resolution of team issues, including leadership wrinkles
- Full commitment from all members to accomplish the task(s) at hand
- Utilizing communication systems effectively
- A solid identity as a team
- Team roles are solid and members reliably follow through
- Outcomes attainment and having the mission accomplished (Tuckman & Jensen, 1977)

Lastly, in the *adjourning stage*, the leader may need to guide team members, especially if the team has been well established and working together for an extended period. Leaders should plan a final celebration to recognize team accomplishments and leave teams feeling proud of what they accomplished, even if the project is ending (Eyre, 2015). Transactional approaches are needed to formalize the dissolution of teams, but as a leader, you will focus your team on the personal and team growth and successes they have experienced and value the accounts of transcendent team lived experiences. During the adjourning phase, some groups will cease to exist, and the team is disbanded. It is important to remember that not all groups become teams, nor do they need to. When adjourning, group/team members experience the following:

- Process of letting go
- Arranging to tie up loose ends and reporting off
- Some members feel sadness during adjournment
- The continuation of some relationships (Tuckman & Jensen, 1977)

Healthy versus Unhealthy Team Climates

Healthy professional practice environments are critical to individual and team performance and job satisfaction. Furthermore, quality practice environments have a positive impact on the delivery of safe, ethical, competent patient care (Aiken, Clarke, Sloane, Lake, & Cheney, 2008; CNA, 2001). Having worked on hundreds of patient care units over the years, we know that a healthy climate is palpable. You can sense something different upon entering a well-functioning, warm space. We suggest that you will find an HPT working there. From the greeting received upon entering, to the buzz in the air, one can sense the positive energy emitted from healthy healthcare workspaces. Bendaly and Bendaly (2012) speak of cool and warm environments and how cool environments manifest in depletion of energy, people operating in survival mode, and harmful conflicts that remain unresolved and fester, bringing negative behaviors. Cool workspaces provide fertile ground for conflict in teams. Moreover, dysfunctional or nonfunctional teamwork is linked to increased patient safety risks (AACN, 2013; IOM, 2010a). Collaborative team practices benefit both healthcare teams and the healthcare system and are considered one of the top factors for creating safer care and reducing healthcare costs (Reeves et al., 2009). Therefore, there is a dire need for HPTs in healthcare to replace our traditional hierarchical and fractured multidisciplinary models and their poor-performing teams.

Barriers to collaboration in healthcare teams stem from numerous places. Barriers include (1) existing professional hierarchies and resulting power and status differentials (real or perceived); (2) long-standing traditions of ranking and competition for status; (3) turfism or territorialism spurred on by changing scopes of practice; (4) the dance of autonomy and interdependence; (5) lack of role clarity and understanding; (6) failure to engage, a fear of communicating for fear of reprisal or ridicule; and (7) a historical culture of nurse subservience to physicians and organization culture (Edmundson, 1999; Kvarnström, 2008; Lichtenstein, Alexander, McCarthy, & Wells, 2004; Martin, O'Brien, Heyworth, & Meyer, 2005; O'Leary et al., 2010; Reeves et al., 2009). Another barrier to building cohesive

relationships in teams is that teamwork in healthcare primarily unfolds in *unbounded teams* where team members are together for a short time with frequent transitions occurring between groups of caregivers (e.g., shift change or patient transfers) (Wageman, Hackman, & Lehman, 2005). Lastly, the authors' claim that the very nature and complexity of human beings, relationships, and personalities can confound a team's ability to gel. It is a well-known fact that there exists a positive correlation between teams that excel in relationship building and the production of positive outcomes. The challenge, therefore, lies in knowing just how to build effective, life-giving teams.

Creating a "Safe Container" for Teams

"We need to recover the soul as a domain of learning." —Julio Olalla

It is the leader that sets the initial tone and conditions for safe learning spaces, and followers then share a collective responsibility to maintain the safe space. **Safe containers**, according to Rudolph, Simon, and Raemer (2014), necessitate that educators create psychologically safe learning spaces for participants in simulation (i.e., group/team members). A safe container is one that encourages and empowers others to engage actively in meaningful professional learning. Feelings of comfort, trust, well-being, security, nurturing, adventure, excitement, and acceptance characterize spaces that allow us to be authentic, especially when we are asked to take risks and be vulnerable in the presence of others. Therefore, safe containers create a supportive milieu for experimentation where trial and error can be experienced without harsh judgement or labeling. Rather, errors are pointed out with honesty and always accompanied by curiosity about the interplay between personal and contextual contributing factors. Successful leaders must do more than manage processes. Leaders also need to create safe spaces for teams that tap into the intrinsic motivation of people, to inspire and motivate them to become their best. Both leaders and followers, as co-creators of safe spaces, truly are catalysts for transformation and in doing so serendipitously transform organizations as well as themselves.

At the start of each new faculty development event, I draw an open empty container on the whiteboard (C. Foisy-Doll, personal communication, 2016). I ask each simulation participant to define their "safe container for learning" by writing words that describe the conditions they require to feel safe when learning. You can also do this anonymously with a jar and pen and paper. This exercise has proven to be an effective springboard for establishing group norms and expected behaviors and provides a foundation for team building with learners, faculty, and our simulation team. Figure 10.5 depicts a compilation of comments I have gathered from safe container activities.

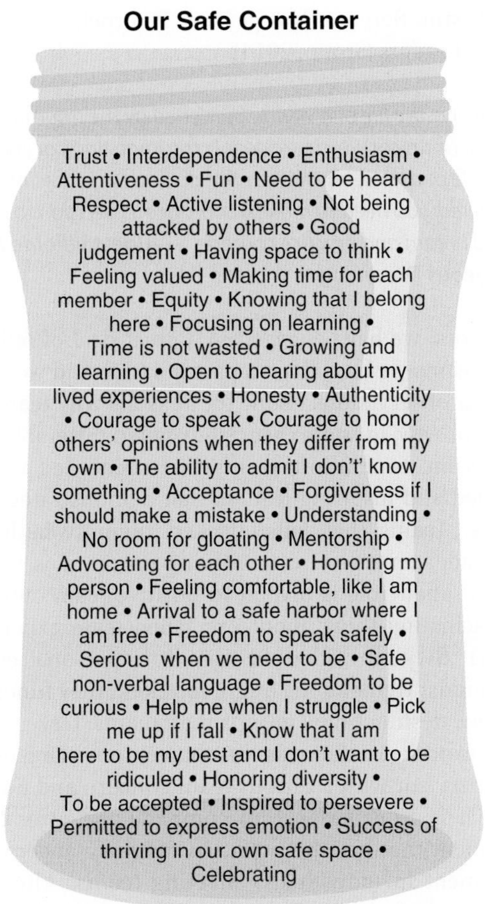

Our Safe Container

Trust • Interdependence • Enthusiasm • Attentiveness • Fun • Need to be heard • Respect • Active listening • Not being attacked by others • Good judgement • Having space to think • Feeling valued • Making time for each member • Equity • Knowing that I belong here • Focusing on learning • Time is not wasted • Growing and learning • Open to hearing about my lived experiences • Honesty • Authenticity • Courage to speak • Courage to honor others' opinions when they differ from my own • The ability to admit I don't' know something • Acceptance • Forgiveness if I should make a mistake • Understanding • No room for gloating • Mentorship • Advocating for each other • Honoring my person • Feeling comfortable, like I am home • Arrival to a safe harbor where I am free • Freedom to speak safely • Serious when we need to be • Safe non-verbal language • Freedom to be curious • Help me when I struggle • Pick me up if I fall • Know that I am here to be my best and I don't want to be ridiculed • Honoring diversity • To be accepted • Inspired to persevere • Permitted to express emotion • Success of thriving in our own safe space • Celebrating

Figure 10.5 Our Safe Container Activity. (Foisy-Doll, C. (2016). This activity is based on the article by Rudolph, J. W., Simon, R., Raemer, D. B. (2014). Establishing a safe container in simulation: The role of presimulation briefing. *Simulation in Healthcare, 9,* 339–349.)

Leadership Lessons: Four Critical Practice Points on Creating Safe, Productive Team Spaces

Note: These next four points transpire simultaneously and are not polarities; they operate together but remain separate concepts. We start with groups and work toward teams.

1. *Trust your individual group members.* Remember that not all groups are teams. Teams must evolve and emerge. Having confidence in other members contributes to mutual respect. Have a clear view of talent and strengths among stakeholders and group members. Take time to build relationships and identify leadership opportunities for each group member. Allow followers to challenge you openly and then to find the courage to share their voice with the group. Validate them and their contributions. These actions will help to build strong team character. Teamness emerges early in groups!

2. *Trust the team!* Trustworthiness begets trustfulness, so be trustworthy and trusting. Whether groups come together for a task or whether persons team around a common goal, success on a long-term basis comes from *team spirit*—the act of putting your heart into what you believe in. High efficacy outcomes will result when team spirit and team motivation are present. As a leader, you must balance your focus on both task and relationship, that is to attend to the work and the social aspects of the team. It is also about balancing leadership and followership to cherish each person on the team. There is no" I" in *team* and no "m" in *we*. If team success is genuine and true, it is a team success, and there is no single hero or single warrior but a team of heroes and a team of fighters.

3. *Make excellence the goal!* Give group members reasonable responsibility and accountability for tasks with the goal of excellence. Make "good judgements" about opportunities that will allow learning moments that challenge and reward your group members in their personal development. *Celebrate* each win and have the group set targets for accomplishments in reasonable time frames ensuring successes are achievable and recognizable. Shared governance will promote excellence as a collective. Take time to laugh! Share the "not so good" times. Be willing to acknowledge failure and collaborate on corrections that are required: be flexible and agile in correcting and changing. Excellence does not occur without great risk management. Make *transparency* your goal in all interactions. "Energy sucking" in the form of denial, criticism, cynicism, false support, and assumption of others' responsibilities is taboo and sets the group up to devolve. Engaging in these behaviors puts you at significant risk of, de*successing your team*. Believe in your group members, and facilitate belief among group members, and excellence on the team will germinate! Hold members responsible for commitments and make sure to meet your own! Sit back and listen. Create and encourage safe containers for learning and doing. Stand back, and let the members go! Patiently hold back and wait! Team excellence under these conditions will flourish!

4. *Build in a communication plan and a sustainability plan.* This is the point in team development at which managership is enacted within the leader/manager roles. Communication and sustainability programs are integral to the change and need to be open, regular, transparent, brief, and inclusive. Be humble; be accountable. Be ready to accelerate and decelerate during implementation phases. Ask for help and honor the suggestions. Think, "if this is...

then what else is ... and why?" and share all proactive plans and reasons for decisions. Listen to others' ideas and incorporate them. Share reasons for decision-making honestly and with integrity. When the project is finished, end it and celebrate. *Give credit to the team.* Ensure that sustainability plans are enacted, established, and reported. Follow up to ensure that the change is working as envisioned by stakeholders and executive sponsors. If you are part of the sustainability initiative, then vision with the team about what will bring growth and strengthening. Stability and equilibrium are not your goals at this point; keeping up momentum is, so don't make the mistake of sitting back on your laurels. Keep the momentum going!

Igniting Moral Courage in Leaders and Followers

*"We are what we repeatedly do. Excellence then is not an act, but a habit." —**Aristotle***

Both leaders and followers must live the values required to build a moral and ethical workplace community. **Moral courage** is a quality and not a gift; it is about willpower and making a choice between two alternatives (Moran, 1967). As a leader, it is not enough to clearly communicate the values inherent in moral and ethical team-based principles; you must embody them. In Rushworth Kidder's classic book titled Moral Courage (Kidder, 2005), the author describes moral courage as the "bridge between talking ethics and doing ethics" (p. 6). In other words, it is one thing to articulate strong moral convictions and to skillfully talk yourself through a mental walk-through, but it is quite another to actually do it! Leaders that can clearly articulate their values and stand up for them through *action* are said to have moral courage. Leaders who fail to act are thought to have a lack of integrity and moral courage and are seemingly not hard to find in corporations, communities, and organizations these days. We all want to enact moral courage, but the truth of it is that exercising moral courage as a core virtue is never easy. We are all called to be courageous and humbly admit to mistakes. It only becomes easier when we choose to make moral courage part of our daily practices, in work and life, such as, through self-development activities like moral imagination: a process where leaders contemplate potentially right or wrong responses in imaginary dress rehearsals.

It is a well-known fact in the study of neuroplasticity that repeatedly practiced behaviors form new neural pathways in the brain, thus rendering us capable of changing, adapting, and reorganizing to build new roadmaps to habitual behavior. As such, nurse educators must support each other in practicing moral courage to build this core

skill (Austin, Bergum, Nuttgens, & Peternelj-Taylor, 2006; Fearless Leaders Group, 2014).

*"You can live the life of a victim, burdened by the traumas of your past [many of which are deeply traumatizing], or you can live the life of a hero, but you cannot do both. If you want to feel empowered, you need to make a courageous decision to create a sacred dream and practice courage" —**Albert Villoldo from Courageous Dreaming***

As authors, we have engaged in a great deal of reflecting on the teams we have been a part of in life and work. Our common observations about the reasons why teams succeeded or why, in some cases, they failed miserably led us to the same conclusion; teams that succeeded were led by skilled and inspiring leaders that demonstrated moral courage. Teams that failed lacked them. Whether the team leader emerges from within a group or is formally assigned, their role is pivotal to positive team outcomes. The fascinating thing about our failed team experiences was that they all evidenced very little personal engagement amidst tremendous fragmentation. They functioned more like dysfunctional groups than teams. Have you had a team experience that was less than empowering or gone to a supervisor with a serious team concern and not been heard? It is an experience of complete and utter disempowerment that has the potential to create anger or disengagement in individuals, affecting teams. Alternately, when people feel heard, they tend to feel less emotional distress, even when facing serious issues (CNA, 2008).

Leaders Creating Moral and Ethical Team Environments

Creating healthy workspaces is complex, multidimensional, and dynamic. Sometimes team conflicts ensue, and leaders will need to engage in conflict mitigation and resolution (Konstantinos & Ouzouni, 2008; Sui, Spence- Laschinger, & Finegan, 2008). A moral workspace is one that places value on relationships so that nurses feel valued and respected, whereas, ethical environments not only recognize and value nurses but also create and support opportunities for nurses to act on those beliefs (CNA, 2003, 2008).

Arenas, León-Pérez, Munduate and Medina (2015) emphasize the crucial roles leaders play through effective use of personal power strategies associated with their formal position. It takes a mountain of moral courage to face conflict and maintain **ethical workspaces**, but it is important for nurse followers to know that they are both heard and supported, even in the midst of distress. The WHO (2011) promotes effective leadership as an essential characteristic of effective teams. Leaders are encouraged to facilitate, coach, and coordinate the activities of teams by accepting and embracing their leadership role. They do this by continuously monitoring situations and asking for help as appropriate. They must set priorities and make good decisions for, and with their teams while utilizing resources to maximize individual and team performance. The leader also needs to balance team workloads, delegate tasks or assignments fairly, and plan for continued team excellence. In conflict situations, the leader must empower team members to speak freely and ask questions that seek to uncover situations and circumstances, and *not exclusively on persons*. Modeling effective communication in critical conversations is inspiring for team members and promotes maintaining a positive group culture. This approach also sets the tone for zero tolerance of abuse and incivility (Clark, 2013; CNA, 2003, 2005, 2009). Dr. Forni (as cited in Clark, 2013, p. 127) lists eight rules for a civil life to help us model civility. They are as follows:

- Slow down and be present in your life
- Listen to the voice of empathy
- Keep a positive attitude
- Respect others and grant them plenty of validation
- Disagree graciously and refrain from arguing
- Get to know the people around you
- Pay attention to the small things
- Ask, don't tell

The Canadian Nurses Association (2010) underscores the importance of quality practice environments for staff and patients. The phrase, "I love being a nurse, but I hate my job" (Duchscher & Myrick, 2008, p. 195) encapsulates much of the uncomfortable emotion that accompanies dysfunctional work environments. Unhappiness spreads like wildfire and negativity can spiral downward very quickly, so it is important to stay on top of it.

The old view of leadership no longer serves leaders or teams well. Old leadership beliefs are evidenced in comments like "Leaders have all the answers"; "Just do what you are told and all will be well"; or, "High risk necessitates high control" (Wheatley, 2011, 2012). New leadership is different. As we examined in previous chapters on leadership, followership, and managership and globalization, the very essence of leadership is undergoing a radical transformation in our increasingly connected, and often broken world. Leaders can no longer rely exclusively on their personal skill sets alone. Leadership structures are flattening, and collaborative leadership is becoming the norm. "Leaders in the future will need new skill sets, greater collaboration skills, organizational architecture ability, and a more flexible style to be open and adaptable to new ideas" (Martin, 2007, p. 3). Martin also challenges us to drop the heroic leader act and to create space, instead of taking up space. The new leader welcomes others in, sees the creative ability in them, and supports them

in fully participating. In turn, followers develop a great deal of autonomy as well as trust in leaders.

"Being a hero is about the shortest-lived profession on earth."
—***Will Rogers***

When Things Totally Break Down: Leading for Higher Performance

Teams comprise living and breathing complex human beings, and as such, are subject the possibility of dysfunction, aka: meltdowns. Organizational leaders in healthcare deal with the human effects of such things as fatigue from shift work, communication breakdowns in unbound teams, dynamic changes in workload and staffing, and diversity in teams (Registered Nurses of Ontario, RNAO, 2012). When things fall apart, it can be very distressing.

Trust can be lost, nasty emails fly, huge differences of opinion about important matters create tension, relationality gives way to hurt feelings, and high team performance gives way to resentment and brokenness. The RNAO (2012) cites that both perceived and actual sources of conflict in health teams are "professional identity; cultural identity; gender; gender identity; nationality; race or ethnic origin; color; religion; age; sexual orientation; marital status; educational background; disability; work values; goals; and interests" (p. 6). Teams themselves can become the victims of the conflict. If left unresolved, the result can be total team collapse. Teams, in fact, can implode to the extent that members abandon their team roles or involvement or may even decide to leave an organization altogether. We have lived this more than once over our combined 70+ years in nursing. Naturally, this extent of dysfunction causes a great deal of personal strife and organizational harm, and organizations and teams should create evidence-based and transparent processes to mitigate "meltdowns."

Warning signs that meltdowns are brewing are often not heeded. Be on the lookout for a loss of team productivity. Watch for things like an increase in team grievances or complaints; mounting user issues over the level of service; overt conflict or hostility between or among team members; continuous and spiraling gossip or backbiting; high levels of confusion about roles and expectations; increased absenteeism or long-term leaves; constant miscommunications or misunderstandings; repeated poorly planned, executed, or communicated decisions; ongoing expressions of complete exhaustion; or a general state of apathy and lack of motivation to engage in work. Layered occurrences will have a compounding effect and should signal to leaders that teams are on the brink of a total breakdown.

To mitigate these dire outcomes, all team members and their leader must commit to the goal of becoming a high-performance team.

Conflict is sometimes presented as being either good or bad in nature, however, conflict, in and of itself, is neither good nor bad. In fact, organizations, teams, and individuals can experience positive effects of conflict, such as the motivation to change behaviors and protocols or an opportunity for personal growth. Bendaly et al. suggest that "differences of opinion in teams can be effectively explored and managed, are essential to team success, and can produce very positive outcomes, and conflict in teams suggests a battle that has no positive outcome." At its core conflict is rooted in differing perceptions and perspectives where dissimilarity or inconsistency between peoples' opinions exits and is a day-to-day reality in HPTs (Adams, 2015; Clark, 2013).

In her wisdom, Oprah Winfrey reminds us that all of life's tsunamis start with a whisper of trouble in the air, followed by a harder hit to the head with a pebble, then a brick—and all of a sudden—there it is, the tsunami! (Oprah's World Tour, personal communication, 2012). We are shocked when the gigantic wave arrives without warning—right? In the same way, overt conflict appears in our lives, and when it does, there is no more ignoring it. Adams states that at its worst, conflict in teams can play out in horrible power struggles where individuals "harass, demean, injure or neutralize another" (p. 162). *Workplace bullying* is understood as the final stage of prolonged, unresolved interpersonal conflict where power imbalance, emotional, and relational problems exist (Arenas et al., 2015; CNA, 2015). Leymann's seminal work on bullying views it as the result of failure to resolve conflict involving "one individual, seldom more, being attacked by one or more (seldom more than four) individuals on a daily basis and for periods of many months" (Leymann, 1996, p. 168). Do you listen for whispers on your team, or do you put off those whispers until the arrival of the tsunami? If you have ever experienced any of the above effects of protracted conflict, you most certainly understand that it can take a tremendous toll on individuals and teams.

So let's say your simulation team has something negative brewing? Based on what you have read so far, think of what can be done to prevent it from spiraling into a meltdown. We suggest to your team gets to work to a plan to attain HPT status. Your team's best chance of staving off team failure is by planning, implementing, and evaluating high-performance team development strategies, principles, and processes.

Grave breaches of trust and human rights issues can also play out in teams and lead to large-scale disastrous outcomes (Adams, 2015). If a team member's actions trouble you to the point of having legal concerns, or include complaints about unethical and immoral conduct, it is time to get help. It is vital that you engage professional or organizational support to lead you through an established process. If, for some reason, you do not feel safe in doing so, there may be alternate routes to deal with these violations, such as seeking police assistance or reporting the behavior under whistle-blower legislation. Either way, team leaders and followers must find their moral courage and report unethical or immoral actions to protect personal and team integrity and safety. If you are the leader faced with such issues, know that the time does come when a person needs to leave. The crossing of ethical boundaries, human rights violations, or the point at which poor performance or persistent negativity are taking down the team, termination is a viable option. In these cases, you must act in the best interests of others and preserve the integrity of teams and the organization. Even though it is never easy, leaders must muster up their moral courage to do the right thing. Zenger and Folkman (2014) list fatal flaws that take teams and organizations down as, lack of honor, failure to deliver and keep promises, untruthfulness, seeks personal gain above needs of others and the organization, lack of ability to learn from mistakes, poor communications skills, not, or lack thereof, open to new ideas, and a lack of drive and accountability.

Facilitating Effective Communication and Transformational Team Change

Communication usually resides at the root of the conflict, but it also is the means by which conflict can be resolved. As such, efforts to improve team communication are essential in team skill development. Ultimately, creating healthy workspaces is about individual and collective commitments to relational practice through developing relational connections. Hartrick Doane (2002) defines *relational practice* as "a humanely involved process of respect, compassion, and authentically interested inquiry into another's experiences (p. 401). *Relational connection*, on the other hand, is "a way of connecting with others requiring that nurses turn to people and family experiences and open themselves up to their fullness and depth" (p. 401). Effective engagement to produce this level of connection also involves a great deal of self-knowledge and the ability to adopt an authentic and genuine stance of curiosity about yourself and others. As Abraham Lincoln once said, *"I don't like that man. I must get to know him better."*

Teams can enhance their collective abilities to resolve conflict or disagreement by using a simple, yet sophisticated debriefing technique called Advocacy-Inquiry (AI), an approach within the Debriefing With Good Judgement model (DWGJ) (Rudolph, Simon, Rivard, Dufresne, & Raemer, 2007). The AI technique is grounded in honest sharing of personal observations and perspectives, with an accompanying and parallel inquiry into another's cognitive frames (i.e., attitudes, values, feelings, needs, past experiences, beliefs, assumptions, observations, understanding, perspectives, biases, etc.). DWGJ using AI allows you to contrast your frames against another's. If you are willing to take the time to explore others' perspectives with a stance of genuine curiosity, at the root of most conflict lies a host of surprising assumptions held on the part of those involved.

It is often the case in disharmonious relationships that people will say "we are simply incompatible" or "our personalities clash." The personality clash approach is not helpful because it focuses on character rather than behavior, personal strengths, perspectives, or beliefs. By taking the focus off of blaming and shaming, or labeling others with personality traits, you can use that energy to uncover differences in opinion, understandings, and perspectives. This approach is more productive and conducive to creating mutual understanding. When uncovering frames, expect to hear the following types of phrases frequently, "Oh really, I did not know that! ... What I saw led me to believe something different" or "Thank you for sharing that, it helps me to understand your strong reaction to this...I did not realize." It has been our experience that consistent use of this approach can, and does transform relationships.

*"Don't Make Assumptions. Find the courage to ask questions and to express what you really want. Communicate with others as clearly as you can to avoid misunderstandings, sadness and drama. With just this one agreement, you can completely transform your life." —**Don Miguel Ruiz***

In our Simulation Program at MacEwan University, we hang large process posters and have printed pocket cards for faculty and students that provide an immediate visual reminder of the process we have adopted for effective communication. Harmful team experiences can be mitigated in many ways. One way is to develop a *zero tolerance* policy to address abusive behaviors, discrimination, and bullying. Other more proactive approaches include staff and team education; modeling professionalism; adopting a team communication process that focus on high performance team indicators; using communication tools like newsletters, email, posters and media monitors; conveying messages of team respect and valuing; building inclusive environments where all have a say in decision-making; and by creating opportunities to foster and reward excellence in teams (Adams, 2015; Clark, 2013).

Organizations can also undertake measures to minimize conflict including the use of regular climate surveys.

The use of quality indicators will contribute to a collective understanding of policy and processes. Climate surveys are also great tools for simulation teams for lack of becoming entrenched in daily practices and mindsets. Modern organizations make an explicit commitment to developing and mentoring transformational leaders with the skills they need to meet and resolve conflict (RNAO, 2012). Ultimately, these changes will fail to take root and unless social transformation involves an integrated approach to organizational cultural change to build capacity, inform and empower individuals and groups, promote relational community building, and institute lasting culture change. Without a change leadership and change management process, many such organizational initiatives do not last.

When Reconciliation Serves Us Better Than Conflict Management

Saying "I am sorry" is only a start. It is however, a good start. Over the past few years, a Truth and Reconciliation Commission (TRC) took place in Canada (1 of 74 TRCs that have taken place throughout the world). Canada's TRC sought to unearth the silenced truths about the violence, extraordinary abuses, genocide, and structural and social injustice that stemmed from Canada's hundred-year history of Indian Residential Schools (Truth and Reconciliation Committee of Canada, TRC, 2015). We offer Simulation Champions a short account of the lessons that we as non-Aboriginal Canadians have gleaned from participating in the TRC as it unfolded across our country.

Sadly, it is through human suffering that the need for healing and reconciliation arises and team members are certainly not immune to hurt and damage. **Conflict management** approaches aim to achieve good outcomes for both parties through five common approaches or strategies: competition, avoidance, accommodation, compromise and collaboration (Blake & Mouton, 1985). Unlike conflict management, **reconciliation** attends to the lived experiences of *the other* instead of on both parties. We contend that the other-centric leader, one that leads by giving voice to others, can effectively employ TRC principles toward reconciliation and healing in teams.

The TRC principles elucidate reconciliation as a multistage process. Reconciliation centers around an acknowledgment and acceptance of the past and a dedication to renewed peaceful coexistence. It is a delicate and intricate process that aims to consolidate peace. Reconciliatory approaches view healing as a nonlinear, ongoing, and sometimes messy process. Reconciliation manifests in other-centric practices that honor human dignity: as such, it gives voice and listens carefully, very carefully. It seeks to uncover the full spectrum of the truth from the injured person's perspective because it knows that healing requires more than a heartfelt apology. Healing from deep wounds involves a long-term commitment to changing attitudes. It also moves forward with a plan to heal through a collective perseverance toward meaningful change.

We can tell you from our painful team experiences that we believe there comes a time when reconciliation trumps conflict management as a way to mend broken fences. It is not as simple as wiping the page clean and starting over. To extend the olive branch requires moral courage, but more so humility to admit one's failings. We do not believe that well-meaning persons wake up each day with the aim of coming to work to hurt each other. However unintended, conflict and subsequent woundedness does happen, and for the high-performance team, healing is the catalyst for growth and transcendence.

Team Spirit: Fostering Mutuality, Trust, and Friendship in Teams

"We are greater than the sum of our parts: I am because you are", Ubuntu.

This South African philosophy places an emphasis on our common humanity, interconnectedness, and interdependence. Simply stated, Arch Bishop Desmond Tutu says of Ubuntu, "I am, because you are" (Tutu Foundation, 2015). Teams that adopt the spirit and underlying principles of Ubuntu commit to the precept of interdependence and to respecting, supporting, and upholding each other, because in doing so, they also do onto themselves.

Teams, as opposed to groups, develop strong cohesion through acts of mutual respect, accountability, support, trust, and friendship. These experiences, in turn, build team resilience. There is nothing that compares to working alongside someone you trust, respect, and can count on through thick and thin. Therein lies the beauty of friendship. We are both very grateful to have developed the best of friendships in our nursing and simulation teams.

Simulation High-Performance Team Assessment

The *High-Performance Simulation Team Discussion Tool* (Toolkit 10-3) is a series of questions that will guide your team through organizational and team assessment. Assemble the team and use these questions to engage members in a thought-filled discussion. Determine a method that works for your team to compile and document the team's collective results. If

you wish to gather anonymous feedback, do so by having individuals provide answers online or have manual responses independently collated. HPTs, however, would welcome the opportunity for open discussion and debate. The discussion questions are divided into four main categories according to Dyer et al.'s Four Cs. Your team will need to consider: context, composition, competencies, and the change management practices of the simulation team. The questions also draw from critical inquiry for teams from Rampersad and El-Homsi's (2007) Total Performance Scorecard. Take the time to flush out each area and provide written rationale for the results. Once completed, examine and analyze the results as a team to ascertain where you are situated overall. Identify strengths and areas of concern. Simulation team responses can serve as a catalyst for team growth.

Summary

We hope that the content and tools provided in this chapter serve to ground your practice in team theory, stimulate thought, and inspire you as a leader and team member to be the best you can be. Simulation Champions need to be effective leaders, followers, and managers but even more importantly, effective team

---

Box 10-3   Turning to One Another

There is no power greater than a community discovering what it cares about.
Ask, "What's possible?" not "What's wrong?" Keep asking.
Notice what you care about.
Assume that many others share your dreams.
Be brave enough to start a conversation that matters.
Talk to people you know.
Talk to people you don't know.
Talk to people you never talk to.
Be intrigued by the differences you hear.
Expect to be surprised.
Treasure curiosity more than certainty.
Invite everybody who cares to work on what's possible.
Acknowledge that everyone is an expert about something.
Know that creative solutions come from new connections.
Remember, you don't fear people whose story you know.
Real listening always brings people closer together.
Trust that meaningful conversation can change your world.
Rely on human goodness. Stay together.

From Wheatley, M. (2009). *Turning to one another.* San Francisco, CA: Berrett-Koehler Publishers, Inc.

members. This chapter has focused on what it takes to become and sustain a high-performance team. We have also elucidated the knowledge, skills, and attitudes that are required to lead teams to higher performance. It takes a firm commitment from all members of the team to building and sustaining a culture of team excellence. Our journey on the road to team excellence has been filled with opportunities for individual and team growth, transformation, and transcendence. We wish for you and your simulation delivery team the profound sense of accomplishment and pride that can only come when a team performs at the top of its game. Team leading and learning brings with it a deep inner knowledge of self and others; a sense of trust, joy, friendship, humility, mutuality, courage, and resilience. We leave you with a poem from Margaret Wheatley that speaks to the inception of teams. We dedicate this chapter to the amazing simulation and healthcare teams that courageously commit to to being difference makers in the world, together! (Box 10-3)

Toolkit Resources

Toolkit 10-1: Levels of Cross-Functionality in Simulation Teams

This document can serve as a template for creating your own cross-functional team levels. This document classifies different levels of simulation delivery relative the to number of team members and functions needed. Is it going to be a level one, two, three, or four day?

Toolkit 10-2: Collaborative Online Team Communication Tool

This tool was developed to help very busy teams communicate using Cloud-based technologies and tools.

Toolkit 10-3: High-Performance Simulation Team Discussion Tool

Take the time to assess your HPT potential. Use team findings to develop a plan to attain HPT status on your simulation team.

11 Managing Simulation Program Operations and Human Capital

Colette Foisy-Doll

Key Terms

Management, Manager, Leadership, Leader, Follower, Administration, Project Management, Strategic Plan, Organizational Chart, Policy, Procedure, Event Flow, SOAR, SWOT, Total Quality Improvement, Return on Investment, Return on Expectations, General Operations, Human Capital Management, Technical Operations, Program Evaluation, Programmatic Assessment, Operating Budget, Metrics, Integrated Data Management, Reports, Inventory Management, Hardware, Software, Simulation Delivery Team, Fiction Contract

Guiding Questions

1 What makes leadership and administration different from management? Does the Simulation Program Manager's role encompass all three? Can you describe your managerial style?

2 What is project management (PM) and how can PM approaches be helpful in Simulation Program operations?

3 What is a Simulation Program and what is involved in managing one?

4 Are you aware of current standards and guidelines that serve as benchmarks for measuring progress and outcomes in a Simulation Program?

5 Would you know where to begin if asked to operationalize a Simulation Program? What processes and tools will you need to do the job well?

6 How do you go about developing policies and procedures to support the smooth functioning of your Simulation Program?

7 What is important to measure in Simulation Programs, and which metrics should you use?

Introduction

Often, a Simulation Program (i.e., Program with a capital "P"—noun) unfolds within a dedicated physical space

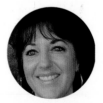

**Colette Foisy-Doll,
MSN, RN, CHSE**

called a Simulation Center, although Simulation Programs also unfold within shared spaces as part of a consortium, as mobile units traveling from place to place, in actual practice settings, and even in virtual worlds. Whatever the context, the basic tenets of management apply, and therefore, this chapter focuses on the stuff it takes to operationalize the "Simulation Program." The simulation manager role, title, and scope of work will vary from place to place depending on organizational structure, program goals, workload distribution, and funding. For this chapter, the *simulation manager* refers to the person charged with the task of operationalizing a Simulation Program, as opposed to a person responsible for the educational or organizational leadership aspects of Simulation Programs.

It is true, however, that for smaller Programs, one person might take on all of these functions, and as such, the manager role frequently encompasses other roles.

In the past, those charged with managing the first Simulation Programs used the *trial by fire* approach because Simulation Programs as we know them today did not exist. In the beginning, pioneer managers engaged in active experimentation to figure out the best ways to operationalize Programs. They also shared ideas by connecting with others from within the simulation practice community. Today, there are various titles assigned to the person with the primary authority and responsibility of running the Simulation Program, including Program Director, Business Manager, Simulation Center Manager, Simulation Program Coordinator, or Simulation Program Director. The simulation community now has many options for training, support, and education that help prepare people for educator roles, but little exists in the way of managerial training for simulation. There is discussion that the Society for Simulation in Healthcare (SSH) creating a credentialing process for the simulation leader/manager; however, to date, this has not yet come to pass. At the 2016 INACSL Annual Conference in Grapevine, Texas, the board of directors announced that a new standard for Simulation Program Operations is in development.

This chapter guides the new simulation manager through a step-by-step approach to operationalizing Simulation Programs. The content is divided into six main sections: (1) The Simulation Program, (2) Administration, Leadership, and Management, (3) Stakeholders and Committees, (4) Educational Programming, (5) General Operations, and (6) Challenges and Opportunities. I provide a host of valuable online resources in the Simulation Champions online Toolkit, including a series of simulation manager guidebooks to help new managers organize, hire talent, develop a team, design and deploy simulation learning, and evaluate various facets of a Simulation Program. Toolkit items are divided into numbered folders and then listed by item (i.e., Folder 1: Item 11.1). Before you begin reading this chapter, retrieve *The Simulation Program Manager's Getting Started Checklist* (Folder 7: 11.7.4) and the *Policy and Procedures Master Categories List* (Folder 4: 11.4.9). Together, these resources will provide structure to frame the content featured in this chapter. A discussion of simulation modalities and typologies is located in Chapters 6 and 7 and therefore, is not included in this chapter.

The Simulation Program

The Simulation Program: What Is It?

The term *Simulation Program* means different things to different people and will vary with context. The "Simulation Program," as per SSH Accreditation, is defined as "an organization or group with dedicated resources (personnel and equipment) whose mission is specifically targeted toward improving patient safety and outcomes through assessment, research, advocacy, and education using simulation technologies and methodologies" (SSH Accreditation Process, 2014, p. 5). The Simulation Program includes "all planned and coordinated healthcare simulation activities in assessment, research, teaching/education, or systems integration that is administered by an organization with dedicated resources for the administration and delivery of such healthcare simulation activities" (SSH, 2014, p. 1). Sadly, and yet all too often, simulators are purchased before there is a sound plan and vision for the Simulation Program (Seropian, Brown, Gavilanes, & Driggers, 2004). Therefore, this chapter aims to help you understand the other aspects of Simulation Program planning and development that should precede simulator purchases. In keeping with the SSH definition of a Simulation Program—I will refer to it here to, as either the "Program" or the "Simulation Program." For a *comprehensive mind map* of the most common aspects of managing Simulation Programs, follow this link (https://www.mindmeister.com/768029206/simulation-program-management).

Naming Your Simulation Program

All Simulation Programs need a name and names are important. The name can provide insight into a Program's identity, purpose, and vision. For example, the name "Centre for Clinical Excellence and Innovation" tells us something about the Program. This statement holds true regardless of whether the Program is delivered from within a purpose-built facility, a mobile unit, or the virtual world. Things to consider in selecting a name are (1) your purpose and the geographic location; (2) the programs served; (3) the population(s) served; (4) your mission, vision, and value statements; (5) donor(s); (6) corporate sponsors (in part or in whole); and (7) the branch of the organization of which you are a part. To garner buy-in from administrators, faculty, and learners—make naming (and logo creation) a fun competition. Alternately, conduct an Internet search to explore the names of other Programs. Be sure that the team is satisfied with the chosen name, as you will likely have it for a long time. Remember, names have associated costs—branding, logos, print material, business cards, signage, and promotional materials such as banners and signage all add up. Also, consider how to protect the name and communicate to staff and others how to use it appropriately within and outside the institution. For example, set a policy to stamp all Program PowerPoint presentations with your logo and Program name. Presentation content can also undergo a review process for quality control. This approach serves to protect and uphold a Program's good name and reputation.

The Program Description—Letting Others Know Who You Are

The Simulation Program description is unique to your Program. Start by giving a brief historical account of how the Program came to be and the populations that it serves. Include descriptions of key relationships to stakeholders within the institution, including photos, images, and a description of simulation innovations. Most important is to tell others about the Program's WHY—the reason it exists. For a sample Program description, see the *Guidebook for Writing a Simulation Program Manual* (Folder 1: 11.1.1).

Benchmarks for Simulation Programs

Unlike 10 years ago, we now have benchmarks from simulation accreditation standards, credentialing criteria, simulation guidelines, position statements, frameworks, theories, and in some cases, discipline-specific regulatory standards. These key documents provide direction to the new Simulation Program Manager for Program development. A brief summary of key benchmarking documents is listed in Table 11.1.

Other key resources include NLN recommendations for the use of simulation in high-stakes assessment projects (Rizzolo, Kardong-Edgren, Oermann, & Jeffries, 2015) and the NLN Vision Series document titled *Debriefing Across the Curriculum* (2015), written and published in conjunction with INACSL. Collectively, these resources provide key points of reference for evaluating overall Program performance. Conduct an environmental scan to identify appropriate benchmarks in your milieu. These can include, but are not limited to, local/regional/national/international regulatory standards, accreditation standards, and educational standards. With benchmarks in hand, articulate your Program goals, and then define strategic actions and implementation timelines for achieving those goals. Remember that actionable and measurable plans are critical for tracking and analysis of Program outcomes.

A Word on Policy and Procedures

Establishing **policy** means to articulate a set of principles, rules, and guidelines adopted by the Simulation Program to bring plans to life. Policies define what should happen within a Program's operational, educational, and technical initiatives. **Procedures** are the processes that are needed to comply with a given policy. For example, if the Program sets a goal to have all educators attain SSH Certified Simulation Healthcare Educator (CHSE), then the Program Manager might create a policy mandating that all newly hired simulation educators in your Program must achieve the CHSE certification requirements within 2 years of hiring. The procedures will list the specific steps they will need to follow to comply with this policy. Typically, workplace rules and practices are collated into one Simulation Program Policy and Procedure (P&P) Manual, made available in either hard or soft copy format. Conducting an Internet search for examples of Simulation Program P&P Manuals is a great strategy. There are many good examples available online. Table 11.2 provides a list of high-level Policy and Procedure categories. Also, access the *Guidebook for Writing a Simulation Program Manual* (Folder 1: 11.1.1) for a comprehensive 300+ item list for consideration in P&P development. Use this resource to begin building your own P&P Manual.

Accreditation and Affiliations

The Society for Simulation (SSH) in Healthcare Accreditation Standards (SSH, 2016c), *Core Standards* document, identifies the major operational standards expected in the operationalizing of all Simulation Programs. To achieve SSH Accreditation, all Programs must attain the Core Standards, along with at least one of four additional standards (see the core standards list below). See Chapter 4 for a complete list of all the Accreditation Standards, or go to the website at (http://www.ssih.org/Accreditation/Full-Accreditation).

Other Simulation Program accrediting bodies do exist and all address the following common elements, "curriculum, instructor/personnel qualifications, equipment and technology, and organization and supporting infrastructure"—where some bodies have specific areas of focus (Fernandez et al., 2010, p. 1094). In addition to the SSH Accreditation Program, other known simulation accreditation programs include the following:

1. American College of Surgeons Accredited Education Institutes (ACS-AEI, 2015)
2. American Society of Anesthesiologists (ASA) Simulation (endorsement)
3. Royal College of Physicians and Surgeons of Canada (2016)
4. The Society in Europe for Simulation Applied to Medicine (SESAM) (2016).

SSH Accreditation (2016a) Core Standards feature seven core functional and operational elements with criterion subsets for each, as follows:

1. **Mission & Governance**

The Program has a clear publically stated mission and/or vision statement, that

a. Specifically addresses the intent and functions of the Program
b. Has an appropriate organizational structure

Table 11.1 Summary of Program Benchmarking Resources

NLN Jeffries Simulation Framework—Now Simulation Theory (Jeffries, 2007b, 2015)	12 Features and Best Practices (2010) for SBME (McGaghie, Issenberg, Petrusa, and Scalese)	INACSL Standards of Best Practice: Simulation^SM (2016, December) (Earlier versions 2011, 2013, 2015)	Simbase Critical Success Factors for Simulation Program Success (Garcia & Guisado, 2013)	Eight Critical Success Factors in Creating and Implementing a Successful Simulation Program (Lazzara, Benishek, Dietz, Salas, & Adriansen, 2014)	SSH Accreditation Standards (SSH, 2016d) (Earlier versions, 2012, 2014). SSH Credentialing Program, (2012–2016)	NCSBN Simulation Guidelines for Prelicensure Nursing Programs (Alexander et al., 2015)	Reporting guidelines for healthcare simulation research: extensions to the CONSORT and STROBE statements (Cheng et al., 2016a)
• Simulation unfolds in context • Background and Design impact the experience • Best Education Practices ground the experience • Environment of Trust, Experiential, Interactive, Collaborative Learner-Centered • Dynamic Interaction between facilitator and participant • Desired output is transformational change of systems, better outcomes for patients, and for participants.	• Feedback • Deliberate practice • Curriculum integration • Outcome measurement • Simulation fidelity • Skill acquisition and maintenance • Mastery learning • Transfer to practice • Team training • High-stakes testing • Instructor training • Educational and professional context	• Professional Integrity • Simulation Design • Outcomes and Objectives • Facilitation • Participant Evaluation • Debriefing • Sim-IPE • Glossary	• Orientation towards healthcare requirements • Integration into the curriculum • Available resources • Design of the training activity • Fidelity in simulation • Team-based learning • Feedback • Deliberate practices • Role of the instructor and training roles • Skills acquisition and retention • Translation to practice • Measurement of results • Organizational and educational context	• Science—maximize your training potential • Staff—recruit champions to promote simulation • Supplies—obtain resources from local facilities and external organizations, agencies, and institutions • Space—think beyond your own walls • Support—network • Systems—match fidelity requirements to training needs and ensure that technological infrastructure is in place • Success—evaluate and share success stories throughout the organization • Sustainability—focus on maintenance not just development	• Core Standards and Measurement Criteria • Teaching/ Education Standards and Measurement Criteria • Assessment Standards and Measurement Criteria • Research Standards and Measurement Criteria • Systems Integration Standards and Measurement Criteria	• Commitment on the part of the school for the simulation program • Program has appropriate facilities for conducting simulation • Educational and technological resources and equipment to meet the intended objectives (Program Preparation Checklist) • Lead faculty and sim lab personnel qualified to conduct simulation (Faculty Preparation Checklist)	• Participant Orientation to the simulator and the environment • Simulator—make, model, functionality • Simulation Environment—location, equipment, external stimuli • Simulation Event—event description, learning objectives, group vs. individual practice, use of adjuncts, facilitator/operator characteristics, pilot testing, actors, SPs, SiPs, confederates • Instructional Design—duration, timing, frequency, repetitions, clinical variation, standards/assessment, adaptability of intervention, range of difficulty, non-simulation interventions, integration • Feedback and/or debriefing—source, duration, facilitator presence and characteristics, content, structure/method, timing, video, scripting

Table 11.2	Simulation Program Policies and Procedures Condensed List
Simulation Program Policies and Procedures List 2017 (See Online Toolkit in Folder 4, Item 11.4.9 for the expanded list)	
The Simulation Program	● General Information ● Program Foundations: Establishing Authority and Transparency
Administration, Leadership, and Management	● Strategy Plan and Directions ● Talent Acquisition and Development ● Fiscal Management ● Sustainability
Personnel and Stakeholders	● Stakeholders: Internal and External ● Simulation Program Personnel: Administration, Educators, and Support Staff ● Human Capital Management ● Simulation Educator Policy ● Course Participant Policy
Educational Operations and Research	● Course Offerings ● Simulation Design Standards ● Remediation ● Research
General Operations (Daily)	● Scheduling ● Security and Safety ● Customer Relations ● General Communications ● Equipment and Supplies ● Tours of the Simulation Center ● Nonparticipant Observers ● Marketing and Media ● Website Presence
Technical Operations	● IT/AV Integrated Systems Management ● Video Recording Management

Adapted from Seropian, M., Driggers, B., & Gavilanes, J. (2013). Centre development and practical considerations. In A. Levine, S. DeMaria Jr., A. D. Schwartz, & A. J. Sim (Eds.). *The comprehensive textbook of simulation in healthcare.* New York, NY: Springer, with permission.

c. Has a process for strategic review and approval of Program activities
d. Has a written plan designed to accomplish the mission and/or vision of the Program

2. **Program Management**
   a. Adequate fiscal resources to support its mission and/or vision
   b. Day-to-day oversight of simulation activities
   c. Ability to prioritize resources as needed
   d. Written policies and procedures to assure Program quality

3. **Resource Management**
   a. Ability to obtain, maintain, and support simulation equipment and relevant technologies
   b. Appropriate physical space for simulation activities
   c. Provides an adequate number and variety of simulation activities to support vision and/or mission of the Program

4. **Human Resources**
   a. The Program is directed by a qualified individual with appropriate authority and time directs the Program.
   b. Adequate Program staff to support the mission/vision of the Program.
   c. Has a process in place to orient, support, and evaluate Program staff.

5. **Program Improvement**
   a. Continually improves the operations of the Program through the use of a quality management system.
   b. Processes in place to identify and address concerns and complaints.

6. **Integrity**
   a. Committed to ethical standards

7. **Expanding the Field**
   a. Have activities that extend beyond the Program, contributing to the body of knowledge in the simulation community (pp. 2–5).

Logistical Information

It is important to communicate key information to patrons about the facility location and how to contact or find it. Include the following on your Program's website, Facebook page, or LinkedIn site:

● *Geographical location:* many sites embed Google Maps into their website or attach downloadable PDFs.
● *Parking:* cost, location, and instructions on how to find the facility from the parking location, availability of parking passes, after-hours access, and accessibility entrances
● *Hours of operation:* statement of business hours (weekday, weekend, and closure times on statutory days or vacation periods); for learners accessing the Center after hours, you will need to create a system for entry with permission (e.g., have security officer open doors)
● *General contact information:* general office (telephone and email address)
● *Facility information:* a list of room types, including room names and numbers, quantities of each room, room capacity, room equipment lists, and simulation or technological services available (include a room diagram or map).

Program Foundations: Establishing Authority and Transparency

High-Level Features of the Simulation Program

Programs must demonstrate established hierarchy, structures, roles, and processes, as well as have people in place to get things done. For smooth operations, the Program manager must also develop policy and procedures, and then communicate and enact them. The next section looks more closely at the dimensions of the Program.

Governance, Oversight, and Organizational Structure

Governance in educational institutions and hospitals refers to the internal structures used to uphold autonomy and how these structures are organized and managed. In simple terms, governance speaks to the way that rules, norms, and actions are established, implemented, sustained, and for which organizations are ultimately held accountable (Hufty, 2011). Governance models vary. *Traditional governance models* are hierarchical in nature because they tend to utilize a centralized top-down authority and decision-making model. In contrast, a *shared governance model* decentralizes decision-making authority to people throughout an organization. Reporting structures, positions, and lines and levels of authority will all stem from the chosen governance model. Simulation Program governance is crucial to positive outcomes because it directly impacts the degree of influence that simulation leaders, managers, and personnel have in organizational and programmatic decision-making. The body that provides oversight, and to which a Simulation Program is held accountable, is termed the governing body. In some cases, oversight will be carried out by a hospital's Board of Directors, and for educational institutions, a Dean's office, or other designated groups. Governance and reporting structures are communicated through organizational charts. The *Guidebook for Writing a Simulation Program Manual* located in the online Toolkit provides you with three examples of organizational charts depicting governance structures in small, medium, and large Simulation Programs (see Folder 1: 11.1). Today, good governance entails looking beyond a singular focus to include regional, national, and transglobal goals and entails adopting a mindset of global citizenship and stewardship. Simulation Programs professionals from around the globe are working together across borders to advance the simulation agenda.

Simulation Terminology

Efforts to create a universal taxonomy in simulation are under way, but there continues to be variation in the terminology used in simulation in healthcare. To determine the terms your Simulation Program will adopt, refer the SSH Healthcare Simulation Dictionary (Lopreiato et al., 2016), the INACSL Standards of Best Practice Simulation^SM (INACSL Standards Committee, 2016, Glossary). and textbook simulation glossaries. The adoption of standard terminology within and across programs facilitates better communication for shared learning and research.

Philosophical and Theoretical Underpinnings

Program philosophy can be likened to the roots of a tree: roots provide stability and nourishment while grounding the entire system. Therefore, articulating philosophy helps your personnel and others to understand what grounds the Program. Optimally, organizational philosophy should inform and be enmeshed with a Simulation Program's mission, vision, and values statements. This step is important because not all organizations hold the same beliefs, think the same way, or act alike.

A Simulation Program's philosophy statement makes explicit core beliefs and professional values as they relate to simulation education, educators, learners, patients, and partners. A philosophy statement gives meaning and direction to all operational and educational practices and processes within a given program (Gaberson & Oermann, 2010). Moreover, the Program philosophy is what drives educational curricula, preferred teaching methodologies, debriefing approaches, and even evaluation. Simulation-based learning is grounded in varied philosophical perspectives, theories, and frameworks. Himes and Schulenberg (2013) explain how philosophy and theory are different, yet perpetually linked. "Philosophy influences how one sees the world [or worldview], theory shapes how one intentionally interacts with that world" (para. 7). For nursing programs, nursing philosophy and theory can form the basis for simulation curriculum development providing the advantage of both a nursing theoretical and philosophical basis for simulation activities (Gaberson & Oermann). However, given that simulation is grounded in many philosophical and theoretical perspectives, a blended approach is often adopted. When examining and adopting theories, seek to understand related frameworks, concepts, constructs, and assumptions, and then to determine the value proposition a given theory brings to your Simulation Program's curriculum. Engage in critical examination of theories and be open to the limitations, biases, prejudices, and weaknesses found within. (For more, see Chapter 16.)

Healthcare Pillars

It is important to articulate core healthcare–related beliefs and goals, or the healthcare pillars of the Program. Healthcare pillars should link to vision, mission, or core value statements. List all affiliations the Program has with the healthcare entities that are tied to those pillars (i.e., simulation associations, patient safety organizations, human factors groups, and interprofessional team training, and so on).

Developing a Vision Statement

A vision statement is a compelling depiction of the institution/organization's future—it communicates what you dream of someday becoming. The vision articulates a visionary plan, speaking to what you aim to become 5 to 10 years from today. This statement helps others to understand what you believe is possible. Dream, but also be realistic. Be clear, visible, audacious, and descriptive about WHERE your Program is heading. Ultimately, you want to provide a vivid idealized description of an outcome that inspires and energizes your team and others. Upon hearing your vision, your patrons should be able to quickly develop a vivid mental picture of your Program's aspirations. Vision statements can be short or long depending on the extent of your goals. The visionary message should mesh well with your mission statement (http://www.samples-help.org.uk/mission-statements/vision-statements.htm). A step-by-step guide to writing vision, mission, and values statements is available in *A Guidebook to Strategic Planning* (Folder 1: 11.2).

Developing a Mission Statement

Whether the Program is a stand-alone entity, or as part of a consortium or partnership, there are core Program functions that must be managed. SSH (2014) states that there must be "a clear publically stated mission that specifically addresses the intent and functions of the Simulation Program" (p. 3). The mission statement is a sentence or short paragraph written by key stakeholders that reflects its core purpose, identity, values, and principle aims. It explains WHY you exist, as opposed to WHERE you are going (vision statement). Sometimes external stakeholders will have input as part of a strategic planning process. Mission statements focus on the present, offering a snapshot of today. In a nutshell, a mission statement describes what the organization does, how they do it, why they do it, and those who are served by the organization, but not where they are headed (Alton, 2016). From the Program's mission statement will flow overall goals and objectives within a strategic plan. A mission statement should align with, and draw upon other institutional, system, campus, college, or university programs' mission statements. Ultimately, it must clearly convey relevant information to internal stakeholders (i.e., students/faculty) as well as to external stakeholders (community partners, clinical affiliations, and others). Lastly, when crafting the mission statement, aim to feature unique aspects of the Program(s) (i.e., field of study, undergraduate nursing, medicine, health faculty, or other), or any particular catchphrase or signature piece that contributes to making the statement a memorable one. Use *A Guidebook to Strategic Planning*

(Folder 1: 11.2) to help you write your vision, mission, and core values statements.

Developing a Core Values Statement

Develop a core values statement based on core institutional values if documented. With that as a starting point, explore how well current or planned simulation endeavors reflect and enmesh with these values. As previously noted, the online workbook (Folder 1: 11.2), guides you through a process that helps you to identify your core values.

Establishing Simulation Program Excellence

"What gets measured, gets improved" Peter F. Drucker (2006)

In simulation, measuring and analyzing Program effectiveness, efficiency, and quality are imperative. Decision-makers and policy-makers at program, organizational, and systems levels, such as a board of governors, steering committees, executive teams, management teams, and accreditation and regulatory bodies, are responsible for a Program's impact and overall success. As competition for resources in organizations increases, quality assessment and quality improvement tools are needed to demonstrate accountability and responsibility in the allocation and use of valuable resources. To accomplish this, we need a variety of measures to assess the many facets that make up a Simulation Program. These specific measures are called metrics.

One of the things I had to learn, and continue to learn as a Simulation Program Director, was business-speak. It was important for me to understand the language of the executive office suite and to be able to express my needs in a language that would be understood. As I had been a nurse educator for my entire career, terms like metrics, value proposition, return on investment, return on expectations, and scorecards and dashboards were foreign to me. I offer you the basics to get you started.

Metrics

Metrics are the "standards of measurement by which efficiency, performance, progress, or quality of a plan, process, or product can be assessed" (Businessdictionary.com, 2016). Trying to grow and improve a Simulation Program without metrics is like shooting blindfolded in the dark. Metrics quantify Program performance and are not just for evaluation of learner performance. Intentional targeted evaluation of key aspects of Simulation Programs is critical to positive outcomes. Today managers can run the risk of *drowning in data and still be staved for information*. So remember, metrics are only valuable when paired with data analysis to inform better decisions. Therefore, be strategic and intentional in metrics selection and don't take on more data processing than you can handle.

Simulation Programs can benefit from the use of metrics in any number of ways, such as to weigh *fiscal performance* (e.g., budgeting, profit, revenue, expenses, cash flow, productivity); track overall *facility and equipment* usage (numbers of users, course registrations, room booking stats, simulation typology use, or simulation modality use); track *research activity*, impact, and outcomes (number of projects funded, funding sources, findings); feature the sim team's *scholarly projects or awards* (journal articles, conference presentations, feature events, etc.); monitor *social media* traffic (the number of Twitter, Facebook, LinkedIn hits and comments); assess *website performance* (Google Analytics is a freemium Google product that tracks and analyzes traffic); and monitor *email performance* and usage (programs like Constant Contact and MailChimp are examples of email systems that have report generating). Metrics and associated analytics can also be used to assess the need for improvements; measure customer satisfaction; track updates to educational offerings; track simulation team development and outcomes; assess marketing and advertising effectiveness; or track technology failure rates, including simulators and other medical equipment.

Tools and Instruments

Program metrics are accompanied by a variety of tools (or instruments) for measurement. Tools with established reliability and validity are especially helpful in decision-making in that they generate trustworthy statistical information. Remember that the ultimate test of tool validity is the consequences that result from using it. If a tool is wrongly applied, the ensuing results and conclusions are also flawed. Today, you can find tools that will help you measure and track any measurable process: employee performance, operational or educational assessment, simulation delivery modality or simulation typology usage, equipment performance and maintenance, customer satisfaction, quality improvement, and patient safety initiatives like hand-washing practices. Be smart and streamline processes so as to carry out more than one function. For example, a well-designed centralized scheduling system can do double duty and collect data about non-scheduling specific items.

All tools contain key performance indicators (KPIs): the performance criteria by which you will measure different aspects of performance.

When choosing tools for Simulation Program metrics, ask yourself the following questions:

- Is the tool you selected being used for its intended purpose?
- Does the tool measure what is important to measure, and not too much?
- Does the tool possess a reasonable level of complexity to give you meaningful measures?
- Does the tool reflect organizational vision and strategy?
- Does the tool align well with existing benchmarks and standards?
- Does the tool clearly itemize a list of key drivers for success (KPIs)?
- Is the workload associated with the use of the tool reasonable and manageable?
- Do you have a person on staff to which data collection, analysis, and reporting are delegated?

Data Collection and Data Analysis

Today, we live in a data-rich world and there is an entire industry with a long line up of the goods and services devoted to data collection and analysis. The number and type of products can be overwhelming. So start small and *measure only what is important.* Organizations also use metrics to tie critical success factors back to organizational strategy, values, and goals. To achieve a sustained level of quality in priority areas, you must tie results back to what you set out to achieve in the first place. Metrics, therefore, should always be linked to a Program's vision, mission, and value statements and strategic plan indicators and targets. Knowing this in advance helps you be clear on what you need to measure. Select and test specific tools for measurement, and then build from there.

Program Evaluation Versus Programmatic Assessment For Learning

Program evaluation involves "a process used to create information for planning, designing, implementing and assessing the results of our efforts to address and solve problems" (McDavid, Huse & Hawthorn, 2013, p. 3). Program evaluation is also known as the process of making a judgement as to the overall value and worth of a program (or components thereof) based on the assessment information gathered (Oermann, 2016). The first step in program evaluation involves (1) knowing your the Simulation Program's WHY; followed by (2) defining strategy and related objectives; (3) tool selection and data collection; (4) data analysis, (5) evaluation, (6) mapping, and tracking; and (7) reporting and disseminating findings. Figure 11.1 depicts a sample process cascade for Program evaluation. Adamson and Prion (2015) suggest that those engaged in Program evaluation for simulation consider the guiding questions listed in Box 11-2.

Distinct from program evaluation is ***programmatic assessment***, an integral approach to the design of an assessment program with the intent to optimize its learning function, its decision-making function and its curriculum quality-assurance function (Van Der Vleuten, Schuwirth, Driessen, Govaerts, & Heeneman, 2015, p. 641,

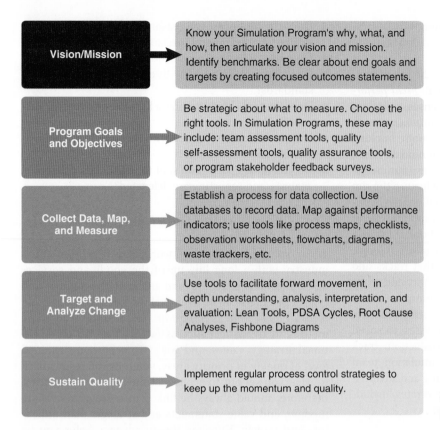

Figure 11.1 Process Cascade for Simulation Program Evaluation.

see Box 11-1). Although many apply the basic tenets of programmatic assessment to Program evaluation, in healthcare education, programmatic assessment is applied to learning and involves developing, deploying, tracking, and evaluating discrete learning assessments across an entire program, where continuous monitoring and measurement of learner progress is compared to pre-established desired learning outcomes. As such, programmatic assessment in this chapter constitutes one of many components included in overall Program evaluation and refers a program of assessment for learning and related outcomes measurement. By its very nature, assessment is evaluation because ultimately, teachers make judgements about performance as a result of discrete assessment moments or as part of a cumulative total of discrete assessments. In the end, all assessments (both formative and summative) should be linked to global performance evaluation and to program outcomes. Educators teaching in Simulation Programs, therefore, require literacy and fluency in both programmatic assessment and program evaluation.

Measuring Value in Simulation Programs

Simulation is an expensive endeavor that requires a significant investment in resources. Global annual expenditures for healthcare provider training are now in the billions of dollars (Walsh, Reeves, & Maloney, 2014). Funding for Simulation Programs generally resides with the public purse and, for some, from private stakeholder donations, while for others, by using a business model to generate revenue (Haines, Kent, & Keating, 2014; Maloney & Haines, 2016; Walsh et al., 2014). More often, Simulation Programs are coming together to share the costs. Bar-on, Yucha, and Kinsley (2013) describe how three entities collaborated to

---

Box 11-1   12 Tips for Programmatic Assessment

1. Develop a master plan for assessment
2. Develop examination regulations that promote feedback orientation
3. Adopt a robust system for collecting information
4. Assure that every low-stakes assessment provides meaningful feedback for learning
5. Provide mentoring to learners
6. Ensure trustworthy decision-making
7. Organize intermediate decision-making assessments
8. Encourage and facilitate personalized remediation
9. Monitor and evaluate the learning effect of the programme and adapt
10. Use the assessment process information for curriculum evaluation
11. Promote continuous interaction between the stakeholders, and
12. Develop a strategy for implementation.

(Van Der Vleuten et al., 2015, p. 641–646).

Box 11-2   **Guiding Questions for Simulation Program Evaluation**

1. What is the need for the program? (i.e., to supplement clinical instruction, provide opportunities to practice)
2. Is the program relevant (i.e., do simulations help students link theory and practice, are they better prepared to provide patient care)?
3. Was the structure/logic of the program appropriate (i.e., does the sequencing of coursework, simulation, and clinical activities make sense)?
4. Was the program implemented as intended (i.e., if there was an implementation plan, was it followed)?
5. Was the program technically efficient (i.e., are resources being used to their full capacity, what resources might improve the efficiency of the simulation laboratory, etc.)?
6. Was the program responsible for the outcomes that actually occurred (i.e., do recent data such as National Council Licensure Examination pass rates or other

metrics reflect outcomes of the simulation program, are there other variables that may account for these outcomes, etc.)?
7. Did the program achieve its intended objectives? What measurements support this?
8. Was the program cost-effective (i.e., in general terms, how did the costs of the simulation program compare with the effects)?
9. Was the program cost beneficial (i.e., in monetary terms, how did the costs of the simulation program compare with the effects)?
10. Was the program adequate (i.e., was the magnitude of the simulation program sufficient, would additional resources enable it to have an even greater impact)?"

(Adamson & Prion, 2015, pp. 505–506).

---

create a successful funding model for sustainability. That said simulation leaders/managers are responsible and accountable to organizations and to the general public for the effective and responsible use of that funding. More than ever, organizations are scrutinizing and weighing the costs and benefits of delivering Simulation Programs versus traditional clinical education models (Haines, Isles, Jones, & Jull, 2011). When asked, "Is simulation profitable?" Or, "What are the costs of simulation?" many find it a struggle to pin down justification for Simulation Programs based on costs alone. Although quantitative measurements like cost are important, we also need to factor in qualitative value and the downstream effects of simulation education. Although these effects are difficult to measure, they nonetheless bring tremendous value that can be expressed as a simulation value proposition (McGaghie, Draycott, Dunn, Lopez, & Stefanidis, 2011).

Value Propositions

Value propositions in Simulation Programs are statements based on the review and analysis of the benefits, costs, as well as, from the overall promise of service you bring to internal and external stakeholder groups. Lanning and Edwards (1988) originally described a value proposition as, "a clear, simple statement of the benefits, both tangible and intangible, that the company will provide, along with the approximate price it will charge each customer segment for those benefits" (Barnes, Blake, & Pinder, 2009, p. 28). McGaghie et al. (2011) state that simulation education has value in that is has "a long and rich research legacy shows that under the right conditions, simulation-based medical education is a powerful intervention to increase medical learner competence" (p. s42). Additionally, the authors note that translational research (T1 to T3) exists to demonstrate improved downstream

results in clinical practice and patient and public health outcomes. However, more T3 type research is needed to understand the downstream impacts of simulation and then to clearly articulate those value propositions (McGaghie et al., 2011).

To date, little exists in the simulation literature specific to Program cost-benefit analyses and value. There are many issues that arise when trying to link simulation education as the upstream cause of downstream patient care outcomes. Haines et al. (2011). underscore the need for more research to create suitable approaches to justify costs versus the educational benefits in the face of demands for sustainability.

Return on Investment

Return on investment (ROI) is a measure that demonstrates investment outcomes within an organization (Rundio, 2016).

A formulaic depiction would be:

$$ROI = \frac{Gains - Investment\ Costs}{Investment\ Costs}$$

When it comes to calculating ROI in Simulation Programs, it is wise to seek the counsel of a financial officer or the person that helps you manage your financial costs. However, ROI through a cost/gains/loss analysis will not necessarily yield those positive fiscal results that the Dean or CEO wants to hear. Seek out help to conduct and understand costs analyses of your Program, and then, work to find strategies so you can at least break even. To enhance the ROI discussion, educate yourself about the real world problems that hospitals and community care contexts experience and know them well (p. 2010). Measure what you can and then tell your story in the boardroom. For example, a decrease in hospital-acquired infection rates in your institution could be linked to simulation training. Or perhaps you can demonstrate that simulation team training resulted in shaving 3 minutes off emergency response times, to result in better patient care with a projected cost savings.

Evaluating *economic efficacy* in healthcare and education involves a "high degree of complexity, uncertainty, negotiation between multiple objectives, and consideration of the varied perspectives of different stakeholders" (Pattillo, Hewett, McCarthy, & Molinari, 2010, p. e188). Maloney and Haines (2016) discuss the importance of *economic evaluation* for Simulation Programs as it "provides a comparison of value...[and looks at] what is it that is being obtained, what do you need to give up to get it, and how does that compare to what you get with the next best alternative" (p. 1). The economic evaluation process for simulation education as described by Maloney and Haines employs four types of *cost analyses*. They are (1) cost minimization analysis, (2) cost-effectiveness analysis, (3) cost utility analysis, and (4) cost–benefit analysis. Choosing the appropriate type of analysis is important when examining cost benefits/effects in Simulation Programs. Maloney and Haines also offer an algorithmic flowchart for cost–benefit and cost-effectiveness analyses (see Fig. 11.2). The authors remind us of the importance of cost and value measures in simulation and how they can "provide information about the viability and

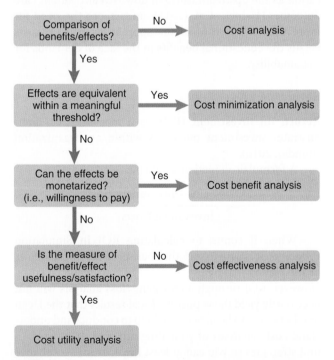

Figure 11.2 Algorithmic Flowchart for Cost/Benefit and Cost/Effectiveness Analyses. (From Maloney, S., & Haines, T. (2016). Issues of cost-benefit and cost-effectiveness for simulation in health professions education. *Advances in Simulation*, 1–6. http://doi.org/10.1186/s41077-016)

sustainability of simulation education, enabling simulation education in healthcare to demonstrate its worth" (p. 1). In educational settings, the primary focus is on creating great learning where this type of outcome is better expressed as a Return on Expectations.

Return on Expectations

Return on expectations (ROE) is believed to be the ultimate approach for measuring the success of any training initiative (Kirkpatrick, 2016). According to Kirkpatrick Partners, the ROE is "the practitioner's approach to creating and demonstrating the organizational value of training... moreover, the degree to which their expectations have been satisfied" (para. 1–8). The steps to measuring ROE in simulation training programs can be based on the Kirkpatrick Model for evaluating training programs: "(1) Focus on the organizational mission (Kirkpatrick Level 4: Results); (2) Identify leading indicators; (3) Define critical behaviors (Kirkpatrick Level 3: Behavior); (4) Determine required drivers; (5) Design learning (Kirkpatrick Level 2: Learning); and (6) Monitor and adjust" (para. 8). The ROE process provides a way to engage stakeholders, tie training results to business results, and help understand stakeholders' perceptions of value (Kirkpatrick & Kirkpatrick, 2010). The reality is that we know intuitively and anecdotally that much of what we are teaching in our Simulation Programs has the potential to impact patient outcomes, but measuring those outcomes is challenging. McGaghie et al. demonstrate that such measurement is possible through well-designed translational research (2011). Even so, ROI alone may not be sufficient to satisfy Boardroom Executives. Perhaps the best approach is to use a blend of financial ROI, healthcare ROI, and educational ROE as a better way of calculating value propositions in Simulation Programs.

Continuous Quality Improvement in Simulation Programs

Everything about designing, deploying, and evaluating simulation involves precision and a high level of detailed monitoring to ensure quality education for learners. It is important for managers to understand how to streamline these processes best. Some of the biggest waste in systems arises from (1) time-waiting caused by delays, (2) lack of readiness, or simple procrastination; (3) partially done work resulting from suboptimal workflow; (4) extra processing or processes resulting from poor organization or bureaucracy; (5) defects and reworks caused by insufficient skills, tools, inspections, or filtering; (6) movement of people or work resulting from physical separation; (7) overproduction or extra features caused by working toward speculative goals; and (8) task switching caused by multiple competing commitments (Rampersad & El Homsi, 2007).

To offer excellence, simulation managers must adopt total/continuous quality improvement frameworks and metrics by which to evaluate outcomes. Many of these approaches and tools arise from other sectors, such as from industry. Toyota Company, the number one car manufacturing company in the world, has created the Toyota Production System (TPS) proven to increase productivity and quality while decreasing inefficiencies.

Toyota Production System and Lean

Lean processes are highly relevant and applicable to Simulation Programs. In 2016, medical error was reported as the third leading cause of death in the USA (Makary & Daniel, 2016). Although safety practices have certainly been enhanced through systems engineering and a recent shift to focusing on safety, system-wide change is not yet realized. In fact, medical errors continue at the rate of 1 out of 10 patients adding astronomical costs to healthcare systems to the tune of over 29 billion dollars per year (2012).

Dr. Frederick Southwick, an American physician, learned about the need for patient safety and quality care through a series of personal tragedies. In his book titled *Critically Ill: A 5-Point Plan to Cure Healthcare Delivery* (Southwick, 2014), he recounts the story of how his wife nearly died from medical and system error and later how he experienced a significant loss due to medical error. Southwick reported that "despite aggressive institution of safety programs in the majority of hospitals [in the USA], there has been no significant reduction in harm to our patients" (p. 20). In years since, Southwick has coupled TPS with the key practices of high-performing athletic teams to create higher reliability in healthcare teams that deliver quality patient-centered care (Southwick et al., 2014). *Lean* is a management system that is core to TPS and continues to be highly utilized today (Spear & Bowen, 1999). Lean processes and tools focus equally on people and process and can easily be applied to managing Simulation Programs. Lean aims to eliminate waste while increasing efficiency and productivity by implementing (1) intelligent automation; (2) just-in-time manufacturing; and (3) and Jidoka, the practice of stopping to notify others of abnormalities to create precision equipment (Bodek, 1988; Womack, Jones, & Roos, 1990).

In TPS, workflow is everything. Toyota referred to workflow in production, as the "value stream." Lean value stream mapping (workflow mapping) is one way of identifying and removing obstacles to progress in project management (Rampersad & El Homsi, 2007). Using *lean value stream mapping*, teams assemble to examine both speed and quality in each step of a given process and then decide if the activity adds value to the end goal, or not. Based on team input, decisions can be made to trial new approaches. Not only can a team eliminate waste and enable greater productivity and creativity but also decrease upset and frustration. Think about how to apply lean thinking to your Simulation Program operations. It could be very useful for many things such as scenario production, minimizing medical supply waste, and to ensure simulator readiness. In simulation, for example, value stream mapping could be applied to the process of creating Simulated Clinical Events (SCE) or scheduling.

Brock and Holtschneider (2016) present an excellent example of the systematic application of value streaming as applied to human performance in a Simulation Program as seen in Figure 11.3. They used the value stream process to ascertain overall organizational impact and value to society by examining human performance–related indicators for "(1) the right people (competence [knowledge, skills, attitudes], capabilities [ability to learn and improve], and commitment [attitudes/motivation]; (2) *organizational required resources* [standards, working conditions, incentives, tools, technology, information, training, education, development]; (3) *tasks on the job* [what they have to do]; (4) *accomplishments achieved* [what was achieved]; (5) *organizational results* [outputs like financial stability, reduced risk, increased readiness and reliability]; and (6) measurable *societal value* to all stakeholders (impact, e.g., measurement of harm reduction, loss of life statistics)" (pp. 58–59).

Using TPS, every single aspect of SCE creation from the time an idea is conceived through to the design, deployment, and final evaluation of the event would be pulled apart, tested, analyzed, and redesigned until the process was 100% efficient and effective. Scenario templates could be considered a lean tool for simulation that aim to streamline the process of scenario writing by providing standardization and structure to produce consistency and promote quality.

Six Sigma

Six Sigma is a distinctive form of quality control and management founded in 1986 by managers at the Motorola Company and later fully implemented and refined by General Motors Electric Company. Today, it is safe to say that achieving Six Sigma means that quality control is

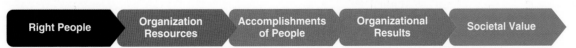

Figure 11.3 The Human Performance Value Stream. (Based on ideas from Brock, T. R., & Holtschneider, M. (2016). Simulation operations, curriculum integration, and performance improvement. In: L. T. Gantt & M. H. Young (Eds.), *Healthcare Simulation: A Guide for Operations Specialist* (pp. 56–67). Hoboken, NJ: John Wiley & Sons, Inc.)

excellent. Six Sigma is an exciting management strategy grounded on three things:

1. Philosophy: the belief that you must know what is important to the customer; defects are costly and can be eliminated; anything less than ideal is an opportunity to improve; understanding processes and improving them is the best way to achieve lasting results; and leader engagement is key to leading organizational change.

2. Process: two main process approaches are used in Six Sigma: DMAIC (define, measure, analyze, improve, and control) to achieve higher performance and DMAD-V (define, measure, analyze, design, and verify) to create a new process.

3. Statistical Tools: strategic use of powerful statistical tools is the hallmark of Six Sigma. These tools allow companies to eliminate error and waste in the production line. The target statistical measure in Six Sigma is 3.4 defects per million (dpmo), which means perfect products, nearing 100% of the time. This level of efficiency results in cost reduction, consistent and quality products, and happy customers.

Six Sigma features an "organized, parallel-mesostructure (it runs like a separate structure, but alongside a company's existing structure) to reduce variation in organizational processes by using improvement specialists, a structured method, and performance metrics with the aim of achieving strategic objectives" (Schroeder, Lindeman, Liedtke, & Choo, 2008, p. 538). One defining characteristic of Six Sigma is its switching mechanism. Six Sigma teaches organizations to be flexible and to switch their structure between mechanistic and organic when needed. For example, flattening hierarchy to bring people from every level of the organization together to generate new ideas and then having them go back to their original roles after having completed the task (Schroeder et al., 2008).

Box 11-3 | Lean and Six Sigma Thinking

Together, Lean and Six Sigma can be used to improve outcomes by:

● Identifying the *value stream* for each product or service and then to challenge (and eliminate) all of the wasted steps currently used to produce it (generally 9 out of 10 steps are found to be wasteful)
● Making the *product flow* continuously through the remaining value-added steps
● Introducing *pull* between all steps where continuous flow is possible
● Managing toward *perfection* so that the number of steps and the amount of time and information needed to serve the customer (whoever the customer might be) continually fall (Rampersad & El-Homsi, 2007, p. 29; Womack, Jones, & Roos, 1990).

Simulation Programs can use Lean, together with Six Sigma by enacting the principles listed in Box 11-3.

The Total Performance Scorecard

The *Total Performance Scorecard* (TPSC) is both a process and tool that your simulation team can use to improve overall team and organizational performance (Rampersad & El-Homsi, 2007). Teams are inextricably tied to organizations and vice versa, so it is logical to view the performance of one within the performance of the other. The TPS concept comprises four individual interrelated elements (as shown in Fig. 11.4). For holism to manifest in the workplace, there needs to be a balance between four closely related management concepts: The Personal Balanced Scorecard, The Organizational Balanced Scorecard, Talent Management, and Total Quality Management. Balance

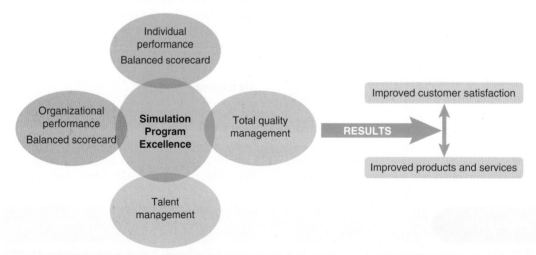

Figure 11.4 Total Quality Improvement Balanced Scorecard. (Adapted from International Standardization Organization. (2015). *ISO: Selection and use of the ISO 9000 family of standards*. Retrieved June 10, 2016 from http://www.iso.org/iso/selection_and_use_of_iso_9000_family_of_standards_2016_en.pdf)

within the TPSC model results in a system that thrives, improves, develops, and learns (Rampersad & El Homsi, 2007). Managers must work to fully develop each element.

Happy, motivated, and fulfilled employees are essential to productive workplaces. The Personal Balanced Scorecard (PBSC) is used to lead individuals through a process of articulating a personal vision, mission, and key roles in life. This vision then informs the development of personal critical success factors that tie to personal objectives, personal performance measures, personal targets, and personal improvement actions by which they will measure their score (Rampersad & El Homsi, 2007). A PBSC requires in-depth reflection on the following four personal dimensions with the overall aim of increasing "awareness, enjoyment, fun, learning, and creativity" (p. 74):

1. Internal perspective—one's physical health and mental state
2. External perspective—relations with your spouse, children, friends, employer, colleagues, and others
3. Knowledge and learning perspective—your skills and learning ability
4. Financial perspective—financial stability

Organizations need equilibrium as it contributes to holistic wellness; therefore, it is important to use metrics that evaluate the overall health of an organization. The Organizational Balanced Scorecard (OBSC) is a "top-down management instrument that is used for making an organization's strategic vision operational at all organizational levels. It includes the overall (corporate) organizational vision, mission, core values, critical success factors, objectives" (p. 16). The OBSC assesses fours dimensions in organizations:

1. "Financial: Fiscal soundness
2. External: Customer satisfaction
3. Internal: Control of primary processes to create value for, and satisfaction in customers
4. Knowledge and Learning: Skills and attitudes of the employees and the organizational learning ability" (p. 17).

Talent Management is "the process of the continuous development of human potential within the organization" (p. 17). Talent management is concerned with attaining maximum employee development to ensure they reach their potential and goals.

Total Quality Management *and Improvement* reflects the extent to which discipline has been ingrained as a way of life through a core commitment to continuous improvement in organizations (Rampersad & El Homsi, 2007). The International Organization for Standardization (ISO) outlines seven ISO Principles of Quality Management principles as Customer Focus, Leadership, Engagement of people, Process approach, Improvement, Evidence-based decision-making, and Relationship Management (http://www.iso.org/iso/pub100080.pdf).

Simulation Programs can work to become an ISO–9001 (2015) accredited Program/Center as a part of their sustainable development and quality management initiatives. The ISO (2015) 5th edition is available for purchase at https://www.iso.org/obp/ui/#iso:std:62085:en. To accomplish this, organizations must follow a comprehensive change leadership and management process to develop, document, measure, analyze, and track improvements in the Simulation Program against ISO requirements to meet core standards (Canadian Standards Association, 2011). Achieving balance among these fundamental elements is key to success for both departmental and organizational improvements. More details are available at (https://committee.iso.org/tc176sc2). Quality and a commitment to excellence are critical concepts in 21st century management.

Dashboards for Continuous Monitoring of Metrics

Dashboards are used to display key metrics. Before assembling your Program's dashboard display panel, know what purpose it will serve, what you will be measuring, and what tools you will use (Lunger, 2017). Only measure what is truly important. A vehicular dashboard has gadgets for displaying and monitoring vehicular performance, such as, speed, gas tank levels, and temperature. In similar fashion, today's corporate dashboards provide managers with an at-a-glance view of select key performance indicators in their program. Likewise, Program dashboards employ visual graphics containing key information about what is going well or can signal problems that need attention and analysis. Low scores on a Balanced Scorecard, for example, can be the sign of a bigger problem. Scores can also be tracked and mapped for trends.

According to Lunger (2017), There are three types of dashboards:

1. *Strategic dashboards* that focus on processes and provide information to leaders by tracking performance against objectives.
2. *Operational dashboards* use processes that inform front-line workers and their supervisors on monitoring and optimizing operational processes.
3. *Tactical dashboards* to inform business managers on how to improve their understanding of internal and external processes and activities for which they are personally accountable and responsible.

Good dashboard design involves five key characteristics: simplicity, minimal distractibility, meaningful timely data, clearly presented visual information, and comfort to the eye (Lunger, 2017). Typically, companies use one of the leading performance management and quality frameworks and tools, such as, the Balanced

Scorecard, Performance Prism, Six Sigma, or economic value evaluations. Ultimately, Lunger suggests using a combination of tools. The online Toolkit provides the

Simulation Program Performance—Data Collection and Tools for Measurement table (Folder 7: 11.7.8). This table contains a list of common categories of data to collect along with the associated data sets required to populate dashboards and generate reports. Creating regular managerial reports is the primary way of communicating both Program's achievements and challenges to internal and external stakeholder groups.

Simulation Program Tracking and Reporting

Reports in Simulation Programs entail all required documented information used to chart progress status and outcomes. Subsequently, reports inform decisions about general operations, educational operations, technical operations, and human capital management. Simulation Programs should include an annual report that features Program leadership, infrastructure, reputation and experiences, and operational data that has been tracked.

Dashboard metrics can be transformed into visually appealing infographics and are great for communicating operations data sets, such as the number of courses offered in a given year, the number of learners, the number and types of stakeholders served, the number of learner contact hours, a summary of Program innovations and developments, total quality improvement outcomes, patient safety, and risk management initiatives, policy and procedure compliance, and updates on personnel (qualifications and simulation training). Also included could be teaching and learning information, such as, curriculum development activities, the number and type of educational offerings, course and educator evaluation, records of simulation event development and revisions, and educational outcomes. Other elements on which to report might include a synopsis of research projects, findings, and publications, and a summary of general scholarship activities conducted by Program members or stakeholders. In the online Toolkit, you will find a great example of summary report using infographics to display stats from a major Interprofessional Education event. (Folder 4: 11.4.11).

Maximizing Use of Computer Software

Brown and Kingston (2009) explain the vital importance of data tracking to provide justification of simulation-related purchase requests and to allow tracking of the effectiveness of very costly simulation resources, as well as, program outcomes. Managers must be organized and use valid and reliable data collection methods and products

to track **hardware** (space, equipment, and other physical resources like simulators, computers and related components, integrated AV/IT systems, medical equipment, consumable supplies), **software** (intangible components of computer systems like a computer operating systems [Gantt & Young, 2016b], and management products and procedures [Cornele & Leland, 2010]). Database-driven management systems are essential tools for Simulation Program management. They provide the user with a platform for concurrent document updating, data integrity protection, and many also have built-in change management performance monitoring and measurement capabilities. Efficient and effective data analysis and reporting can only happen if you have systems and processes in place to enact detailed data entry, storing, and tracking. **Integrated data management** systems contain database engines and data-driven apps to allow data to be stored, articulated, accessed, locked, and modified (http://www.ibm.com/). Consider purchasing an integrated management system that attends to both operational and educational data. Many simulation vendors now provide database driven management products. Moreover, many of these products feature LDAP integration (Lightweight Directory Access Protocol) to create a seamless single log-in access point that serves both your Program and the institution. LDAP integration links the vendor product to your institution's population and course databases (including Learning Management Systems [LMS]) and to web authentication systems. Whenever possible, purchase complementary products, such as inventory barcode systems and labeling software/apps that can sync with your database. Seamless and simple is what you should aim for. If you are not in a position to purchase the total system solution, Microsoft Access, or simply using Microsoft Excel are options.

Managing Risk—Integrated Risk Management

Simulation Programs are primarily public organizations and institutions that are educating, training, and populating our healthcare systems (HIROC, 2014). As such, they are accountable to the public for effective, responsible, and efficient use of public dollars. Part of this process involves creating an organizational mindset that seeks to identify and manage potential threats to the Simulation Program and the organization at large. Managers must therefore be forward thinkers and engage in processes to (1) identify risks, (2) assess risks, (3) manage risks, and (4) report risks. By asking the right questions and planning ahead, Programs will be in a better position to mitigate the harmful effects of poor risk management. In short, managers must do everything they can to avoid threats to the Simulation Program.

Integrated risk management (IRM) starts at the top as part of organizational culture where people are conditioned to be vigilant and on the lookout for problems. Recall the aviation organizational cultural shift that Captain Sulley described in Chapter 1. He explained how airlines experienced a marked culture shift where identifying, assessing, managing, and reporting risks became more important than retaining the right to punish individuals when things failed. Simulation Program managers must do the same by providing risk oversight, coordination, and monitoring. Let's face it, nobody likes nasty surprises or significant losses, and everyone appreciates the smooth functioning of organizational systems and resources. Interestingly, successful simulation programs are wise to guard against the effects of success, listed by Francis (2013) as "complacency; inattention; and the development of tunnel vision and blind spots."

The Canadian Standards Association (CSA) (2011) offers a comprehensive list of potential benefits associated with IRM including:

- Improved identification of threats
- Improved organizational learning
- Minimization of losses
- Improved controls
- Increased likelihood of achieving objectives
- Better decision-making and planning
- Improved loss prevention and incident management
- Effective allocation and use of resources for risk treatment
- Improved operational effectiveness and efficiency
- Improved governance
- Improved stakeholder confidence and trust
- Compliance with relevant legal and regulatory requirements and international norms
- Improved financial reporting

Simulation Administrators, Leaders, and Managers: Roles and Functions

To thrive, Simulation Programs must exist within a framework that ensures adequate and sustainable efficiencies in fiscal, human, and material resource management to meet programmatic goals and objectives. Managing a Simulation Program involves managing people, money, and material resources. In order for Simulation Programs to offer vibrant and responsive learning and clinical practice environments, we must attend to each of the functions found within leadership, administration, and management. **Leadership** unfolds at all levels of an organization and involves visioning, inspiring, and communicating clear messages around transformation. **Administration** involves determinative functions such as making key decisions, creating objectives for

transformation, and formulating crucial policies. **Management** on the other hand, concerns executive functions and is a subset of administration. Simply put, **leaders**, create and communicate a vision for the organization as a whole; **administrators**, often referred to as bureaucrats, work with leaders to determine a plan and a framework (i.e., policies and procedures) to manage the larger organization; **managers** execute those plans by implementing these plans and frameworks at various levels within the organization; and **followers** at all levels, follow. In smaller centers or with entrepreneurial endeavors, the administrator and manager—and the leader—can be one person. Kerr (2015) contends that organizations must leverage the functions of leaders, managers and followers in organizations for greater success. "The best leaders lead and let others manage; the best managers [and followers] understand their leader's vision and work with their teams to achieve it" (para.15). Regardless, it is important to understand and include in your plan the key people functions and activities needed for leadership, administration, and management (Hatherly, 2011). Table 11.3 features a summary of people functions for simulation operation success.

Management Functions

Let's return to the concept of management itself. Koontz and O'Donnell's (1972) seminal work on managerial functions has continued relevance for today's manager. They identified five core functions of management: planning, organizing, staffing, directing, and controlling. Together, these five functions form the management process as seen in Figure 11.5. Capable healthcare providers and educators often manage Simulation Programs, but these people are often inexperienced in management or leadership. This next section provides a brief overview of management functions for the Simulation Champion as manager.

Planning

Planning for Simulation Programs involves determining the "program's philosophy, goals, objectives, policies and procedures, and rules" (Marquis & Huston, 2017), then to set and execute plans to attain Simulation Program goals. Planning also involves managing change effectively by making short- and long-term projections and determining a fiscally responsible plan to execute action(s) (Marquis & Huston, 2017).

Organizing

Organizing involves establishing the structure needed to facilitate reaching Simulation Program goals. The structure is important as it impacts a Program's position and level of authority within the organization. A Program's

Table 11.3	People Roles and Functions for Simulation Operations Success		
Leadership Role "Doing the Right Thing"	**Administrative Role** "Doing Things"	**Management Role** "Doing Things Right"	
Path Finding	*Path Clearing*	*Path Following*	
● **Forges** future directions and new paths through creative imagination and abstract thinking ● **Transforms** through authority that emerges by transforming and achieving follower critical mass (formal and informal power) ● **Leads** visioning with knowledge of context ● **Communicates** the vision with conviction and inspires others to act ● **Maneuvers** complexity and finds ways to adapt ● **Intervenes** with confidence in the face of chaos ● **Accountable** to the whole organization and takes reasonable risks	● **Determines** a strategic master plan and implementation framework ● **Establishes** goals, sets targets, and evaluates outcomes ● **Creates** positions for people ● **Delegates** authority ● **Develops** policy, procedures, and rules ● **Maintains** regulatory enforcement ● **Ensures** consistency and stability ● **Accountable** to the organization and to stakeholders	● **Achieves** organizational goals by operationalizing the vision ● **Manages** - the "Doer" manages transformation through planning, organizing, staffing, directing, and controlling ● **Enacts** the vision in day-to-day operations by empowering others to act ● **Acts** through delegated authority and specifically assigned responsibilities ● **Improves** through measurement, data analysis, and interpretation ● **Knows** how to get things done right within the organization ● **Enacts** and enforces procedures and processes ● **Clarifies** roles and responsibilities ● **Accountable** to the team	

Adapted from Hatherly, A. (2011). *ECE Online: Leadership and Management—Core Education*. Retrieved from http://eceonline.core-ed.org/groupcms/view/13898/leadership-and-management and from Kerr , J. (2015). *Leader or manager? These 10 important distinctions can help you out*. Retrieved November 16, 2015, from http://www.inc.com/james-kerr/leading-v-managing-ten-important-distinctions-that-can-help-you-to-become-better.html

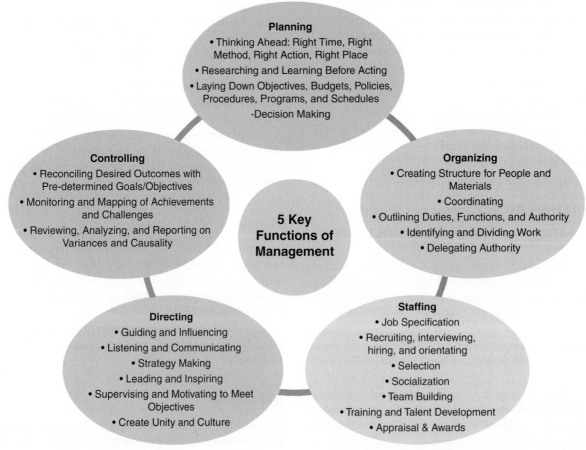

Figure 11.5 Five Key Functions of Management. (Based on ideas from Koontz, H., & O'Donnell, C. (1972). *Principles of management: An analysis of managerial functions*. New York, NY: McGraw-Hill; Marquis, B. L., & Huston, C. J. (2017). *Leadership roles and management functions in nursing: Theory and application* (9th ed., p. 44). Philadelphia, PA: Wolters Kluwer.)

position within an organization directly impacts power distance in relationships and the manger's ability to influence decisions and outcomes (Koontz & O'Donnell, 1972; Marquis & Huston, 2017).

Staffing

Staffing the Simulation Program involves acquiring quality talent to lead, manage, teach, and support activities within the Program. Staffing also requires determining key positions for the Program and hiring the best-suited talent. Once talented people are on the team, provide a comprehensive orientation and maximize opportunities to promote socialization to the team and the simulation community of practice. It is important also to manage and develop talent on the simulation team. Both individual and team talent development are key to maintaining a positive culture and climate.

Directing

Directing entails motivating people to implement and successfully execute day-to-day operations of the Simulation Program. The directing function entails the everyday human resource management functions of managing conflict, delegating responsibilities, communicating, and keeping the team productive and on target (Marquis & Huston, 2017).

Controlling

Lastly, controlling denotes measuring, modifying, and tweaking to ensure that the plan is carried out successfully. This function includes things like talent appraisals, "fiscal accountability [such as, managing the budget], quality control, legal and ethical control, and professional and collegial control" (Marquis & Huston, 2017, p. 44). Whether you are a one-person show running a small program, or you are managing a large team with a gargantuan facility, managing a Simulation Program is a huge undertaking (Fig. 11.5).

Strategy and Future Directions

It is the work of the manager to operationalize the greater institution's **strategic plan**. However, whether Simulation Champions serve in leadership, administrative, or managerial capacities, at some point they will likely need to write a strategic plan for the Simulation Program and in some cases, a business case/proposal(s). The next section offers a synopsis of the main elements in strategic planning and outlines key components of a business case. For additional process information and templates, refer to A Guidebook to Strategic Planning (Folder 1: 11.1.2).

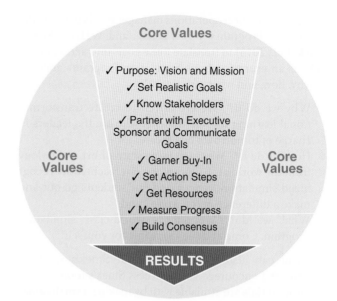

Figure 11.6 Ten Step Strategic Planning Process. (Based on ideas from Marquis, B. L., & Huston, C. J. (2017). *Leadership roles and management functions in nursing: Theory and application* (9th ed., pp. 169–170). Philadelphia, PA: Wolters Kluwer.)

Strategic Relations: Garnering Buy-In

Strategic planning should never unfold in a vacuum. Doing so sets you up for stakeholder failure to buy-in. Engage all key stakeholders in an iterative process that unearths valued perspectives and gathers vital information, and then work toward a unified strategic vision and plan. This approach will help to garner acceptance of the plan, or *buy-in*. Any strategic process begins with knowing your purpose. Think back to the first time you were introduced to simulation. What moved you? What connected for you? Passion and drive are fueled by connections that are formed in the heart. Connecting with the heart ultimately allows us to transmit our values to others. In the process of making binding connections, the intellect may be captivated, but more importantly, the heart is hooked. That is what is meant by *total buy-in*. Conrad, Guhde, Brown, Chronister, and Ross-Alaolmolki (2011) address the need for transformational leadership practices when implementing Simulation Programs (Lucas et al., 2007).

Simulation leaders must inspire and lead followers toward a common mission, vision, and strategies that lay out direction and priorities. They must work to cocreate a culture that supports articulated values and to enact operational functions and processes that align with the requirements of a Simulation Program. Lastly, leaders work to put in place the requisite infrastructure for effective, efficient operations (i.e., information technology and human resources) (Lucas et al., 2007).

The simulation operations manager needs to know the Simulation Program's WHY, HOW, and WHAT (Simon Sinek, Inc., 2015) to translate these goals into action plans. Here is an example of one Simulation Program's answers to why, how, and what questions.

- Why we do it? "We are driven to create transformational learning for our students who are the leaders in charge of tomorrow's healthcare."
- How we do it? "We teach using state-of-art technology from the world's top innovators, our teachers are recognized simulation leaders, and our students go out and make a difference in the world," and
- What we do? "We offer a world-class simulation Program. Come and see the magic for yourself!"

You can also learn more about Sinek's work in Chapter 9. I encourage you to access Sinek's tools online. Many materials are available with by making a small donation at (https://www.startwithwhy.com/default.aspx).

The Art of Influence: Getting Others to Follow Your Vision and Mission

Values are the fuel that gets the fire in us started, but more importantly, our values are what will fuel us when the flames start to die out. This premise also holds true for the people you will need to influence on your journey as an operations manager. Remember that when interacting with a senior administrator, a vendor, a hospital President, or non–healthcare–oriented external stakeholders, their values will likely differ from yours. As Simulation Champions and healthcare providers, our common values include safe patient care, person- and family-centered care, compassion, empathy, commitment to clinical excellence, competence, a spirit of inquiry, and an altruistic commitment to improving health in the world. So, to garner buy-in, one must seek to connect with the heartstrings and passions of others while effectively communicating their own. Once that emotional connection is made and continuously fueled, it is less likely that change will fail (Kotter, 1996; Kotter & Cohen, 2002; Kouzes & Posner, 2014). Knowing what all involved parties value most also enables better decision-making when it comes to prioritizing in Simulation Programs things like equipment purchases, or resolving conflicts, or engaging in strategic planning.

As a nurse educator and Simulation Champion, I was passionate about simulation-based learning but unable to speak the language my superior used with her direct reports and key stakeholder groups. I was lacking knowledge of business and organizational leadership acumen. So the day inevitably arrived when my altruistic values clashed with my administrators' values, and the result was a resounding no to my request! I shook my head, and asked myself, "What do they not get here? We are talking about peoples' lives." This event was particularly painful for me because that person was the decision-maker and purse string holder. In retrospect, had I been able to make my pitch in business terms, the outcomes might have been different. So the lesson here is: learn the language of the boardroom and develop fluency to communicate about such topics as economic efficiencies including return on investment, cost of investment, and rate of return on investment, long-term cost projections, and value propositions. In truth, you are more likely to connect with the heart of the CEO when you at least try to speak the language.

Elements of a Strategic Plan

All organizations want to know if they are doing the right work, how to make better decisions, and how to get superior results. A strategic plan is intended to help accomplish these goals. Strategic planning comprises the following elements: organizational philosophy mission, vision, values, and purpose statements, and overall goals and objectives with corresponding strategies to achieve them. Organizational planning can be for the long term (3 to 7 years; Marquis & Huston, 2017) or the short term (2 to 3 years). The long-range organizational planning process is "deliberate, premeditated, and intentional" …and focuses on "purpose, mission, philosophy, and goals related to the external environment" (Marquis & Huston, 2017, p. 101). Generally speaking, the frontline simulation manager will be more involved in short-term operational, strategic planning, whereas administrators tend to be more involved in long-term planning for the larger institution. The strategic planning process can be enhanced with the use of a model, such as the Strategic Logic Model to provide structure and process to strategic planning efforts (Ritala & Huizingh, 2014). A sample is found in the toolkit item listed below.

Simulation Managers are charged with the process of developing a Program's strategic plan. The process can be broken down into ten steps (Marquis & Huston, 2017; see Box 11-4). Remember that good strategic planning requires inviting the right people to the discussion, gathering the right information, and using the right process. No vacuums allowed. See the *A Guidebook to Strategic Planning* in the online Toolkit (Folder 1: 11.1.2).

Elements of a Business Plan

As part of the strategic planning process, the need for writing a business plan (sometimes referred to as a business case) may arise. A business plan comprises several core elements, one of which is the strategic plan itself (Kahrs & Harmer, 2013). *Business plans* are written to help secure funding for larger initiatives, such as special projects that require the acquisition of material

Box 11-4	The Strategic Planning Process: Ten Steps

1. Clearly, define the purpose of the organization.
2. Establish realistic, attainable goals that align with the existing mission, vision, values, and goals of the greater organization. When creating a brand new Simulation Program, include vision, mission, and core values statements.
3. Identify external constituents or stakeholders and know their WHY! Find out what they know about simulation and set out to bring them into your camp. It will not happen by osmosis.
4. Partner with your executive sponsor to clearly and concisely communicate the vision by articulating your Simulation Program's goals and objectives to internal and external stakeholders.
5. Garner buy-in and take ownership of the plan.
6. Identify strategies to meet and measure goal attainment.
7. Plan to make the best use of the resources available and seek out additional resources.
8. Adopt and consistently use systems that measure progress and outcomes.
9. Use change leadership and management models to inform the change process.
10. Build consensus around your WHY! Write and disseminate your plan to others.

Based on ideas from Marquis, B. L., & Huston, C. J. (2017). *Leadership roles and management functions in nursing: Theory and application* (9th ed., pp. 169–170). Philadelphia, PA: Wolters Kluwer.

and human resources, like a Simulation Program. Tom Doyle, a nurse, entrepreneur, businessperson, and fellow Simulation Champion offers a synopsis of the key elements of a business plan.

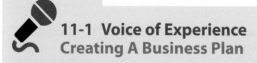

11-1 Voice of Experience
Creating A Business Plan

Thomas J. Doyle, MSN, RN

The Challenge

Writing a business plan can be daunting. However, a detailed business plan of activities is a roadmap for business success in Simulation Programs. A business plan is a living document that projects 3 to 5 years ahead and outlines the route a company or program intends to take to grow revenues. In Simulation Programs, the business plan can map out how to grow the adoption and use of simulation within an existing educational program or it could be a map to revenue generation. Make your business plan stand out. Describe what is unique to your Program and makes you distinct from others. For example, consider that any given city has numerous restaurants, all offering a basic commodity, which is food. However, each targets a niche market (e.g., Italian, Mexican, Arabic, Fine Dining). Describe and illustrate what sets your Program or business apart from others.

Meeting the Challenge

To make life easier for you, I am listing the key components of a business plan. They are summarized as follows:

- *Executive Summary:* "Your executive summary is a snapshot of your business plan as a whole and touches on your company" or program's profile and goals (https://www.sba.gov/starting-business/write-your-business-plan). It provides an executive with a quick summary of the proposal. Think of it as the pitch in miniature that will take up only 5% to 10% of the space of your document. Include key elements of your Program's strategic plan, such as a Program description, mission, vision, value, and purpose statements, that describe what your Program is all about. Also, include historical company information, such as when the Program was formed. Briefly describe the Program products and services. Include a brief summary of plans. Use language that is accessible—simulation specific jargon may not serve you well here. The executive summary should end with recommendations, justification, and conclusions.
- *Program or Business Need Description and Desired Outcomes:* The next step involves articulating your business needs: this is what you want and when you want it. Clearly describe the need, the key drivers for the change, any high-level requirements, overarching assumptions, constraints, or dependencies of the project and a clear statement of outcomes and the exact scope of the project and any projected timelines.
- *Company Description:* Your company or program's description provides information on what you do, what differentiates your business

(Continued)

11-1 Voice of Experience (*Continued*)

or program from others, and the markets your business or program serves. This synopsis provides a high-level review of the different elements of the business [Program]. Think of this as the "30-second elevator pitch."

- *Organization and Management:* Every business or program is structured differently. This section should include your company or program's organizational structure, details about the ownership of your company or program, profiles of your management team (include past accomplishments), and the qualifications of your board of directors or advisory board for a simulation program. An easy way to do this is to include an organizational chart. Include ownership information in this section.

- *Market Analysis:* Before launching the business or program, it is essential to research the business industry, market, and competitors. Include a description of the industry, any outlooks or projections, as well as information about your target market and estimated size, your pricing, and gross margin targets, and provide a competitive analysis.

- *Risks:* Every business venture has risk. Be honest and upfront. Describe any impacts associated with either proceeding or NOT proceeding. Describe the likelihood of risk occurring and any impact to internal and external stakeholders, or operational impact.

- *Service or Product Line:* Identify what you have to sell or have to offer? How does it benefit your customers? What is the product lifecycle? Note any existing, pending, or any anticipated copyright or patent filings, and list them here. Outline any research and development (R&D) activities that you are involved in or are planning. Note the results of future R&D activities you expect to see on the horizon. Be sure to analyze the R&D efforts of not only your own business but also of others in your industry.

- *Marketing and Sales:* Identify how you plan to market your business or program. How will you penetrate the market? What is your strategy for growth? What is your strategy for reaching potential customers? What is your sales strategy? Also, include outlining your sales activities.

- *Funding Request and Fiscal Recommendations:* If you want to fund the business or program, use this section to outline financial requirements. Include the amounts needed now, any incremental funding over the next 5 years, and plans for the use of the funds. Also describe historical information and financial projections. Develop the financial projections section only once you have analyzed the market and set clear objectives. At this point, think about making a plan to allocate resources efficiently. Since a picture speaks louder than words, use graphical representations of any projections.

- *Final Recommendations:* The final message involves articulating a clear, concise summary of priority recommendations. List key financial and strategic factors, cost summaries, critical success factors, and a brief implementation plan.

- *Appendices:* This section is optional and provided on an as-needed basis. It could include items such as the resumes of key players, letters of reference, and legal documents. You should also keep track of the distribution of your business plan so as it is updated you will be sure and include everyone that initially received it.

Outcome

As you can see, there are many components to a successful plan that requires a significant amount of research, analysis, and strategic thinking. Assumptions have to be made, such as financial projections, which are tied directly to the marketing and sales strategies.

Most Valuable Lessons Learned

After writing the initial business plan, one should reflect on what has been written and make any necessary changes. A business plan is not created the night before it is due and should be revised, at a minimum, on an annual basis. See the online Toolkit for a Business Case template (Folder 1: 11.4).

Consortia, Coalitions, Partnerships, Alliances, and Networks

Simulation-based education, when properly deployed, is often expensive. One cost containment strategy is to collaborate and share valuable human and material resources. Increasing demands for current and innovative programming, the advent of new technologies for learning, the need for increased patient safety outcomes, limited access to resources, and shrinking availability of funding form the impetus for educators and administrators to explore alternate options to building stand-alone Simulation Programs. Increasingly, we are seeing the emergence of consortia, alliances, coalitions, formal partnerships, and networks in the simulation practice community (Jeffries & Battin, 2012; Maxworthy & Waxman, 2015).

An *alliance* is typically a longer-term relationship that is described as "a union between people, groups, countries... a relationship in which people agree to work together or allied for some activity or effort" (Merriam-Webster Online Dictionary, 2016). Maxworthy and Waxman describe an alliance as "a purposeful relationship between organizations, often focused on a particular mission or issue" (p. 424). In an alliance, members retain their organizational identity and agree to donate institutional time, talent, and resources toward the attainment of common goals. Waxman states the central component in simulation alliance success is a focus on sustainability planning. This type of resource donation is called in-kind. There are many simulation alliances that have formed throughout the world. In the United States, there are simulation alliances in Oregon, Florida, Tennessee, Mississippi, Hawaii, and Indiana (Waxman, 2016, as cited in Palaganas et al., 2015).

A *coalition* stems from an alliance or a union between groups that is usually temporary (ad hoc) in nature and for a specified purpose (Freedictionary.com).

A *consortium* (plural consortia) is a formal entity. It is described as "an agreement, combination, or group (as of companies) formed to undertake an enterprise beyond the resources of any one member" (Merriam-Webster). A consortium, therefore, is greater than the simple sum of its parts. One member has something the other member needs and wants, and vice versa. Consortium members share a common purpose and will often articulate a unified vision and mission.

A *partnership* is considered a legal relationship and usually involves "close cooperation between parties having specified and joint rights and responsibilities" (Merriam-Webster). A consortium may, or may not chose to enter into a formal partnership agreement that contains binding legal requirements for each member.

A *network* involves an "informally interconnected group or association of persons" (as with friends or professional colleagues) (Merriam-Webster); however, networks have also been known as formal entities. For example, the National Simulation Network has successfully used simulation to "achieve wider dissemination and sharing of information, institutional collaboration around research, and action programs" (Dauphinee & Reznick, 2011, p. 94). Networks can also be used to share developmental and operational costs of new products of services and are able to reach multiple partners joined by technology that crosses geographic boundaries (Dauphinee & Reznick, 2011). As you see, there is flexibility in the types and models for collaboration. Before jumping in head first, think about which approach best fits the intended purpose.

In the book *Building Successful HealthCare Education Simulation Centres: The Consortium Model* (Jeffries & Battin, 2012), the authors offer advice to those embarking on collaborative endeavors at a regional, state/provincial, or national level. They describe a step-by-step approach

that uses cooperation and collaboration to build a consortium. Key steps in the consortium building process comprise (1) building networks, trust, and commitment; (2) establishing leadership with vision and purpose; (3) organizing governance structure and committee work; (4) planning for roles and responsibilities; (5) enacting management principles; (6) establishing mechanisms for communication; (7) establishing priority strategies, principles, and goals; (8) strategic evaluation; (9) building professional development programs; implementing total continuous improvement; and (10) creating a plan to keep the momentum for change and growth.

Consortia have the potential to reap many benefits, such as the potential for safer patient care, sharing of financial and educational resources, synergistic professional development for simulation educators, increased opportunities for team development across institutions, opportunities for increased educational programming, a greater capacity to train large numbers of professionals in times of expanding job markets and nursing shortages, and providing space for learning that bridges the gap between theory and practice (Jeffries & Battin, 2012). Challenges or barriers to consortium models include the lack of well-defined models for training students, conflicting schedules that lead to competition for space, colearning scheduling conflicts, differing assessment and evaluation practices, encountering a lack of flexibility in conflicts, and the use of simulation, a little-known pedagogy (Jeffries & Battin). Should you decide to explore using a consortium model approach, know that consortia must be designed to meet the needs of the all its members and constitute coming together to form a unique identity, vision and mission, groups and teams, and shared dollars and outcomes. As noted above, many sharing models exist so do invest some time to determine which approach best suits your needs.

When developing formal agreements between partners, remember to engage your organization's contract and procurement services for assistance in developing contracts and to explore institutional policies and liability coverage. It is also prudent to involve legal council when drawing up formal agreements, memoranda, or ownership documents. Many relationships start off well and end in disaster, not because of lack of good intentions, mostly because of lack of planning. Ask the tough questions from the outset to avoid disappointment and discord, and then begin the task of building a collaborative consortium team. Gratton and Erickson (2007) describe the elements required for building collaborative teams (see Box 11-5).

Simulation Programs may be situated in one locale or distributed across many locations. Consortia can also deliver programming via mobile simulation units or by transporting low-cost learning events from one place to another (distributed simulation). Currently, there is a lack of Practice-Education partnership models from which

Box 11-5	**Building the Consortium Team**

- Ensure that you have *executive support* who themselves have an investment in social relationships and collaborative behaviors. Create opportunities for top executives to meet each member of your simulation consortium.
- Work to create a *gift culture* that sees team members embrace team interaction as precious gifts: something that is valuable and generously offered to others. Create opportunities for consortium members to teach each other (featured presentations from the team, for the team).
- Invest in *signature* relationship practices: your unique brand. Work to develop practices that are difficult for others to replicate and are specific to your environment. This exercise might involve something as basic as office space layout— for example, high-efficiency teams love to work closely together and to rub shoulders frequently so collaboration can manifest as shared offices spaces. If staff comes from different sites, then build capacity to communicate via technology—give these meetings a fun name and make them enjoyable, that is, "Our Weekly Sim Connect Conference." Make this activity a part of your unique identity.
- Make your *honor code* visible to others. For example, postcollaborative behavior norms and practice what you preach, or let the team see top executives in action that models collaboration by making arrangements to rotate one simulation consortium team member through meetings with the executive leadership team.

- Ensure requisite *training and skills* to collaborate: We were not all born collaborators. Teach team members how to build relationships, model how to communicate well, and invest in developing in each member the tools they need to resolve conflicts.
- Connect with the community: Build a *strong sense of community* by encouraging the entire team to engage in simulation community of practice in multiple ways. Create conditions for this to happen.
- Assign *team leaders* in the consortium who are both task and relationship oriented; both are needed: to do the right thing and to do it the right way. Strike a healthy balance of dreamers and doers.
- Build *heritage relationships*: These are established long-standing relationships. When a new team comes together, these tight relationships can be a source of exclusion and sometimes leave people feeling left out. Leave no staff member behind and work to create new heritage relationships by pairing people who have like interests and strengths. Create opportunities for people to get to know each other, their unique roles and gifts, and bring them up to collaborate in different ways.

Gratton, L., & Erickson, T. J. (2007). 8 ways to build collaborative teams. *Harvard Business Review, 85*, 100–109. Retrieved from https://hbr.org/2007/11/eight-ways-to-build-collaborative-teams

to draw, but anecdotal evidence supports the use of this approach. Further research is needed to clearly identify benefits and drawbacks. The authors report positive outcomes as an increased sense of collegiality, teamwork, and appreciation for contributions from each discipline (Senger, Stapleton, & Gorski, 2012, p. e478). Antecedents to successful outcomes were believed to be "a shared mission, dedicated nurse leaders, supportive administration, and innovative thinking led to the establishment of a hospital-based simulation lab and a multi-institutional simulation experience" (p. e481). Challenges in this endeavor included the time and effort it took to plan and organize the event, increased participant interaction, and increased clarity in the process to participants.

Partnering across Practice Sites

Several healthcare institutions and nursing colleges are developing either formal or informal partnerships to address budgetary constraints, the nursing workforce shortage, and insufficient clinical learning experiences (American Association of Colleges of Nursing [AACN], 2002). Senger and colleagues offer an interesting account of the development of a Practice-Academe partnership that brought partners across disciplines to learn together (2012).

Multisite collaborative approaches can benefit through shared educational offerings. The Idaho Simulation Network (ISN) featured the ISNs Tele-Sim, In-Situ

Neonatal Resuscitation Program (NRP) education feasibility project on May 6, 2015, via webinar hosted by Education Management Solutions (EMS) (https://youtu.be/RvMxibDPBPw). The webinar presenter Marion Constable described how the ISN leveraged expertise and resources to roll out training across several clinical practice sites. Simulation-based learning via Tele-Health technology was used to deploy team training; practice new protocols; enrich technical and teamwork skills; identify clinical and teamwork performance gaps; and to uncover and correct system, process, and equipment issues across multiple hospital sites throughout Idaho. Outcomes were cited as increased collegiality, stronger relationships, an increased knowledge and comfort level with resuscitation technology, and increase confidence in the trainees' abilities to better manage NRP. A copy of the presentation can be viewed through the EMS site at: http://SIMULATIONiQ.com. A consortium model holds promise for shared fiscal and human resource sharing in the future.

Project Management: A Manager's Friend for Creating Change

Performance optimization in organizations is more important now than ever; however, today's organizations are highly complex and often reside on the edge of chaos. What we need to help pull us back from the edge of chaos are new approaches to leadership and management. One approach to Simulation Program management is **Project Management** (PM) (Duffield & Whitty, 2015). PM is a staged process of engaging, planning, implementing, monitoring, and sustaining a desired change or strategy through work tasks and groups to accomplish an immediate desired task or goal or outcome. Using PM, the Simulation Program could be considered one large project that is then further broken down into a myriad of smaller projects, that each must be managed. Using a project management approach for managing Simulation Programs then, makes perfect sense. A mind map that demonstrates how Simulation Programs can be divided into project-focused sub groups is located at (https://www.mindmeister.com/76802920). Because of the dynamic nature of simulation, Simulation Programs are in a constant state of flux and must therefore, constantly and effectively manage change (Ramazani & Jergeas, 2015). Sometimes PM involves hiring external consultants. It is wise to develop a

process for hiring consultants and to work with institutional HR representatives to facilitate this. Refer to *The Project Manager's Guidebook* (Folder 1: 11.1.3). This resource also includes the following tools:

● Brainstorming for Idea Generation
● Fishbone/Ishikawa Diagrams for Cause and Effect Analysis
● **SWOT** Analysis for Strategizing
● **SOAR** Analysis for Planning for Growth
● Delegation for Increased Efficiency and Effectiveness
● Critical Path Analysis Flow Diagrams for Chronological Chunking
● Gantt Charts for Mapping Events and Targets
● The Good Ole Whiteboard
● PDSA Cycles for Total Quality Improvement

Fiscal Management

Fiscal management entails financial controlling and reporting, financial projection and retrospective analysis, asset lifecycle management, and travel and expense management. A sound financial planning process involves financial goal setting; information and data gathering; analysis of the data; making recommendations and submitting plans for approval; implementing the plan; and finally measuring outcomes against established goals.

Budget Basics

Simulation Program managers set fiscal goals to align with the vision, mission, values, and overall goals and objectives of the Program. The **budget** is a "formal, quantitative expression of management's plans, intentions, expectations, and actions to control results"

(Rundio, 2016, p. 5). It serves to forecast the resources needed to deliver services, to plan for coordinating the financial goals of an organization, and to "yield a return on investment to sustain and maintain the viability of an organization" (p. 6). Designing the budget should be done in collaboration with experienced personnel from the finance or senior administration department. Established Programs rely on historical budgets from previous years to build new budgets. Dollar amounts are

projected based on historical and projection data for the coming year. See the Toolkit for a *Hypothetical Simulation Program Budget Template* (Folder 4: 11.4.1). Once approved and developed, the budget is closely monitored (monthly, quarterly, and annually) and often adjusted. Financial reports are then generated to give information on performance and financial position. According to Rundio, the budget-development workflow consists of six steps: "(1) collecting relevant data; (2) planning the services you will deliver; (3) planning the activities you will undertake; (4) implementing the plan; (5) monitoring the budget; and (6) taking corrective measures when necessary" (pp. 61–62). In conjunction with the finance department Simulation Program managers are responsibility and accountability for budget performance and compliance.

Getting the entire team on board is an essential part of compliance. Making the budget available to the team helps to create cost awareness, promotes transparency and shared accountability, and facilitates measuring productivity.

Budget Types

Commonly, budgets are divided by type as follows: Master budgets, Operating budgets, Capital budgets, and Program budgets. Budgets contain three major components: assets (owned and provides future economic benefit), liabilities (money owing), and equity (excess of assets over liabilities—as in being in the black or in the red) (Rundio, 2016). Assets are further broken down into

● *Current assets:* assets expected to be used up or converted to cash within 1 year (e.g., cash, investments, receivables, inventories, supplies, and prepaid expenses like rent or leasing) (Kimmel, Weygandt, Kieso, Trenholm, & Irvine, 2012).
● *Fixed assets* (Plant, Property, and Equipment): include land, buildings, equipment, and furniture. These items have a long life span and as such, have estimated useful lives referred to as amortization (or item's lifecycle) (Kimmel et al., 2012). Note: Archival processes are part of lifecycle management and are an important consideration in operational sustainability. For example, upon purchase of any fixed asset, a predetermined percentage of the overall replacement value of the item is paid from

the operating budget to a lifecycle fund that is carried forward from year to year over the lifetime of the asset. When the lifecycle matures, funds are released to purchase updated assets.

- *Noncurrent assets* are intangibles that cannot be seen but are still of great value. These include such things as patents, copyright, trademarks, trade names, licenses, and goodwill or in-kind donations (Kimmel et al., 2012).
- *Liabilities:* can be divided into current liabilities and long-term liabilities.
  - ○ *Current liabilities:* must be paid within on year period (wages, taxes)
  - ○ *Long-term liabilities:* debts that are due beyond a 1-year period (leases, loans, archival payment on lifecycle replacement programs) (Rundio, 2016).
- *Equity:* is an expression the of overall net worth of a given entity. It is determined formulaically by calculating **Equity = Assets – Liabilities**.
- *Revenue:* the amount charged to users in Simulation Programs for goods and services. This can include course fees, consultation fees, space rental, personnel hiring, etc.

- *Fiscal Year and Year End*: a predetermined cut-off date whereby an organization's accounting period ends. The year-end date will vary between institutions.
- *Expenses*: an overall expression of all costs incurred in the process of doing business.

Fee Structure and Fee Schedules

The first time the phone rang with these questions, I was a bit stumped. "Hello. I am making a movie and would like to use your hospital spaces. How much do you charge?" Or, "I want to run a simulation event in your space with your staff running it. How much will that cost?" I learned quickly that the answer to those questions was complicated and what ensued was a 2-year project that involved reviewing insurance policies, creating legally binding user-agreement forms with liability clauses and waivers, and building a fee structure and schedules. Jamal, Wallin, and Arnold (2015) offer a five-step process for generating a fee structure. Figure 11.7 depicts the five phases and the recommended activities for each. I also learned although it would have been nice to generate extra revenue, those

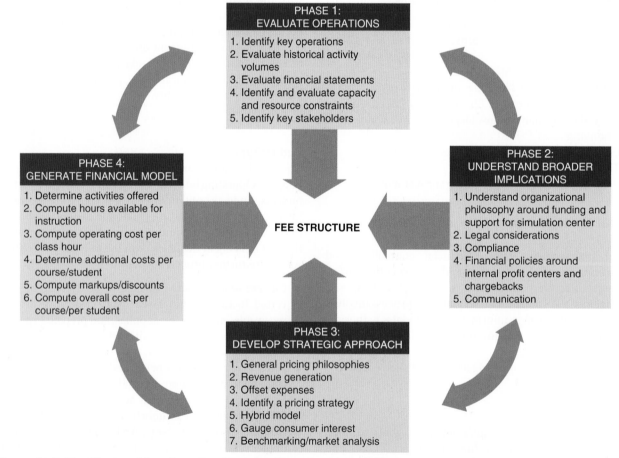

Figure 11.7 Five Phases of Creating a Fee Structure. (From Jamal, A., Walling, K. D., & Arnold, J. L. (2015). Creating a fee structure. In J. C. Palaganas, J. C. Maxworthy, C. A. Epps, & M. E. Mancini (Eds.), *Defining excellence in simulation programs* (p. 293). Philadelphia, PA: Wolters Kluwer.)

requests did not align with our overall mandate and the capacity of our staffing complement. A sample *Fee Schedule and Outside User Booking Agreement* document is found in Folder 4: 11.4.10.

Conflict of Interest

Individual and institutional relationships between academia and industry are long-standing and you will need to make provisions to ensure ethical interactions and dealings. Conflict of Interest (COI) policy is aimed at "preventing compromised decision making rather than to try to remedy its consequences" (Institute of Medicine [IOM], 2009, p. 216). Conflict of Interest can pose a serious threat to the integrity of a Program and its personnel. Consider the impact on institutional COI of patents, equity positions, or stock options in medical industry companies or the practice of giving or receiving gifts or grants from companies. Personnel in the Simulation Program need to consider all personal financial interests that could impact work related decisions or impact work performance (IOM, 2009). For example, acting as a consultant for an outside vendor may pose a COI depending on established employer rules for external consultancy. Ensure that the Program P&P are squarely aligned with institutional policy. There may be requirements for personal declarations and official forms needed documenting COI, or disclaimers to denounce COI. Programs, as part of an annual performance review, may have employees sign an official declaration of remuneration from all relationships with outside companies, and then detail how activities comply with COI policy. Consider also stipulating any consequences of noncompliance.

Financial Reporting

Many organizations use accounting software or some version of a unified/integrated resource management program. These programs can automatically generate ledgers and also conduct financial report analytics. Tools make it easier for managers to produce timely, visually pleasing and easy to read reports; increase efficiencies; promote budgetary compliance; and make adjustments to the plan if needed. See the online Toolkit for an example of a monthly, quarterly, and annual budget breakdown (Folder 4: 11.4.1).

Procurement: Supplier Relations and the Supply Chain

Digitization and the marked shifts in global social, political, and economic forces over the past 25 years have revolutionized procurement practices (Daft, 2012). My grandmother managed and owned a children's clothing store, and I recall the realms of paper, logbooks, and binders vividly. How times have changed. Back then, nothing was automated—everything in the supply chain wheel depended on manual processes. We are now living in technology-driven workplaces, and procurement practices have evolved immensely, including how computers, emails, and automated online purchasing have impacted supplier relations. Today, just the task of computer-based asset purchasing can be a full-time job.

Supply chain management and maintaining healthy supplier–customer relationships are important manager functions. Working to build strong relationships with your suppliers is key to receiving timely and satisfactory service, and creates favorable interpersonal conditions for when problems arise. Invest and make time for getting to know your supplier company representatives and welcome them as collaborators on your team. Sales and service professionals from the simulation industry are keen to offer flexible solutions and to help customers meet operational and educational goals. Don't hesitate to ask for their assistance; they are the experts in product knowledge, operations, maintenance, and servicing.

Supply chains represent the flow of products starting with the supplier and ending with the customer. In a basic supply chain model, suppliers furnish goods to manufacturers; manufacturers sell goods to distributors, and distributors resell goods to retailers; retailers sell to the customer (Daft, 2012). *Supply chain management*, therefore, means to manage the "sequence of suppliers and purchasers, covering all stages of processing from obtaining raw materials to distributing finished goods to consumers" (p. 51). For example, it is important for managers to understand and think about the many steps involved in creating a simulator before it arrives on your doorstep. Effective and efficient procurement of goods takes time and planning. *Inventory* refers to all Program assets, including hardware and requires inventory management that ensures the optimum number or amount of each inventory item to provide uninterrupted production, sales, and/or customer-service at a minimum cost (Businessdictionary.com, 2016).

There are many levels of decision-making and approvals tied to new purchases in a Simulation Program. Make friends with internal procurement department representatives and senior administrators. They have knowledge and skills regarding procurement processes like sourcing out a prime vendor; initiating the tender process and issuing a request for proposal (RFP) for large ticket items (usually anything about $75,000.00 or more); leading procurement selections procedures; providing assistance with asset lifecycle replacement; and inventory tagging and tracking. The following questions provide food for thought regarding procurement practices in your Program:

● How will requests for the acquisition of new equipment or supplies be processed?
● What is the budget source for the purchase? Do you have the dollars you need?

- What is the prioritization process for purchases?
- Who has the right to get what, and when? Who pays?
- How will you source out your purchases? Do you need to engage your procurement department? Is there a group or committee whose input you require (i.e., faculty)?
- Who makes the final decision to purchase? Do you need the approval of other individuals/groups/departments?
- Do you have or need a prime vendor service agreement/provider?
- Who will be responsible for generating new purchase orders to suppliers?
- What is your approval mechanism for purchases in your Simulation Program? Is there a maximum dollar allowance that will trigger the need for higher-level approvals? Where will requests go for approval?
- What process will your Program use for tagging and tracking equipment?
- Will you have asset lifecycle management process to archive old equipment and upgrade to new?
- Is there an institutional policy for procurement (RFPs or other competitive processes such as issuing tenders to potential vendors)? What is the dollar value assigned to initiate the competitive bidding process (also known as tendering)?

For detailed information on asset management, see the Chapter 27 online workbooks. There is a wealth of information and resources available to you there. Included is a sample *Inventory Template* to get your Program inventory tracking started off on the right foot (Folder 4: 11.4.3).

Invoicing and Collections

The task of invoicing and collections is critical, and especially so for Simulation Programs that use a revenue generating business model for viability and sustainability. Develop policy and procedures for both. If you don't have integrated program management software that automatically generates invoices, consider developing of electronic forms. Clearly articulate the process for billing, issuing, tracking, closing, and acceptable methods for contacting and collecting payment. Think about consequences that may ensue for nonpaying customers. A sample *Invoice for Simulation Program* is located in (Folder 4: 11.4.4).

Managing for Sustainability and Complexity

Managing for some may be intuitive, but in today's highly complex environments, managing itself has become increasingly complex. Simulation Program managers are no exception and require management knowledge and skills to do the job well. Managers must forge good relations with the principal stakeholders, competitors, customers, marketers, vendors, and of course their leaders and employees. Today, managers are called to employ more human-centered management approaches. To achieve this end means being relational, having moral and ethical courage, and being culturally sensitive within populations that are increasingly diverse. Ethical management is now "accepted as a fundamental skill" (Marcelino-Sadaba, Gonzalez-Jaen, & Perez-Ezcurdia, 2015, p. 12) and ethics has become increasingly important with increases in environmental complexity (Daft, 2012). Therefore, whether you are a Simulation manager, or you are searching to hire one, ensure that the incumbent treats employees fairly and supports them to perform at their best.

Organizational and Simulation Program Stewardship

Sustainability is a cortical concept that is vital in 21st century management. Humanity has reached a crucial turning point in a world that is experiencing exploding populations, extreme poverty, and unprecedented positive and negative environmental challenges (United Nations General Assembly, 2012). Our planet is going through sweeping climates changes, accompanied by a lack of fresh water, the continuous demise of living species, changes in the chemistry of oceans and land, and unparalleled technological advancement that is putting our world under unprecedented stress (Rockstrom et al., 2009; Sachs, 2016; The Royal Society, 2014). Sustainability, however, is not just something for scientists to figure out. Each of us has an important part to play in turning the tide for the future of all humanity.

The term *sustainability* means being able to use resources without completely depleting or destroying them so as to last or continue for a long time (Merriam-Webster Online Dictionary, 2016). Sustainable development practices entail the interplay of three complex systems: the world economy, the global economy, and the Earth's physical environment (Rockstrom et al., 2009; Sachs, 2016). Sustainable development also focuses on "social interactions of trust, inequality, and social support in communities" (Sachs, p. 1). To be sustainable, Simulation Program personnel must engage in critical inquiry using scientific- and moral-based problem solving approaches toward sustainable practices that will benefit the both the Program, as well as our planet. The term "simulator graveyards" comes to mind. Industry, academics, and healthcare providers need to come together to find solutions to these problems. For example, some vendors provide options for simulator recycling and repurposing of parts.

Increasingly, we are called to do more with less and to be good stewards of our financial and social environments (Pattillo et al., 2010). But what does it mean to be a good steward? According to Sachs (2016) good stewards stem from good societies that are fashioned upon four basic pillars: "economic prosperity; social inclusion and cohesion; environmental sustainability; and good governance" (p. 3). Programs, using the four pillars, can work toward building economic, social, environmental, and governance sustainability. Each of us has a part to play in leaving a smaller footprint behind. Contemporary managers must embrace and put into practice an, "act local but think global" perspective.

To accomplish sustainability, managers also need to enact *knowledge translation* (KT) in their work and Simulation Programs. KT involves the syntheses, dissemination, exchange, and ethically sound application of knowledge to improve (the organization and its outcomes) (Canadian Institutes of Health Research [CIHR], 2015). Both sustainability and KT are now standards that are considered a part of corporate social responsibility. As dollars are squeezed and competition for projects increases, sustainability and KT are weighty criteria in project selection and funding allocation.

Pattillo et al. (2010), created The Capacity Building for Simulation Sustainability Model (CBSS) (see Fig. 11.8). Employing a complex systems approach, the CBSS Model maps a Program's inputs, throughputs, and outputs to build capacity in their Simulation Program. *Inputs* in this Program were considered nursing infrastructure (technologies, lab space, simulation equipment and supplies), university infrastructure (technologies and personnel), and national standards (National League for Nursing, simulation resources, literature, conferences, best practices [INACSL Standards of Best Practice Simulation^SM

(INACSL Standards Committee, 2016)]); *throughputs* were collaborative relationships (Idaho Simulation Network, needs surveys, personal interviews), teaching strategies (existing, literature review, faculty research), and organizational relationships (workshops, resources sharing, satisfaction surveys, continuing ed. courses); and *outputs* were faculty outcomes (participation in simulation, internal website and evaluation tools for simulation), student outcomes (pre-, posttests, knowledge surveys, quizzes, satisfaction surveys); and community outcomes (personal interviews, written surveys). The intrinsic feedback that shaped the model came from student, faculty, and administrative evaluation. External feedback comprised community evaluation, accrediting agencies, contributions, and additional simulation development). This model provides a good example of how Programs can employ a complex systems model to evaluate simulation activities (Pattillo et al., 2010). In education, capacity building links to any strategy that closes the student -learning gap where learning of competencies and attitudes are measurable. Sustainability, in this model, is tied to both educational and revenue-generating successes.

Fiscal Sustainability

Fiscal sustainability in Simulation Programs begins with securing sustainable funding sources. It also involves the responsible use of valuable resources. Business models rely on revenue generation for profit, whereas, cost recovery models used in most academic institutions access

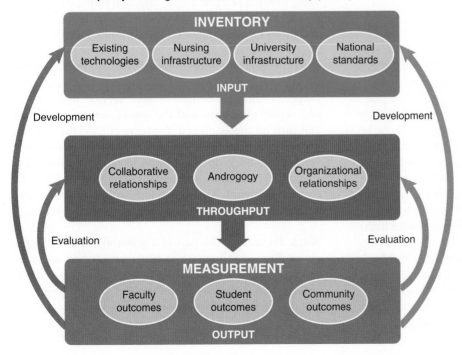

Figure 11.8 The Capacity Building for Simulation Sustainability Model (CBSS). (From Pattillo, R. E., Hewett, B., McCarthy, M. D., & Molinari, D. (2010, September). Capacity building for simulation sustainability. *Clinical Simulation in Nursing, 6*(5), e185–e191. doi: 10.1016/j.ecns.2009.08.008, with permission.)

operating funds through course fees, student material fees, or via the allocation of a percentage of the organizational operating budget. Fiscal sustainability also requires a strategy for asset management; practices to ensure equipment longevity (such as powering down equipment procedures); maximizing value through vendor buy-back programs for retired simulators; and responsible equipment surplus and donation programs. Read along as Kim Leighton describes a cost cutting measure her institution used.

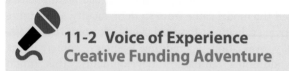

11-2 Voice of Experience
Creative Funding Adventure

Kim Leighton, PhD, RN, CHSE, CHSOS, ANEF

The Challenge

Finding funding for the early, more expensive, versions of the patient simulators was not easy for nursing schools and their tight budgets. In 2003, our college president asked me to attend a conference, "check out" the human patient simulator, and then let her know whether we should buy one for our school. The price tag, at that time, was an approximate $218,000. From where in the world would that money come?

Meeting the Challenge

Phylis Holloman, former President of Bryan College of Health Sciences had a plan and vision. She had been saving money for several years just for this purpose. How? Well, a fashion show and silent auction! While most think that a price tag that large needs to be covered with a grant or substantial donor gift, Phylis knew that if she kept at it, the money would build. Each year the college (a diploma school of nursing, at that time) hosted its annual *Flair for Care*, a fashion show with models that included nurses, physicians, and their children modeling clothing from the high-fashion district of Lincoln, NE. While we partook in eating our delicious meals, the silent auction of hundreds of items continued in the background. Student nurses working the crowd let people know when they were overbid so that they could increase their bids. Husker football tickets for a big game can command

a high price! So can a week at someone's vacation home. Sometimes the greatest treat was seeing a puppy that got to go to a new home after the event.

Outcome

These events continued over the years and averaged around $35,000/year in revenue for a 4-hour event. Not a bad return on investment!

Most Valuable Lessons Learned

I urge leaders not to be overwhelmed by the cost of simulation and instead, to think of practical—and fun—ways to meet your ongoing needs.

Environmental Awareness and Monitoring

Green initiatives to support both environmental and economic sustainability include such things as: energy efficiency (sensors and monitoring systems to conserve electricity, and energy use; air quality monitoring; the purchase and monitoring of low-energy AV and IT equipment; using Leadership in Energy and Environmental Design [LEED]) certified building construction; actively implementing a Three-R program to reduce, reused, and recycle equipment and medical supplies, printer cartridges, and plastic ware whenever possible; limiting photocopying and printing to essential only; converting to electronic and cloud-based data storage to limit paper-based documents; and being conscious of transportation costs by limiting deliveries between campus sites or service providers, using group travel and carpooling, and riding your bicycle or walking to work. Other ways to promote fiscal health and promote environmental sustainability include the use of green practices. Examples include initiatives like (1) the use of responsible procurement practices like asset life-cycle management programs; (2) promoting equipment longevity through comprehensive service maintenance and repair programs, and the use of automatic shut on and turn on mechanism to conserve energy; (3) reducing waste by advocating for equipment donation programs or vendor buy-backs as opposed to having it surplussed or stockpiled in a warehouse, and (4) executing measures for cost containment. More content to come on green practices later in this chapter section on fiscal management.

Waste Prevention: As part of a green mindset, Programs are challenged to manage and prevent medical and non-medical waste. The World Health Organization (2015c) reports that nonmedical waste generated by healthcare activities accounts for approximately 85% of total waste, with the remaining 15% consisting of hazardous materials that may be infectious, toxic, or radioactive waste (WHO,

2015c, para. 1). In our simulation Program, we put great effort into implementing waste prevention strategies. One example is to issue skills kits that learners can retain and reuse for the duration of the program. We sponsor a medical equipment-recycling program for used kits that allows learners to come and refresh kit components as needed.

 We also offer a Medical Waste Management Reduction Program populated by student volunteers. Go to the online Toolkit for a sample (Folder 4: 11.4.12) and a sample *Student Volunteer Request Form* (Folder 4: 11.4.13).

Stakeholders and Committees

Defining Stakeholders: Who Are They?

A *stakeholder* is a person or group that is affected by or has a vested interest in the Simulation Program's operations or services, such as the employees, customers/students/faculty, local community, local businesses, or agencies/organizations. Typically, internal stakeholders are those that exist within your organization. External stakeholders are those who exist from outside the organization. When identifying stakeholder groups, consider that relationships and affiliations with stakeholders play a key role in the strategic development of your Program. Relationship building is key. Be proactive to aligning yourself with the following types of stakeholder individuals/groups: (1) persons with the authority to make decisions about the Program; (2) persons that deal directly with program operations such as management; (3) funding groups or funding agencies; (4) contributors that can add credibility and visibility your efforts or program(s), either internally or externally; (5) others who impact day-to-day implementation of the activities and are part of the Simulation Program; (6) advocates for, or those that authorize changes to the program and contribute to recommendations for change; and (7) those affected by the Program such as patients or clients, advocacy groups, community members, and

 elected officials. See *A Guidebook to Strategic Planning* in the Toolkit (Folder 1: 11.1.2) for a comprehensive list of Simulation Program Stakeholders.

Simulation Program Committees

This question often surfaces, "Which committees are needed to operationalize a simulation program?" In response, it is best to underscore the importance of assembling strong core teams, as opposed to having a certain number or type of committee. Although there are commonalities in committee types and structures

between Simulation Programs, no two entities will look the same. To start the process of building your simulation committee types and structures, pull out the *Simulation Program Committees Pick and Pull Chart and Terms of Reference* sample (Folder 7: 11.7.5). The pick and pull chart provides sample committee types, potential functions, and suggested membership ideas.

Committee Types

At times, mandates for committee structure and membership are prescribed by the organization. For example, there may be an organizational protocol that stipulates when to strike a standing committee, ad hoc committee, versus needing an advisory committee. Other organizations are more organic and allow groups the freedom to create what they think they need. Be sure to verify this before assembling your teams. Committee types vary considerably so invest time to discern which type will help achieve your specific goals. Meakim (2007) used Kotter's eight steps to change model and a Guiding Coalition to bring about positive organizational change. Kuiper and Zabriskie (2013) describe how they struck a Simulation Learning Committee as one of the phases in building a new Simulation Centre to advocate for best practices in curricular integration before the space was ready. The following is a list of common committee types that might be used in or alongside Simulation Programs:

- *Board of Directors:* found in large organizations where smaller bodies are given the authority to make decisions, spend or allocate money, approve budgets, and take actions (Walker & Bauser, 2012).
- *Governance Committees*: to review the performance of the board of directors and to review board policy as well as nominate candidates for the board (Walker & Bauser, 2012).
- *Advisory Committees* assist and advise a board of directors or other larger committees/groups to fill gaps or provide expert advice (e.g., policy). Members can supplement and guide the work of the board by bringing unique knowledge and skills to guide an organization. An advisory committee can be granted decision-making authority, however, often will focus on advising rather than enacting decisions.
- *Steering Committees* can also be called advisory committees. They are "usually made up of high-level stakeholders and/or experts who provide guidance on key issues such as company policy and objectives, budgetary control, marketing strategy, resource allocation, and decisions involving large expenditures" (http://www.businessdictionary.com). If the projects are long-standing, the committee structure might change to a more permanent one. For example, when a research grant was awarded, a Steering Committee was struck to

oversee, guide and control the expenditures and large decisions (McLeod & Schnell, 2006). Once the grant was expended, the committee evolved into a permanent operations committee.

- *Standing Committees* are permanent and formal, and operate with standing rules, by-laws or regulations within (or outside) your organization (i.e., Simulation Curriculum Development Committee). These committees function within a particular scope as defined by key guiding documents of the larger organization. Standing committees usually make recommendations or advise those that have ultimate decision-making authority, such as, a Board or Executive Committee members (Robert, Honemann, & Balch, 2011).
- *Sub-Committees:* smaller sub-sets of a larger committee. They can be long-, or short-term in nature. Any committee can have sub-committees to accomplish work or the greater committee in smaller teams (Robert et al., 2011).
- *Ad Hoc Committees*: are appointed as temporary bodies for a specific reason and have a short-term mandate. Once the committee has served its function, the committee is dissolved and disbands.

Number of Committees

The number of committees you form will depend on many factors, such as the size of your Simulation Program, the population(s) you serve, the amount and type of simulation offered, and the outcomes the Program is aiming to achieve. For example, if your Simulation Program serves just one faculty (a single discipline), rather than forming an entirely new set simulation specific committees, consider forming simulation sub-committees that branch off of existing committees, such as, a standing nursing curriculum committee. If you have a larger Simulation Program, it is wise to have Program specific committees for ease of planning, tracking, and reporting on committee work and results. Know what is vital for the group to achieve, and then design your committee structure and membership requirements from there. It has been my experience that having one or two high functioning committees with active members is better than spreading yourself too thin between a greater number of committees. Often in simulation, the same Simulation Champions reappear on several committees, so it might be better to consolidate and conquer as part of one entity.

Committee Power and Authority

Beware of the "death by committee" syndrome. There is nothing worse than asking people to donate their time, generate fabulous ideas, and then have absolutely no power to enact those ideas. Make sure you have the people you need to make things happen on your committee. Create the committee terms of reference and membership inclusion/exclusion criteria. Think about the committee's mandate, its specific goals, and objectives, and reporting and approval mechanisms for the committee's work. Start the search for the Simulation Champions in your midst and invite them to membership on a committee. Think about who will comprise your core simulation team and what decision-making authority they will need to have.

Representation on Institutional Committees

Carefully examine where you will need Simulation Program representation on institution-wide or external committees, such as a Campus Technology Committee. Your presence may be required on a variety of internal and external committees or with simulation associations or networking groups. There is a broad range of possibilities. Consider how will you network with other groups to facilitate simulation initiatives with other working groups/committees at the local, provincial/state, national level, or international levels?

Read Carol Huston's account below of how a Simulation Integration Committee was able to meet the needs of an underfunded Simulation Program by forming a *Simulation Integration Committee.*

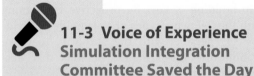

11-3 Voice of Experience
Simulation Integration
Committee Saved the Day

**Carol L. Huston,
MSN, DPA, FAAN**

The Challenge

In light of competition for clinical sites that required students to commute up to 200 miles per day for clinical, the results of the NCSBN study (2014) suggesting simulation could be as effective as traditional clinical in promoting student learning, and the availability of a top-notch simulation center locally, the faculty at Chico School of Nursing (CSU) located in California, USA, voted to increase their utilization of simulation. They immediately doubled the amount of clinical time in simulation from 5% to 10% and began to phase in a plan that would increase this to 25% over a 5 year period.

Meeting the Challenge

The excitement faculty felt about using more simulation as a pedagogy gave way quickly to the recognition that implementation would be challenging. The program Director needed to find fiscal resources to support the change, faculty needed additional training in simulation and had to revise courses accordingly, and our small, underfunded simulation center had to figure out how to accommodate what sounded like a minor change. In reality, the change resulted in a very significant increase in clinical hours.

Outcome

We formed a *Simulation Integration Committee* of faculty across semesters and programs. The committee established strategic planning goals related to simulation, created a "roll-out plan," and leveled learning objectives related to simulation as a teaching pedagogy across the curriculum. Funding mechanisms were identified and implemented. Implementation challenges did occur; some faculty members were reluctant to give up traditional clinical time while others wanted to opt out of having an active role in scenario development or teaching in the simulation center. Often, this reflected a lack of self-confidence in their ability to use simulation effectively.

Most Valuable Lessons Learned

Involving those most likely to be impacted by the change was key to reducing and eventually overcoming resistance to this change. For faculty "buy-in" to occur, faculty across semesters and programs need to participate in the planning process and be actively involved in using simulation. To achieve this required ongoing faculty development in simulation principles and practice as well as significant leadership and coordination by Simulation Center staff.

Inspiration for Simulation Champions

"We may all be born average, but staying average is a choice."

Simulation Program Personnel

Staffing a Simulation Program

Unlike 10 or 15 years ago when staffing a simulation initiative often involved allocating partial workload to one person, staffing today involves building and developing highly empowered and skilled teams of individuals. Of course,

not all nursing (or other healthcare) programs offer fully integrated simulation curricula, and therefore many do not have dedicated full-time staff. However, it is crucial that leaders that are developing new programs or expanding current ones, be mindful of current evidence that outlines the conditions under which simulation programs should optimally unfold (Alexander et al., 2015; Hayden, Smiley, Alexander, Kardong-Edgren, & Jeffries, 2014). In response to the 2014 NCSBN Study, came the development of the NCSBN Simulation Guidelines for Prelicensure Nursing Programs. These guidelines are designed to help "boards of nursing (BONs) evaluate the readiness of prelicensure nursing programs using simulation as a substitute for traditional clinical experience...(meaning practice in an inpatient, ambulatory care, or community setting where the student provides care to patients under the guidance of an instructor or preceptor)... and for nursing education programs in the establishment of evidence-based simulation programs for the undergraduate nursing curriculum" (Alexander et al., 2015, p. 40). The guidelines serve as benchmarks from which you can begin to plan your Program needs for staffing. Needs assessments can be carried out in a number ways. In *The Project Manager's Guidebook* (Folder 1: 11.1.3), you will find sample SWOT and SOAR analyses to help in conducting a needs assessment. The *Guidebook to Staffing a Simulation Program*

(Folder 1: 11.1.6) offers information on staffing needs assessment; position description writing, sample position descriptions, sample staffing models, and sample interview questions.

As the simulation program in my workplace has grown over the past 20 years, so has the need for increasing the number and diversity in positions. I began as one full-time simulation and lab coordinator with one administrative assistant, and we now have seven full-time simulation employees. In my experiences and my travels around the world, I have witnessed many understaffed simulation programs: all resulting in overstretched, overworked, and exhausted employees. I have come to learn that successful Simulation Programs need excellent leadership and the backing of administrators and executive sponsor(s). Also needed are dedicated lead faculty and other qualified educator champions to spearhead curricular integration and the skilled facilitation of simulation. There is a need for support personnel prepared to assist such as simulation operations specialists and appropriate facilities equipped with the necessary educational, technological, and equipment resources. Additionally, good governance is needed to develop and enact policies and

processes (Alexander et al., 2015; García & Guisado, 2012; Gallagher & Issenberg, 2007). For additional information and tools, refer back to the *Guidebook to Staffing a Simulation Program* (Folder 1: 11.6).

Staffing Models for Simulation Programs

It is critical to design a staffing model to support plans for simulation learning. Without adequate numbers of trained staff, Programs will fall short of reaching established goals. The staffing model and corresponding staffing complement you choose is dependent on many factors but is driven primarily by the size and the scope of your Simulation Program. As demands for more simulation mount, you will invariably find yourself short of staff. Back in the day, we had very basic staffing models. The typical model being one person working alone that may, or may not be assigned formal workload to deliver simulation. Since then, the world has changed and thankfully, so have simulation-staffing models. It is now recognized that simulation requires a skilled team of trained individuals to effectively deploy simulation (Alexander et al., 2015; Dongilli, 2016; Gantt & Young, 2016b; Huang & Dongilli, 2008; Riley, 2016; Seropian, Brown, Gavilanes, & Driggers, 2004a). However, it is acknowledged that while smaller Programs with smaller student numbers and one simulator might require partial workload release for simulation, other larger full-scale simulation centers will need a dedicated simulation team.

When developing your Simulation Program staffing model, think about the following three key development areas: (1) administration and operations needs; (2) simulation education needs; and (3) support needs. Within each development area, five skill sets must be present with a Program's staffing model: "project management, educational design, advanced clinician, technology support, and administrative support" (Denning et al., 2010, p. 340). Cheney and Josey (2014) offer a role-based approach to determining staffing in Simulation Programs. They suggest a variety of roles that apply: Administrator/ Leader/Coordinator, Simulation Scenario/Curriculum Development, the Subject Matter Expert, Programming Operations, Facilitator, Debriefer, Evaluator, Researcher, Data analyst, Technical support, Audiovisual, Scheduler/ Administrative Assistant, Human Factors, Clinical Educators, and Simulated patient educators. Knowing your Simulation Program focus will also help to determine staffing needs. Brock and Holtschneider (2016) identify the purposes of simulation operations as, (1) Training and Clinical Research; (2) Education and Advocacy; (3) Research and Development; (4) Assessment of Competence; and (5) Improvement in Patient Safety and Quality. Build your team around core Simulation Program goals. At a minimum, plan to include three streams of personnel in your staffing model: administrative, educational/ clinical, and technical expertise.

- *Administrative expertise* entails a background in leadership and management. Functions include creating and operationalizing the strategic plan, managing the budget and many projects, and managing human capital.

- *Technical expertise* includes a background in information systems, audio-visual, electronics, biomedical engineering, and computer graphics where functions include simulator installation, care, maintenance, and repair, to scenario programming or developing virtual simulation. Some larger Programs have created specific positions for each of the background areas noted above.

- *Educational and clinical expertise* include a background in teaching and learning, specific clinical disciplinary knowledge and skills, and especially simulation educator knowledge and skills. Functions include facilitation, simulation design, assessment and evaluation of learning. For a comprehensive list of common positions and roles common to many Simulation Programs, see the *Guidebook to Staffing a Simulation Program* (Folder 1: 11.6).

Little has been written about staffing models for simulation. However, Berro and Knowsel (2016) wrote of their innovative use of new graduate nurse volunteers in their Program as a means of extending resources. The volunteer nurse served as "support person during simulation sessions, and responsibilities included the setup and break down of simulations, assisting with technical aspects of running the computer program, maintenance of human patient simulators, managing the video recording system, portraying the voice of the patient, and assisting with the observation of student participation during simulations" (p. 53). Faculty perceived this position to be an invaluable resource and quickly upgraded it to a paid simulation nurse intern position. Other programs have leveraged existing resources by offering students a variety of volunteer opportunities with the laboratory setting.

To date, I know of no magic formula to determine exact staffing requirements. What I can tell you is that determining your staffing needs is a complex task that involves some degree of experimentation using various staffing combinations. Fundamentally, you must consider your specific needs based on population size and type, space and equipment availability, the nature and number of planned and projected simulated clinical immersion events, the needed resources, and expectations for support. Three staffing models and organizational charts, one for each of small, medium, and large Programs are in the online Toolkit— *Guidebook to Staffing a Simulation Program* (Folder 1: 11.6). Also, there is a sample *Simulation Team Scheduling Template* we created using Google Docs (Folder 4: 11.4.5). This team schedule planner provides and example of how closely simulation teams must work together to enact simulation. The form resides in the Cloud and each team member inputs their own information so that we are aware of each other's needs. Many Cloud-based calendar and scheduling products offer similar capabilities.

Allocating Workload and Workload Hours

Eisert and Geers (2016) conducted a recent study examining how much faculty time is required to enact simulation activities. Although the findings are not generalizable due to a small sample size, interestingly they found that approximately 26.9% of time went to pre-scenario learning, deploying the simulation scenarios, and debriefing. Other elements such as simulation design, evaluation, and cleanup accounted for 73.1% of time reported by faculty. These findings have implications for administrators when allocating workload for those engaged in simulation education. It would be faulty to allocate workload based only on time spent in the Simulation Center. Administrators must also consider the tremendous amount of time it takes to design, deploy, and evaluate simulation-based learning. For example, the setting up of supplies, room staging, application of moulage, and taking down of props and equipment alone requires masterful planning for simulation to be well-executed. This fact holds true whether the simulation educational modality unfolds in the sim suite, the classroom, on the road, or in situ. Kardong-Edgren and Oermann (2009) underscored the challenges faced by Deans and Chairs of nursing programs, suggesting that administrators need to get in step with the additional time and skills faculty need to deliver an effective simulation, as well as, the need for other personnel to enact simulation. Each Program will need to develop their unique approach to workload, but it is clear that it must happen if Simulation Programs are to succeed.

Expanding the Team—It Starts by Asking for New Positions

If you are not starting a brand new Program, invariably the need to expand your staff will surface. It is important to collect data that supports the need for a staffing increase. Consider the following questions to guide data collection:

- What is the current use of simulation in your Program?
- Which disciplines are currently using simulation and plans to expand? What are the current and projected group sizes for each?
- What is the probability that you will receive additional fiscal support for simulation? Are you anticipating new funding sources?
- How many full time dedicated positions are exclusive to simulation?
- Is there clarity regarding faculty roles in simulation Curriculum planning and simulation design? For example, computer operation? Voice of the patient? Will faculty be inside or outside the simulation room? Prebriefing and debriefing?
- What are current event flow patterns and how many staff are required to deliver simulations using that configuration (timing, group size, room allocation, flow of people)? Event flows take into account the following:
  - Number of rooms used for each simulation event
  - Number of students per simulation event
  - Total length in hours/minutes of the simulation events
  - Timing breakdown of the simulation event (length of preparation, prebriefing, simulation, debriefing) aches the simulation repeated, or not
  - Turn around time between events (room re-staging, moving people, prop resets) how often you use
- What is the current staffing pattern simulated patients, for running simulations (will vary depending on scenario)? Consider embedded actors, patient voice, computer operator, etc.
- What is the maximum number of hours* per faculty member in simulation per day—(anecdotally, we have found our faculty limit to be 6 hours in the simulation lab, allowing for an additional 1-hour lunch and short coffee breaks, for a total of 8 hours/day). Working more than 6 hours/day has proven to be very draining and faculty communicate a decrease in the quality of facilitation. This timeframe might also drop further, especially when facilitating simulations with emotionally charged content.
- How will you plan for additional coverage in the case of absences (i.e., illness)? How much sick time is incurred for staff/faculty? What is your plan B? Or C? Are staff working additional unpaid hours, or are you consistently paying staff overtime? Are people complaining of exhaustion and being overworked?

Personnel in the MacEwan Clinical Simulation Centre (CSC) (my place of employment) serve approximately 1,300 undergraduate students in its healthcare programs (primarily nursing). The current simulation staffing model includes seven designated full-time employees comprising: 1 Full-time (FT) Director, 3 FT dedicated Simulation Educators, 1 FT Administrative Assistant, 1 FT Lab Assistant - materials/resource manager, 1 FT Simulation Technologist, and several student volunteers. Additionally, we have 80+ faculty trained as simulation facilitators (the majority of theory/clinical/lab instructors engage). At MacEwan, learners take part in simulated clinical immersion events several times per course offering throughout the nursing program (in the classroom/labs/clinical orientation/seminar). We run approximately 20 curricular integrated simulations for all students in nursing programs. These simulations unfold within varied spaces, including a dedicated simulation suite, a standardized patient exam suite, classrooms, and laboratory learning spaces. Our staffing model hence involves a blend of dedicated simulation staff and trained faculty from the BScN program.

Today, there are more Programs that have full-time **simulation delivery teams** to design, deploy, and evaluate the entire Simulation Program and therefore, have 100% of their full-time workload dedicated to simulation. The Bachelor of Nursing Program at the University of Calgary in Alberta, Canada uses this model. They have a simulation delivery team comprised of full-time continuing or tenured faculty employed as full-time dedicated simulation educators. The dedicated sim team fills all roles for simulation-based learning, such as simulation design, facilitation (prebriefing and debriefing), assessment and evaluation, patient voice, embedded actor, computer operators, and setup and take down (P. Morgan, personal communication, 2016). Using this model fosters conditions that promote consistency and quality in simulation deployment while having the team readily available for simulation-specific operational and educational sessions.

Inexperienced managers may find it stressful to ask for new positions and therefore may shy away from asking. Take solace in the fact that the need to expand personnel is common to all developing Simulation Programs, so prepare ahead. The ask is usually precipitated by mounting demands and subsequent stress on employees without adding extra people; adding new simulation modalities or typologies without knowledge of what is involved (i.e., a Simulated Patient Program); or having personnel leave accompanied by a failure to implement succession planning. The later instance however, does create an opportunity to reconfigure your current staffing model.

To ascertain staffing needs, start by conducting a *needs assessment*. If you have a team in place, start by tracking operational requirements, staff hours, and functions (including documentation on the need for cross-functionality). Inquire as to current workload demands and record them using quantifiable statistical data such as sick time or overtime that is, staff are working in excess of 12.5 hours each per week for a total of 200 hours in overtime payment monthly equaling $6,000.00/month or $72,000.00/year. This could be the equivalent of one full-time position. You may also want to include statistics on outputs or results. Consider whether employees are working outside their current scope of practice (e.g., simulation educator is spending 60% of daily hours engaged in technology support), then decide on a position that would be a better fit, such as a simulation operations specialist. If you do not have an existing Program, you might start by gathering data from other Simulation Programs related to numbers of students, numbers of simulation events run, staffing complement, and average workload hours in simulation, outside of simulation. Do a comparative analysis and based on the results, make a determination of your projected staffing needs.

Gather data on the new position and include a list of tasks and related competencies. Begin by grouping tasks into larger roles or areas of responsibility: Leadership role, academic role, administrative role, scholarship, service, etc. Explore the current budget and look for synergies or

flexibility. For example, we decided to change our reception front desk hours to ½ days only to accommodate that person working in a different capacity within our Program for the afternoons. This created a domino effect that freed up dollars in other areas. If you budget doesn't allow for a new hire, you are going to need to write a proposal for allocation of new dollars to the budget or get creative. Once the new dollars have been earmarked, you can proceed with the HR processes.

Position Descriptions, Scope of Work, and Classification

In recent years, there has been an increasing acknowledgment of the need for specially trained personnel to successfully run simulation programs (Alexander et al., 2015, National League for Nursing—Simulation Innovation Resource Centre, 2016; SSH Credentialing, 2016b). The rapid expansion of SBL resulted in the increased differentiation and diversity in the types of personnel we now see staffing Simulation Programs. Refer to the *Guidebook to Staffing a Simulation Program* (Folder 1: 11.6) in the online Toolkit. Additionally, INACSL and SSH both offer a job description repository and job postings site for their members-only websites.

Project far in advance for simulation expansion because as the use of simulation expands, so does the need for staff. Remember to engage your Human Resources department in the hiring process from the outset. HR personnel are invaluable when it comes to writing position descriptions and classifying job descriptions to determine salaries/pay rates. Staff position descriptions could be written as expected outcomes with measureable behaviors that each employee is expected to achieve. This facilitates an approach that enables outcome-based **performance appraisals** to be realistic, objective and achievable. The CHSE, CHSE-A, and CHSOS CHSOS Credentialing Standards are a very useful guide when determining expected performance outcomes (SSH, 2016b).

Your HR rep brings essential knowledge of organizational hiring practices and policies. For example, in a unionized environment, it is helpful to discuss position classifications and evaluate how each would fit within institutional collective agreements. Some positions are hired within the scope of a collective agreement, while others may reside outside a collective agreement—or out of scope.

Who is Who? Personnel on the Simulation Team

People are the number one resource in Simulation Programs and the number of personnel required to support simulation-based learning is substantial (Jones, Hennessey, & Deutsch, 1985 as cited in Gantt & Young,

2016b). Programs do run the risk of having a fantastic, fully equipped state-of-the-art facility that sits unused or misused without the right people to run it. Be sure to create an organizational chart **organizational chart** that features employee roles and responsibilities. See the *Guidebook to Staffing a Simulation Program* (Folder 1: 11.6) in the online Toolkit for *sample job descriptions*.

Administrative, Leadership, and Management Personnel

According to the Society for Simulation in Healthcare accreditation process (SSH, 2016d), leaders and managers of Simulation Programs must possess the academic, clinical, leadership, managerial, educational, and simulation skills and experience that match the needs of the Simulation Program. Typically, this entails a position titled Program Director, Coordinator, or Manager. Larger Programs with more capacity for staff can separate formal leadership and managerial roles whereas smaller Programs may have one person assuming more than one role and assume many functions.

It is important to place an emphasis finding and hiring leaders with *relational* and *ethical strengths*. That is a person that is consciously and intentionally invested in building honest and open human relationships that are grounded in respect, compassion, and authentic interest in others (Hatrick Doane & Varcoe, 2015). For a leader and simulation professional to be relationally and ethically strong, they must possess the ability to take a critical account of their own assumptions and values and then take action by balancing those in consideration of professional values, as well as the values of others (Hartrick Doane & Varcoe, 2015; Rudolph, Simon, & Raemer, 2015). A relational and ethical leader has a keen sense of what constitutes doing good, or doing harm in a given situation. That person will also work to "protect personal boundaries to preserve the ethical sanctity of relationships" (Austin, Bergum, Nuttgens, & Peternelj-Taylor, 2006, p. 81). As was stated in Chapter 10, high-performing teams thrive within clearly established boundaries, respect, caring, and generous collaboration.

Educational Personnel

Simulation Educators

In the early days, simulation educators in nursing and other healthcare programs were for the most part, the individuals tasked with every single aspect of simulation. Today, new positions and the roles and functions that accompany them have carved out a distinct niche for the simulation educator. Simulation-specific educator training, formal education, and credentialing have become commonplace and in many cases, serve as a hiring criterion for employment. In 2012 the Society for Simulation in Healthcare (SSH) launched its professional credentialing program for the Certified

Healthcare Simulation Educator (CHSE and CHSE-A [Advanced]). The SSH website reports that there are now more than 700 CHSEs from 19 countries around the world. Additional information is available in Chapter 4 and on the SSH website (http://www.ssih.org/Certification/CHSE). Socialization to the simulation practice community in addition to providing quality opportunities for education and training is vital. The NCSBN Guidelines (Alexander et al., 2015) feature a faculty checklist that is helpful when developing a learning plan. Alexander et al., state that faculty members should know and follow the INACSL Standards of Best Practice: Simulation^SM (INACSL Standards Committee, 2016), and be able to "create a learning environment that encourages active learning, repetitive practice, and reflection and to provide appropriate support throughout each activity" (p. 41). Additionally, the program must provide "a means for faculty members to participate in simulation-related professional development, such as webinars, conferences, journals, clubs, readings, and certifications such as Certified Healthcare Simulation Educator (CHSE), and participation in NLN Sim Leaders/Sigma Theta Tau International (STTI) Nurse Faculty Leadership Academy (NFLA) with a "focus on simulation... and collect and retain evaluation data regarding the effectiveness of the facilitator" (p. 41). These are important considerations for the Simulation Program manager as you formulate a plan to develop talent on the team. The SSH Accreditation Core Standards (2016a) and Teaching/Standards also lay out provisions for educators in Simulation Programs, as follows:

"An expert in simulation education oversees the Program's educational activities" (SSH, 2016c, p. 4). Sub-criterion 1.d.i. States, "The Program must document or demonstrate the qualifications of a simulation expert. These can include, but are not limited to: post graduate work in simulation education training; evidence of accumulated experience in simulation in healthcare education for at least 2 years; continuing education (CE) courses in simulation; and simulation certification" (p. 4). The document also denotes that "in many cases the simulation expert who oversees the educational activities is the same person as the Program Director" (p. 4).

Simulated/Standardized Patient Simulation Educators

A specific subset of simulation educators entails training as a Simulated/Standardized Simulation Educator. Apart from the SSH simulation educator credentialing process, there are multiple opportunities for acquiring the fundamental knowledge in SP methodology required to facilitate learning using simulated/standardized patients (Heine & Ferguson, 2015). The Association of Standardized Patient Educators (ASPE) offers a Core Curriculum Program and features a web page that lists other SP educator learning opportunities and certificate programs (http://www.aspeducators.org/node/100). The National League for Nursing, Simulation Innovation Resource Center offers an online module on Simulated/Standardized Patients (http://sirc.nln.org/mod/page/view.php?id=842), and INACSL offers fellowship and mentoring opportunities. If you are planning on integrating the use of simulated patients in your Program, it is strongly advisable to access education and training for new hires prior to starting their new role, or at a minimum plan for this training immediately upon hiring.

Technical Personnel

Simulations Operations Specialists

The simulation operations specialist (SOS) has emerged over the past 10 to 15 years in response to clinical and healthcare education program increasing demands for technological expertise in simulation-based learning environments (Gantt & Young, 2016b). The title itself includes many variations such as, "simulation technician, simulation specialist, simulation technology specialist, simulation operator" (Gantt & Young, 2016b, p. 6), and simulation technologist, or simulation technology specialist (STS) among others.

More and more, Simulation Program teams recognize the value of the SOS and the need for technical expertise to manage the vast technological infrastructure required to deploy simulation (Nicholas, Spain, Lopez, & Walker, 2015). The SOS provides essential support to the sim team, possessing expertise in computer operations and programming of technological systems such as simulators, web-based recording system, and virtual learning platforms. More specifically, they:

● Lead in the preparation, use, maintenance, and repair of simulators
● Manage, program, and operate web-based audio-visual recording and storage systems and related information technology systems
● Assist with room preparation including setup, take-down, and moulage
● Support event flow during simulation events
● In some cases, provide assistance with prebriefing and debriefing (Bailey, 2016; Dongilli, 2016; Young, 2016)

Today, the SOS is recognized as an essential and as a unique sim team member that complements the simulation educator role. Simulation educators are content experts that focus on the design, deployment, and evaluation the simulation program curriculum and are skilled at simulation facilitation. More recently, the status of the SOSs on the team has been bolstered by a new professional certification offered by the SSH starting in 2014 to 2015: the Certified Healthcare Simulation Operations Specialist (CHSOS).

As the sole simulation educator and simulation lead for our program, I found myself increasingly overwrought with mounting demands of the job and therefore, I eventually reached out to someone with the technological expertise I lacked. I now laugh at the things I had my faculty doing. For example, all faculty members (20+) in our program received training in programming the simulator's physiological modeling software. Say what? For many, the sheer complexity of that one task proved to be too much, while others thrived. I was also doing much of the simulator maintenance and some of the repairs. Although we had purchased vendor warranties, the first simulators we bought required cross-border shipping for all repairs. This made my ever-expanding role as simulation lead even more complicated. I couldn't keep up and it was clear that needed help! The SOS (aka life saver) we hired came to us with a computer programming and graphic design background and without previous experience in healthcare.

Not all Programs however, have this level of technological support and it continues to fall within the scope of other positions, including the faculty role. Initially, the SOS role often emerged as part of simulation clinician and educator roles. Today, the SOS professional stems from diverse healthcare backgrounds such as, allied health, nursing, medicine, and other healthcare professions; as well as, nonmedical backgrounds like engineering, computer programming, information technology (IT), audio-visual technology (AV), and project management (Gantt & Young, 2016b). Young (2016) suggests that there are two critical background areas required of the SOS: (1) experience in healthcare, and (2) comfort (and skill) with computer and audio-visual technology. Detailed information on the SOS is available in Chapter 21.

Ideally, the SOS will have both healthcare and technological knowledge and skills, but this is not always the case nor is it realistic. Dongilli points out that many SOSs have become involved in "academic, operations, administrative, and research sides of simulation" (2016, p. 164). The trend towards increasing integration of the SOS on sim teams is tied to budget cuts to educational programs, program demands for more simulation, and the need for more data on simulation outcomes (Dongilli, 2016). Knowing this, you will need to consider the division of labor and the scope of each position that best suits your chosen sim team-staffing model. There are many potential areas of *cross-functionality* between them. See the online Toolkit in Chapter 10 for Cross-Functional Team Tool.

The SSH—CHSOS credentialing requirements listed on the SSH website are as follows (SSH, 2016b). Applicants must demonstrate: "(1) participation in healthcare simulation in an operations role; (2) focused simulation expertise on learners in undergraduate, graduate, allied health or healthcare practitioners; (3) a Bachelor's degree or equivalent experience; and (4) have 2 years of experience in a healthcare simulation operations role" (para. 2). In the years to come, I believe that it will be feasible to expect formal SOS education to emerge. However, it will be a challenge to develop and offer programs for SOS training that provide current and relevant industry knowledge, as well as, best practices in technology and simulation education (Dongilli, 2016). Onboarding the SOS with a nonmedical background is a process that can require extensive orientation to the language of medical simulation and perhaps, education. Training and education for sim techs is available in many locations using a variety of educational delivery platforms. See the *Guidebook to Simulation Team Talent Development* (Folder 1: 11.1.5) in the online Toolkit for a long list of learning opportunities for sim team training.

Simulation Moulage Technicians

The word moulage refers to the "art of applying mock injuries or conditions for the purpose of training (healthcare) students and other medical personnel" (Schleicher, 2014, para. 1). Moulage is often a function of many staff members in Simulation Programs; however, today moulage technicians/artists possess specialized skill sets that require training in the art of moulage. Many resource books and training opportunities exist, and depending on the extent to which moulage is used in a Program, teams may hire part- or full-time moulage technicians. Refer to Chapter 19.

Simulation Assistants and Administrative Support Personnel

Consider the type and amount of general and administrative support you will need run your Program and deploy simulation. The need for support ranges depending on Program scope and size. Assistive personnel can include full-time, part-time, or casual lab assistants, administrative assistants, and custodial staff. Based on your Program's configuration and size, you might need a receptionist to meet and greet customers/students/faculty, and to do computer processing, organizing, and scheduling. Depending on the budget and the division of labor in your Program, the number of assistive personnel will vary, as will their roles and functions. For example, institutional custodial staff will usually cover basic cleaning requirements, but may not dust or clean all audio-visual equipment. You will need to define who is responsible for cleaning and maintaining simulators, computers, screens, cupboards, and desktops.

Clerical support is vital to smooth functioning so where possible, plan for dedicated administrative positions. Secretaries fill basic clerical duties and administrative assistants fill more complex clerical functions, including project management responsibilities. Simulation Programs require an extensive list of administrative assistance, including bookkeeping, scheduling, coordinating meetings, facility maintenance, repair booking, vendor communications,

connecting to the larger institution, participant registration, borrower services, office supply management, simulation supply and equipment management, organization and maintenance, procurement, shipping and receiving, minute taking, answering, transferring and setting up calls (e.g., teleconference), answer emails, manage incoming and outgoing mail, prepare and send out packages, maintain filing systems, create and manage spreadsheets to enter data, and manage and enter data into databases. So, if you initially thought that having one person oversee the administration, technical, educational, and support needs of your Simulation Program would be sufficient, stop and think again. It will not be long before you find yourself on your knees voicing a desperate plea for help.

Other positions emerging rapidly in Simulation Programs include Biomedical Engineers, Human Factors Engineers, Patient Safety Specialists, Data Analysts, Systems Analysts, Healthcare Team Trainers, Clinical Specialists, and Subject Matter Experts, to name a few.

Managing Human Capital

"Managers today focus on developing, not controlling people to adapt to new technologies and extraordinary shifts, and thus achieve high performance and total corporate effectiveness" (Daft, 2012, p. v).

People are the number one resource in Simulation Programs and the number of personnel required to support the use of simulators is substantial (Jones, Hennessey, & Deutsch, 1985 as cited in Gantt & Young, 2016b). **Human capital management** is defined by Bersin (2013b) as the process of "attracting and engaging highly talented people, developing global leaders, improving and sharing new skills, and keeping people aligned and working together in a highly connected way" (p. 1). You could have an amazing, fully equipped state-of-the-art facility that sits unused or misused without the right people to run your programs. Unlike 10 or 15 years ago when staffing a simulation initiative involved allocating partial workload to one person, today it involves building and developing highly empowered and skilled teams of professionals. Of course, not all nursing (or other healthcare) programs offer fully integrated simulation in their curricula and therefore may not have full-time dedicated staff. However, it is crucial that leaders developing new programs or expanding current ones, be mindful of current evidence that outlines the conditions under which simulation programs should optimally unfold (Hayden et al., 2014). In response to the Hayden Study, the NCSBN formulated the Simulation Guidelines for Prelicensure Nursing Programs. These guidelines were developed to help "boards of nursing (BONs) evaluate the readiness of prelicensure nursing programs using simulation as a substitute for traditional clinical experience…(substitute meaning: practice in an inpatient, ambulatory care, or community setting where the student provides care to patients under the guidance of an instructor or preceptor)… and for nursing education programs in the establishment of evidence-based simulation programs for the undergraduate nursing curriculum" (Alexander et al., 2015, p. 40).

As the Simulation Program in my workplace grew over the past 20 years, so have the needs for increased and more diverse staffing. I began as one full time simulation and lab coordinator with one administrative assistant, and we now have seven full-time simulation employees. In my own experiences and in my travels around the world I have witnessed many understaffed Simulation Programs: all resulting in overstretched, overworked, and exhausted employees. Simulation Programs need the backing of administration, champion executive sponsor(s), appropriate facilities, educational, technological, and equipment resources, lead faculty and simulation personnel that are prepared to lead simulations, and policies and processes to support consistent quality in simulation (Alexander et al., 2015).

Recruiting Talent in Today's Global Market

"In looking for people to hire, you look for three qualities: integrity, intelligence, and energy. If you don't have the first, the other two will kill you."–Warren Buffett

Recruiting involves a process that aims to find the right people for your Simulation Program (see Box 11-6).

Box 11-6	**Steps for Recruiting New Talent**

The steps involved in recruitment include

- Creating a recruitment advertisement (job ad)
- Posting the add via multimedia
- Creating an candidate evaluation screening tool to assess suitability for the position
- Screening and scoring the candidates' submissions to qualify for an interview
- Selecting and confirming the interview panel members
- Scheduling candidates' and interview panel meeting times for interviews
- Creating a list of interview questions, or use a preexisting candidate scoring tools
- Creating a communication strategy and correspondence to reply to unsuccessful candidates
- Generating a formal employment offer for successful candidate—including salary and benefits; be prepared to negotiate terms
- Establishing start dates
- Ascertaining preemployment activities or requirements that must be met with time frames
- Deploying your new talent by arranging for orientation to the Simulation Program and the Organization

It sounds easy, but recruitment processes are becoming increasingly complex as human resources departments work to keep abreast of technology, the pace of change, and shifting demographics in the workforce. Remember that staff recruitment processes must be aligned with institutional practices and protocols. Whether you are asking for a new position that did not previously exist or you are adding additional positions, you will need to justify adding the new member.

Refer to the *Guidebook to Staffing Simulation Programs* for a host of recruiting information and tools like job adds, positions descriptions, interview questions, and more.

Deploying New Talent on the Team

New talent requires the support of a great manager and a welcoming team. Onboarding is a critical time for new employees and sets the tone for what it to come. I have provided you with a list of pre-employment and onboarding strategies to help you plan for the arrival of your new talent. For a pre-employment and orientation checklist for new talent, see the online Toolkit for the *Guidebook to Staffing Simulation a Program* (Folder 1: 11.6).

Developing Talent on the Team

"Train people well enough so they can leave, treat them well enough so they don't want to" Richard Branson (Twitter feed @ richardbranson)

Developing the talent on your team is the key to happy people and positive outcomes. Simulation Champions are by nature curious, motivated, and eager to continue learning. Therefore, it is important that Simulation Programs promote active engagement and life-long learning for their personnel. As far back as 2005, Senge has reported that engagement is a huge part of entire employee value proposition today. It is not just skills building. Simulation Champions want to be a part of something bigger: our mission is to improve the quality of education our learners receive and to shift healthcare culture for safer patient care.

Creating a culture of engagement means encouraging learning through ongoing education and training. Engagement and culture ranked number one among the corporate needs identified by top executives in 2016 (Bersin, 2013b). As much as possible, load the budget for learning but also seek out low-cost, high-impact learning from within your organization and maximize the talent that surrounds you. We don't' have to travel long distances to learn when we have skilled people in our own backyard. How often has your in-house simulation champion been referred to as a sim guru outside of your workplace? Consider interinstitutional, shared learning. Also, search for free online education. MOOCS, or Massive Online Open Courses and other open source learning is readily available online. This past year, I completed three Coursera courses (two specifically related to simulation, and one on leadership) and several other Lynda.com courses in management. One of those

courses had 340,000 learners registered. See the online Toolkit item *Guidebook to Simulation Team Talent Development* (Folder 1: 11.1.5) for a comprehensive list of talent development learning resources.

In learning organizations, teams share what they are learning for the benefit of all. Think of each Simulation Program initiative as an opportunity to promote learning and scholarship. Actively promote team presentations at professional conferences and workshops, and encourage publications to disseminate research findings, program outcomes, and innovative and creative uses of simulation, or share systems improvements within your organization. Make learning a part of all that you do. Create team and individual learning-related goal setting. Encourage your simulation personnel to create *stretch goals* by having them articulate a pie in the sky goal, then knocking that goal down a couple notches to one that is more doable, yet still ambitious. STRETCH but don't throw yourself out of kilter.

As the manager, you will need to create policies and procedures for talent development. These include (1) travel; (2) requests and approvals for learning activities; (3)

reporting back on learning; and (4) performance appraisal that reflects new learning. See the online Toolkit for a sample *Expense Report Template* (Folder 4: 11.4.2) and a *Sample Staff Time Sheet* see (Folder 4: 11.4.6)

The Performance Appraisal and Performance Assessment Criteria

Individual and team *performance appraisal* in Simulation Programs is key to ongoing quality improvement. As a manager leading others, it is important that you help to develop the whole team, as well as, each individual on the team by tracking competencies, skills, and accomplishments. Zenger Folkman (2009), state that "leaders who are able to create positive development experiences for their team members are more apt to create an inspired and motivated team" (p. 1). The manager/leader, therefore, takes on the roles of *coach*, *mentor*, and *motivator*. Zenger and Folkman's *Developing Others Checklist* itemizes the things that team members appreciate:

- Regular, honest, supportive, and ongoing formative feedback on performance with follow-up
- Weekly check-ins with the team for issues and needs assessment
- Make strengths visible and align work and needs for development accordingly

- Encourage team members to create individual development plans, then to share with each other to make team development plans
- Challenge people in new and exciting ways that align work with their passions
- Seek out training and education that clearly align performance outcomes with criteria and activities that scaffold learning for success to motivate and inspire
- Delegate tasks to individuals and partner team members with each other to develop new competencies for career development (e.g., present at conferences, write articles for publication, engage in research)
- Hold social events, such as, lunch and learns
- Increase credibility by making accomplishments visible
- Make challenges and mistakes opportunities for growth and to ensure that people are doing the right things for the right reasons (e.g., hard-working, well-meaning team members can spin their wheels doing the wrong things)
- Lead by example. Share your personal professional development plans and successes with employees.

It is important to use valid and reliable measures for performance appraisal and to do so while upholding organizational protocol. Check with your human resources personnel or administrators for information on how the performance appraisal process plays out in your milieu. Many organizations now rely on the use of *unified/integrated resource management programs*, like PeopleSoft (now marketed by Oracle). These management programs comprise software packages and tools to enable core global management of an entire organization's human resources, as well as, financial management, supplier relationship management, enterprise services automation, and supply chain management. Within these systems, organizations can custom-build key *human capital performance criteria and indicators*. Processes are designed to help managers implement a strategic end-to-end management system to attract, retain, and motivate top talent; map and track individual goals alongside organizational goals; access talent management analytics to increase team visibility (Missildine Martin & Calabrese, 2011). Built-in metrics include such things as Impact of Loss, or Risk of Leaving measures. Using a systems approach to talent management is beneficial, however, these systems are complex and both training and experience are needed to develop proficiency.

Awareness of, and enforcing labor rules is an important part of a manager's roles. It is essential to become well versed in collective bargaining agreements or workplace agreements and policy, and to interpret them correctly. Seek out guidance with this from experienced and knowledgeable individuals.

Compensation, Benefits, and Rewards

Employee *compensation* comes in the form of promotions, financial rewards for accomplishments, incremental salary increases, and benefits packages. Some organizations even offer stock options as compensation or reward. *Financial compensation* involves the use of pay grade matrices to facilitate forward movement up the pay ladder (usually based on hours worked), while other formal compensation systems are based on meritorious accomplishment. Managers need to create a compensation strategy and plan to clearly communicate how a team member can receive increased compensation. Work with your HR Department to facilitate pay grade placement, reviews, and promotions. Items you will need to consider include developing policy for time and remuneration. Think about how to compensate overtime (OT) hours. Can OT be taken in the form of time back or involve payment based on incremental rates?

Rewards and incentives in organizations exist as formal and informal talent recognition. There is consensus in the literature that recognition and acknowledgment of individual or team behaviors not only increases an organization's profile but that it creates a whole host of benefits that are often overlooked (Bersin, 2013b; PBrun & Dugas, 2008; Salie & Schlechter, 2012). Formal awards are often based on personal recognition; recognition of results; recognition of work practice; and recognition of job dedication (PBrun & Dugas). Salie and Schlechter, cite opposing views on recognition programs, reporting that rewards often result in temporary employee compliance to organizational values and are, therefore, not reliable predictors of sustained performance. Moreover, some employees see rewards as manipulative and unfair, where selection processes of recipients can create a perception of awards as punishment rather than motivation. Interestingly, factors that most often contribute to employee motivation are tied to the person's sense of job fulfillment and in knowing that they are making a difference by contributing to organizational success. In other words, "rewards are typically seen as a poor substitute for genuine feelings of accomplishment and satisfaction" (p. 3). What is suggested, from both supporters and refuters of recognition programs, is that when care and attention are taken to design and implement recognition programs, they have the "potential to offer benefits like improved retention, effectiveness, and loyalty" (p. 4).

Formal *recognition* processes should be tied to the organization's vision, mission, and core values and involve formal, transparent processes that are accessible and based on clear criteria for selection. It is important to be cognizant of the messaging inherent in awards and recognition and the nuances they carry with them. Awards then should be carefully created and reinforce organizational values by featuring employees whose work embodies those same values. For example, the INACL and SSH award categories and selection criteria are enmeshed with the organization's vision, mission, and values. I encourage you to submit your team and team members for awards.

As a manager, should you choose to create team or individual recognition awards, consider the need for transparency and fairness in the development of criteria and recipient selection. Reward items can include: issuing of tangible memorabilia like trophies, certificates; and hosting gala events such as an awards night banquet. Ensure that you celebrate and mark these significant individual or team milestones together in ways that are known to be meaningful. Suggestions include having a celebration where all can share in another's success, or publishing important accomplishments in newsletters, or other publications (locally, regionally, or internationally) to increase the visibility and profile of the team. Work to enmesh praise and celebrating success into your everyday workplace etiquette and organizational culture and the payoffs will be palpable and rewarding for all.

Informally, managers and team members can encourage each other and build a more positive work climate in a number of creative ways. Small gestures can go a long way to enhance team members' perceptions of being valued on the team. Consider anonymously leaving someone a small gift card or a sticky note on their coffee cup; making visible employee accomplishments, ideas, and innovations (paper or electronic medium—e.g., INASCL Linked In platform); create a Celebrating Talent section in your Program manual to feature the team's significant accomplishments; start a suggestion board/box and make a point of thanking the individual whose idea you implemented; acknowledge birthdays and culture-related celebrations of team members; arrange a special lunch with the Dean to celebrate big milestones; or host open public ceremonies to recognize accomplishments such as PhD/Masters degrees, or other academic accomplishments such as CHSE, CHSE-A, or CHSOS designations, or certifications. Get the endorphins flowing and have some fun!

Employee Hour Tracking

Employees are accountable and responsible for their attendance and performance in the Simulation Program, whereas managers must create, implement, and monitor systems to track attendance and approve overtime, time back in place of overtime, sick time, and leaves of absence. It is important that policy and procedures be clearly articulated and that reporting mechanisms are reliable. Equity in applying a policy to all team members is essential if you want to be known as a fair manager. See the online Toolkit for a *Sample Staff time Sheet* (Folder 4: 11.4.6).

Drug and Alcohol Policy

In the current safety in healthcare climate, many institutions are implementing a drug and alcohol policy to ensure the safety of patients and the integrity of high-performance healthcare teams. The impacts of employee alcohol and drug use on teams are profound and can affect employee health, workplace and public safety, and operational productivity in the Simulation Program. In the absence of institutional policy, each Program will need to create its own standards for expected behavior policy. This means creating policy that "balances between measures to control or deter use (standard investigation tools and discipline) and prevention measures (education, training, and assistance) appropriate to the nature and size of the business" (Minister of Public Works and Government Services Canada [PWGSC], 2011, p. 1).

Succession Planning

The truth is that employees on the team will come and go. Succession planning for Simulation Programs involves strategizing to ensure smooth transitions in and out of key roles in organizations and is supported by continuous attention to talent recruitment, development, and retention (Oracle, 2016). Our workforce is top heavy with Baby Boomers that are starting to retire in huge numbers. To roll out a succession plan, start by ensuring that the members of your sim team are not islands onto themselves. Have team members work together and encourage them to teach each other about their roles and key function. In essence, you are building a cross-functional talent pool while encouraging capacity building on the team. Ultimately, this approach makes it easier if a team member must leave without notice, as with unexpected illness. To further facilitate cross-functionality and smoother succession should the need arise, have each team member (or group by position type) document a detailed account of his or her roles and functions. I suggest this information in shared computer folders or online. Ensure that team members have access to each other's shared folders for timely access to vital information. Teams can also capture their work by creating screen capture videos or computer screen shots, or by using other multimedia to lessen the workload of documenting their roles.

Although global succession planning is typically the work of organizational administrators, front-line managers also have an important role to play in planning for operational sustainability. One person departing the team can leave behind a gaping hole that can be challenging to fill. Many of the positions held in Simulation Programs require years of development to acquire the requisite knowledge and skills. Moreover, fierce competition for simulation talent in the marketplace makes the job of finding the right people time consuming. As much as you can, build in time for your new hire to be mentored by the person leaving. Don't shy away from having career building discussions with your team members. Ask them to share their career goals and plans for moving up or out of the organization. Hopefully, you can entice them to stay, but the reality is that today, people are mobile and do not often

stay with one company for an entire career. Also, individuals realize higher levels of education and training; they are more apt to seek out work that aligns with new credentials and skills sets. For the new employee, a manager will engage in creating a talent development plan with goals and milestones to achieve, and built-in target dates.

Employment Termination

Although unpleasant, termination of employees is part of ensuring Program quality. Termination is rarely, although can be at times, related to a single event. Ideally, there should be a clear record of performance management to support termination. Ask for assistance from your organization's HR department or senior administrators if you have an employee that is struggling to meet expected performance criteria so that you can follow the appropriate performance tracking and measurement processes. There are specific institutional policies, procedures, and protocols that must be followed to the letter in these situations. For example, the actual process for termination, the calculation of mandatory severance pay, and issuing of official documents. When the termination process is grounded in best practices in performance management, the person will likely self-identify their lack of success before termination arrives. They will understand that they have been unable to meet expectations and termination will, therefore, not come as a surprise. As a matter of fact, the servant leader will go so far as to help the team member move to a more suitable position inside or outside the institution to support their strengths and overall wellbeing. However, this is not always the case, and if the process has been acrimonious, seek out the assistance of someone with experience in managing conflict. Terminations should never be implemented alone with an employee, and at the very least, an HR representative ought to be present. You will need to articulate policy and procedures related to required data, conditions of terminations, and documentation for the same.

Travel and Meeting Attendance

In the Simulation Program, travel for business, academic affairs, professional development or scholarship is required or desired. As a manager it is vital to establish policies and procedures for staff travel that are fair, equitable, and transparent. People are more accepting if they understand the reasons why one person's request was approved over another. If one person was the last to attend a conference, they are often more than happy to let another team member have a turn. There is often competition for limited funds, so making these decisions open and transparent will go a long way to perceived fairness. Meetings could be held locally, or may involve booking flights, accommodations, and the use of your own vehicle, parking, among other costs. Expense reimbursement is simple when organizational systems are in place for booking travel. If absent, formulate P&P for allowable expenses and reimbursement procedures. Also, consider the need for employee activity reporting on presentations once the learning activity is complete. For a *Sample Expense Report*, see the online Toolkit (Folder 4: 11.4.2).

Simulation Educator–Specific Policy

There are multiple policy and procedure development considerations for educators in your Simulation Program. Consider the different needs and contracts of continuing faculty versus sessional or part-time staff. P & P should clearly outline performance expectations, support for talent development, and logistical expectations of educators. Areas to consider when developing educator-specific policy and procedures include:

Minimum Standards and Requirements, and Proficiency Maintenance

Create a clear statement of expectation for professional development (e.g., approved on-site training program, or other quality educational activities/programs). The Educator/Facilitator Readiness for Simulation Self-Assessment Survey is a tool designed to help educators identify areas of focus when creating a plan for professional development (see online Toolkit, Chapter 20-1). Consider charting a course towards attaining the knowledge (content), skill (ability), and attitudes (motivation) required to achieve CHSE, or CHSE-A credentials. Include the following in your plan:

- INACSL Standards of Best Practice Simulation^SM, (INACSL Standards Committee, 2016), and SSH Accreditation Standards (2016a). Standards (other benchmarks as appropriate)
- Simulation pedagogy; grounding theories and philosophies; simulation modalities (delivery platforms); simulation typologies (tools for enacting simulation modalities)
- Educator preparedness (e.g., attendance at dry-runs for teaching in simulation; room and equipment orientation, skilled and appropriate use of simulation technologies, functions, and operating systems [simulators, laptops, patient voice systems, room paging, recording systems, etc.])
- Validation of learner readiness, and preparedness for simulation, and support for learning needs (builds supportive learning environment to empower students and lessen anxiety and fear)
- Standardized simulation deployment practices (e.g., scripted prebriefing, following predetermined event flow, timing, etc.)

- Simulation design (INACSL Standards of Best Practice Simulation^SM) (required process, format, template)
- Socratic, guided reflection approaches to debriefing
- Assessment strategies and evaluation of learners (formative, summative—including High stakes testing, tool development, etc.)
- Facilitator evaluation approaches and tools

Educator Performance Assessment

Develop a policy and a process for self-, learner-, peer-, and expert performance review, mentorship, and coaching. Adopt specific performance measurement tools, and be explicit about the frequency of use, benchmark attainment, and proficiency maintenance. For example, if you adopt the DASH or FACE tools for assessment of faculty in debriefing and giving feedback. Plan for training on the proper use of these tools (Center for Medical Simulation, www.harvardmedsim.org, 2016) to promote a common understanding of, and approach to giving feedback. Use formative tools to support educator development by encouraging ongoing feedback from a variety of sources (student, peer, and experienced facilitator) that aims to correct misconceptions and missteps, motivate, and facilitate self-regulating behaviors. Make explicit the expectations for faculty use of such tools and articulate a clear plan for ownership and sharing of faculty feedback. Consider tying into existing processes already in place in your institution and then make them explicit for your program.

Distressed Participants in Simulation Experiences

Simulation events can produce anxiety and heightened stress for many learners, so be intentional about adopting strategies that might lessen participant anxiety, such as having evaluators or other observers situated outside the simulation room in remote locations like as monitor/control rooms via one-way windows, or remote video recording (Horsley & Wambach, 2015). Facilitators have an ethical imperative to implement processes that uphold participant integrity while mitigating the potential for harm to participants, embedded actors, or educators as part of simulation best practices (INACSL Standards Committee, 2016, Facilitation; Debriefing; Professional Integrity). When a simulation includes emotionally charged content, it is wise for the facilitator to be candid and disclose the potential for strong emotional responses to participants prior to engaging in the learning event. Plan ahead for additional participant supports in these circumstances, should the need arise.

Good simulation design should also attend to cognitive load demands on participants to ensure that the learning event provides opportunities for optimal learning by adhering to the golden rule that working memory is limited to learning seven things at any given point in time (Reedy, 2015). When high stakes testing is employed, the need for participant support is even more acute (Tagher & Robinson, 2016). Consider implementing policy around the need for support measures like early identification of at-risk students, implementation of an integrated faculty-led remediation, or the development of individual learning plans. Clear remediation and skills testing policies will also ensure that participants understand the implications of unsuccessful performance in high-stakes testing events (Tagher & Robinson) underscore the importance of having a skilled facilitator take measures to lessen stress before, during and after debriefing (Janzen et al., 2016). Consider things like adopting "safe space" only environments in your Program and then consistently attend to building elements of psychological safety for participants in simulation (Rudolph, Simon, & Raemer, 2015). For example, some participants report a fear of mannequins (Pediophobia) where various strategies could be implemented by the facilitator in advance of simulation to lessen the stress inducing effects of working with simulators (Macy & Schrader, 2008).

Process for Creating New Simulation Events or Changes

Consider the type of request and approval process you will use when developing new simulation events. Make the process clear and transparent and attach specific timelines to the simulation development process. Visit the online Toolkit for a sample *Simulation Approval Pathway* (Folder 7: 11.7.1). Decide on key requirements such as the required use of the INACSL Design Standards (INACSL Standards Committee, 2016). Also, clearly articulate expectations for internal and external stakeholder roles and levels of engagement in the simulation development process.

Course Evaluation

Gleaning course evaluation feedback from a variety of sources and using different methods is an important aspect of TQI. Evaluations should include student feedback on the course itself, the scenario, the learning environment, and educator/facilitator performance. Look at adopting the use of valid and reliable tools for measuring the various aspects of courses offered in the Simulation Program. You will also need to consider how evaluation data are to be accessed, stored, and disseminated appropriately. Visit the online Toolkit for a comprehensive list of *Simulation Program Performance—Data Collection and Tools for Measurement* categories, data to collect, and tools for measurement (Folder 7: 11.7.8).

Code of Conduct

Provide a clear statement of expectations for *professionalism*: communication, preparedness, timeliness, dress code, equipment use, confidentiality: uphold *participant integrity*—positivity, honesty, good judgement, authenticity; *scenario integrity*—sharing, and storage, authorship; consent/permissions; *ethical conduct*—disclosure, research, media access, storage, sharing, and publishing; or *consequences* for nonconformity. Articulate the conditions under which a participant can be asked to leave the Simulation Center (e.g., violation of honor code). Such incidents, will require a process for documenting tracking any follow-up contact.

Use of Forms and Permissions

A master list of forms commonly used in Simulation Programs is located in the online Toolkit (Folder 3: 11.3.2). Many standardized forms are either used by educators or distributed to participants. The following samples are provided in the online Toolkit: *Media Permissions Form* (Folder 6: 11.6.5), *Confidentiality Pledge Forms* (Folder 6: 11.6.2), *Simulation Participant Honor Code Form* (Folder 6: 11.6.9), *Fiction Contract Forms* (Folder 6: 11.6.3 and 11.6.4), *Code of Professional Conduct for the Simulation Lab* (Folder 6: 11.6.1 and 11.6.8), and a *Code of Conduct Form* (Folder 6: 11.6.1). Additional course, scenario, and healthcare related forms (e.g., copies of the scenario, event flow, schedules, patient chart, patient Kardex, simula- tion event evaluation forms, educator assessment forms, etc.) and other required documentation are listed throughout the chapter. For a comprehensive list of Chapter 11 toolkit items, refer to the *Toolkit Master List,* item 11.0. Decide how and when forms should be made accessible to the participants before during, and after learning events.

Educator's Role(s) and Functions for Staging

Create a plan and then communicate expectations for simulation educators/facilitators roles and responsibilities in the Simulation Program. Articulate clear expectations for room staging, equipment preparation, the setup and takedown of equipment, and for simulator or actor moulage. Take pictures of staged rooms or setups so that it can be easily duplicated. Consider processes for events that are internal versus external (e.g., weekend course offerings versus weekday). No one appreciates inefficiencies or having to deal with cleaning up someone else's mess. Create standard forms or scripts for tasks that educators will use time and again include an *Orientation to Simulation Room Script* (Folder 6: 11.6.6), *Simulator Orientation Checklist* (Folder 6: 11.6.10),

Remedial Session Educator Request Form (Folder 6: 11.6.7), *Plus Delta Gamma Debriefing Template* (Folder 6: 11.6.11), and a *Safe Space for Learning Norms Poster* (Folder 6: 11.6.12).

Access to Simulation Equipment, Personnel, and Spaces

Specialized equipment requires specialized care and maintenance. Creating a list of Do's and Don'ts for the care and use of equipment and supplies and for the maintenance physical spaces can help. Patrons also need to understand how to go about accessing equipment, people, and spaces. For example, rules for simulator use, setup, cleaning, operating, and transport can be posted in room(s) where they are housed. To encourage compliance, strategically post clear signs. "No food and drink in this area", or "Live Cameras Streaming—Please Keep Quiet."

Priority Use

Establish a priority use policy to promote the appropriate allocation of, and equitable access to valuable resources of these valuable resources, To accomplish this, invite key stakeholders to co-develop a priority use guideline, decision-tree, or policy that takes in account physical space requirements, technological requirements, staffing requirements, specialized equipment, room capacity, required preapprovals, field of study, curricular integration, revenue generation, funding source, or other criteria needed to make fair and equitable decisions.

Travel and Meetings

Outline a process for requesting and approval of travel to conferences and meetings. Identify what constitutes approved and non-approved expenses, and the process for expense reimbursement. Also consider developing a process in the case that simulation equipment needs to be shipped as part of an event that requires off-site travel. In this case, you will need to plan for secure crating and shipping of the products.

Reporting Absences/Leaves

Provide a clear statement of who to call, and the process for educator replacement or course cancellation. Many simulation events occur in the early morning before regular office hours. It is sometimes necessary for faculty and participants to reach personnel in the Simulation Centre before or after hours. Make sure that information is accessible and easy to locate.

Course Participant–Specific Policy

Similar to the need for educator-specific policy, learners must also be aware of, and have clarity about expected behaviors. Learner policy and procedure provide vital information that will promote learner satisfaction and success in simulation.

Consider the following the information in the following sections when developing learner P&P.

Knowledge of Simulation-Based Learning

Create a plan to educate participants about the basic elements of simulation-based learning and their role as learners prior to their experience. Orientation to SBL could include the use of didactic presentations, online modules, video review, discussions, sim lab tours, or even via classroom simulation. Alfes (2008) describes the making and use of an introductory video to set the stage for learning about clinical simulation.

Preparation for Simulation

Provide a clear statement of standard expectations for preparation (required prereading/video review/skills review/self-assessment/etc.) and consequences for noncompliance (e.g., will they be able to participate if unprepared?) Also, consider what constitutes appropriate attire for simulations and how students will access this information for each event. Plan ahead for space and equipment orientation needs.

Code of Conduct

Articulate clear expectations for professional behaviors including agreeing to an institutional requirements for: course preparation, honor code, confidentiality, timeliness, media access, use, viewing, and sharing (cell phone/video use); dress code; team learning; equipment use; effective communication, including supportive, honest feedback; consequences for noncompliance, etc.), contacting someone in the case of absences, and appropriate routes for reporting concerns.

Supports for Learning

Articulate exactly what learners can expect in terms of support before, during, and after the simulation (e.g., non-punitive approach, honesty, good judgement, assessment, authentic interactions, ability to start or stop a scenario if in trouble [phone a faculty, time out for team huddle, or other supportive measures or strategies]). Also, see above under the distressed participant section.

Assessment and Evaluation

Outline a process and clear expectations on how to advise learners of evaluation strategies and associated tools, checklists, and grading rubrics. As well, articulate requirements for including assessment/evaluation information in the course syllabus.

Forms and Permissions

Many different types of forms are used in Simulation Programs. Provide users with a list of forms and accompanying rules for completing them. For example, fiction contracts media permissions, video access and use, research, equipment sign out, waivers, or other required forms. Consider if you will use web-based applications, hard copies, or a combination of these and then create a plan for secure storage.

Engagement and Team Learning

Simulation involves extensive team learning. Therefore, learner engagement and commitment to team learning are important. State your expectations for adherence to facilitator/learner agreements like the **fiction contract** (learner is informed of variations in fidelity and asked to engage as though it is a real event), or expectations for enacting positive team behaviors to support others' learning. When one learner fails to treat the simulation as serious learning, it can have a negative effect on their peers' ability to learn.

Active Observers

Learners can learn by watching others do. Hober and Bonnel (2014) found that observers do learn through "recognizing individual and team patterns of patient care through noticing, interpreting, responding, and reflecting" (p. 16). Make clear your expectations for the observer role in simulation and note the need to develop learner supports, for example an observer form or checklist. Also consider adopting a common approach to giving peer feedback in debriefing for those in the observer role. Make explicit the best practices you endorse to engage learners in peer-to-peer observation. (e.g., use of rubrics to guide observers). See the online Toolkit for a sample *Active Observer Form* (Folder 3: 11.3.7).

Reporting Absence/Leave

Plan ahead for missed experiences. Regardless of whether this type of decision is made at the individual course level, or at the Program level, you will need a process to manage missed simulation time. Be clear and tell students exactly what is expected of them should they be unable to attend. Strategies for making up missed time will vary based on existing Program policy, the nature of the absence, participants' track record, and the feasibility and availability of alternate learning experiences. Missed learning can be made up in a number of creative ways for example, by repeating the simulation experience or having a student view peer video recordings with permission and write an assignment. Ensure that you provide learners with telephone numbers, email addresses, and the names of the personnel they should contact to report an absence. You may also need a way of tracking or reporting such absences.

Course Communication

Participants need to have ready access to important materials for simulation-based learning. Communicate expectations for the learner to access course information, or stipulate requirements for learner participation in course platforms via email, Learning Management Systems (LMS), telephone calls, email, or other prearranged posting sites. Ensure that all participants have access to a location map and parking information if courses are delivered onsite.

Policy for Educational Programming

At the heart of all Simulation Programs are course offerings. Course offerings require forethought and detailed planning for simulation development, deployment, and evaluation. Before investing significant time and energy in new course development, ensure that you have the capacity, the resources, and the required approvals to run the event. Develop policies and procedures related to course offerings in the following areas.

Course Requests and Approvals

The course approvals and simulation development process will look different for every Program. Determine the process the best suits your Program needs and establish a workflow for requests and approvals. See the online Toolkit for *Sample Simulation Program Integration Pathway—Approval Process* (Folder 7: 11.7.1). Articulate the following: Who needs to approve the simulation activity? Who will approve the content of the simulation? Who will approve and pay for the cost of the event? Which benchmarks or key development documents will be required to promote quality simulation? I suggest formally adopting the INACSL Standards of Best Practice: Simulation^SM (INACSL Standards Committee, 2016) as one means designing, deploying, and evaluating quality programming.

Course Offerings

Whether you are a stand-alone Program that develops and deploys in-house course offerings, or you take simulation on the road, you will need to publish a current list of course offerings. Ensure to use a standardized approach to course titling and numbering (aligned with organizational standards), and determine how and where you will host this information (website, LMS calendars, AV monitors in hallways, Program publications, front office whiteboard, other).

Certification, Recertification Courses

Many Simulation Programs are certified or designated as an official site for offering certification courses like ACLS, BLS, TNCC, etc. As such, the Program must demonstrate compliance with the external body's protocol for course offerings. Establish internal P&P to uphold the required standards for registration, attendance and completion tracking, exam results, payment, invoicing, and reimbursements, and issuing of certificates.

Continuing Education

Specific disciplines in many countries, such as the United States, use a post-licensure continuing education credit system (CE credits). CE credits are a requirement to maintain professional licensure. Develop processes to ensure that CE educational and operational requirements are met, that, participants' hours are tracked, and that course credits are issued.

Course Registration

Simulation Programs sometimes offer courses for which participants must register and pay in advance. Alternately, for some courses, course fees are not collected by the Simulation Program. Today, most programs will employ computer-based registration platforms. See the online Toolkit for a sample online course registration form built using JotForm. (*Note:* When using online platforms that store information offsite, (e.g., Google Forms) seek out institutional permissions and have forms vetted through the appropriate approval process).

Master Course Syllabus (MCO) Standards

The Master Course Syllabus or Outline (MCS/MCO) is a standardized document that specifies intended learning outcomes and serves as an educational road map for course delivery in the Simulation Program. MCS Simulation format and content will vary from program to program. If you do not have a standardized template then take time to create one for your Program. Clearly articulate the required components of course syllabi for your Program. Included below are sample headings (University of Washington, 2016):

- *Program Identifier:* branding (i.e., logo, colors, etc.)
- *Course Description*: course content, learning objectives, simulation modalities (e.g., Procedural Simulation,

Simulated Clinical Immersion, Just in Time Learning, Virtual Simulation) and list simulation typologies (mannequins, simulated patients, avatars, etc.); and other learning activities (prebriefing, debriefing, peer discussions, online blogs, video review); logistics (instructor name(s), contact information, what to wear, location of facility, location of course)

- *Access to Course Materials*: how and where to access precourse material, day of the course materials, and postcourse materials (in person or online)
- *Course Topics and Assignments*: schedule of main themes/topics in the course; required and recommended readings; list and schedule of assignments by date: explanation of goals of learning from assignments; value of assignments (participation marks, percentage of course grade, formative—no grades, etc.)
- *Course Policies and Values:* explain the core values that shape and underpin the simulation experience; expectations for team learning, inclusiveness, integrity, confidentiality, responsibility and accountability, and measures of success

Course Cancellations and Notifications

You will need to determine under which conditions courses will be cancelled permanently, rescheduled, and how to issue cancellation notifiers to participants. Consider blanket statements directing users to the institutional main website for global announcements like campus closure due to severe weather. Also think about including disclaimers on your registration forms stating that cancellations may occur related to equipment failure, staff shortages, or inclement weather.

Course Design and Deployment

Simulation is a resource-heavy endeavor with a million moving parts. Be sure to plan well in advance. For example, allow a reasonable time frame for course development. Our Program requires a 6-month development timeframe to develop new simulations. For some Programs, there may be the need to involve others in the simulation approval process such as the Dean or finance officer. Be sure to obtain all required approvals prior to starting the work of course development. Consider what you will need to make available to learners, educators, other faculty, and the simulation team and which mechanisms to use for sharing that information. Divide simulation course development into precourse, day of course, and postcourse phases to facilitate planning. Consider the following key areas for preparation below. In our Program, we host all of these planning sheets in the Cloud in shared folders using Google Docs. This has proven to be very effective. In the Toolkit, you will find the

Master Simulation Design Intake Form (Folder 7: 11.7.2) that pairs with the *Master Simulation Design Template* (Folder 7: 11.7.3). These tools feature a comprehensive, sequential simulation design process that is grounded in the INACSL Simulation Design Standard (INACSL Standards Committee, 2016). If you are new to simulation design, you will find these exceptionally helpful.

Booking Rooms, Personnel, and Equipment

Well thought-out and well-executed scheduling and booking systems can be a thing of beauty, or if done poorly, the bane of your existence. For the purposes of this chapter, I refer to scheduling as a complex system and/or process by which an organization or Simulation Program coordinates and books people, equipment, and spaces to deliver learning events. Typically, simulation-learning events are scheduled in advance as either single, one-time bookings, occasional bookings, or regular curriculum integrated bookings. Depending on the event type, you may need to schedule up to one semester, or even one year in advance to ensure the necessary resources. Book far enough ahead so as to leave sufficient time for all the steps in simulation design. See the online Toolkit for a sample *Simulation Event and Room Booking Form* (Folder 8: 11.8.10).

- *Key People:* Plan ahead for key people that will need to be involved and remember to allow time for any training needs: simulation team, learners, and other faculty. Ensure that these people are qualified and ready to participate. Think of the need for dry runs (pilot runs), simulation and medical equipment orientation, orientation to spaces, and instruction on the proper use of assessment tools and rubrics. Sometimes it is helpful for each member of the simulation team to have their own intake and planning form. See the online Toolkit for a *Sim Ops Tech Event Intake Form* (Folder 5: 11.5.1).

- *Key Technological Systems*: Using technological systems demands time, effort, and coordination. For example, simulators may need special setup or testing. Scenarios may need to be programmed into the software, -and then tested. Many technological systems used in simulation have back end administrator functions, such as the need to upload learner and faculty names with associated passwords for integrated AV/IT video recording systems. Monitoring stations require a monitor and computer setups. Electronic evaluation forms need to be designed, assigned, and uploaded. Lastly, room staging and moulage need to be completed. An *Integrated AV/IT Orientation Checklist* (Folder 5: 11.5.3) and a *Simulator and Technological Systems Orientation Guide* (Folder 5: 11.5.4) are available in the online Toolkit.

- *Key Spaces:* Your space and room type requirements will vary depending on the selected simulation delivery platform (modality); simulation typologies (mannequins, task trainers, embedded actors, simulated patients, etc.); the number of participants; and the timeframes available. Mobile simulation and In situ simulation, for example, have entirely different requirements.

Simulation Staff Scheduling Matrix

A scheduling matrix is a table that contains detailed information about simulation personnel, event timing, and learner group information. When scheduling large numbers of people, you might consider placing your scheduling matrix on a Cloud-based server platform. This approach allows many people access to collaborate in event planning. This practice increases efficiency and saves a lot of time. See the online Toolkit for sample *Sim Event Schedules* (Folder 8: 11.8.7 and 11.8.8) and a sample *Master Simulation Event Planning Sheet* (Folder 8: 11.8.9).

Event Flow Maps

Event flow maps provide a visual critical event pathway map depicting how an event will unfold. They are very useful and for many, are easier to understand than tables and charts. Refer to the online Toolkit for several samples of Event Flow Maps (Folder 8: 11.8.2—11.8.6). There is also an *Event Flow PowerPoint Template* (Folder 8: 11.8.1).

Standardized Equipment Planning Lists

Organized and well-laid out equipment lists, supply bins, and spreadsheets are essential in Simulation Programs. In order to achieve fiscal sustainability, keep an accurate cost sheet for each simulation event. You should be able to say to the nearest dollar, how much each event will cost to run. Detailed cost breakdowns are required for effective budgeting and to make accurate cost projections. See the online toolkit for a sample equipment cost breakdown list (Master Simulation Event Planning Sheet, Folder 8:11.8.9, Tab 2).

Course Print Materials Planner

Photocopy handouts and post reading lists or articles to LMS folders, etc. Include the need for standard Program forms (media permissions, confidentiality agreement, fiction contracts, debriefing tools, observation tools, or assessment tools), or for other course specific forms and handouts. See the online Toolkit for a *Master Simulation Event Planning Sheet* with multiple planning tabs (Folder 8: 11.8.9).

Issuing of Certificates

Certificates (hard or soft copies) will be required for CE credit courses, as well as, other offerings for which you may issue certificates of attendance. Determine requirements for mailing and electronic processes. Design a template with preembedded eSignatures to create digital certificates.

Simulation Design Standards

The INACSL Standards of Best Practice Simulation[SM] (INACSL Standards Committee, 2016, December, Simulation Design) offers an evidence-based process for

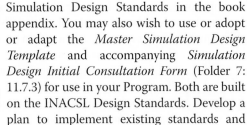

designing simulations. Refer to the INACSL Simulation Design Standards in the book appendix. You may also wish to use or adopt or adapt the *Master Simulation Design Template* and accompanying *Simulation Design Initial Consultation Form* (Folder 7: 11.7.3) for use in your Program. Both are built on the INACSL Design Standards. Develop a plan to implement existing standards and guidelines and the need for creating related policy and procedures. Consider the following:

- Guidelines for the use of, or adaptation of preconfigured (purchased) scenarios
- Documentation requirements such as the use of a standardized template, logo use
- Scenario storage and access; authorship and sharing or editing permissions
- Curricular mapping requirements for scenario concept or content mapping
- Use of valid and reliable tools for assessment of learners/simulation events/scenarios
- Simulation Quality Control (QC) measures: adopt standardized process for scenario content validation, expert validation of content, scenario revisions, and updating
- Access to video recordings postcourse for reflection, annotation, assessment, or analysis
- Fee structure and fee schedules for courses

Remediation as Deliberate Practice

The purpose of remediation is to assess and improve individual or team competencies. Formative remediation is primarily employed to achieve the timely correction of faulty techniques and raise the student's knowledge and ability to perform skills. Ideally, learners will self-identify and follow through with the need for learning assistance, but if not, be prepared to have that conversation. When learning is grounded in a Deliberate Practice and Cognitive Load theory, regular remediation after simulation experiences should be a way of life, and not the exception (Josephsen, 2015; Joseph & Juwah, 2015; McGaghie, 2008). Mastery learning is not a singular event. To master

a skill and maintain competency requires repeated skills practice in different contexts, over an entire career (Griswold-Theodorson et al., 2015). Oermann, Kardong-Edgren, and Odom-Maryon (2011) found that with only 6 minutes of CPR practice per month, students demonstrated continued proficiency over a 12 month period. A key underlying assumption in Deliberate Practice (DB) is that given the right opportunities for practice accompanied expert coaching and formative feedback, all learners can achieve success. Remedial sessions grounded in DB require, (1) clear learning objectives and goals with a clear minimum standard for competency; (2) baseline performance measurements from which to gauge progress; (3) varied learning activities for targeted skills practice; (4) regular and rigorous formative assessment and coaching by a skilled tutor to facilitate goal attainment; and (5) learner engagement in the process of attaining mastery.

Either the learner or the educator can initiate a remediation session. Sometimes all that is required to remobilize a learner is the focused review of a concept or skill component. Sustained performance, however, requires ongoing practice at regular intervals. Consider offering faculty supervised open practices times to encourage learner self-managed remediation. Simulation has long been viewed as an excellent platform for remedial sessions and for assessment and evaluation of learner competencies, such as, clinical judgement (Haskvitz & Koop, 2004; Lasater, 2007b). When developing a remediation P&P for your Program, consider the following:

- Will your program support learners by providing remedial sessions and performance assessments for learners?
- If so, what will the process be? Who can request remediation? Faculty? Students?
- How can requests be submitted? Will you require a written referral?

See the online Toolkit for an *Remedial Assessment and Session Request Form* (Folder 6: 11.6.7).

- Who will complete the assessments? Will documentation be required? Who will have access to this information if a learner is struggling and falling below minimum performance criteria?

A policy and associated procedures related to the sharing of learner performance in any simulation-learning event, is required. Interpreting and applying freedom of information and right to privacy legislation to educational programs will need to factor into creating this policy.

Research in the Simulation Program

As an emerging field, simulation has many unanswered questions. Not so long ago, there was a paucity of research in healthcare simulation but that has changed. In fact, research in simulation has made great strides in the past ten years. The healthcare simulation community now has two major journal peer-reviewed publications featuring quality research findings. Recently, there are newly released Simulation Research Reporting Guidelines (Cheng et al., 2016a). In simulation we engage in two forms of simulation research: research where the research is about simulation itself, and research that investigates another entity using simulation (Kardong-Edgren, Dieckmann, & Phero, 2015). To that end, teams and individuals in Simulation Programs can also conduct research *on* simulation, or *with* simulation, inside or outside of the Program. Simulation periodicals focus on content that features research on simulation.

In 2011, the first Research Consensus Summit in Simulation was held in conjunction with the annual IMSH meeting and SSH conference. The Summit proceedings reflected great hope for increasingly sophisticated levels of inquiry in years to come, a greater volume of inquiry, more synthesis-oriented inquiry, new dissemination routes with evolving digital scholarship capabilities and platforms. Goals for future research were established as follows:

- To optimize the use of simulation through relevant research
- To broaden the scope of simulation and research
- To provide guidance in terms of research topics and methods, and to
- Describe state of the art and future directions for simulation research.

The 2011 SSH International Meeting on Simulation in Healthcare (IMSH) Research Summit reported the need to focus scientific inquiry in the following areas: Individual learning, team learning, systems development, human factors studies, human factors tools, outcome studies (T1–T3), formative and summative assessment/evaluation, and research reporting. The 2017 IMSH Research Summit highlighted an impressive collection of more than 30 presentations to spotlight current research in the field.

Determine how your Simulation Program will engage in research or research related activities by asking:

- How will your simulation team contribute to research and scholarship activities?
- How will you maintain currency in simulation? How will you disseminate new findings in the advancement of simulation to the team, or how will your team contribute?
- How will research and scholarship be promoted within your Program and on the team?

Consider P&P development in the following areas:

- General Guidelines for conducting research (if different from institutions guidelines, don't reinvent the wheel if you don't need to): Provide links to institutional policy.

- Ethics Approval and Participant Consent: Establish Program-specific policy, or align with institutional policy.
- Collection, Security, and Storage of Data: See security section.
- Funding: Grant funding accounts for the vast majority of research income and must be managed and accounted for. Writing a grant proposal is key to success. See the *Tips for Research Grant Proposal Success* (Folder 7: 11.7.7), and also review the list of current *Research Questions* (Folder 7: 11.7.6).

- Authorship: Set clear expectations for first, second, etc. authorship and acknowledgments.
- Dissemination of Evidence: Articulate the required number of publications/presentations and rules for use of a Program's Brand.

Policy for General Operations

General operations pertain to the logistics of running the the Simulation Program day in and day out. In the *Simulation Champions: Ten Steps to Design Workbooks* in Chapter 27, you will find a vast amount of information that will also be helpful in developing your operational P&P.

Daily Operations

Daily operations include attending to the basic daily operational needs and are to discussed in the sections that follow.

Facility Access (Daytime, After Hours)

Simulation centres are busy places. Determine the entrance and exit permissions you will assign for facility and equipment access. For example, for electronic key card entry, you will need to assign levels of access for each person using the space: full access, partial access, or no access. In our facility, we assign partial keycard access to all instructional faculty for teaching spaces only to teaching spaces only, and full access only for full time Simulation Program personnel. Create a process for after-hours access for staff, learners, or customers renting your space in the evenings or on weekends.

Facility Standards (Physical Spaces, Equipment and Personnel)

Maintaining clean, safe workspaces is everyone's responsibility. However, in the absence of clear expectations facility standards will slide. When developing policy, be clear of what is expected of personnel, users of the facility, and custodial staff. Consider the use of visible room maintenance checklists to promote compliance. See the online Toolkit for a sample *Equipment Repair Tracking Form* (Folder 2: 11.2.6) and a *Room Occupant Responsibility Checklist* (Folder 2: 11.2.7).

Start up and Shutdown of Operations

As of yet, simulators do not have the ability to start up, or shut themselves off. This operational function is a good opportunity to develop capacity and cross-functionality on the team. As far as I am concerned, nearly all simulation personnel should be able to turn a simulator on, and off. This holds true for operating other critical equipment in the Program. It has been the case on more than one occasion that someone has forgotten to turn off equipment and a staff member has been able to help out. The same holds true for simple start up functions. Simulators, and other medical equipment will overheat and can be damaged if run for too long. These types of P&P may seem mundane, but are critical to providing quality service, and optimal equipment functioning. Some Programs will also train teaching faculty to do this.

Scheduling Systems and Processes

Scheduling is a vital operations process in the Simulation Program. I liken it to assembling one of those 1,000 piece puzzles. Paying attention to detailed policy and procedures for scheduling will facilitate smooth day-to-day operations.

Integrated Scheduling Systems

Times have changed and today there are integrated scheduling software products that can provide us with end-to-end scheduling solutions. These web-based solutions can generate, receive, and track scheduling requests; automatically notify users of double-bookings and cancellations; allow for customization; send meeting and event reminders; and auto-generate statistical reports about scheduling. Users can be assigned permissions for view-only access or be granted online booking privileges. Schedule view at-a-glance features even allow internal and external patrons to view schedules on mobile devices. Some scheduling software programs also interface and sync with other products like Facebook, Google Calendar, or Outlook. Additionally, most simulation vendors offer integrated systems solutions. For example, our Cloud-based recording system has video capture and distribution capabilities, and provides for curriculum, operations, and inventory management. Through LDAP integration, this system is connected to our university web-, and database systems. LDAP capability provides all internal users with a seamless single point of entry for access to university and Simulation Program web-based programming. Program patrons and staff will

need to know, or have ready access to information about how to schedule simulation events or booking meetings/conferences. Lay out clear expectations for all scheduling processes.

Automated Scheduling Systems

Make a determination of whether the Program will use institutional scheduling software, integrated LMS scheduling, integrated Simulation Program management software; or other commercially available software. Look for the features described above, and remember to program automatic confirmations, notifications, and reminders. Note that nearly all software-based scheduling programs today are customizable. Customization allows you to build layers of scheduling headings and subheadings to suite your specific needs. For example, each scheduling booking can be broken down into such headings as: program type, discipline, year in the program, course name, set up blocks, sim event, number of learners in each event, take down time, room hold time, modality usage (platform used to deliver simulation - simulated clinical immersion, classroom sim, procedural sim, In Situ, etc.), typology usage (tools used to enact the modality—SP, mannequin, avatar, volunteer actor, student role player, etc.), equipment bookings, or event type (meeting, learning event, faculty development, student remediation, etc.). By taking the time to build the administrative back end of your scheduling software, you can optimize the scheduling program functionality. Most scheduling systems also contain built-in analytics and the ability to generate detailed reports that will save valuable time and money.

Booking Request Submissions and Forms

Booking request forms should be detailed enough to give you the information you need to complete a booking. I encourage the use of automated systems because they provide you with seamless end-to-end scheduling management. See the online Toolkit for an example of a sample *Simulation Event and Room Booking Form.* (Folder 8: 11.8.10) (Folder 9: 11.9.3). Consider what constitutes appropriate use of the facility by staff and outside users. For example, use for personal financial gain might be disallowed.

Posting the Schedule

Deidentifiers should be used for public posting of schedules or other notifications. Ensure that you are aware of privacy legislation when formulating your scheduling P&P. To post the schedule, use codes or number systems to represent individual users or user groups. There are many local or remote options for posting scheduling information, such as monitor displays with scrolling schedules, server-based online viewing, or even wall-mounted or freestanding whiteboards. Many still like the flexibility and large surface a whiteboard offers.

Priority Use

Establish priority use policy and/or guidelines from the outset. It is essential to have decision making parameters in place before conflicting requests for people, space, and equipment arise. For example, you receive competing requests for the a fully equipped debriefing space where one user wants to hold a meeting, and the second wants to conduct a debriefing. The first requires zero use of technology, the second requires full access to technology. Your priority use criteria can then be used to clearly stipulate that priority will always be given to educational activities, allowing you to legitimately to decline the first request.

Booking Cancellation

A cancellation policy is important for many reasons. If events are booked and not cancelled, this will have a trickle-down effect on other Program resources. Planning for simulation events is labor intensive, so Programs may incur losses in income, time, and the use of other valuable resources if cancellations are not received in a timely fashion. Also, failing to capture cancelled events in the booking system will affect the accuracy of booking statistics. Assign a time frame and clear process for cancelling not only spaces, but also people, and equipment.

Dispute Resolution

When competing requests for the simulation facility, personnel, and equipment occur, clear processes are required for disputing and resolving scheduling decisions. Think carefully about who might need to be involved in dispute resolution and who will have the final say in resolving the matter. Remember that transparency, negotiation, and fairness are key. Most problems can be resolved by thinking out of the box, and coming up with creative solutions.

Security

Accessing to your simulation facility may require the issuing of visitor badges and/or giving out parking passes. You facility and Program also has many other valuable moving parts such as, key documents (research data, exam data, personal identifiers); expensive equipment (laptops, simulators, pumps); things with monetary value (parking passes, lunch passes, gift cards); personal items (in offices); and a host of valuable teaching resources.

Document and Data Storage and Cloud-based Applications: You will need rules in place to protect valuable resources that are stored on hard drives, as soft copies, or in Cloud-based spaces. For example, consider using document encryption or password protected secure storage, and then be sure to lock up all data backups. Also, create a secure process for tracking and storing all software licenses, and program specific passwords. Consider how will these will be labeled, stored, accessed, and monitored. For example, if one person on the team has access to equipment-specific password lists and for some reason is unavailable or away from work, the team will be unable to function. Shared online spaces are wonderful tools that have the capability to revolutionize work flow and organize data, however, sensitive information in the wrong hands can put your Program at risk so plan ahead. An institution's private server is a great place to start building your shared spaces and folders. Off site Cloud-based options are available, however, institutional permission may be required. For example, when creating forms or surveys that gather personal data and store it on off site servers. Ensure that you include all required identifiers for documents available in the public domain online.

Security Monitoring: It is a good idea to work with your institution's security department to ensure the safety of the Simulation Center. You may need to install extra security cameras or supplemental locking systems for certain types of equipment. For example, one evening, all 10 of our mannequin laptops were stolen from our Center. You can only imagine the horror of coming in to find them missing. It was an operational nightmare! We have since installed individual laptop security devices and have not since experienced the same issue. There is a need to develop processes for when and how to report missing equipment, or in some cases, to report theft to the authorities.

Lost and Found: Consider what you will do when things are left behind. Determine where lost items will be stored (valuables should be locked—but not a water bottle), Who will be responsible for contacting the owner? How long valuables are kept before disposal? It is good practice to link your Program's Lost and Found policy to that of the greater institution.

Safety

Safety in the Program is paramount. Create clear and visible instructions for reaching EMS in your facility and clearly mark all and that you run drills to promote compliance and proper use telephone stations. Some places have safety panic buttons installed that send an emergency response request directly to security. Make sure you communicate clear expectations for how to use these systems.

At some point, you will likely need to administer First Aid. What if someone falls and fractures an ankle or cracks their head after fainting, or suffers chest pain? I have called the ambulance many times over the years, even for an SP on one occasion. The Program must be prepared to initiate a timely, appropriate response. Consider the need to have a qualified first aid provider on your staff to deliver care to deliver First Aid. If you don't have an institutional grade first aid kit, Huang and Dongilli (2008) suggest the following basic contents to make your own kit: (1) smelling salts, (2) AED/defibrillator, (3) ice packs in freezer, (4) flashlight, and (5) bandages and dressings.

For hospital settings, other medical equipment should be earmarked. Remember to clearly mark all *functional* and *nonfunctional* equipment (e.g., LIVE defibrillator) to avoid untoward incidents, and ensure that the equipment is labeled with servicing and maintenance dates. Managing medical equipment in your facility requires that you comply with regulatory standards. Make provisions for managing and monitoring product updates, equipment maintenance, product recall repairs, and regular service calls. See the online Toolkit for a sample *Code Blue Cart Contents Checklist* (Folder 2: 11.2.5).

Simulation Programs need to document safety incidents and therefore, need dedicated forms (e.g., First Aid report, incident reports, and equipment maintenance labels/stickers). Emergency P&P must also address fire prevention and response practices, as well as, fire marshaling for emergency evacuations. Consider all requirements for safety training, certification, and tracking (e.g., Fire Marshall role, live shooter response, ladder safety training, WHMIS, etc.).

Unusual Physical Findings During Simulation Events: Sometimes, during examinations involving live human subjects like embedded actors, simulated or standardized patients, and even peers, unusual or abnormal findings are uncovered. Sometimes the reverse is true when an abnormal finding exists but is not found. In either case, it is important to consider the need for waivers and disclaimers to avoid liability in situations where participants are learners and are not yet practicing professionals. *Waivers* release participants, faculty, and the organization from liability in such cases. A waiver is a signed legal document involves the act of waving, releasing, or giving up an individual's right to something to which they would normally be entitled (in this case, within the context of student learning, the individual gives up the right to sue for wrong doing, harm, or malpractice). A *disclaimer* on the other hand, is the act of denouncing, denying, or relinquishment of title, claim, estate, or trust. Educators, for example, will include disclaimers on course documents advising prospective live human participants in learning events that the educator or institution will not assume any liability for missed physical findings. Another instance is the use of a disclaimer to protect the integrity of the Program for external stakeholders bringing information into your institution that may not be aligned with, or endorsed by the Program. Disclaimers can be part of a formal legal and binding contract between parties to prevent being sued (Schultis, Domenech, Fritz, Starry, & Winton, 2006).

Disposal of Medical and Nonmedical Waste

All Programs generate large volumes of medical and nonmedial waste. Some Programs also generate pathological waste from the use of living animal or human tissue, or by allowing learners to carry out medical care procedures that may generate biohazardous waste. Care and attention to proper hazardous waste disposal is important for harm reduction and needs to be properly managed according to Workplace Hazardous Materials Information System (WHMIS) regulations, or other regulations for the management of biohazardous waste. Biohazardous materials require secure storage in proper containers (sometimes even a locked room/cupboard), and then must be incinerated. If you are not located within a health facility that already has these systems in place, you will need to source out a local waste disposal service. Each region/country has Laboratory Biosafety Guidelines that stipulate the provisions for compliance for biological safety and handling of infectious substances, as well as, for safe storage and storage devices. Become acquainted with these and other occupational health and safety guidelines, such as WHMIS for safety in the workplace (http://whmis.org/).

Linen Management

Linen management entails the ordering, payment, receiving, storing of clean and soiled linen, and shipping out for laundering. You will need to establish processes to ensure safe lifting and back care, and the safe handling and storage of soiled linens. Some Programs do their own laundering. If this is the case, articulate the process. Consider compliance to code for safe storage of soiled linens in your geographical area.

Customer Relations

Service First Mentality: A mission to provide quality, timely, and efficient customer service goes a long way to making the workplace a happy place. Customer service is not a department, it is a culture. Expectations for service-provider dependability, availability, responsiveness, and quality must be articulated and communicated to your personnel and made visible to customers. Adopt service standards and abide by them. Consider how you will communicate to customers the level of service they should expect, as well as, the behaviors you expect of customers. Also develop processes for formal partnerships, contracts, or other memoranda of understanding with external entities.

Customer feedback is a required component in Program evaluation. Develop processes to regularly collect feedback (complaints or kudos) using clearly defined and accessible systems. Consider anonymous feedback strategies like placing suggestion/feedback boxes in strategic locations throughout the facility, or the use of online feedback surveys. Celebrate good news! Work to correct customer identified issues and track actionable improvement plans and outcomes.

Customer service is only as good as the processes that are in place to uphold it. There is nothing more frustrating for an educator than arriving to broken equipment or rooms not ready for use. All the smiling in the world won't fix that. Ensure that you have human and resource management strategies in place to support demands. Establish an in-person or online complaint/compliments process for all customers and have a system to compile and track these data. An sample *Simulation Program Customer Feedback Form* is provided in the online Toolkit (Folder 4: 11.4.8).

Vendor Relations

Vendor relations abound in the simulation world and it is important to forge healthy working partnerships. See the online Toolkit for a *Vendor Contact List Template* (Folder 4: 11.4.7). When it comes to vendor-related policy development, consider developing practices in your relationship that are fair and equitable. Consider these key aspects of relationship building and the need for boundary setting with vendors:

- Beta testing: Are you going to be testing new products? If so, clearly outline a process that includes contractual obligations for each party and who is responsible for each part of implementation;
- Accepting and giving gifts;
- Product showcases;
- Accepting grants or sponsorships dollars;
- Vendor access to facilities; and
- Dispute resolution process when conflict arises.

General Communications

Information dissemination, making announcements, issuing newsletters, publishing annual stakeholder reports, messaging on display monitors, emails, shared drives, voicemails, social media (e.g., Facebook, Twitter, Linked In, Instagram, Snapchat), website content, team meetings and face-to-face encounters are all important modes of communication. Your Program will need to consider each of these modes and determine the need to develop policy for each. Standardization of communications is important and also serves to build brand recognition.

Cell Phone Issuing, Usage, and Billing

The issuing of cell phones, tablets, or other technological equipment like laptops, requires developing related policy and procedures. While these devices increase an organization's connectedness to their employees, they can also result in exposing an organization to corporate liability related to employee misuse or negligence. Also, there has been more than one scandal of late involving cell phone users receiving gargantuan data and roaming fee bills, or the inappropriate accessing or sending of top secret documents over public servers, as opposed to private servers. To avoid these nightmares, ensure that you have thought through the following as part of a signed use agreement: appropriate use of the device while on the job (e.g., will you allow student or faculty cell phones to be turned one during simulations); use of devices in unsafe working conditions (e.g., hospital policy states not at bedside); expectations while driving or operating a motor vehicle (e.g., no texting) versus hands-free technology; use of devices for personal versus company business; appropriate use of camera phones in simulation spaces; posting of images to the Internet (private or public sites); review of monthly charges; updating or upgrading of devices (timing, frequency of replacement); right to purchase if leaving; and rules regarding breakage or misuse.

Hospitality

Hospitality means to create a welcoming, inviting space and experience for those entering your facility. Determine how you will greet visitors to your facility, or host others during outside events. Clearly stipulate what constitutes an allowable expense and assign spending limits for allowable hospitality expenses. Consider gift purchases, or rules for purchasing food in restaurants or via catering services. Alcohol purchase is most often not an allowable expense. Predetermine set amounts that require additional levels of approval (e.g., any amount exceeding $200.00 must be preapproved). You may wish to articulate the types of expenses that are NOT covered such as staff lunches during working meetings with internal stakeholder, as opposed to a corporate working group lunch for external stakeholders). There may also be institutional policy that requires the use of specific prime vendor caterers, or the requirements to order specific types of foods (vegetarian, nut-free, Kosher or Halal prepared foods or other culturally appropriate food choices).

Hosting Conferences and Special Events

It is inevitable that you will be planning and hosting events in your Program. Engage your conference department very early in the process, as well as, any other departments and stakeholders that have a vested interest in the success of the event (i.e., marketing, administration, media, fund development, faculty teams, etc.). The online Toolkit contains a *Special Event Planning Template* (Folder 7: 11.7.10) and a sample *Special Event Planner Gantt Chart* (Folder 7: 11.7.11) that have proven helpful for event planning.

Procuring Equipment and Supplies

This next section refers specifically to P&P related to equipment and supply procurement. See the Chapter section on fiscal management for information specific to that topic. Ensure that P&P are developed for each aspect of procuring and managing equipment and supplies. Consider each of the sections that follow.

Procurement

The procurement process involves equipment requesting, obtaining quotes, tendering process, the equipment selection, receiving, and asset management through equipment inventorying and tracking. Equipment selection is an overwhelmingly complex process and it is helpful to have tools to assist you with expensive purchases like simulators, virtual platforms, and integrated IT/AV systems.

The *Simulator Value Index Tool.* As technology advances and becomes increasingly sophisticated, simulation professionals are faced with difficult challenges to determine which simulators are best suited to a particular use. With the growing list of features and characteristics to consider, aligning needs with simulator features and characteristics, while taking into consideration the factors that influence our decisions, can be daunting. To minimize these associated challenges, Rooney et al. (2017) have developed and evaluated a tool called the Simulator Value Index (SVI) tool intended to facilitate and standardize the simulator evaluation and purchase process. See the online Toolkit for the SVI tool description and worksheet. In a multi-phase process, they identified and refined the top factors that should be considered during the simulator purchase process, then created the *Simulator Value Index* (SVI) as a for making simulator purchase decisions. You will find an SVI worksheet (Folder 2: 11.2.1) and descrip-

tion (Folder 2: 11.2.2) in the online Toolkit. The authors evaluated the practical value of the tool by offering the tool to targeted simulation professionals. Using responses from participants (*n* = 80), Rooney and her colleagues evaluated the tool's practical value by calculating its sensitivity to predict a preferred simulator. Findings indicated the SVI tool was able to successfully predict the preferred simulator with 87% sensitivity. The majority (73%) of participants agreed that the SVI tool was helpful at guiding simulator purchase decisions and 88% agreed the SVI tool would help facilitate discussion with peers.

Keyin is a community comprising peer professionals that post product reviews on virtually every simulation product, manufacturer, supplier, and service providers. To join, go to (http://get.keyin.to/). Another idea is to use a simulator comparison table. Build them from the specs on product sheets, and then send them out for review to the team. Additionally, some Simulation Programs will

publish an online list or soft/hard copy catalogue with images of all their equipment provide online access to the equipment inventory and provide equipment booking or borrower services.

Product Returns and Reimbursement Process

Consider how will you process product returns to vendors. It is important that you obtain a product return number from the vendor and then consider choosing a shipping method that will track your package. Identify the process you will follow, required paper work and how returns will be sent back.

Equipment Breakage and User Liability

Develop processes to deal with, and replace equipment breakage that happens through misuse, abuse, or accidental mishaps.

Equipment Repairs

Equipment breaks down. Consider how to identify and track and monitor repairs, costs, and warranty coverage for repairs. Consider using an "Equipment Needing Repair" clipboard in each room that is checked on a regular basis. You will find assorted equipment and maintenance forms in the online Toolkit: *Equipment Repair Tracking Form* (Folder 2: 11.2.6), *Room Occupant Responsibility Checklist* (Folder 2: 11.2.7), *Room Equipment Maintenance and Repair Tracker* (Folder 2: 11.2.8), and *Room Maintenance Checklist* (Folder 2: 11.2.9). It has been my experience that you need to have a system in place that allows people to write the

problem down quickly or it is often forgotten and not reported. An actual toolbox with real tools is an essential piece of equipment. See the online Toolkit for a *Sim Ops Tech Toolbox List* (Folder 5: 11.5.2).

Warranty Management

It is very important to track and monitor product warranties. Each purchase and corresponding warranty amounts must be tracked and then budgeted for on an annual basis. Keep copies of all purchases and associated warranties and invoices in one location. It is smart to post warranty renewal dates with notifiers pop-ups into your scheduling program. There are some Programs that opt for in-house maintenance and repairs and do not purchase extended warranties. If you are considering this, do verify all options for simulator repair training as well as access to parts for repair from the vendor. Tech simulator training courses, when available are expensive and usually involve travel to vendor manufacturing headquarters. Engage in a cost–benefit–risk analysis and make your decision from there. Remember that simulator repairs and parts are costly. One breakdown can set you back a large sum of money. Also consider what would happen if you had one trained technician, and that technician chose to leave your Program. What then? There are risks—so look at the big picture. Some vendors are now offering leasing options through third party lenders that come with 24-hour guaranteed simulator replacement. Things to consider in decision making are the value and age of the product, ease of repair (modular versus complex), the cost of simulator repair training programs, and the level of training required to become a qualified technician.

Product Registration and Licenses

For every product you purchase, complete a product registration form. This is an important step in the procurement process and provides proof of date of purchase. Also, software and hardware license agreements will need to be managed and stored. Develop a system to keep track of the registration numbers, serial and product numbers, and the storage location for software. Track all products license renewal dates.

Equipment Replacement Programs

All equipment has a shelf life. Immediately upon purchase, even before the product arrives, product depreciation begins. Consider how you will manage the asset lifecycle, depreciation, archiving, surplussing, and donation of outdated equipment. Refer to the section on asset management addressed earlier in the chapter. Engage your in-house procurement department representative or asset manager/officer in this process.

Day-to-Day Equipment and Supply Handling

Equipment entails hardware that is reused time and time again. These are things like task trainers, medical equipment [AED, ECG], and mannequins. *Supplies* on the other hand are not reusable and are consumed and then discarded after use during operational, educational, and technical activities. There is an overwhelming amount of stuff to manage. Together with the team, determine standardized processes for equipment and supply management. Establish clear guidelines and rules for the organizing, storing and packing, stocking and re-stocking, maintenance, cleaning, and use and re-use of all inventory items. Having ample storage space is critical to effective supply and equipment management. Dorney, Walston, and Decker (2014) state that between 35% and 50% of a simulation facility's footprint should be designated as storage space. See Chapter 27 for the *Simulation Champions: Ten Steps to Design Workbooks* for detailed information and pictures on equipment and supply management.

Loaning Equipment

If you have it, they will want it, but only if they know you have it! Determine a process for equipment borrowing that includes: sign-out forms (hard or soft copies—online borrowing forms work great); waivers and liability forms (e.g., statement to address replacement and cost of the item if lost or damaged); note the value of the item; care and maintenance needs; timeframes for loans; equipment that can or cannot be loaned, on and offsite loans (e.g., what is safe to take to the clinical area, or to a primary school for teaching); and consequences if returned late. For sample *Internal Equipment and Supply Loan Request Form and an External Equipment Loan Agreement Form*, see, see the online Toolkit (Folder 2: 11.2.3 and 11.2.4).

Tours in the Simulation Center

Touring Simulation Centers has become commonplace: simulation learning facilities are brimming with interesting and fascinating unconventional learning spaces filled with neat things like simulators, cameras, and other impressive equipment. They are also full of people with valuable experience from having worked in the trenches. For the simulation manager, tours are opportunities to connect with other professionals to learn about how they run their Programs, or to share with others your knowledge, skills, and experiences. Having said that, tours can take up a significant amount of time and energy. Determine the following P&P: process for requesting a tour; leading a tour (I suggest the use of a standardized script); tour cancellations; and explore options for creating virtual tours. Follow this link to see a sample of a virtual tours that features one suite in MacEwan University's Clinical Simulation Centre, Bodnar High-Fidelity Suite (https://youtu.be/XmtkPKioGI8). Some Programs opt to create a fee structure and fee schedule for tours: especially the larger centers that may be bombarded with tour requests. When offering tours, consider the need to include personnel from other departments in your institution, such as those from Facilities, Project Management, and AV and IT departments. Often, there is a need to explain systems and equipment in more detail.

Nonparticipant Observers

A long time ago, I experienced the dire outcomes of having a nonparticipant observer be unprepared to witness a simulation unfold while providing a demonstration for a external stakeholder event tour. One of the observers quickly exited the viewing gallery in obvious distress. I later learned that this individual had lost her husband only 2 weeks prior from the same condition we were depicting in the scenario. I learned a hard lesson that day about the value of disclosing scenario content to nonparticipants and about the need to obtain consent before proceeding. Had I properly introduced the event and prepared the group, the observer would have had the chance to bow out of the experience.

Consider the need for obtaining the permission of the learners who are being observed. Having strangers watch might not be sit well with them. Develop the following P&P:

- *Event Disclaimers:* The use of disclaimers for nonparticipant observers. It is essential that all observers be aware of required confidentiality around what they observe in your facility. You may wish, also, to use disclaimers for tour participants.
- *Permissions:* Consider the need to obtain permission from the learners and faculty for any type of tour.
- *Video:* Also consider whether noncourse participant observers can view videos (e.g., conference presentations, in-house training).

Marketing and Media

Marketing is a viable, organization-wide function that should be integrated into everyday Program operations. Marketing strategies range from simple to complex and can entail the use of loyalty programs for frequent users, branding initiatives, and all communications via internal and external multimedia advertising campaigns. Effective marketing strategies aim for maximum customer impact. Developing your *Brand* is a very important business strategy that tells your customers verbally, in writing, and through visual imagery what you promise to deliver. While developing your vision, mission and value statements, you were engaged in a key aspect of branding: that is to define your purpose - or your WHY. Other aspects of branding include designing a great logo, the use of key messaging, and integrating your brand into all aspects of the Program (e.g., answering phones or stamping emails with key messages or taglines, or adding logos to all print and online material, and presentation formats) (Williams, 2016).

Simulation Program Brand Use and Acknowledgements

Many Programs invest in branding as part of a strategic marketing initiative. Brand components like a logo, catch phrase, or other identifiers that facilitate Program recognition. Articulate clearly when, where, and how the brand must be used. For example, presentations by Program personnel should use a standard presentation slide template or letterhead. To ensure quality and consistency with communications, it is important to determine the need for an internal vetting approval process for all offerings inside and outside the Program. Often, simulation professionals

are asked to participate in consultancy work outside their place of employment. This practice has been especially true during the past 10 years with the rapid proliferation of Simulation Programs. Ensure that you formulate a process for approval of such activities (if allowed by the organization). Consider any institutional requirements for disclosure of external work, and the need for any disclaimers for information or presenters coming to your facility from outside the Program (Dongilli, Shekhter, & Gavilanes, 2015). Also consider the need for *required acknowledgements* when you have official Program or special event sponsors, or donors.

Remember to allocate time and resources to promoting special events. Develop processes to manage sponsorship, advertising, and marketing materials for these events.

Simulation Programs in the News

Employing multimedia publicity is a value-added activity for your Program. Whether you are planning a grand opening event or a baby shower for your new simulator, you should consider going public. Public recognition can bolster stakeholder engagement and positive outcomes by making the Program more visible to others. Initiate discussions with your institutional Media Relations department to strategize. Also, potential donors are actively seeking great causes to sponsor, so do not hesitate to engage your Fund Development team. You will want to shed the best light on your initiatives, so don't hesitate to bring in the specialists. Develop P&P for news

- Media spokesperson(s) for media interviews or local publications
- Outside use of logos
- Approvals for publicity ads and events (i.e., script and news item reviews), and
- Engaging institutional stakeholders in multimedia publicity

Website Presence

The Internet is the single most effective marketing tool and is critical to building relationships with internal and external stakeholders, and the public at large. Simulation Programs need them for public relations, recruitment, promotions, way finding, hosting valuable shared and private resources. Consider best practices in website development. Work with your institution to ensure website protocol alignment and adherence to institutional P&P. Huang and Dongilli (2008) and Healthysimulation.com (2016) suggest the following key areas for inclusion when developing content for Program websites (See Box 11-7).

Box 11-7	**Website Content for Simulation Programs**

- **Homepage with Vision, Mission, and Value Statements:** Post other documents you want viewed in the public domain. For example, an Internet search revealed more than thirty many Simulation Program P&P manuals.
- **Facility Description:** Include pictures, floor plans, and functions of each space.
- **Faculty and Staff Information**: include photos, bios, and high-level position descriptions for all personnel, and abbreviated curriculum vitae, a summary of scholarly works or research projects for faculty.
- **Directions and Maps:** ensure that people have the information they need to get to your facility. Links to online geolocators like Google Maps is very helpful. Institutional maps and parking instructions are essential.
- **Contact Information:** Too many websites make you dig to find contact information, so make this information highly visible.
- **Course Catalogue and Syllabi:** If you are offering courses to externals, ensure that necessary information is included on the website.
- **Calendar and/or Scheduling:** Post course calendars to showcase booked events or provide links to other important events. Posting important simulation conferences and dates for example, can be very useful.
- **Educational Resources:** Websites are often designed with an administrative back end or private site that is accessible by user name and password only. Such permissions only access sites are a great place to host internal documents that you may not want to reside in the public domain.
- **Virtual tour and Photo Gallery:** Showcase your Center via the use of multimedia. Work with your institutional IT/AV department or hire out multimedia productions to outside vendors to create virtual tours or take quality images.

- **News Links and Events:** Be sure to keep breaking news and attention grabbers on your front page. The use of ticker taping or rotating images across the web page are effective attention grabbers. Don't' be afraid to feature innovations in research and programming.
- **Simulation Reference Area:** Simulation communities of practice are known for sharing resources, so include a resource sharing section on your website if possible.
- **Research Initiatives:** Publish lists of research studies and resulting publications including all peer-reviewed publications and contributions to other research-related publications, peer-reviewed publications, in addition to all scholarly works completed by Program faculty and collaborative partners.
- **Acknowledgments:** Ensure to give credit to all Program sponsors. You can include donors and corporate sponsor logos or levels of sponsorship as appropriate. For example, we hold an event that advertises sponsors and one of three sponsorship levels.
- **Course Work:** It is possible to link websites to learning management systems (LMS) via web-link so consider where such links are appropriate and build them in.
- **Search Engine Capabilities:** Internal search functions are handy for site users, so wherever possible, build this feature into your website.

   Consider website-related P&P for the following:

- Website content development and maintenance
- Social media integration and use
- Firewall protected areas on your site (permissions, or members only sections)
- Violations of privacy or posting inappropriate content in public discussions on the website (List Servs, blogs, internal discussion forums, etc.)

Technical Operations

IT and AV Systems Management

Technical operations involves managing a host of Informational Technology (IT) and Audio Visual (AV) systems with the Program. IT department personnel "manage network security, computers, servers, and credentials (logins and permissions)" (Gantt & Young, 2016b, p. 10). Audiovisual Communications (AV) departments concern themselves with many forms of communications technologies, including sound, video, lighting, display and projection systems in institutional classrooms and meeting spaces. Telecommunications departments are generally housed as a separate entity and oversee wired and wireless communication, including the setup of landlines and cell phones. The Simulation Program personnel and IT/AV department personnel should work together to formulate a plan to integrate simulation and institutional systems. This

process often gives rise to conflicts between systems that will need to be resolved for smooth technical operations. For example, it took us nearly 1 year to achieve Lightweight Directory Access Protocol (LDAP) integration between our Cloud-based video-management vendor and our IT/AV departments. The two directory systems did not mesh well and we had to work together to find solutions to make it work. Most technological systems in Programs today involve intensive back end administration (inputting data and setting up events) and management (planning, organizing, staffing, monitoring, and controlling). The Program manager, simulation educator(s), and SOS personnel must work together to create a cohesive and effective management plan.

Simulator Maintenance, Repairs and Warranties

Establish a regular simulator maintenance plan and repair processes. Unless you have a biomedical engineer on staff, you will need to access external service providers or companies to carry out this type of work. They can do the work onsite, or it can be taken or shipped offsite. Other options include having your SOS or other staff trained to provide regular scheduled maintenance. Many simulator companies now provide onsite maintenance and repair. Articulate the process that you will use in your Program. Simulators come with a limited warranty and options for extending them. When making the decision about whether or not to purchase warranties, consider that the cost of one of major component failure along with replacement parts, repair fees, and travel costs might put you over the cost of an extended warranty package. Other Programs purchase service and maintenance kits, and has their in-house trained technicians complete mannequin maintenance and repairs. See the online Toolkit for a sample *Equipment Repair Tracking Form* (Folder 2: 11.2.6).

Hardware and Software Management

Inventory management and tracking of technology-related hardware and software is essential. Determine asset management requirements like tagging, replacing, and repairing hardware, and software updating, password storage, and the maintenance hard or soft copies. These processes should be based on institutional practices. Before setting up inventory spreadsheets for example, find out how institutional asset management officers log inventory, and then build on those same systems. Simulation facilities often subscribe to simulated electronic healthcare record systems (EHR). Hanberg and Madden (2011) view these EHR systems as a unique simulation modality, and consider them only one of many modalities that can be effective in teaching nursing informatics. Integration of a simulated EHR into high-fidelity simulation has shown to improve student speed and accuracy in the use of EHRs (George, Drahnak, Schroeder, & Katrancha, 2016). Greenawalt (2014) speaks of their importance of teaching students how to maneuver technology-rooted challenges of "access, security, privilege, availability, authentication, oversight, and technique" (p. e199). Some Programs use simulated healthcare records while others have the capacity to tap into existing hospital training with actual patient documentation systems (often access is limited). Others use a homegrown version, while some may still use paper charting. Visit the online Toolkit for sample paper charts you would commonly need to build a simulated patient chart (Folder 3: 11.3.1 through 11.3.31).

Video Recording Management

Video-recording management (VR) involves the use of extensive Cloud-based, or local server-based video recording and storage systems. Managing these systems involves

establishing P&P in the following areas: confidentiality; security of media content and files; assigning logins and permissions; video and image recording and storage; video release, distribution, and destruction; information management using databases, forms, and logs; as well as, the monitoring functions to upkeep and maintain these complex systems. You will need to consider consequences for noncompliance. I suggest that it is always better to establish proactive rather than reactive approaches. For example, ask learners and faculty to agree to and sign a media agreement that clearly stipulates expectations and what constitutes a breach of policy. For more information on technical operations, see Chapter 21.

Challenges and Opportunities for Simulation Managers

A large-scale initiative such as opening a Simulation Program and facility does not come without its fair share of challenges. Those leading the charge have experienced many limitations and challenges, however, the issues are shifting as technology and pedagogical approaches for simulation continue to evolve. For example, 10 to 15 years ago, there was no clarity around what led to Program success. Today, things look different and managers can access relevant, evidenced-based information to bolster implementation efforts and stave off troubles.

Baily, Bar-on, Yucha, and Snyder (2012) recount their experiences in the planning and operationalizing of a multi-institutional, interprofessional Simulation Center. They identified six areas of challenge as follows: "(1) the actual move into new physical spaces; (2) fluctuating needs in staffing and shifts in position descriptions over the 1st year of operations; (3) scheduling of the spaces; (4) collaboration and integration of three institutions; (5) incorporating simulation itself into curricula; and (6) faculty development and interprofessional training" (p. e1). We know a lot more than we did 20 years ago and subsequently, there are benchmarks, guidelines, and standards that serve as guides to Program development. Box 11-8 features a list of hot topics and burning issues that was recently generated during a meeting of local Simulation Program managers.

Summary

Many years ago when I first conceptualized and began writing this book, my key goal was to help others have a smoother journey than my own. This chapter aimed to provide the new Simulation Manager with important information and key resources needed to operationalize a Simulation Program. Simulation Programs need inspired, capable, and skilled managers that are also able to engage in leadership roles and managerial and administrative

Box 11-8	Hot Topics and Burning Issues for Simulation Program Managers

- Funding for sustainability and organizational leadership support
- Capacity building for faculty, staff, and the organization
- Curricular integration
- Program evaluation: measuring ROI, ROE, value, and other methods of value propositioning and economic evaluation
- Space and staffing: needs to expand with growing demands
- Faculty buy-in, professional development opportunities, and funding
  - Breaking down traditional attitudes and beliefs
- Infrastructure and technological issues
- Organization of equipment/supplies

    The list of opportunities that was generated is encouraging. The list included the following:

- A distinct shift in the evolution of simulation theory, pedagogy, and research

- Positive effects of simulation on patient safety and team development in healthcare
- Amazing evolution in standards, guidelines, and recommendations for Program success
- Tremendous synergies that have been created within members of the simulation practice community
- Publication of excellent peer-reviewed simulation journals
- Evolution of technologies, especially in virtual reality, 3D and 4D augmented reality industry
- Global sharing and conference opportunities with professional associations that are growing in membership
- A strong sense of purpose and a shared vision for patient-centered care that that is more visible in our day-to-day workplaces and in our Simulation Programs
- The shared belief that we are all better people and professionals for contributing to the simulation revolution.

functions. Remember to access the online guidebook series and the many individual Toolkit items. I hope you will take the time to analyze your managerial style to create a personal performance plan that builds on your strengths. It is important for each of us to model the way through a personal commitment to growth and through transparent, actionable plans for continuous self-improvement. The last

Toolkit item I want to share with you is an account of my most glorious mistakes and successes over the years (Folder 7: 11.7.9). Enjoy reading about my many learning points on this journey.

    This chapter introduced project management as a key approach to managing nearly every facet of day-to-day Simulation Program operations. Metrics were defined, and assorted tools were provided to help you measure Program and project outcomes. Cortical concepts for 21st century management included discussions about sustainability, effective human capital management practices, especially the importance of talent acquisition and team development. We covered the many facets of managerial responsibility and accountability including fiscal, educational, and technical operations management. This chapter placed an emphasis on the need for effective change leadership and management practices to enact strategic planning, benchmarking, and Program evaluation. As well, we discussed the importance of embedding

existing simulation standards and guidelines required for Simulation Program success. We then navigated our way through a sea of information for the development of policies and procedures. I wish you every success in reaching your Simulation Program goals. Enjoy the journey!

Toolkit Resources

Over 100 different tools are available in the following categories:
Toolkit Item 11-0 Master Toolkit List
Toolkit Folder 11-1: Simulation Manager Booklets - Guidebook Series
Toolkit Folder 11-2: Equipment and Supply Management
Toolkit Folder 11-3: Simulated Patient Care Forms
Toolkit Folder 11-4: Simulation Manager Templates
Toolkit Folder 11-5: Simulation Operations Technical Tools
Toolkit Folder 11-6: Forms for Simulation Program Events
Toolkit Folder 11-7: Simulation Scenario Development Manager Tools
Toolkit Folder 11-8: Simulation Event Scheduling

12 Managing Simulated/Standardized Patient Programs

Pamela Rock, Petra Duncan

Key Terms

Standardized Patient, Simulated Patient, Simulated Clinicians, Formative Learning, High-Stakes Testing, Licensure Examinations, SP Teaching Methodology, SP training, SP Performance Evaluation, Sustainability, Hiring, Recruitment, SP Script, Strategic Planning, Organizational and Program Structure

Guiding Questions

1 If you were asked to initiate and manage a Standardized Patient or Simulated Patient Program, where would you begin?

2 How do organizational structure, governance, and strategic planning impact an SP Program?

3 Can you identify core elements in managing an SP Program? Which policies and procedures would you need to develop for the Program?

4 Can you identify the key components of an SP script and how you would go about training an SP?

5 What are the fiscal and sustainability issues related to running SP Programs?

A **standardized patient** (SP) or **simulated patient** (SiP) is a healthy person trained to portray the personal history, physical symptoms, emotional characteristics, and everyday concerns of an actual patient. As you see in Figure 12.1, SPs/SiPs are used as a dynamic educational tool for a variety of settings. In this instance, the SP is portraying the wife of a patient (mannequin) in end-stage heart failure in an emergency room setting. As explained in Chapter 6, a distinction can be made between an SiP and an SP. The Healthcare Simulation Dictionary (Lopreiato, Downing, Gammon, Lioce, Sittner, et al., 2016) states that the terms simulated and standardized patient are interchangeable "in the USA and Canada, but in other countries simulated patient is considered a broader term than standardized patient because the simulated patient scenario can be designed to vary the SP role in order to meet the needs of the learner" (Lopreiato et al., 2016, p. 32). Churchouse and McCafferty (2012) suggest that there are significant differences between the SP and the SiP because their use requires different structures in their preparation, development, and delivery of simulation. We established our Program as an SP Program and, therefore, will use that term throughout this section acknowledging that there are sometimes differences in interpretation between the terms.

Evidence from subjective and objective data supports the use of SPs to improve students' critical thinking and assessment skills (Slater, Bryant, & Ng, 2016). SPs are valuable for teaching communication and clinical skills (May, Park, & Lee, 2009) and increasing self-efficacy and learning motivation that affect knowledge and clinical skill acquisition (Oh, Jeon, & Koh, 2015). Comprehensive **SP training** can yield standardized reproducible patient

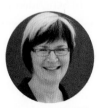

**Pamela Rock,
BSc, PT**

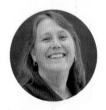

Petra Duncan

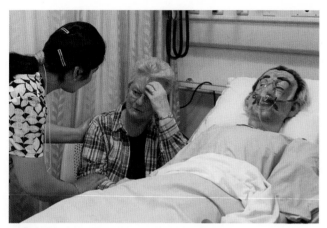

Figure 12.1 SP Playing the Role of the Distressed Wife of a Patient in End-Stage Heart Failure in an Emergency Room Simulation. (HELP! Save Stan, 2013 in Edmonton, Alberta Canada, used with permission.)

depictions for assessment purposes (Boulet & Errichetti, 2008); therefore, SPs, primarily used for **formative learning** and participant evaluation in healthcare programs, are also included in summative high-stakes certification and **licensure exams** (Boulet & Errichetti, 2008). Glaseroff (2015) encourages educators and clinicians to adopt more innovative uses of SPs, such as training SPs as **simulated clinicians** to assist with teaching and healthcare team training. Literature exists that highlights an evidence-based approach for using SPs in medical education (Cleland, Abe, & Rethans, 2009); however, more rigorous research is required to establish best practices in **SP teaching methodology** (May et al., 2009; Oh et al., 2015).

Managing SP Programs is a challenging endeavor that has increased in complexity over the years. Key challenges identified by Nestel et al. (2011) include (1) recruitment, categories of SiPs, and performance and training; (2) faculty development; (3) organizational structure and context, including funding models and changes in funding, contractual arrangements, databases, upsizing, downsizing, and regulatory and institutional requirements; and (4) quality assurance. Boulet and Errichetti (2008) emphasize that setting up SP Programs involves several steps including center design; detailed content development by creating, validating, and administering standardized educational events and trainee assessments and requisite tools (rubrics, rating scales, checklists, etc.); faculty training; and the recruitment and training of SPs. For SP physical space and learning environment design information, refer to Chapter 27 and corresponding online tools.

This chapter outlines the key considerations for developing and managing a comprehensive SP Program and covers the following areas: strategic plan and organizational structures, staffing, policies and procedures, tips for developing a learning experience using SPs, booking and scheduling, the child SP, accreditation, and financial considerations.

Getting Started—Strategic Plan and Organizational Structures

A well-formulated strategic plan and organizational structure with supporting policies and procedures will guide and support the implementation of SP Programs and the management of SPs. The **organizational structure** for your program will identify the various personnel and associated roles required by your program, their positioning in the organization, and their function and/or relationships to each other. It is very common today to see SP Programs integrated into larger simulation centers that include the use of multimodal simulation using an array of simulation typologies, while others operate programs as stand-alone SP-only entities. The organizational structure for the SP Program is tied to an institution's organizational structure, such as in a university, hospital, or government-based organization where structural requirements can vary significantly (Heine & Ferguson, 2015). Also, funding source(s) for SP Programs will significantly impact organizational structure. For some, the institution will fully fund their program, while others may operate using cost recovery or revenue generating models or the program will use a combination of these. Therefore, depending on the financial resources, the ability to hire and develop SP Program staffing teams will vary. More on the financial considerations of managing SP Programs is outlined later in the chapter.

Strategic planning and related goal for SP Programs are essential components of running efficient and effective operations. Make your overall SP Program goals visible through your mission, vision, and value statements to provide both structure and direction for the program, which will in turn support day-to-day decision-making. The development of a directional strategic plan and targeted timelines should include input from a broad variety of internal and external stakeholders and would be dependent on your associated institution and client group. The information gathered from stakeholders will support the decisions made surrounding the nature and scope of SP Program development. An advisory board or executive committee can provide direction and support to an established or developing SP Program and can also provide the SP manager/director with insights and ideas that are distanced from the day-to-day operations.

Staffing a Standardized Patient Program

Staffing an SP Program is dependent upon many things, including organizational structure and size, program goals, business plan, funding model, and institution. Each program will establish their staffing needs based on these factors where needs do vary considerably. Depending on the extent of SP usage and demand, you may or may not be required to hire employees. For example, smaller programs often choose to involve SP volunteers (Husson & Zulkosky, 2014) from the community at large or have staff volunteer from other areas of the organization. Sometimes, SP Programs will train students from inside or outside the institution to perform SP roles (i.e., high school drama students or students from undergraduate Performing Arts programs). In our SP Program at the Health Sciences Education and Research Commons (HSERC) at the University of Alberta, we operate as a shared resource with a database of over 350 SPs for seven internal health science faculties in addition to providing SP services for several external health education programs and institutions. It would be nearly impossible to provide the level of clinical expertise required for each of these areas, so we depend on clinical faculty and their departments to co-develop scripts and checklists and manage measurement and psychometrics of their SP activities.

The following sections describe the various roles common to successful SP Programs that may be over and above the typical staffing you would expect in simulation centers.

SP Program Manager/Director

The role of the person in this position is to provide leadership and direction, as well as to and manage the program and staff based on the program's goals and strategic plan. This will include day-to-day program administration, supervision of personnel, and fiscal management including the development and management of an annual budget and creating and supporting an environment that enables the program to support all aspects of SP methodology.

Standardized Patient Educator/Trainer

The best fit for this role would be a person with a background in clinical education with SP knowledge and experience, a background or knowledge in adult educational theory, and experience in theater. That said, there are many training programs available for SP trainers, and many successful educators do not start with the qualifications mentioned above. The SP educator duties often include recruitment, hiring, training, and supervising SPs. Once experienced, many SP educators seek out credentialing through the Society for Simulation in Healthcare (SSH) as Certified Simulation Healthcare Educators (CHSE) (2016c) (http://www.ssih.org/Certification/CHSE).

Standardized Patients

When recruiting your SPs, you will want to recruit individuals who are intelligent, reliable, and adaptable, have good communication and memorization skills, and are willing and able to learn new things. SPs are professionals trained to accurately simulate medical problems and conditions,

document and assess skills, and provide feedback (Boulet & Errichetti, 2008; Husson & Zulkosky, 2014).

Administrative Support

A person in this role provides administrative support for the program. Duties may include scheduling SPs for training, managing requests for use of the simulation or SPs, data entry, and being the first point of contact for the program and event setup and teardown. Administrative supports also play a key role in creating and maintaining complex SP event schedules, props lists, and event flow planning. Toolkit 12-1 features an **SP script** for a health assessment learning event; Toolkit 12-2 features our SP Program's script template; and Toolkit 12-3 offers a tabbed Excel spreadsheet with two sample SP event schedules, event flow maps, and a props list.

Technical Support

The role of this position is to support the simulation centers technology. This includes a vast array of skill sets and involves managing and monitoring everything from a computer program desktop application to managing and operating highly sophisticated technology-based learning environments. This individual may also be certified as a CHSOS through SSH (2016b) (http://www.ssih.org/Certification/CHSOS).

Clinicians

These persons have the appropriate clinical knowledge and background in healthcare and simulation using SP methodology. Clinicians can provide consultative and professional practice expertise for events using SPs in the development of learning objectives, scripts, and assessment checklists/rubrics. Knowledge and understanding of simulation and, in particular, SP methodology is a bonus in this role. However, knowledge and skill can be gained through faculty development programs either within the Simulation Program, through external resources, or through the support of the SP manager or SP educator.

Policies and Procedures

The development of a policy and procedure manual serves to define the intentions of your Program and the functions that must be carried out. You must carefully consider and correctly implement policies and procedures to reduce the risk of your organization making errors or failing due to a lack of focus (Anderson, 2013).

A policy and procedure manual will provide information for your clients or business partners and employees about what they can expect. It also defines clear expectations of them. Clearly articulated policies can improve communication, business processes, and employee training, as well as guide all employees to operate according to consistent prearranged formulae. A well-developed policy and procedure manual will reflect your program's "best" practice. There is a list of *Simulation Program Policy and Procedure Categories* you might require in an SP Program in the online Toolkit for Chapter 11.

Ten Tips for Developing a Learning Experience Using Simulated/Standardized Patients

Student learning experiences can be enhanced by using SiPs or SPs. SP educators provide support and aid in how best to approach the integration of SPs into courses, as well as scripting roles, delineating learning objectives, training SPs, providing faculty development opportunities, and debriefing the simulation experiences. Box 12-1 features ten tips for developing a learning experience using SPs. The ten tips echo the INACSL Simulation Design Standard (INACSL Standards Committee, 2016).

Booking and Scheduling

A comprehensive SP booking process will provide the educational program (or course), and your client with the tools needed to inform SP and event requirements. Depending on the size and supports available in your Program, the process can be either digital or paper-based. Clear processes and well-developed policies and procedures will inform your client of what is expected of them and what the SP Program will provide in return. Using this approach goes a long way to establishing an effective and efficient working relationship. Ensure to collect information in the booking process that will expedite SP recruitment and training and ensure that all aspects of the SP booking requirements are managed. Your booking process and request form can be used to provide your client/faculty confirmation of the booking, including the names of the scheduled SPs and can be used to support your payroll and billing process if required. See the online Toolkit 12-4 for a *Sample Booking Form* that also serves as a payroll generator. Booking policy and procedures will look very different from program to program. Toolkit 12-5 features a sample of one Faculty SP Booking policy and procedures manual. Make sure you receive your SP requests with sufficient notice to allow you the time to schedule and train the SPs before the event. Our Program requires a 3-week minimum time frame for all SP requests.

Box 12-1 | **Ten Tips for Developing a Learning Experience Using Simulated/Standardized Patient**

1. **Identify the need for a simulation learning experience**
   Can you fill that practicum experiential learning gap? If you cannot get the experience in real life, then something needs to be put in place.

2. *Formulate learning objectives*
   What is it that you want the students to experience and learn? Choose a maximum of three learning objectives.

3. **Recreate a suitable event**
   Some of the best scenarios have been based on real-life experiences. Perhaps there are past situations where you would have liked to perform your first exercise in a safe environment such as a simulation lab.

4. **Draft the script**
   There are many script templates available. Choose a template that suits your program and health profession.

5. **Train the SPs**
   The SP educator will train the SPs to portray the patient in the role that you have developed, paying particular attention to condition, movement, character, and mannerisms and focusing on your learning objectives.

6. **Dry run the simulation**
   Run the scenario with the SP educator, a facilitator or with each other. Make any necessary changes, additions, and revisions to the script and document those changes.

7. **Pilot an inauguration program**
   Start small—organize an official pre-event practice with SPs, facilitators, and students Which benchmarks or standards will you base changes on? (if available).

8. **Feedback**
   Explore the many different types of feedback resources that are being used to assist in today's learning activities. Choose the right feedback tools for your simulation. Common types offered in SP simulation include peer feedback from student participants or observers, expert instructor feedback, and SP feedback from the patient's perspective.

9. **Debrief the event**
   Remember that the SP scenario is a teaching tool for the preceptor and that the next phase of learning begins after the role has been played out. Documenting and recording the simulation will help in research and building future programs.

10. **Debrief the debriefing session**
    What went well? What could be done better next time? Reflection is a powerful tool.

By Petra Duncan, Pam Rock, Sharla King, Renate Kahlke, Health Sciences Education and Research Commons, Health Sciences Council, University of Alberta.

Managing Your SPs

Managing the SP involves timely and effective **recruitment**, hiring, training, performance appraisal, and the use of quality improvement processes to achieve and maintain excellence. The next sections provide information related to these aspects of managing SPs.

Recruitment

Recruitment is an ongoing activity for SP Programs. It is important to maintain a diverse compliment of individuals in your SP database who are capable of portraying a variety of roles and character portrayals. Requests for diversity in SPs, such as age, gender, past experiences and backgrounds, size, race, languages spoken, etc., will vary depending on end-user educational requirements, and levels of fidelity in the portrayal of SP roles. Figure 12.2 depicts an example of SP realism when portraying a bariatric patient that falls. Focus and carry out your SP talent search within local and regional organizations and groups, including community groups, theater companies, schools, and health-related facilities (Hart & Chilcote, 2016; Hussan & Zulkosky, 2014). Networking with other SP Programs in your region to share SP human resources can promote the effective and efficient use of resources. Print, the web, and other electronic media sources are effective methods to reach a broad range of demographics. Your existing SP pool is a fantastic resource.

Selection and Retention

Of paramount importance to your Program's success is hiring high-quality SPs who are enthusiastic, intuitive, and capable. Actors have incredible strengths and skills that are vital to enacting diverse, sometimes emotionally charged, roles (Hargraves, 2012); however, never discount the value of other potential candidates, such as stay at home or retired parents, teachers, firefighters, police officers, students, and retired health professionals. All have talents, personal qualities, and life experience that can make for a great SP. Determine your *selection process* and base it on the SP core competencies that you desire. Errichetti (2015) categorizes SP core competencies as foundational and advanced competencies. Look for acting ability and keen observation skills, those with experience in giving feedback, and people with the ability to retain accurate details of interactions (Cleland et al., 2009). SPs must possess a high level of accountability and responsibility: they must be able to follow the policies and procedures exactly as set out for them and be a supportive and reliable team member to other SPs. Often, SP events involve

high-stakes testing, where there is no room for tardiness or lack of compliance to requirements. Retention of your SPs becomes your next major concern. According to Schegel, Bonvin, Rethans, and Van der Vleuten (2016), SPs have a strong desire for recognition for performing successfully, and the well-being of your SPs is impacted by the affirming behaviors of SP trainers. Included in the online Toolkit is a series of interview questions that have proven to be helpful (see Toolkit 12-6). Your challenge will be to determine the selection process that will best meet these needs. Read on to hear from Peter Jarvis as he shares with us the qualities he deems essential for a simulated/standardized patient.

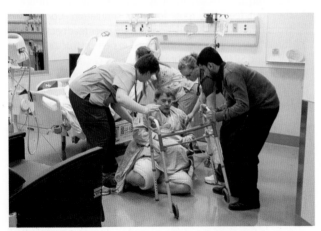

Figure 12.2 SP in Bariatric Suit Playing the Role of a Patient who Falls and Can't Get Up. (HELP! Save Stan, 2013 in Edmonton, Alberta Canada, used with permission.)

12-1 Voice of Experience
A Standardized Patient's Heartfelt Script

Peter L.L. Jarvis, BA, MVA

The telling moment sought by the experienced SP while scanning a fresh script is surely, "The Heart of the Story"! The SP asks him or herself, "Has the scriptwriter managed to envision the "whole person" compassionately?" Today's aspiring scriptwriters learn their craft through online Internet courses or in-person workshops, such as

Robert McKee's seminar and book "Story" or the local Film and Video Arts Alberta (FAVA). New or inexperienced writers, however, may be tempted to create a "Character Arc" or "Story Arc." That is to say, developing a character or situation to effect change—dramatically. Such screenplay or theater scriptwriting tactics are "overkill"; for the "SP Script" demands simplicity—written with ordinary words, clear and pertinent. The scriptwriter's efforts may present as a flat, lifeless body if the highs and lows of pertinent thoughts and emotions are absent. From the greeting through the main complaint, basic history, family background, etc., the author must be mindful to ensure that "The Heart of the Story" embodies care and compassion for the person—not the character. The ambitious scriptwriter desiring to create "The Great Standardized Patient Script" is well advised to "Just Tell." Simple words containing a "Key Opening Line" and a few "Must Tell" or "Must Not Tell" expressions, along with some key prompts or cues. The thoughtful writer composes the script to reveal the SP's concern in a "Heartfelt fashion." This strategy proves superior to anything grander written for the stage or screen. A good script provides the essential information. A better script includes an emotional ambiance. The superior script enables both participant and SP to become engaged with the essentials while reaching for the "Heart of the Story" in an exchange involving wits and emotional intelligence most "Heartfelt"!

SP Training

Preparing your newly hired SP for their role requires a planned approach. Develop and implement an orientation process that will provide the SP with the tools they need to perform their role. It is common for SP Programs today to provide an electronic version of an orientation manual or policy and procedure manual on their website. Box 12-2 provides you with a potential list of topics you might want to include in your manual.

The SP educator must take an engaged role in SP training, making sure to facilitate the learning of the scenario by using a learner-centered approach based on adult learning theory. The approach to preparing SPs who are children will be different. The number of trainings required for a case will depend on the complexity of the case (portrayal of emotions, responses to physical maneuvers, checklist completion, and providing feedback), the number of SPs being trained for the role and their level of experience

Box 12-2	**Suggested SP Training Manual Topics**

1. Standardized Patient Program overview
   a. Overview of program
   b. Overview of the facility
   c. Staff list and contact info
   d. Committees
   e. Communication (website and email)
2. What is a Standardized Patient?
   a. SP job description
   b. Lead SP role
   c. Confidentiality
   d. Disclosures and waivers
   e. Responsibilities/expectations
   f. SP feedback for students/participants
3. Type of SP work
   a. Regular
   b. High-stakes examinations
   c. Video productions
4. Procedures
   a. Booking procedure
      i. Regular roles
      ii. High-stakes exams
      iii. Video productions
   b. Quality reports
      i. Faculty/client
      ii. SP trainer
      iii. SP quality report about training
      iv. Video review
   c. Performance management
5. Payroll information
   a. Regular
      i. Contract and addendum
      ii. Electronic funds transfer
      iii. Invoice
      iv. Address change form
      v. Fee schedule
   b. High-stakes exams
      i. Contract and addendum
      ii. Electronic funds transfer
      iii. Invoice
      iv. Address change form
      v. Fee schedule
6. Recruiting new SPs
7. Complaints/issues/concerns
8. Continuing education/resources

as an SP (Wallace, 2007). The objective is to ensure that adequate time is devoted to the process to ensure that all aspects of the role are addressed and that SP performances are standardized (full replication between SPs). Therefore, if multiple SPs are performing the same role, they should be trained together (Wallace, 2007). According to Baig, Beran, Vallevand, Zarrukh, and Monory-Cuadros (2014), we need to continue to strengthen and ensure standardization of training and place additional focus on the emotions, facial expressions, and body language of the SPs during training. SPs who are experiencing difficulties with any aspects of a given role, including feedback or checklist management, will need additional coaching or may need to be replaced to ensure the integrity of performance outcomes. Dr. Harold Barrows, the father of SPs, offers the following advice:

During training, give copious feedback to the SPs about their performances in a very positive manner. If they get it right—celebrate! (Cheer, pat on the back, etc.) If they come close to being right, tell them. "Wow, that's almost it!" and then "Now, just try it a little more this way (or whatever)." If they get it wrong, tell them in essence, "You are trying hard, but that's not quite what we want; it is difficult I know, now let's try it this way (or words to that effect)." Coaching with clear, unambiguous, continuous, and positive feedback is essential to successful training (1999, p. xviii).

12-2 Voice of Experience
The Healthy Standardized Patient

Petra Duncan

Once the SP has completed the simulated event, it is important that you equip the SP with the tools to come "out of character" and safely leave the scenario behind. The SP trainer should always be ready to debrief with the SPs, but for some experienced SPs, self-debriefing is preferred. Here are some techniques and anecdotal lessons learned to consider using with SPs in the scenario termination phase or role exit phase:

● If more than one SP portrays the same role, consider having them decompress and debrief together after the event to let off steam—cry, or laugh, and joke.

● The use of a structured debriefing approach such as advocacy inquiry has proven to be helpful in uncovering frames and stimulate meaningful discussion.

● Sometimes, writing out their thoughts, concerns, and feedback can help them with "letting go" the role. Also, if they are willing to share their notes, this can be a handy tool for you.

● SPs can better switch off the emotions and step out of character by changing contexts. This might be to visit family or friends and talk about upbeat, unrelated topics.

● Sometimes, a role can be physically challenging and emotionally draining and all you want to do is sleep. Falling asleep, listening to some soft music, or turning on the television to a cartoon or comedy has proven helpful.

● Get engrossed in a good book.

● Engage in some form of physical activity.

● Allow SPs time and space to chat with fellow SPs and share experiences and self-preservation techniques. Keep a list of such strategies posted in your SP training area (Wallace, 2007).

Remember, it is just as important for the SP to step sensibly out of the role, as it is to prepare and learn its portrayal.

SPs and Feedback

Feedback is described as the "information given or dialogue between participants, facilitator, simulator, or peer with the intention of improving the understanding of concepts or aspects of performance" (Van de Ridder, Stokking, McGaghie, & Ten Cate, 2008). Also, feedback is cited as the most important variable in the use of simulation-based medical education to promote learning (McGaghie, Issenberg, Petrusa, & Scalese, 2010, p. 52).

There are many different techniques for training SPs to provide feedback to participants, both written (paper or computer based) and verbal. These include corrective, instructive, reflective, and formative techniques. SP feedback to students involves a process that offers them insight into a patient's unique perspective (Howley & Martindale, 2004; Wallace, 2007). Cofacilitation with your client for training SPs to give feedback helps to ensure that SPs provide targeted and appropriate feedback to meet the learning objectives for the simulation activity. Giving effective feedback is one of the most complex skills that your SPs will need to master. According to Errichetti (2015), "not every SP is appropriate for delivering debriefing or feedback activities. These tasks require maturity, psychological awareness, and discernment" (p. 212). Onello, Rudolph, and Simon (2015) have developed the Feedback for Clinical Education (FACE) tool. This tool is designed to facilitate clinical instructor giving of feedback and can be used within a wide variety clinical contexts.

You can either develop or use existing training programs to support the development of this skill. Hatchett, Haun, and Goldenhar (2004) offer an extensive list of resources for SP training in addition to an SP Feedback

Survey (http://www.aspeducators.org). SPs need to practice giving and receiving feedback according to best practice. Feedback should be given using *good judgement* (Rudolph, Simon, Dufresne, & Raemer, 2006) and be honest, relevant, accurate, and descriptive (Dudley, 2012), thus making this a positive and valuable learning experience for the learners. We suggest the use of an evidence-based feedback tool, such as the Harvard CMS Feedback Assessment for Clinical Education (FACE) (https://harvardmedsim.org/).

Child SPs

You can design incredible simulation experiences for learners using child actors as SPs. However, there are serious considerations that must be taken into account when using children as SPs. Issues such as parental consent, time off from class, training time, behavioral compliance, and state or provincial regulations or laws concerning the use of child actors. Seeking legal counsel is advisable if you are going this route.

The use of child actors also warrants examining ethical questions, such as "Who will benefit and who might be at risk of being harmed?" Developmental stages in children create vast differences in their cognitive and psychosocial capacity. Do consider the age and developmental level of the child and their ability to grasp what is transpiring within a scenario. Ask if possess the capacity to separate fiction from reality? Be intentional about a child's developmental stage when planning training and scenario design (Woodward & Gliva-McKinley, 1995). For example, think about how their participation could imprint them or shape lasting perceptions, and perpetuate stereotypes or misconceptions. Accordingly, develop a plan to mitigate harm (Woodward & Gliva-McKinley, 1995) and policy for full disclosure of all event specifics to parents. For all minors, you will need to obtain parental consent and consider the level of parental involvement you need. For high school students, it might be as simple as a consent form, while for younger children, it will involve a more extensive plan for screening before recruitment followed by debriefing post event (Lane, Ziv, & Boulet, 1999). Other aspects of child SPs to consider include what to do if a child becomes upset or tired: that is, the effect of repetition or scheduling times might have on the child and have a plan in place to manage any issue that might arise.

Performance Management and Quality Improvement

SP performance is a reflection of the time and effort you put into recruitment, selection, script development, and training. Setting standards for recruitment, professional conduct, training, and communication skills, including performance feedback, will define the quality measures for your SP improvement process. This process can include the use of client satisfaction surveys, and various forms of ongoing **evaluation of SP performance** using a mixture of self-reflection, client, learner, supervisor, and peer reviews (Perera, Perera, Abdullah, & Lee, 2009). The use of SP performance feedback is recommended to promote SP development, offering the SP increased opportunities to learn and advance to a higher level of performance (Schegel et al., 2016).

High-quality and timely *performance management* is key and is best supported by clearly laid out policies, procedures, expectations, and information sharing. In addition to extensive opportunities for formative performance assessment, we use a *three-strikes you're out* approach to talent management. There is little room for a lack of accountability and responsibility when running SP events. The SPs know our expectations clearly, and unless there are extenuating circumstances for lack of performance, there are times when it is best to terminate the working relationship with an SP.

The key to a successful quality improvement program or program evaluation is the development of a process to review the data or information collected and implement changes in practice based on the outcomes of this information. It takes an enormous effort on the part of the SP team in consultation with educators to design, implement, and evaluate excellence in simulation learning events.

Accreditation

One mechanism that sets your organization apart and identifies your SP Program as a best practice site is achieving accreditation. The Society for Simulation in Healthcare (SSH, 2016d), offers accreditation for SP Programs operating within simulation centers. The SSH website provides informative and helpful tools (as well, see Chapter 4) that can guide you in the process of assessing readiness and preparing for accreditation (http://www.ssih.org/). ASPE, the Global Network for Human Simulation Education (http://www.aspeducators.org/), offers a Core Curriculum Program for SP educators that are grounded in best practices in SP-based education.

Financial Considerations for the SP Program

Financial considerations are critical to the successful management of the SP Program. SP Programs are implemented using various funding models, and the model you choose will depend on the needs of your organization, strategic goals, and organizational structure. A variety of funding models exist, such as funding through the organization or institution's annual budget using a cost recovery approach or revenue generating model, or a combination of the these. Each funding model presents its challenges, and creating a fee structure can be complex, requiring you to develop a process to monitor and review its fiscal effectiveness at regular intervals. Diligent fiscal management of your SP Program will provide **sustainability** and support on future growth opportunities.

Fee structures are vital to cost containment and are a key aspect of your fiscal health. Things to consider when developing your fee structure are

1. Cost recovery or revenue generating or a combination of both
2. Single or tiered fee structure. Will your fee structure be the same for all your clients or will particular groups receive a discounted price?
3. Will you develop a fee structure that costs out a price for each service or will you set a flat rate for bundling your services? Bundling services may reduce your administrative expenses for invoicing but may also reduce your ability to do a cost analysis.
4. The systems you use to manage your financials may dictate the type of fee structure you choose. For example, you may want to purchase or purpose build applications that allow you flexibility in billing (single or batch billing options with built-in calculation ability).
5. Will you purchase an off-the-shelf data management system or will you create a customized database using an Excel spreadsheet?
6. Establish an hourly wage for SPs including both training and performance time.
   a. Will the fees be the same for both training and performance?
   b. Do you need to consider travel or parking costs?
   c. Be sure to include the cost of employee benefits into the wage.
   d. Will you pay the SP different wages based on the complexity of role or have a pay structure that provides the experienced SP with a higher rate?
   e. Will you establish a minimum hourly booking? For example, the SP rate will apply for a minimum of 4 hours, even if the client only requires the SP for 3 hours.
7. How will you bill the costs associated with the SP educator/trainer in regard to recruitment, scheduling, and training of SPs? Are these costs that you want to recover separately?
8. Consider costs associated with consulting, preparing user reports, and revising cases/scenarios. Will fees be required for these activities and if so who will be performing them will impact the rate charges?
9. Think about the usage of facility fees. Some programs only charge facility fees when the user group is external to their program or institution and others charge for all users, but different rates apply for groups external to their institution or program.
10. Technology support and use—will there be additional fees based on technology requirements?
11. How will you recover administrative support costs such as setup and take down time, assistance with Objective Structured Clinical Examinations (OSCEs), or other type events? Will you allow the customer to provide those services in kind? If so, how will this unfold and be accounted for?
12. How will you track and bill for equipment, supplies, and material costs?
13. How are you planning on making your fees and fee structures known to customers/users? Consider publishing your fee structure online or create a brochure.

Summary

The need for an evidence-based approach to teaching in health professional education requires developing meaningful and impactful learning experiences and robust assessment strategies. Integrating SPs into learning experiences and assessment practices can provide a rich learning environment for students. However, the creation of these learning experiences demands a thoughtful, well-planned approach based on best practices. Additionally, managing an SP Program also requires detailed planning, strong institutional support, and clear financial accountability to ensure a sustainable educational resource.

Toolkit Resources

Toolkit 12-1: SP Script for Health Assessment - sample script for your use.
Toolkit 12-2: HSERC Script Template
Toolkit 12-3: Tabbed Excel spreadsheet with two samples of SP event schedules, event flow maps, a props list, and a sample script
Toolkit 12-4: SP Event Booking Form - Sample
Toolkit 12-5: Sample Faculty SP Booking Policy and Procedures
Toolkit 12-6: Sample SP Interview Questions

13 | Competencies for Simulation Champions Leading in a Globalized World

Renee Pyburn, Joanne Lorraine Davies, Colette Foisy-Doll

 Key Terms

Globalization, Simulation Centers, Simulation Programs, Superdiversity, Intercultural, Transcultural Neocolonialism, Post-Colonialism, Cultural Safety, Ubuntu, Ethical Principles, Equity, Health Disparities, Social Responsibility, Social Justice, Distributive Justice, Transition Shock, Culture bubbles, Cultural Brokering, Global Citizen, Reflection and Reflexivity, Low-, Mid-, and High-Income Countries, Virtual Reality Simulation

 Guiding Questions

1. Where is the fastest expansion of simulation predicted in global markets?

2. What theoretical perspectives inform my personal ethic for building positive relationships?

3. How are ethical principles of global distributive justice, social responsibility, and equity an obligation of Simulation Champions originating from higher-income countries and working low-, or mid-income countries?

4. In what ways can Simulation Champions be effective global citizens?

5. What is Ubuntu? How can this philosophical stance enhance encounters with people from diverse backgrounds?

6. How can reflection and reflexivity contribute to creating relational and ethical spaces when building relationships in foreign contexts?

7. If you were moving to another country on work assignment or for a permanent job, would you thrive working within an environment that is very different from your own? How would you prepare yourself for such a move? Are you aware of the challenges inherent in working in foreign countries?

**Renee Pyburn,
MS, RN, CHSE**

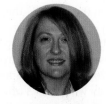

**Joanne Lorraine Davies,
MSc, RM, CHSE**

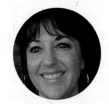

**Colette Foisy-Doll,
MSN, RN, CHSE**

251

This chapter describes the burgeoning global expansion of simulation centers, simulation programs, and the successes and challenges experienced by Simulation Champions working to integrate simulation around the globe. There is a paucity of evidence specific to simulation in global contexts, and therefore, we offer you a melding of current evidence, related theory, and personal insights derived from many years of living and working as simulationists in foreign contexts.

In this chapter, we begin by exploring the expansion of simulation, its prevalence, and the use of consortia in global contexts. We then introduce culture theory and related practices in the nursing profession, however, for more detail, see Chapter 14. We describe alternative viewpoints and offer what we believe constitutes healthier approaches to fostering positive intercultural encounters as global citizens. We introduce proven approaches to fostering relationality that include enacting Ubuntu, personal reflection, reflexivity, and the creation of safe and ethical interpersonal spaces for relationship building. As you read along, we invite you to consider the roles you might play in international simulation initiatives, as well as the responsibilities you have in working and interacting with diverse populations.

We conclude by addressing the more personal aspects of global work, offering practical strategies and approaches for the simulationist working on foreign assignment. As such, you will note that the images in this chapter stem primarily from learning contexts and collaboratives where we have worked. The global perspectives sections that follow this chapter depict simulation in many parts of the world. We accompany these strategies with tools to facilitate transitioning to new and unfamiliar environments.

Expansion of Simulation in a Globalized World

Globalization can be defined as the unification and interconnection of the worlds' economic, political, cultural, and social dimensions (Chen & Berlinguer, 2001). We are currently witnessing the explosion of simulation in healthcare due, in part, to globalization. As our world becomes increasingly globalized, countries are experiencing migration patterns that according to Vertovec (2010) are leading to "superdiversity." "**Super-diversity** is a term intended to capture a level and kind of complexity surpassing anything many migrant-receiving countries have previously experienced" (p. 87). Fueled by improved methods of transportation, people now travel, work, and study abroad more often than in the past. Migration-driven diversity as well as dislocation of refugee citizens are increasing yearly, resulting in more diverse populations around the world (global migration has increased 33% from 2000 to 2013) (UNPF, 2013). Kingma (2006) states that today, the vast majority of international migrant workers are highly skilled professionals moving from lower-income countries to live and work in industrialized nations: nurses are one group of professionals that migrate extensively. The

author points out that this contradicts the popular notion that immigrants are born of extreme poverty. Additionally, there are increasing numbers of people who temporarily relocate to other countries for many reasons, be it for study, business, or healthcare employment. In our changing world, all individuals must work to develop cultural competency to strengthen relationships within emerging *superdiverse* populations. Diversification from globalization has created this need, whether you are residing in your country of origin or you are temporarily or permanently relocating to another country.

Globalism is characterized as the world's overall global economic system and generally involves the integrated efforts of business operations and production across boundaries, borders, and local, regional, national, and global levels (Edberg, 2013a). For example, in simulation, parts for a computer-driven mannequin could be produced in Korea, China, and Taiwan and then installed and assembled in Canada; however, the company headquarters resides in the United States where company communications and customer service are outsourced to India. It is in this dynamic context that simulation program development is advancing at a rapid pace worldwide. No longer confined to **high-income countries**, there is an increasing presence of simulation in **low- and mid-income countries**. The World Bank (2015) categorizes high-income countries has having an annual per capita income of greater than $12,475 USD, mid-income $4,023-12,475 USD, and low-income $1,026-4,035 USD. Within global simulation expansion, there are endless opportunities for simulationists and colleagues from diverse backgrounds to meaningfully and genuinely connect. With the common goal of attracting and developing local talent and global leaders in simulation, simulationists from around the world are working together in highly connected ways to share new knowledge and skills. Additionally, a younger global workforce is demanding new models for engagement and integration of social technologies to serve a borderless workplace (Bersin, 2013). Therefore, the global expansion of simulation transpires through a combination of in-person and technology-mediated encounters. Simulation educators and operators, project managers, learning space designers and developers, and institutional administrators are engaging in the creation of mutually beneficial relationships to build stronger global communities and a stronger global learning economy.

Bersin reports that "Skills are the new arms race" and that "nearly 70 percent of international organizations feel they lack the required skills to compete, and those who thrive are those who continuously build deep skills". Developing productive cross-cultural partnerships is best accomplished through cultural immersion within a foreign milieu, as opposed to having episodic and sporadic encounters that often yield poor results. *Design and Dash* approaches are not helpful and contribute to negative outcomes like vast resources that sit unused, poorly prepared educators and a lack of skill to operationalize simulation programs. Fly-in, fly-out meetings are useful for focused information sharing and instruction but fail to promote more collaborative, lasting change. Therefore, planning longer-term stays of 2 to 5 years or more versus 1 to 2 weeks is mutually beneficial. There are employment models using multiple shorter-term contracts (i.e., weeks, months, or 1 year) and/or a combination of on-site and remote consulting. Longer stays abroad also serve to provide opportunities for reciprocal self-reflection, something often overlooked in cross-cultural relationships (Boutain, 2005). As Foster (2009) stated, "The fruit of good partnerships is the trust that deepens our connections with each other, and it is these connections between [people]...despite the challenges, that sustain the motivation to improve" (p. 105). Forging lasting international partnerships, therefore, takes a reciprocal commitment to personal and moral courage, caring, and connection.

The Prevalence of Simulation around the World

According to Rosen (2008), various types of medical simulation have been used for centuries, but the widespread use of simulation has only gained real momentum since the mid-1990s and into the 2000s. Currently, the majority of clinical simulation activity is still centered in mid- and high-income countries. See Table 13.1 for a summary of the over 500 **simulation centers** across the globe.

Simulation program development is expanding to many regions including Africa and the Middle East, Asia Pacific, Latin and Central America, and the Caribbean. To date, North America has been the major medical simulation market and is expected to continue to dominate the market in coming years followed closely by Europe and the Asia Pacific region. However, in the Asian market, maximum growth is anticipated over the next 5 to 7 years in India and China due to stronger levels of economic development. Today, many factors contribute to the heightened use of simulation including an increased awareness of the need for patient safety, more interprofessional education opportunities, and quality evidence that supports what constitutes best practices in simulation (Meticulous Research, 2015). As there is no definitive global list of simulation centers, this list represents known simulation programs along with data collected from websites searches as well as personal communications and knowledge of established programs (Society for Simulation in Healthcare [SSH], 2016e; Davies & Alinier, 2010; Meticulous Research, 2015). What we do know from personal experience is depicted in Table 13.2. This is not a complete list but illustrates that the largest concentration of simulation centers is, at this time, in mid- to high-income countries.

Simulation program development in low- and mid-income countries often requires simulation expertise from outside the country (Davies & Alinier, 2010). This approach necessitates the hiring of full-time staff or consultants with prior knowledge and skills to help build the programs, especially in the initial stages and often beyond. Both Qatar and Rwanda are examples of countries that have successfully created their programs with assistance from professionals originating from mid- to high-income nations (Chapter 15 offers detailed simulation stories about Qatar and Rwanda).

Table 13.1	World Simulation Center Locations	
World Simulation Center Locations—MedSim (2015, January)		
United States of America	432	
Canada	58	
Other	10	
Self-identified Simulation Centers—Society for Simulation in Healthcare Website (2015)		
Asia	9	Middle East	3
Australasia	6	South America	5
Canada	13	Central America	0
Caribbean	4	United States	432
Europe	29		

Table 13.2	Locations Simulation Centers by World Region
Locations Simulation Centers by World Region	
Africa	Ethiopia, Ghana, Malawi, Nigeria, Rwanda, South Africa, Tanzania, Uganda, Zambia, and Zimbabwe
Asia Pacific	China, India, Japan, Kazakhstan, Singapore, and Korea
Australasia	Australia and New Zealand
Caribbean	Dominica, Grenada, and the Dominican Republic
Europe	Germany, France, the United Kingdom, Italy, Spain, and other
North America	United States and Canada
Middle East	Egypt, Jordan, Kuwait, Lebanon, Saudi Arabia, Qatar, Israel, Turkey, Egypt, and the UAE
Asia Pacific	China, India, Japan, Kazakhstan, Singapore, and Korea
Latin America	Mexico, Brazil, Chile, and Costa Rica
North America	United States and Canada

In Africa, Rwanda's model for using international assistance in building simulation programs involved establishing partnerships with educational or healthcare entities located in Belgium, Canada, and the United States. Initially, outside partners provided funding for setup costs such as equipment, facilities, and staff training. Later, funding was provided via ongoing operating budgets of simulation programs. The ultimate goal from the outset was to build a self-sufficient, sustainable program that would be able to stand alone without outside assistance.

Countries with little or no internal expertise in simulation are finding it necessary to rely on outside expertise to build their programs, thus creating opportunities for experienced simulationists from other countries to work in their simulation programs, especially in the start-up phase. The initial project phases often require that workers, typically from high-income countries, commit to long-term employment, typically accepting 2- to 5-year employment contracts.

Multicountry alliances such as the EU (European Union) now allow simulation experts to move from one employer to another within those countries that form the alliance. There are similar alliances elsewhere, for example, the GCC (Gulf Cooperation Council) in the Middle East and the East African Alliance in Africa, that allow workers to move more freely between countries. Moreover, in recent times, there has been increasing migration of healthcare workers to initiate simulation, in particular with the movement of healthcare workers from higher-income to mid- and low-income countries. As the shortage of healthcare workers grows in mid- to high-income countries, there is a growing need to train and hire workers from lower-income nations. According to Klokkerud (2008), of the 57 nations who have a critical shortage of healthcare workers, 36 are found in sub-Sahara Africa. Africans educated abroad, as is often also the case with low-income nations, do not return to their countries origin to work upon graduation. For many years now, "opportunity is the driving force of migration" (Saravia & Miranda, 2004). This reality contributes to the "brain drain effect" through the loss of valuable talent in those countries, and the "brain recirculation effect" as talent moves in an out of the country for employment (Saravia & Miranda). Klokkerud underscores the need to stop the brain drain and recirculation from lower-income countries to ensure sustainable healthcare delivery and a sufficient healthcare workforce. This is why it is so important for simulationists to acknowledge an ethical obligation to engage in collaborative capacity building in the host country.

Simulation Consortia: Solutions for a Globalized World

Simulation consortia are being developed on a regional, state, national, and international level (see Table 13.3 for examples). These alliances are growing in number as simulation programs are increasing at an exponential rate, and

Table 13.3	Simulation Consortia around the World

Simulation Consortia Around the World

Regional Consortia

Bay Area Simulation Collaborative (Waxman et al., 2011)

British Columbia Interprofessional Model for Simulation-Based Education in Healthcare (Qayumi et al., 2012).

Southeastern Indiana Simulation Consortium ("Southeastern Indiana Simulation Consortium," n.d.)

State Consortia

Oregon Simulation Alliance (Oregon Simulation Alliance, n.d.)

Mississippi Healthcare Simulation Alliance ("Mississippi Healthcare Simulation Alliance," n.d.).

National Consortia

Scotland (Glavin, 2008); Qatar (the Qatar Simulation Consortium); Rwanda (National Simulation Program); Israel Center for Medical Simulation (Ziv, Erez, Munz, & Vardi, 2006; Ziv et al., 2008).

International Consortia

MENA User Simulation Network (Middle East) (MENA Simulation User Network, n.d.) (https://www.linkedin.com/topic/group/mena-simulation-user-network?gid=6948474) SESAM (Society in Europe for Simulation Applied to Medicine) (SESAM, n.d.) (http://www.sesam-web.org/)

healthcare recognizes the value of collaborative efforts (Waxman, Nichols, O'Leary-Kelley, & Miller, 2011; Ziv, Erez, & Berkenstadt, 2008).

Theoretical Perspectives on Building Healthy Relationships in Global Contexts

In this section, we feature both traditional and emerging nursing theory to provide a framework for the simulationist working in international contexts. This involves processes needed to build individual, organizational, and systems capacity for simulation-based learning at local, regional, and national levels. Simulationists on international work assignments are often immersed in contexts where they operate outside their comfort zones. On a personal level, simulationists must learn how to maneuver their way through unfamiliar environments while adapting to foreign languages, dissimilar interpersonal relationship norms, unique traditions, customs and beliefs, and unknown structures, organizations, and systems

(Herberg, 2012). From a systems perspective, they must work to introduce and integrate simulation within existing governmental structures and policy, organizations and institutions, and health professions. We offer various theoretical perspectives as foundations for relationship and capacity building with new partners in new environments.

Perspectives on International Nursing

International nursing as a specialty consists of a "unique body of knowledge with specific problems and domains of practice" (Herberg, 2012, p. 439). Nursing has a long-standing history of participating in efforts in response to global needs for improved health. This is accomplished through coordinated efforts to support education, health, and humanitarian assistance and to enhance government efforts at local levels (Herberg, 2012). Herberg categorizes external assistance entities as follows, with examples in each category:

- *Major government aid/donor agencies* (country based) (e.g., U.S. Agency for International Development [USAID], Department for International Development DFID in the United Kingdom, Canadian International Development [CIDA], Centers for Disease Control and Prevention [CDC], Clinton Health Access Commission [CHAI])
- *Major intergovernmental organizations* (e.g., International Monetary Fund, the United Nations, the World Health Organization, the Pan American Health Organization)
- *Major nongovernmental organizations* (NGOs) (e.g., Project HOPE, Doctors Without Borders/Médecins Sans Frontiers, Amnesty International, Save the Children, the International Committee of the Red Cross, and International Federation of the Red Cross and Red Crescent Societies)
- *Professional organizations* (International Council of Nurses [ICN], Sigma Theta Tau International Society of Nursing [STTI]).

The work of simulationists can be tied to such organizations (see the Global Exemplars in Chapter 15), while in other instances, a simulationist might serve as an independent consultant, a permanent or temporary employee of a host country, or, for example, as part of an interinstitutional research collaborative or educational partnership.

To function effectively in host countries, simulationists as part of the growing stream of global workers should use proven approaches to prepare for and frame these experiences. An adapted version of Herberg's Characteristics of International Nursing (2012) in Box 13-1 offers guidelines to help prepare simulationists for working abroad.

Box 13-1	**Herberg's Characteristics of International Nursing**

Simulationists traveling to foreign host countries and wanting to build positive relationships should:

- Gain knowledge of organizational culture, climate, structures, and mechanisms for communication and decision-making regarding health and nursing: such as policies, procedures, and regulations at local, regional, and national levels.
- Learn about healthcare and nursing in context.
- Recognize that within dominant expressions of culture are unique expressions of that culture both individually and collectively.
- Learn about dimensions and expressions of the dominant culture such as perspectives and norms for handling conflict, family obligations, roles of family members, personal hygiene, cross-cultural communication, touch, etiquette, clothing and accessories, time orientation, interpersonal relationship, gender and sexual orientation, history and rivalries, and moral and religious beliefs (Andrews & Lugwig-Beymer, 2012).
- Employ the concepts of collaborative development and shared capacity building.
- Work as a partner and collaborator with the host country and unfamiliar systems to functional safely, ethically, and responsibly.
- Demonstrate capabilities to face challenges inherent in working with unfamiliar environments and systems. This includes knowledge of and compliance with requirements for work, exit and entrance visas, immunizations, insurance, residency applications, location of embassies, and host country laws and regulations (p. 438).

Adapted from Herberg, P. (2012). Perspectives on international nursing. In M. M. Andrews & J. S. Boyle (Eds.), *Transcultural concepts in nursing care* (6th ed.). Philadelphia, PA: Wolters Kluwer, Lippincott Williams & Wilkins.

Perspectives on Transcultural Nursing

Madeleine Leininger, a cultural anthropologist and nurse, conceptualized and introduced her *Theory of Culture Care Diversity and Universality* in the early 1960s and later founded the *Transcultural Nursing Society*, the *Journal of Transcultural Nursing*, and the *Sunrise Model* (2006). Over the past 50+ years, this framework has also informed other culture care paradigms and related cultural competence models of practice. Refer to Chapter 14 for a more detailed account of this theory. In this segment, we review key criticisms of the theory and offer suggestions for an expanded view of culture arising from current needs and contexts. Healthy debate within the profession is important because it gives voice to dissenting opinions born of fundamental differences in philosophical, historical, socioeconomic, cultural, religious, and political ideology (Andrews & Boyle, 2012b).

The limitations associated with transcultural nursing and related theory are described by Andrews and Boyle (2012) as follows: the use of ambiguous or ethnocentric terminology (e.g., ill-defined differences between cultural competence, awareness, sensitivity, and cultural congruence); use of terms by the nurse that infer judgement and a negative bias such as client noncompliance; too little focus on morale agency and the role of the nurse as advocate and negotiator of public policy to effect change in the realms of politics, economics, and social justice; a lack of recognition of power distance and power imbalances inequitable social relations in healthcare; and inattention to the complexities of transcultural encounters such as racism, prejudice, and discrimination (Andrews & Boyle, 2012; Browne et al., 2009). Andrews and Boyle point out that many of these criticisms are defensible and that others may simply persist as irreconcilable disciplinary or worldviews.

We believe that nurses are at an important juncture in the evolution of our professional identity. As leaders in the 21st century, we must listen, hear, and respond to powerful voices from civil rights movements that are demanding change to overcome societal racism and discrimination (Vertovec, 2010). As a profession, nursing must take pause to reflect on and examine the causal relationships between past healthcare systems, health policy, nursing practices, and the health outcomes of those we have served, especially ethnic minority and low-income populations. The journey of our past and the lessons contained therein must inform future directions for the profession.

Why is this important for the simulationist working within diverse populations to know? In response, it is important that Simulationists working abroad be informed of both the historical and current contexts to better foster new connections. They must engage in critical **reflection** and analysis about the impact of past and current professional practices, health structures and models of care, and related public policy. This reflective approach affords each of us the opportunity to shift our thinking about how we enter into and build **intercultural** relationships, meaning those relationships existing between two or more cultures. Newer culture theories, frameworks, and models posit that nurses working within diverse populations in all contexts must shift their stance from nurse-centric to client- and context-centric approaches (Ridenour & Trautman, 2009). Long ago, Ball (1994) described the shift in *power dynamic* that is needed to crush oppression and abuses of power as "a relation in which people are not dominated but empowered through critical reflection leading to shared action" (p. 23).

Perspectives on Post-Colonial Theory

Post-colonialism is the study of the cultural legacy of colonialism and imperialism. Although the world has been affected by conquests and takeovers since the beginning of time, the *Colonial Era* specifically took root in the late 14th century during an age when Europeans set sail to conquer and build settlements in other worlds. These voyages by explorers and merchants involved the deliberative process of shaping the belief of indigenous peoples to one that saw white Europeans as superior to themselves (Ertan, Putterman, & Fiszbein, 2012). Indigenous people, in turn, were regarded by these explorers as savages, incapable of attaining the status of their white colonizers (Nelson, as cited in McMullin, 2010). Portugal, Spain, the Dutch Republic, France, and England led conquests as early as the late 1400s that eventually led to the spread their culture, people, and dominant perspectives (McGibbon, Mulaudzi, Didham, Barton, & Sochan, 2014). **Neocolonialism** (new colonialism) includes "all forms of control of prior colonies or populations, such as Indigenous people who continue to live under conditions of internal colonialism" (Reimer-Kirkham & Brown, 2009, p. 334). There is also evidence that supports the positive effects of colonialism, such as local and international economic benefits or increased security and stability in high-risk countries (Auerbach & Hoffenberg, 2016), more rapid routes of dissemination and communication, increase life expectancy, and decreased morbidity from infectious disease (Edberg, 2013a). "To appreciate the benefits of colonization, it should be considered in its relation, not to a single country, but to the collective economic interests of the human race" (Mill as cited in Halsall, 1998, para. 2).

Today, the negative effects of colonialism and the ever-present results of neocolonialism (some refer to as the insidious effects of globalization) persist, resulting in the continued substandard lifestyles and **health disparities** of affected populations (a health inequality that is closely linked with social or economic disadvantage). Other examples of the negative effects of colonialism include increasing safety challenges related to clashing worldviews in increasingly diverse contexts, reduced control over labor conditions in global market economies, increasing complexity in environmental regulations and responsibility, and rapid spread of disease (e.g., SARS) (Edberg, 2013a). This is true in particular in Canada, the United States, and Australia where the dire effects of neocolonialism prevail (McGibbon et al., 2014). It is important for simulationists, therefore, to understand and recognize the presence of these long-standing effects (i.e., lost cultures, languages, and identities, and grave health disparities)—and the potential for lingering unresolved sentiments. In such instances, colleagues from differing backgrounds can collaborate to create shared strategies for simulation initiatives that honor and give presence to the need for local ownership and control and the many unique needs of the host community and country (Greenwood, de Leeuw, Lindsay, & Reading, 2015). To turn the tide, there is a dire need for nurses to critically reflect about how colonialization impacted the evolution of the profession and how it has shaped current mental models, nursing theory, and professional practices and the consideration of these factors when designing educational curricula and simulation programs.

Nursing literature in recent decades signals a growing and urgent call for the decolonization of nursing and nursing education toward building healthier human relationships in healthcare (Aboriginal Healing Foundation, 2002; Adelman, Fortier, Smith, Stange, & Strain, 2008; McGibbon et al., 2014; Truth and Reconciliation Commission of Canada [TRC], 2015; Vertovec, 2010). Many now advocate for a transition to **cultural safety** as the basis for intercultural encounters. At its core, "Cultural Safety is not about the cultural practices of the nurse but is about engaging in a recognition of the social, economic, and political position of certain groups within society" (Gerlach, 2012, p. 152). This approach seeks to root out unsafe cultural practices and comprise "any action that diminishes, demeans or disempowers the cultural identity and well-being of an individual" (p. 152). Transitioning to culturally safe practices involves a philosophical shift and adopting a stance of critical inquiry to promote reflexivity in practice. Browne et al. propose that to enact this shift; nurses must learn about culturally safe practices at individual and institutional levels (2009).

At its core, cultural safety involves a commitment to cocreate and engage in culturally safe practices that aim to transfer the power away from the nurse and back to the client. A simulationist working with healthcare colleagues can adopt culturally safe practices by acting as moral agent with a central emphasis on distributive justice, ethics, and equity in the development of simulation programs. Additionally, simulationists can act as change agents to root out and resolve inequities where and when they are encountered. By focusing on strengths and motivations, the host client can determine what constitutes appropriate approaches for their context. In that same light, simulationists working with diverse groups should adopt a model of *caring about*, rather than *caring for* others. As equal colleagues the focus then shifts away from the goals of the simulation expert to one of host goal attainment. See Table 13.4 for examples that depict a shift from simulationist-centric to host-centric approaches.

Perspectives on Interculturality and Human Connection

In Africa, the word **Ubuntu** describes our human interconnectedness in a way that English words cannot. Archbishop Desmond Tutu (2015) professed, "You can't exist as a human being in isolation. Ubuntu is translated as "I am because you are." "In essence, you can't be human all by yourself, and when you have this quality—Ubuntu—you are known for your generosity. We think of ourselves far too frequently as just individuals, separated from one another, whereas you are connected, and what you do affects the whole World" (Tutu Foundation, 2015, para. 4). Ubuntu also implies entanglement (intertwining with another): a concept that does not necessarily sit well with

Table 13.4	Cultural Safety: Shifting the Focus and Locus of Power in Intercultural Relationships
Visiting Simulationist-Centered Approach	**Host-Centered Approach**
"I understand simulation and what you need for successful integration and implementation. Let me teach you."	"Help me understand what you already know and would like to learn about simulation."
"I know exactly what you need to learn, so let's get started."	"Teach me about your environment and this context so we might collaborate to make better decisions."
"As the expert and I can clearly see that you are lacking key supports to make simulation work for you here."	"I have something very valuable to learn from you about how simulation might work differently. Please tell me about your vision."
"Your teaching practices are very different from mine, let's set out to fill those gaps with my expert knowledge of best practices."	"Let's explore your educational approaches and how best practices in simulation can be adapted or applied here."
"I know how simulation can work for you."	"Tell me about your goals and aspirations for better educational experiences using simulation."

individualist mentalities where people see themselves as independent and self-reliant (Wheatley, 2012). The challenge in the entanglement of western and eastern ways lies in how to bridge differing and sometimes opposing philosophies and cultural truths. The realities of interfacing cultures involves a process that searches for meaningful connections that bind us. From its collectivist roots, Ubuntu means having a profound respect for our connectedness to other people: a place inside you where joy, pain, sadness, home, food, accomplishments, happiness, and all of life are for sharing. This approach to life provides spiritual principles through which strong international partnerships can flourish. It is in the spirit of Ubuntu that Simulation Champions can work to promote intercultural learning and simulation expansion (see Fig. 13.1).

Wulf (2010) suggests that two dominant tendencies are playing out in globalization today: "one that moves towards a universal standardization of the world, and the other that makes provision for cultural diversity in the process" (p. 33). He predicts that the approaches we choose to human interaction have an enormous role to play in whether we move forward in peace, or at war. Therefore, it is with intentionality that today's Simulation Champions must strive to create positive intercultural encounters guided by principles of intercultural learning. While cultural diversity is a proven

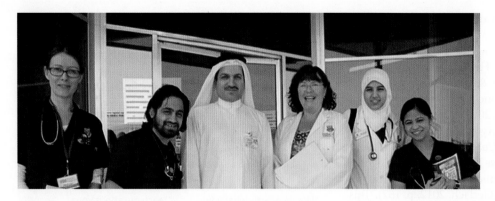

Figure 13.1 Learning Across Cultures, University of Calgary Qatar 2010. (Photo by John Gulka, used with permission.)

source of enrichment, it can also lead to the emergence of counterideologies, putting social cohesion under severe stress and strain. This outcome is certainly evident today as new forms of inter- and intracultural warfare erupt all over the globe. Intercultural learning grounded in **social justice** with peace as its aim can help to mitigate these dire effects (UNESCO, 2013; Wulf, 2010). Social justice involves actioning to resolve the inequitable distribution of wealth, opportunity and privilege in a given society.

According to Aldridge, Kilgo, and Christensen (2014), **transcultural** (often referred to as intercultural) education is central to positive outcomes. Transcultural education transpires through a process called *transcendent culturing,* which is the use of purposeful and positive interaction to overcome barriers that result in limited human interaction across borders. This educational approach seeks to "foster interculturality [and interconnectedness] to develop cultural interactions in the spirit of building bridges among peoples" (Wulf, 2010, p. 34).

To that end, intercultural learning using simulation can be achieved in a variety of innovative ways. For example, national organizations like the National League for Nursing's Simulation Innovation Resource Center (SIRC) and Laerdal Medical have collaborated with stakeholders from Australia, Canada, Chile, Japan, Norway, and the United States to integrate international perspectives into SIRC online learning modules for simulation educators (Kelly, 2009). Additionally, Kelly adds that there is promising potential for international collaboration in patient safety and interprofessional learning tied to national government agency initiatives like patient safety agendas.

More and more students and educators are exposed to people from diverse backgrounds through travel, work, volunteering, and studying abroad. Face-to-face exposure with other cultures permits learning on a firsthand basis. However, we believe that physical immersion is not the only means of developing cultural competency. We suggest that simulation can be an effective method of teaching cultural competency and promoting intercultural learning. Pyburn and Bauman (2013) state that virtual reality and game-based simulation can also be useful to teach and learn cultural competency. Communication in virtual worlds

happens in different and often more engaging ways than traditional person-to-person interactions, such as landline telephone calls. With increasing diversity and modern technologies, human interaction has evolved to be highly mediated, interactive, and very much under our control. Today, all Internet users can create and brand a personal professional image, allowing individuals to market and/or share professional services and resources. It is important to be mindful of how we maintain that professional image in technology-mediated encounters, for example, when representing ourself as an avatar in virtual learning. These are realities in our mediated connections with others that require intentional management (Wheatley, 2012).

Technology now offers us the luxury of language translation apps on mobile devices, so as long as you have connectivity, you can communicate via your smartphone app. Recently, the use of such an app helped us as foreigners to better maneuver new territory and languages. Today's technological advances can also facilitate the sharing of common interests and resources among international colleagues (Mill, Ogilvie, Astle, & Gastaldo, 2010).

Ethical Principles and Global Simulation Program Development

Many simulationists are also healthcare professionals and educators and, therefore, have a moral responsibility to adhere to **global ethical principles**. The INACSL Professional Integrity Standard states that all those engaged in simulation "are responsible for acting with professional integrity and developing self-awareness of how one's personal and professional behavior affects those around him or her" (INACSL Standards Committee, 2016, p. S30). We must collaborate with colleagues to uphold these principles and to develop a sense of ethical and professional responsibility in those we educate. Below, we discuss three fundamental ethical principles in global development: social responsibility, distributive justice, and equity. We then discuss how to incorporate these principles into simulation program development.

Social Responsibility

The International Bioethics Committee report, On Social Responsibility and Health (UNESCO [IBC], 2010), describes **social responsibility** as "responsibility that is extended from individuals to groups and communities, but also from private to public institutions and corporations to produce effects that are potentially beneficial or harmful for workers, suppliers, customers, other concerned persons or the environment" (p. 19). Social responsibility can also refer to the duty of each person to act for the benefit of society as a whole, as well as when choosing ethical frameworks used to make those decisions. As trusted healthcare educators and clinicians, simulationists have a heightened ethical, legal, and moral obligation to promote the learning of social responsibility and related ethical and moral obligations in our programs. Learners must know that social responsibility is what we expect of them as individuals and employees. To be a socially responsible healthcare provider means to always ask, "In what ways can I commit to promoting the health and well-being of others?" Therefore, designers of simulation learning should develop experiences that afford students the opportunity to make socially responsible choices. Examples include scenarios where students must speak out to avoid harming the health of others, protect the environment, ensure sustainable use of resources, avoid producing and marketing of harmful goods and substances, safeguard individuals, and promote equity-focused policy and program development (WHO, 1997). Patterson and Hulton (2012) reported that with proper planning, organization, and reflection, simulation experiences designed to have participants learn about poverty can offer impactful, lifelong learning about civic engagement and social responsibility.

Distributive Justice

Distributive justice can be defined as "the apportionment of privileges, duties, and goods with the merits of the individual and in the best interest of society [the global society]" (Merriam-Webster Dictionary, n.d.). Armstrong (2012) distinguishes between global distributive justice in a general sense and principles of distributive justice. Global distributive justice describes *the need* to share the benefits and burdens of our lives among members of a given society or community. Principles of distributive justice, on the other hand, provide guidance on *how* to go about sharing of benefits and distribution of burdens. For example, when we work to develop international collaboratives, we need to ask important questions like, "In a global economy, what constitutes a 'fair share'?"; "What belongs to who?"; and "Between the the low-income and high-income groups, who handles what part of their fair share?" Easy answers to these questions do not exist, but asking them is vital to developing fairness and goodwill in international simula-

tion program development. As education continues to transform globally, simulation educators and healthcare providers must aim to create new practices through which we can better discern the concept of fairness.

Equity

The WHO defines **equity** as "the absence of avoidable or remediable differences among groups of people, whether those groups are defined socially, economically, demographically, or geographically" (2015, para. 1) (http://www.who.int/healthsystems/topics/equity/en/). Equity, unlike equality, means fairness, not sameness. Health inequities, therefore, speak to more than inequality with respect to health determinants. Equity also involves having access to the resources needed to improve and maintain health and health-related outcomes (UNESCO, 2013). Additionally, governance models are needed to ensure that processes are in place that position countries around the world for greater integration within the world economy. Such models promote the "movement of goods and services, capital, technology and (to a lesser extent) labour" in light of global realities (Solar & Irwin, 2010). As educators and healthcare providers at the forefront of global healthcare education, we are called to ensure that education and collaborative partnerships influence equitable global development.

Simulationists can apply and enact principles of social responsibility, distributive justice, and equity in simulation program development in global contexts in a number of ways (Corbett & Fikkert, 2009). The first approach encourages those involved in simulation programs that originate from high-income countries to reach out and assist those in low- and mid-income countries. Assistance, in this context, is understood as a fully engaged community-based learning process where doing together, as opposed to doing for, is key. All countries, regardless of levels of economic prosperity, have a great deal to teach other nations. Simulationist partners are well positioned to provide assistance in the form of financial help for building facilities and purchasing or sharing of equipment and supplies, curricular integration of simulation, training faculty and simulation staff, and operationalizing simulation programs. Moreover, the technological explosion throughout the world enables us to share educational resources and learning sessions across borders, such as with the NLN-SIRC initiative (Kelly, 2009). It is essential to share resources and teach known best practices in simulation and to apply those practices while being mindful of context, diversity, and particular needs.

In January 2016, three INACSL representatives traveled to Istanbul, Turkey, to teach 400 nurse educators over two full days about the INACSL Best Practices in Standards: Simulation^SM, (INACSL Standards Committee, 2016). Lori Lioce from the United States, Matthew Aldridge from the United Kingdom, and Colette Foisy-Doll from Canada shared their knowledge and experience and numerous resources to advance simulation in nursing in Turkey. In return, the Turkish nurses engaged in lively debate about current teaching methodologies in nursing, followed by discussions on how we could proceed to work together. The enthusiasm, national patriotism, professionalism, and commitment were inspiring and contagious. Sharing of human resources and intellectual capital through educational offerings is happening with increasing frequency, and so it should (personal communication, C. Foisy-Doll, 2016).

The second way is to use simulation methodologies to promote the development of cultural competency, safety, humility, and sensitivity in learners within simulated patient encounters. Simulation has been shown to be an effective method for teaching where students must apply principles of cultural competence in context (Foisy-Doll, 2013). To ensure authenticity and accuracy of diversity- and culture-focused simulations, educators should seek validation of scenario content through consultants or individuals familiar with that cultural context. For example, a simulation team designing a simulation scenario on end-of-life care for the Muslim patient in the Middle East consulted with a local Imam (see Fig. 13.2). Ozkara San (2015) conducted a literature review to understand better the use of clinical simulation to enhance cultural competency in nursing students. Although the author identified gaps in the overall effectiveness of simulation to improve cultural competency in nursing care, the results revealed that the use of simulation does support its development "by providing a safe environment to conduct a cultural assessment, elicit students' attitudes toward cross-cultural situations... recognize cross-cultural issues in interviewing... so [and by] providing treatment and nursing care for patients from diverse ethnic and racial backgrounds" (p. 228). There is more content to follow on cultural competence in simulation in Chapter 14.

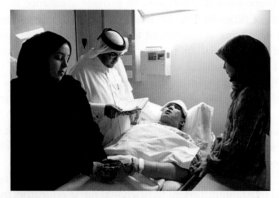

Figure 13.2 University of Calgary Qatar Students Participating in End-of-Life Care of the Muslim Patient— Simulation—Family Member Holding Patient Hand (Simulator), 2012. (Photo by John Gulka, used with permission.)

Together, with a united front and a commitment to shared international goal setting for best practices in simulation and healthcare, we hope to achieve the ultimate goals of improved patient safety and improved patient outcomes within local and global communities.

Simulation to Engage Learners as Global Citizens

"The more active global citizens there are, the more progress in the world we make will be" (Gates & Gates, 2015). As people around the world become increasingly connected through ease of transportation, the Internet, and technology, so too does the mounting impetus for us to become responsible **global citizens**. As citizens of an emerging borderless world, we are called to be active agents in political, social, environmental, and economic realms. Braskamp (2008) tells us that future citizens and leaders of tomorrow must possess an "understanding of the world's cultures, languages, religions, economics, sciences, and technologies... and a sensitivity and respect for all cultural traditions" (p. 2). Currently, 1.3 billion people still do not have access to adequate and affordable healthcare, and low- and mid-income countries bear 93% of the world's disease burden, yet account for only 18% of the global income and 11% of global health spending (Bale, n.d.). According to the WHO Commission on Social Determinants of Health, the reduction of health inequities is an ethical imperative for this generation (Commission on Social Determinants of Health [CSDH], 2008). As simulationists and healthcare professionals, we are positioned to assist in improving healthcare in remote or lower-income remote parts of the world.

Levintova, Johnson, Scheberle, and Vonck (2011) list the learning outcomes that students believed to be critical global competencies. These competencies include knowledge and skill in (1) international politics, (2) global connectedness, (3) global improvement, (4) environmental responsibility, (5) social skills, (6) team work, (7) negotiation skills, (8) collaboration, (9) diversity, and (10) tolerance. It is evident that today's students are aware of the importance of learning how to be an engaged global citizen. Learning to be a global citizen can either be achieved at home or away through international employment, volunteering, studying, or traveling abroad (volunteer tourism). However, travel is not the exclusive means of developing the competencies required of global citizens. It must and should be developed locally and globally.

Global connectivity has increased our ability to connect exponentially. More healthcare programs are providing students with opportunities to work, study, and volunteer abroad and to connect with each other while doing so within classrooms that unfold on a global stage. Simulation-based learning can include innovations like telebroadcasting simulation and teleconferencing for collaborative debriefing. Other opportunities include "service-learning, internships, community research, journaling, blogging, wikis, fieldwork, experiments, and active learning in class—to create students who are global citizens and useful neighbors to everyone, including those in our own communities" (Levintova et al. 2011, p. 2).

Cultural Brokering: Becoming Active Global Citizens

Cultural brokering can be defined as "a healthcare intervention through which the professional increasingly uses cultural and health science knowledge and skills to negotiate with the client and the healthcare system for an effective, beneficial healthcare plan" (Wenger, 1995, as cited in Bronheim (2011), p. 3). For example, when healthcare workers from host countries provide care for foreigners that fall ill, they are in fact acting as cultural brokers. Imagine a simulation that requires students to act as cultural brokers for a newly landed immigrant patient and his/her family. Brokering is a cultural competency that is increasingly required of us all. Based on personal experience, cultural brokers are also vital to the well-being of foreign workers.

Kirkham, Van Hofwegen, and Pankratz (2009) suggest a framework for international learning experiences for students traveling abroad or receiving foreigners that includes the following guiding principles:

- Maximize transformative learning
- Create equitable partnerships (attending to power relations)
- Organize the experience
- Generate knowledge

Simulation can serve as a useful approach to teach the principles of global citizenship and cultural safety and prepare learners for international experiences by replicating lifelike experiences they might expect to encounter in the host country. Braskamp, Calian Trautvetter, and Ward (2008) tell us that developing an understanding of global citizenry is possible when using a synergistic blend of both experiential and traditional academic education. Doing so immerses students in rich experiences that are rooted in community and social issues to cultivate conscientiousness, compassion, and relationality. Simulation educators today are creating simulated clinical experiences with those outcomes in mind. Waite and McKinney (2016) remind educators of the vital need for nurses to learn and develop emotional and social competencies, both requisites for effective leadership and followership in nursing. For example, Bachen, Hernandez-Ramos, and Raphael (2012) developed a computerized simulation game called "REAL LIVES" in which the players were able to assume the roles of other people in different countries around the world. They found that students who played the simulation game as part of their curriculum expressed more global empathy and greater interest in learning about other countries. Together, with a united front and a commitment to shared international goal setting for best practices in simulation and healthcare, we may achieve the ultimate goals of improved patient safety and improved patient outcomes within local and global communities.

Virtual Simulation for Global Learning and Sharing

The Internet and technology are making it increasingly possible to maximize accessibility of simulation and to share resources and learning opportunities globally. Two rapidly developing areas in simulation are virtual reality and gaming, which make it possible to access training and exercises from any place, anytime (see Fig. 13.3). In addition, several countries have developed mobile simulation units that are able to go to outlying rural areas without their own simulation facilities, thus enabling simulation to be brought to remote areas where it would otherwise not be available. An example of this is the Clinical Skills Managed Educational Network (CS MEN) in Scotland (Laerdal, n.d.). With the use of this mobile unit, rural areas in Scotland who do not have their own simulation centers can deliver simulation education programs by using this mobile unit. Further examples of this can be seen in Australia where remote areas are supported by larger public programs such as the work in Queensland by the Clinical Skills Development Service Center (Clinical Skills Development Service, 2015).

Telehealth is playing a larger role in the future of healthcare, allowing healthcare providers to interact with patients in remote and underserved areas. For example, teleconferencing equipment in each simulation room equipped with medical scope attachments could allow students to gain experience examining patients in a home or rural clinic setting while consulting with a physician or assessing home health patients remotely.

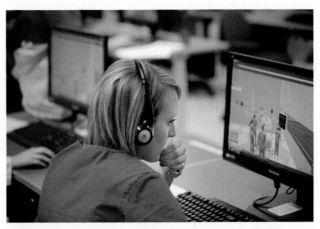

Figure 13.3 Example of Virtual Simulation at HELP! Save Stan—Learning in Second Life. (From University of Alberta Health Sciences Education and Research Commons, with permission.)

There is great potential for enhanced global learning with platforms such as those used by the Oregon Health and Science University, which is now using Tele-OSCEs (Palmer, 2014). Simulated/Standardized patients (SP) connect with the students via a teleconference interface. Not only do the students learn how to deliver patient-centered care by interacting with simulated patients, but they also learn how to interact with to a patient via teleconferencing, which may be increasingly used as a method of interacting with real patients. It is not hard to envision how telehealth applications could be used to remotely deliver the same quality of simulation education in low-income countries or in rural or inaccessible areas as in more densely developed, urban areas. For example, students could participate in simulation sessions in one location and be debriefed remotely by debriefers at another location. Simulation education sessions could be delivered to simulation staff or faculty remotely. Additionally, clinicians in training can use a virtual reality simulator (e.g., a surgical training simulator) while being coached by an instructor using the same simulator in remote location.

As we move ahead, the use of computers and personal mobile devices, as well as virtual and cloud-based applications will only increase, as will their integration within simulation in healthcare.

Global Workers in Simulation

An *expatriate* is historically known as a person that has relocated to a country other than his/her country of origin, often abbreviated as *expat*. Essentially, the term is derived from the root words *ex* (out of) and *patria* (country, or the fatherland) (Koutonin, 2015). In practice, the term has been applied to professionals, skilled workers, or artists from affluent countries, often transferred by companies, rather than referring to the broader category of immigrants in general (Castree, Kitchen, & Rogers, 2013). It is very interesting to note that in the lexicon of human migration, the word expat is not applied equally across the board. Koutonin contends that expat exclusively refers to the person of privilege (often Western white people) traveling to work *ex patria*. Take pause to consider why nonwhite people leaving their country of origin to resettle and work in other countries are referred to as immigrants? Orsini (2015) describes the mental images conjured up by the term expat as "luxury... shiny desks in multinational corporates and privileged lifestyles...On the other hand, when it comes to the term 'immigrant,' we tend to think about dreams, hopes and cardboard suitcases" (para. 1). As a result, many consider the use of the word *expat* as outdated and highly inappropriate (Koutonin, 2015; Orsini, 2015). Ossowski (2015), on the other hand, states that it is not the color of one's skin that fuels the expat impression; rather, it is the governments that issue the passports and visas that are unfair and result

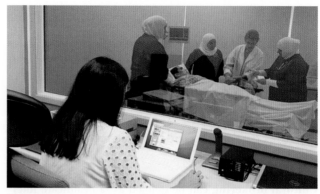

Figure 13.4 University of Calgary Qatar Simulation Educator and Students in the Clinical Simulation Learning Center. (Photo by John Gulka, used with permission.)

in systemic inequities that perpetuate racist perceptions. In some countries, for example, it is much easier for some individuals to obtain work visas. Whether born of systemic inequities in government policy or a specific ideology of privilege, for the purposes of this chapter, we intentionally avoid the use of the term expat. Simulationists from high-income countries should be mindful of language and recognize the power gradient inherent in this type of verbiage and then work to eliminate such disparities. See Table 13.4 for examples of how one might shift the focus and locus of power within intercultural relationships.

Across the globe, there is a rapid expansion of Simulation Programs, and as a result, there are more full-time jobs and consulting opportunities available for those with expertise in the field. Countries with little or no internal expertise in simulation are finding it necessary to rely on outside assistance to build their programs, thus creating opportunities for simulationists to work in their Simulation Programs, especially in the start-up phase (see Fig. 13.4).

Simulationists, many of whom originate from high-income countries, are well positioned to assist in reversing this trend by lending our assistance in developing sustainable simulation programs with locally trained workforces in low- and mid-income countries. However, having worked in both high- and low-income countries ourselves, we think it is crucial to consider diversity through a lens of cultural humility. It is important to view these encounters as partnerships and opportunities to celebrate intercultural diversity. Through the intentional use of a more humanistic lens, we can encourage perceptions of each other as equal, capable, and valuable members of one team.

Downward Trending for High-Income to Low-Income Migrant Workers

Interestingly, the days of workers emigrating from high-income countries to resettle and work in low-income countries are trending downward. Companies are now investing huge dollars in building local leaders who identify with local culture and workforce dynamics (Bersin, 2013). The Qatarization program is one such example where the state of Qatar is developing tomorrow's leaders through succession planning aimed at local talent development to fill key leadership positions. When good succession planning happens, the national leadership pipeline is strengthened, thereby decreasing the country's reliance on an external workforce (Qatar Foundation, 2015). When asked to assist with simulation endeavors, it is crucial to collaborate with a mindset of capacity building and empowerment and also to ensure sustainability and transfer of skills.

Calling out Privileging

The literature suggests that fruitful intercultural exchanges stem from a stance of critical reflection and an acknowledgment that one's knowledge of another is always partial, incomplete, and inevitably biased (Ausland, 2010; Wear, 2008). For example, as a woman from a high-income country arriving to work in a low-income country, one could take the time to understand others' perceptions and beliefs of oppression, marginalization, and privilege. Simulationists from mid- to high-income countries working in low-income countries can also make a conscious choice to acknowledge and be critical of acts of *privileging* (granting certain individuals rights because of certain conditions, i.e., color, money, status, etc.). Moreover, they can make every effort to eradicate manifestations of privileging in their encounters with others by politely turning down privileges as they arise. One example from our collective personal experiences was being asked to move to the front of a queue because of perceived status or skin color. In that instance, we simply chose to smile and decline the offer. These actions are powerful and can speak louder than words. In systems where privileging is the norm, locals are often treated as less worthy (for example, being placed in a separate queue) - a perception that can be abated through our actions, however small.

The Ups and Downs of Working on Foreign Assignment

For many nurses, international work becomes a lifelong career bringing with it both highs and lows. While foreign workers are party to amazing adventures and life-shaping experiences, they also face immense challenges and significant emotional stresses that typify work abroad (Bolton, 2004). Findings from several studies regarding the experiences of foreign workers revealed that stress stems from both personal and organizational factors that can either contribute or detract from stress levels. Of course, extended and chronic stress will affect a migrant worker's resilience and their capacity to endure in unfamiliar settings (Connor & Miller, 2014; Yao, 2015). Personal factors that can

contribute to stress include age, gender, health, education, nationality, personal ideologies, experiences of loneliness, independence and industriousness, presence of family members, and personal finances, while organizational factors include unexpected or unsatisfactory social and living conditions, language barriers in the workplace, having organizational outsider status, the stressors of immigration processes, and unfamiliar cultures and climates (Connor & Miller, 2014; Pocnet et al., 2015; Yao, 2015).

Ethical Dilemmas in Foreign Contexts

Harding (2013) describes the ethical dilemmas that can arise when nurses interact with individuals or groups from diverse backgrounds. Often, they will attempt to apply universal notions of ethics, such as the right to autonomy and justice only to be met with resistance. These terms, from a global perspective, are highly relative and are subject to contextual interpretations. Historically, these ethical concepts are born of privileged whiteness, predominantly rooted in western philosophy and could, in fact, unwittingly perpetuate a colonialist mentality (Harding, 2013). The challenge is to learn the art of confronting our personal frames and assumptions in these situations and to explore how to enact principles of cultural safety and humility in our interactions with other cultures. For example, when interacting with a woman who self-identifies as the second of four wives to one husband, a simulationist that is unfamiliar with this custom can choose to get curious and learn more, rather than impose judgement based on personal beliefs. To recap, a culturally safe stance requires that we consider others' viewpoints and then engage in thoughtful reflection about how tensions might stem from power distance, equity, and social responsibility when building relationships in culturally diverse settings.

Developing a Relational Ethic through Reflective Practice

*"The focus of relational ethics is on people (whole persons) and the quality of the commitments between them."—**Vangie Bergum and John Dossetor, from Relational Ethics (2005)***

Life and relationships, in whatever context, bring us the opportunity for learning and growth and to come to a deeper understanding of one's own relational ethic—that is to say, the essence of how I choose to enter into relationship with myself and others. Relationships flourish in relational and ethical spaces: such spaces are "found both between people as well as within each person" (Bergum & Dossetor, 2005, p. xviii). Bergum and Dossetor's seminal work on relational ethics maintains that relational and ethical spaces continuously evolve through thoughtful intention and a commitment to fostering ethical encounters in those spaces. Indeed, each of us is the shaper of mutuality, engagement, embodiment, and respect within ourselves and our relationships with others.

Working abroad involves living in unfamiliar environments with people yet unknown from diverse backgrounds. Perhaps the only way we as healthcare providers can ethically approach our differences is to intentionally give equal voice to our differing values, beliefs, cultures, ways of knowing and being, and so on (Bergum, 2012). Entering into authentic exploration of these differences can make us feel uncomfortable. Foisy-Doll (2013) refers to the experience of discomfort that stems from such differences as *cultural dissonance* and embraced it as "daily occurrences that caused me to stop and marvel at our differences" (p. e4). This is, in fact, a catalyst toward Praxis—the juncture where "reflection facilitates a dialogue between theory and practice to develop a new understanding of the world of practice, and a new ability to change practice" (Nairn, Chambers, Thompson, McGarry, & Chambers, 2012, p. 190). In everyday terms, nursing praxis emanates from reflection and learning, and ultimately is that place where the rubber meets the road in clinical practice.

As a species, humans are in search of a space where they feel at home with a sense of love and belonging (Maslow, 1943). In a study of Latino immigrant workers' needs relative to Maslow's hierarchy of needs, workers expressed their greatest need as love and belonging, especially because they tended to experience social isolation and loneliness from being separate from their families (Eggerth & Flynn, 2012). To that end, intentional reflective practices can serve as a catalyst to critical reflection, critical analysis, and critical action informed by our experiences of cultural dissonance. Inner harmony and harmonious relationships can be realized through mutuality and respect between people (Bergum & Dossetor). Erasmus+, a European Union programme that encourages the international mobility of learners believes that individually and collectively, we have the capacity to imagine and cocreate a better future through mutual decision-making to pursue our common goals (http://ec.europa.eu/programmes/erasmus-plus/node_en) and to achieve lifelong learning, health, and wisdom for all.

"The greatest challenge to the world community in this century is to promote harmonious relations between peoples of disparate origins, histories, languages, and religions."—**George Erasmus (2002): from Why Can't We Talk?**

Our call as professionals is to seek a deeper truth and, in doing so, to develop disciplinary knowledge, skills, attitudes, values, and wisdom. One approach to deeper reflection is through a process known as reflexivity. **Reflexivity** differs from reflection in that reflection involves a unidirectional process that looks back on previous action to gain insight (Engward & Davis, 2015). Reflexivity, on the other hand, involves a bidirectional process that entails self-transparency and intensive self-examination. The reflexive approach, therefore, supports intense self-scrutiny of one's thoughts, actions, and emotion to build self-conscious awareness and promote self-development. Although reflexivity can involve others, it does not require their input to take place. In reflexive thought, individuals examine their own actions, assumptions, beliefs, philosophies, and perceptions, as well as those of others,' to reshape and inform new ways of being and doing. (McDermott and Vareene, 2010 as cited in Engward and Davis, 2015).

To be reflexive also involves reflecting on your feelings and reactions in a given situation and is an important aspect of critical reflection and reflective practice for nurses. Browne et al. (2009) encourage that we ask ourselves challenging questions, warning that there are risks in engaging in open dialogue about "culturalism, racialization, or institutionalized racism and discrimination" (p. 174). This process does not come naturally and requires that we give presence to vulnerability in the process; it is a learned process that takes time to develop. Take, for example, the following questions to foster reflexivity:

- What are my deeply entrenched notions of difference? Of privilege? Of color? Of status?
- What are my beliefs about others from diverse backgrounds?
- Where do these beliefs come from? Who or what instilled them in my psyche as part of my value and belief structures?
- Do I feel guilt, anger, or other emotions when exploring the concepts of privilege versus disadvantaged minorities? Do I ever take part in, or tolerate racializing discourses (those that perpetuate negative stereotypes, bias, and misconceptions), either knowingly or unknowingly?
- What are the assumptions I hold about influences on health and social inequities? In what ways have I contributed? Impacted change? Actively sought out the perspectives of others?
- How do I react when I see or hear something that does not fit with my mental models? If I am angry, do I take pause to consider more than what I observe? Do I examine personal assumptions, beliefs, and value structures?

Admittedly, it takes both vulnerability and honesty to open oneself up to this level of self-scrutiny. It also takes commitment to understand how personal frames may unwittingly cause imbalance or even harm, and then to work to change those cognitive structures (Kumashiro, 2000). Therefore, it is through a strengths-based approach to relationship building and adopting a stance of cultural humility that we can create inviting and safe spaces to learn with and from each other. Ausland (2010) offers a framework for such encounters that comprises building honest relationships through active listening and acknowledgment of assumptions, holding a deep affection for others while keeping people at the center of the process, identifying a community vision based on others' values, and actively putting pride aside to make room for others. Based on personal experiences, we believe that it is through a mutual reflexivity and the building of relational and ethical spaces that simulationists around the world can cocreate vibrant and sustainable simulation programs.

Planning a Move Abroad

For some, the lure of adventure and working in far off lands is powerful, but there are very real challenges that come with accepting an international assignment. Whether you are the traveler, or you are receiving someone from abroad, it takes a considerable amount of time and energy to plan for a longterm move. Are you considering a move to work abroad? There is a lot to think about when you are moving to a foreign country. From our collective years of experience working in foreign countries, we offer you the simulationist's relocation prep sheet, which can be found in the Toolkit (Toolkit 13-1).

Many factors impact the ease of transition to a new country and its people, culture, politics, and social systems and structures. Cleary, Walter, Siegfried, and Jackson (2014) encourage meaningful reflection on things such as your *personality traits* (i.e., are you flexible and adaptable in nature, tolerant of uncertainty, embrace diversity, or intolerant of perceived inequities or injustices). The World Traveler's Self-Assessment Tool, also found in the Toolkit (Toolkit 13-2), is a short series of questions we have assembled based on our collective lived experiences and the typical struggles we and others have faced in work abroad. Your answers to these questions can provide some insight into your degree of risk for transition shock.

Transition Shock

Transition shock (sometimes referred to as culture shock), or a rocky period in adaptation, can often occur after the excitement of relocation wanes (Cleary et al., 2014). Foreign workers suffering intense homesickness and feelings of isolation will often spend time in **culture bubbles**, mostly choosing to socialize with others from a similar or familiar background. A reality also referred at homophily - the tendency to associate and bond with those similar to ourselves. Others, in contrast will dive right in and immerse themselves in local culture, people, and traditions (Cleary et al., 2014). Whatever the assignment, remember, a period of time to adapt and settle into the new environment is essential, and it can often take several months before foreign workers feel a sense of familiarity and belonging. Take time to explore the Internet and tap into online blogs, learn about the country and its culture, read all contract offers carefully, talk to people who have experienced working in that environment, and be clear on expectations while setting some realistic initial goals. Above all, have an open mind and heart and carry a spirit of adventure. Choosing to step outside of your culture bubble can bring the most unanticipated, memorable life-giving experiences.

Summary

By virtue of our changing world, we are now connected global citizens in an increasingly diverse and connected world. Today, Simulation Champions are working on the ground throughout the world and often via technology-mediated platforms to cocreate strong relationships and build simulation centers and programs. In order to facilitate the ethical and responsible global expansion of simulation, we all have a role to play in upholding the principles of distributive justice, social responsibility, and equity by keeping them forefront of program development. Simulation Champions everywhere also have a responsibility to foster culturally safe relationships within a framework that empowers both parties in relational and ethical spaces. Together, we can forge a stronger global simulation practice community through collaboration, such as the development of consortia at local, state, national, and international levels. Whether you are currently a simulationist working abroad or you are considering migrating to work in another country, we hope you find this chapter, the packing list, and the self-assessment tool helpful. Finally, it is our sincere desire that nurses and other healthcare professionals working as Simulation Champions throughout the world lead by upholding the principles of global citizenship and Ubuntu: demonstrating care for others, generosity of spirit, hospitality, friendliness, caring, and compassion to promote global excellence in simulation.

 Toolkit Resources

Toolkit 13-1: The Simulationist's Relocation Prep Sheet. This extensive relocation to-do-list will help plan any type of longterm move, but is especially designed for relocation abroad.

Toolkit 13-2: The World Traveler's Self-Assessment Tool. This self-assessment tool is designed to help you consider how your personal characteristics and circumstances affect your suitability and potential for success when working and living abroad.

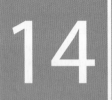

14

Cultural Competence, Safety, and Humility in Simulation Education

Cynthia Foronda, Sandra M. Swoboda, Nasreen T. Bahreman, Colette Foisy-Doll

Key Terms

Culture, Cultural Competence, Linguistic Competence, Cultural Safety, Cultural Sensitivity, Cultural Humility, Cultural Diversity, Inclusion, Simulation, Cultural Sensibility

Guiding Questions

1 Which nursing culture care approach is most aligned with your personal and professional values (cultural competence, cultural sensitivity, cultural safety, cultural humility and linguistic competence, or cultural sensibility)?

2 How can you enact culture and diversity within your teaching practice, curriculum, or Simulation Program?

3 How can you champion ethical and authentic depictions of culture, diversity, and linguistic competence in your Simulation Program?

4 Have you considered barriers in your environment that may pose a threat to enacting cultural best practices in your Simulation Program? If not, how could you plan to anticipate and address challenges?

Introduction

One of the driving forces behind simulation as a preferred pedagogy is the use of experiential learning to better prepare nurses for the provision of safe, quality, and holistic care. To that end, nurses must not only be competent in attending to the biomedical needs of clients, they must also be competent in spiritual, psychosocial, socioeconomic, environmental, and cultural dimensions of patient care (Roberts, Warda, Garbutt, & Curry, 2014). Rapidly changing demographics require that nurses all around the world be properly prepared to care for culturally diverse client populations. Historically, these populations comprised marginalized and silenced populations—such as racial and ethnic minorities, immigrants, and economically disadvantaged communities that were not given the same access to treatment in healthcare (Alberta & Wood, 2008; Carpenter-Song, Nordquest Schwallie, & Jonghofer, 2007).

Nurse educators employing simulation to teach culture care must be equipped to design, deliver, and evaluate culturally diverse experiences in simulation. Todaro-Franchesci (2012) believes that social, ethical, and moral role development in nurses is just as important as teaching and learning

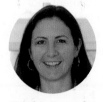

Cynthia Foronda,
PhD, RN, CNE, CHSE, ANEF

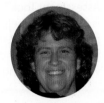

Sandra M. Swoboda,
MS, RN, FCCM

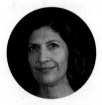

Nasreen T. Bahreman,
MSN, RN, PCNS-BC

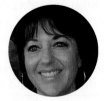

Colette Foisy-Doll,
MSN, RN, CHSE

nurse think skills, such as critical thinking, clinical reasoning, and clinical judgement. Moreover, simulation educators must possess and demonstrate skill in addressing culture themselves. In doing so, they need to model excellence in cultural competence and other culture-related competencies to ensure that culture-focused simulation experiences are administered and debriefed in a safe and inclusive manner (INACSL Standards Committee, 2016, Debriefing). To that end, incorporating culture and diversity into nursing education must extend beyond the enactment of one or two token simulation scenarios. Culture and diversity must thread throughout the broader nursing curriculum.

In this section, the term **cultural diversity** is interpreted within the broadest context and describes

"Differences in ethnic or racial classification and self-identification, tribal or clan, affiliation, nationality, language, age, gender, sexual orientation, gender identity or expression, socioeconomic status, education, religion, spirituality, physical and intellectual abilities, personal appearance, and other factors that distinguish one group or individual from another."—**Bronheim & Goode, 2013a**

In current contexts, we must also consider factors, such as immigrant or refugee status, educational or literacy levels, health literacy, and the profession or discipline, in addition to individual differences and factors that distinguish one group or individual from another.

This chapter offers Simulation Champions a brief introduction to culture-related concepts and theories. We describe how simulation educators can enact and advocate for creating culturally safe and sensitive learning environments in their Simulation Programs. Since culture is context driven, it is important to share that three of the authors of this chapter are nurse educators from the United States, and the fourth originates from Canada; thus, all suggested practices may not be culturally relevant or applicable in other contexts (i.e., international locations). Note that the definitions of culture and related concepts do vary somewhat across contexts as seen through differing worldviews, disciplines, and practice settings. We are very excited to offer Simulation Champions tools and activities to facilitate the integration of culture and diversity in your Simulation Program, curriculum, and organization. Let's begin the journey with our preferred definition of culture.

Culture

There are as many definitions of **culture** as there are dimensions of it. Culture is not an easy concept to define. When you hear the word culture, you automatically think "oh, yes I know what that is," and yet when it comes to articulating its meaning, we struggle and consensus seems elusive (Edberg, 2013b). Edberg explains that many of us come to see culture though stereotypical conceptualizations, often

expressed through "the differences in the way people look, act, talk, and carry out their daily lives" (p. 9). Here, we refer to culture as "the totality of socially transmitted behavioral patterns, arts, beliefs, values, and customs, life ways, and all other products of human work and thought, characteristics of a population of people that guide their worldview and decision making… these patterns are shared by most (but not all) members of the culture and are emergent phenomena that change in response to global phenomena… culture is largely unconscious and has powerful influences on health and illness" (Giger et al., 2007, pp. 6–7).

Culture-Related Theories and Definitions

When terms such as *cultural competence, cultural awareness, cultural sensitivity, cultural safety, cultural humility,* and, most recently, *cultural sensibility* arise, most will experience confusion as to what distinguishes them. These terms describe distinct cross-cultural capabilities and approaches; yet, interpretations do vary based on geographical location, the populations they reference, as well as individual knowledge, context, or personal and professional experiences and interpretations. To provide clarity and a foundation for understanding, we address the most prevalent theories and related concepts.

Cultural Sensitivity, Awareness, and Sensibility

The concept of **cultural sensitivity** first emerged in the mid-1990s (Adams, 1995). It refers to a person's knowledge and subsequent acceptance of the differences and similarities that exist among cultures. Cultural sensitivity adopts a stance that is free of value-laden judgements like good or bad, better or worse, and right or wrong (Texas Department of Health, National Maternal and Child Health Resource Center on Cultural Competency, 1997). Becoming a culturally sensitive person also requires the pursuit of cultural knowledge regarding the "characteristics, history, values, and belief systems, and behaviors of members of another ethnic group" (Adams, 1995, p. 5).

Cultural awareness, on the other hand, speaks to the process by which a person develops cultural sensitivity. The premise here is that you must first develop deep self-awareness of your culture and related traditions, beliefs, values, and assumptions and how they impact your thoughts, feelings, and behaviors. Only then are you able to recognize the differences and similarities that exist between yourself and other groups or individuals. The culturally sensitive healthcare provider, therefore, adopts a neutral stance toward patients and their significant others; one that is free of labels and judgement. The aim is to value and honor diversity and to tailor relational approaches to ward more effective communication, interventions, and mutual satisfaction (Foronda, 2008).

Similarly, Ellis Fletcher (2015) describes **cultural sensibility** as "a deliberate, proactive behavior by healthcare providers to examine cultural situations through thoughtful reasoning, responsiveness, and discreet actions" (p. 3). The author reminds us that each individual must be mindful of the positive and negative effects of our personal history and how those experiences have shaped our attitudes, values, and beliefs.

Cultural Competence

The origins of **cultural competence** are broad with primary influences stemming from medicine, nursing, psychology, anthropology, and social work. Madeleine Leininger (1978), a nurse anthropologist, and Arthur Kleinman (1981), a medical anthropologist, spoke first of

the need to shift to client-centered care that was inclusive of the patient's culture. Although it is well known that culture impacts a patient's health-related beliefs, behaviors, and values, many healthcare providers still struggle with how to define cultural competence and, therefore, fail to operationalize it well in healthcare education and clinical practice (Kleinman, 1981; Racine, 2014).

It was Madeline Leininger who first coined the term **transcultural nursing**. Transcultural nursing, a term often used interchangeably with cross-cultural, intercultural, or multicultural nursing" (Andrews & Boyle, 2012a, p. 3). Transcultural nursing informed the foundation for what we know of today as *cultural competence*. The constructs of transcultural nursing, cultural competence, cross-cultural care, and culture care work are also used interchangeably within the context of her work. Leininger also developed the Sunrise Model (1988) depicting her Theory of Cultural Care Diversity and Universality (see Fig. 14.1).

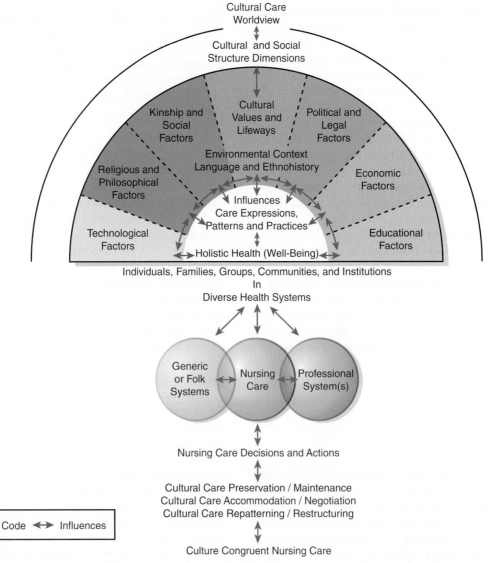

Figure 14.1 Leininger's Sunrise Model Depicts Her Theory of Cultural Care Diversity and Universality. (From Leininger, M. M. (Ed.). (2001). *Culture care diversity and universality: A theory of nursing.* New York, NY: National League for Nursing Press.)

Within this theory, she defines culture as "the learned, shared, and transmitted values, beliefs, norms, and life practices of a particular group that guides thinking decisions, and actions in patterned ways" (Leininger, 1978, 1988, p. 156). Leininger also acknowledged the unique influences of social structures, such as "religion, politics, economics, cultural history, life span values, kinship, and philosophy of living; and geo-environmental factors, as potential influencers of culture care phenomena" (Leininger, 2007, p. 9). In essence, what Leininger describes is the source of one's cultural identity: an ever-changing, paradoxical process of self-preservation and evolution, driven by our human need to know and understand who we are in this world. Leininger's model (1995) features three dominant modes as follows:

1. Cultural care *maintenance or preservation* (seeking to maintain cultural integrity of the patient within a given culture)
2. Cultural care *accommodation or negotiation* (creative nursing actions that help others attain the shared goal of optimal health)
3. Cultural care *restructuring and repatterning* (therapeutic actions of a nurse[s] or family to modify personal health behaviors toward beneficial outcomes) (Sitzman & Eichelberger, 2011)

These three modes serve as guides for nursing decisions and actions in the provision of culturally congruent care. Their use can also steer the nurse away from using "largely inappropriate, routine, unsafe, traditional, or destructive actions that fail to fit or to be acceptable to cultures" (Leininger, 2007, p. 11). By merging anthropology with nursing, Leininger developed a new way for nurses to understand individuals, families, and cultures (Leininger, 1988, p. 155). Furthermore, her work provided the first framework for nurses to incorporate the various domains of diversity into curricula and practice. Cultural competence, therefore, involves the nurse's focus on acquiring the requisite knowledge, skills, and attitudes to provide care to diverse populations to eliminate health disparities. It also involves the ongoing process of respecting differences, actively acquiring new knowledge and skills to fill gaps, and the understanding that others' personal beliefs and worldviews may differ from our own.

Since the time that Leininger introduced her transcultural nursing theory, many other theories, frameworks, guidelines, and best practice standards for cultural competence have emerged from many countries (AACN, 2008a; Bronheim & Goode, 2013a; CNA, 2010; Douglas et al., 2009; Goode, 2013; Goode & Bronheim, 2012; RNAO, 2007). One prevalent theory is the Purnell Model for Cultural Competence developed in 1991, which is classified both as a conceptual framework and by some as a grand nursing theory (2005) (see Fig. 14.2). Another important theorist, Campinha-Bacote (2002), whose work is deemed critical to

understanding the process of cultural competence, developed a model for care called The Process of Cultural Competence in the Delivery of Healthcare Services. Campinha-Bacote also developed the *Inventory for Assessing the Process of Cultural Competence among Healthcare Professionals-Revised* (IAPCC-R), a valid and reliable tool that is designed for healthcare educator, clinician, and student self-assessment of cultural competence and is available for a nominal cost at the following link (http://transculturalcare.net/iapcc-r/). She defined cultural competence as "the process in which the nurse continuously strives to achieve the ability and availability to work effectively within the cultural context of a client individual, family or community" (Campinha-Bacote, 1998, p. 6). This interpretation of cultural competence features the nurse as being humble and open to the process increasing his or her cultural awareness, cultural skills, and cultural knowledge to practice client, family, and community-centered cultural encounters. Being open to others with a sense of cultural desire is the first and most critical step to invoke the entire process.

Professional entities tend to depict cultural competence within the larger context of ethical, safe, competent nursing practice. The International Council of Nurses (ICN) states that nursing care decisions (concerning culture) must not result in substandard nursing practice or be in "contravention of professional codes of ethics, nursing practice standards, legal frameworks or United Nations human rights conventions" (ICN, 2013, p. 1). The ICN position statement on cultural and linguistic competence stresses that nurses have "an obligation to safeguard, respect, and actively promote people's health rights at all times and in all places...especially with respect to vulnerable groups such as women, children, elderly, refugees and stigmatized groups" (p. 1).

Although cultural competency is now widely adopted, Kleinman (1981) suggests that cultural competence in healthcare contexts has become a technical skill for which clinicians are trained and where culture narrowly relates to ethnicity, nationality, and language. Therein lie inherent dangers that foster assumptions and generalizations about faith, fixed traits, and beliefs that can lead to a prescriptive set of practitioner *do's and don'ts*. It is important to be aware of overgeneralizing and labeling, that is, "the Chinese always..."; "the Africans do that because..."; "Americans are..."; and so on. Making such generalizations can jeopardize building therapeutic relationships and impact patient safety. Cultural competency has also been criticized for being too nurse centric and for failing to take into account the many structural forces that shape individuals' experiences and opportunities (Fisher-Borne, Montana Cain, & Martin, 2015, p. 165). To contrast, we briefly explore newer approaches and frameworks, such as cultural humility and cultural safety. These more contemporary approaches account for some of the gaps that are thought to be present in cultural competency by "giving presence to the fluid

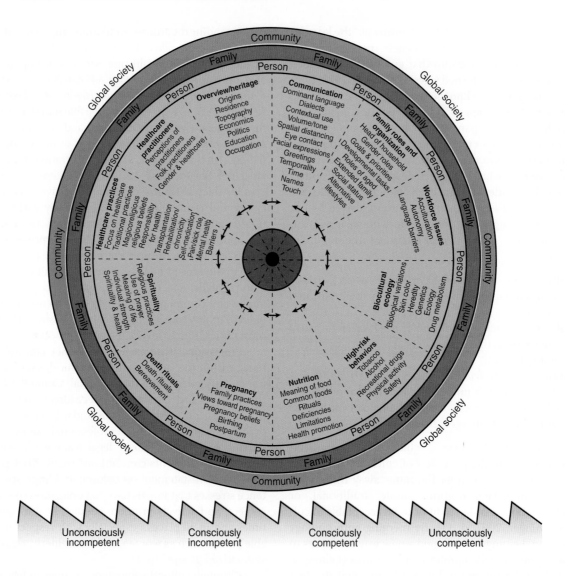

Figure 14.2 Purnell's Model for Cultural Competence. (From Purnell, L. (2005). The Purnell model for cultural competence. *Journal of Multicultural Nursing and Health, 11*(2).)

nature of culture while challenging both individuals and institutions to address inequalities" (p. 165). Goode (2004) proposes an enhancement to cultural competence with The Continuum of Cultural Competence. The continuum ranges from cultural destructiveness at the bottom, through cultural incapacity, cultural blindness, cultural precompetence, and cultural competence, and culminates in cultural proficiency at the pinnacle. Cultural proficiency in organizations can be reflected in organizational philosophy, systems, talent development, policies and processes, marketing, publications and dissemination, and advocacy to hold culture in high esteem. Most recently, the Blanchet Garneau and Pepin (2015) propose a Constructivist Cultural Competence Development Model. The authors offer a constructivist theoretical proposition for the development of cultural competence that is grounded in reflection and

action. Learners using this framework engage in self-exploration and critical thinking to draw upon prior knowledge, integrate new knowledge, and explore disorienting

dilemmas that result from clinical immersive experiences, whether they are real life or simulated (Blanchet Garneau, 2016). See the online Toolkit for a tool that helps learners to prepared for culture-focused simulation.

Cultural Safety

The construct of **cultural safety** first emerged in the late 1980s in New Zealand and has since been refined and embedded as a standard in healthcare education in the region and throughout the world (Nursing Council of New Zealand, 2005; 2008). Unlike cultural competence, awareness, and sensitivity, "cultural safety is not about cultural practices of the nurse, but it is about engaging in a recognition of the social, economic, and political position of certain groups within society" (p. 152). Its introduction into nursing education was highly contentious and political, challenging long-standing paternalistic structures, power, distance, and authority in relationships between healthcare providers and indigenous peoples. Today, its use in nursing education serves to root out unsafe cultural practices that comprise "any action that diminishes, demeans or disempowers the cultural identity and well-being of an individual" (Gerlach, 2012, p. 152).

Cultural Humility

Similar to cultural safety, **cultural humility** incorporates "a lifelong commitment to self-evaluation and critique, to redressing the power imbalances in the [healthcare provider]-patient dynamic, and to developing mutually beneficial and non-paternalistic partnerships with communities on behalf of individuals and defined populations" (Tervalon & Murray-Garcia, 1998, p. 123). Whereas cultural competence suggests a static notion of competence—a skill that one acquires through training—cultural humility is an ongoing, courageous, honest, and reflective process. Cultural competence assumes an achievable goal or terminal state, while cultural humility is "a process of openness, self-awareness, being egoless, and incorporating self-reflection and critique after willingly interacting with diverse individuals. The results of achieving cultural humility are mutual empowerment, respect, partnerships, optimal care, and lifelong learning" (Fig. 14.3; Foronda, Baptiste, Reinholdt, & Ousman, 2016, p. 4). As such, we suggest cultural humility as the desired direction for healthcare providers.

As you can see, there are numerous interpretations of culture-related concepts and constructs within various nursing theories, frameworks, and approaches. Though covered in brief, we hope that this content will serve as a starting point and catalyst for Simulation Champions to formally integrate culture and diversity into teaching practices. Simulation educators require knowledge of definitions and theories as well as a clear understanding of the terminology related to culture and diversity. Selecting a designated theory, definition, or model is advantageous when integrating these cultural concepts into Simulation Programs. Table 14.1 provides a synopsis of key terms and points.

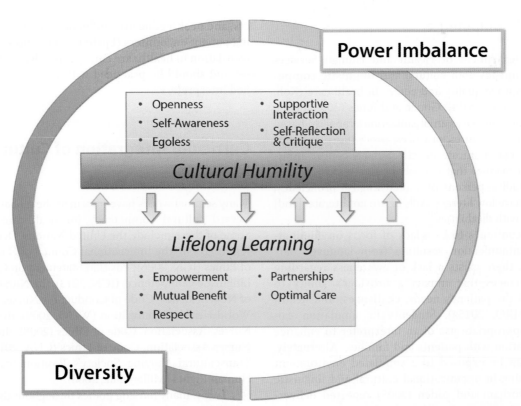

Figure 14.3 A Concept Analysis of Cultural Humility. (Reprinted by permission of SAGE Publications (2015). From Foronda, C., Baptiste, D., Ousman, K., & Reinholdt, M. (2016) Cultural humility: A concept analysis. *Journal of Transcultural Nursing, 27*(3), 210–217. doi:10.1177/1043659615592677.)

Table 14.1	Comparison of Terms Related to Culture	
Term	**Definition**	**Key Features**
Cultural Sensitivity	"Employing one's knowledge, consideration, understanding, respect, and tailoring after realizing awareness of self and others and encountering a diverse group or individual" (Foronda, 2008, p. 210)	Infers a level of awareness and attempt for an optimal communication or intervention
Cultural Competence	"The process in which the nurse continuously strives to achieve the ability and availability to effectively work within the cultural context of a client individual, family, or community" (Campinha-Bacote, 1998, p. 6)	Acknowledges the importance of being open to others' differences as a step in a process. Designed for specific encounters
Cultural Safety	"Engaging in a recognition of the social, economic, and political position of certain groups within society" (Gerlach, 2012, p. 152)	Acknowledges power differentials and importance of recognition and respect of client rights to self-determination and self-directed healthcare
Cultural Humility	"Cultural humility incorporates a lifelong commitment to self-evaluation and critique, to redressing the power imbalances in the physician–patient dynamic, and to developing mutually beneficial and nonpaternalistic partnerships with communities on behalf of individuals and defined populations" (Tervalon & Murray-Garcia, 1998, p. 123)	Acknowledges a mindset embracing critical self-reflection and lifelong learning in a dynamic context. Cultural humility is a way of being, and a mindset.
Cultural Sensibility	"A deliberate, proactive behavior by healthcare providers to examine cultural situations through thoughtful reasoning, responsiveness, and discreet actions" (Ellis Fletcher, 2015, p. 3)	Acknowledges the need for deep self-reflection and an acknowledgement of how past positive and negative experiences have shaped our life and our interactions with others

Linguistic Competence

The U.S. Department of Health and Human Services (HHS) encourages both cultural and **linguistic competence** to improve quality and equity in healthcare (Koh, Garcia, & Alvarez, 2014). Goode and Jones (2009) define linguistic competence as an organization's capacity, based on "its policy, structures, practices, procedures" and personnel, "to communicate effectively, and convey information in a manner that is easily understood by diverse groups including persons of limited English proficiency, those who have low literacy skills or are not literate, [and] individuals with disabilities".

There continues to be a lack of focus on eliminating miscommunication resulting from language barriers. Also, there exists a lack of awareness regarding cultural nuances that impact a provider's ability to understand the patient's needs, challenges, and health beliefs (AHRQ, 2015a). Students in simulation can learn the appropriate use of an interpreter to enhance communication with patients and families. Alternately, students can be exposed to a simulated environment that is lacking in organizational cultural and linguistic support. Durham and Alden (2008) reported delivering a scenario focusing on the use of an interpreter for a non–English-speaking patient and family. Differing perspectives on the patient, family, healthcare provid-

ers, and health educators influence communication during patient encounters (Epstein, 2006). Interpreting and translation in healthcare contexts involves a defined skill set and should be practiced with competent and qualified interpreters.

Curricular Integration of Culture and Diversity

Many seminal works have informed the global movement toward cultural competency for healthcare providers. Some of these include the United Nations' Declaration of Rights (2008), the International Council of Nurses - Code of Ethics (ICN, 2006); Position Statement on Cultural and Linguistic Competence, (ICN, 2013), the Nursing Council of New Zealand - Code of Conduct for Nurses (2008), the World Health Organization (WHO, 2009), the American Nurses' Association, Code of Ethics (2008), the Canadian Nurses Association, Code of Ethics (CNA, 2010), and the Transcultural Nursing Society's Position Statement on Human Rights (Miller et al., 2008).

Today, many nursing bodies throughout the world list cultural competency as a graduate outcome in undergraduate and graduate nursing programs. For example, the AACN Advisory Committee for Cultural Competence (2008a) outlines the need for the development of cultural competencies in undergraduate and graduate nursing education. Unfortunately, existing curricular models in baccalaureate education struggle to incorporate culture competencies for the care of diverse individuals and groups. Just acquiring knowledge about cultural competence or other cultural approaches is not sufficient; clinicians must also be able to apply the knowledge, skills, and attitudes of culturally competent approaches (Roberts et al., 2014). To do so requires hands-on practice. Roberts et al. (2014) acknowledge that academic institutions are making some ground by attempting to integrate "some semblance of cultural competence" into their curricula. However, there continues to be a lack of application in practice, and cultural competence remains scarcely evident (Racine, 2014).

Today, **culture-focused simulation** offers educators a viable alternative for engaging students in learning about the care of patients from diverse backgrounds. Students can also practice and develop culture-related skills in a safe learning environment to minimize the risk of inappropriate and culturally incongruent behaviors in real patient encounters. Teaching cultural competence in the classroom may increase the learners' knowledge; however, the learner must be able to apply this foundational knowledge within an authentic patient encounter. The simulated environment provides the ideal opportunity for context-relevant immersion in culture-focused experiences where students can experiment with recently acquired skills in a controlled setting (Jeffries, 2012b; Ndiwane, Koul, & Theroux, 2014). Through the strategic integration of culture-focused experiences at all levels of the simulation curriculum, students can gain comfort and acquire the requisite skills needed to interact capably with diverse patients and colleagues. We believe that knowledge, skills, and attitudes about culture and diversity gained through the use of all simulation modalities and related typologies can improve the quality of patient care, patient outcomes, and care provider satisfaction. More importantly, we believe that simulation provides students with space and time they need to explore their thoughts, feelings, and reactions to dealing with diverse populations and complex situations. Additionally,

 (INACSL Standards Committee, 2016, Sim-IPE) can introduce interprofessional teams to collaborative approaches using relevant, and authentic representations of the frontline lived experiences of culture and diversity in the workplace. Research has emerged suggesting that differences in values, language, poor communication and lack of teamwork is resulting in sentinel events and poor patient outcomes (Interprofessional Education Collaborative Expert Panel, 2011; The Joint Commission, 2012; Pronovost & Vohr, 2010). To address challenges of location, time, and space in facilitating interprofessional simulations, emerging technology including virtual simulation may be an option (Foronda & Bauman, 2014).

The **inclusion** of culture requires the use of a thoughtful, intentional process grounded in theory and best practices

in education and simulation. The NLN's (2015b) Vision for Teaching with Simulation recommends that faculty "(1) purposefully integrate simulation into the curriculum making clear connections toward achievement of student learning outcomes (which would include teaching of culture and diversity); (2) incorporate simulation standards of practice in the design, implementation, and evaluation of simulation-based experiences; (3) use theory-, and evidence-based approaches consistently to ensure competence in debriefing; (4) partner with faculty from other disciplines to create interprofessional simulation experience; and (5) pursue the development of expertise as a simulation leader" (pp. 5–6). Adding to this mandate are the challenges for educators that are inherent in a culture-focused simulation. These challenges include the sensitive nature of the topics, stereotypes, biases, teachers who cling to traditional instructional techniques, incongruent cultural environments, a potential lack of faculty self-awareness, and a lack of knowledge or comfort on how to facilitate scenarios with culturally sensitive topics.

When facilitated by a knowledgeable and skilled facilitator, the simulation setting can provide an environment conducive to exploration and practice improvement in areas like communication skills and empathy development (Roberts et al., 2014). While student experiences in traditional clinical placements vary significantly, simulation-based learning about specific client populations or situations can reach the entire student body. Through the curricular integration of culture-focused scenarios, nursing programs can offer a standardized and comprehensive approach to learning about culture. Of course, the capstone of any Simulated Clinical Immersion is a facilitator-led, structured debriefing that allows learners to explore and experience growth in culture-related competencies (INACSL Standards Committee, 2016, Facilitation; Debriefing; Roberts et al., 2014).

Threading Culture Themes

To create a simulation that parallels or mimics population-specific patient encounters like those experienced in traditional, clinical practice settings require that educators introduce a wide array of persons and topics that reach well beyond race and ethnic differences. Threaded themes of culture and diversity within a simulation curriculum should include most, or all, dimensions of culture, such as age, gender, socioeconomic status, non–English-speaking persons, and issues of substance abuse, elder abuse, child custody issues, religious or faith-based diversity, gender and sexual identity issues, and individuals who are lesbian, gay, bisexual, or transgender (LGBT). Also, persons who experience disabilities, mental health disease, intimate partner violence, divorce, single-parent families, military families, teen pregnancy, the homeless, imprisoned persons, people with genetic disorders, or situations unique to particular ethnicities. One should also consider other dimensions of culture such as organizational culture, professional and interprofessional culture, or healthcare culture. Moreover, educators can expose learners to differences in cultural beliefs, traditions, and normative practices around birth, death, illness, and family. Clarity of the intended learning outcomes coupled with sufficient time and opportunity for repetition supports learners who can benefit from ongoing exposure to culture concepts. Designers of simulation must introduce these topics incrementally so as not to overwhelm students. Alternately, overexposure could potentially lead to students becoming immune to the intent of the culture-related learning.

Simulation Scenario Development and Testing

To create educationally sound culture-focused simulation, use an evidence-based approach to simulation design (INACSL Standards Committee, 2016, Simulation Design), coupled with current evidence on teaching and learning about culture. In brief, the Simulation Design Standard comprises these criterion: "(1) perform a needs assessment; (2) construct measurable objectives; (3) structure format of simulation; (4) design scenario or case; (5) use various types of fidelity; (6) maintain a facilitative approach that is participant centered and driven by the objectives, participant's knowledge or level of experience, and the expected outcomes; (7) begin simulation-based experiences with a pre-briefing; (8) follow simulation with a debriefing and/or feedback session; (9) plan to evaluate the participant(s), facilitator(s), the simulation-based experience, the facility, and the support team; (10) provide preparation materials and resources to promote participants' ability to meet identified objectives and achieve expected outcomes of the simulation-based experience; and (11) pilot test simulation" (p. S6). Additionally, the Master Simulation Design Template and Intake Form© (Foisy-Doll & Leighton, 2017) is available in the online toolkit (Toolkit 20-3 and 20-4) in Chapter 20. Also, consider creating a template to document and map various aspects of culture contained in all simulations by tracking key concepts and themes addressed in cultural experiences. A sample Diversity Variables Mapping Grid is available in your online Toolkit (Toolkit 14-1).

This holistic approach will reveal gaps in the curriculum for quality improvement purposes and assist in developing a comprehensive simulation curriculum. Several authors cite curricular innovations for embedding culture in the literature. Butteris, Gladding, Eppich, Hagen, and Pitt (2014) explain the use of simulation to prepare students for international experiences. They trained facilitators using case studies with culturally specific information about health, safety, and language unique to countries where students were to have an international clinical rotation. This activity provided students the opportunity to explore personal beliefs and emotions they may encounter while working abroad and at home with culturally diverse populations.

Although there is a lack of consensus and a dearth of research on how best to teach culture and provide useful learning experiences, Roberts et al. (2014) cited approaches that have been used to feature culture using simulation. These include the use of clinical scenarios in practicums, computerized scenarios, the integration of cultural competence training throughout the entire curriculum, the delivery of a particular classroom scenario(s) dedicated to the instruction of cultural competence, and cultural immersion experiences, usually abroad. The National Center for Cultural Competence (NCCC) website hosts an extensive assortment of tools and checklists to assist assessment, development, and research of cultural and linguistic competence https://nccc.georgetown.edu/training/.

Simulation educators can access the following NCCC checklists at for use in building culture-focused simulation by engaging in self-assessment and examining your Simulation Program in the following areas:

- Applying Cultural and Linguistic Competence to a Framework for Creating Learning Spaces for the Enhancement of Experiential Learning (https://nccc.georgetown.edu/training/NCCC_Learning_Table.pdf)
- Climate of the Learning Environment: Cultural and Linguistic Competence Checklist for MCH Training Program (https://nccc.georgetown.edu/training/NCCC_Climate_Checklist.pdf)
- Promoting Cultural and Linguistic Competency Self-Assessment Checklist for Personnel Providing Primary Healthcare Services (https://nccc.georgetown.edu/documents/Checklist%20PHC.pdf)
- Research: Cultural and Linguistic Competence Checklist of MCH Training Programs (https://nccc.georgetown.edu/training/NCCC_Research_Checklist.pdf).

The Ethical Imperative in Culture-Focused Scenario Creation

It is vital that simulation educators take the time to stop and think about the situations they are creating from an ethical viewpoint. The educator designing culture-focused scenarios should consider population-specific student needs before deploying the simulation experience. For example, oppression experienced by students from marginalized or silenced minorities in real life could be exacerbated when entering an event that, yet again, portrays persons from minority populations as such. Therefore, facilitators must be intentional when preparing students for cultural content that might ring a little too close to home for students. We recommend engaging learners in preparatory activities that build on prior learning before the day of simulation (INACSL Standards Committee, 2016, Simulation Design); such activities could include preparatory questions, readings, an overview of the patient case and background, and relevant videos or written reflections. Implementing preparatory activities and a pre-briefing to prepare participants for the simulation-based experience are a standard of practice (INACSL Standards Committee, 2016, Facilitation). A student who is participating in an LGBT scenario, for example, may experience a wide array of emotions before attending the simulation. Perhaps, he or she is not personally comfortable with openly discussing the topic or, alternately, is a member of the LGBT community and fears that the simulation could exacerbate misconceptions or stereotypes with peers. In creating such experiences, it is important to be mindful that we do not perpetuate unhealthy stereotypes of culture; therefore, careful preparation of the learner and the provision of context is a critical dimension of culture-focused scenario preparedness. It is also important to review key information and provide context to students about the nature and intent of the learning experience. To mitigate harm to learners and promote healthy cultural encounters, consider the following strategies:

- Engage in deliberate conversations, readings, and specific preparation that will help the students uncover their perspectives and feelings ahead of time, specifically around experiences of the marginalized and vulnerable.
- Acknowledge that everyone in the room feels vulnerable, some more than others, but most do.
- Establish group norms to support safe and inclusive language (verbal and nonverbal).
- Celebrate the uniqueness of each student in simulation, especially in the debriefing phase.
- Use a culture framework that ties the experience from theory to practice, creating a bridge for practical application.
- Ensure that the scenario reflects believable and accurate depictions of culture.
- Validate your scenarios with content experts for all cultural content.

Standardized Implementation Processes

When facilitating simulations, nurse educators must ideally use the same educational process for purposes of continuity and consistency. For example, cultural considerations could become standard practice for the preparatory, prebriefing and debriefing phrases. Other suggestions include hanging posters with culture cues in the debriefing room to remind students of the value of diversity or asking guided reflection questions that pertain to culture (Williamson & Harrison, 2010). When we routinely acknowledge cultural differences, the act of recognizing and attending to diversity becomes normalized or, even better, part of the organizational culture. Including culture concepts can be as simple as discussing patient data such as the patient's age and background, where simulation facilitators can prompt students to consider any differences between the patients and themselves as a standard practice. "So, was there anything in this particular case that created a moment of cultural dissonance for you?" is an excellent guiding question. In reply, a facilitator might say, "I hear that this situation caused unease for you and I understand that feeling from my own personal experiences. If you are willing, let's unpack that experience together". There are many different debriefing techniques from which to choose, and depending on the type of simulation, the topic, and the depth of discussion required, certain frameworks may be preferred over others.

Modes of Thinking and Cultural Fidelity

Dieckmann, Gaba, and Rall (2007) urge creators of simulation to "engage our participants deeply in simulation [underscoring] the need to recognize that humans think about reality in at least three ways." The authors feature three modes of thinking that include the (1) physical mode, (2) semantical mode, and (3) the phenomenal mode. When developing the many dimensions of culture-focused simulation, it is helpful to explore culture using the various modes of thinking (Fig. 14.4).

Physical Mode

The *physical mode* (environmental fidelity) is an important dimension when creating an effective simulation and involves paying attention to physical properties of the simulation such as space and equipment (Dieckmann et al., 2007). First consider that the physical space itself can evidence culture and diversity by emanating inclusivity through the use of signs, images, or displays. We suggest it as desirable to feature visuals that represent local diversity from populations represented within your regional context, or alternately that are transglobal in nature. Secondly, consider the use of a wide array of accouterments with mannequins, simulated/standardized patients (SPs), or virtual patients in the form of props that provide sensory cues. For example, when designing a scenario, reproduce the physical environment to include cultural content such as clothing specific to the culture, religious items at the bedside, or the use of foreign languages by SPs or embedded actors (Roberts et al., 2014).

If funds are available, establishing diversity in your mannequin inventory is recommended to include diverse skin tones, available all age ranges from infant to elderly. When

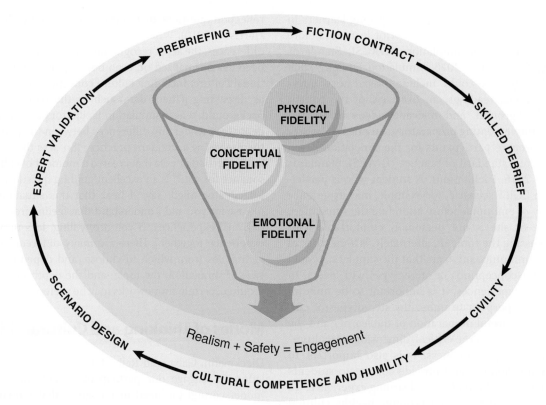

Figure 14.4 Diagram to Illustrate Creating Dimensions of Fidelity in Culture-Focused Simulation Creating Cultural Fidelity in Simulation.

the entire inventory of simulators is white, students of color may feel excluded (Foronda & MacWilliams, 2015). Graham and Atz (2015) studied how students who self-report as a minority feel about their experiences with high-fidelity simulation. Students described the lack of diversity in simulation when interacting with white-only mannequins—they expressed feeling underrepresented by not having mannequins of color. Alternately, Fuselier, Baldwin, and Townsend-Chambers (2015) found that students of color expressed a sense of inclusiveness and validation at having mannequins of color at their disposal in the simulation center. However, students did indicate a desire to see mannequin features that resembled those of persons of color rather than mannequins with European features and dark skin tones. It is important to provide this feedback to the creators of simulation products toward the development of more helpful tools.

The same holds for the use of simulated/standardized patients where a broad demographic should be accessed to portray patients from varied backgrounds as appropriate to the context you are creating. Intentionally depicting culture in any form must, of course, be tied to core learning objectives (INACSL Standards Committee, 2016, Objectives and Outcomes). Virtual simulation products should be screened to assure a diverse array of patient depictions (see Fig. 14.5). To achieve environmental fidelity related to the cultural dimensions of the experience, you should consider

which items are essential to engage the physical mode of thinking: things like artwork, clothing, artifacts (traditional/religious symbols), mannequin skin tone, and images that provide the learner with specific visual cues (Wyrostok, Hoffart, Kelly, & Ryba, 2014).

Semantical Mode (Conceptual Fidelity)

Regardless of the simulation modality and typology selected, care should be taken to ensure that cross-cultural encounters with patients (mannequins, SPs, embedded actors, or avatars) are conceptually realistic. Careful planning must go into building "if" and "then" conceptual relationships during scenario development and relational aspects of the simulation need to be piloted. For example, one would not present a patient as having English as another language (EAL) only to have them speak fluent English with a local accent. Therefore, IF the learners read a given patient description in the case stem, THEN the patient they encounter should mirror that story. In other words, the learners should not have to do too much pretending, or you risk compromising realism. Consider verbal, nonverbal, spoken language, speech patterns, and alternate ways of communicating such as hand use, and voice inflection or intonation. The dimension of spoken language presents a challenge for scenario creators. You should explore hiring SPs that are multilingual. New technologies featuring voice changers,

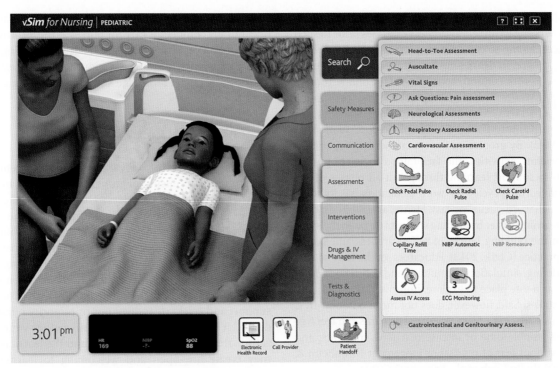

Figure 14.5 Screenshot from vSim for Nursing | Pediatric showing nursing care of a virtual pediatric patient. (Courtesy of Laerdal Medical. All rights reserved.)

such as the VOX BOX™, allow for the transmitting of the female voice as a male voice, or a child's voice, and vice versa. The use of such aids will enhance conceptual fidelity. Other ideas to consider are nonverbal elements such as cultural norms around physical distance and eye contact, words used in scripting, and even the amount and level of information required to build the overall desired reality (Hober, Manry, & Connelly, 2009). We encourage you to be intentional about which elements constitute the most salient aspects of those conceptual relationships to increase learner fidelity modulation (the student's ability to maneuver between what is real and what is not within a scenario).

Phenomenal Mode (Emotional Fidelity)

Thinking in this mode involves the learner's ability to modulate effectively within a complex real-time situation with the prior knowledge that the encounter is not with a "real patient". When simulation "works," students buy into the scenario and experience real emotions in response to "real" situations. Creating *sociological fidelity* involves thinking about how to recreate social dimensions in simulation, such as hierarchy, power relations, culture, gender, conflict, and identity aspects of a given situation (Heinrichs, Bauman, & Dev, 2012; Sharma, Boet, Kitto, & Reeves, 2011). Simulationists are challenged to replicate social realities, and so must pay attention to character development, context, and social interactions. According to Dieckmann (2012), a simulation "works" when the modes of thinking work together allowing the learner to buy into the learning

event as a valid means of learning (culture in this case). Time should be taken to develop ethically responsible and accurate depictions of culture in the process of character development (i.e., race and ethnicity, gender, etc.), cultural norms, religion and spirituality, folk traditions, and special days of celebration or practices. Also, consider consulting an expert and authority on the topic, or a member of the culture being portrayed for content validation.

Facilitation and Facilitators: Creating Safe and Inclusive Learning Environments

Psychological Safety for Learners and Educators

In addition to offering learners a rich variety of simulations, it is imperative that students feel safe, especially since simulation is sometimes linked to promoting anxiety in learners (Foronda, Liu, & Bauman, 2013). Suboptimal learning occurs when individuals are under conditions of stress, so harm reduction strategies are necessary. Simulation standards recommend that you uphold the integrity of participants by preparing learners for simulation (INACSL Standards Committee, 2016, Simulation Design; Professional Integrity). To accomplish this, the facilitator must work to create psychologically safe spaces and group conditions that are conducive to open participation. When dealing

STANDARDS

specifically with culture and diversity, we encourage you to have learners engage in self-awareness exercises prior to such experiences. Doing so can help to spark meaningful discussion in debriefing around perceived and actual cross-cultural capabilities. In the online Toolkit, you will find a preparation and prebriefing activity worksheet: Preparing Students for Culture-Focused Simulations Worksheet (Toolkit 14-2). By grounding the experience in preparatory and prebriefing activities, the facilitator can enact guided reflection to support learning throughout all phases of the simulation learning cycle. The word facilitation has its roots in the French word "facile" or easy. Hence, a facilitator's job is to make learning easier by guiding students through the steps that form the building blocks of self-awareness and skilled cultural practice (Clark, 2013). Educators set the tone so that the prebriefing, simulation encounters, and debriefing activities provide a safe place to explore, improve one's skills, and make mistakes. Safe, however, does not mean emotion-free. Rather, a safe space is a place where participants can feel free to express troublesome or intense reactions, thoughts, and feelings without fear of reprisal or judgement (Bronheim & Goode, 2013b; Rudolph et al., 2006, 2007; 2014).

Although civility may not appear related to cultural humility, civil conduct within a simulation event is essential to creating safe learning spaces. Clark (2013) defines civility as an authentic respect for others requiring time, presence, engagement, and an intention to seek common ground. This premise holds especially true for sensitive topics related to culture and diversity that permeate social and political realms. Learners in simulation can benefit from clear expectations and ground rules regarding civility in culture-related encounters and debriefing, that is, the facilitator should use a framework for uncovering personal frames around culture and diversity employing rules of engagement that promote respect, active listening, and openness to others' point of view. The atmosphere should evidence mutuality, tolerance, curiosity, civility, and respectful processing of conflicting viewpoints. Students must feel supported by facilitators and comfortable enough with peers to actively engage in experimentation during simulations, as well as express themselves openly during the debriefing. As such, facilitators will need to monitor the debriefing environment and stave off bullying or incivility by modeling better ways to handle differences (Milesky, Baptiste, Foronda, Dupler, & Belcher, 2015).

As individuals and teams of simulationists, each of us is accountable for the ethical learning of culture and diversity in our professional practice. As such, it is incumbent upon educators to root out bias and the potential for any discriminatory behavior on our part. It takes time and intentionality to become well versed in the language of cultural competence and related terms like linguistic competence, cultural diversity, inclusion, prejudice, bias, discrimination, oppression, superiority, healthcare disparity, and stereotyping. Monteneny, Jones, Perry, Ross, and Zoucha (2013) found

that faculty have great potential to facilitate the provision of culturally competent care for nurses at the local, national, and global level. They also state that the learning of cultural competence for nurses is a journey, not a destination. Together, through knowledge and capacity building, we can learn to do this well.

Organizational Culture

One crucial aspect of delivering cultural content in the curriculum is to ensure alignment of cultural safety with internal institutional practices. That is to say, the culture of your organization plays a significant role in the successful integration of inclusivity and diversity in your Simulation Program. For example, would you anticipate either acceptance or push back from your peers at the suggestion to include diversity elements in simulations? Penn (2014) challenges us to think about institutional structures that support and celebrate indigenous or minority nursing students. It is important to reflect on whether your organization, the people you work with, and the learning spaces they create are open and welcoming to learners from minorities or marginalized groups. Safe learning spaces uphold the uniqueness that each participant brings to the teaching and learning environment. Consider how your institution imbues openness and inclusivity through (1) physical environments and resources (i.e., access to related journals, books, videos, posters); (2) marketing, branding, and communication; (3) professional development; (4) culture and diversity departments, groups, or initiatives; (5) cultural expressions in written, imagery, and video forms; (6) mission, vision, and values statements; (7) policies, that is, zero tolerance for incivility or abuse; (8) research in this field; or (9) a diversity hiring policy. These are important questions to ask about your work environment and will help you to prepare for barriers when embedding culture and diversity in the simulation curriculum.

Evaluation and Assessment in Simulation Learning

It is important to assess student performance and evaluate learning outcomes related to cultural competence, as well as to evaluate the depiction of culture within scenarios. Using reliable and valid instruments is ideal (Adamson, Kardong-Edgren, & Willhaus, 2013; Mikasa, Cicero, & Adamson, 2013). In a 2013 systematic literature review on the use of clinical simulation to enhance culturally competent nursing care, Ozkara San reported the use of several tools for evaluating culture learning in a simulation. Among those listed were

- Cultural Awareness Scale (CAS) (Rew, Becker, Cookston, Khosropour, & Martinez, 2003)
- Attitudes Towards Healthcare Teams Scale (ATHCTS) (Curran, Heath, Kearney, & Button, 2010)

- Transcultural Self-Efficacy Tool (TSET) (Jeffreys, 2010)
- Cultural Competence Assessment Tool (CCA) (Dorrenbos, Schim, Benkert, & Borse, 2005)
- Cultural Assessment Survey (Godkin & Savageau, 2003)

Dr. Marianne Jeffreys is a scholar in transcultural competence. Her website hosts a variety of culture-related measurement tools that can be accessed at http://www.mariannejeffreys.com/culturalcompetence/questionnnaire.php, as does the Center for Cultural Competence at Georgetown University.

In the quest for continuous quality improvement, administrators and educators should seek to evaluate their teaching environments, simulation scenarios, and simulation educators for outcomes. Franklin, Burns, and Lee (2014) have studied and endorsed the use of the NLN Simulation Design Scale (2004) (http://www.nln.org/docs/default-source/professional-development-programs/nln-instrument_simulation-design-scale.pdf?sfvrsn=0) as a valid and reliable tool for educational research, and although not specific to culture, it could be used to evaluate design elements of the simulation. It is important for educators and students using simulation-based learning to have the opportunity to provide feedback to inform change.

 Using a grid chart to plot out the curriculum and track evaluation results for the presence and strength of culture and diversity content and learning is helpful (see Toolkit 14-1).

Simulation Champions: Promoting Culture, Diversity, and Inclusivity

One effective way to ensure that culture, diversity, and inclusivity are continuously infused, updated, and evaluated in the curriculum is to enlist diversity champions or teams and to create an institutional or simulation diversity committee. To that end, we suggest that simulation teams have at least one member dedicated to embedding diversity and culture in learning. In the absence of a formal sim team, consider creating a program-related scenario committee. Ideally, the larger organization will have a diversity committee to monitor and drive future efforts and with whom Simulation Champions and teams can collaborate. All educators involved in the creation and implementation of nursing curricula must attend to building cross-cultural capacity with each other and in educational experiences for learners.

Summary

Simulation is an ideal platform to provide learners the opportunity to learn and practice culture-related skills with diverse populations. To foster learning environments that are welcoming, inclusive, and safe, the Simulation Champion must have a solid understanding of fundamental concepts related to culture. Simulation holds great promise for enacting high-impact culture and diversity-focused content. Therefore, educators should set a priority agenda for curricular integration and leveling of learning about culture and diversity. This endeavor requires a commitment to uphold simulation best practice standards in the design, delivery, and evaluation of culture-focused simulation (INACSL Standards of Best Practice: Simulation[SM], 2016, Simulation Design; Evaluation). Through the appropriate use of simulation and the vigilant monitoring of physical, conceptual, emotional, and sociological fidelity, simulationists can produce authentic and relevant culture-focused simulation.

Simulation Champions are well positioned to prepare learners for culturally safe nursing care. Expressions of culture and diversity need to extend beyond the ethnically diverse patient, to include culture and diversity of all forms. Moreover, simulation educators have an ethical and moral obligation and relevant to appraise all simulation offerings to ensure ethical and authentic depictions of diversity and culture.

In this section, we provided an introduction to culture theory, and many concepts and constructs related to culture: namely, cultural competence, cultural awareness, cultural sensitivity, cultural sensibility, cultural safety, and cultural humility. It is our hope that this information and the online toolkit resources will stimulate thought, discussion, and planning on how, why, where, and when culture and diversity best fit in your nursing curriculum and, more specifically, within your Simulation Program. We believe that cultural humility and safety offer more contemporary approaches to cultural education in nursing programs. Preparation for success in the nursing profession involves not only a significant paradigm shift but also a new prism through which we clearly see each other's uniqueness and vulnerabilities. It is our collective responsibility as nurse educators to build a better world by creating experiential learning that helps students to enact culturally safe encounters that mirror our core nursing and humanistic values. We wish you all the best in your culture-related endeavors!

 Toolkit Resources

Toolkit 14-1: Diversity Variables Mapping Grid.
Toolkit 14-2: Preparing Students for Culture- Focused Simulation Worksheet.
Toolkit 14-3: Master Simulation Design Template
Toolkit 14-4: Master Simulation Design Companion Intake Form

15

Global Perspectives on Simulation
Colette Foisy-Doll

Preface

For decades, inter-cultural exchanges have contributed to the enhancement of nursing education and professional practice worldwide. In the past, nurses traveled to far off places to learn about diverse ways of being and doing, while today, our media- and technology-rich world offers a plethora of ways to connect in meaningful ways that don't involve relocating. When I was a child, I remember watching the TV show, *The Jetsons*. I would daydream about communicating through a screen-based TV just like the one George Jetson used. "How remarkably amazing," I thought. Well, we have lived to see that day become a reality. Telecommunications have evolved to the point where most have access to the Jetson experience by using a cellphone. When working and living in the Middle East accompanied by my two boys, ages 13 and 15, my husband would join us daily for breakfast (his supper) via Skype. How amazing is that? As I continue my work overseas, I am cognizant of how privileged we are to have access to technology that connects us with our colleagues, friends, and loved ones around the world. Technology-mediated communication also brings together simulationists from around the world, providing our community of practice with unprecedented access to other healthcare professionals with the ability to view video-zoom right into each others' workplaces and share our stories.

While simulation-based education was taking root in North America, other members of the global simulation practice community were also busy transforming nursing education and practice in other parts of the world. Today, international simulation associations bring us together to collaborate in the simulation revolution, and we are richer as nurses and educators for knowing one another. We are

so pleased to offer you a sampling of global perspectives from Simulation Champions working in eight different parts of the world. These perspectives are not intended to cover everything that is happening in simulation everywhere. Rather, these stories serve as exemplars to provide snapshots of simulation in different regions of the world. As with simulation, context and immersion are everything, so authors situate their simulation stories within a given country's history, people, and systems. We hope you enjoy learning about their journeys in simulation and the countries where they carry out such inspiring work.

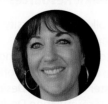

Colette Foisy-Doll, MSN, RN, CHSE

15A Global Perspectives on Simulation: Africa (Rwanda)

Renee Pyburn, Philomène Uwimana

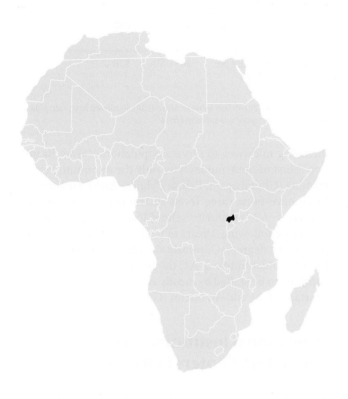

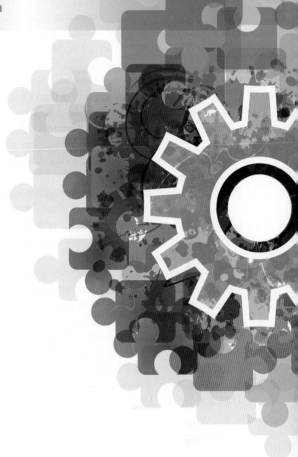

Rwanda: Profile

Rwanda has had a turbulent history. In 1959, the ruling majority of Hutus overthrew the government, and over the next few years, many of the Tutsis were killed or exiled. Rwanda gained independence from Belgium in 1962. More recently in 1990, a civil war transpired between the ruling Hutus and the Tutsi-led rebel Rwandan Patriot Front (RPF). Tensions escalated, culminating in the 1994 genocide in which approximately 1 million people (about

¾ of the Tutsi population) were killed. The next few years were still turbulent, but since 2000, President Paul Kagame has led the country and it has enjoyed relative peace and prosperity, and the country has made remarkable progress since 1994 (Central Intelligence Agency [CIA], 2015). The tropical savanna climate is dry in the winter months and wet in the summer months with temperatures ranging from 16°C to 28°C year round (WeatherSpark, 2015).

Currently, the population is approximately 12 million, and it is the most densely populated country in Africa with a median age of 18.7 years. The government is a republic, governed by an elected president, with a multiparty political system. The official languages are English and Kinyarwanda, although French is widely spoken. The predominant religion is Christianity, with Roman Catholics comprising approximately 49.5%, Protestants 39.4%, other Christian 4.5%, Muslim 1.8%, animist 0.1%, other 0.6%, none 3.6%, and unspecified 0.5%. Rwanda's population is primarily rural with 90% of the population engaged in subsistence

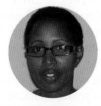

Renee Pyburn, **MS, RN, CHSE**

Philomène Uwimana, **MSN, RN**

agriculture. Rwanda's main sources of income are tourism, minerals, coffee, and tea. The country's main exports are coffee, tea, animal hides, and tin ore, while its main imports are foodstuffs, machinery and equipment, steel, petroleum products, cement, and construction materials (CIA, 2015). The average annual *gross domestic product* (GDP) growth since 2003 is 7% to 8%. In 2006, 56.7% of the population lived below the poverty line. This number has since been reduced to 44.9% in 2011 (The World Bank, 2014).

Rwanda has joined the East African Community (EAC) and is aligning budget and trade policies with its regional partners. The government is working diligently to try to reduce poverty by improving education and healthcare infrastructure and increasing foreign and domestic investment. Rwanda is also seeking to become a regional leader in information and communication technology (CIA, 2015).

Rwandans practice unique cultural traditions such as Girinka Munyarwanda (owning a cow as a sign of prosperity), Gacaca (a council of elders or wise people in the community who convene to reach a fair settlement when crimes are committed or disputes arise), Ubudehe and Umuganda (similar traditions where community problems are solved as a collective), and Itorero (passing on of traditional culture and values, now done formally through Itorero programs), among others. National holidays include New Year's Day, National Heroes' Day, Good Friday, Tutsi Genocide Memorial Day, Labor Day, Independence Day, Liberation Day, Assumption Day, Eid El-Fitr, Christmas Day, and Boxing Day.

Healthcare in Rwanda

Rwanda has made remarkable strides in improving its healthcare and education since the genocide in 1994. The current literacy rate is 68.3%, and average number of years of school attendance is 10 years (CIA, 2015). Life expectancy is currently 59.26 years, up from only 28 years in 1994 (Drobac & Naughton, 2014). The primary infectious diseases encountered are bacterial diarrhea, hepatitis A, typhoid, malaria, dengue fever, and rabies (CIA).

The health system in Rwanda comprises four tiers of health services (Ministry of Health and Human Resources, 2014): 34 health posts (outreach activities), 442+ health centers, 48 district hospitals, and 4 national referral hospitals. Table 15A.1 shows other key healthcare statistics for Rwanda compared to sub-Saharan Africa.

Physicians, Nursing, and Midwifery

The majority of Rwandan physicians are general practitioners. As of February 2011, there were 470 Rwandan general practitioners, 133 Rwandan specialists, and 58 specialists from foreign countries working in Rwanda (Drobac & Naughton, 2014). Immediately after the genocide, there were only 346 nurses remaining in Rwanda, and currently, there are approximately 11,500 nurses (of all levels),

Table 15A.1	Rwanda Health Indicators		
Indicator	**Rwanda**	**SSA**	**Other**
Doctors per 1,000 population	0.06	0.19	
Nurses per 1,000 population	0.66	1.02	
Under 5 mortality per 1,000 live births	91	70	USA—6.8
Maternal mortality per 100,000 live births	540	640	USA—24
Health expenditure per capita (% of GDP)	$48 USD	$76 USD	

The World Bank. (2014). Sub Saharan Africa (SSA). Retrieved from http://data.worldbank.org/region/sub-saharan-africa.

including midwives to serve a population of over 10 million. Most of these nurses have only the minimum level of training (Gitembagara, Relf, & Pyburn, 2015). Historically, there have been three levels of training for nurses and midwives: A2 (secondary school level), A1 (an advanced certificate following 3 years of tertiary education), and A0 (bachelor's degree). Currently, the minimum requirement for a Rwandan nurse is A1, though many health facilities continue to be staffed by mostly A2 nurses due to a serious shortage of A1 and A0 nurses (Gitembagara et al., 2015).

Educational Institutions and Simulation Centers in Rwanda

The University of Rwanda College of Medicine and Health Sciences (UR-CMHS) provides the majority of clinical education in Rwanda and consists of the following schools: School of Medicine and Pharmacy, School of Health Sciences, School of Public Health, School of Nursing and Midwifery, and the School of Dentistry. The UR-CMHS School of Nursing and Midwifery program is offered on six different campuses: the UR-CMHS in Kigali (formerly the Kigali Health Institute (KHI), as well as in Nyagatare, Byumba, and Kibungo (public institutions), and at Kabgayi and Rwamagana (faith-based institutions). In addition, there are several other private schools of nursing that are not part of UR-CMHS.

Given that Rwanda is classified as a low-income country (The World Bank, 2014), it has a remarkably well-developed national simulation program. Rwanda's primary simulation center is located at UR-CMHS in Kigali (the capital city) (Fig. 15A.1), but there are several other smaller centers in schools and hospitals outside Kigali. In 2014, the University of Rwanda (UR) amalgamated all regional nursing schools into its organization in an attempt to standardize curricula, assessments, clinical

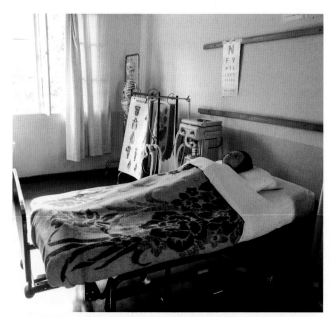

Figure 15A.1 Simulation Lab at Nyarugenge Campus (Kigali).

placements, and the use of simulation throughout the programs of nursing and midwifery nationally.

Emergence of Local Simulation Leaders

In 2001, simulation planning was initiated by Dr. Kamanzi (then Head of the Department of Nursing and Midwifery), and a candidate from the Seychelles. At the time, both were working two days per week in the skills lab, allowing them to gain insight into needed resources. They approached KHI (now the UR-CMHS) management to make videos on nursing procedures available in addition to other essential resources. Several leaders at KHI then visited the University of Natal in South Africa, which resulted in the signing of a

"Memorandum of Understanding" between the School of Nursing of the University of Natal (now called KwaZulu-Natal) and KHI. The School of Nursing of Natal University then used its position as a WHO Collaborating Center to obtain funds for the project from both the WHO and the African Development Bank. The proposal was approved for funding through Rwanda's Ministry of Foreign Affairs.

Based on the identified needs, the KHI Rector approached various international agencies, ultimately selecting the Flemish Association for Development Cooperation and Technical Assistance (VVOB) to establish a new skills lab at KHI. VVOB is a nonprofit organization whose aim is to sustainably improve the quality, efficiency, and effectiveness of education and training in developing countries. VVOB organized a mission to KwaZulu-Natal to learn more about the design and development of nursing skills labs. Various people from KHI and VVOB then contributed to the establishment of our current skills lab (Dr. Kamanzi, personal communication, 2015).

The Rwandan program was built from three external partnerships with Western entities. These partnerships are outlined in Table 15A.2. The main strategic partnership was formed with VVOB who then organized a field trip to KwaZulu-Natal to learn more about simulation and then work with staff from KHI to establish the first and current skills lab at KHI (Dr. Kamazi, personal communication, June 2015). Other key partnerships are detailed in Table 15A.2.

Key factors in our success have included the following:

- A strong commitment from university/hospital leadership (including the principal, deans, head of departments, and hospital CEOs)
- Providing the necessary space for the skills lab
- Providing long-term required staffing for program sustainability
- Providing a trained technician to help service and repair equipment

Table 15A.2	**Key Partnerships for Simulation in Rwanda**	
2003–2010: KHI (now UR-CMHS) and VVOB (Belgium)	**2010–2012: Central University Teaching Hospital of Kigali (CHUK) and the Canadian Anesthesiologists Society International Education Foundation (CAS-IEF)**	**2012–Present: University of Rwanda and Human Resources for Health Programs— Rwanda (HRH)**
• Simulation education plan formulated • Budget developed and approved • Governance model built • Rooms for skills labs and offices outfitted • Equipment purchased • Simulation staff trained • Simulation integrated into nursing curriculum • Skills lab opened at KHI 2004 • Recruitment and training of standardized patients • Program operated 2010–2012 independently by KHI	• Skills lab (one room) outfitted for purpose at CHUK for use of medical students, residents, practicing physicians • Equipment purchased • Skills lab staffed with one Full time equivalent (FTE) and opened • Program now operated independently by CHUK	• Extension of KHI skills lab activities to allied health and nursing schools countrywide • Training of faculty in use of simulation • Assistance in setup of skills labs outside Kigali • Assistance with computerized booking and inventory • Assistance in setup of CPR training • Further training of simulation staff • Purchase of substantial amount of new equipment and training sessions for this equipment

- Collaboration between the various campuses and schools, and between the university/schools and public hospitals to work toward common methodologies, standardizing curriculum and evaluation methods, and a continuing program for faculty development
- Commitment to ongoing faculty education in simulation methodology and equipment training

In 2003, KHI spearheaded the development of a formal simulation program and the setup of an initial simulation skills lab. The skills lab was opened in 2004 and initially served only the School of Nursing and Midwifery. At that time, Objective Structure Clinical Examinations (OSCEs) were used to assess nursing and midwifery. A Standardized Patient Program was initiated in 2008, with full implementation taking place by 2010. Also by 2009, the overall Simulation Program had expanded to include the Schools of Health Sciences and Dentistry, and in 2010, the Schools of Medicine and Pharmacy. In addition, in 2009 to 2010, the KHI simulation staff began to teach and build capacity in other nursing and midwifery schools outside of Kigali. Also, in 2009 to 2010, three hospitals, the Central University Teaching Hospital of Kigali (CHUK) (public university teaching hospital), the Military Hospital (public), and King Faisal Hospital (private), began to incorporate simulation into their education programs.

In 2010, simulation funding and administration of the budget shifted from VVOB to a local entity, UR-CMHS in order to ensure sustainability. With the assistance of the Canadian Anesthesiologists Society International Education Foundation (CAS-IEF), a simulation lab was set up and opened at CHUK (Fig. 15A.2), the largest public referral hospital in Rwanda. Finally, in 2014 to 2015, a partnership with the Human Resources for Health Program—Rwanda, made it possible to purchase a substantial amount of new simulation equipment. The new equipment was distributed to clinical schools and hospitals throughout Rwanda with training provided for faculty in these locations.

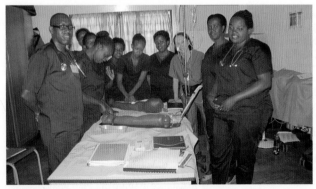

Figure 15A.2 CHUK Hospital (Centre Hospitalier Universitaire de Kigali). Skills Lab at Central University Teaching Hospital of Kigali (CHUK Hospital, or Centre Hospitalier Universitaire de Kigali). Used with permission.

Prevalence and Extent of Use of Simulation in Rwanda

Currently, Rwanda's simulation programs are part of a national simulation program that includes the UR-CMHS (Colleges of Nursing and Midwifery, Medicine, Health Sciences, and Dentistry) as well as some of the public and private hospitals. Altogether, the national simulation program has 13 operating simulation centers including the schools and hospitals. There are also simulation programs operated independently at other schools and hospitals outside of the national program. Currently, the country's simulation centers do not have affiliate status with larger simulation organizations, such as SSH or the International Nursing Association of Clinical Simulation and Learning (INACSL).

At present, simulation is most widely used in the College of Nursing and Midwifery and is integrated into the curriculum. It is primarily being used to teach and assess students' practical skills in preparation for going into the clinical setting. Simulation is also being used to a lesser degree in academe as a component of educational programs for anesthesia, medical imaging, physical therapy, mental health, dentistry, ophthalmology, and clinical medicine. Clinical medicine is a 4-year program that is roughly equivalent to a physician's assistant in North America. After graduating from this program, students practice independently at a level somewhere between the scope of practice of a nurse and a physician, performing general medical duties such as diagnosis and treatment of diseases, minor medical and surgical procedures, giving medications, ordering and interpreting diagnostic tests, and making referral to other physicians. Often, clinical medicine practitioners practice alone or with nurses and midwives in rural health centers where there are no physicians available. This specialty is common in East and Southern Africa and some countries in West Africa. Simulation is also being used in the hospital setting to train medical students, residents, staff nurses, and physicians.

To date, simulation has been most effective in Rwanda for improving clinical skills in nursing, midwifery, and allied health undergraduate students; clinical skills of residents, medical students, and physicians in surgery, anesthesia, emergency medicine, and in OB/Gyn; and in life support training. Simulation Programs are collaboratively working toward the integration of interprofessional education and professional communication in both clinical practice and academic programs over the next 2 to 3 years.

Today, the UR-CMHS in Kigali houses the primary simulation center serving the UR-CMHS healthcare programs and sometimes the staff/faculty from public and private hospitals. The most common types of simulation activities conducted at the university are skills demonstrations and practice and skills assessments (in the form of OSCEs) (Figs. 15A.3 and 15A.4). Standardized patients are also used but primarily in mental health, dentistry, and

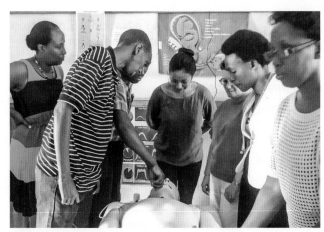

Figure 15A.3 SimMan Training Session 1.

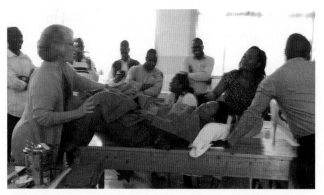

Figure 15A.5 Simulation Session with Standardized Patient Portraying a Mother Giving Birth, at the Byumba Campus.

physical therapy programs (Fig. 15A.5). Student class sizes are usually large—from 60 to 100+ students. Hospital staff access the Simulation Center for teaching medical students, residents, and staff. The most common types of simulation activities include skills practice and assessments, as well as the deployment of unidisciplinary simulation scenarios. These groups are usually much smaller—typically 5 to 20.

The Kigali Simulation Center is also used to run life support training (primarily BLS, Helping Babies Breathe

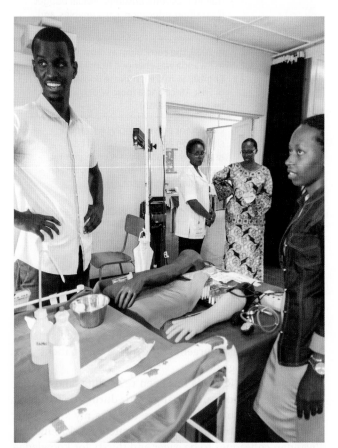

Figure 15A.4 Sim Lab 8: Simulation Lab at Nyarugenge Campus (Kigali) Open House 4.

[HBB], and Helping Mothers Survive [HMS]) for university faculty, students, and hospital staff. HBB is a neonatal resuscitation program developed in 2010 by the American Academy of Pediatrics, and Jhpiego (an international, non-profit health organization affiliated with Johns Hopkins University). Both are simple but effective programs with low-cost training kits available that are best suited for low-resource settings and are endorsed by the WHO. Life support training is also conducted in public and private hospitals using simulation equipment.

Other well-equipped simulation centers are located in Nyamishaba (where all first year nursing, midwifery, mental health, and allied students study), in Butare (where the school of medicine and pharmacy are located), and in various other nursing schools outside of Kigali. In addition, a number of public and private hospitals both in and outside of Kigali have simulation programs, however the extent to which they are developed and equipped varies widely.

The simulation staff is just beginning to expand professional development and scholarly work. Faculty have delivered poster presentations at several international conferences and recently submitted several peer-reviewed journal articles as well as a book chapter for publication. To date, Simulation Programs have not undertaken formal research, although there are plans for this in the next academic year and grant proposals are in process.

Simulation Program Funding in Rwanda

Today, the University of Rwanda (UR) primarily funds simulation programs at the UR-CMHS with substantial support from their international partners. Hospital-based simulation programs, on the other hand, are mostly self-funded. However, there are exceptions and at CHUK, the simulation center received substantial funding from the Canadian Anesthesiologists' Society. To our knowledge, there are currently no educational cost-recovery (tuition-based) models or business-for-profit (fee-for-service-based) models used in simulation programs in Rwanda.

Barriers and Challenges Encountered in Simulation Integration

On our journey, we have encountered various barriers and challenges in implementation and continued development of simulation programs. Table 15A.3 summarizes some of the key challenges we faced and the solutions we successfully implemented. We hope that these suggestions derived from lived experience, will assist others that are seeking to develop simulation programs in low-resource settings such as Africa.

Foreign and Local Simulationists' Perspectives

In the next segment, Renee Pyburn, an American citizen having worked in Rwanda for the Human Resources for Health Program, and Philomène Uwimana, the Acting Director of Simulation for the UR-CMHS) describe their personal experiences of working as simulation collaborators that originate from culturally diverse backgrounds.

Renee Pyburn

At the time of writing this chapter section, I was employed by the Human Resources for Health Program—Rwanda (a US government-funded program to assist Rwanda in the development of clinical education and clinical staff expertise). I was partner to the Director of Simulation at UR-CMHS. Prior to coming to Rwanda, I had accumulated over 21 years of international experience working and living in Saudi Arabia, Kuwait, Qatar, and Thailand. In contrast to the Middle Eastern countries where I had previously worked, Rwanda's fiscal resources were very limited. In our simulation program, we were a small staff of four (an acting director, an assistant, a simulation technician, and myself) delivering simulation with limited equipment and small supply budget with very large class sizes and a faculty that have heavy workloads and limited time for faculty development in simulation.

Upon my arrival in Rwanda, I experienced quite an adjustment to the fiscal realities of my new work environment. I also faced a significant culture shift with new language barriers and differences in ways of being and doing that impacted me in various ways. For example, the primary spoken language in Rwanda is Kinyarwanda, a very difficult language to learn! In the work place local people were more comfortable speaking French than English, so I had to work hard to improve my Kinyarwanda and French in order to facilitate better communication. With my inability to speak the mother tongue(s), it was particularly helpful that Rwandans characteristically maintain a polite

Table 15A.3	Developing a National Simulation Program in Rwanda: Our Challenges and Solutions
Challenge	**Solution**
Limited funding	Partnerships with outside entities (VVOB, Canadian Anesthesiologists Society, HRH) who provided large amounts of funding.
Lack of local simulation expertise	Assistance was provided during partnerships to train local staff, since this ongoing training has been provided by Rwandan faculty.
Lack of equipment	Substantial donations were made by various partners.
Curricular integration	Begun during partnership with VVOB and very successfully done in nursing and midwifery; continues to be ongoing in other programs. Supported by senior leadership at UR-CMHS. We are continuing to try to improve curricular integration in other programs and to introduce it into the Master's in Nursing Program.
Ensuring sustainability of programs	Has been accomplished by training Rwandan education faculty and technician, having regular workshops and other training sessions; ensuring annual budget for staffing, education, consumables, and equipment.
Language barriers	In 2009, the curriculum at most schools in Rwanda was changed from French to English, to make it more in line with the rest of East Africa and a more widely spoken language (English).
Accessibility to technological systems/ infrastructure to support simulation programs	Consistent power supply to support simulation activities can be an issue, especially in rural areas. Consequently, we have focused primarily on low-tech simulation equipment.
Differing values and traditions	Integration of Western evidence-based educational and simulation best practices within Rwandan culture and educational traditions have been implemented in a way that will be be sustainable to Rwandans.

and nonaggressive way of speaking and a relaxed sense of time with decreased urgency. They were very patient with my steep learning curve.

Working in Rwanda has been rewarding, and I experienced tremendous personal growth during that time. It has been a pleasure and privilege to bring my knowledge and skills to contribute to positive outcomes. I found my Rwandan colleagues to be eager and thirsty for knowledge about simulation. I feel so privileged to have been in a position to collaborate professionally with this team. As a rule, it has been my experience that Rwandans are a gentle and kind people that quickly form deep personal relationships with others. They are also a hardworking and committed people. I am profoundly moved and impressed by the extreme challenges they have overcome as evidenced by the advancements they have made since the devastating 1994 genocide. It is nothing short of amazing to witness their resilience. I am also in awe of how much learning can be accomplished in simulation with very little equipment and few staff. Below is a list of what my partner and I accomplished together in one year by setting a list of shared goals:

- Reorganization of all consumable supplies and equipment
- Development of an electronic booking form and database for tracking skills lab usage
- Completion of a 13-module workshop for UR-CMHS faculty on "Writing for publication" (co-taught with another HRH colleague)
- Distribution and training for large equipment donation made by HRH
- Delivery of simulation workshops to several groups of faculty
- Acceptance and presentation of two conference posters; one article and one book chapter currently being reviewed for publication (authored by simulation staff)
- Assisting with the development of curriculum for the new Masters of Science Degree in Nursing and the A1 (3-year) nursing program
- Assisting with development and delivery of life support training

 Employees of the University of Maryland stay connected by telephone and by submitting a monthly written report to program leads describing the challenges we faced, what we think went well and what did not, what we would do to try to overcome these challenges and improve our outcomes, and whether or not we expected these challenges to continue (See Toolkit 15A-1). I have experienced many rich cultural experiences such as attending my first traditional Rwandan wedding and going on a sightseeing trip where, of 22 women, I was the only non-Rwandan in attendance. I have come to know Rwandans as a people that value loyalty family, friends, and colleagues. They are creative and resourceful and therefore can accomplish a lot with very little. Being respectful and practicing deeply held cultural traditions are important to them. I also marvel at how they maintain a palpable cheerfulness and joie-de-vivre, even through their many struggles and the lingering ghosts of past traumas.

Compared to other struggling nations in Africa, I appreciated the stability the Rwandan government provided, as well as its commitment to economic improvement

and the elimination of corruption, and a commitment to healthcare and education. I enjoyed living in a perfect climate, a politically safe and stable environment, and noticeably clean surroundings.

I believe that through key collaborative partnerships, Rwanda has been able to build a remarkably sustainable national simulation program with very few resources. By combining the strengths and expertise of our collaborating partners and upholding Rwandan culture and educational traditions, together we have been able to set realistic goals and make remarkable strides. I feel very proud to have been a part of this journey, and it was certainly an experience I will always cherish and remember.

Philomène Uwimana

I am a registered nurse, and currently the Acting Director of the Simulation Program at the University of Rwanda College of Medicine and Health Sciences. I have been working in the Simulation Center for almost 10 years, first as a skills lab assistant until 2008 and thereafter with the Rwandan partner to the VVOB as coordinator of the center. Since its inception, the Simulation Program at CMHS has been benefiting from partnerships with Western institutions. As such, I have had the opportunity to work with people from varied contexts with cultural backgrounds and educational resources that differ from my own. When I joined UR-CMHS, the VVOB, a Belgian organization, was operating as funding partner to build a skills lab center. One of the important assets I brought to that partnership was my ability to speak the French language. French, at that time, was still the primary teaching language at KHI.

In Rwandan culture, planning and timeliness are more relaxed than in Western cultures, so at first I found it challenging to work with our Belgian partners who had very different expectations in terms of detailed advance planning and adhering to strict time schedules. In 2010, I was appointed as Coordinator of the Simulation Program and took on the responsibility for planning, organizing, and managing all activities of the other KHI Simulation Center as well as helping to develop simulation programs in schools and hospitals outside of Kigali. Around that time, we transitioned away from our partnership with VVOB, and I was in a better position to be able to adapt our processes to match the local cultural norms. In 2009, the UR-CMHS shifted their primary language for curriculum delivery from French to English. It was very challenging to change our entire curriculum from French to English, but with practice, I became more confident in English. Throughout the years I have worked with three foreign employees in the development of simulation. This reality is challenging because of the coming and going and the need to continually establish new working relationships while adjusting to personal and cultural differences.

Most recently, I was working with our third foreign simulation employee, Renee Pyburn. We spent a year working hand in hand towards collaboratively established goals. Fortunately, we continued to work as partners for one more year. I have gained a lot from this partnership, as the ultimate goal of the twinning process is to transfer skills—in this case for the learning of managerial and organizational skills needed to operationalize a Simulation Program. HRH employees working in Rwanda are paired with a Rwandan "twin"—a Rwandan who is working in the same specialty or education area as their HRH counterpart. The primary objective of this "twinning" model is transfer of skills/knowledge to the Rwandan twin in a way that will ultimately be sustainable by Rwandans alone. Through this partnership, I feel that I have greatly improved my management and organizational skills, as well as developed professionally through collaborative scholarly writing and submitting and presenting at conferences. In my work with people from other parts of the world, I have developed a better understanding and appreciation for our cultural differences.

Most Important Lessons Learned in Implementing Simulation In Rwanda

We believe that the partnership model that was used successfully in Rwanda serves as a model for other low-resource nations working to integrate and implement simulation. We are both proud of the tremendous strides made here in Rwanda, accomplished through a shared vision to make simulation an essential and increasing presence in Rwanda's education and healthcare sectors.

Toolkit Resource

Toolkit 15A-1: Monthly Written Report. Example of a report used to communicate challenges faced, successes, and proposed strategies to overcome challenges and improve outcomes.

15B Global Perspectives on Simulation: Australia

Michelle Kelly, Jonathan M. Mould, Tracy Levett-Jones

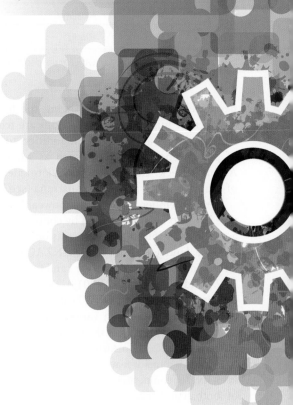

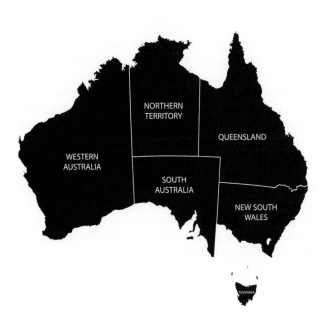

Australia: Profile[1]

With a landmass of approximately 7.6 million square kilometres, Australia is the sixth largest nation in the world (after Russia, Canada, China, the United States of America [USA], and Brazil). Australia has a population of 23.5 million, and the average age is 38 years. The majority of the population is concentrated along the eastern seaboard with 70% of people living in the 10 largest cities.

The traditional owners of the land are Indigenous Australians. The Aboriginal people are the oldest surviving generation in the world and their presence in Australia dates beyond 60,000 years. There are numerous tribes or "mobs" within the Indigenous population but irrespective of geographical location across the vast land mass and differing dialects, all have a fundamental, strong connection with the land. Their culture is expressed through painting, song, dance, and storytelling (Creative Spirits, 2015). Aboriginal and Torres Strait Islanders constitute 2.2% of the population. While two thirds of Australia's Indigenous people currently live in towns and cities, others live in rural and remote areas, and some still have a traditional way of life.

Contemporary Australia is one of the most culturally diverse countries in the world with four out of ten

[1]Note: Information within this section has been adapted from the Australian Government Department of Foreign Affairs and Trade.

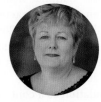

Michelle Kelly,
PhD, MN, BSc, RN

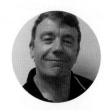

Jonathan M. Mould,
PhD

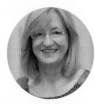

Tracy Levett-Jones,
PhD, MEd, RN

Table 15B.1	Range of Religions (And Percentages) Practices in Australia		
Religion	**Percentage**	**Religion**	**Percentage**
Protestant	35%	Muslim	2.2%
Catholic	25%	Hindu	1.3%
Buddhist	2.5%	Other or unspecified	34%

Table 15B.3	Key Aspects of the Australian Economy
Strengths	Mining (iron-ore, gold); agriculture (livestock, meat, wheat, wool); energy (liquefied natural gas, coal); manufacturing and service sectors (education, training, health, transport)
Economic partners	Global, but particularly East Asia countries

people either born overseas being the first-generation children of migrants, half of whom are from non-English-speaking backgrounds. In addition to English, 77% of people speak languages such as Mandarin, Italian, Arabic, Greek, Cantonese, and Vietnamese. A number of religions are practiced in Australia (see Table 15B.1).

As a member of the Commonwealth, Australian culture has also been influenced by contributions to military activities. A strong allegiance exists between Australia and New Zealand as a result of the ANZAC tradition particularly evident during World War I and the events at Gallipoli (DVA and BOSTES NSW, 2015). "Mateship" is a hallmark of this Australian and New Zealand culture. Those who defended our country in various military campaigns are acknowledged every year during the ANZAC Day National Holiday (April 25th in Australia).

Sport is a major feature of Australian culture. There is a keen level of competitiveness across the States in three codes of football and soccer (English football), and with England and New Zealand, particularly in cricket or rugby union.

History

European settlement commenced in the years after Captain James Cook charted the east coast of Australia in 1770 and claimed the "new found area" for Britain. Penal

Table 15B.2	Summary of Influences and Current Government Organization
Westminster influences	● Six separate colonies initially established ● Declared a Federation in 1901 ● Currently—six States and two Territories
USA influences	● Federal government body—with relationships between national and state
Australian Constitution	● Executive powers of government vested in a Governor-General ● Federal Government—defence, foreign affairs, trade and commerce, taxation, customs and excise duties, pensions, immigration and postal services ● Other powers—States and Territories

colonies were then established in New South Wales, Tasmania, and Western Australia but by 1830 free settlers outnumbered convicts who had been transported to Australia, often as punishment for menial crimes. The discovery of gold in the 1850s and post WWII infrastructure projects brought an influx of migrants from all over the world and began to shape Australia as a country of diverse cultures.

Australia remains part of the Commonwealth with ties and allegiance to Britain; however, the establishment of a Republic has been debated for many years and may be introduced in the future. In the meantime, the Governor-General of Australia remains the representative and figurehead of Her Majesty Queen Elizabeth II.

Government and the Economy

Table 15B.2 provides a summary of influences and the current government organization. Over the past 50 years, Australia has developed a highly diversified economy, as outlined in Table 15B.3.

Employment Location and Setting—Simulation

The preparation of healthcare practitioners is predominantly embedded within bachelor degree programs offered at universities. Exceptions exist with some colleges of technical and further education (TAFEs) that provide a Bachelor degree for registered nurses in addition an 18-24 month program for enrolled nurses (similar to licensed practice nurses [LPNs] in the USA). Accreditation of curricula is based on the national health profession's Standards and Competencies for practice (Australian Health Practitioner Regulation Agency, 2010) in addition to the specific university processes and Australian government regulations (Australian Government Department of Education and Training, 2011).

Interest in using simulation as a contemporary teaching and learning strategy has occurred at all levels across the health professions in Australia. Uptake has been dependent on knowledge about and interest in this learning approach and more recently access to resources including equipment, space, and personnel. Influenced by international activities, contemporary simulation first emerged from hospital centres or facilities, led by anaesthetists and surgeons (Cregan & Watterson, 2005; Flanagan, Nestel, & Joseph, 2004; Watterson, Flanagan, Donovan, & Robinson, 2000) to address issues related to safe practice in operating theatres. In relation to nursing and midwifery, strategic directions for simulation in Australian higher education institutions have aligned with the Australian Safety and Quality frameworks (Australian Commission on Safety and Quality, 2015), the professional standards for practice (Nursing and Midwifery Board of Australia) and Australia's national health priorities (Australian Institute of Health and Welfare, 2015). Other factors that influence the approaches and context of simulation learning experiences are the cultural diversity across student cohorts, the healthcare workforce, and healthcare consumer demographics.

Evolution of Simulation in Australia and Emergence of Leaders

In the 1990s, clinicians in Australia were beginning to recognise the potential of simulation-based education (SBE) as a valuable teaching and learning methodology. In healthcare, this was undoubtedly as a result of work done in anaesthesiology in the United States (Gaba, 1992; Gaba & DeAndra, 1989). There were local examples of innovation, for example, in Perth Western Australia, Dr. Richard Riley was a driving force in the establishment of one of the first skills and simulation centres and in South Australia, Professor Harry Owen developed the Flinders University medical simulation centre. Both of these early champions were initially focussed on medical and procedural education rather than healthcare education per se. Without any policy directives, in healthcare, the progression of SBE at a national level was slow.

Despite early innovations, it was nearly 20 years after Australian physicians developed the Manbits Perfusion Simulator (Rosen, 2008) that SBE was adopted at a national level. Anaesthetists were the main professional group to utilise simulation in healthcare with examples of training centers being set up in many states. For example, the Sydney Simulation Centre in New South Wales (NSW) was initially established in 1997 under the directorship of Dr. Leonie Watterson. Recently, the Centre combined with the Clinical Skills Centre and co-located into a new purpose-built facility (Sydney Clinical Skills and Simulation Centre, 2010). In Western Australia (WA), the Centre for Anaesthesia Skills and Medical Simulation opened in the late 1990s prior to moving into a purpose-built Centre in 2000 (Riley, Grauze, Trewhella, Chinnery, & Horley, 2003). In South Australia (SA), Flinders University's Department of Anaesthesia

and Intensive Care developed their STructured Airway Teaching (STAT) laboratory in 1999 with airway trainers for anaesthesia and intensive care physicians.

Similar initiatives emerged in Victoria (VIC) with the Monash Simulation Centre becoming operational in 1997 led by Dr. Brendan Flannagan (Monash Simulation, 2015) and now offering a range of interprofessional courses and innovative educational strategies. Development, training, and use of simulated patients have been a particular area of expertise and scholarship emerging from Monash University's Professor Debra Nestel and Dr. Margaret Bearman (Nestel & Bearman, 2014). From these notable beginnings, staffing and initiatives have expanded and numerous other centres have commenced operations in metropolitan, urban, and in some instances, rural settings.

The incorporation of simulation into university nursing and midwifery curricula and collaborations between leaders and scholars from these disciplines (nationally and internationally) has contributed in significant ways to simulation practice, evaluation, and research (Arthur, Kable, & Levett-Jones, 2011; Bogossian et al., 2012; Buykx et al., 2012; Cant & Cooper, 2010; Kable, Arthur, Levett-Jones, & Reid-Searl, 2013; Kelly, Forber, Conlon, Roche, & Stasa, 2014; Kelly, Hager, & Gallagher, 2014; McKenna et al., 2014; Mould, White, & Gallagher, 2011; Neill & Wotton, 2011; Orr, Kellehear, Armari, Pearson, & Holmes, 2013; Rochester et al., 2012). More details about the range of simulation scholarship and research are provided below.

A somewhat different model of simulation operations is seen in the Queensland Health Clinical Skills Development Service (CSDS), established in 2004 (Clinical Skills Development Service, 2015) as a result of multimillion dollar funding from the State Government. Unlike the centres in other states, the CSDS offered state-wide services based on a "hub and spoke" approach. Although many of these early groups commenced with a focus on education and training for medical and surgery, course offerings have extended to incorporate other health disciplines and interprofessional simulation activities.

Subsequently, the remaining States and Territories have been able to offer SBE following earlier innovations and interest in the other cities. Tasmania is developing SBE in healthcare and has increased the capacity for SLEs for clinicians (Tasmanian Government, 2014). There has also been an increase in SBE in healthcare for undergraduate education in Tasmania. The Northern Territory opened a Sim Lab in 2013 at the Royal Darwin Hospital (The Northern Territory Regional Training Network, 2013) and similar activities are offered in the Australian Capital Territory (ACT).

As can be seen, all of the states and territories have established simulation programs to a greater or lesser degree, and the vast majority now have an interprofessional approach to SBE. It is somewhat difficult to identify specific local champions across the country because many areas have developed pockets of expertise to suit their immediate demands. Some groups have shared their resources and expertise through networking at national (ASSH; SimHealth; NHET-Sim) and international levels (IMSH; SESAM, etc.) and numerous individuals have served on committees and boards of ASSH, Simulation Australasia and the Society for Simulation in Healthcare (SSH). Exemplars of simulation champions in nursing and midwifery are featured below.

National Initiatives

Outside of the healthcare sector, SBE was being formalised at a national level and innovations and developments in SBE were increasingly being shared (Simulation Australasia). Academics and industry partners collaborated with the Defence Science and Technology Organisation (DSTO) to form the Simulation Industry Association of Australia (SIAA). This national body established an annual conference (SimTecT) and in 2010 introduced a name change to Simulation Australia, then to Simulation Australasia in 2015 to reflect growth in the field and geographical partnerships. The goal of Simulation Australasia is to be an all-inclusive organisation with government, business, education, and health. A simulation health division commenced in 2007—the Australian Society for Simulation in Healthcare (**ASSH**) (Australian Society for Simulation in Healthcare, 2015). The seven divisions of Simulation Australasia are now called **specialist communities**. From the outset, ASSH has promoted an interprofessional approach at all levels of activity—membership, committee work, and the annual conference, **SimHealth**. Figure 15B.1 features the SimHealth 2015 Organising Committee enjoying the Simulation Australasia Awards Dinner. ASSH (through the legal entity of Simulation Australasia) has been an affiliate of the Society for Simulation in Healthcare since 2010. Leaders from both Societies share a close relationship and collaborate on projects at organisational and personal levels. ASSH also contributes to meetings and project work of the Global Network for Simulation in Healthcare (GNSH). In 2015, the then Chair of ASSH, Kirsty Freeman, and immediate past Chair, Michelle Kelly, participated in the discussions and group work at the GNSH meeting in Stavanger, Norway.

The Health Workforce Australia Era

A significant drive to expand the use of SBE at a national level was the formation of Health Workforce Australia (HWA). HWA was established by the Council of Australian Governments to build a sustainable health workforce and improve education on a national level (Commonwealth of Australia, 2009). One area of collective reform under HWA's mandate was simulated learning environments (SLEs), which received $94m in funding in 2011 (Health Workforce Australia, 2014). Following discipline-specific surveys of

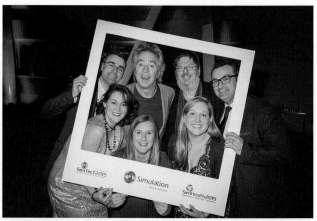

Figure 15B.1 SimHealth 2015 Organising Committee Enjoying the Simulation Australasia Awards Dinner with MC Brian Nankervis. L-R (**back row**): Julian Van Dijk, Co-Convenor; Brian Nankervis, Cyle Sprick Workshop Convenor; Robert O'Brien, ASSH Chair and Scientific Convenor. L-R (**front row**): Kirsty Freeman, Co-Convenor and Immediate Past Chair ASSH; Jessica Stokes-Parish; Sarah Verdonk, ASSH administrative officer. Courtesy of Simulation Australasia, with permission.

the current status of simulation and areas for future growth, one of the main projects to emerge from the HWA era was a national simulation training program. Phase one of this project was the establishment of the Australian Simulation Educator and Technician Training (**AusSETT**) Program. This program was developed by a consortium of Australian universities: Edith Cowan University (WA), Flinders University (SA), Monash University (lead), The University of Melbourne (VIC), The University of Queensland, and Queensland Health (QLD) (National Health Education and Training in Simulation Program, 2012).

The AusSETT program provided a national standardised approach for simulation educators, technicians, and coordinators of SLE. The inaugural workshop in December 2011 involved 15 participants from diverse professional groups. These experienced simulation educators helped to develop and then deliver the program at a local level to over 230 train-the-trainer personnel. Phase 2 of this project, the National Health Education and Training in Simulation (**NHETSim**) program, had a different focus—to support simulation educators and technicians to work directly with simulation-based education. At the recent 2015 SimHealth conference, the NHETSim program was recognised with a Simulation Australasia Project Innovation Award.

What is significant about the approach to SBE in Australia is that the aforementioned programs were free to healthcare educators. This unquestionably led to a huge increase in simulation education hours across Australia. Before HWA closed in 2014, it funded a significant number of projects that resulted in increased use of SBE and collaborative partnerships at a national level.

Another national initiative that arose from HWA funding was the creation of **SimNET**—a simulation in health directory, which is a repository for educational resources (Simulation Australasia and the Australian Society for Simulation in Healthcare, 2012). Finally, the Quality Frameworks for Simulation project is focussed on determining the standards, indicators, and support tools for simulation programs and educators in relation to accreditation and certification processes. Reporting of deliverables from the consultant group is expected by the end of 2015.

Prevalence of Simulation in Australia

Students within nursing and midwifery degree programs, like several health disciplines, are required to complete a set number of clinical hours to be eligible for registration and to graduate. Under the present legal and regulatory conditions, simulation is not able to be used as a substitute for clinical hours. A national research project to determine the impact and outcomes of simulation within Australian nursing and midwifery programs is under way. A large national study involving six universities investigated the impact of simulation for physiotherapy practice. Physiotherapy students need to meet competency standards, rather than a set number of clinical hours, to meet degree course requirements. Within two randomised controlled trials, the group determined that SLE could replace 25% of students' clinical time with real patients (Blackstock et al., 2013; Watson et al., 2012). These robust local studies provide good direction for other disciplines in this endeavor.

Areas of Simulation Expertise in Nursing and Midwifery

Use of simulation in nursing and midwifery has grown exponentially in Australia, particularly in the university sector (McAllister, Levett-Jones, et al., 2013). Predominantly, simulation is used to prepare undergraduate (UG) students for upcoming clinical practice experiences or for specialty areas such as paediatrics, critical care, and mental health placements.

Exemplars of innovative work and substantial scholarship and research are now featured. However, significant others lead and contribute to simulation initiatives through use in hospital new graduate programs and continuing professional development activities.

Preparation for Practice: Large and Diverse Student Cohorts

Simulation is used in many universities as a segway to prepare students for the health setting. This approach is helpful in many ways. Students gain insight into areas that need further development (knowledge and skills); the expectations from the workforce about their role and contribution to patient care; and the professional behaviours important for the nursing role (Rochester et al., 2012). Through featuring the importance of clear communication with patients, relatives, and the healthcare team within simulation scenarios (Disler, Rochester, Kelly, White, & Forber, 2013), educators can gain insight into students' communication abilities and in some instances delay clinical placement experiences until remediation has been undertaken. One successful initiative, to support the large percentage of international students in Australian nursing courses, is the Clinically Speaking program at the University of Technology Sydney (see http://www.uts.edu.au/current-students/health/clinical-practice/clinically-speaking). Online modules modelling communication interactions and role play together with student practice aim to reduce potential miscommunication and errors in the clinical setting (San Miguel & Rogan, 2009).

Recognising and Responding to the Deteriorating Patient

Several authors have developed and incorporated simulation scenarios around this important issue and embedded the experiences specifically in the final years of the UG programs. Dr. Simon Cooper and colleagues from numerous Australian states and the UK used their program of research in this field (Buykx et al., 2012; Cooper et al., 2010, 2012; Endacott et al., 2010, 2012; McKenna et al., 2014) to create an online portal—First2Act http://first2actweb.com/—with supportive materials to enhance these critical skills (First2Act, 2015). Access to the site is free of charge and is suitable for any health professional or student. Other evaluations of specific simulations to boost final year students' skills of noticing and responding to patient deterioration (Kelly, Forber, et al., 2014) have corroborated the work of Cooper and colleagues, which illustrates agreement on this important direction for simulation.

Outstanding Realism—MASK-ED™

An initiative from Professor Kerry Reid-Searl, to maximise the authenticity and participant interaction with a "simulated patient", saw the emergence of bespoke silicone masks (and other body parts) paired with a character, to create the concept of the masked educator—or MASK-ED™. Here, the educator assumes the persona of the character and deliberately guides learning with probing questions about students' actions and thinking (McAllister, Reid-Searl, & Davis, 2013; Reid-Searl, Levett-Jones, Cooper, & Happell, 2014). Kerry has expanded the range of artefacts to include child-like puppets to assist students and nurses to refine techniques for age-appropriate interactions with paediatric patients and their families (see https://www.cqu.edu.au/about-us/structure/schools/nm/simulation/mask-ed).

Pedagogy and Quality Indicators for Simulation

Australian nurse academics have been mindful of the need for robust pedagogical frameworks as foundations for the development and delivery of simulation. A program of work led by Professor Tracy Levett-Jones and colleagues created *Quality Indicators for Simulation* as part of a nationally funded project. The indicator statements address pedagogical principles, fidelity, student preparation and orientation, staff preparation and training, and debriefing (Arthur, Levett-Jones, & Kable, 2013). These principles are similar to the INACSL Standards of Best Practice: Simulation[SM] (INACSL Standards Committee, 2016), and offer frameworks to develop and deliver contemporary healthcare simulation activities.

More recently, Dr. Michelle Kelly has engaged with experienced education academics to elicit different and broader perspectives regarding simulation pedagogy. Agreement was realised on the key approaches and concepts, which underpin impactful simulation learning experiences—the sociocultural and sociomaterial frameworks of learning (Hopwood, Rooney, Boud, & Kelly, 2014a). Simulation enables ways of engaging with other learners and artefacts in the context of real-world scenarios to learn of and about practice (Hopwood, Rooney, Boud, & Kelly, 2014b). In challenging simulation participants to become keen observers no matter what role they assume, the intent is to foster agile learners who will become agile practitioners (Rooney, Hopwood, Boud, & Kelly, 2015).

The keen focus on pedagogy resulted in a special issue in August 2015 in *Clinical Simulation in Nursing* with five invited papers presenting a range of theoretical frameworks, which experienced users have found applicable for simulation. Australian authors featured in three of the five publications (Husebø, O'Regan, & Nestel, 2015; Kelly & Hager, 2015; Smith, Gephardt, & Nestel, 2015).

The "Thinking" Aspects of Practice—Clinical Reasoning and Judgement

Experienced simulation users have extended the domains of research to explore the "thinking" aspects of practice, to determine how simulation contributes to the holism of practice and subsequent clinical encounters. Levett-Jones and colleagues (Levett-Jones, 2013; Levett-Jones et al., 2010) explored in detail the components of clinical reasoning to align with learning in simulation and assist students to make informed decisions about patient care. Similarly, influences from Tanner (2006) and Lasater (2007a) directed Kelly (2014) to explore how simulation could attune students to the dimensions of clinical judgement, and then to follow nine new graduate nurses into practice to determine the impact on subsequent clinical encounters.

Mental Health Simulations

Role-plays have been used in mental health education for decades; however, the resurgence of contemporary simulation strategies has helped in some ways to repurpose teaching and learning strategies in this clinical specialty. Two specific initiatives are the Hearing Voices simulation and rehearsing interviews in triads to uncover the importance of recovery from episodes of acute mental illness. Key to these contemporary initiatives is the partnership with mental health consumers—those who have lived experiences of this health disruption (Orr, Kellehear, Armari, Pearson, & Holmes, 2013).

Academics who are leading this work believe that mental health consumers are able to provide more authentic responses and perspectives when interviewed by simulation participants, more so than actors or experienced clinicians.

Difficult Conversations—Requesting Organ and Tissue Donation

As a component of a renewed national program relating to approaches for requesting organ and tissue donation (http://www.donatelife.gov.au/health-professionals), a specific simulation role-play initiative is offered to those undertaking the program in NSW (http://newsroom.uts.edu.au/news/2014/04/requesting-the-gift-of-life?utm_source=life_gk6&utm_medium=gk&utm_ca). Intensive care doctors and nurses training for the role of "designated organ donor requestor" rehearse the conversation with actors who play the roles of the patient's relatives. Debriefing by those experienced in the newer techniques incorporates AV playback of defined moments in the conversation where the spoken word or body language may need attention. Evaluations and research continue, to determine the impact of the new approach on subsequent practice, donation rates, and the satisfaction of relatives about the process for making informed decisions during these stressful occasions (Potter et al., in press).

A Research Agenda

A national research agendum for healthcare simulation (Nestel, Watson, Marshall, & Bearman, 2014) was informed by a summit following the annual SimHealth

Box 15B-1	Themes for a National Healthcare Simulation Agenda

- Using simulation to support student and clinician learning
- Debriefing and simulation
- Using simulation for performance assessment
- Establishing standards for simulators and simulated environments
- Modelling healthcare systems
- Using simulation to address education and workforce issues
- Considering simulation in the broader world
- Theorising simulation
- Translating research outcomes to education and healthcare
- Conducting healthcare simulation research and evaluation

conference in 2013. The summit had a broader scope than education as stakeholders from outside the education community were invited to provide perspectives. The agendum is intended to guide the development of research programs and individual researchers in framing their projects. Ten themes were generated from analysis of the feedback from summit participants. The role of simulation in leading to better patient outcomes underpins most themes. The themes, as reported by Nestel et al. (2014) are outlined in Box 15B-1.

More detailed discussion and reporting are forthcoming in an edited text on healthcare simulation practice, education, and research due for publication early 2017 (Nestel & Kelly, in press).

Barriers or Challenges Encountered Integrating Simulation

For nursing, large and diverse student cohorts (e.g., 600 students per year) provide challenges in offering more intimate simulation experiences. However, strategies reported by Rochester et al. (2012) and Disler et al. (2013) provide guidance in how to manage large numbers while maintaining a quality student experience. The large percentages of international students whose cultural beliefs in learning differ from the Socratic discussions expected in Australian educational culture provide further challenges. Encouraging students to engage in discussion, rather than expect exclusively didactic content, and identify areas for improvement is an evolutionary process.

Casualization of teaching faculty puts strain on permanent academics in ensuring "quality control" over the delivery of simulation activities. Like in other countries, sustainability of simulation initiatives requires commitment from management for designated leadership and specific technical support.

Large Distances—Supporting Simulation in Rural and Remote Areas

Due to large distances within States and across the country, health services and educational facilities are heavily populated in metropolitan and urban areas. Some of the HWA "bricks and mortar" funding helped with the building and equipping of regional simulation centers (e.g., Coffs Harbour on the NSW mid coast). This area services local and regional simulation requirements while also collaborating with urban groups.

Another strategy, similar to initiatives in the United Kingdom, involves using mobile simulation buses equipped with dedicated equipment and resources that travel to more distant areas to provide simulation education.

Sustainability for Simulation: A Global Challenge for Funding

Following the change from the HWA era, a division within the Federal Ministry of Health has managed responsibility for simulation recurrent funding. While some projects (e.g., NHET-Sim) have received funding until the end of 2015, there is uncertainty about future funding and which sources may provide such funding. Foresight from the simulation community in Victoria led to development of a program to create sustainability by developing a user-friendly business-planning module to guide simulation operations and business processes (Victorian Department of Health and Human Resources, 2014).

Most Important Lessons Learned

Through the engagement and commitment of the healthcare simulation community and injection of funding by Government, predominantly through the HWA, Australia is well placed and well regarded for the current state-of-play in this field. With a research agenda to guide further investigation and scholarship in simulation, there is a solid plan for future directions. However, sustainability and quality control of simulation activities continue to be a risk for quality outcomes.

Collaborating with others at local, national, and international levels is key to ensuring that strong evidence about the benefits of simulation is articulated and delivered to governments and businesses who influence funding and resourcing.

Global Perspectives on Simulation: Canada
Nicole Harder

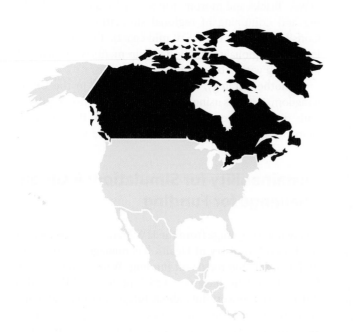

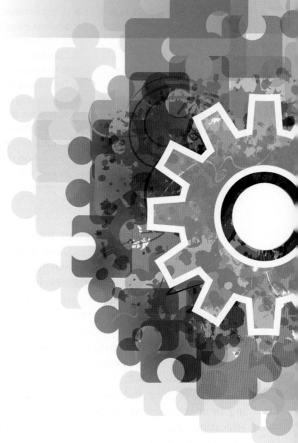

Canada: Profile

The indigenous peoples inhabited Canada before being discovered by Europeans. While the first Viking explorers reached Canada in 1001, no colonies were established, and Canada remained a relatively forgotten land. In 1497, King Henry VII of England sent the Italian explorer Jean Cabot on an expedition that resulted in the discovery of Atlantic Canada. In 1534, Frenchman Jacques Cartier also sailed to Canada and arrived via the St. Lawrence River in current day Québec City, Québec. Even with these

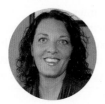

Nicole Harder, PhD, RN

two expeditions resulting in the discovery of Canada, no permanent European settlements were established until the early 17th century. In 1608, the French created settlements in the region now known as the city of Montréal as well as in surrounding areas. The new colony was named New France, and by 1685, the population grew to approximately 10,000.

Diseases from Europe accompanied the new inhabitants of the colonies such as smallpox, to which the indigenous people had no immunity. During that period, the English were also interested in the new colony with explorers Henry Hudson arriving in Canada in 1610 and Thomas James in 1631. Rivalries mounted between the English and French over control of the new colony and several disputes erupted resulting in the control of Montréal changing hands between the two nations. Tensions between the English and the French escalated during the War of the Spanish Succession (1701–1713) and the Seven Years War (1756–1763), which ultimately led to the English capture of Québec and resulting Treaty of Paris. This Treaty required the French to surrender all their territories to the British, including New France (Canada).

English rule in Canada continued into the 19th century. In 1791, many Canadians, both French and English were dissatisfied with their governments and elected a legislature. The legislature, however, was not a true democracy in that the King had executive powers and appointed council. These circumstances led to a rebellion of French Canadians in 1837, as well as an uprising in Upper Canada (Toronto). The rebellion was crushed, but during the uprising the Toronto Mayor, William Lyon Mackenzie was slain. Years later, Canada became a real democracy in 1867 with the signing of the *Constitution Act*. Today, Canada is both a parliamentary democracy and constitutional monarchy as one of 53 members of the Commonwealth with The Queen of England as Sovereign.

Healthcare in Canada

The establishment of the current healthcare system in Canada has evolved significantly since the *Constitution Act* in 1867. Under the *Constitution Act*, the provinces were responsible for establishing, maintaining, and managing hospitals, asylums, charities, and charitable institutions, and the federal government was given jurisdiction over marine hospitals and quarantine. Before the *Medical Care Act* in 1966, healthcare services were, for the most part, privately delivered and funded. Between 1947 and 1966, the provinces created universal healthcare plans that provided publically funded inpatient hospital services. In addition to these programmes, the Federal *Hospital Insurance and Diagnostic Services Act* in 1957 provided for publicly administered universal coverage for a particular set of services under uniform terms and conditions. The advent of the Act of 1957 created the foundation for the new *Medical Care Act* to follow. Saskatchewan introduced a universal, provincial medical insurance plan to provide doctors' services to all its residents in 1962. The federal government passed the *Medical Care Act* in 1966, which offered to reimburse, or cost share, one-half of provincial and territorial costs for medical services provided by a doctor outside hospitals. Within 6 years, all the provinces and territories had universal physician services insurance plans.

Since then, funding formulae and fiscal arrangements have changed, as did the needs and priorities of the provinces. In 1984, the *Canada Health Act* was passed. This legislation replaced the Federal hospital and medical insurance acts and consolidated their principles by establishing criteria on portability, accessibility, universality, comprehensiveness, and public administration. Since then, several reforms have occurred that have seen changes in services provided and cash transfers from the federal government to the provinces. Ultimately, however, Canada still has a publically funded healthcare system that provides and funds the large majority of all healthcare services for Canadians (Health Canada).

Nursing Education in Canada

In the early years, nursing education offered inexpensive programmes for the well-disciplined labour force. Little education or training took place at the time, and the emphasis was on domestic skills development. In 1874, physician Dr. Theophilus Mack opened Canada's first nursing school in St. Catharines, Ontario. Two nurses trained in the Nightingale system were brought in to set up the training programme. Subsequently, several other nursing schools in eastern Canada were established. By the end of 1902, there were 70 nursing training programmes right across the country.

In the early years of nursing education, training programmes were either 2 or 3 years in length and were located in the hospital setting. For the most part, physicians determined the clinical practice of the nurse and hospital administrators led educational programmes. Back in the day, attempts to improve nursing education standards frequently involved didactic lectures provided by physicians at the end of very long clinical days. These were not always well attended. Meanwhile, there was growing dissatisfaction from nursing educators who were advocating for a change in the structure of nursing education. By 1908, 16 organized nursing bodies from across Canada met in Ottawa to form the Canadian National Association of Trained Nurses (CNATN). By 1924, the CNATN membership grew to include nine provincial associations from across Canada, changing its name to the Canadian Nurses Association (CNA, 2016).

In the late 1920s, the Canadian Medical Association in collaboration with the CNA commissioned a report to address all aspects of nursing and nursing education. The Weir Report, released in 1932, recommended the removal of nursing programmes from hospital control and the closure of smaller programmes. The report also suggested that education in a university setting was an essential part of the professional progress of nursing. By 1920, only five Canadian universities had begun to provide nursing education. In earnest, administering of nursing programmes did not transfer to educational institutions until 30 years later in the 50s. While training schools still existed, the shift to educational institutions was the beginning of a movement that would eventually see all nursing education programmes moved out of hospitals and into colleges and universities (Kirkwood, 2005).

Currently, all nursing education in Canada is at the baccalaureate level except in the province of Québec—a predominantly French-speaking province. In the Québec nursing education system, students can either complete a 3-year diploma in nursing programme at a CEGEP (*Collège d'enseignement général et professionel*), and in most cases after completing at least 1 year in a college setting, students can continue their education by transferring to a university baccalaureate nursing programme. Universities and colleges are largely public institutions, with only one nursing baccalaureate programme being offered at a private university. Upon completion of a nursing programme, all new graduates are required to write and pass an examination. From 1970 to 2014, the exam was developed by and in partnership with the Canadian Nurses Association. In 2015, the provincial jurisdictions determined that the National Council Licensure Examination (NCLEX) developed by the National Council of the State Boards of Nursing in the United States would be the new entrance exam for Canadian students. This exam includes input from Canadian content experts. In Québec, students write a different French language examination developed by nurses and nurse educators from the province of Québec.

Simulation in Canada

Geographically speaking, Canada is a vast country. Despite its size, most of the education and healthcare institutions across the country offer very similar experiences. Health and education are publically funded entities, where collaboration and sharing of resources are encouraged. Developing a simulation centre can be a costly endeavour, and many academic institutions with links to hospitals share both their physical and human resources. While sharing is evident in some regions, there is a growing interest and subsequent recognition of the growing need for more high-fidelity simulation centres. Moreover, the early centres tended to focus on simulation with specialty groups, and as time passed and simulation adoption increased, it became evident that additional simulation facilities were required.

Simulation as a teaching methodology and training tool is not new to nursing in Canada. Since the 1950s, using low-fidelity simulators (task trainers) to teach clinical and psychomotor skills has been commonplace. What has changed since then is the availability and capabilities of technology. Moreover, after the 1970s, the technical skills required of nurses increasingly grew in number and complexity. With a greater reliance on technology in both learning and healthcare, the skill set of nurses required them to expand the growing repertoire of psychomotor skills. Concurrently, newer mannequins and task trainers emerged (Bradley, 2006). As technology evolved, nurse educators increasingly adopted simulation-based learning as it allowed students needed immersive practice and application of nursing skills in context.

Additionally, during the 1970s, nursing and medicine placed more emphasis and value on technology and critical care skills associated with technology (Toman, 2005). A key factor when discussing simulation is the importance that nursing placed on acquiring more advanced skills during this decade. Transfer or delegation of functions and skills from medicine to nursing was becoming more common (Toman, 2005). There was also a perceived sense of personal

importance in advanced skill acquisition, and the use of simulations and adjunct technologies was emerging as useful learning tools to achieve this. So while accessibility to simulation technology remained an issue, technical advances and interest in simulation teaching and learning approaches grew. While some individuals explored the use of high-fidelity simulators, it was not until the technology became more readily available in the late 1990s and 2000s that any large-scale adoption of high-fidelity simulation (also known as Simulated Clinical Immersion or Full Mission Simulation) became an integral part of health professions education.

Simulation in the Hospital and Education Setting

The Sunnybrook Canadian Simulation Centre in Toronto, Ontario, was the first large-scale simulation centre in Canada when it opened in 1994, followed in 1995 by the Telus Telehealth and Simulation Center at the Royal Alexandra Hospital in Edmonton, Alberta. The Sunnybrook Centre initially included high-fidelity simulations for undergraduate medical education having since become a multidisciplinary simulation centre. Between that time and the early 2000s, many nursing and medicine programmes introduced high-fidelity simulation in their schools. In the mid-2000s, the Ministry of Health and Long-Term Care of Ontario made funds available to all nursing programmes in the province to establish a simulation centre. Most nursing schools took advantage of this funding. Ontario is the only province to date to allocate specific dollars for all nursing programmes to purchase simulation equipment. Currently, Canada does not have an updated comprehensive directory of simulation centres. However, the SSH directory currently lists 21 centres in Canada (http://www.ssih.org/Home/SIM-Center-Directory). A Canadian Patient Safety Institute simulation special interest group cites the early key players in simulation development in Canada as "deans and leaders of Canada's academic health science centres, community colleges, professional colleges (in particular the Royal College of Physicians and Surgeons, College of Family Physicians of Canada), certifying & regulating bodies, and others" (CPSI, 2008).

Since the mid- to late-2000s, a large majority nursing programmes across Canada have an established simulation presence in their schools and faculties of nursing. With the exception of Ontario, most of these centres have been funded through a combination of University or College dollars, supplemented by grants and private or corporate donations. In addition to creating simulation centres, there has been a growing recognition of the need for developing simulation human resource specialties, such as professorships and fellowships engaged in research in the area of simulation and nursing education, and certified simulation educators and technical operators. Investments in both the technology and human resource aspects of simulation have led to furthering the understanding of the uses of simulation in healthcare education.

Large- to small-scale simulation centres offering educational and accreditation programmes have emerged across all health disciplines in Canada. In Vancouver for example, the Centre of Excellence for Simulation Education and Innovation (CESEI) offers a multidisciplinary and interprofessional facility for education and training based out of the University of British Columbia (UBC) and Vancouver Costal Health Authority (VCH) (Qayumi, 2010).

With the expanding growth of simulation centres and programmes, organizations and groups have also emerged to support simulation. Many provinces have organizations that support simulation in their respective regions. In large part, these are interdisciplinary groups that include medicine, nursing, and other allied healthcare team members. Examples of these include the following:

- British Columbia and Alberta Lab Educators Group (http://www.bcit.ca/health/labedconference/)
- Canadian Association for Schools of Nursing (CASN): Simulation Interest Group (http://www.casn.ca/professional-development/nurse-educator-interest-groups/)
- Canadian Network for Simulation in Healthcare (CNSH) (http://www.cnsh.ca/)
- eSim Alberta Health Services (http://www.albertahealthservices.ca/info/esim.aspx)
- Ontario Sim Alliance (OSA) (http://ontariosimalliance.ca/)
- Saskatoon Institute for Medical Simulation (SIMS) (http://www.sasksims.ca/)
- SIM-one—Simulation Network (http://www.sim-one.ca/)
- The Royal College of Physicians and Surgeons of Canada, Simulation Accreditation through the Centre of Excellence for Simulation Education and Innovation (CESEI) (https://www.cesei.org/simulators.php) and
- The Interdisciplinary Healthcare Education Partnership (IHEP) in Edmonton, Alberta (Fig. 15C.1) (https://sites.google.com/site/ihepsavestan/aboutIHEP)

With several academic and healthcare institutions across the country housing large and fully equipped simulation centres, there is no lack of opportunity to provide simulation-based experiences to both students and experienced healthcare providers alike. In 2008, the Canadian Patient Safety Institute (CPSI, 2008) examined the need for a Pan-Canadian body and strategy to lead Canada's Simulation efforts. Following the 2008 report, the *Canadian Network for Simulation in Healthcare* (CNSH, 2012) was formed but has yet to gain traction and a large national presence. In January of 2017, Sim-ONE and CNSH announced their intent to amalgamate and establish a new Pan-Canadian interprofessional healthcare entity for simulation in Canada. Meanwhile, Canadian nurses and fellow

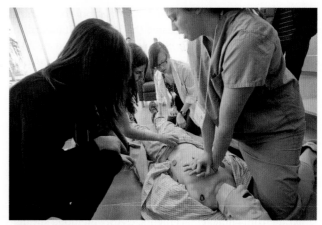

Figure 15C.1 HELP Save Stan Saturday, IHEP 2014 Flash Sim. Used with permission.

healthcare providers continue to be substantive contributors to other major international simulation associations.

Simulation Regulation and Practice Guidelines

In most provinces, the inclusion of simulation in nursing education programmes has been poorly identified. When it comes to recognizing simulation-based learning experiences as a replacement for traditional clinical practice hours, most regulatory bodies across the country are either silent on the issue or explicitly deny this option to nursing programmes. In Canada, it is the provincial regulatory bodies that approve nursing curricula. As such, they yield a significant amount of power regarding the use of simulation in nursing education. The release of the American study by the National Council of State Boards of Nursing on the use of simulation in nursing education (Hayden et al., 2014) created additional evidence for the inclusion of simulation-based experiences in clinical courses. In 2014, the College of Registered Nurses of Manitoba and the nursing programmes/schools of Manitoba formed a provincial working group to address how and where to include and count simulation-based experiences. Subsequently, Manitoba became the first province to recognize simulation-based experiences as valid replacement for clinical time within a clinical course offering. They also underscored that at least 25% of clinical courses include simulation-based experiences. Evaluation of this new clinical model is ongoing. Most recently in 2016, the Nursing Education Program Approval Board (NEPAB) in Alberta set out criteria for the replacement of traditional clinical hours with simulation-based learning, provided that programs demonstrate adherence to evidence-based best practices in simulation education, while continuing to provide quality practical experiences in traditional settings.

In 2011, the International Association for Clinical Simulation and Learning created the INACSL Standards of Best Practice: Simulation^SM updated in 2013 2015, and again in 2016 to reflect the evolution of simulation. Several Canadian nursing programmes use the standards to assist in developing their simulation programmes; however, with provincially based nursing programmes, this is largely accomplished on an individual programme basis. In 2015, the Canadian Association for Schools of Nursing (CASN) released a document titled "Practice Domain for Baccalaureate Nursing Education: Guidelines for Clinical Placements and Simulation." Rather than treat simulation separate from clinical placements, CASN included simulation as a practice environment and created guidelines that encompassed all areas of clinical practice (http://www.casn.ca/wp-content/uploads/2015/11/Draft-clinical-sim-2015.pdf).

Challenges Integrating Simulation

Simulation has evolved significantly since the early beginnings. Currently, in the world, there are over 50 simulation centres that are accredited by the Society for Simulation in Healthcare (SSH, 2016b) (http://www.ssih.org/Certification), more than 1,000 individuals from over 26 countries who are Certified Healthcare Simulation Educators (CHSE, and CHSE-A [advanced]), with many more qualified as Certified Healthcare Simulation Operations Specialists (CHSOS). Given the geography of Canadian, it was initially challenging to share resources and ideas, however as new centres emerged, they also created local networks and sharing platforms. A spirit of open sharing characterized simulation development and expansion across Canada, providing support for emerging centres to optimize their equipment and resources.

Canada faces similar challenges as others surrounding funding and using clinical time for simulation. Funding for equipment and human resources continue to be an issue for academic institutions, and funding, in general, has been cut in recent years. Programmes in remote areas such as Nunavut, the North West, and Yukon Territories may find it difficult to procure and maintain their simulation equipment, as well as to attract and retain qualified and competent educators and staff for simulation-based activities. Rural and remote nursing programmes also have smaller numbers of students making simulation expensive and unaffordable for some institutions.

Funding for research in nursing education, let alone for simulation in nursing education, has been difficult to secure. National agencies typically fund larger multisite, multidiscipline studies, making it difficult for smaller centres or new researchers to obtain funding. This reality is not exclusively characteristic of simulation research funding.

However, it seems to be more of a challenge to obtain funding than it is with recognized priority research areas.

In regard to allocating simulation-based activities as clinical time, there needs to be continued dialogue between the academic institutions and the regulatory bodies as well as a recognition of the conditions under which simulation can legitimately and effectively replace learning in traditional clinical settings. In doing so, we also need to leverage our common goals to promote patient safety, system change in healthcare, and interprofessional learning by keeping this at the forefront of the discussions. Using the Manitoba example, it is more likely to have positive outcomes that benefit the learner, achieve the regulatory body requirements, and improve patient safety.

Understanding how to teach in simulation-based experiences continues to be both a national and international issue. Most educators were not educated using this pedagogical approach and therefore lack knowledge and skill in teaching using simulation. For some, this reality can contribute to an aversion or fear of using simulation. There are core concepts that are based on philosophical and theoretical underpinnings for teaching with simulation, and these need to be understood by the facilitator before they engage in facilitating simulation-based experiences. Preparation, facilitation, and debriefing each includes various strategies that assist in maximizing learning in simulation. Those involved in simulation should be educated or trained in these techniques before engaging in simulation. There are local, national, and international workshops that can assist new facilitators in developing these skills. With many opportunities for ongoing development, there is no need to a simulation facilitator to be ill prepared to teach in simulation.

Canada has two official languages, French and English. Given this, there are additional issues when collaborating nationally on simulation projects. Many scenarios or guidelines have been initially created in the English language, thereby requiring translation if they are to be used across the nation. The province of Québec has subsequently developed a local simulation network that allows nursing programmes to share scenarios and resources in the French language. Additionally, healthcare education programs such as l'Université de Montréal, McMaster University, and McGill University in Québec have well-established simulation centres and programs. Outside of Québec, other Francophone nursing programmes collaborate with schools and faculties of nursing in Québec. However, ongoing collaboration is required to create a national agenda.

Moving Forward

Simulation in Canada is a strategy and pedagogy that is now firmly rooted in most nursing education programmes. Programmes in remote areas are no longer excluded simply due to geography, and many have established partnerships with other larger academic institutions. We need to further such partnerships to allow for simulation-based experiences in the remote regions of Canada. With access to the Internet and video, geography can be removed as a barrier.

In general, the simulation community is one that openly shares. This is a past trend that needs to continue if we are to achieve best educational outcomes for all. Creating scenarios, for example, is often one of the first things that new simulationists embark upon, however, is the piece that is often the easiest to share. Creating and affiliating with networks to share scenarios, learning objectives and simulation strategies must continue on regional, national, and global fronts. Additionally, Canada must work to strengthen a National research agenda that includes multidisciplinary research groups. With limited funding opportunities for research in simulation, working in larger groups that include both seasoned and new researchers could allow for a more efficient use of resources, as well as provide valuable research experience for the novice researcher.

Ultimately, there needs to be a recognition at all levels of nursing education that simulation is an established tool and pedagogy with benefits to learners and patients alike. Just as the discipline of nursing values evidence-based practice, it also values evidence-based nursing education. The evidence strongly points to simulation-based experiences being able to promote critical thinking, clinical judgement, and prioritization skills. The evidence also suggests that our current models of clinical practice do not achieve what educators intend (Harder, 2015; Hayden et al., 2014).

My hope for the future of nursing education is that the use of simulation continues to expand in all areas of curricula (clinical, theory, and lab) and that simulation becomes a core teaching and learning strategy for all areas of nursing practice.

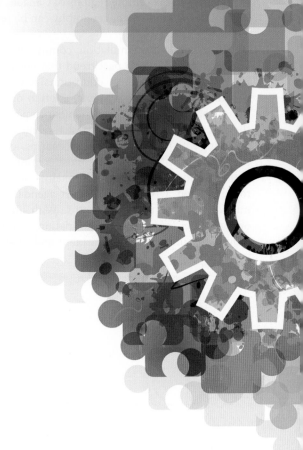

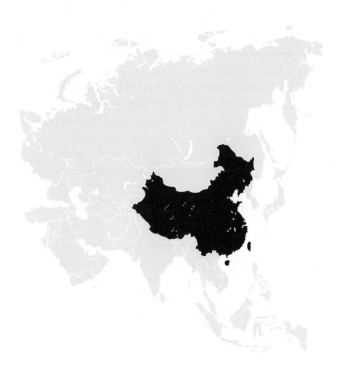

China: Profile

Dating back nearly 4,000 years, China is one of the oldest civilizations in the world. It has a complex history, with evidence of written script carved on bones and bronze as early as the Shang Dynasty in 1600 BCE (Asia for Educators, 2013). To understand the evolution of healthcare and healthcare education in China, one must

first consider the impact of Chinese cultural beliefs, philosophy, and social structure in a historical context (Goldschmidt, 2009).

For centuries, China flourished during the era of dynastic rule. Most scholars consider the Qing (Ch'ing) Dynasty (1644–1912) the beginning of Chinese modern history. China's status began to change during the long period of peace in the 17th century, when its population doubled from about 150 million to over 300 million. By the middle of the 19th century, the Chinese population reached 450 million. The inability to cope with rapid growth gave rise to inefficiency and bureaucracy, which was further amplified by rampant opium addiction (http://afe.easia.columbia.edu/).

In 1839, China's attempt to ban the British sale of opium in the port city of Canton gave rise to the Opium Wars. The country suffered a number of military defeats and was forced to relinquish territorial control to Western powers. By the late 19th century, China was beset by war

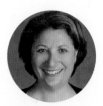

Susan A. Schory,
MEd, BSN, RNC-OB

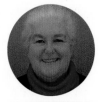

Marcia A. Petrini,
PhD, FAAN

debts and exploitation by foreign governments (https:// www.cia.gov/library/publications/the-world-factbook/ geos/ch.html). During this time, there was a decentralization of government, and military splinter groups and rebelling farmers gained power at the local level. Between 1876 and 1879, famine and drought reduced food production, and starvation claimed an estimated 9.5 million lives.

The National People's Party assumed control in the wake of the collapse of the Qing Dynasty in 1911. The Chinese Communist Party (CCP) was formed in opposition to the Nationalist Party; the CCP's leader, Mao Zedong, promoted Marxist ideals and rural revolution.

The already divided nation became engulfed in World War II when China was invaded by Japan in 1937. The Chinese people were subject to torture, murder, and destruction of their homes and cities at the hands of the Japanese invaders. Following the defeat of Japan and the liberation of China by the allies, the conflict between Chinese Nationalists and the Communist Party resumed, eventually leading to the defeat of the Nationalist Party. In 1949, communist leader Mao Zedong established the People's Republic of China (PRC).

Mao ruled under an autocratic socialist system. Though his leadership ensured sovereignty, he also exercised harsh restrictions on the daily lives of the Chinese (https://www.cia.gov/library/publications/the-world-factbook/geos/ch.html). Workers were relegated to "work units" where the boss of each unit had unlimited influence over the daily lives of those who lived and worked in the community. The party monitored the movement and behavior of individual citizens, and the consequences for disobedience served as an effective deterrent to many who might otherwise seek autonomy or independence (Spence, 2001). In 1959, Mao Zedong created a plan known as the "Great Leap Forward" to rapidly increase the country's agriculture production and industrialization. The plan had disastrous consequences and ended in hardship and famine, resulting in 20 million deaths (Spence, 2001).

During the Cultural Revolution, between 1966 and Mao's death in 1976, education was seen as a threat and many schools and universities closed. Intellectuals were persecuted and beaten, and many lost their lives. It is estimated that more than 1.5 million people were killed during this 10-year period, and many more were tortured, imprisoned, and had their property seized. By the end of this period, China's education system, public works, and healthcare were in shambles (Spence, 2001).

Following Mao's death, the economic system began to move to a more market-oriented model and slowly opened to the outside world. Foreign trade and investments followed, and there was rapid growth of the Chinese economy. Education and social infrastructure also began to change. Universities were reopened, national exams were instituted, and intellectuals returned to academia (Chow, 2004).

China Today

The People's Republic of China is the most populous country in the world and the fourth largest nation in area, after Russia, Canada and the United States. It is composed of twenty-two provinces, five autonomous regions including Tibet, four self-governing cities, and three special zones. Ninety-two percent of China's over 1.3 billion people are of Han descent, and the Chinese government recognizes more than 50 ethnic groups, many of who live as they did centuries ago. The average life expectancy for women is 73.7 years and for men 70.4 years, and the official language is Mandarin, though Cantonese is widely spoken in the South and each province has many local dialects (Central Intelligence Agency [CIA], 2015).

In the past 25 years, China has made tremendous strides in the decline of extreme poverty. Between 1981 and 2005, the national level of those living on less than $1.25 a day declined from a high of 84% to a low of 16%. By 2011, that percentage had dropped to 6.1%. It is important to note, however, that China has changed its poverty line to RMB 2,300 per year, which is approximately US $400 per year (US 1.03 per day) and is below the poverty line designated by the World Bank. China's explosive growth has also resulted in a significant gap in income. While the elite in Chinese society continue to enjoy greater consumer choices and an open market economy, 98 million Chinese still live on less than 2,300 RMB per year, and the nation is second only to India in the number of those considered "poor" (http://www.worldbank.org/).

The country's ruling party is the Communist Party of China (CPC) led by a president who is also the general secretary of the CPC. The leadership is considered authoritarian; and stringent restrictions on things such as Internet use and mobility continue to be enforced. The current administration has, however, proposed sweeping positive reforms including the relaxation of China's one-child law, the closing of labor (reeducation) camps, and comprehensive restructure of the healthcare system. China is currently the second largest economy in the world.

Healthcare in China

According to the World Health Organization (WHO), China's total health expenditure in 2010 was 199.80 billion RMB (about US $29.51 billion). It accounted for 5.1% of GDP, lower than the average for all middle-income countries (6.6%). Per capita health expenditure is 1,490 RMB (about US $220). As of 2011, China had nearly 900,000 healthcare facilities. It currently has a three-tiered medical system with services provided at the national, provincial, and county level. Healthcare coverage is a combination of self-pay, government and employer-subsidized insurance, and private insurance. The WHO reports that there are approximately 3.8 hospital beds per thousand people; however, this number is lower in rural areas (http://www.wpro.who.int/china/mediacentre/factsheets/health_sector_reform/en/).

History of Nursing, Medical Education, and Simulation in China

The earliest written record of Chinese medicine dates back to about 5,000 years. The 18 volumes of *Huangdi Neijing* are said to contain conversations between Huangdi (the Yellow Emperor) and his physician Qibo. The manuscript's 162 chapters are thought to comprise the oldest medical text in the world.

Physicians in ancient China were trained in traditional Chinese medicine (TCM) by serving as apprentices. Formal medical education was established between 420 and 589 AD with medical schools training physicians chiefly to provide care for the Imperial family (Lam, Wan, & Sau-Man, 2006). Nonphysician "scholar-officials" (Goldschmidt, 2009, p. 45) led the way in promoting medical and public health policies during the Song Dynasty (960–1279).

The origin of healthcare simulation in China also dates back to the Song dynasty. In 1026, the famous acupuncturist Wang Weiyi wrote the block printed book *Illustrated Manual on the Points for Acupuncture and Moxibustion on a New Bronze Figure*. A year later, in 1027, two bronze figures designed by Wang Weiyi were manufactured, with the internal organs set inside and the meridians and points engraved on the surface for visual teaching and examination. The acupuncture model (Fig. 15D.1) is, in fact, the world's first known medical simulator (Goldschmidt, 2009).

American and European missionaries introduced Western medicine to China in the early 19th century. According to Schwarz, Wojtczak, and Zhou, (2004), "Western science–based medical education" (p. 215) began to become the norm early in the 20th century and relied on collaboration with Western benefactors and medical schools. Chinese medical education in the 20th and 21st century has been heavily influenced by politics and is generally viewed in terms of its state before, during, and after the Cultural Revolution (Wu et al., 2014).

In the 1950s and 1960s, 80% of China's half a billion citizens lived in rural areas. The principle method of dispensing healthcare in the countryside was through work camp or village health teams who lived in the communities they served. The members of the health teams had 3 to 6 months' medical training and provided education on sanitation and prevention and were able to deliver basic treatment—mostly with traditional medicine. The term "Barefoot Doctors" emerged in the 1970s during the Cultural Revolution and described the young health workers who walked through the rice paddies without shoes to deliver care to farmers and peasants (Wei, 2013). The growth in the number of community-based barefoot

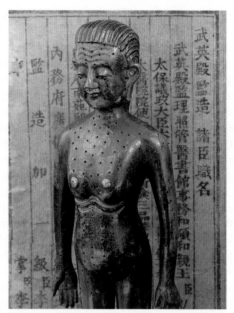

Figure 15D.1 Bronze Simulator Used for Acupuncture and Moxibustion Training. (Credit: Science Museum, London. Wellcome Images. Image retrieved from https://commons.wikimedia.org/wiki/File:Bronze_acupuncture_figure,in_silk_covered_box_bearing_text_Wellcome_L0057614.jpg. Copyrighted work available under Creative Commons Attribution only licence CC BY 4.0 http://creativecommons.org/licenses/by/4.0/)

doctors came at a time when formal medical and nursing education had essentially ceased (Wu et al., 2014).

When Universities began to reopen in the early 1970s, the emphasis was on producing as many physicians and nurses as possible, with minimum investment in education. Vocational and practical training were stressed, rather than scientific problem-based teaching and learning (Lam et al., 2006). The vocational nurse-training framework established in the 1950s resumed (Eddins, Hu, & Liu, 2011). Medical school curricula prior to 1980 consisted of just 3 years post-ninth grade education, and graduates, while trained in primary healthcare, lacked instruction in basic medical sciences and research (Lam et al., 2006, p. 942).

As discussed earlier, Traditional Chinese Medicine (TCM) has also played a role in shaping attitudes toward medical education. It is rooted in the ancient philosophy of Taoism and dates back more than 2,500 years. The goal of TCM is to restore harmony (Carteret, 2011) and is based on the supposition that good health is maintained only when man maintains good relationship with heaven and earth, balancing Yin and Yang.

Though western medicine has become dominant in physician training, the integration of western and TCM is again gaining favor. Medical and nursing students whose background and frame are grounded in traditional medicine are now exposed to both Western and traditional medical education programs, and some of those programs have begun to include simulation as a learning modality. The work of Li et al. highlights simulation as an activity that is patient centered and emphasizes problem-solving, communication, and "summing up" (2012, p. 3). In their study on the application of simulation teaching methods in Chinese (Traditional) Medicine, Li concluded that, "In clinical teaching of Chinese medicine, simulation teaching methods are significantly better than conventional ones, and worth spreading" (p. 1).

Prevalence of Simulation

Currently, China has three the Society for Simulation in Healthcare (SSH) accredited simulation centers: two in Hong Kong, and one at the Peking University People's Hospital Clinical Skill Simulation Training Center. These centers are leading the way in meaningful use of simulation as a learning modality. Simulation-based learning is increasing throughout the mainland; however, its utilization is inconsistent and rarely interdisciplinary. While there are most certainly many academic centers and medical facilities that have purchased simulators, most appear to lack coordinated efforts to provide formal simulation training for faculty and educators.

Barriers and Challenges Encountered in the Integration of Simulation

The description and interpretation of simulation in Chinese medical education lacks consistency. The term simulation is often used to describe skills training; there is scant published English-language literature describing simulation as a learning tool to improve communication or patient safety. Wang, Liu, and Wang discuss the advantages of using Simulated/Standardized Patient to provide "a standardized experience for all students in a safe environment" (2012, p. 83); however, the authors seem to place a significant amount of weight on improving "scores" and mastery (p. 83) and do not discuss debriefing.

Further development and expansion of simulation as a teaching/learning modality has been limited in some cases by economic capacity, but more significantly by social and cultural beliefs. One of the most significant barriers is the slow reform and transformation of China's philosophy and approach to education (Shen & Liu, 2011). Traditional Chinese culture has always been, and remains, hierarchal and patriarchal. The measured acceptance of simulation as an integrated, interdisciplinary teaching modality reflects the cultural roots of education in China dating back to Confucius. Confucianism emphasized proper conduct and submission to authority. Even today, this notion dictates the relationship between teacher and student.

Customary education methods in China are passive, are theoretically based, and encourage rote learning rather than creativity and critical thinking. Most medical and nursing education programs continue to follow a didactic, teacher-centric model with students as passive rather than active learners. The focus in the classroom is on the concrete, with examinations as the primary motivator for learning. This teaching/learning style also has a practical application; information and basic skills can be communicated to a large number of students in an orderly and digestible fashion (Zhenhui, 2001). The cultural emphasis on harmony and balance, community before individual, and respect for position validates this educational structure. According to Kennedy, Chinese students may be uncomfortable working in groups and are hesitant to challenge and critique their peers (2002). This paradigm is also reflected in the clinical setting.

In the healthcare work environment, the nurse is passive and subservient to the physician. This perspective is exemplified by the Chinese saying "The doctor's mouth directs the nurse's legs" (Eddins et al., 2011, p. 30). In China, nursing is considered a lower-status profession despite increasing numbers of highly educated nurses entering the workforce (Zhou, 2014). The role of the registered nurse in many Asian nations is simply to carry out the physician orders. In his observations on transcultural nursing, Yu Xu points out the difference between the "doer" versus the "critical thinker plus doer" (Xu, 2006, p. 422). In the United States and other Western nations, clinical reasoning and collaborative decision making are fundamental elements of quality and safety in the clinical setting. As professionals, Western educated nurses are expected to assess the patient, make clinical recommendations to providers, advocate for patients and families, and provide comprehensive, expert care. There is a tangible accountability, and the entire care team shares the responsibility for outcomes. The Chinese nurse's role is very different. While many nurses in Asia have extensive education and advanced degrees, they may be limited to tasks rather than caregiving. The transition to independent thinking and problem solving is a slow one (Xu, 2006).

The concept of "face" is also a significant driver of behavior where status in the eyes of others is essential in maintaining dignity (Chin, 2005). This societal norm has the effect of suppressing an individual's confidence, creativity, and risk taking in the professional realm (Lam et al., 2006). This norm, in some cases, conflicts with some of the most basic constructs of simulation-based learning: teamwork, interdisciplinary communication, and flattening the hierarchy. While these cultural differences pose a formidable challenge, simulation-based learning in nursing and medical education particularly in an interdisciplinary setting presents the ideal opportunity to impact quality of care, patient safety, and change while placing value on Chinese cultural frames.

Employment Location and Setting: Wuhan University and the HOPE School of Nursing (WUHSON)

Wuhan, China, is the capital of the Hubei province and a city of more than 10 million people. It is located between Shanghai and Chengdu and is the most populous city in the province. Wuhan is comprised of three cities: Wuchang, Hanyang, and Hankou, combined in 1927. The city is more than 3,500 years old and has survived multiple wars and occupations. During the Second World War, Wuhan became the headquarters for the Japanese forces. It is bisected by the Yangtze and Han Rivers and is the transportation hub of central China.

Wuhan University (Fig. 15D.2) traces its history back to the late Qing Dynasty. It was founded in 1893 and has undergone multiple mergers and name changes. The University is ranked as one of the top 10 universities in China and offers baccalaureate, masters, and doctorate programs. It currently serves approximately 55,000 residential and commuter students (http://en.whu.edu.cn/).

The founding of the HOPE School of Nursing was China's first international academic nursing collaboration. In 1983, the Hubei Medical College introduced an evening undergraduate nursing program. It enrolled its first class of full-time diploma students in 1986 and in 1988 became the education and training center of nursing in the Hubei province. A 5-year full-time nursing undergraduate program followed in 1993. Wuhan University and Hubei Medical College combined in 2000, and in 2002, and the partnership between the US-based nongovernmental organization

(NGO), Project HOPE (Health Opportunities for People Everywhere), and Wuhan University resulted in the formation of the Wuhan University HOPE School of Nursing (WUHSON).

In 2003, the school underwent a major curriculum revision and adopted a concept-based Western model of nursing education. Master's and PhD programs began in 2006 and a BSN international program followed in 2010. Since 2007, WUHSON has been awarded three American Schools and Hospitals Abroad (ASHA) and USAID grants totaling 2.7 million USD. The grants were utilized for the development of a long-distance education center, the HOPE School of Nursing Simulation and Research Center, and the HOPE School of Nursing Comprehensive Simulated Rehabilitation Center.

Simulation at Wuhan University Hope School of Nursing

The HOPE Nursing Simulation and Research Center (http://www.hopenursing.cn) was one of the first nursing education simulation labs in China and is considered a model for centers throughout Mainland China. The simulation center includes seven simulation rooms and two practice labs, three conference rooms equipped with live streaming, and a central control room. In addition, the lab has a variety of technologically advanced mannequins (see Fig. 15D.3). The school employs a full-time simulation technologist and two physician simulation coordinators. Graduate assistants also provide simulation support during the school year.

As a leader in simulation-based nursing education in Mainland China, the HOPE School of Nursing is committed to research as well as the growth and integration of its simulation programming. The very first study of the impact of simulation-based learning on Chinese undergraduate nursing students was conducted by Wang et al., at HOPE. The study included 50 sophomore participants in the health assessment course and utilized validated evaluation

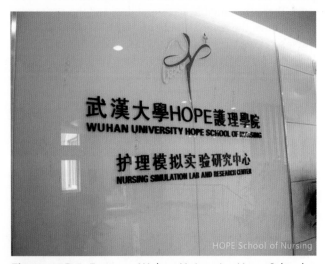

Figure 15D.2 Entrance Wuhan University, Hope School of Nursing, 2015. (Image courtesy of Hope School of Nursing, Wuhan, China, Marcia Petrini, Dean. Image retrieved from http://www.hopenursing.cn/.)

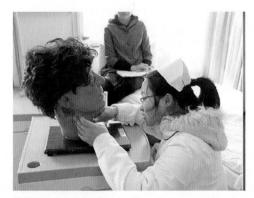

Figure 15D.3 Student Nurse Practicing on Head and Neck Trainer, Wuhan University. (Image courtesy of Hope School of Nursing, Wuhan, China, Marcia Petrini, Dean. Image retrieved from http://www.hopenursing.cn/.)

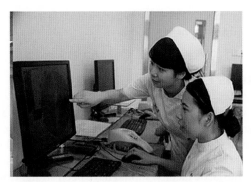

Figure 15D.4 Student Nurses Learning on Virtual IV Trainer, Wuhan University. (Image courtesy of Hope School of Nursing, Wuhan, China, Marcia Petrini, Dean. Image retrieved from http://www.hopenursing.cn/.)

instruments. Students reported overall satisfaction with the simulation learning process and an increase in self-confidence. Clinical supervisors reported that students were more confident when performing physical assessments (Wang, Fitzpatrick, & Petrini, 2013).

Nursing programs throughout China attend simulation conferences hosted by the university. Conferences are facilitated by the coordinators of HOPE's simulation center and provide faculty development workshops in scenario writing, meaningful use of simulators, and debriefing, as well as networking opportunities. Simulation center faculty members have authored over 200 scenarios that are culturally appropriate and in the native language and are specific to clinical situations in Chinese healthcare. Currently, most Chinese simulation centers use only the standard scenarios published by simulation equipment vendors. Publication of the HOPE center cases will provide an extensive library that will be for use by other programs throughout China. In addition, the center has recently applied for National (China) Virtual Simulation Center designation. The HOPE faculty has received grants and funding for projects and research that include the creation of an evaluation system for simulation education, the integration of disaster response virtual simulation into the nursing curriculum, and the utilization of simulation education on the critical care unit (Fig. 15D.4).

Foreign Worker Experiences In China

I have spent the majority of my career in women's and children's health: specifically in obstetrics (OB) as a staff nurse and later a clinical educator (S. Schory, personal communication, 2016). Five years ago, I became a volunteer with Project HOPE. HOPE has a long and respected history as an organization that not only provides disaster and humanitarian relief but also focuses on sustainable programs and education. As an educator, HOPE's emphasis on sustainability and creating partnerships appealed to me. My first experience was an assignment in Cameroon in

the summer of 2011. This was followed by a semester-long teaching appointment at the HOPE School of Nursing in Wuhan, China.

The HOPE administrators reported that while their simulation laboratory was a large, very well resourced space, they recognized a need for improvement in capacity, meaningful use, and further integration of simulation into the curriculum—particularly in obstetrics and women's health. I viewed the opportunity as a wonderful chance to collaborate, learn, and contribute. I was also very eager to experience China from the expatriate perspective.

I arrived in Wuhan in early March and was met at the airport by a graduate student named "Cindy." I was reasonably sure that her given name was not Cindy; her use of an English name was the first example of the efforts made by the students and faculty to meet MY cultural/language needs. After a brief introduction to the facility, several faculty members, and their ("English") names, I had the opportunity to observe several simulations as well as debriefing sessions.

In my initial observations, I was very impressed with the organization and operation of the simulation center. Clinical instructors were responsible for designing scenarios, facilitating, and debriefing cases with support from the simulation staff. Students were oriented prior to each simulation and the cases were well organized. I did notice however that scenarios appeared to be task driven, communication among participants was limited, and the students seemed "frantic" in their attempts to problem-solve. Debriefing often resembled a didactic lecture—some instructors used a PowerPoint in the debrief session. While the cases were written, facilitated, and debriefed in Chinese, it was not difficult to comprehend that some of the students were unsure about how to interface with the mannequin and had a difficult time "suspending disbelief." I could see that there were many opportunities for growth.

I met first with the obstetrics team. The OB clinical instructor was committed to providing the students a rich experience despite some limitations in her knowledge of obstetrics. Students attended a preconference lecture given by the clinical instructor the day before each clinical. Prior to the preconference day, we discussed the best way to prepare them for the OB clinical. We both felt that a formal simulation might escalate their anxiety. Instead, we involved a willing graduate student and used Laerdal's "MamaNatalie" birth simulator. Natalie is a pack worn over the abdomen of a volunteer or Simulated/Standardized Patient. The "uterus" in the simulator can be filled with "blood" and "amniotic fluid," and the operator can manually deliver the baby; it is a wonderful tool for flipping the classroom. About 5 minutes into the lecture, the graduate student entered the room appearing very pregnant and complaining that her "water broke." As our actress escalated her discomfort, the students, at first confused, began to engage with the "patient" and assess her condition by asking appropriate questions (in Chinese). We concluded by delivering the baby and debriefing the group following the experience. Students reported that the unexpected, impromptu simulation was "fun," "crazy," "amazing," and a "great learning experience." Most importantly, they were looking forward to future simulation experiences.

We went on to write an unfolding scenario beginning with a preconception counseling appointment and concluding with a postpartum assessment. Instructors served as embedded actors in the vignettes, and students observed via live stream with a reflection tool. A basic plus/delta method of debriefing was utilized, and facilitating the debriefing in Mandarin encouraged participation. The following week, we ran an OB hemorrhage drill simulation (Fig. 15D.5). During the exercise, the students performed professionally and interacted appropriately with the facilitator/simulator and their peers. The simulations continued for each clinical group through the second semester, and we received positive feedback from the participants. In addition, the instructor noted that they appeared more confident in the clinical setting. Many of our students were accustomed to motivation by examination and grades. We worked diligently to stress the learning (formative) value of simulation and to ensure a safe and nonthreatening environment.

Lessons Learned

In my work in China, the charge was to encourage a standardized integration of simulation learning into the school's curriculum, with emphasis on communication and teamwork. This was a goal, which given the school's resources and enthusiastic faculty, should have been straightforward and fairly simple. I did not, however, consider the fact that culture impacts every facet of Chinese life. Cultural beliefs are the very essence of Chinese identity. The students and faculty exemplified this in the way they interacted, the way they taught, and the way they learned. The realities of this identity in nursing practice did not necessarily coalesce with my perspective on how simulation was supposed to "look" and the impact I assumed it would have on collaborative practice.

In her study on Chinese immigrant nurses in Australia, Yunxian Zhou talks about "reconciling different realities" (Zhou, 2014, p. 9). She goes on to explain that nurses growing up in China developed "systems of meaning" (p. 2), which were shared by other Chinese people and reflected societal social norms. Zhou noted that even Chinese nurses who had lived aboard for quite some time found it difficult to understand and embrace the Australian practice model (caregiving, independence, and collaboration) and often felt ambivalence in their decision to emigrate despite better status, pay, and more autonomy (Zhou).

As my experiences in Wuhan unfolded, I became more mindful of the lack of shared experience between us. I learned to listen to what my colleagues and students said they needed, and then meet them where they were so that we might advance together. Using this approach proved to be the most effectual way to begin the process of making incremental but sustainable modifications in the school's approach to simulation. I also had the opportunity to work with several graduate students on their research proposals, one of which will examine senior nursing and medical student satisfaction and learning when collaborative, interdisciplinary simulations are included in the final year curriculum.

Finally, I encouraged faculty to embrace the notion that our work as educators in mentoring future nurses and physicians can be far-reaching and transformative. It is the widespread adoption of a collaborative culture in medical and nursing education that can, in time, impact culture in the clinical environment as well. Not only will the meaningful use of simulation in the prelicensure environment enhance the clinical reasoning and decision-making skills of soon-to-be professionals, it will help create future leaders who can be agents of change.

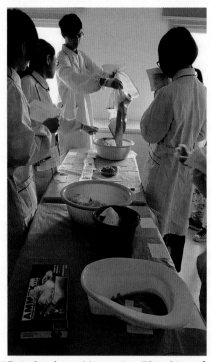

Figure 15D.5 Students Measuring Blood Loss from Postpartum Hemorrhage Scenario, Wuhan University. (Image courtesy of Hope School of Nursing, Wuhan, China, Marcia Petrini, Dean. Image retrieved from http://www.hopenursing.cn/.)

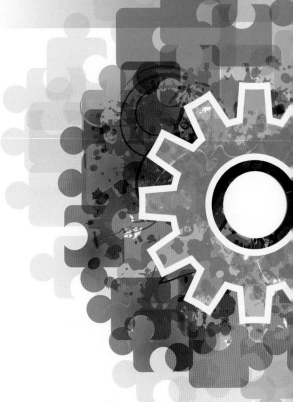

15E | Global Perspectives on Simulation: Europe
Amanda R. Wilford

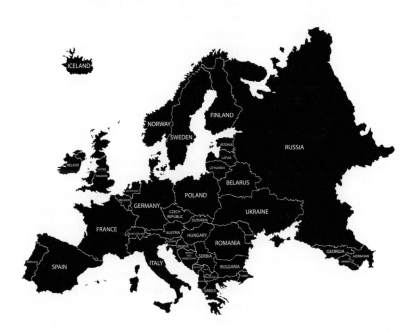

Europe: Profile

Herodotus, the Greek Historian, divided the world into three parts Europe, Asia, and Libya (Africa). More recently in 1730, Philip Johan von Strahlenberg (1676–1747), a Swedish geographer in 1730, classified Europe as countries west of the Ural Mountains to the United Kingdom and Ireland. Today, geographers now generally define Europe as the western part of Eurasia, with its boundaries marked by large bodies of water to the north, west, and south (Hamilton, 2011). Europe today includes 51 independent states. Russia, Kazakhstan, Azerbaijan, Georgia, and Turkey are the five transcontinental countries, partially located in both Europe and Asia. Armenia

and Cyprus politically are considered European countries, though geographically they are situated in the West Asia territory. Europe's largest country is Russia (37% of total continent area), and the smallest one is Vatican City, in Rome, Italy (List of Countries in Europe in Alphabetical Order, n.d.). Within Europe, there are currently 23 officially recognized languages, for example, Russian, Dutch, and Italian, and if regional and minority languages such as Catalan and Maltese are included, this rises to over 60. The most widely spoken languages are English (38%), French (12%), German (11%), Spanish (7%), and Russian (5%), and this vast array of languages are discussed relative to nursing simulation education (EU386, 2012).

What Is the European Union?

In the 20th century, Europe was transformed and changed irrecoverably due to the two World Wars, and this continues to the present day. These changes impacted people on personal, political, cultural, healthcare, education, and socioeconomic levels. One of the major changes that affect many Europeans on a daily basis including healthcare and education is that of the formation of the European Union or EU. The EU was created after the second world war to

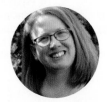

Amanda R. Wilford,
RGN (Hons), Dip ANC, ENB 254, ENB 998

Table 15E.1	The EU Member States with Year of Entry		
Austria (1995)	Estonia (2004)	Italy (1958)	Portugal (1986)
Belgium (1958)	Finland (1995)	Latvia (2004)	Romania (2007)
Bulgaria (2007)	France (1958)	Lithuania (2004)	Slovakia (2004)
Cyprus (2004)	Germany (1958)	Luxembourg (1958)	Slovenia (2004)
Croatia (2013)	Greece (1981)	Malta (2004)	Spain (1986)
Czech Republic (2004)	Hungary (2004)	The Netherlands (1958)	Sweden (1995)
Denmark (1973)	Ireland (1973)	Poland (2004)	United Kingdom (1973)

European Union (2015). Retrieved from http://europa.eu/index_en.htm.

foster economic cooperation: the idea being that countries who trade with one another become economically interdependent and so are more likely to avoid conflict—history will in time determine if this holds true (European Union, 2015).

Initially, the EU consisted of six member states; today, this has raised to 28, the last one joining being Croatia in 2013. Albania, Macedonia, Montenegro, Serbia, and Turkey are on the road to EU membership at present (European Union, 2015). Table 15E.1 charts the entry of EU member states by date. The EU member states are leading the way in the implementation of simulation education, and this will be discussed; many of the non-EU member states are following the changes in healthcare education and are adopting their recommendations as many in the future are seeking to join the union.

Nursing Education in Europe

Nurses and midwives have a unique role in patient care, as they are the only profession who are there 24 hours a day. Nurses act as advocates for patients and their families and are in a privileged position to address their physical, psychological, spiritual, and social needs. In 2000, the World Health Organization (WHO) European Region adopted the Munich Declaration of Nurses and Midwives: A Force for Health often referred to as the "Munich Declaration." This is an international policy focusing on the contribution that nurses and midwives contribute to healthcare and suggests unified financial and policies across the European region as a whole (WHO, 2009). One area of focus from the "Munich Declaration" was a focus on nurses' undergraduate training in Europe. The EU decided to direct its member states to implement the Munich Declaration, and this was a key strategy in the development of simulation in nursing education. The EU wrote a policy that was to ensure that all countries that are in the EU have common elements concerning content and practice. The underpinning philosophy was that nurses could if proficient in the language of another member state could practice as a registered nurse, so, for example, a nurse who trained in Spain if proficient in the Dutch language could practice in the Netherlands and vice versa.

European Union (EU) requirements apply to both nursing and midwifery. The nursing requirement is titled Directive 2005/36/EC (WHO, 2009). These requirements focus on themes such as the length of training, and the type and level of qualification awarded at the end of training to try and provide consistency and ultimately patient safety across the EU. One part of Directive 2005/36/EC focuses on the theoretical and practical knowledge and skills that all undergraduate nurses who are training in the EU are mandated to have, and these are illustrated in Tables 15E.2 and 15E.3 (WHO, 2009).

Furthermore, this directive states that all nurses within the EU undergo training that is at least 3 years in

Table 15E.2	Illustration of the Theoretical Components of Directive 2005/36/EC		
	Nursing	**Basic Sciences**	**Social Sciences**
Theme	• Nature and ethics of the profession • General principles of health and nursing • Nursing principle • General and specialist medicine • General and specialist surgery • Child care and paediatrics • Maternity care • Mental health and psychiatry • Care of the old and geriatrics	• Anatomy and physiology • Pathology • Bacteriology, virology, and parasitology • Biophysics, biochemistry, and radiology • Dietetics • Hygiene: preventive medicine; health education • Pharmacology	• Sociology • Psychology • Principles of administration • Principles of teaching • Social and health legislation • Legal aspects of nursing

World Health Organization (WHO). (2009). *European Union Standards for Nursing and Midwifery* (2nd ed.). Denmark: Author.

Table 15E.3	Illustration of the Clinical Components of Directive 2005/36/EC
Nursing clinical instruction	General and specialist medicine General and specialist surgery Child care and paediatrics Maternity care Mental health and psychiatry Care of the old and geriatrics Home nursing

World Health Organization (WHO). (2009). *European Union Standards for Nursing and Midwifery* (2nd ed.). Denmark: Author.

length or 4,600 hours of a combination of theoretical and clinical training: the split between theory and practice varies according to the country. These EU requirements have assisted the implementation of simulation in nursing across Europe, and these are discussed below. Those countries not in the EU have in part implemented some of these directives as they are seen to be of best practice examples include Kazakhstan and Turkmenistan, who are implementing simulation education for nurses at undergraduate and postgraduate centres by creating national simulation centres and rolling out the concepts across individual countries' regions. The Ministry of Health in Turkmenistan have implemented a policy called "Saglyk," which is to lower morbidity and improve health for the population (Saglyk Info, 2015), and to do this, they have built a seven-story building to train all the professions using surgical, endoscopy, human patient simulators, and standardized patients (Turkmenistan, 2015). Similar schemes are being built in Turkey and Russia with simulation being offered at undergraduate and postgraduate level for nurses for technical and nontechnical skills. These national schemes to improve health are benefitting nursing education at all levels and are one of the key drivers in promoting simulation education across Europe in conjunction with the EU directives.

Simulation Nursing Education in Europe

The challenges facing nurse education across Europe in the 21st century are numerous. Nursing education across all of Europe at the registered nurse level is university based; 50 years ago, many were in nursing school attached to hospitals (WHO, 2009). Universities offering nursing and midwifery are facing increased intakes, decreased clinical placements, and a shortage of patient availability. Student nurses and midwives are competing with other learners in the workplace, for example, medical students and physiotherapists, to gain the essential knowledge and skills to become a registered practitioner (Wilford & Doyle, 2009). This is not a European phenomenon and is happening in Asia Pacific, the Middle East, and the Americas. With the increased use of technology and advances in drugs and medical care, patients are in the hospital for shorter stays. Thus, there are more students trying to access fewer patients and struggle to meet EU requirements. For example, in maternity, mental health, and critical care, student nurses may not gain as much "hands-on" time and may not see many aspects depending on the type of patients available when they are in practice (Aiken et al., 2014). Although the EU directive states that there should be 4,600 hours, the practice hours are not defined per se; Sweden, United Kingdom (UK), offer a 50/50 split with 2,300 hours of each, respectively; Italy and Germany are offering 1,600 theory and 3,000 hours practically, so there is variation in the EU. The amount of exposure to real patients in nursing programmes is difficult to assess as it depends on patient availability and the extent to which students spend time in active patient care being difficult to document. Outside of the EU, nurses are trained to a minimum degree standard where there are also variations among institutions in the amount of required clinical hours despite the Munich Declaration, a declaration that sought to strengthen the status of nurses and midwives and make full use of the potential in healthcare (WHO, 2009). Non-EU member states have similar problems with increased numbers of students and fewer accessible patients.

Within Europe, the United Kingdom has taken the lead in exploring simulation education in an effort to tackle the issues cited earlier. One final issue that has limited student nurses' experiences is the implementation of the European Working Time Directives that have affected rosters creating reduced hours and opportunities for patient care experiences (DoH, 2003) (Fig. 15E.1).

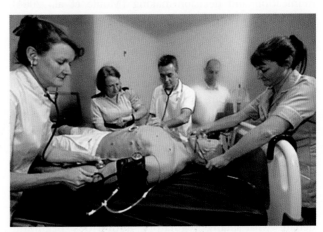

Figure 15E-1 Some of the early adopters of simulation, lecturers from University of South Wales, University of the West of London and Bristol Medical Simulation Centre, UK. Reprinted with permission from CAE Healthcare.

Simulation in the UK Revolutionizing Nursing Education

The regulatory body for nurses in the United Kingdom is the Nursing and Midwifery Council (NMC). The NMC in 2005 reviewed whether nursing students were fit for practice at the point of registration, that is, were they prepared to be a registered nurse (NMC, 2005). Students, lecturers, mentors, and preceptors were interviewed and surveyed and highlighted many concerns. These included concerns regarding the variation in competence in such areas as communication, medicine administration, and decision-making (Wilford & Doyle, 2006). Many students commented that they felt they did have enough experience and were nervous about the role of the registered nurse. The NMC stipulates that the 4,600 hours from the EU directives be split 50/50 with 2,300 hours of theory and the same in practice.

Following this review and acting on feedback from students, practitioners and lecturers support for the use of simulation has grown to assist nursing students in consolidating their learning. The NMC in March 2006 asked for expressions of interest from higher education institutions to investigate the use of simulation: the Simulation and Practice Learning Project for Preregistration Nursing Programmes (NMC, 2006a). Thirteen universities reported their findings to the NMC in early January 2007. The research study responses indicated that those programmes using combinations of e-learning, standardized patients, human patient simulators, and the virtual world had overwhelmingly positive remarks from both educational and satisfaction perspectives (Hope, Garside, & Prescott, 2011; Moule, Wilford, Sales, Haycock, & Lockyer, 2006). The students involved in the research ($n = 6,300$) gave robust feedback that simulation education did contribute to their learning and competence in areas such as communication and decision-making (Moule et al., 2006). Following the review of the data, the NMC announced in November 2007 (NMC, 2007) that institutions training nurses could use up to a maximum of 300 hours of the 2,300 hours practice component to provide clinical training within a simulated practice environment in support of providing direct care in the practice setting. This was and remains a landmark decision not just in Europe but also worldwide. It was the first regulator of any healthcare regulatory body to mandate that an entire country was permitted to use simulation in all its forms could replace practice hours (Fig. 15E.2).

The work in Europe, particularly data from the United Kingdom, is fuelling further discussion and debate with many regulatory authorities beginning to address whether simulation can be a substitute for clinical practice hours in traditional practices settings. Countries are assessing and actively researching, and

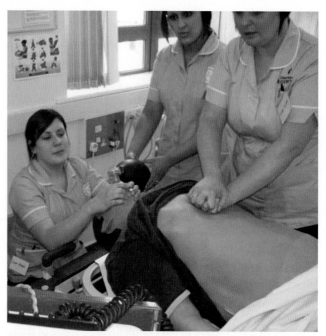

Figure 15E-2 Third Year Student nurses practicing advanced life support at Huddersfield University, UK. Reprinted with permission from CAE Healthcare.

over the next few years, more regulators will make such announcements.

One final factor that has increased support for simulation is the large numbers of experienced nurses leaving the profession due to reported lack of exposure to particular patient populations, and therefore, fewer opportunities to develop required clinical competencies (Aiken et al., 2014). In Europe, the differences in pay and career prospects have allowed for much movement across borders (WHO, 2009). This movement has brought pressure in practice as nurses from different healthcare systems across the EU are working together to bring differing approaches to learning patient care.

Even though student nurses may be in putting in time in practice settings, they may not be learning what they need to learn. Simulation grounded in best practices is holding great promise as one viable way of ensuring that learning experiences are relevant and required in practice (NCSBN, 2014, 2015). Furthermore, it is of concern that newly qualified nurses may not have all the requisite skills and knowledge to support the student nurses they are mentoring and supervising. Within Europe to date, only the United Kingdom has stipulated that simulation may be used to replace clinical time. This issue will need to be addressed when with the next update of the EU nursing directives, so that clear regulatory mandates make it easier to embrace simulation as an educational technique. In 2015, the WHO published their strategy for nursing and midwifery towards 2020, and key elements including transforming education and training with the concepts of innovation, teamwork, and leadership were mentioned, but not the use of simulation-based education, which may be a missed opportunity.

Simulation Societies in Europe

Europeans were early adopters of simulation as an educational technique with the first two centres set up in 1997 with interactive mannequins in Bristol, United Kingdom, and a few months later in Mainz, Germany. Both centres focused on medical training. In Europe, other institutions were beginning to extend traditional skills-based training, for example, the Netherlands and Denmark, into what today we would call simulation-based education by teaching technical and nontechnical skills training. Many of these early adopters wanted to join forces to share best practice and provide peer support. In the end, two societies were formed: the first was the Society in Europe for Simulation Applied to Medicine or SESAM with the first president serving 1994 to 1998 (SESAM, 2015). At this time, the focus was heavily influenced by medicine with few nurses attending these meetings. The early UK centres (Bristol, Liverpool, London—St. George's and St. Bartholomew's) formed an alliance in the late 1990s, and in time, this transformed into the National Association of Medical Simulators (NAMS). In 2009, NAMS joined with the Clinical Skills Network (CSN) to become the Association for Simulated Practice in Healthcare or ASPiH with its first president being a nurse (ASPiH, 2015). This change in 2009 was to include nursing and allied health as at that time simulation teachers who were medics tended to be part of NAMS and nurses and allied health CSN. By merging the two societies, the organization became truly interprofessional and reflects changes in simulation education for all professions involved in healthcare at community, military, disaster care, hospital, or academia. SESAM, for example, presents in English, and as there are over 60 languages spoken in Europe, many individual countries have formed their own national societies conducted in heritage or multiple languages, for example, SPSIM, Portugal; ROSOMED, Russia; MEDSIM, Romania; and SASH, Switzerland (SESAM, 2015).

Nursing education across Europe tends to be delivered in the heritage language, whereas some of the education for medicine is delivered in English. This may account for why there are still fewer nurses represented at SESAM. In national society meetings, nurses are well represented and are undertaking research and advancing nursing simulation at all levels as seen by those societies' programmes and abstract booklets. Simulation societies can provide support for nurses starting out and have a key role to play and is an important driver in adopting simulation at the national level. One international society that is addressing this local need is INACSL (International Nursing Association for Clinical Simulation and Learning). Although based in the United States, the association touts Chapter Europe as one of its international chapters. Language and the multilingual dissemination of findings is one area that European and International Societies need to address to be truly international. Societies such as SESAM and SSH (The Society for Simulation in Healthcare) based in the United States are gaining affiliate membership and, as such, support localised meetings in Europe, Middle East, Asia Pacific, and Latin America. These conferences encourage new adopters as the meetings are held in local languages with local leaders presenting and sharing their experiences and research (SESAM, 2015). Although there are many simulation societies all over Europe, other meetings are also offering a simulation focus, for example, the Turkish Nursing Association and British Association of Critical Care Nurses where there are simulation tracks. This growing number of papers and workshops being presented in academic and societal meetings is another driver for implementing simulation into nurse education.

Simulation Progressing in Europe

Europe's population in 2013 was estimated to be 742.5 million (European Union, 2015). This large population will require an exponential increase in the need for nursing care in year to come. Simulation in nursing education has been gaining traction since the late 1990s where there is a difference in implementation between EU and nonmember EU states. EU states tend to have stronger profession-specific adoption, perhaps relating to funding streams as the professions are funded separately. Interestingly, non-EU member states such as Turkmenistan have followed along later yet appear to be more progressive. Having seen what has happened in the EU, they have chosen to implement large interprofessional national programmes with significant government support and funding. The impact of this on the population's health and welfare is too early to tell. In broad terms, from west to east, simulation programmes in nursing education are still primarily uniprofessional, whereas from east to west, nursing programmes are beginning to be educated interprofessionally.

In June 2016, the United Kingdom (UK) voted in a referendum to leave the European Union. The actual exit strategy is slated to start unfolding in 2017. Today, nurses all across Europe are being affected by political and socioeconomic reform-changes that will most assuredly impact the profession at all levels. Even so, during this tumultuous juncture in Europe's history it is safe to say that simulation education is here to stay (Fig. 15E.3).

Europe is integrating simulation education across all the healthcare professions, and nursing is leading the way!

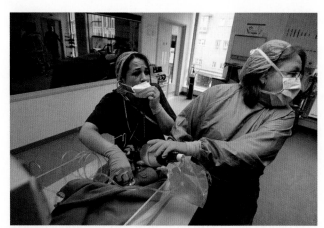

Figure 15E-3 Post graduate interprofessional training at Bristol Medical Simulation Centre, UK. Used with permission.

The UK regulator was an early leader, and organizations, such as INACSL with the Standards of Best Practice: Simulation[SM] first published in 2011, revised in 2013, added to in 2015, and updated again in 2016, are providing the world with evidence-based approaches simulation education (INACSL Standards Committee, 2016).

The key drivers promoting the integration simulation-based education into nursing have included patient safety, the EU directives, the working time directives, and the growing number of simulation societies. Barriers to integration include the funding streams as previously discussed. Language also continues to be a barrier for nurses, as many do not feel confident in their language abilities to attend and present their work at meetings where English is the dominant language. Professional simulation associations can do much to assist by providing official translations of key documents in other languages.

Final Thoughts

I feel that nursing is at the forefront of leading the way in simulation education. Europe with its early nursing pioneers continues to lead the way in countries such as the United Kingdom and Turkmenistan, both at different ends of the continent yet taking steps to implement simulation as a proven education technique. As the lady of the lamp said in 1860 (she might as well have been referring to simulation):

"So never lose an opportunity of urging a practical beginning, however small, for it is wonderful how often in such matters the mustard-seed germinates and roots itself."

Florence Nightingale—1860

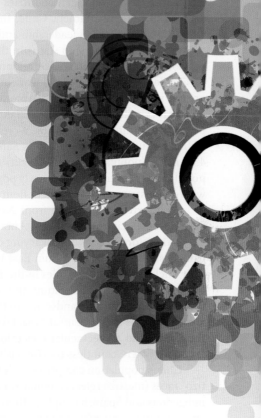

15F

Global Perspectives on Simulation: Latin America (Chile)

Eliana Escudero Zúñiga

(Translated from Spanish by Stéphane C. Erickson)

Latin America and Chile: Profile

Latin America comprises 20 countries in the Americas that originated in 19th century and evolved with strong influences from France, Spain, and Portugal. The predominant

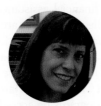

Eliana Escudero Zúñiga, Msc.NU

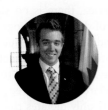

Stéphane C. Erickson, BCom, LLL, JD (Translator)

language is Spanish, save Brazil, Latin America's most populous country, where the official language is Portuguese. Contrary to what many may believe, Latin America is a very diverse part of the world in terms of the people, the food, the economy, social policy, as well as its models and levels of education. It is also diverse in climate, geography, and health systems. People and sociocultural behaviors in Latin America, therefore, vary considerably from region to region. Nonetheless, Latin Americans share many common traits, such as their warm and welcoming approach to others, historical background, and artistic uniqueness, namely, in music. Latin American people are very traditional valuing cultural customs and practices that run deep. As such, Latin Americans are often characterized as strongly independent and protective in nature. However, at times, Latin America is viewed as conservative and slow to change, especially in the face of current challenges or failures of the past. For example, there are still many socioeconomic disparities that exist in this part of the world, and many countries struggle with poverty and gender- and discrimination-related issues. Despite this fact, some Latin American countries have made significant advancements, namely, Chile. In the past 30 years, Chile has shown strong leadership and growth, which led to its current membership status in the Organisation for Economic Co-operation and Development (OECD).

Chile, the country where I work and reside, is located on the southern tip of South America and is home to nearly 17.5 million inhabitants (Eliana Escudero Zúñiga, personal communication, 2016). Women outnumber men (INE, Census, 2012). Its capital is Santiago, where about 43% of the population lives. In fact, most of the Chile's population is centralized in densely populated urban areas where industry and development flourish.

Chile extends 4,270 km from North to South, with Peru bordering in the North and Antarctica in the South. Chile, therefore, has a widely varying climate and terrain. Chile also extends 445 km from East to West, geographically enclosed in by the Andes in the East and the Pacific Ocean in the West. Chile features the Atacama Desert and its barren and beautiful landscapes in the North, vineyards and fruit farms in the Central Area, lakes and volcanoes in the South, and a spectacular collection of glaciers in the far South where countless tourists visit each year.

Chile's population comprises both the white and "mestizo" races (mestizo refers an ethnic mix from the Mapuche indigenous and Spanish peoples). There is also a large presence of immigrants who came from Spain, Italy, Germany, and Yugoslavia, among others, adding to Chile's rich heritage of mixed races and ethnicities. According to the latest census, Christianity, more specifically Roman Catholicism, is Chile's predominant religion, but many other religions are also practiced and respected. Chile has a stable democracy and a free-market economy, one of the most reliable in the region. Its demographic indicators are becoming increasingly similar to those of developed countries, with a continuously decreasing birth rate of 13.9 pmp (National Institute of Statistics of Chile [INE], 2015) and an average life expectancy of 79 years of age (76.5 for men and 81.6 for women). From a medical perspective, Chile's aging population means that there has also been an increase in chronic conditions, creating a need for changes in healthcare policies.

Higher Education in Chile

Chile has a complex model of higher education. All institutions charge student tuition; entirely publicly funded postsecondary institutions do not exist in Chile, unlike some other countries in Latin America. Before the 1980s, Universities belonged to the Chilean Traditional Universities (CRUCH), which is an independent organization that coordinates the country's universities. Some member universities of CRUCH receive substantial funding from the State, but this funding, unfortunately, does not allow the universities to support the entire student population. Financial assistance in many cases is secured through scholarships. In the late 1980s, Chile passed the *Higher Education Act* (La Ley Orgánica de Educación Superior [LOCE]) (Congress of Chile, 2005) that established three types of educational institutions: technical training institutes, professional institutes, and universities. Universities were allowed to establish programs, confer academic degrees, and focus on research. This law had many shortcomings because it did not guarantee the quality of teaching. However, it did permit the establishment of many private universities and gave Chile's youth a greater opportunity to access higher education. For this reason, the rate of Chilean youth accessing post-secondary jumped from approximately 4% or 5% before 1986 to about 40% today (Servicio de Información de Educación Superior [SIES], 2014). One example of this success is the University of Finis Terrae, an institution founded in 1988. Throughout this chapter, I will refer to the Finis Terrae School of Nursing and the experiences I have lived working there. To date, Chile has experienced the greatest advancements and developments in simulation-based education and leadership.

In the past, governments have failed to find solutions to increase accessibility and educational opportunities for youth, which is problematic and undoubtedly affects the development of the country. However, when looking at the general indicators and comparing them with the rest of the region, it is important to recognize that remarkable achievements have been made thanks to the many contributions of private universities, as well as technical and vocational training. Generally speaking, students start postsecondary education at 17 or 18 years of age, after completing the University Selection Test (PSU). University degree programs take between 4 and 7 years, institute run programs less than 4 years, and only 2 years for technical institutions. After meeting certain requirements, universities have complete autonomy over the management of their academic programs. This means that every degree program's curriculum, including nursing programs, is determined according to each institution's respective criteria. Contrary to many parts of the world, including Latin America, there is no state-based financial assistance for any of the degree programs in Chile. As a result, areas of spending and academic projects vary from institution to institution, and projects related to simulation, patient safety, and human factors are not mandated nor are they standardized in degree programs in Chile. Chilean law currently only dictates that medical programs be accredited. Accreditation allows graduates to apply to work in the public sector or apply for specialization scholarships granted by the Ministry of Health. Accreditation requirements, however, do not apply to nursing education programs. While each program remains unique, all share a common foundation of the basic sciences and related theory, as well as core content in areas of adult medical–surgical practices, pediatrics, mental health, community family health, and clinical nursing practice. It is also common to see varying emphasis and importance accorded to complementary courses such as administration, research, public health, emergency care, and ethics. Required hours of placement or internship also vary. Currently, all placement hours must be done at health institutions with which Universities have legal agreements that set out costs and reciprocity agreements for clinical teaching. Therefore, clinical activities come with a high price tag, making healthcare degree programs very expensive. This reality is motivating many educational institutions to evaluate their situation and consider the creation of simulation centres and the integration of simulation pedagogy.

Nursing and Nursing Education in Chile

For more than 100 years now, universities have run nursing programs in Chile. Program influences in the development of nursing education and practice in Chile stem primarily from the United States. As such, nursing programs in Chile are grounded in nursing theory and clinical practice principles derived from rigorous research methodology (ACHIEEN, 2006). In the 1950s, Chilean nurses who travelled to the United States returned to establish the first independent university nursing degree program. Today, the Chilean nurses' scope of practice extends to many areas of healthcare. Nurses are respected, highly valued, and held in high esteem both socially and economically. But this reality does not hold true in all parts of Latin America. In neighboring countries, for instance, nursing education and training have not reached comparable levels, where the nursing profession lacks professional autonomy and adequate remuneration. According to the Pan-American Health Organization (PAHO), this creates a situation of grave concern as there is a pressing need for nurses in these regions.

There has been a been high demand for nurses in Chile, which led to the creation of University postdegree masters and doctoral programs to respond to market needs. Still, it is unfortunate that State policies and the need for recognition of nursing specializations have not followed suit.

Another significant problem is a surge in the number of nursing schools that have opened in past years and a lack of control regarding the quality of training at these institutions. The trickle-down effect of unregulated schools and the lack of educational standards are now of significant concern to employers. This shifting situation has motivated university-based programs to review their programs of study and

educational methodologies. As such, it is now becoming apparent that simulation may be an excellent opportunity to better educational outcomes. Moreover, as is the case in the developed world, the health system in Chile is now legalized and patients are able to be more vocal and assert their rights as healthcare consumers (Law 201584).

Simulation in Chile and Latin America

Having covered the framework governing Chilean healthcare education, we can move on to the history of simulation in Chile and Latin America. Corvetto et al. (2013) describe the inaugural arrival of simulation in Chile at the Pontifical Catholic University where medical students interacted with actors (simulated patients) for practice interviews and assessment of patients' medical history. Later, in 2004, its School of Health also adopted this nontraditional approach to education and a curriculum based on technical skills and active methods of teaching and learning. It was while observing these changes in medical education that nurse educators were first inspired to introduce this disruptive innovation to the discipline of nursing. After all, the School of Health already had simulation-like environments for other career paths, such as culinary arts and car workshops for automotive technicians, and it therefore, made sense to design and build a simulated hospital for nurses. Many did not understand the need for simulation in nursing at the time, but with the help of the only simulation company on the ground and the assistance of Dr. Hernando Matiz and Dr. Adalberto Amaya of Colombia, simulation would find its place in nursing in Chile. In March 2004, the School of Health at the Pontifical Catholic University opened two modest simulation centres in separate locations. They adopted a student-centered model allowing the student to learn from his or her mistakes and improve accordingly. Nurses that were leading the first simulation design and build projects attended the 2006 Technology Conference in Baltimore, USA. A team led by Dr. Pamela Jeffries and the National League for Nursing (NLN), USA, organized this conference. Our attendance at this conference planted the crucial first seeds of change and resulted in making life-changing professional connections. It was an excellent learning opportunity, after which time the energized and enthused nurse educators returned home, bound and determined to develop the first full-fledged simulation centre in Chile!

The next significant event occurred in 2007 when simulationists from the National League for Nursing - Simulation Innovation Resource Center (SIRC) (http://sirc.nln.org) provided consultation and assistance to Chile as part of the group of international development experts. This group focused on the creation of "education standards" and developing courses in a virtual platform. This collaborative initiative made it possible for nursing programs to incorporate educational standards into existing curricula, namely, to implement high-quality teaching and learning using simulation.

During this time, there was increasing interest in featuring simulation in related conferences, seminars, and postgraduate programs. Other universities also became more interested in the subject, which led to further financing for simulation projects, including state funding. Alongside the growing interest, medical education was also developing simulation capacity. It was no longer enough to be a good nurse or doctor, you had to be a better teacher. Therefore, teaching professionals needed to learn about and better understand how to enact simulation pedagogy. This trend is also starting to emerge in other parts of South America, but the response is slow, leaving much work to be done to bring about further change.

The Pontifical Catholic University of Chile, known for its quality and leadership in education, decided as early as 2005 to conduct a pilot project, introducing two simulation-based courses in medicine. I had the pleasure of creating and delivering one of the programs. Simulation innovation called for new approaches to education with a need for clinical professors to learn together and be taught by experts in the field of interdisciplinary education and practice.

Growth and Expansion of Simulation

The Latin American Association of Clinical Simulation (ALASIC) contributed significantly to the growth and development of simulation in the region. In 2007, five professionals, Dr. A. Amaya, Dr. R. Alasino, Dr. A. Scalabrini, Dr. D. Champin, and the Mg. E. Escudero, (as seen in Fig. 15F.1), signed a ground-breaking partnership at the notary's office in the city of São Paulo, Brazil. This partnership aimed "to promote scientific research, application, and development of clinical simulation, as a training

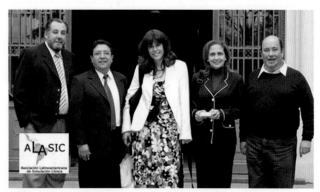

Figure 15F.1 First Director of the Latin American Association of Clinical Simulation (ALASIC), 2007. Photo courtesy of Eliana Escudero Zúñiga, with permisison from ALASIC.

strategy for health sciences professionals in Latin America" (ALASIC, n.d., para. 1). With members from Colombia, Argentina, Brazil, Chile, and Peru, they formed a collaborative partnership in the region that established the foundations for simulation in the future of South America.

Today, ALASIC is an organization with members from many countries (www.alasic.org). It has hosted four major conferences, with the last one held in November 2015 in Santiago de Chile, where 16 countries were represented and with many internationally renowned guest speakers in attendance. This conference is currently the largest of its kind in Latin America, allowing for the emergence of new leaders, the recognition of work and research, and the achievement of remarkable progress and development in the field of simulation.

Simulation's Evolution and the State of Progress

In Latin America, Colombia was the first country to pioneer simulation, taking the first steps to integrate simulation into the curriculum of health programs throughout Latin America. Chile and Brazil followed with the adoption of simulation and the development of national organizations that gave momentum to the simulation movement. Mexico and Costa Rica soon followed, and in the past 5 years, Argentina and Uruguay have followed suit. Argentina and Uruguay are now working to incorporate simulation and to educate and train professionals with the support of foreign professors and by creating a strong collaborative network. Peru, Ecuador, Paraguay, and Bolivia are the most recent countries to join this movement.

Generally speaking, simulation developed within universities, but in some cases, like Brazil, medical institutions such as the Albert Einstein Hospital and the Hospital of São Paulo have developed on-site simulation facilities, no doubt, as the result of mounting concerns about "patient safety" in the health professions. In Argentina, efforts to improve patient safety in neonatology and obstetrics are underway. There, the Garrahan Foundation has recently sealed an agreement with the Simulation Program at Children's Hospital Boston for simulation education and training (http://www.fundaciongarrahan.org.ar/). Unfortunately, we have yet to see this level of integration and partnership develop in the rest of Latin America.

Leaders in Simulation in Chile

Steady progress in health and healthcare education in developed nations is also fueling the advancement of simulation in Chile. However progressive, there remains considerable resistance to change in Latin America where the voices of tradition continue to yield significant power. Unfortunately, this has been a major barrier to innovation

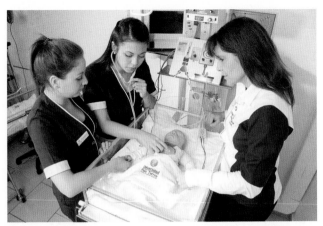

Figure 15F.2 Finis Terrae School of Nursing: Students are Giving the First Nursing Care to a Newborn with the Teacher. Photo courtesy of Eliana Escudero Zúñiga, Director, Finis Terrae School of Nursing.

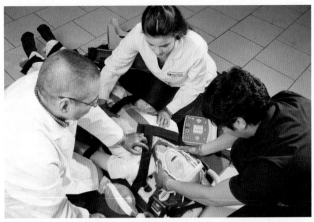

Figure 15F.4 Finis Terrae School of Nursing: Students and the Lab Technician are Preparing a Patient with Multiple Traumas for his Transfer at the Emergency Room. Photo courtesy of Eliana Escudero Zúñiga, Director, Finis Terrae School of Nursing.

and to the successful integration of simulation in prelicensure and postgraduate programs.

Despite the contextual barriers, the University of Finis Terrae took up the challenge and created its first School of Nursing (http://facultadmedicina.finisterrae.cl/escuelas/enfermeria). In 2008, the University invited Dr. Pamela Jeffries, a "Simulation Champion" from the National League for Nursing (NLN) to help establish its curricular programs launched in 2010 (UFT, 2008 archives). It would be the first nursing program in Chile and the region to integrate simulation-based education (Figs. 15F.2–15F.4), where assessment would be part of the educational process and where 40% of the student's final accreditation exam would employ simulation. This change also meant that the University had to train teachers in simulation pedagogy and invest in simulation learning spaces to meet standards and ensure quality education (http://www.ssih.org/Accreditation). Since

its inception, Dr. Pamela Jeffries has continued to participate and collaborate closely with the school's management team to incorporate the skills set out by "*The Quality and Safety Education for Nurses*" QSEN (http://qsen.org/). The nursing program was also the first to integrate the topics of patient safety and safety culture and quality. Their motto is "Services of Safety for Safe Patients" (http://facultadmedicina.finisterrae.cl/escuelas/enfermeria).

For the past 6 years, the teaching staff from Finis Terrae has grown and now collaborates within a multidisciplinary body of professionals (nurses, doctors, psychologists, physiotherapists, etc.). There, my role is to lead simulation development and integrate simulation standards of best practice (INACSL Standards Committee, 2016, INACSL Standards of Best Practice: Simulation[SM]). Many leaders of the Chilean Society for Clinical Simulation and Patient Safety, SOCHISIM, originated from this university and contributed to the furtherance of national and international training programs, research, courses, and degree programs, which have resulted in the continued expansion of simulation.

SOCHISIM's mission is:

To collaborate with the academic community and healthcare professionals in the area of clinical simulation; promoting and contributing to the scientific and methodological development of an evidence-based simulation model, and with a firm commitment to meet the objectives that support simulation for quality and safety in the care of our patients (SOCHISIM, n.d.) (http://www.sochisim.cl/mision/).

Our mission is geared to grow simulation in the country and within a framework that promotes collaboration and agreements with other simulation organizations (i.e., ALASIC and SSH), and to work together toward quality of care for our patients.

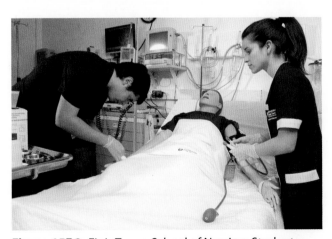

Figure 15F.3 Finis Terrae School of Nursing: Students are Evaluating the Patient and Taking Blood Tests. Photo courtesy of Eliana Escudero Zúñiga, Director, Finis Terrae School of Nursing.

Barriers to the Growth of Simulation

As noted previously, the road has not been easy and so much remains to be done in the field of simulation. The greatest barriers are the policies of countries that do not understand that positive change needs to come from developing discipline-specific and team competencies and by adopting approaches that serve to improve healthcare systems. Punitive models should cease, and government members need to step up to the plate as advocates for change in scientific and post-secondary communities. Vital decisions that will shape our nation's future healthcare should involve the whole of the country. Furthermore, healthcare professionals must uphold the guiding principle in person-centered care that the patient has a right to be part of the team and the decision-making process. Nurses are powerful advocates for change and must encourage patients and their families to participate proactively in the campaign for improved quality of health and quality patient care.

Lessons Learned

I would like to share a message to those who are starting in simulation. The road is complicated, but brings great satisfaction. Students value this form of learning and educators are transformed by teaching using simulation. Strong scientific evidence exists to support simulation and networks in the simulation practice community are becoming increasingly fruitful. Indeed, it is always easier to achieve our goals together, as a team. A global team! Simulation is here to stay. We will continue to research and publish our findings in Latin America, and together, we will build a better society equipped and with greater awareness and capacity in the provision of safer patient care.

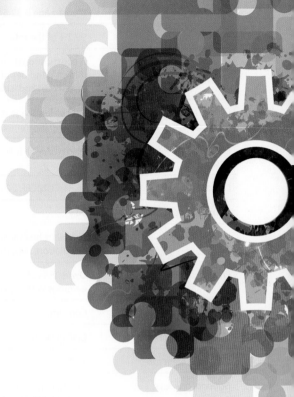

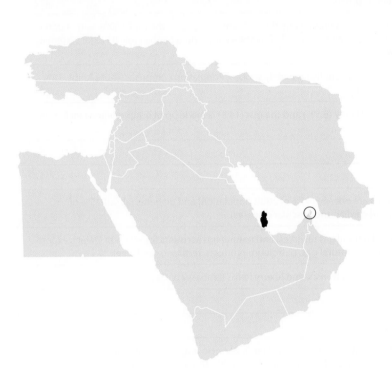

15G | Global Perspectives on Simulation: The Middle East (Qatar)

Renee Pyburn, Joanne Lorraine Davies

Qatar: Profile

The growth of simulation programs and facilities throughout the Middle East is expanding and none more so than in regions such as Qatar. This exemplar explores facts about the country and simulation developments to date. We will also share the efforts of our simulation colleagues countrywide: all inspiring innovators who have worked tirelessly to realize the expanded use of simulation in healthcare and post-secondary education. Qatar is a small country, a peninsula surrounded by the water of the Persian Gulf. The climate is desert-like, mostly flat and covered with desert sand, dunes, and gravel. See Table 15G.1 for more information on Qatar.

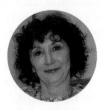

**Renee Pyburn,
MS, RN, CHSE**

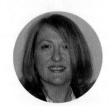

**Joanne Lorraine Davies,
MSc, RM, CHSE**

From 1972 to 1995, the country was ruled by Emir, Sheikh Khalifa bin Hamad Al Thani, but in 1995, the country was overtaken in a bloodless coup by his son, Hamad bin Khalifa Al Thani. Since then, the economy has developed rapidly (CIA, 2015a). By early in the 21st century, Qatar's vast natural gas revenues had led it to becoming one of the countries with the highest per capita income in the world (World Atlas, 2015).

Qatar Healthcare and Postsecondary Education

Qatar has an excellent healthcare system that is overseen by the Supreme Council of Health, established in 2005. The majority of healthcare falls under the auspices of Hamad Medical Corp (a public corporation that operates a total of five hospitals and centers, as well as numerous primary care centers). There are also private facilities and one publicly funded hospital that is currently in the developmental stage (Sidra Medical and Research Center) (http://www.sidra.org/). Healthcare is the responsibility of the State and therefore comes at little or no cost to Qatari

321

Table 15G.1	Fast Facts on Qatar
Population of Qatar	~2.2 million Only 15% of the population is estimated to be native Qatari (CIA, 2015a).
Median age	Median age is 32.6 y, with 70% between 25 and 54 y.
Urban/rural population	99.2% of the total population is urban.
Government	A constitutional monarchy that has been ruled by the Al-Thani family since the mid-1800s, with a prime minister and deputy prime minister and a council of ministers appointed by the Emir. Its legal system is mixed civil and Islamic law.
Official language and ethnic groups	Official language is Arabic, although English is widely spoken. Population comprises ~40% Arabs, 18% Indian, 10% Iranian, and 14% other.
Predominant religion/faith base	Islam (77.5%), followed by Christianity (8.5%) and the rest (14%) is made up of other religions including Hinduism
Literacy rate	96.3% (UNICEF, 2015)
Number of years in school	14 y
Primary disease	Prevalent healthcare concerns are obesity (41% of adult population) and diabetes (about 15% of population, hypertension, and cardiac and vascular diseases).
Primary exports	Owns 13% of the world's total natural gas reserves, and natural gas accounts for ~92% of Qatar's export earnings with exports in liquefied natural gas, petroleum products, fertilizers, and steel.
Primary imports	Consumer goods, vehicles, food, electronics, and luxury items (Embassy of Qatar in Rome, 2015)
GDP growth rate	GDP growth rate is ~6.1%.
Unemployment rate	1.3%
National holidays	Jan. 1, New Year's Day; Feb. 10, National Sports Day; Mar. 1, Bank Holiday; Eid Al-Fitr (date varies); Sept. 34, Eid Al-Adha (date varies); Dec. 18, National Day; Dec. 31, and New Year's Eve
Unique cultural practices	Qatar has a rich tradition of music, poetry, handicrafts, and Islamic art and calligraphy (Qatar Investment Authority, n.d.). Perfume and incense are important in Qatari culture and also used as a sign of hospitality. There are many perfume shops for men and women in Qatar. Frankincense, Myrrh, and Oud (agar wood) are also used in incense burners (Qatar Culture and Traditions, 2015).

citizens and residents. For recent healthcare data, see Table 15G.2. The Qatar Foundation for Education, Science, and Community Development built Education City, a 14 square kilometer region in Doha that houses numerous educational facilities, including nine of the world's top Western universities offering many academic programs. Post-secondary healthcare education in Qatar features the University of Calgary, Qatar (UCQ), a Canadian School of Nursing and the College of the North Atlantic-Qatar-(CNAQ), a Canadian School of Allied Health and Technology.

Qatari Traditions

The majority of the population in Qatar is Muslim, therefore, both State and Church are seamlessly woven into the fabric of all public systems, including healthcare and education. The Qatari dress conservatively in traditional garments comprised of a head covering and full body garments. Conservative, modest dress is also expected of foreigners. A large percentage of the Qatari population descended from Bedu (or Bedouin) tribes, a desert nomad people; therefore, Qataris still have strong tribal identities. Camels were traditionally a large part of the Bedouin culture, and previously, most nomadic people lived in tents traveling throughout the desert. Many Qataris still enjoy camping and spending time in traditional tents in the desert, and some also keep herds of camels. Camel racing remains a popular sport (Qatar Culture and Traditions, 2015). Arabian horses are prized, horse shows are well-attended premiere events, and Qatar is home to several riding academies. Falconry is also a traditional pastime of Arabs in the Gulf region, where these prized birds are used for both sport and hunting. Arabs, and falcons were used both for sport and hunting. Qataris are very

Table 15G.2	Qatari Health Indicators (SSA)	
Indicator	**Qatar**	**Other**
Doctors per 1,000 population	7.74	2.54 per 1,000 people
Nurses	10,615 nurses	2.93 million nurses
Under 5 mortality per 1,000 live births	7.00	USA—7.0
Infant mortality per 100,000 live births	6.0	USA—6.0
Health expenditure per capita (% of GDP)	2.2%	17.90
Hospital beds per 1,000 population	12.0	30.0
Life expectancy	79.00	79.56

Quandl.com. (2016). Health Indicator Data. Retrieved from https://www.quandl.com/

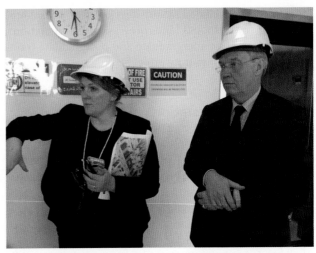

Figure 15G.1 Jo Davies and Dr. Joachim Dudenhausen, Touring Simulation Centre Construction Progress. Used with permission.

family-oriented and honor longstanding culture, and faith-based traditions and practices. In the past 20 years, huge investments in urban planning and design have brought modern day building advancements and an impressive Doha city sky scape. Locals enjoy leisure time in beautiful shopping malls, attend cultural events in theaters and museums, eat out in local restaurants, and frequent green park areas.

Qatar Simulation Employment Setting

Authors, Joanne Davies and Renee Pyburn have served as employees of the Sidra Medical Research Center in Doha, a new 400(+)-bed women and children's academic medical center hospital project in Doha. The original hospital space plan allocated only one room for simulation. Following consultation with SimHealth (an American-based consultant group), the design was altered. In the process of building the simulation program and associated simulation learning spaces, the project team recognized the need to expand the size of the facility as it would become the on hub for training thousands of new hospital staff. Relatively early in simulation program development, a team of simulation specialists was hired including six simulation technologists, four simulation specialists, and a very experienced operations manager. This strategy greatly reduced the need for external consultants to support the program.

Sidra is a Greenfield hospital project, a process where untested innovations are designed, tested, and evaluated as the project unfolds. Delays are a reality in this process and the main simulation center that has yet to open is planned for the spring of 2017. Figure 15G.1 depicts Joanne Davies

touring the Sidra construction site. However, this has not prevented the simulation team from concurrently building a robust simulation program. This has been accomplished by opening a temporary simulation center that has four simulation suites and access to a large classroom. The primary focus of the simulation program to date has been curriculum development, piloting faculty development programs, and readying resources to deliver a simulation program that can support the opening of the large women and children's hospital.

Despite delays in construction and occupancy have also provided a unique opportunity for on-boarding and orientating using in situ simulation for a diverse healthcare workforce. The simulation team has had the advantage of being able to carry out individual, team, and system testing and training.

Using a blended approach to curriculum design, the simulation team, in collaboration with our education department and clinical experts, have developed e-learning, skills stations, and simulation scenarios that have been rigorously piloted in the temporary space. The primary simulation modality will be in situ and mobile simulation with the simulation team deploying scenarios in actual clinical practice settings with real clinical teams. Additional programs under development include a technical training program that all staff and simulation core faculty are required to complete. Pre- and posttesting is conducted to determine learning progression and close performance gaps, and also to ensure that we are evaluating the effectiveness of the teaching program.

The Sidra Medical and Research Center simulation teams have collaborated on projects with local partners including UCQ, WCMC-Q, Qatar University School of Pharmacy, HMC, and CNA-Q. Inter-institutional initiatives have included faculty development workshops, debriefing workshops, interprofessional simulations, research projects, undergraduate and postgraduate training events, and community projects.

Evolution of Simulation in Qatar

Prior to 2009, simulation had already begun with a well-developed Standardized Patient Program at Weill Cornell Medical College-Qatar (WCMC-Q) and to a much lesser extent at the College of the North Atlantic-Qatar (CNA-Q), the University of Calgary in Qatar (UCQ), and Qatar University School of Pharmacy. Brief descriptions of each of these programs are included at the end of this exemplar. The use of simulation in Qatar has expanded very rapidly since these early efforts. It is now being used extensively within the four college-level clinical programs, with a commitment to move toward interprofessional simulation education at the undergraduate level. Additionally, the public healthcare system in Qatar (Hamad Medical Corp.) has also embraced simulation as a primary mode of education to support the development of healthcare teams. As capacity-building efforts ramp up for simulation educators from both practice and academe, so does the uptake of simulation. Plans for a state-of-the-art simulation center are underway to support this large public healthcare system and include a Pediatric Emergency Clinic to implement interprofessional simulation-based education for emergency teams with support from Sidra Medical and Research Center. The Sidra Medical and Research Center and Hamad Medical Corporation initiated the TeamSTEPPS program using simulation in 2015. The Qatar Robotics Surgery Center (QRSC) officially opened in 2010 (Ministry of Information and Communications Technology, Qatar, 2015) offering programs focused on teaching minimally invasive surgery to practicing surgeons in the region in specialties such as cardiology, urology, and OB/Gyn. These programs have greatly expanded to include teaching basic and specialized skills and other specialized surgical skills to medical students, interns, and residents in Qatar.

Today, Qatar's National Health Strategy vision is to improve and expand healthcare education and encourage more interprofessional educational opportunities (Qatar National Health Strategy, 2015). As a result, the need for simulation-based education has never been stronger. Hamad Medical Corp. (HMC), in collaboration with Sidra and others, has rapidly expanded their use of simulation for healthcare providers, and a large new simulation facility is planned.

Growth in simulation in Qatar has occurred in two main sectors—in undergraduate education and in hospital-based education. Staff development has also

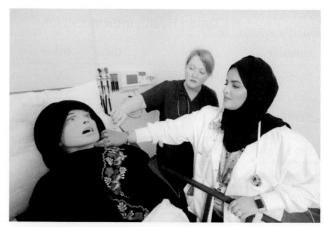

Figure 15G.2 Jo Davies and Nouf Al-Kuwari engaged in a simulation-based learning event. Used with permission.

been strongly supported where staff from simulation organizations in Qatar have taken a very active role in attending international simulation conferences including International Meeting for Simulation in Healthcare (IMSH), International Association for Clinical Simulation and Learning (INACSL), and the International Pediatric Simulation Society (IPSSW). Staff at the various simulation centers in Qatar have been very active in pursuing professional development opportunities, both individually and in collaborative partnership with one another. Many have attended and/or presented scholarly work at premiere international simulation conferences including IMSH, INACSL, and IPSS. They have also presented as inter-institutional teams at local health education forums and conferences and a number of articles have been accepted and published in peer-reviewed journals. For example, the Qatar Simulation Consortium presented at the first United Arab Emirates (UAE) simulation conference as a team. Figure 15G.2 depicts health professionals engaged in a simulation training session.

Institutional leaders strongly endorse simulation programs offering dedicated positions for simulation teams. They also strongly support collaboration through the Qatar Simulation Consortium to facilitate the development of simulation programs and general resource sharing. Through this consortium the members have collaborated in many areas including curriculum development, facility design, faculty and staff workshops, SP training programs, conference presentations, and technical planning and training. Additionally, during the second UAE Clinical Simulation Conference (http://uae-csc2015.com/) in collaboration with SESAM- the Society in Europe for Simulation Applied to Medicine, in February of 2015 the MENA Region Simulation User Network was formed. The purpose of this network is to have an interprofessional group that can promote, encourage, and develop simulation-based education, research opportunities, collaborative partnerships, and innovations in simulation within the MENA region.

Funding for Simulation Programs in Qatar

Post-secondary-based simulation programs are self-funded. Hamad Medical Corporation's simulation program is a government state-funded program while Sidra Medical and Research Center's Program receive state funding through the Qatar Foundation or other State departments.

Barriers or Challenges Encountered Integrating Simulation

When developing simulation programs in this region, we encountered challenges similar to those experienced by all start-up programs. Such challenges include gaining leadership buy-in, securing funding, delays in planning and construction, recruiting team members with experience in simulation and retaining them, developing a capacity of faculty to support the program, developing effective collaborations, collecting and analyzing of data, continuous program improvement and maintaining a motivated cohesive team. With strong leadership, dedicated team members, collaborative partnerships, and a unified goal to make improvements in patient care and healthcare systems, we have found immense support for simulation-based education in this region.

Adapting Simulation to Local Culture

The simulation development model in Qatar is primarily fashioned after, and influenced by Western institutions and by the teaching and learning approaches adopted by the faculty and healthcare professionals working within them. It is precisely because Western standards, best practices, and simulationists predominate in the region that there must be deliberate attention to how best incorporate simulation in a predominantly Muslim country. Designing authentic simulation experiences requires engaging with our Muslim counterparts in a culturally competent, sensitive, and respectful way. Adopting a stance of cultural humility is vital to understanding how Muslims live out their faith from birth to death. It is important to remember that the rigor and accuracy of simulation-based education are based on how "real" scenarios feel to the learners. Other important adaptations have included adjusting to the use of video or filming, accommodating delivery times to allow for prayer rituals several times daily, and being mindful of gender-specific needs in some cases (Foisy-Doll, 2013). HMC's simulation development, in contrast, has been led primarily by local Qataris under the advice of Western staff/consultants.

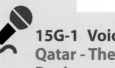

15G-1 Voice of Experience
Qatar - The Pearl of the Gulf Region

Renee Pyburn, MS, RN, CHSE

Fortunately, before moving to Qatar, I had worked in Saudi Arabia and Kuwait for 13 years so I was familiar with Arabian Gulf culture and lifestyle. However, the organizational culture of the Sidra project was very different, so the bigger adjustment was to the new organizational culture. It was a relatively complex project with multiple stakeholders, so I spent a lot of time in the beginning trying to understand the structuring of the project and learning about the Qatar Foundation, the Qatari healthcare system, and state-based decision-making processes and getting to know key influencers. I also took time to understand the differences between Qatari culture and the cultures in Saudi Arabia and Kuwait as each Arab country is quite different.

My position at Sidra was that of a senior level manager charged with overseeing the development of the simulation project for the hospital. As part of that work, I had the honor of working with several high-ranking officials in the public healthcare system; gaining great respect for the work that they did, their expertise, and the multiple challenges they overcame. I also grew to appreciate Qatari values of loyalty, respect, and warmth. It was fascinating to learn about the work of these officials and the systems within which they operate.

I also found great pleasure and fulfillment in working collaboratively with leadership and simulation personnel from the various clinical schools in Qatar. I learned so much by being involved in the planning of a large simulation center/program from the ground up and the unique opportunity to integrate simulation into a hospital orientation program. We were fortunate to be generously funded, so I had the opportunity to hire some very qualified staff and to design an impressive state-of-the-art simulation facility and order the very best in simulation equipment. In many ways, it was like the Simulation Champion's dream job. I was able to expand my knowledge of simulation by attending international simulation conferences. I was able to meet many prominent figures in the world of simulation and learn from them and was struck by their generosity and willingness to share.

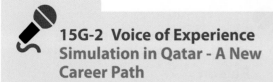

15G-2 Voice of Experience Simulation in Qatar - A New Career Path

Joanne Lorraine Davies, MSc, RM, CHSE

Although originally from the United Kingdom, I have worked and lived in a few countries in the Middle East including Saudi Arabia and the UAE, so I feel that my adjustment to living in Doha was somewhat straightforward. I think my biggest challenge was in adopting a new professional role, that of working on a large project after being primarily in obstetrical clinical, education, and management roles. I also observed a difference in the culture of the Qatari locals compared to Saudi and UAE, understanding that these countries have a lot of similarities but unique differences also. What struck me the most was the incredible drive that the Qatari healthcare teams had for improvement in education and healthcare, especially for women and children. This vision aligned with my professional motivations. Today, I am extremely proud to lead a talented and motivated team toward our goal of implementing quality simulation sessions into the clinical healthcare education programs to improve patient, environmental, and system safety.

Another huge challenge was finding simulation professionals with the requisite expertise to design and deliver quality simulation. Transient work populations often means a shorter time for professional development and mentorship to attain mastery. Retraining is an ongoing reality in this environment. At times, I have been completely overwhelmed by the enormity of the task that lay before me. However, with the many small wins I have seen over that last 5 years, I have come to learn that with persistence, the right people, and commitment, anything is possible.

I have also been impressed by the commitment of the State of Qatar to embrace and adopt simulation and strive toward improvements to standards in the region. I am proud to say that this project has afforded me the opportunity to grow as a leader, innovator, and champion in the field as I helped to shape some of the programs and projects that are currently in place within Qatar and the MENA region. I have been the lucky beneficiary of the generosity of the staff from local healthcare institutes and academic institutions to collaborate and share knowledge and resources. Examples are the use of a digital curriculum management system and the use of technology to embrace a paper-light environment (Hansen & Davies, 2015).

Most of all, I am inspired by our wonderful learners. I feared that the implementation of simulation into a traditional education system would be met with skepticism. Instead, what I have found is that learners have cried out for more of this educational approach, embracing it with open arms. The Qatari students are hardworking, genuinely enthusiastic, and committed to excellence. To our team's credit, we have supported the implementation of many programs, and the results are starting to reveal significant improvements in knowledge, skills, and attitudes in the delivery of healthcare. As we move forward, we look forward to making a positive impact with the opening of a new simulation center, outpatient clinic, and a state-of-the-art women and children's hospital in Qatar.

Most Important Lesson Learned

We think that one of the most important lessons learned is the power of collaborative simulation efforts on a national scale. We believe that all institutions have benefited tremendously from these collaborative efforts and the sharing of resources on a national scale. Institutional partners are committed to continue these collaborative efforts, focusing on faculty and staff development, increasing integration of simulation into clinical education at all levels, completion of several of the large facilities under development, and research development. Simulationists will continue to have a strong presence in local and international simulation organizations such as SSH, INACSL, IPSS, and the MENA simulation network. Simulation in the Middle East and particularly in the GCC (Gulf Corporate Council of Arab States) is exploding. As such, we are committed to becoming leaders in simulation-based learning and education at local, regional, and international levels in the coming years. We also believe that credentialing for simulation professionals, accreditation of simulation centers, and the implementation of evidence-based standards of best practice are important steps toward high-quality simulation program development. We have been honored to be a part of working toward realizing Qatar's vision (Personal communication, R. Pyburn and J. Davies, February 2017).

Feature Simulation Centers and Programs in Qatar

This section presents snapshots of three additional simulation centers and programs currently operating in Qatar.

Weill Cornell Medicine - Qatar—Clinical Skills Center

Mohamud Verjee, MBA, MBChB, BSc(Hon), DRCOG, CCFP, FCFP

The earliest adopter in Qatar, Weill Cornell Medicine - Qatar (WCM-Q), had a state-of-the-art Clinical Skills Center built in 2004. Custom designed from the outset, it boasted six complete office-setting consulting rooms, with full support training, audiovisual, equipment, and recreational areas. Standardized Patients (SPs) are trained to reproduce thoroughly crafted clinical scenarios simultaneously, strictly following a learned script. SP recruitment has proven successful in the Gulf region, but mostly comprises spouses of foreign working professionals (see Fig. 15G.3). The turnover of help necessitates constant SP recruitment and training. WCM-Q's Clinical Skills Center SP Trainer trains all SPs for clinical scenarios. SPs are also taught to give nonmedical feedback to students or residents, predominantly on communication and interpersonal skills. Some clerkship groups hold OSCEs on a formative training or summative basis, for example, primary care (family medicine), obstetrics and gynecology, and pediatrics.

Thorough preparation for the U.S. Medical Licensing Examination (USMLE CS) step 2 assessment is also provided to all 3rd year MD students annually. Undergraduate learners in all 4 years of their MD studies undergo progressively more developed assessments as their clinical experience increases. In-house training on medical mannequins such as *Harvey*, a product of the University in Florida, continues throughout the year. Basic life support training is now integrated

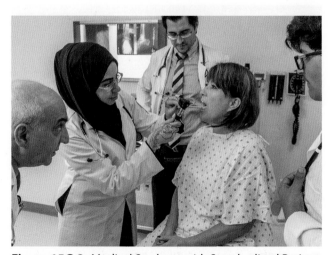

Figure 15G.3 Medical Students with Standardized Patient. (Used with permission of Weill Cornell Medicine - Qatar.)

into the clinical curriculum. Residents from Hamad Medical Corporation, a regional-affiliated tertiary care teaching hospital, also undergo vigorous formative and summative OSCEs, for example, professional ethics, pediatric, psychiatric, and internal medicine scenarios. To date, WCM-Q graduates have achieved 100% success in their obligatory STEP 2 CS examinations prior to taking up a residency.

Knowing that a significant amount of undergraduate clinical skills mastery and assessment relies on simulation with a modern, fully equipped clinical skills and simulation center, WCM-Q strives for more efficient integration of innovative clinical methods for teaching in the undergraduate medical curriculum.

College of the North Atlantic-Qatar (CNA-Q): Simulation Programs

Charlene Mercer, MALAT, RRT, CHSE

The College of the North Atlantic (CNA) is one of the leading educational institutions offering technical training in Canada. In 2002, through a partnership with the State of Qatar, CNA opened its first international satellite campus in Qatar. The school offers programs in various disciplines including business, security, and information technology. However, the School of Health Sciences is where simulation began at the institution.

The School of Health Sciences offers programs for various healthcare professions including respiratory therapy, medical radiography, dental assisting, emergency medical sciences, environmental health, and a pharmacy technician's program. Most of these programs deliver the same curriculum as what is offered by their Canadian counterparts and since opening have achieved and maintained internationally recognized accreditation status. As with many colleges and universities offering a healthcare curriculum, the College of the North Atlantic-Qatar (CNA-Q) made plans to utilize simulation as an educational modality from the time of opening its doors. The instructors from various programs integrated simulation training into curricula where applicable, and most simulation conducted during the initial stages was done in an "on-the-fly" format and primarily using a unidisciplinary approach. In general, audiovisual capture was not incorporated.

Later, in 2009, the first skills competition was conducted in the School of Health Science. This initial competition was unidisciplinary and involved the emergency medical sciences. The competition involved students taking part in various simulations where they were assessed on their clinical management. In 2010, the skills competition evolved into an interprofessional competition where teams including the six professions within the school competed in a combination of scenarios; some of which were discipline specific and one was a team-based scenario that incorporated all of the professions. The following year the skills competition became a college-wide event and the School of Health Science expanded their competition and the interprofessional makeup of their teams to include students from other health programs in Qatar. In 2010, CNA-Q joined with Qatar's other healthcare institutions in the Qatar Simulation Consortium (QSC), which is discussed earlier in this chapter. After more than 12 years in Qatar, the College of the North Atlantic-Qatar (CNA-Q) is one of the largest postsecondary institutions in the country with over 650 staff and more than 4,600 students. Simulation continues to be recognized as a key modality to support the internationally recognized curriculum in the School of Health Science.

The University of Calgary in Qatar: Clinical Simulation Centre

Julie Hoffart, MN, BScN, RN

Jayne Smitten, PhD, MEd Dipl. AdultEd., BA, RN, CHSE-A

Leanne Wyrostok, MN, BN, RN(r)

Colette Foisy-Doll, MSN, RN, CHSE

In 2011, the University of Calgary in Qatar (UCQ; Fig. 15G.4) became the first Canadian baccalaureate nursing program to be internationally accredited outside of Canada with the Canadian Association of Schools of Nursing (CASN). The Faculty of Nursing at the University of Calgary in Canada is known for its excellence in clinical practice and family healthcare education. It is at the forefront of health promotion and disease prevention in Qatar.

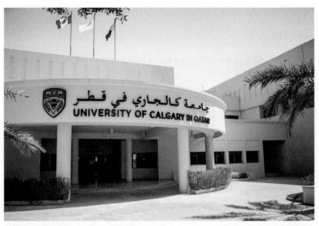

Figure 15G.4 The University of Calgary in Qatar Campus Front Entrance, with permission.

The vision of UCQ is to enrich health and wellness in Qatar and the Gulf region through world-class education of nursing leaders and practitioners. Its mission is to excel in (1) educating nurses who will become renowned for excellence in practice, (2) preparing nurse leaders who will contribute to the development of emerging healthcare systems, and (3) research and educational initiatives that will contribute to health and wellness of the citizens of Qatar (http://www.qatar.ucalgary.ca/).

In 2007, the State of Qatar launched UCQs undergraduate nursing program. The following year, three nursing faculty members taught the first lab groups of students with limited equipment and supplies. This necessitated their creativity in crafting basic teaching tools and spaces for skills acquisition (see Fig. 15G.5). In 2009, over a 10-month period and under the project leadership of a simulationist, the first high-fidelity state-of-the-art simulation center for undergraduate nursing

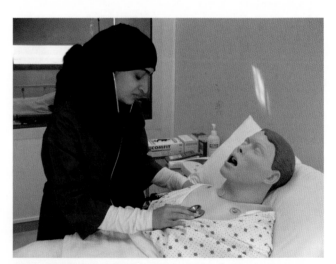

Figure 15G.5 Student in Clinical Simulation Learning Centre, The University of Calgary in Qatar, 2010, with permission.

education in the Gulf region was constructed. The UCQ Clinical Simulation Centre (CSC) initially served a group of 36 undergraduate nursing students, most with English as an additional language. In preparation for the CASN international accreditation process in 2010, the UCQ simulation directors collaborated with nursing faculty to design, develop, and integrate simulation scenarios within all 4 years of the undergraduate nursing program. Simulation provided nursing students an excellent platform for a wide range of experiences from acquiring nontechnical skills like applying their nursing language in English with patients to very technical clinical skills to be replicated in the healthcare environments within Qatar.

Over the past 10 years, the UCQ Clinical Simulation Centre (CSC) has expanded its spaces and curricular programming to accommodate over 500 undergraduate and graduate nursing students. The current CSC is a state-of-the-art facility, rich in advanced technological equipment and innovation to support the integration of all simulation learning modalities (mannequin based, standardized patient [SP], virtual/haptic, and hybrid). A resource web portal can be accessed within the CSC, providing a venue for expanding simulation education, practice, and research. Additionally, the center also offers flexibility and built-in capacity for the delivery of interprofessional (IPE) learning experiences. Currently, UCQ and the CSC are immersed in IPE, most notably with the Faculty of Pharmacy at Qatar University. In future, the CSC proposes a faculty-supervised, student-led health promotion clinic area for general Qatari public access. Under the direction of the State of Qatar and UCQ administration, the CSC simulationists have prioritized the development of strategic partnerships with local stakeholders for simulation-based educational initiatives and resource sharing.

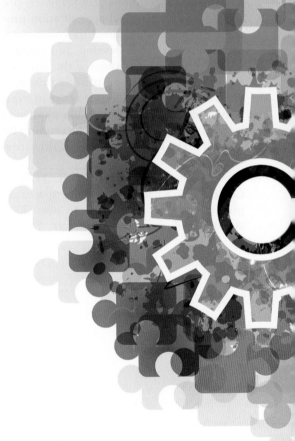

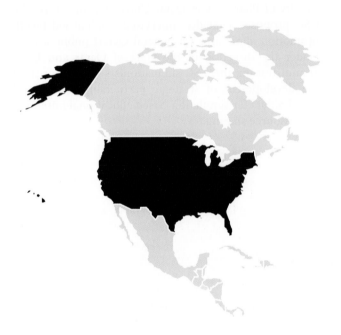

United States of America: Profile

The United States of America (US) achieved independence as a nation after winning the Revolutionary War against Britain in 1776. We celebrate this date with our national Independence Day on July 4. The official recognition of this country took place in 1783 with the Treaty of Paris. The nation began with 13 original states located in the northeastern part of the country. Over the next two centuries, another 37 states were added. Forty-eight of these states are located in what is called the continental United States, which covers the largest single land mass.

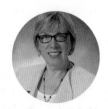

Wendy M. Nehring, PhD, RN, FAAN, FAAIDD

Two additional states, which were added last, Alaska and Hawaii, are not connected by land to the other 48 states. Two events in our country's history have served to define our country. The first was the Civil War (1861–1865) in which 11 southern states fought to form a separate union. One of their seminal issues was the right to possess slaves. The second event was the Great Depression of the 1930s. In those years, approximately 25% of the working men and women lost their jobs. Our economy has remained strong since then and unemployment and inflation are controlled. Among other things, the United States is recognized for its education and technological advances (Central Intelligence Agency, 2015b).

The people of the United States are diverse and free to celebrate their traditions. According to the 2007 estimate, 79.96% are Caucasian, 12.85% are Black, 4.43% are Asian, 0.97% are Amerindian and Alaska natives, 0.18% are native Hawaiian and other Pacific Islanders, and 1.61% are of two or more races. As of 2015, it is estimated that there are 321,368,864 residents of the United States, placing us as the fourth largest country. Our residents primarily speak English (79.2%), followed by Spanish (12.9%). Today, the greatest proportion of the population is between 25 and 54 years of age (39.76%), followed by birth to 14 years (18.99%), 65 and over (14.88%), 15 to 24 years (13.64%), and 55 to 64 years (12.73%). The median age is 37.6 years. There are more males than females from birth to age 24, but after age 25, there are more females. The birth rate is 12.49 births per 1,000 population, which ranks the United States as 150 in the world. The infant mortality rate is 5.87 deaths per 1,000 live births. The death rate is 8.15 deaths per 1,000 population with a ranking of 94 in the world. Life expectancy is 79.68 years with males at 77.32 years and females living longer at 81.97 years. We also rank 40th in the world for migration with 3.86 migrants per 1,000 population. The population of the United States is primarily Protestant (51.3%) or Catholic (23.9%), although several other religions are practiced freely (Central Intelligence Agency, 2015b).

The government of the United States is a democracy and is a constitution-based republic. The constitution was first written in 1781 and was effective in 1789. Several amendments have been added over the years. We have a president, and the national capital is Washington, DC. There are three branches to our government: executive, legislative, and judicial. Four political parties are recognized: democratic, green, libertarian, and republican, the majority belonging to either the democratic or republican parties (Central Intelligence Agency, 2015b).

In 2015, the gross domestic product (GDP) per capita for the United States in millions was 54,800. Health expenditures made up 17.1% of the GDP in 2013, and education expenditures were 5.1% of the GDP in 2011. Our top three exports in 2008 were technology (49.0%), industrial supplies (26.8%), and consumer goods (15.0%). Our top three imports in 2008 were industrial supplies (32.9%), consumer goods (31.8%), and technology (30.4%) (Central Intelligence Agency, 2015b).

Employment Location and Setting: College of Nursing at East Tennessee State University

In the United States, simulation takes place in academic and practice settings. It is quickly becoming standard practice in all health disciplines, predominantly in medicine and nursing, to provide simulation, in a variety of forms, to students in undergraduate and graduate, including continuing education programs (pre- and postlicensure) for skill, synthesis of care, and interprofessional team development. Many hospitals have also invested in simulation programs for skill and team performance assessments. Academic simulation champions have also taken simulation into primary and secondary education settings to educate students on health conditions, such as drug overdoses, and to illustrate healthcare of patients Figures 15H.1 and 15H.2 depict introductory simulation technologies used by the author in the late 90s.

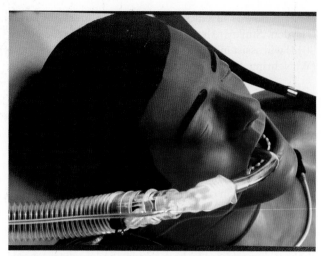

Figure 15H.1 Simulation mannequin, 1999. (Photo by W. Nehring.)

I am the dean of the College of Nursing at the largest nursing program in the state of Tennessee at East Tennessee State University. We use many forms of simulation primarily in our undergraduate nursing programs. We use standardized patients in our nurse practitioner concentrations in our Doctor of Nursing Practice (DNP) program to teach the male and female examination. Our college is one of five health sciences colleges that comprise our Academic Health Science Center. We have two rooms in our building that are dedicated to medium- and high-fidelity patient simulation. We also have a large skills laboratory. In 2018, we will open a newly renovated historical building that will house interprofessional education and research. One floor will be dedicated to standardized patients and another floor to high-fidelity simulation. The College of Nursing will be very involved in these programs, and this will enable us to enhance our simulation experiences. Clinical placement is a barrier in our area and the results of the National Council

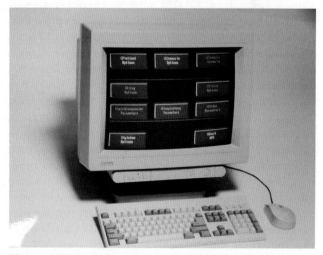

Figure 15H.2 Early computer interface for simulation. (Photo by W. Nehring.)

of State Boards of Nursing's (NCSBN) Simulation Study (Hayden, Smiley, Alexander, Kardong-Edgren, & Jeffries, 2014) will assist in impacting our student's clinical learning (W. Nehring, February 2017).

Evolution of Simulation in the United States of America

Simulation has been used in medical and nursing education for over a century, and as technology has developed, so has the sophistication of the simulation products. Perhaps the earliest form of simulation were cadavers, which were used by medical schools in the late 1800s (Harper & Markham, 2011), anatomical skeletons from cadavers, and models of limbs that were used by both nursing and medical schools (Harper & Markham, 2011; Nehring, 2010). Since these early years, categories of simulation have included anatomical models, task trainers, role-playing, games, computer-assisted instruction, standardized patients, virtual reality and haptic systems, and low- to high-fidelity mannequins. Bradley (2006) discussed different movements across time that has influenced not only the education of health professionals but also the development of simulation as a field and the products of simulation in the United States. These movements include resuscitation, anesthesia safety and competence, and medical education reform. Each of these movements has also been affected by political accountability, workforce shortages, ethical considerations, social expectations, and professional regulation (Bradley, 2006; Nehring, 2010).

A historical review of the literature, including the research literature for each of the categories of simulation can be found in the nursing and medical literature (see Chapter 1; Bradley, 2006; Harper & Markham, 2011; Nehring, 2010; Nehring & Lashley, 2009; Palaganas, Epps, & Raemer, 2014; Rosen, 2008, 2013; Schaefer et al., 2011; Slone & Lampotang, 2014). A number of books on simulation have also provided a historical overview of the field across time (Dunn, 2004; Jeffries, 2007b; Kyle & Murray, 2008; Loyd, Lake, & Greenberg, 2004; Nehring & Lashley, 2010; Palaganas, Maxworthy, Epps, & Mancini, 2015). Of note is the August 2011 supplemental issue of *Simulation in Healthcare* in which monographs from the *First Research Consensus Summit of the Society for Simulation in Healthcare* (SSH) were printed. In each article, the state of the science of that topic was presented. Across time, cost, accessibility, quality, and technology have affected progress. The advances in technology, coupled with lowered costs based on demand, and political and societal pressures for safety and competence in the past two decades have seen the greatest adoption and use of simulation in the United States in the health professions.

So, what has impacted the education of health professionals in the United States in the past two decades that has resulted in such growth and use of simulation? In two words, safety and competence. Two seminal documents from the Institute of Medicine (IOM), *To Err is Human: Building a Safer Health System* (Kohn, Corrigan, & Donaldson, 2000) and *Crossing the Quality Chasm: A New Health System for the 21st Century* (Institute of Medicine, 2001), focused the country's attention on safety concerns, workforce supply issues, and the emergent need to reform our healthcare delivery system.

This focus directly affected health professions schools and their need to produce competent and safe graduates. The availability of medium- and high-fidelity patient simulators boomed and the field of virtual reality and haptic systems began in both nursing and medical schools. The use of standardized patients also grew and more nursing schools adopted the use of these types of patients. Simulation was used for formative and summative evaluation, and the use of simulation for high-stakes evaluation was discussed (Boulet, 2008).

Several surveys of nursing and medical schools have been done over the past 11 years. In 2004, Nehring and Lashley surveyed the nursing programs at 18 universities and 16 community colleges in the United States and six international simulation centers that were using Medical Education Technologies, Inc. (METI, now CAE), high-fidelity simulators. They found that these programs were using the high-fidelity simulators in less than 5% of the curriculum and when found were used in foundation, physical assessment, and medical–surgical courses. The community college programs used the high-fidelity simulators for assessment, technical skills, critical events, and certain disease conditions most often. In the university setting, high-fidelity simulators were used for airway management, technical skills, critical events, and physiology.

Two follow-up studies were done in 2010 (Katz, Peifer, & Armstrong, 2010) and 2012 (Kardong-Edgren, Willhaus, Bennett, & Hayden, 2012). In 2010, the sample was 60 BSN nursing programs, an increase of over 300% from 6 years when the earlier study was published. The same courses were using simulators and also pediatric and maternity courses were mentioned. The growing lack of clinical placement sites pushed the need for more use of simulation to replace time in hospitals and other healthcare agencies. Additional reasons to use simulation were delegation, critical thinking, transition, and prioritization. The study by Kardong-Edgren and colleagues (2012) 2 years later involved all prelicensure nursing programs ($n = 1,060$), and the researchers found that approximately 1/3 used standardized patients and more than half used simulators. Courses and use of simulation were similar to the earlier studies. It is interesting to note the growth of simulation in nursing programs.

Surveys have also been completed for medical schools (Huang et al., 2012; Torre, Aagaard, Elnicki, Durning, & Papp, 2013). Huang and colleagues surveyed all North

American schools and teaching hospitals and found that simulation was used to evaluate core competencies and was used more in medical school than at the teaching hospitals. Torre and associates (2013) found that in the internal medicine clerkships in the United States that 84% (*n* = 72) use simulation to teach history taking, diagnostic reasoning, and clinical skills. Simulation was used to formatively and summatively evaluate core competencies. Standardized patients were used more often than simulators.

In medicine, simulation has been used to test competence as part of their licensing and certification. Since 2004, standardized patients have been used as part of the US national licensing process for Step II Clinical Skills (Rosen, 2008). The American Society of Anesthesiologists (ASA) mandated the use of high-fidelity simulators for Maintenance of Certification in Anesthesiology Programs (MOCA) in 2006. As of January 1, 2016, this mandate will no longer be required, although it will still be highly valued and can still be used for the Part 4: Improvement in Medical Practice requirement (ASA, 2015).

Simulation has been discussed for use in nursing licensure and certification and has not been adopted, but regulation of the use of simulation has been addressed. In 2008, Nehring surveyed the state boards of nursing in the United States to ascertain what regulations concerning simulation were in place. At that time, five states and Puerto Rico had regulated the substitution of clinical time with simulation, but Florida was the only state that had indicated a percentage of substitution (25%). Several states were giving approval for substitution and many more were considering such approval. This led to the landmark longitudinal, multisite study by the National Council of State Boards of Nursing (NCSBN) (Alexander, 2014). Five associate degree nursing programs and five university baccalaureate nursing programs representing the United States participated in this 3-year study in which the students were evaluated to see if simulation could replace 10%, 25%, or up to 50% of clinical time. The authors found that up to 50% of clinical time could be replaced with simulation. This finding will result in a significant change in the next several years for nursing programs. Additionally, in October 2015, the NCSBN published the study follow-up Simulation Guidelines for Prelicensure Nursing Programs (Alexander, Durham, Hooper, Jeffries, Goldman, Kardong-Edgren, et al., 2015).

The International Nursing Association for Clinical Simulation and Learning (INACSL) published seven standards of best practice in 2011, which were revised in 2013 (see Chapter 3) (INACSL, 2011, 2013; Rutherford-Hemming, Lioce, & Durham, 2015). Two additional standards covering the use of simulation in interprofessional education (VIII; Decker et al., 2015) and simulation design (IX; Lioce et al., 2015) were introduced in 2015. The topics of these standards are not unlike the dimensions of simulation first discussed by Gaba in 2004. In December of 2016, the most recent version was published-the INACSL Standards of Best Practice:

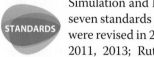

Simulation^SM (INACSL Standards Committee, 2016) is available at (www.inacsl.org).

In October 2015, NCSBN, after a review of their study results, the INACSL standards of practice, and the research literature regarding simulation, determined that it was time to issue simulation guidelines for all prelicensure nursing programs in the United States. These guidelines will need to be in place for a nursing program to be able to substitute up to 50% clinical time in simulation and state that:

1. There is a commitment on the part of the school for the simulation program.
2. Program has appropriate facilities for conducting simulation.
3. Program has the educational and technological resources and equipment to meet the intended objectives.
4. Lead faculty and sim lab personnel are qualified to conduct simulation.
5. Faculty are prepared to lead simulations.
6. Program has an understanding of policies and processes that are a part of the simulation experience (Alexander et al., 2015, p. 40).

Simulation, in many forms, has been a strong component of medical and nursing education for greater than a century, but the growth of the use of simulation has not been greater than in the past 20 years.

Emergence of Leaders

The primary users of simulation in the United States have been medicine and nursing, and its use in the military has led the technology advances that result in the equipment that we have available for use in educational and healthcare settings today. There have been many pioneers and leaders in the field of simulation, and different individuals have led the different areas of simulation and users have been noncompetitive. The most examined area currently is that of high-fidelity simulation. A review of the literature in both nursing and medicine since the late 1990s will illustrate the early pioneers and their achievements to those individuals leading the field today. Two names among the many pioneers that are most recognized are David Gaba (Gaba, 2004; Gaba & DeAnda, 1988) in medicine and Pamela Jeffries (2007b) in nursing.

Prevalence of Simulation-Based Education in the United States of America

The prevalence of different forms of simulation have been adopted by health professions faculty and healthcare agencies for use in education depending on cost and a champion(s) for its use. This is very true in nursing in the use of high-fidelity simulation. Many nursing programs acquired this technology when it was first introduced at meetings and through word of mouth. However, for programs that lacked a faculty champion there are many stories of the box holding the simulator remaining in storage and not used. Likewise, student experiences differed depending on the organization's ability to purchase different types of simulators from medium to high fidelity. As we know, simulators are not all created equal. But, it is safe to say that the use of medium- and high-fidelity simulators is here to stay in the United States for the education of health professionals. With the development of standards of practice (Decker et al., 2015; International Nursing Association of Clinical Simulation and Learning^SM, 2011, 2013; Lioce et al., 2015; Rutherford-Hemming et al., 2015) and guidelines for prelicensure nursing programs (Alexander et al., 2015) as well as certificate programs for simulation educators (e.g., Wright, Kim, Ross, & Pellegrini, 2011), the use of simulation to measure competency and safety is quickly becoming a standard part of the educational programs in the health disciplines, predominantly now in nursing and medicine.

National Agenda for Simulation

I believe that there is an informal agenda for simulation in the education and continuing education of health professionals in the United States, especially for nurses and physicians. Back in 2004, the Center for Telemedicine Law and Telemedicine and the Advanced Technology Research Center, US Army Medical Research and Materiel Command, sponsored a conference, inviting the leaders of simulation in medicine to present their work and discuss building a national agenda for the use of simulation in medical education. Rationales for this move were patient safety, ability to react quickly to public emergencies, competency of providers, and minimizing healthcare costs. Participants addressed the need for funding, the availability of simulators to meet need, curriculum development, increased research to show efficacy, buy-in from professionals in the field as well as organizations, and communication across different networks (Eder-Van Hook, 2004). The aims of this conference are still applicable and many of their recommendations have been realized.

Primary Users of Simulation in Healthcare in the United States

Today, simulation is being used in the classroom (at all levels), the clinical skills laboratory, the simulation lab, out in the field for such activities as disaster drills, in hospitals, and in other healthcare agencies. It is a tool for health professions education and continuing education as well as for exercises to measure patient safety. In the United States, besides the health fields, simulation is used in the air-

line industry and in nuclear energy fields (Bradley, 2006; Rosen, 2008).

The Prevalence of Simulation Programs in the United States

There is not an exact number of simulation programs in the United States. I would estimate that the majority of medical and nursing programs have at least one medium-fidelity simulator, and a large percentage of university-based nursing programs and medical programs have a high-fidelity simulator. The majority of medical schools use standardized patients. I would estimate that all health professions programs use task trainers. Many universities, especially those with academic health centers, have or are constructing simulation centers to be used for education across health disciplines. Several large hospital systems have also developed "virtual hospitals" for the use of their staff and area health programs. There are 264 simulation centers in the United States listed on the webpage for SSH (http://www.ssih.org/Home/SIM_Center_Director/Area/US). The MedSim Directory lists 423 simulation centers in the United States (http://MedSimdirectory.com).

Healthcare Sectors Experiencing the Most Growth in the United States

Education in medicine and nursing has seen the greatest growth for high-fidelity simulation. Medicine leads in the use of high fidelity, in the development of tools to measure competency in the use of the simulators, and in research to measure efficacy of the use of simulation in education to teach competency. Nursing follows, but, due to cost, use more medium-fidelity simulators across all programs, and the research has not been as sophisticated. Nursing has led the field in the development of standards and guidelines for use in education (Decker et al., 2015; Hayden, Smiley, Alexander, et al., 2014; International Nursing Association of Clinical Simulation and Learning, 2011, 2013; Lioce et al., 2015; Rutherford-Hemming et al., 2015). The other health professions are further behind.

As far as the use of simulation with specific specializations in healthcare settings, simulation is most often written about in critical care, anesthesiology, and emergency departments, followed by the other specializations as all have been written about. The simulators were manufactured with recommendations from physicians and nurses in those primary areas. See Chapter 1 for background on the development of the first high-fidelity simulators for use in anesthesiology and cardiac care. Subsequent simulators have been designed for obstetrical and pediatric purposes.

Examples of How Simulation Has Been Most Effective in the United States in Addressing Health or Educational Issues

Patient safety and competency of healthcare providers, namely, physicians and nurses, have been the primary motivators for the development of the simulators. As their use became more widespread, users asked for more specificity in the simulators, such as skin changes, bowel sounds, and the ability to seize. Early high-fidelity simulators had the capacity to compute different types of individuals, such as the overweight, middle-aged alcoholic who has a cardiac arrest, but the outward appearance of the simulator looked the same for all of these different individuals, so the ability to "morph" the simulator into different people had to be possible. As users asked for help from the vendors to address different clinical situations, such as end of life, their clinical educators addressed these issues. An example was the nursing curriculum designed by the team at Medical Education Technologies, Inc. (2010).

National and Regional Simulation Organizations in the United States

The SSH is considered the national simulation organization. Although originally the SSH was US based (see Chapter 4), it now has a strong international mandate (http://www.ssih.org/). The International Nursing Association for Clinical Simulation and Learning (INACSL; http://www.inacsl.org) also serves as a national organization for nurses and nursing educators in simulation (see Chapter 3). The National League for Nursing (NLN) has a Simulation Innovation Resource Center (http://www.nln.org/sirc) (see Chapter 5). In addition, simulator manufacturers such as Laerdal and CAE, offer regional and national meetings for users.

The United States is a known leader in the field of simulation. Through the educational programs, simulation centers, and organizations, including those organizations that regulate professional education and practice, simulation has evolved to be an integral part of measuring competency and assuring patient safety. Organizations also publish journals, such as the *Journal of Association of Standardized Patient Educators,* Cureus, the online journal of *International Pediatric Simulation Society, Simulation in Healthcare,* and *Clinical Simulation in Nursing,* that publish state-of-the-art best practices and research. Besides those activities already mentioned, many universities and their simulation centers and organizations offer degree programs and/or certificate programs for simulation educators and technicians (also see Chapters 10, 11, and 21).

Scholarly Works in Simulation in the United States

The literature on simulation is vast, especially in the past decade. The disciplines of nursing, medicine, and allied health in the United States have made significant contributions toward the advancement of simulation in recent years. Currently, interprofessional education and practice, educational efficacy, faculty development, and patient safety are areas of importance.

Funding for Simulation Programs in the United States

Funding for simulation programs greatly varies. Federal research funding has been low with only two grant cycles available from the Agency for Healthcare Research and Quality (AHRQ) (Huang et al., 2012). Many health professions programs charge a technology fee that provides funds for purchase and maintenance of simulators and use of standardized patients. Simulation centers charge for their services. Sustaining simulation centers has been the subject of articles (Baily, Bar-on, Yucha, & Snyder, 2013; Jeffries et al., 2013). Besides the articles listed above, the reader is encouraged to read the chapters on these topics in *Defining Excellence in Simulation Programs* (Palaganas et al., 2015). (See Chapter 11 for detailed information on simulation program management.)

Simulation is less accessible in many rural areas, but some rural schools have invested in simulation since clinical placements are scarce. The articles cited for sustaining simulation centers address the accessibility of simulation for rural areas and rural states.

Barriers or Challenges Encountered Integrating Simulation

The two major challenges today for integrating simulation in health professions education and practice in the United States are costs and faculty development. Costs have been mentioned throughout this chapter, but the need for faculty development in simulation is just as important. Nehring, Wexler, Hughes, and Greenwell (2013) summarized the literature on faculty development and the use of high-fidelity simulation. The growth of educational degree and certificate programs will help, but funding for this area of need is warranted.

Most Important Lesson Learned and Vision for Simulation

The most important lesson that I have learned as a dean of a College of Nursing is that it takes time and money to develop faculty to lead and to use simulation in their courses. The field of high-fidelity simulation is almost 20 years, and some would say more, but the integration of simulation into health professions education has been slow. Recent contributions to the field, such as the standards, guidelines, research results, development of tools, growth in the simulation organizations, availability of journals on the topic, and greater accessibility to lower priced simulators have all helped and should assist in advancing the field.

My vision for the future includes much change and disruption. Due to changes in healthcare delivery, advances in science, and changes in higher education due to technology and funding streams, a faculty "redesign" is evident. The traditional model of imparting wisdom and knowledge, both in classroom and in clinical settings, has become out of date. Students are also vastly different than the faculty; generational differences are great. Deans must rethink their budgets and the personnel makeup for their school to address the use of technology and learning styles. Virtual reality will also gain importance, along with simulators and standardized patients. In fact, advances in virtual reality should eventually replace standardized patients. Wearable technology will also dictate how health information is gathered for the population. Interprofessional education will be mandatory and omnipresent, and other disciplines will be greater partners with the health disciplines as never before. For example, engineers will join with health professionals to design the smart homes for the near future where the majority of healthcare will take place. Funding and faculty development will continue to be major challenges as will the need for research to sustain the evolution of this field.

16 Theoretical Principles to Effective Simulation
Timothy C. Clapper

Key Terms

Andragogy, Cognitive Load Theory, Cognitive Overload, Competence Constructivism, Deliberate Practice, Expertise, Facilitator, Fidelity, Imposter Syndrome, Just in time Training, Kirkpatrick's Educational Outcomes, Kolb's Experiential Learning Theory, Mastery Learning

Guiding Questions

1. Which practices may be best suited for assisting our learners with reaching the highest levels of clinical competence?

2. Why is it important to ground simulation-based education in theory?

3. How is reflection used in the learning process known as constructivism?

The Importance of Naming Your Practice

Name your practice, or *naming your practice*, "may be an American phrase used in academic circles that implies that a practitioner should be able to identify the theory(ies) that support or provide the basis for what they do in practice" (Clapper, 2015a, p. 134). As educators and researchers, it is important that we can *name our practice* for a number of reasons. First, we need to be aware of our educational philosophy of learning. Gutek (2004) suggested that a philosophy of education examines the meaning and purpose

of education (p. 2). We may strongly believe that an education experience should be an active one, but in practice, we may put our learners to sleep with a boring lecture. Argyris and Schön (1992) observed this discrepancy that often exists between a person's *espoused theory* and that theory put into practice referred to as the *theory-in-use*. At those moments when we might stray from our *espoused theory*, we can remind ourselves that is not who we are and what we stand for. When we know what we stand for and can name it, we also become aware of our bias, which is not necessarily a bad thing. In this chapter, I make it clear in a few places that I have my own bias that is based on years of research and practical experience. I let you, the reader, know about them so you can understand where I am coming from and you can make informed decisions about your own practice.

Another reason why we need to *name our practice* is so we can accurately justify the reason for what we do. For example, you will hear many in the simulation community making statements, such as Malcolm Knowles suggesting

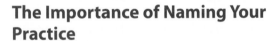

Timothy C. Clapper, PhD

that adult learners need to see that the instruction is relevant. If they read Knowles' books published in 1968/1980 (many did not, but they pass along this phrase/belief in periodicals, conferences, and conversations), they would know that Knowles did state the importance of relevance for adult learners, but in 1984, he published another book where he recognized that even younger learners need to know *why* they are learning something. We'll explore the important work of Knowles a bit more in this chapter.

Let's look at another reason to *name your practice*. Many of those educating with simulation are excellent clinicians, technicians, and leaders in their field. Some were moved into simulation with few education credentials and have been operating by what they think are best education practices (Clapper, 2014a), many for years now. Many serve or have served on education and certification committees in simulation organizations without the education credentials to support membership in those positions. Like the Knowles example above, their own beliefs, practices, and misconceptions get passed along to others and we end up with people who really want great educational outcomes that impact patient safety, but cannot get there. When you can *name your practice* and understand how people truly learn, you can design powerful simulation sessions that *will* make a difference. You can see why it is important to follow a simulation framework that allows a learner to go through the entire transformation process that is involved in learning and not piecemeal the session as is too popular today. It will also help you with becoming, as I like to refer to it, a **facilitator** *of learning* (Clapper, 2009). Rather than putting out facts through a lecture, you provide the environment and resources that provide learners with an enriching opportunity for change to occur. In this chapter, you will find that many researchers share this belief and have put it to practice.

Finally, in being able to *name your practice*, you will understand how important the term *best practice* really is and how it is lacking in the clinical and simulation community. Part of designing effective simulation sessions is looking at both the research and the needs of the organization you support. It makes no sense to include equipment and practices in your instructional plan and objectives that have been replaced or are viewed as inferior. You have to look at where the clinical errors are occurring and be able to research viable solutions so your learners receive quality sessions and you and your team can be seen as critical to the organization's success.

We begin our exploration with a brief overview of some thoughts on *expertise*. You might say it is a look at our ideal state or goal for learning so it is important to look at what some leaders in the field say about the subject. Following some insight on *expertise* and the professional path to reaching it, we will explore how people learn and of course,

we will look at what it means to facilitate good learning experiences. It is also important to look at how simulation in healthcare is currently being conducted. After exploring how people learn, you will be able to decide for yourself which framework is most suitable for your learners when you really want to make a difference. Finally, we will put it all together with some suggestions for implementation.

On the Road to Expertise

I do not like to use the term *expert* very often. To me, an *expert* is one who has learned everything in their field or craft. I am passionate about learning theory and how people learn and yet I always look forward to another curtain opening and being exposed to additional concepts, principles, or research that cause me to reflect on my practice and what I know. In this day of the Internet, we have no shortage of new or republished material, so we are ever learning, ever changing. Right up front I will state my personal bias/belief, and it is that we never reach expertise, but as professionals, we should strive to achieve it. Benner, Tanner, and Chesla (2009) wrote, "With expertise comes fluid, almost seamless performance" (p. 138). This is a desirable goal, but unlikely to be reached when we consider that every patient situation cannot be treated in the same way (Benner et al., 2009) and it is difficult to measure expertise because the variables differ greatly (Ericsson, 2006).

However, I agree with Benner et al. (2009) that as "experts," we can reach a state of practice where we can quickly see the big picture and get to work on the obvious in a situation, albeit as we will soon discover, this can come with a cost. Benner (1982) suggested that quality education and working experiences led the nurse from a *novice state* up to the desired *expert state* that we would like our professionals to attain. Using the Dreyfus Model of Skills Acquisition as a foundation, she developed the *five stages of clinical competence* generalized for nursing (Table 16.1).

Benner (1982) emphasized that experience is not based on time in a position or in a particular field. This statement is critical for you as a facilitator because again, I provide you with a preview of part of Knowles' (1984) position, which recognized that adult learners may have a vast amount of experiences, but they may not be quality ones. While Benner posits that experts no longer rely on guidelines, it might be that they have difficulty with doing so. Ericsson (2015) cites research where surgeons reported that they could only execute the most straightforward laparoscopic surgery cases according to simple rules. The surgeons found that they had to rethink how they would perform the procedures. Other cases and procedures also have several steps that must be taken by clinical care teams. Gawande (2009), surgeon, and author of the well-known

Table 16.1	Five Stages of Clinical Competence
Novice	Lacking experience, novice workers depend on context-free rules to make decisions.
Advanced	Operates on general guidelines. Needs assistance prioritizing what is most important.
Competent	Lacks speed and flexibility, but feels a certain sense of mastery. Develops new guidelines to coincide with existing rules. Achieved in 2–3 years.
Proficient	Looks at the whole picture rather than the parts. Through their experience, they consider less options and zoom in on the specific task. Achieved in 3–5 years.
Expert	No longer relies on guidelines and an assortment of possible solutions. Through their vast amount of experience, the expert considers fewer options and focuses on the task. Achieved in 5+ years.

Adapted from Benner, P. (1982). From novice to expert. *The American Journal of Nursing, 82*(3), 402–407.

book, *The Checklist Manifesto*, tells the story of a 3-year-old girl who became lost in the Alps while walking with her parents and fell through an icy pond. She became lifeless and was under the ice for 30 minutes before her parents reached her. For hours and days, teams of healthcare providers worked around the clock, performing thousands of tasks that brought this child back to a full recovery. But as noted by Gawande, many other drowning stories are not told because the patient did not make it. The patients did not recover for many reasons, including the difficulty of orchestrating and following the many critical steps that need to be taken in these cases.

With so many changing variables and perishable skills in the healthcare field, particularly if not used often and consistently, one's performance and knowledge of the task can decline. As such, you need to know that while *experts* can streamline their action process and go right to work on a clinical case, this same process can lead to clinical errors, which is why checklists and timeouts are important. From education to years of practice, many nurses know the importance of checklists. It was nurses who embraced the idea of checklists in the 1960s and entered into a routine of recording and checking vital signs at regular intervals (Gawande, 2009). Yet, I have worked with many nurses on education projects, including the development of central line maintenance procedures for 11 public hospitals in New York City (Clapper, 2012), who collectively acknowledged the necessity of a checklist for central line maintenance and other skills because the steps are easy to forget if not used or revisited often. All of the nurses working on this project were educators who later recognized how

valuable the project and the new checklist would be when teaching their own learners correct ways of performing maintenance on the lines. The expert may also leave out a large amount of information when teaching others. Let's look at a few specific cases:

A study by Crispen (2010) focused on the number of surgical experts it would take to teach a surgical resident to perform a cricothyrotomy. In this study, each individual surgery expert was asked to state the steps needed to perform a gold standard open cricothyrotomy, but Crispen found that the surgery experts *were only able to provide 56% of the total steps*. In another study, Canillas (2010) found that surgeons *omitted 30% of the action steps* and *35% of the decision steps* when describing the placement of a central venous catheter. Still other researchers (Clark, Pugh, Yates, & Sullivan, 2008) found that surgeons who described events, decision-making strategies, and problem-solving tactics used in emergency surgical situations omitted *65% of the procedural steps*. In yet another study, involving 50 senior nursing students, 100% of the participants committed errors in identifying rule-based errors, including failure to communicate assessment of respiratory status, confirming patient identity, errors related to allergies, recognize abnormal findings, and delayed or incorrect intervention/treatment (Henneman et al., 2010). While Henneman et al. recognize the need to identify strategies for reducing rule-based errors committed by the nursing students, they do not address the root cause of the 100% error rate, which may include inadequate or incomplete teaching of strategies by their clinical instructors to reduce rule-based errors.

As one who may have moved from the clinical setting to the educator setting, I am sure you can add volumes of examples based on observations of professionals or experts in action. Consider how healthcare professionals use the term *best practices* to describe what is done in clinical settings. Given the research provided above, we must consider whether professionals in any of the stages described by Benner really received the latest research as part of their instruction and whether or not they learned everything they were supposed to know. Research on why errors occur in the clinical setting show inadequate performance at the individual and team level (Box 16-1).

We might be able to define in some way what an expert is or what they might be able to do in practice. However, in the healthcare fields, we rarely have a plan to get the professional to that point, and as a result, patient safety can be negatively affected.

Bloom (1968) introduced teaching for mastery or **mastery learning** while looking at individual differences in the achievement of our school children. Mastery is set at a particular level and learners receive opportunities for practice, often including repetitive practice, along with practical feedback. With so much information to cover and a

---

Box 16-1   Clapper's Conflict Theory of Medical Errors

Based on what we know today, medical errors can occur because of

1. Inappropriate or inadequate skill performance at a particular time (conflict with themselves)
2. Inappropriate or inadequate team performance and communication at a particular time (conflict with other people)
3. Human factors issues: conflict between humans and their equipment (conflict with their clinical environment)
4. A combination of any of these variables

Adapted from Clapper, T. C. (2013a). In situ and mobile simulation: Lessons learned … Authentic and resource intensive. *Clinical Simulation in Nursing, 9*(11), e551–e557. doi:10.1016/j.ecns.2012.12.005

---

timeframe to graduation, most medical, nursing, and other healthcare learning institutions do not have the time and resources to enable mastery learning to occur. As previously noted, it is easy for anyone in the five stages of clinical competence to forget, especially regarding those tasks that do not present themselves very often in clinical settings. However, when we look for targeted solutions to common clinical error, mastery learning can be one solid solution and can occur in a simulation laboratory for learners at any stage of clinical competence. Mastery learning can be most beneficial through something referred to as **deliberate practice**. In the simulation community, *deliberate practice* is very often confused with *repetitive practice*. *Deliberate practice*, a *noun*, can include bouts of repetitive rehearsal or practice, a verb, but here is another example of not properly naming one's practice. *Deliberate practice* occurs when the learner recognizes the need to find safe opportunities to practice a skill(s) that they feel that they cannot do very well any longer (Clapper & Kardong-Edgren, 2012). That is, the learner makes "deliberate efforts to improve one's performance beyond its current level" (Ericsson, 2008, p. 991). Simulation educators allow the learner to practice as often as necessary to refresh or master a skill. The facilitator includes immediate feedback to the learner, reflection, and correction, until the skill can be completed with consistent success (Ericsson, 2008). There is a growing amount of evidence that deliberate practice may be very beneficial for improving the practice of healthcare workers. For example, Sullivan (2015) conducted an integrative review of the literature from three major research databases to explore effective training methods to improve retention of cardiopulmonary resuscitation (CPR) skills for nurses. Sullivan found that brief simulation sessions and deliberate practice provided the strongest evidence for practices that led to retention of CPR skills.

When providing opportunities for deliberate practice, it is important that the learning conditions, including the accuracies of the simulator, closely mirror or provide the same cues that the learner will encounter in the clinical setting (Ericsson, 2015; Kyaw Tun, Alinier, Tang, & Kneebone, 2015). Later in this chapter, in the section on *how we learn*, I will address multiple reasons why this is important to learning and practice.

One form of deliberate practice is something referred to as just-in-time training (JITT). With JITT, learners refresh on a particular skill immediately prior to performing it in a clinical setting. For example, a newer surgeon that plans to remove a gall bladder later in the morning might stop by the simulation lab and practice the procedure on a laparoscopic simulator. Likewise, a surgeon who has not performed this or many other procedures may do the same, so we can see how this technique may benefit novice and experienced professionals. The JITT may include other forms of multimedia in addition to a simulator. For example, a nurse may watch a video on how to perform maintenance on a catheter while also practicing on a central line catheter trainer. When we think about simulation, full-scale simulation comes to mind, where learners move through a clinical case or scenario using a patient simulator. However, as noted in Box 16-1, we have to remember that many of the errors that are created in healthcare are caused by inappropriate or inadequate skills. We can improve patient safety by encouraging and providing opportunities for *deliberate practice* and JITT for professionals at all five of the stages of clinical competence suggested by Benner. Both deliberate practice and JITT opportunities may be set up in skills labs or training rooms and depending on the type of simulator may not involve a lot of cost or attention from the simulation staff. Deliberate practice can produce a return on investment for your organization by increasing test scores for students and reducing errors for professionals. Of course, getting your learners into the simulation lab or center to take full advantage of the learning opportunities can be a challenge. As well as the long hours devoted to patient care, adult learners may have some other unique characteristics you need to know about to fully reach them.

Understanding the Adult Learner

As we transition into the topic of how people learn, it is appropriate to introduce some concepts and ideas pertaining to those who will likely be your #1 participants in your simulation center. In 1968, Malcolm Knowles proposed a theory that he referred to as an andragogy, which means "the art and science of helping adults learn" (p. 43). At that time, Knowles felt that his theory differed from preadult pedagogy because adults, he posited, possessed certain characteristics that made them unique learners. Some of these characteristic include:

- Self-directedness
- An accumulated reservoir of experience that becomes a resource for learning
- Readiness to learn and growing orientation to the developmental tasks of the learner's social roles
- Application of knowledge that is increasingly tied to application and problem centeredness (pp. 44–45)
- Internal motivation to learn
- The need to know why something should be learned (Knowles, 1984, p. 12)

I ask you to look at the list again and reflect on how much these characteristics are really isolated to adults (or not). We can think of some high school students who are certainly more focused, motivated to learn, and self-directed than some of our college-level learners. In addition, when we think about one's experiences, we have to ask, how, and where did they learn what they know. Are their experiences quality ones? The news is filled with stories of how teenagers knew exactly what to do in emergency situations, including calling 911 and performing CPR, while adult bystanders stood by in shock or awe. Further, look again at the last characteristic. Those of us with children and who work around them know what many children will say when we tell them to do something or teach them something ("why"?). While these characteristics are indeed important and very much applicable to adult learners, Knowles (1984) changed his position to recognize that andragogy is situation specific and not unique to adults.

As a facilitator in the simulation community, I keep hearing others around me referring to the work of Knowles. I always smile and suggest to them that there is more to adult learning than that observed by Malcolm Knowles. Based on a rich literature review, I suggested that adult learners possess six factors that we should consider as course developers and facilitators (Clapper, 2010a):

1. Adult learners may have had bad learning experiences in the past.
2. Adult learners prefer learning that is active, and they want to be assisted with making meaning of the information.
3. Learning is an emotional event.
4. Adult learners prefer assessment and improvement to evaluation and failure.
5. Adult learners want to leave the lesson with a better understanding of the content.
6. Adult learners have many other priorities in their lives.

While some of these characteristics may be self-explanatory, I will address them briefly and collectively. When my son was 7 years old, we were on an evening walk when he said out of the blue, "I love school." He attends a great school that is very supportive and nurturing and this caused me to reflect on my own learning experiences. Like him, first grade through fourth was some of the best times for me. The son of a military man, we moved a great deal, but we were geographically stable during those years. The teachers were supportive and kind. We read and were read to passively, but we seemed to have a vast number of hands-on experiences as well. I don't recall ever being ridiculed by a teacher or a fellow learner in those years and errors were opportunities for more learning. Like most others, we took examinations, but the teacher seemed to use several forms of assessment far more often than exams to observe where we were in our understanding. If we were on the wrong road, we were gently guided back to the learning objectives. I loved school too! Unfortunately, for many of our youth, especially young males (Whitmire, 2010), school experiences change greatly after the third grade and tend to transition from active learning centers to rote-memorization, testing places. From that point on, we seem to be competing more with one another than learning with and from one another. This pattern even continues into healthcare education as learners compete to get into certain schools, are educated in silos, but then expected to perform in a physician-nursing clinical team (Clapper, 2014b). What does this mean? It means that you can become a **facilitator** of learning and prepare full lessons that include strategies and activities that bring the learner to a fuller state of understanding that also leads to accomplishment of the objectives (Clapper, 2009). During the lesson, right from the start, we must also respect the knowledge and experience that the adult learner brings to our learning environment and ensure that we do not put them on the spot, call them out, or embarrass them. MacLean (1990) referred to this as keeping the learner in a positive learning state. In his *triune brain theory*, MacLean suggested that the brain consists of three sections where learning takes place: the neocortex, related to higher-level learning, the limbic system, where memories and emotions are processed, and the reptile or r-complex where the brain is concerned with survival, fight, or flight.

Most learning occurs in the limbic system in the center of the brain, and when the learning environment is a positive one, many connections are made in the neocortex through the process of reflection. However, when the learner feels they are threatened emotionally, they can *downshift* to the r-complex and have a difficult time focusing on the subject. In addition, as noted by Brookfield (1995), we always run the risk of exposing ourselves as the imposters that we feel we are, referred to as the **imposter syndrome**. That is, when we gather among other professionals like ourselves, we may feel like imposters, who are not supposed to be in that setting.

We may not ask questions or provide input because if our response is not 100% accurate we do not want others to think that we slid through the system somehow and are not really supposed to be there in that learning session (Clapper, 2010a, 2010b). Also, as learners, we do not want to follow along with a PowerPoint presentation and receive an examination or be thrown into a simulation scenario and evaluated. Instead, we want to have an opportunity to share and compare our experiences, learn new knowledge and skills in an active learning environment while receiving feedback on our performance, and be able to try out the new skills and knowledge. More directly, we are coming to your center or simulation lab to learn in a *psychologically safe and supportive environment* that is conducive to learning (Clapper, 2010b). Yet another thing that is important for you to know is that as adult learners, we have a lot going on (Clapper, 2010a). McClusky's (1963, 1970, 1974) *Theory of Margin* recognizes that adult learners take on more and more responsibilities as they mature and there is a struggle between power, load, and margin.

We have the ability or *power* to handle a certain amount of load, with *load* being all the tasks and responsibilities in our personal and professional lives. When the number of tasks (load) increase, we have less margin to take on additional ones. So when the learner comes into your simulation center, be mindful that they may not be immediately 100% tuned into urinary catheters or whatever the subject is for that particular session. They are very likely thinking about a number of things such as *did the kids get on the bus? How's my patient in room 302? Will we have a test after this course and will I be out in time to catch the train to work for my shift?* Please remember also that your learners may have had some bad learning experiences or heard horror stories about "scare and talk about it" methods of simulation (as described in Clapper, 2014a). The learners are thrown into a simulation scenario, with little to no active instruction beforehand, and then humiliated in a debriefing process. They may not be looking forward to going through a learning experience where they might be embarrassed or put on the spot. As an administrator and facilitator of a simulation center or lab, Thorndike's Law of Effect (1928) becomes very telling. Thorndike posited that behaviors followed by pleasant consequences will be more likely to be repeated in the future. That is one of our goals: to be seen by our learners as creators of enriching learning experiences and not as grim reapers looking for an "I got ya" moment. As a *facilitator of learning*, you will also be seen as one that can help them gain interest and focus on the subject to enhance the learning process (Clapper, 2009).

How People Learn

In describing how people learn, I could go all the way back to the work of Socrates and Plato, but I'll stay with author-researchers from the past 100 years or so. Since the late 1960s, we have increasingly placed labels or names on our practice, based on converging ideas emerging from research and practical educational practice. Most knowledge about learning stays the same but is always subject to investigation and the arrival of newer evidence. Through the years, many author-researchers may have offered a variation of the concepts, but I stay with descriptions of time-tested, and very often, research-supported practices involved in education.

My great-great uncle, Horace Mann, might be one of the first pioneers of what we know of the **constructivism** philosophy. According to Mann, the role of the teacher is to create relevance for the learner until the learner can find it themselves (Brooks & Brooks, 2001, p. 35; Cremin, 1957, p. 39). The need for relevance is applicable to both children and adult learners. Just as relevance is important to the learner, interest generated through the learning process may stimulate enough effort to allow learners to persevere through the lesson (Clapper, 2014a; Dewey, 1913). What Mann and Dewey described is something referred to as *situational interest*. *Situational interest* is generated in the learning environment and includes the attention and the reaction of the learner that may or may not last over time (Hidi, 1990; Hidi & Baird, 1986). Some learners may come into the learning environment with an *individual interest* or even a *passion* for the subject, but in many cases, we have to create *situational interest* in the topic. For example, I love learning and reading about almost anything related to learning theory and how people learn best. Years ago, in a workshop on brain-based learning, the facilitator created *situational interest* in the topic that lasted throughout the entire session. I can say that I was a bit hesitant in the first part of the workshop so he did not have the fishhook set, as they say. But as the days went on, I was sold on this method of learning. Following the workshop, when opportunities came for me to acquire more about how people learn and how to support those beliefs, I jumped on them. I enrolled in a graduate program and just kept going. That is to say, that workshop created *situational interest* in learning theory and practice, which progressed to an *individual interest*, and as is known to many now is a *passion* of mine. As soon as situational interest was established, *effort* followed (Dewey, 1913).

As well as emphasizing interest, Mann posited that information cannot be poured into a learner's head and each person played an active role in constructing their own learning, which may be scaffolded and aided by others (Clapper, 2011a; Cremin, 1957, p. 37). As well as serving as the basis of *constructivism*, Mann's emphasis for scaffolding and aiding others in the learning environment to help them reach new levels of understanding would later be supported by Vygotsky's (1978c) *Zone of Proximal Development* (ZPD) theory (Clapper, 2015b).

The concept or philosophy of *constructivism* holds that knowledge is constructed by the learner, sometimes with the assistance of others (Montessori, 1949; Piaget, 1962, 2008; Vygotsky, 1978c). Although Dewey and Piaget can certainly be credited with building much of what we know about *constructivism*, Maria Montessori is perhaps the only one to consistently emphasize the term *construct*, as it refers to the process of learning. Just as Piaget discovered while conducting research under the supervision of Montessori on learners many thought were hopeless and could not be reached, we all have an inner teacher within us. It is the facilitator's role to step aside from one of being a teacher and instead master the "method of non-intervention" (Montessori, 1949, p. 146). The facilitator's job is to prepare an enriching environment for learning to occur and to intervene only as much as necessary (Montessori, 1949) to assist the learner with achieving the learning objectives. As I tell my learners that are developing their facilitator skills, I cannot change a person or teach them anything. Instead, I can provide the resources and create the conditions for the person to consider the need to change (Clapper, 2014a). If a learner changes a behavior or belief, it is because of intrinsic motivation and identifying the need to change what they know or do and not because I asked them to change (Argyris & Schön, 1992; Clapper, 2014a). As noted by Montessori, children learn difficult tasks such as language all on their own (Montessori, 1949) and seeking information and knowledge is a lifelong endeavor for us all. Everything we learn becomes a schemata or *frame of reference* (Piaget, 1962) or ways of knowing, which are very unique to each learner (Clapper, 2010a). Learners will enter a learning environment with these *frames of reference* that can be built upon or restructured (Piaget, 1962)—that is of course *if* the learner sees a reason to change (Argyris & Schön, 1992).

To illustrate the effect of mental models or frames of reference, think of the movie *Slumdog Millionaire* (2008, Screen International Films). The participant is going through India's version of the television hit, *Who Wants to be a Millionaire*. Each time the game participant is asked a question, he *reflects* back to very real-life situations that cause him to know the answer that he will provide to the game host. What the learner knows or holds as *frames of reference* are very real to them and often formed by experience. The learner may reflect upon what they know and consider new information and *assimilate* easily. Alternatively, they may go through a *state of disequilibrium*, where the new information contrasts with information that is not associated with anything the learner currently knows (Clapper, 2015b; Piaget, 1962). The learner may be in what Vygotsky (1978c) described as the *Zone of Proximal Development* (ZPD). In the ZPD, the facilitator, and other learners as well, can scaffold or support the learner and scaffold them with learning more than they might have on their own. This process may include assisting the learner with working through

the *disequilibrium process* and moving toward a level of *accommodation*, where they make the new information or behavior their own. Active learning *experiences and reflection* throughout the learning process are important elements of *constructivism*.

As I share with my newer facilitators, for learning to occur, we have to do something with the information and reflect upon it. Montessori (1949) noted that the mind is always active and the learning environment should be as well. Consistent with everything we described to this point, Dewey (1938) emphasized the importance of learning through continuous cycles of *experience and reflection*. Like Montessori, Dewey posited that the learner should be involved in active learning opportunities or experiences to construct their knowledge, but each also needed time *during* the learning process to reflect on what has been gained during the active learning experience (Dewey, 1938). This *reflection-in-action process* (Argyris & Schön, 1992) assists the learner with altering or building the frames of reference they came into the environment with and should not be confused with a debriefing or *reflection-on-action* process (Argyris & Schön, 1992) that should occur following the entire learning session. Through our individual reflection and the thoughts shared by others in the learning environment, we can sort and process even the most difficult information.

Based much on the work of John Dewey, Kolb developed his cycle of *Experiential Learning Theory* (Fig. 16.1), which he suggested was "a combination of grasping and transforming experience" (Kolb, 1984, p. 41). *Experiential learning* begins with the learner being involved in an experience (concrete experience). The learner may reflect on the experience (reflective experience) and try out

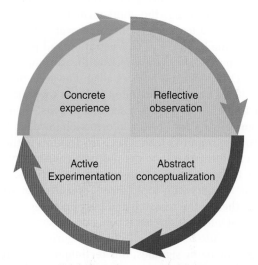

Figure 16.1 Kolb's Cycle of Experiential Learning. (From Kolb, D. A. (2015). Experiential Learning: Experience as the Source of Learning and Development, 2nd Ed. Reprinted by permission of Pearson Education, Inc., New York, New York.)

the new skills/knowledge (abstract conceptualization). Completing the cycle, the learner may learn from the experience and try out what they have learned (active experimentation).

In a cycle of learning, I cannot overemphasize the power of collaborative and social learning. While some learners may prefer to work alone (Dunn & Dunn, 1978), researchers such as Albert Bandura suggested that we can learn quite a bit more by working with others. Bandura (1977b) observed that learning can take place directly and vicariously, meaning through the experience of others. Let me explain with a bit of depth how Bandura's *Social Learning Theory* works in real instructional settings using simulation. When I facilitate team-based courses, I almost always train more than one team at a time. For example, a shoulder dystocia course would include two teams, with each team sitting together at separate tables in the same classroom. I do not lecture very long to the class or provide mountains of reading materials. From what you have read so far, we know that long lectures are not the way to go since the learner would likely be in a passive state and is not doing anything with the information that could assist them with altering their existing frames of reference. If I am lecturing a long time, the learner also may be still thinking of something on slide 9 and I am now on slide 26. If I pass out mountains of articles, especially if I do so along with a heavy lecture, I may overload the *information processing* abilities of the learner. This overloaded mental state is best described in **cognitive load theory**, introduced by Sweller (1988), who suggested that we need to consider the way that we as humans process information. Sweller noted that the brain can only process so much information at a time in short term memory. When the learner experiences too much information concurrently or when the information cannot be readily sorted to enable processing, the short-term memory is overloaded and the learner may become overwhelmed. The result for the learner can be frustration and poor learning outcomes. *Cognitive overload* of the working memory can affect experts and novices alike; however, the latter would likely be more frustrated because they may have fewer frames of reference or schema to assist them with problem-solving and sorting information (Sweller, 1988).

To ease cognitive load, I keep my lectures in the very intense, informative shoulder dystocia course very brief. Rather than providing the mountains of articles, I provide the learners with topic sheets organized by subject that synthesize the research and best practices. The vast amount of information that is being processed is grouped or *chunked* into brief, but effective categories of information. As the name signifies, this technique is referred to as *chunking*. Chunking assists the learner with sorting and categorizing the information so they can process the information more readily. It also enables the learner to make quicker connections with existing *frames of reference* they currently hold in their minds (Williams & Dunn, 2008).

Each learner reads through the topic sheet and is free to reflect, highlight, and place notes in the margins. Remember why this is important: the learner must *reflect and do something* with the information. Everything the learner will do in the instructional plan requires them to think about what they know, consider alternatives and new knowledge, and then do something with it, such as discussing it or putting it to action. Once they have completed that task, they talk freely to the entire group at their table and share what they learned, found interesting, and even express their disagreements. Keep in mind that if I lectured for a long period of time and I was someone that the learner looked up to (and perhaps somewhat feared), the learner may never speak up and voice their disagreement with the content or something I said. But in these smaller groups, the learners tend to speak openly and express themselves more. Here is where the ZPD and Piaget's description of the *disequilibrium state* arise and why *Social Learning Theory* is so important. I have witnessed very seasoned clinicians expressing disagreement (*disequilibrium state*) over some new evidence presented in a topic sheet. It was others in the group (or myself) that assisted them with working through this *disequilibrium* state and helping them to *accommodate* the new information in the ZPD (Fig. 16.2). Another cognitive load–based intervention, worked out modeling (WOM), is described by Josephsen in the Voice of Experience that follows.

16-1 Voice of Experience
Meeting the Challenge with Worked out Modeling (WOM)

Jayne Josephsen, EdD, RN, CHPN

The Challenge

Simulation can be a complex and challenging instructional intervention that can overwhelm students with the multitude of interactive elements, emotional aspects of the experience, or unfamiliarity with the topic or setting. This can cause cognitive overload and detract from student learning. Cognitive load theory (CLT) examines and applies the various aspects of cognitive architecture, such as working memory, long-term memory, schema development, and cognitive load to instructional design. The learning process is affected by each of these aspects. Common simulation design features include the use of several extraneous distractors or requiring the student to determine the correct intervention with little guidance. This can cause overloaded working memory and lead to inaccurate knowledge being gained or the inability of the student to transfer knowledge gained into a schema for future application. To create an optimum learning environment, nursing educators need to be cognizant of the impact of cognitive architecture and load in simulation design and implementation.

Meeting the Challenge

CLT-based interventions can assist with this challenge. Worked out modeling (WOM) is one such technique that models a skill or procedure by a nurse paired with verbal/gestural descriptions of critical thinking processes and pathophysiological connections to the content. WOM can be used for imitation, comparison, or as representation of a standard of practice. WOM provides students a schema concerning multiple element interactivity and a problem-solving framework to use in their nursing practice. WOM was offered in video form to senior level nursing students participating in a two patient simulation, where one patient has multiple issues related to a nasogastric tube and another patient experiences a fall.

Outcome

Posttest evaluation identified that the group that received the WOM video prior to simulation participation scored significantly higher on post fall management knowledge. Students indicated that viewing the video assisted in decreasing simulation anxiety and found that the explanations the nurse gave concerning thought processes assisted their learning.

Most Valuable Lessons Learned

Use of WOM could be enhanced if used in a less complex simulation with the focus on a few aspects of care. The patient with the nasogastric tube issue had many interacting elements and various schemas that needed to be utilized in decision making. The patient fall scenario was more specific and the students took away a schema that can be applied to the clinical setting as evidenced by posttest scores.

Providing a version of WOM prior to simulation participation has a positive effect on student learning by decreasing mental load/anxiety and increasing schema development that can be translated into the student's future nursing practice.

Inspiration for Simulation Champions

"A mind when stretched by a new idea never regains its original dimensions."
—Oliver Wendell Holmes, Sr.

Applying diverse educational theories and interventions to nursing simulation can assist in meeting cognitive architecture and student learning needs. The integration of CLT and interventions such as WOM can provide a framework for the educator to create a safe and supportive learning environment with quality outcomes.

But Social Learning Theory does not stop there in these sessions. Let me continue the example so you can see how it can affect other portions of the learning plan, including the subsequent simulation case or scenario. Following what I refer to as the *gather phase* of learning, where learners are provided demonstrations, receive information as described above, and have opportunities to practice, they are placed into a scenario. One team goes through the scenario while the other stays with me in the classroom/control room and *actively* observes. This means they follow along with a rubric and take notes of what went well and not so well with the first group based on what they learned in the gather

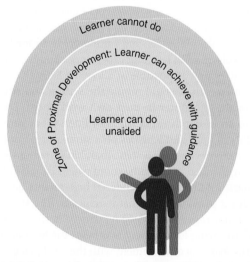

Figure 16.2 Vygotsky's Zone of Proximal Development. (Adapted from Vygotsky, L. S. (1978). *Mind in society: The development of higher psychological processes*. Cambridge, MA: Harvard University Press.)

phase. After the first group has completed the case or scenario, the second group assists me with a debriefing by sharing some of their observations. Following the debriefing, the second group will go through a scenario. Who do you think performs better? You got it—the second group. In line with *Social Learning Theory*, they look on and learn *vicariously*, or *through the actions and feelings of others*, brought out in a robust objective-based reflection process.

When both groups have completed the scenarios and the second group is debriefed on the scenario they went through, I conduct a classroom-wide debriefing. Just because the learners went through a realistic scenario does not imply that they will be able to connect the learning experience(s) they went through with their actual clinical settings. Dewey (1938) recognized that learning is often *situational* or is often situated, existing between the person and the situation, something referred to as *situated cognition*. *Situated cognition* helps us understand that each learner's experiences are very unique to them and they need to be assisted with *transferring* that knowledge to other settings (Bransford, Brown, & Cocking, 2000, Dewey, 1938). *Transfer* (from one *phase of learning to another* or from *learning environment to work environment*) is facilitated much easier when we consider Thorndike's (1923, 1924a, 1924b, 1932) *theory of connectionism*. Thorndike suggested that the closer the elements are to one another between situations or environments, the more likely the stimulus–response mechanism will remain the same (Clapper, 2013a). In the world of simulation, *connectionism* is everything and we must consider **fidelity** as an important tool for helping us connect the learning environment to the working environment. Kyaw Tun et al. (2015, p. 164) present the best definition of fidelity when they suggest that fidelity is "An intrinsic property of simulation and can be defined as the degree of accuracy to which a simulation, whether it is physical, mental, or both, represents a given frame of reality in terms of cues and stimuli, and permissible interactions."

The tools, materials, and simulators used for learning in all levels of a full learning experience should be as close to the real thing as possible or allow the learner to receive efficient *cues* that would mimic the setting and situations they might encounter in their own workplaces. I will not go into an in-depth explanation of fidelity, but remember this: lots of bells and whistles on a simulator do not imply high fidelity. I can have a static manikin or patient simulator lying in a bed in the same room where I am conducting a scenario and it can be considered high fidelity because of the cues it provides and what it achieves. The static mannequin may represent a sleeping patient in the same room that I am caring for a patient and helps the learner to connect the learning environment with the workplace.

As we have seen, many theories support our practice in the learning environment. I will move on to an overview of some of the frameworks involved in simulation, but before I do, I would be remiss if I did not include a couple more final

concepts that are important when considering simulation and instructional design. With everything we have read, we can appreciate the need for *active and reflective* learning experiences, but learners also need to make numerous connections with the materials that can lead to better understanding and superior learning outcomes. You may have read or heard that we possess certain *learning styles* or *learning preferences*. The Dunn and Dunn learning styles model (1978, 1992) included three modality preferences that affect the way a person learns: auditory, visual, and tactile/kinesthetic. If we were to subscribe to the many surveys, we would believe that we have a preference for a certain modality, and in some cases, this is true. For example, males tend to be more visual, tactual, or kinesthetic, prefer to move around, and prefer to work alone (Dunn, 1996; Marcus, 1979), while females generally tend to be auditory learners (Dunn, 1996). However, we should not fall into the trap of thinking that we have to cater to a learner's preference. What is important to remember is that the more ways a person can *see it, hear it, and do it*, the more you can help them make better connections with the content (Clapper, 2012). The learning styles or preferences were updated in 2009 according to international findings and now consist of six perceptual modalities including (1) auditory, (2) visual/picture, (3) visual/print, (4) tactual, (5) kinesthetic, and/or (6) verbal/kinesthetic (Dunn et al., 2009, p. 136).

Remember that gather phase I described earlier when I provided an example from a shoulder dystocia course? Through the demonstration, brief lecture, topic sheets, and opportunities for practice, I incorporate every one of these learning preferences and in doing so provide numerous ways for learners to use the six perceptual modalities or learning styles to make some nice connections with the content (Table 16.2).

Lastly, something to consider is the order for presentation of learning materials. A nurse I worked with was assigned a task to build a teamwork course for surgeons. I asked him about his plan and he said that he would show them a video of bad teamwork and an airline disaster, provide them a lecture on some crew resource management concepts, place them in a scenario with a surgical case, and then debrief them. If you followed along with the chapter, you will pick out several things that conflict with what we know about good learning principles. You may say that the learners will have a difficult time with *connectionism* and *transfer* because they may struggle with connecting teamwork in an airplane with the simulated case or with their own workplace. You may also say that they were only provided the video and the lecture so they were not able to *construct* or alter existing *frames of references* through *action and reflection*. You may also reflect and note that there were likely few opportunities for the learners to activate all the *learning styles* and make numerous connections with the content. In addition to many possible ways that this plan could lead to poor learning outcomes, there is a

Table 16.2	Six Perceptual Modalities Applied to the Shoulder Dystocia Course

Goal: Activate All of the Learning Styles to Make More Connections with the Content

Learning Style	Method
Auditory	Lecture and discussion of what occurs during a shoulder dystocia and how the clinician manages it
Visual/Picture	Anatomical drawings of what occurs during a shoulder dystocia
Visual/Print	Topic sheets or readings from textbooks or journal articles
Verbal/Kinesthetic	Flow diagrams and algorithms about shoulder dystocia management
Tactual Kinesthetic	Participating in shoulder dystocia simulation

Adapted from Dunn, R., Honigsfeld, A., Doolan, L. S., Bostrom, L., Russo, K., Schiering, M. S., …, Tenedero, H. (2009). Impact of learning-style instructional strategies on students' achievement and attitudes: Perceptions of educators in diverse institutions. *The Clearing House, 82*(3), 135–140.

chance that we could leave the learners struggling with the learning goals for the session. Described as *contextual or cognitive interference* (Clapper, 2011b), learners who are exposed to correct and incorrect information during the learning process in simulation-learning events can leave struggling to remember the correct information. If we did want to show a video to establish *situational interest*, we can show one that is related to surgical cases or the topic being studied. But as it relates to learning material, it is far better to show the video of things that went well first. After they have an opportunity to actively work through the learning materials of a well-developed lesson plan that includes simulation, we can show the incorrect information and ask the learners to identify why it is not ideal for their work settings. In this way, they have made new connections and strengthened others and they are now applying what they have learned. This also provides you, the facilitator, with another opportunity to *assess* your learners and not wait until an end of course evaluation that might come too late to correct misconceptions in learning. Please remember that each of your learners will come into the learning situation with varied expertise levels and levels of knowledge. They will leave your simulation center with experiences that are very unique to each of them. We want those experiences to be quality ones so we can maximize the chance that they will have good clinical outcomes at the patient care level. To do so, you will need a philosophy of learning, which hopefully you have started to acquire at this point, and a *framework for simulation* that matches your new *espoused theory* and *theory-in-use*.

Frameworks for Simulation: Things to Consider

As described in Table 16.3, the simulation community currently uses many variations, models, and I hesitate to say, frameworks for simulation-based instruction. The simulation community lacks a framework for conducting simulation-based instruction (Chiniara et al., 2013). The healthcare simulation community often refers to Jeffries's (2007) theoretical framework as a framework for simulation, something that I argue it is not. What Jeffries describes in the nursing education simulation framework are good education practices. Some of these practices recognize the need for collaboration and the necessity to consider important issues such as the knowledge level of the students going through a simulation experience (p. 23). Like the simulation design standards developed by International Nursing Association for Clinical Simulation

Table 16.3	Models or Frameworks for Simulation Currently in Use
Scenario	Learners are brought into the environment and placed in a case-based clinical scenario.
Lecture + Scenario	Learners receive a lecture on the content before being placed in a case-based clinical scenario; the lecture may occur weeks, days, hours, or minutes in advance. The case-based clinical scenario may last 2 min or 2 hr.
Scenario + Debriefing	Learners are brought into the environment and placed in a case-based clinical scenario. The scenario is followed by a debriefing that may occur weeks, days, hours, or minutes after the scenario.
Lecture + Scenario + Debriefing	Learners receive a lecture on the content before being placed in a case-based clinical scenario; the lecture may occur weeks, days, hours, or minutes in advance. The scenario is followed by a debriefing that may occur weeks, days, hours, or minutes after the scenario.
Clapper's Brain-Based Learning Framework for Simulation	**Inquire Phase:** Learners transfer in existing knowledge and establish situational interest. **Gather Phase:** Learners examine new skills and facts, receive demonstration of evidence-based practices, and try them out. **Process Phase:** Learners use their new skills in a case-based clinical scenario that lasts only as long as it takes to achieve specific learning objectives. **Debriefing-Apply Phase:** Learners receive debriefing immediately after the scenario, to help learners solidify and transfer the new skills and knowledge to their clinical settings.

STANDARDS

and Learning (INACSL) (INACSL Standards Committee, 2016) and the framework proposed by Chiniara et al. (2013) and many others in the simulation community, the literature too often specifies a good theoretical framework for conducting *the case or scenario* or how to conduct a debriefing. By themselves, the *case-based clinical scenarios* may not provide the complete learning experience that is necessary for a learner to modify or add to their existing *frames of reference*.

If we are to really make a difference for patient safety, we must make the time to incorporate best instructional and learning practices. That is, we must use a more complete framework that moves beyond using only a scenario and debriefing model, or the lecture, scenario, and debriefing pattern.

At the beginning of the chapter, we noted that our learners have received instruction that was in many cases incomplete and not based on best practices. They deserve an opportunity to move through a complete learning experience that provides them with an opportunity to learn new skills and knowledge and work through the disequilibrium state that often accompanies reframing what we know. As noted, many instructional design models are available today. I will caution you to do some research and select one that was developed by educators using good instructional design principles. Just because it may be popular in the simulation community does not mean it should be considered best practice. It may mean that a vast number of people are following the wrong path paved by well-meaning pioneers in healthcare simulation. The one I use for my own sessions is modified from the Williams and Dunn (2002, 2008) four-phase lesson plan, which coincides with the way that the brain prefers to process information. As shown in Table 16.3, I establish *situational interest* and transfer in existing knowledge with an *inquire phase*, provide a demonstration of correct application of skills and rich sources of information in a *gather phase*, allow the learners to go through a realistic scenario in a *process phase*, and provide a debriefing in the *apply phase* to assist the learners with transferring the new knowledge and skills to their workplace.

I will argue that the *gather phase*, very often left out of a learning plan, is the most important phase of learning for all the reasons we addressed in this chapter. Learners can review the evidence, practice new skills, and see a reason to change almost immediately *before* moving into the scenario. Rarely is a professional with years of experience going to change their skill or behavior because you helped them reflect upon the need to do so. Debriefing is an important part of an instructional plan, but far from a magic wand, far better to get the learner's *buy-in* prior to the scenario. The *unfreezing process* that often occurs in a learning plan as described by Kurt Lewin occurs in the *gather* or "fact finding" phase of learning (1947, p. 13) when learners "practice with new information and skills and consider adopting them for their own theory-in-use" (Argyris & Schön,

1992; Clapper, 2014a, p. 173). The simulation scenario that follows the *gather phase* assists the learners with applying the new skills and information in a realistic manner to help them transition to new levels of understanding. The debriefing that should follow the scenario is conducted with a goal of helping the learners to "refreeze their performance" to the new standard (Clapper, 2014a, p. 173; Lewin, 1947, p. 35) and transferring the new behavior to their clinical settings. Remember: very few opportunities exist for a group of learners to go back through a simulation scenario following a debriefing (Clapper, 2014a), so understanding how one really learns helps us to appreciate the importance of that *gather phase* of learning and a *complete framework for learning*.

Multimedia and Learning Theory

Why discuss multimedia? Because in this day and age, you will very likely incorporate the use of multimedia in your presentations. In addition, hybrid simulation incorporates more than one simulation modality. We can bring standardized patients into our scenario, incorporate 3D virtual simulators, or most any combination of simulators to achieve the most realism in the experience.

We may even ask the learners to complete some coursework ahead of time. This can be as simple as providing articles for peruse or more complex coursework that they must complete prior to entering your classroom. A word of caution, recall what we learned from McClusky (1963) and his *theory of margin*. From my vast experience and the experiences of many simulationists I know, I can state that many of your learners will probably not complete the precourse work. Of those that do, many of them will skim the material at best. Some educators place an examination at the end of the coursework to ensure that the learners complete the assignment. As well as what we have shown to this point on how people learn best, these facts should also be considered. If the material can be covered in class, in collaborative learning communities where learners can assist one another, and there may be less distractions, you may find more benefit by moving the content into the classroom. In addition, some learners may not have reached the level of self-directed learning we would like them to be at and they may require additional scaffolding. When you do incorporate the use of precourse work or simply incorporate the use of multimedia, use it wisely and effectively.

Moreno and Mayer (2000) conducted a vast amount of research into how to best incorporate the use of multimedia. I will not reprint them, because the content in Figure 16.3 is self-explanatory. However, I ask you to observe how relevant the Dunn learning styles are to Moreno and Mayer's findings. Remember when it comes to learning, whether through digital means or face to face, help your learners *see it, hear it, and do it* in many ways so they can make multiple connections with the content. In addition, notice how the research supports best practices for reducing *cognitive load* while enhancing the learning process.

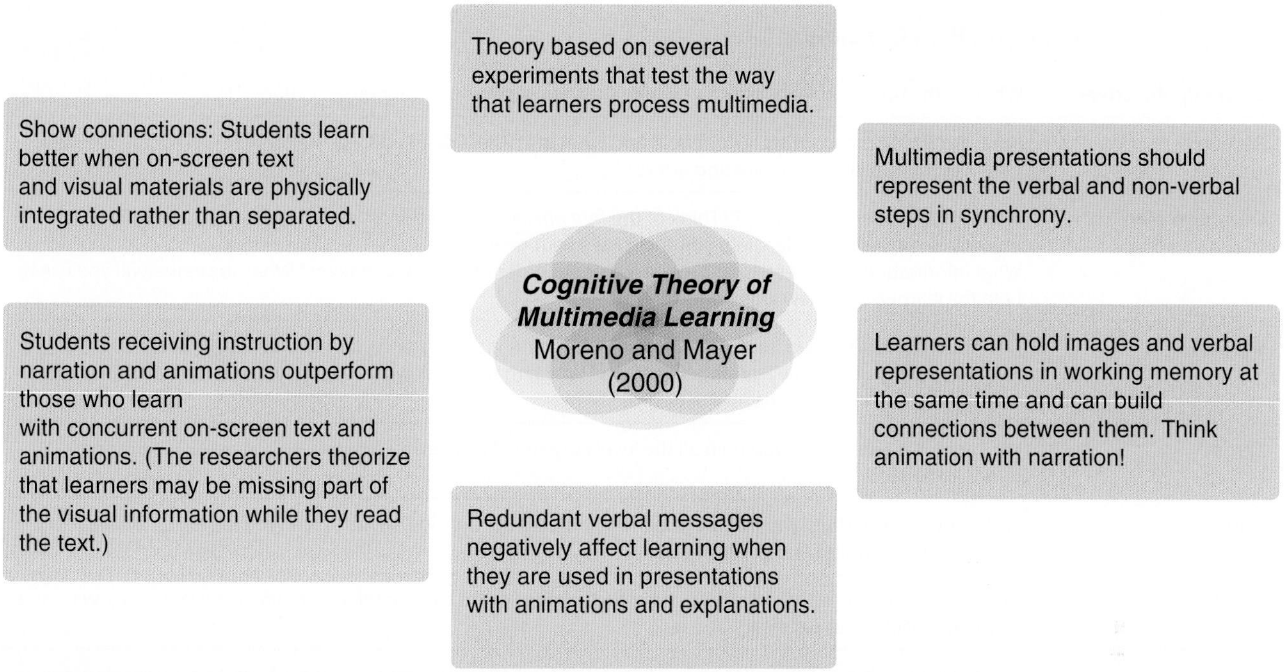

Theory based on several experiments that test the way that learners process multimedia.

Show connections: Students learn better when on-screen text and visual materials are physically integrated rather than separated.

Multimedia presentations should represent the verbal and non-verbal steps in synchrony.

Cognitive Theory of Multimedia Learning
Moreno and Mayer
(2000)

Students receiving instruction by narration and animations outperform those who learn with concurrent on-screen text and animations. (The researchers theorize that learners may be missing part of the visual information while they read the text.)

Learners can hold images and verbal representations in working memory at the same time and can build connections between them. Think animation with narration!

Redundant verbal messages negatively affect learning when they are used in presentations with animations and explanations.

Figure 16.3 Cognitive Theory of Multimedia Learning. (Adapted from Moreno, R., & Mayer, R. E. (2000). A learner-centered approach to multimedia explanations: Deriving instructional design principles from cognitive theory. *Interactive Multimedia Electronic Journal of Computer-Enhanced Learning, 2*(2). Retrieved from http://imej.wfu.edu/articles/2000/2/05/index.asp)

Summary: What This Means to You... Putting Theory to Practice

The Kirkpatrick's (1994) educational outcomes model serves us well as a training evaluation tool. As shown in Table 16.4, the Kirkpatrick model presents four levels, including two that are training or classroom based and result from the learning experience and two levels that result in changes in practice or behavior within the organization.

Although simulation in healthcare is still relatively new, we have seen more than 20 years of growth in the use of simulation, but very little research that moves past the first two levels (Clapper, 2013b; Sullivan, 2015). This state of research may be the result of inadequate instructional practice and a lack of understanding of how learning occurs (Clapper, 2013b).

Based on what you have learned in this chapter, you have an opportunity to make a real difference at the patient care level. I offer some additional suggestions (Table 16.5) of how to apply some of what you learned in a learning plan. Notice in the resources section that time is a consideration. I can bring new learners through a rapid session that makes little difference and puts my simulation center in jeopardy because I cannot make a difference in patient care. Alternatively, I can be a major part of finding real solutions to problems in my organization and present sessions that take a bit longer to facilitate, but may reach the last two levels of Kirkpatrick's educational outcomes.

Most of us will choose the second option, but still too many do not reach that goal because they are stuck in the status quo or do not have a plan to put this belief to practice. Recall that at the beginning of this chapter, I mentioned that you will have to develop your own philosophy of learning and be able to name your practice. Now that you know how people learn and can name your practice, what will it look like?

Table 16.4	Kirkpatrick's Educational Outcomes		
Reaction	**Learning**	**Behavior**	**Results**
Course evaluation	*Pretest/ posttest*	*Observable application in work setting*	*Impact on organization goals*
Learner likes instructor; learner likes course; instruction is useful	Learning is quantified; one or more means of assessment.	Behavior transferred from the classroom to the workplace	Observable change in practice that affects patient care
Learning		Change in behavior and practice	

Adapted from Kirkpatrick, D. L. (1994). *Evaluating training programs: The four levels*. San Francisco, CA: Berrett-Koehler Publishers.

Table 16.5	Learning Plan Considerations
Learning objectives	Where is the need? Look at errors and where they are occurring in your organization.
Research	What are the common errors in your field and what did others do to address the problem? What are the best practices for reducing or eliminating errors?
Develop a plan	What will be your learning plan? (Think of the *four phases* or something similar). Based on the learning objectives, how will this plan help you to achieve your goal? What information/skills need to get to the learner in order to change behaviors? What strategies will you use to help the learners gain new knowledge and skills?
Resources	How much time is needed for the instruction? What amount/types of equipment do I need to achieve the right level of fidelity to reach the learning objectives? Which materials do you need for your instructional plan? Who will facilitate or assist with the instruction?
Target	Who are my learners? Can you train all the levels together? How many sessions do you need to train your target audience?
Scenario	Which scenario will help you reach the learning objectives? Consider a useful scenario template, available on several simulation sites and publications.
Assessment	How can you assess the learner throughout the session so you can reinforce or redirect the learners toward the learning objectives as necessary?
Pilot	When will the rehearsal and pilot course occur? Who will the pilot course include? Note: this is important for tweaking your instructional plan and addressing shortcomings before you roll out the course to your audience.

17

Key Strategies for Enhancing Evidence-Based Practice in Simulation

Oralea A. Pittman, Carolyn Schubert, Lisa Rohrig,
Bernadette Mazurek Melnyk

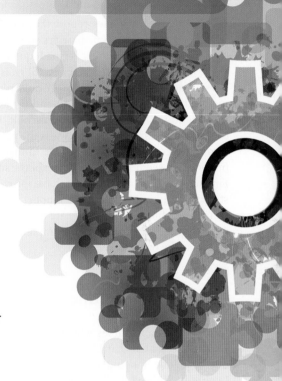

 Key Terms

Evidence-Based Practice, Simulation, Facilitation, Debriefing,
Faculty Development, PICOT, Validity, Reliability, Applicability

Guiding Questions

1 How do you ensure the use of the seven steps of evidence-based
practice in your simulation program?

2 What is the importance of the use of evidence-based practice in
simulation programs?

3 In what ways do you apply best practices in simulation facilitation
and debriefing?

4 Are you aware of different ways to use evidence-based strategies for
preparing faculty to teach simulation?

Evidence-Based Practice Overview

Evidence-based practice (EBP) is a problem-solving
approach that combines a systematic search, appraisal and
synthesis of relevant research data, clinical expertise, and
patient preferences and values to answer clinical questions (Melnyk & Fineout-Overholt, 2015a, 2015b). The
EBP process provides a systematic step-by-step method
that can be employed by any practitioner wherever they
may practice. Have you ever asked a colleague "Why do
we do it this way?" and received the response "Because
we've always done it that way?" If we are honest, we can
all admit to having been on both sides of this scenario.
Increasing demands on nurses can cause them to fall into

survival mode trying to keep their
heads above water. Over time, it is
common to become content with the status
quo. Though you may have an inkling that there might be
a better way to do something in your practice, you may not
know where to begin to make a practice change.

EBP is a way of approaching professional practice that
provides nurses with a sense of ownership and meaning in
their work. Rather than being viewed as adding to the pile
of a nurse's responsibility, EBP should be the foundation that
supports excellence in nursing practice (Melnyk, Fineout-
Overholt, Stillwell & Williamson, 2009). Wouldn't you like to
work in a place that routinely examines their practices looking for ways to do it better? Wouldn't you look forward to a

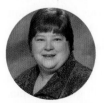

Oralea A. Pittman,
DNP, FNP-BC, FAANP

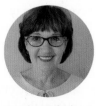

Carolyn Schubert,
DNP, CNE, RN-BC

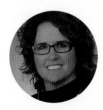

Lisa Rohrig,
BSN, RN

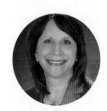

Bernadette Mazurek Melnyk,
PhD, RN, CPNP/PMHNP,
FAANP, FNAP, FAAN

job where you felt you could make an improvement in the care that you provide? With the proper support, every nurse can make a difference through the use of the EBP process.

EBP is one of the five core competencies mandated by the Institute of Medicine to be incorporated into healthcare education (Institute of Medicine, 2003). However, even though most nurses report that they believe in evidence-based care, multiple barriers still exist in full implementation of EBP, including (1) inadequate knowledge and skills; (2) lack of needed resources; (3) resistance by peers, nurse leaders, and managers; (4) cultures and environments that do not support EBP; and (5) lack of access to EBP mentors (Melnyk, Fineout-Overholt, Gallagher-Ford & Kaplan, 2012). The EBP process is the pathway for tested ideas to become common practice. Embarking on an EBP project can seem daunting, but experts such as Melnyk, Fineout-Overholt, and others have provided simplified steps and multiple resources to support nurses as they navigate through this process. We are grateful for their efforts in paving the way for nurses to implement best practices and raise the bar of excellence.

EBP in Nursing Education

In order to shape nurses who are prepared to implement EBP, it is essential that EBP be taught and used throughout academic nursing programs at all levels (Fineout-Overholt, Stillwell, Williamson, Cox & Robbins, 2015). In this chapter, the steps of EBP will be detailed, the evidence that supports simulation as an evidence-based education practice will be reviewed, the evidence for best practices in simulation will be discussed, faculty preparation for simulation will be reviewed, and ideas for including the clinical evidence base during simulation scenarios will be proposed.

Step Zero: Developing a Spirit of Inquiry

Nursing staff committed to excellence and who feel a sense of ownership at work are ready to embark on an EBP journey. However, without an environment that supports the curiosity and courage needed to challenge the status quo, EBP will not occur (Melnyk et al., 2009). Incorporating the EBP process in healthcare decision-making does take more time and effort initially, so minimizing roadblocks for those interested is essential to it occurring at any institution. But how is this spirit of inquiry cultivated? EBP implementation in a workplace is accomplished through shoring up the values, knowledge, skills, tools, and mentorship (Melnyk & Fineout-Overholt, 2015a, 2015b), especially by leadership. Individuals interested in implementing

EBP also can get the process started by asking their own questions such as (Melnyk et al., 2009):

- Who can help me enhance my EBP knowledge and skills?
- Which of my practices are EBP and which are not?
- When and with whom do I question current practices?
- Why am I doing what I am doing in my practice?
- How can I become more skilled and mentor others in EBP?

EBP progresses when an institution's underpinning supports a spirit of inquiry combined with essential EBP tools. That spirit of inquiry is the foundation for step one: asking specific clinical questions.

Step One: Asking Clinical Questions in PICOT Form

Using the **PICOT** format for asking practice change questions assures that all necessary elements are included and, therefore, will more likely result in better "answers" to those questions (Fineout-Overholt & Stillwell, 2015). It helps narrow down the main issue and reveal key terms for database searches. Components of the PICOT format are

- (P) Population of interest
- (I) Intervention or area of interest
- (C) Comparison intervention or group (if applicable)
- (O) Outcome
- (T) Time (optional)

For example, if a clinical question was asked about bedside handoff reporting by nurses on a medical–surgical unit would help patients, the specific foreground PICOT question might read "In (P) patients on a medical-surgical unit, how does bedside handoff reporting by nurses (I) as compared with the current practice of reporting outside the patient's room (C) have on (O) patient's active participation in their care?" This question like other foreground PICOT questions is more specific and relates to a particular practice. In comparison, background questions are more general and open ended.

A background PICOT question related to the topic above might be stated as "In (P) patients on a medical-surgical unit, what are the (I) most effective methods to (O) engage patients as active participants in their care?" While there are several types of PICOT questions (intervention/therapy, etiology, diagnosis/diagnostic test, prognosis/prediction, and meaning), most nursing-related PICOT questions will be intervention/therapy or meaning. The type of PICOT question you choose will depend on your situation, but all PICOT questions will guide the next step of the EBP process, which is searching for evidence. See the online Toolkit 17-1 for a Template for Asking PICOT Questions.

Step Two: Evidence Search

Internal evidence is the results of practice initiatives within your institution. In contrast, external evidence is the body of evidence found through rigorous research studies that present results to be applied more generally (Melnyk & Fineout-Overholt, 2015a, 2015b). Once you have constructed your practice problem into PICOT format, you will begin to search for external evidence to answer your question by searching health science databases for research articles related to your topic. If you are not proficient in performing database searches, you can consult a colleague or ask a library assistant to help you in this process. Health science databases including PubMed, CINAHL, and Cochrane Library should provide you with the data you seek to answer your question. Since each database has a unique focus, you should search at least three databases to find a good representation of the evidence. Some database search strategies include (Stillwell, Fineout-Overholt, Melnyk & Williamson, 2010) the following:

- Search with key words/phrases individually, and then combine all of them in the last searching step.
- Use database controlled vocabulary.
- Apply search limitations such as "humans" and "English search reference lists of articles for other sources."

Once you have uncovered a list of research articles related to your practice question, your next step is critically appraising the worth of each one.

Step Three: Critically Appraise the Evidence

You can examine each study for its value in answering your PICOT question by asking these study appraisal questions (Fineout-Overholt, Melnyk, Stillwell & Williamson, 2010a, 2010b):

- What is the level of evidence on the hierarchy?
- Are the results valid (as close to the truth as possible; are the methods used rigorous)?
- Are the results reliable (do the results matter, and can I get similar results in my practice)?
- Will the results help me in caring for my patients (study applicability)?

A study's abstract can provide a lot of the necessary information used to examine the type of study, how it was conducted, and what the results were. Reading the results and conclusion section will help you glean much information as well. Keep a good research term glossary nearby as you search and appraise each study as well such as this one from Colorado State University (http://writing.colostate.edu/guides/guide.cfm?guideid=90). As you review the studies, you can organize the answers to the analysis questions in a table or spreadsheet for easier comparison

later. From there, you can decide which studies will serve you the most in answering your PICOT question. Those that are not relevant to your question can be removed from consideration. Keep in mind that a practice change should only be made when both the level and quality of the evidence are high (Melnyk & Fineout-Overholt, 2015a, 2015b). See Toolkit 17-2 for a Checklist for Conducting an Evidence Review for Initiating Practice Change.

Evidence Level

As you evaluate evidence pertaining to your PICOT question, consider that all evidence is not created equal (Fig. 17.1). As you can see in Table 17.1, level one evidence is the evidence that best demonstrates the best methodological rigor and lowest bias and that can be applied more generally. Level one evidence is found in systematic reviews, including meta-analysis reports, which summarize and analyze multiple randomized controlled trials related to the subject. Note that not all PICOT question searches will uncover a coveted systematic review (level 1 study) so do not be discouraged if your evidence is lower level evidence on the pyramid. Even though the hierarchy of evidence situates quantitative research methodologies (e.g. randomized controlled studies) at the high end of the pyramid, it is more important to choose the evidence that answers your PICOT question best. All evidence levels can add value and help support your practice change. Though expert opinion is also valuable, standing alone, it may not compel someone to make a practice change independent of higher evidence levels.

Validity

Research **validity** addresses the degree to which a study's methods were conducted with rigor (Melnyk & Fineout-Overholt, 2015a, 2015b). A valid study reduces bias and confounding variables. Though a much more detailed discussion of research validity can be found in any nursing research guide, some basic strategies that increase study validity include (Fineout-Overholt et al., 2010a, 2010b) the following:

- Randomly assigning subjects to intervention and control groups
- Keeping group assignments concealed from subjects
- Retaining most or all of subjects in a study
- Conducting follow-up evaluations long enough after the intervention to determine long-term outcomes
- Using valid and reliable assessment tools

What Are the Results? (Reliability)

Reliability of a study indicates whether the results matter and whether you can get similar results with your patients. For example, two questions to ask in evaluating

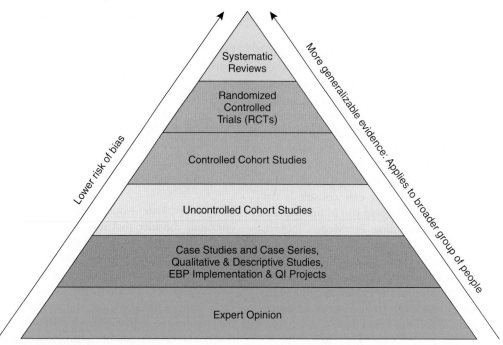

Figure 17.1 Hierarchy of Evidence for Intervention Studies. (Used from Melnyk B. M. & Fineout-Overholt, E. (Eds.). (2015). *Evidence-based practice in nursing and healthcare: A guide to best practice* (3rd ed.). Philadelphia, PA: Wolters Kluwer Health, with permission.)

Table 17.1	Hierarchy of Evidence for Intervention Studies	
Type of Evidence	**Level of Evidence**	**Description**
Systematic review or meta-analysis	1	A synthesis of evidence from all relevant randomized controlled trials
Randomized controlled trial	2	An experiment in which subjects are randomized to a treatment group or control group
Controlled trial without randomization	3	An experiment in which subjects are nonrandomly assigned to a treatment group or control group
Case–control or cohort study	4	**Case–control study:** a comparison of subjects with a condition (case) with those who don't have the condition (control) to determine characteristics that might predict the condition **Cohort study:** an observation of a group(s) (cohort[s]) to determine the development of an outcome(s) such as a disease
Systematic review of qualitative or descriptive studies	5	A synthesis of evidence from qualitative or descriptive studies to answer a clinical question
Qualitative or descriptive study	6	**Qualitative study:** gathers data on human behavior to understand *why* and *how* decisions are made **Descriptive study:** provides background information on the *what*, *where*, and *when* of a topic of interest
Expert opinion or consensus	7	Authoritative opinion of an expert committee

Reprinted from Melnyk, B. M., & Fineout-Overholt, E. (Eds.). (2011). *Evidence-based practice in nursing and healthcare: A guide to best practice* (2nd ed.). Philadelphia, PA: Wolters Kluwer Health/Lippincott Williams & Wilkins, with permission.

reliability of intervention studies is what is the effect size of the intervention (i.e., did it impact the outcomes) and how precise was the effect. This assessment requires some familiarity with common research statistics so reviewing those will be helpful. Rapid critical appraisal checklists also can assist with the appraisal of studies (see Melnyk & Fineout-Overholt, 2015a, 2015b).

Applicability

The final step in critical appraisal involves examining the **applicability** of the evidence. You will need to ascertain the extent to which the study subjects are similar to your population, weigh the benefits and potential for harm, assess the feasibility of implementation in your practice setting, and determine the patient's desire to participate in the intervention (Melnyk & Fineout Overholt, 2011). The final questions might include, is, will the results help me in caring for my patients? Is the body of evidence compelling enough to make any practice changes? This more subjective analysis includes questions about how useful the study results are to your particular practice population. What are the values of the population identified such as patient cultural or religious values? You must also consider the effect of proposing the practice change at your facility. Would it be realistic and feasible? For example, if implementing the use of a new piece of expensive diagnostic equipment would improve care of patients but your facility just announced a spending freeze, the intervention wouldn't be realistic. Once you have determined the answers of validity, reliability, and applicability of the evidence you have collected, you are ready for the next EBP step: implementing a practice change.

Step Four: Integrating the Evidence with Clinical Expertise, Patient Preferences and Values, and Stakeholders

The next step in the EBP process is implementing the practice change at your facility. This step of the process will require you to anticipate how stakeholders and patients who may be affected by the change may receive the change. Active stakeholders include those that will carry out the plan and who will be your focus for education and support throughout implementation. Passive stakeholders are those not directly involved but whose support or lack of support can determine if the plan succeeds. Spending the time to obtain their endorsement of the practice change and maintaining communication throughout the implementation phase is key to the project's sustainment (Fineout-Overholt, Williamson, Gallagher-Ford, Melnyk and Stillwell, 2011b).

Conducting informational meetings, surveys, and focus groups are some examples of including stakeholders as collaborators on the project. Once the project is defined with stakeholder support, develop an implementation plan through task force committee meetings. The plan should be in writing and address creating or revising necessary documents, communication measures, budget needs, and outcome measurements. As the implementation commences, communicating potential outcomes, addressing glitches in implementation quickly and effectively, and offering continued support for stakeholders demonstrate leadership and keep morale high during the process.

You will want to collect baseline data that will be used to determine success or failure of the project after implementation. Internal data sources can include routinely collected information such as incident reports, satisfaction surveys, or expense reports. In preparation for baseline data collection, investigate who holds the data, what is the process for obtaining it, and how it will be managed throughout the project (Fineout-Overholt et al., 2011a, 2011b). During this phase, you may decide you need IRB approval to collect the data, especially if you will want to publish the project's results. Start by conducting the project on a small group of patients to minimize any unforeseen negative outcomes and help you adjust the plan quickly prior to institution wide implementation. As you execute the practice change plan with your team, remember to be flexible, set a positive tone, and know that your efforts will pay off in the end when you move into the next phase, evaluating the project outcomes.

Step Five: Evaluation of the EBP Project

Once you have implemented the practice change for your population and gathered outcome data, someone will need to analyze the data to determine the strengths and weaknesses of the project. If that is not your strength, consider who in your organization might assist you in processing the data. Having someone skillful in data analysis from the beginning will help you to more quickly evaluate and report on the project's success. As you review results, if some outcomes were negative and some were positive, support the positive results and mitigate the negative. As you did throughout the implementation process, getting feedback from stakeholders at the end is also important in making future adjustments in regard to the practice change.

Sustaining the New Practice Change

Your EBP project has been completed and shown some positive results. Though no project is without problems, you see that the change was needed and you feel satisfied with how you have improved your practice. Now what? If the project was successful, you will want it to be continued. Sustaining the change will take communicating the positive outcomes institution wide and may even dictate a policy change. Addressing any remaining barriers to change and supporting the project champions is important during this phase. Strengthening the values, knowledge, and skills in EBP will pave the way for others in your institution to question the status quo and initiate their own practice improvement projects. With your experience, you can now become an EBP mentor to others.

Step Six: Disseminate Results

Not only do you want the change to continue at your facility, you will want to disseminate the results externally as well. Doing so can help others to benefit from your efforts in making similar changes. It can also prevent the proverbial "reinventing the wheel" for those who had the same concerns as you about the practice. This is accomplished through presentations at local, state, or national professional meetings and/or submitting a paper of the project to a peer-reviewed journal, professional newsletter, or other publications. To ensure a successful presentation (Fineout-Overholt, Gallagher-Ford, Melnyk & Stillwell, 2011a):

- Stick to your stated objectives.
- Use simple bullet points (don't write everything you plan to say on a slide).
- Use font large enough to see in the back of the room.
- Use pictures when possible.
- Use the one slide per minute guide.
- Practice in front of others.

An oral presentation can be a springboard to write for a publication as your thoughts are already organized. Since public speaking is reportedly the greatest fear ranking higher than death, however, some might choose to start the dissemination by submitting a journal abstract rather than a presentation abstract. Many institutions have writing centers or library services if you don't know where to begin. Here is a general flow of events in embarking on journal publishing (Fineout-Overholt et al., 2011a, 2011b):

- Establish the purpose and audience you are targeting.
- Choose an appropriate journal for your subject matter and review their author guidelines (found on their website).
- Send a query letter to the editor.
- Start with an outline for your manuscript.
- Have peers review your drafts as you progress toward the final submission.

EBP and Simulation

The above steps of EBP just discussed may be familiar to faculty in academic programs. Many programs now include content about EBP and EBP change projects, but it is essential to weave the use of EBP throughout academic curriculum, including simulation. In the following sections, simulation as an evidence-based teaching strategy will be discussed as well as how to implement the steps of EBP into a simulation program.

17-1 Voice of Experience
RNAO's Best Practice Guidelines (BPG) Program: Clinical Evidence to Inform Simulation

Doris Grinspun, PhD, MSN, RN, LLD(Hon), O.ONT

Irmajean Bajnok, PhD, MScN, BScN, RN

The Challenge

Evidence that is current and relevant is at the core of improved population health outcomes, as well as patient, organizational, and health system outcomes. As such, the emergence of the INACSL Standards of Best Practice: Simulation[SM] is a very important step in the journey to simulation excellence. (INACSL Standards Committee, 2016). Together, these standards form a powerful foundation for the design, implementation, and evaluation of simulated clinical immersion experiences.

Meeting the Challenge

To meet the challenge, the Registered Nurses' Association of Ontario (RNAO) in partnership with the Ontario Ministry of Health and Long-Term Care (MOHLTC) launched in 1999 the Best Practice Guidelines (BPGs) program (http://rnao.ca/bpg). Today, RNAO's BPG program is a flagship on the provincial, national, and international stages, leading BPG development, implementation science and practice, and the emerging area of clinical and healthy work environment evaluation. The program enables organizations and health systems to focus on patient care and clinical excellence, using the latest research to inform practice and optimize outcomes.

Outcomes

The BPG program is recognized the world over for its rigorous guideline development, implementation science approaches, and robust evaluation methodology. The following sections describe its components.

Best Practice Guideline Development

The best practice guideline (BPG) development process involves a rigorous methodology, including (1) identification of the BPG topic, specific purpose, and scoping of the guideline; (2) systematic literature review identifying the best and most current evidence; (3) selection of expert panel of nurses, other health professionals, and patient/public representatives; (4) development of clinical, organizational, educational, and system-level recommendations derived from the evidence; (5) guideline-specific input from external stakeholders to refine the guideline; and (6) publication of the final guideline with graded recommendations. All guidelines are reviewed every 5 years to assess the currency of the evidence and recommendations. Those guidelines selected for updating undergo the full guideline development process and are published as new editions.

Best Practice Guideline Dissemination and Implementation

The BPG program focuses on individual, organizational, and system-level strategies to ensure effective, sustained, and scalable implementation of best practice guidelines in clinical and management practices. The following lists four EBP initiatives for you to consider:

BPSO: Best Practice Spotlight Organizations

RNAO established in 2003 the BPSO designation as its signature model for BPG implementation, sustainability, and evaluation. To date, RNAO counts with about 500 health and academic organizations that are formally engaged in the BPSO designation provincially, nationally, and internationally. BPSO designation enables health organizations to formally partner with RNAO over a 3-year period. Together, they work to make an impact on patient care, organizational performance, and health system outcomes by facilitating and advancing EBP among nurses and other health professionals. Academic institutions and programs have also attained BPSO status. Once designated a BPSO, the partnership is renewed biennially (http://rnao.ca/bpg/bpso).

There are two BPSO designations to consider for organizations interested in applying to become a BPSO: the *BPSO Direct Designation*, best suited for single organizations that wish to apply to RNAO to engage in the 3-year partnership, and the *BPSO Host Designation*, suited for organizations that have the capacity to serve as an RNAO agent in running the full BPSO designation program for a group of health and/or academic settings within a country, region, or community.

NOS: Nursing Order Sets

RNAO's nursing order sets are evidence-based interventions and clinical decision support resources derived from RNAO's clinical BPGs. They enable the integration of the best available evidence into daily clinical practice using technology to facilitate access at the point of care.

Best Practice Champions Network

The Best Practice Champions Network was established in 2002. It consists of thousands of nurses and other health professionals in all roles and health sectors that are passionate about evidence-informed practice and improving persons' health and care. These champions are dedicated practitioners who raise awareness of BPGs, support understanding, and influence their uptake among peers in their workplaces.

Best Practice Guidelines Institutes

RNAO delivers weeklong institutes locally, nationally, and internationally that focus on guideline implementation and evaluation. To date, there are 10 different institutes, including 2 that provide foundational and advanced knowledge about using RNAO BPGs to create evidence-based cultures; and 8 that focus on specific clinical topics such as wound care, mental health, chronic disease prevention and management, and primary care.

Best Practice Guideline Monitoring and Evaluation

NQuIRE (Nursing Quality Indicators for Reporting and Evaluation) consists of a database, a data dictionary, an online data entry system, and a set of organization-level structural, process, and outcome indicators for each BPG, as well as data quality monitoring, collection, and reporting processes. Through NQuIRE, RNAO collects, analyzes, and reports quality indicator data submitted by health service and academic organizations participating in the BPSO designation.

National and International Partnerships

RNAO is actively engaged with provincial, national, and international partners. We welcome opportunities to collaborate in building a strong nursing community to optimize health outcomes for everyone and everywhere.

(Continued)

17-1 Voice of Experience (*Continued*)

ICNP R&D Centre—International Classification for Nursing Practice Research and Development Centre

RNAO is accredited as an ICNP R&D Centre, one of 11 such centers around the world and the only one in North America. The accreditation recognizes RNAO's ongoing contribution to ICN's eHealth program through the development of ICNP codes derived from RNAO's nursing order sets and BPG outcome measures.

RNAO eHealth Program

The mandate of RNAO's nursing and eHealth program is to facilitate the nursing profession's involvement in the eHealth agenda and to support nurses to take a leadership role in the design, implementation, adoption, and sustainability of integrated digital health systems (e.g., electronic medical records) in all healthcare sectors and schools of nursing in Ontario. The program has resulted in an active engagement of nursing leadership in all aspects of eHealth, increased eHealth expertise among nurses to participate effectively in shaping eHealth in their organizations, and greater efficiency in the utilization of digital health systems for the delivery of safe, high-quality evidence-based care.

Inspiration for Simulation Champions

As Florence Nightingale said in 1914, "Unless we are making progress in our nursing every year, every month, every week, take my word for it, we are going back." We at RNAO know that together, we are making progress for nurses and those who we nurse. We invite you to think about the ways you can incorporate the RNAO BPG Programs and Guidelines, as well as the INACSL Standards of Best Practice: Simulation into your simulation program.

The Development of Simulation as a Teaching Strategy

Simulation is widely used as a teaching strategy in nursing education. Interest in simulation has grown rapidly, due to the increasing demand for competent nursing graduates, the intensifying competition for clinical sites, and the limits placed on faculty and students in the clinical arena. Simulations are considered by many to be cutting-edge pedagogy to aid in the quest for more nurses (Hallmark, 2015). Studies show that when faculty develop a well-constructed and well-facilitated simulation, it will bring about improvements in skills, knowledge, critical thinking abilities, and confidence in nursing students (Cant & Cooper, 2010; Halabi Najjar, Lyman, & Miehl, 2015; Stroup, 2014). Simulation is considered to be an effective, uniform way of preparing students to deliver quality care and provides experiences that education programs cannot always provide for students in a clinical setting (Simington, 2011).

The Need for Simulation

Because of the realism of high-fidelity patient simulators simulation can be viewed as an equally valuable clinical learning experience to those gained in traditional, hospital-based clinical teaching environments (Richardson, Goldsamt, Simmons, Gilmartin & Jeffries, 2014).

The additional challenge of finding quality clinical placements for patient care experiences is creating a significant need to replace traditional clinical time with high-fidelity simulation experiences (Jeffries, Thomas-Dreifuerst, Kardong-Edgren & Hayden, 2015). Utilization of simulation as an acceptable substitute for clinical time is an increasing trend in the United States, with many state Boards of Nursing defining, monitoring, and advocating for simulation experiences. A survey in 2014 found that 22 Boards of Nursing support simulation as a clinical substitute, while others define more specific requirements and indications for its use (Hayden, Smiley, & Gross, 2014).

Why Simulation Works

High-fidelity simulation utilizes the latest in technology to provide realistic manikins that mimic actual physiological functions. Such capabilities include breathing, speaking, possessing audible heart and lung sounds, demonstrating palpable peripheral pulses, and responding physiologically to interventions. These high-tech attributes will allow you to foster a realistic and immersive experience for students, which allows for "engagement with the patient" through a scripted and evidence-based simulation scenario (Fig. 17.2).

Advanced technologies associated with simulation increase the potential for more accurate reflections of the clinical environment for your students and facilitate clinical application (Shin, Park, & Kim, 2015). The use of simulated clinical immersion in nursing education allows students to identify good and bad practice within the confines of a safe environment and is an effective strategy for cognitive gains, skills development, and self-confidence ratings (Stroup, 2014). Such interactions occur in a simulation lab where patients cannot be harmed, no safety or quality issues are real, and you as faculty are present to support the learner. Simulation content then can bridge the gap

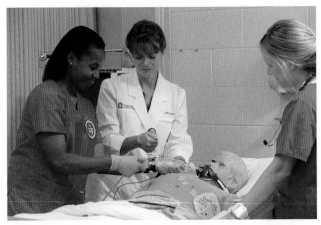

Figure 17.2 Ohio State University Nursing Students Participate in Interprofessional Simulations. (© The Ohio State University College of Nursing. Used with permission.)

between theory and EBP in a controlled laboratory setting. Low- and medium-fidelity simulation, standardized patients, and role-playing can also be effective depending on the scenario and objectives.

Evidence-Based Practice and Simulation

The IOM identified the use of EBP as one of five essential core competencies for healthcare educational programs. Three important nursing organizations—the American Nurses Association, the American Association of Colleges of Nursing, and the American Association of Critical Care Nurses—concur that all nurses should practice from an evidence base. EBP must be incorporated into every aspect of health sciences education, including simulation (Fineout-Overholt et al., 2015). The integration of EBP into simulation as well as throughout the entire academic curricula will assist students in meeting the new EBP competencies for practicing nurses (see Box 17-1). These competencies were formulated by a national consensus panel of EBP experts and then confirmed by a two-round Delphi study with EBP mentors across the United States (Melnyk, Gallagher-Ford, Long, & Fineout-Overholt, 2014). EBP competencies should be integrated into academic programs to establish and continuously

---

Box 17-1   Evidence-Based Practice

Competencies for Practicing Registered Professional Nurses

1. Questions clinical practices for the purpose of improving the quality of care.
2. Describes clinical problems using internal evidence.* (Internal evidence* = evidence generated internally within a clinical setting, such as patient assessment data, outcomes management, and quality improvement data)
3. Participates in the formulation of clinical questions using PICOT* format. (PICOT* = Patient population; Intervention or area of Interest; Comparison intervention or group; Outcome; Time).
4. Searches for external evidence* to answer focused clinical questions. (External evidence* = evidence generated from research)
5. Participates in critical appraisal of preappraised evidence (such as clinical practice guidelines, evidence-based policies and procedures, and evidence syntheses).
6. Participates in the critical appraisal of published research studies to determine their strength and applicability to clinical practice.
7. Participates in the evaluation and synthesis of a body of evidence gathered to determine its strength and applicability to clinical practice.
8. Collects practice data (e.g., individual patient data, quality improvement data) systematically as internal evidence for clinical decision-making in the care of individuals, groups, and populations.
9. Integrates evidence gathered from external and internal sources in order to plan evidence-based practice changes.

10. Implements practice changes based on evidence and clinical expertise and patient preferences to improve care processes and patient outcomes.
11. Evaluates outcomes of evidence-based decisions and practice changes for individuals, groups, and populations to determine best practices.
12. Disseminates best practices supported by evidence to improve quality of care and patient outcomes.
13. Participates in strategies to sustain an evidence-based practice culture.

Evidence-Based Practice Competencies for Practicing Advanced Practice Nurses

All competencies of registered professional nurses

14. Systematically conducts an exhaustive search for external evidence* to answer clinical questions. (External evidence* = evidence generated from research)
15. Critically appraises relevant preappraised evidence (i.e., clinical guidelines, summaries, synopses, syntheses of relevant external evidence) and primary studies, including evaluation and synthesis
16. Integrates a body of external evidence from nursing and related fields with internal evidence* in making decisions about patient care. (Internal evidence* = evidence generated internally within a clinical setting, such as patient assessment data, outcomes management, and quality improvement data)
17. Leads transdisciplinary teams in applying synthesized evidence to initiate clinical decisions and practice changes to improve the health of individuals, groups, and populations

(Continued)

Box 17-1 **Evidence-Based Practice** (*Continued*)

18. Generates internal evidence through outcomes management and EBP implementation projects for the purpose of integrating best practices
19. Measures processes and outcomes of evidence-based clinical decisions
20. Formulates evidence-based policies and procedures
21. Participates in the generation of external evidence with other healthcare professionals
22. Mentors others in evidence-based decision-making and the EBP process

23. Implements strategies to sustain an EBP culture
24. Communicates best evidence to individuals, groups, colleagues, and policy-makers

Used from Melnyk, B., Gallagher-Ford, L., Long, L., & Fineout-Overholt, E. (2014). The establishment of evidence-based practice competencies for practicing registered nurses and advanced practice nurses in real-world clinical settings: proficiencies to improve healthcare quality, reliability, patient outcomes, and costs. *Worldviews on Evidence Based Nursing, 11*(1), 5–15, with permission.

reinforce EBP as the foundation of practice (Melnyk et al., 2014).

Teaching undergraduate and graduate students the processes and skills necessary to access, appraise, and integrate evidence into practice is essential to professional nursing in the 21st century. Using simulation scenarios from clinical practice, students can work through the EBP process by doing the following: (1) developing clinical PICOT questions; (2) collecting information from a variety of sources, including clinical experiences, encounters with patients, and peer-reviewed journals to answer questions; (3) evaluating the strength and relevance of the evidence; and (4) applying and integrating this information with previously learned knowledge (Winters & Echeverri, 2012).

Preparing Faculty to Teach Simulation

The gap between practice and teaching in nursing education is particularly evident in simulation teaching, where many faculty learn to do simulations from other faculty who have also had no formal training. Guiding a simulation effectively clearly requires proper training, but there is very little evidence that any formal training occurs for nursing faculty. In fact, inexperienced faculty are often fearful and lack confidence in simulation (Elfrink, Kirkpatrick, Nininger, & Schubert, 2010). An international survey found that nursing faculty perceived their disinterest in simulation to be directly related to a lack of formal training in its use (Nehring & Lashley, 2004). Such poor preparation was also linked to feelings of fear and dread about having to be involved in a simulation (Dowie & Phillips, 2011; McNeill et al., 2012).

Faculty remain "undertrained, practices are inconsistent, and both can lead to poor results in simulation pedagogy" (Hallmark, 2015, p. 389). Nursing programs using simulation are typically "underbudgeted for faculty development and curricular integration" (Taibi & Kardong-Edgren, 2014, p. e48). Poor pedagogy potentially leads to poor learning outcomes for students.

Best Practice for Faculty Development

Evidence-based teaching is essential to quality of outcomes for students and for faculty. Nursing education includes a steadily increasing number of simulation experiences. Ideally, all nursing simulation programs utilize faculty who are well developed in the strategy, and who are knowledgeable, skilled, and prepared to execute a quality program (see Fig. 17.3). However, this is often not the case according to current literature findings. Despite the fact that evidence-based teaching exists in many educational settings, it has not traditionally existed in nursing academia. Simulation is yet another strategy that nurse educators "pick up" from other more experienced colleagues, and this results in a lack of standardization and a lack of quality.

The need for EBP guidelines for simulation teaching "parallels the emphasis on evidence-based nursing practice" (Oermann, Yarbrough, Saewert, Ard & Charasika, 2009, p. 64). **Faculty development** has been defined as activities that "improve knowledge, skills, and behaviors as teachers and educators" (Rogers, Peterson, Ponce, White & Porterfield, 2015, p. 729). The integration of evidence-based standards

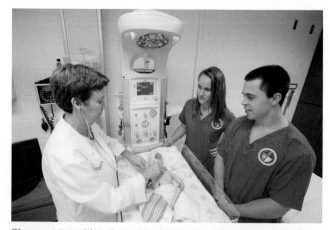

Figure 17.3 Ohio State Health Science Students Conduct Simulated Patient Rounds Led by Faculty. (© The Ohio State University College of Nursing. Used with permission.)

for faculty development has historically been lacking in nursing education, where expert nurse clinicians step into the teaching role with little or no formal preparation.

Nursing faculty often have little or no background in teaching, including the principles of teaching and learning, nor any knowledge of curricular development and evaluation. Conversely, the National League for Nursing's core competencies for nurse educators specify that faculty development is essential to the role and that competencies facilitating learning and employing a variety of strategies, such as simulation, to effectively teach and evaluate students is key to their success (NLN, 2005).

The Gap between Best Practice and Actual Practice when Teaching Simulation

All nurses who practice are formally prepared, while most nurses who teach are not. Recognition of a deficiency in nurse faculty skills and preparation has led to many recommendations for evidence-based and structured programs that educate and train nursing faculty to teach, particularly in the area of simulation. New and advanced technology in simulation has placed the emphasis on the high-fidelity simulators rather than on the preparation of faculty who participate. More faculty have been trained by manikin vendors than by academic experts despite the increasing body of evidence regarding best practice in teaching simulation (Jeffries et al., 2015; Kardong-Edgren, Willhaus, Bennett & Hayden, 2012). To address the deficit in teaching readiness, Jansen et al. (2010) recommended that a "train the trainer approach" and the creation of "simulation super users and champions" would prepare faculty to implement simulation standards and to mentor others for readiness to do so (p. e14). Adamson (2010) found that faculty wanted ongoing training from these "champions and super users" (p. e80).

Very few "simulation training" programs exist to prepare faculty in such evidence-based standards and best practices (INACSL Standards Committee, 2016, INACSL Standards of Best Practice: Simulation^SM). Research that focuses specifically on faculty anxieties or attitudes about simulation as a teaching strategy has not been conducted, despite the fact that simulation challenges educators' knowledge, skills, and attitudes and leads to reluctance to use it as a learning tool (Dowie & Phillips, 2011). A survey in 2008 revealed that 73% of nursing faculty had no simulation preparation, that educational program interventions resulted in significant ($p < 0.05$) and positive changes in attitude and readiness for its use, and that a majority of faculty perceived a need for formal training (Akhtar-Danesh, Baxter, Valaitis, Stanyon & Sproul, 2010; Dowie & Phillips, 2011; Nguyen et al., 2011). This well-documented gap between expectations and preparation is a barrier to effective teaching and learning and impedes growth and experience gained from an effective simulation.

Evidence-Based Solutions: Training the Trainer

Training programs for faculty need to be developed using best practice if outcomes for faculty and students are to be optimal. Support of this is evident, as many state Boards of Nursing, as well as many nursing programs, are requesting information about best practices in simulation teaching and are seeking guidance to develop faculty who can effectively create and implement a simulation-based curriculum (Jeffries et al., 2015).

Strategies for Developing Novice Simulation Teachers into Experts

The few published studies on "best practice" in the teaching of simulation include the need for faculty to facilitate and debrief effectively and to possess particular attributes and approaches that foster learning. The INACSL *Standards of Best Practice: Simulation^SM*, published by the International Nursing Association for Clinical Simulation and Learning (INACSL), provide a valuable framework for faculty development in the conduct of simulation (INACSL Standards Committee, 2016). Evidence-based standards define best practice and provide guidelines for Simulation Design, Outcomes and Objectives, Facilitation, Debriefing, Participant Evaluation, Professional Integrity, Simulation-Enhanced, Interprofessional Education, and a Simulation Glossary. Threaded throughout this framework is the recommendation that experts must assist novices in learning and implementing the nine standards. Such assistance could include formal training, mentoring with coaches, viewing recordings of expert-led simulations, coleading a debriefing, and recording/critiquing a novice during a simulation (INACSL Standards Committee, 2016, Debriefing). In response to the largest and most comprehensive simulation study in nursing to date, the National State Boards of Nursing (NCSBN) published the NCSBN Simulation Guidelines for Prelicensure Nursing Programs (Alexander et al., 2015). Quality research supplemented by expert knowledge in the field translated in to evidence-based guidelines and information to help nursing programs enhance their readiness and preparation and planning for simulation.

Critical Faculty Skills in Simulation

Simulations are executed by faculty who can follow EBP guidelines related to the process. Effective simulation teaching skills are learned and not inherent (Simington, 2011). Furthermore, national standards for simulation require "proficient facilitators who have been prepared through formal coursework, continuing education offerings, and targeted work with a mentor" (Boese et al., 2013, p. S23). In a review of the National Council of Schools and Boards of Nursing's comprehensive simulation study initiated in 2011, Jeffries et al., Hayden (2015) recommend that faculty development be conducted by simulation experts "to ensure quality and best practices" (p. 20). Further recommendations for faculty development include education on the evaluation tools that may be used, as well as the specific competencies to be met by faculty at the end of the development sessions. Faculty should also be instructed on how to select scenarios, write objectives, use a standardized debriefing tool, and evaluate outcomes based on learning objectives.

Developing a Simulation Community

To enhance simulation quality, a simulation team should be comprised of faculty who are trained and enthusiastic about implementing simulations, have a designated coordinator or leader to oversee preparedness and cohesiveness, and develop a "simulation learning community" where simulation faculty meet and share knowledge and updates regarding best practice in simulation (Jeffries et al., 2015, p. 20).

To summarize, the following are recommendations for faculty development from the National Council on State Boards of Nursing's National Simulation Study initiated in 2011 (Jeffries et al., 2015):

1. Use simulation experts to conduct initial core training to ensure quality and best practice.
2. Set aside time for faculty to train, with 3- to 4-day workshops optimal.
3. Develop a simulation team that is enthusiastic and up to date on best practice.
4. Designate a simulation coordinator to ensure preparedness and monitor outcomes.
5. Develop a simulation learning community that includes major stakeholders and innovators.

EBP and Faculty Role in Scenario Development

Using best practices begins in the scenario development phase of simulation. When faculty choose the topic of a simulation, it is important to remember that scenarios are more effective if they fit into the overall curriculum as one of multiple teaching strategies (Cant & Cooper, 2010; Paskins & Peile, 2010). The content of the scenario should also be evidence based and tied to key references. These references may include current clinical guidelines, information from systematic reviews, or appraisal of evidence in research

reports (Waxman, 2010). Scenarios should also have an appropriate "signal-to-noise ratio" (Parker & Myrick, 2012, p. 369). This means that the scenario should not include too much information that is extraneous to the learning objectives such as increasing acuity or psychosocial and interpersonal complexity that may distract the junior learners from the purpose of that particular simulation.

Faculty Role in Facilitation

Skilled **facilitation**, including **debriefing**, is key to student learning in simulation. There is little research that examines in detail what facilitation practices best foster learning. Most studies of facilitation up to this point have been qualitative descriptive studies. Many are from the students' perspective of what constitutes facilitation that promotes learning. Promotion of learning requires that faculty demonstrate and explain the reasons for nursing interventions during simulation.

The teacher must have a profound knowledge of the subject matter. This dynamic process results in a sense of direction and the ability to reformulate the goals of the teaching interaction as the simulation progresses (Simington, 2011). INACSL Standards of Best Practice: Simulation include specific skills for educators, such as allowing a simulation to progress uninterrupted and providing coaching/cues at preplanned intervals in the scenario (INACSL Standards Committee, 2016, Simulation Design).

In their grounded theory study of simulation, Walton, Chute, and Ball (2011) found that students moved through stages of learning through simulation experiences. They also found that there were faculty strategies that students perceived as supporting each stage. Overall, these strategies included welcoming students, being willing to provide or facilitate repetition of key skills or scenarios, role modeling, tolerance for student humor that often masked fear on the student's part, patience, sensitive correction of errors, and specific individualized feedback (Walton et al., 2011). These themes were similar to those found in a study of medical students who felt that deliberate practice (repetitive practice for mastery of skill), reflection, feedback, and teamwork were important aspects of facilitation (Paskins & Peile, 2010). The authors also noted that both positive and negative feedback could have significant impacts on confidence for some students.

In another study, nursing students appreciated a simulation that was extra credit and not part of their grade. This contributed to a low-stress environment, which they felt, was key to learning along with support from faculty during the simulation (Mahoney, Hancock, Iorianni-Cimbak, & Curley, 2013). In a qualitative study of the facilitator role in air ambulance training for physicians and paramedics, feedback both during and after simulation (debriefing) was important to trainees. As the course progressed, they needed less feedback during simulation. Faculty felt that it was important to give feedback during the simulation to keep it on track and not waste time in unproductive training (Usman, Sood, & Goodsman, 2015).

Parker and Myrick described their theory of facilitation as "empowering through fading support" (Parker and Myrick, 2012, p. 367). In this model, faculty, who must know the learners in their group, provide "adaptive scaffolding" to learners. Adaptive scaffolding means that faculty support students where they are learning something new or growing more independent, but gradually withdraw that support as the students become more proficient. At that point, the support may be needed elsewhere wherever the leading edge of the student's skill is now. Key to understanding this model is the work of Vygotsky (1978 as quoted in Parker & Myrick, 2012, p. 367) and the idea of the "zone of proximal development" (ZPD). Parker and Myrick explain this as "the distance between the actual developmental level as determined by active problem solving and the level of potential development as determined through problem solving...in collaboration with more capable peers." The authors suggest that expanding the ZPD is the outcome of excellent facilitation.

Faculty Role in Debriefing

In addition to the facilitation process, debriefing is a crucial part of the simulation experience. Debriefing is a discussion between a group of individuals who are reviewing a simulated activity, with the purpose of assessing and analyzing actions, thoughts, emotions, and information so that performance improvement occurs in real settings; active participant engagement is a sign of a strong debriefing and will intensify learning and its transfer into practice (Simon, Raemer, & Rudolph, 2010). Leading an effective debriefing is learned and not inherent and is the most important part of a simulation (Cant & Cooper, 2011). Debriefers should involve all participants, be supportive and open, maintain confidentiality, and encourage students to transfer learning to the "real world" (Decker et al., 2013). Questions such as "how has this changed your practice" allow students to reflect on what they will do differently if faced with the same patient tomorrow. To achieve successful outcomes during debriefing, the following must occur during debriefing (Cant & Cooper, 2011; INACLS Board of Directors, 2015):

- A competent and trained debriefer who observed the entire simulation must lead successful debriefing.
- Based on the evidence.
- Based on a structured framework for debriefing.
- Based on objectives, learners, and outcomes.

- Be conducted in an environment that supports confidentiality, trust, open communication, self-analysis, and reflection.

To implement best practices for debriefing, OSU College of Nursing faculty use a tool that incorporates the Debriefing Assessment for Simulation in Healthcare (DASH) as well as the INACSL Standards of Best Practice: Simulation (INACSL Standards Committee, 2016; Simon et al., 2010). Faculty are then guided through the five phases of debriefing as defined by INACSL Standards of Best Practice: Simulation. The three-column table includes sample questions for each of the five phases of debriefing. Phase 1 (reflection) asks students to "rehash" or review the events of the scenario, while phase 2 (emotion) asks students to describe how they felt during the simulation. Phase 3 (reception) calls for students to analyze what went well and what they would do differently, while phase 4 (integration) has students evaluate what they've learned and what their greatest "take away" was from the scenario. Finally, phase 5 (assimilation) asks how students will care for similar patients in the future and how their practice has changed.

Practical Applications of EBP into Simulation

At the OSU College of Nursing, we developed a formal training program based on the original publication of INACSL Standards of Best Practice: Simulation (2011) and key documents from the American Association of Colleges of Nursing (AACN). These standards were updated and expanded in 2013, 2015, and again in 2016. The standards specify that faculty must be trained to do simulations, must actively guide students through, and must conduct a methodical debriefing as the most crucial part of the process (INACSL Standards Committee, 2016, Debriefing; Facilitation). The OSU training program included procedural knowledge, decision-making ability, documentation, communication, and time management skills required in the simulation. Two experts in simulation developed an education session on simulation teaching. Faculty were invited to attend the session, and it has been an annual event for all new faculty during orientation. In addition, the materials are posted on the college website and are available at all times to any interested faculty member. The education session included instruction on simulation principles, facilitation methods, and debriefing techniques. In addition, we formed a "simulation community" by developing the OSU College of Nursing Simulation Committee, comprised of administrators, faculty, and staff closely involved with the simulation program. The committee meets monthly to review best practices and innovative strategies in simulation, and members developed a set of standards that was approved by faculty in 2009 to guide the conduct of simulations. The committee regularly collaborates with faculty and content experts to insure that EBP is reflected in the scenarios' details.

Scenario Exemplar

In order for students to adopt EBP as essential to their future nursing practice, they must see it as a normal and valued part of their problem-solving in patient care. Below is an interdisciplinary scenario where students experience problem-solving through EBP.

The scenario concerns an adult trauma patient with multiple fractures, respiratory distress, and internal bleeding. The patient presents to the emergency department with hypotension, tachycardia, and severe pain. Eventually, the patient requires intubation, aggressive fluid replacement, vasopressors, and emergent surgery for a ruptured spleen. In the pre-simulation period, we provide this brief description of the scenario to the students along with pertinent assessment and lab data. Students then process that information in a manner that models the steps of EBP according to:

1. Step Zero: Cultivate a spirit of inquiry.
   a. Students are questioned as to why the patient suddenly experiences respiratory distress, decreased PaO_2, and increased $PaCO_2$.
   b. Students are asked why the patient becomes severely hypotensive despite large volumes of IV fluids (crystalloids).
   c. Students are asked to anticipate what treatments will be ordered for that patient.
2. Step 1: Ask clinical questions in PICOT format.
   a. Appropriate PICOT questions for this scenario would be as follows:
      i. In trauma patients with hemorrhagic shock, are crystalloids more effective than colloids in improving and maintaining vascular volume during the emergent phase of care?
      ii. In patients with respiratory distress secondary to trauma, how does rapid sequence intubation compared to standard intubation impact airway maintenance in the emergent phase of care?
3. Step 2: Search for the best evidence.
   a. OSU CON students must seek the latest literature on the details of the scenario.
   b. This "presimulation" assignment or "prep" work focuses on pathophysiology, pharmacology, and interventions ordered and involves a 10-item question/answer assignment that must be literature based and formally referenced.
   c. Students are then encouraged to choose a specific item of interest in the scenario (such as respiratory

failure in a trauma patient, splenic hemorrhage, or fluid resuscitation), find a recent study on that problem, and prepare an annotated bibliography to summarize the evidence presented.
4. Step 3: Critically appraise the evidence.
   a. Students share their research article with the group at the end of the debriefing.
   b. Faculty provide individual feedback on those annotated bibliographies.
5. Step 4: Integrate the evidence with clinical expertise with patient preferences and values.
   a. Students apply the presimulation information to the trauma/respiratory distress/internal hemorrhage patient when making clinical decisions and judgements about the plan of care (e.g., students will or should question why morphine sulfate is ordered for the patient's pain as it may cause respiratory depression in an already hypoxic patient).
6. Step 5: Evaluate the outcome.
   a. Faculty immediately debrief students when the simulation is completed, focusing on and assessing the effects of clinical decisions made.
   b. Students share what they would do differently if repeating the simulation, allowing them to evaluate actions and decisions in a safe, supportive environment.
7. Step 6: Disseminate EBP results.
   a. Faculty ask students to consider and share how new knowledge gained will change the care of future patients.
   b. We utilize the Simulation Effectiveness Tool (SET) developed by Elfrink Cordi, Leighton, Ryan-Wenger, Doyle and Ravert (2012) to evaluate all simulations, and all students complete online prior to leaving the simulation area.
   c. Members of the Simulation Committee, along with course faculty, review evaluation results at the end of each semester and make recommendations for change.

Additional Practical Ideas

In the above scenario, students use EBP as part of their preparation for the simulation and could also practice EBP during a simulation. What if students paused to check evidence for or against alternative courses of action during a simulation? For this kind of practice, the use of evidence synthesis information like Cochrane or UpToDate, which can be quickly accessed, on mobile devices at the bedside is ideal. Perhaps one student role in the simulation could be the evidence-based practitioner who would anticipate questions and look up evidence about the care dilemmas as the simulation progresses.

Another possible EBP application would be for senior prelicensure or graduate students to develop a formal PICOT question posed by faculty as their preparation assignment for simulation. A properly designed PICOT question would lead to students reviewing several articles, appraising the evidence and deciding how they might answer the question posed. Prior to beginning the simulation, students could discuss their findings and compare and contrast their plans if multiple plans are present. This process could help develop their expertise as clinicians. The students could then experience the next phase of the EBP process during the simulation by experiencing patient preference with the simulated patient.

Summary

EBP is essential to the quality and safety of nursing care. Best practices assure best outcomes for our patients. To assure that these optimal results are achieved, EBP provides a framework of six steps that begin with a clinical question and end with a clinical answer based on valid, reliable, and applicable evidence (Melnyk & Fineout-Overholt, 2015a, 2015b). With these simple steps, nurses who are novices in the EBP process can embark on projects that improve current practices wherever they are employed. In addition, EBP champions can support nurses and nurse educators to create a spirit of inquiry at their facilities.

The practice of EBP must be embedded into nursing academia and introduced to nursing students early in their academic careers (Melnyk & Fineout-Overholt, 2015a, 2015b). A teaching learning strategy where EBP can be clearly exemplified is simulation. Simulations are increasing in frequency in nursing education programs and are becoming a standard approach to learning nursing practice. Evidence-based guidelines and protocols now exist for their implementation. Simulation is an effective teaching–learning strategy that illustrates the EBP process in action, and effective evidence-based simulations equip students with skills, knowledge, and confidence in their current and future practice. Efficacy in simulation denotes the need for knowledgeable and skilled simulationists to conduct the entire process of simulation to optimize learning and promote critical thinking and synthesis of new concepts.

Despite the evidence regarding best practices and faculty preparation, there is often a lack of readiness to fulfill the simulation teaching role. Faculty development calls for guidance and role modeling from simulation experts who practice evidence-based simulation teaching, who are familiar with the INACSL Best Practice Standards: Simulation^SM , and who seek optimal outcomes for students (Jeffries et al., 2015). Faculty must be prepared to integrate EBP into simulation through a structured process for preparing, executing, and evaluating the simulation program. Academic centers are called upon to invest in their faculty in this manner and to recognize that effective simulation teaching is not an inherent skill, but a learned and practiced process that requires faculty development.

Toolkit Resources

Toolkit 17-1: Template for Asking PICOT Questions.
Toolkit 17-2: Checklist for Conducting an Evidence Review for Initiating Practice Change (Intervention).

18 Leading the Science: Research in Simulation

Teresa W. Atz, Trisha Leann Horsley

Key Terms

Simulation Research, Program of Research, Scientific Rigor, Research Funding, Grant Writing, Simulation Researcher, Reliability, Validity

Guiding Questions

1 What is the state of the science in nursing simulation research?

2 How do I develop a research question and design a research study?

3 How do I begin to develop a simulation research program of excellence?

4 What are strategies for success in grant writing and finding funding opportunities for simulation research?

Simulation research is becoming even more important with the recent increase in simulation use in nursing education. We know from previous research of high-fidelity patient simulation (HPS) that simulation provides an excellent realistic and interactive learning experience (Weaver, 2011). Despite the growing popularity of simulation education, there exists a relatively small body of literature examining learning outcomes or the translation to patient outcomes. This leaves many gaps in knowledge (Murphy, 2015; Shinnick, Woo, & Mentes, 2010). This is significant in that simulation is both time-consuming and expensive. Previous research about simulation education has been plagued with single site studies, small participant numbers, less than rigorous study designs, lack of randomization, absence of control group, and a lack of reliable and valid instruments to measure important outcomes such as

knowledge, skill acquisition and critical thinking (Alexander et al., 2015; Doolen et al., 2016; Shinnick et al., 2010). With the recent results of the National Council of State Boards of Nursing (NCSBN) study revealing acceptable outcomes when up to 50% of traditional clinical time is replaced with simulation, it is crucial to perform rigorous research of simulation to inform best practice and assure positive educational outcomes (Hayden, Smiley, Alexander, Kardong-Edgren, & Jeffries, 2014).

This chapter will discuss the state of the science in nursing simulation research: past, present, and future. In addition, we will provide the foundation to help you plan for and develop a research project, get it funded, and start your own simulation research program of excellence.

Nursing Research

Nursing research is a systematic inquiry to develop evidence that answers questions, solves problems, and is generalizable to all aspects of the nursing profession including clinical practice, education, administration, and informatics (Polit & Beck, 2012). The first and most important step in any research is defining the question or problem that warrants an answer. Research questions aim to answer or address a

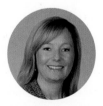

Teresa W. Atz, PhD, RN, CHSE

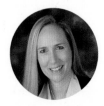

Trisha Leann Horsley, PhD, RN, CHSE, CNE

problem and guide the types of data to be collected in the study. Some questions ask for the problem to be better understood, and some may make a prediction or hypothesis about how a particular problem will be answered.

A common format for creating either an evidence-based or research question is PICO: (P) patient or population of interest, (I) intervention/issue of interest, (C) comparison of interest, and (O) outcome of interest. This format assists the simulation researcher in forming a focused question. Often, researchers add a (T) for time making it a PICOT question. An example of a simulation research PICOT question is the following: Will a medication administration simulation scenario (I) with fourth semester undergraduate nursing students (P) yield higher medication administration test scores (O) in the students who participated in the scenario compared to those who had lecture only (C)? The (T) could represent the time when the medication test occurs.

Once a specific research question is conceived, it is critical to look at what is already known about the topic. Searching the literature is key in order to examine existing research and determine what gaps still exist. A librarian can assist in accessing common databases. Some examples of databases that include simulation literature include, but are not limited to, PubMed, Cumulative Index to Nursing and Allied Health Literature (CINAHL), PsychINFO, Medline, and Ovid. One of the challenges for simulation researchers is the fact that because the field is relatively new, some journals may not yet be indexed. New journals must accomplish certain steps, over time, in order to be accepted for indexing. Therefore, it is crucial to also intentionally search simulation-specific journals that you can identify through simulation organizational websites and simple Internet searches. Based on the results of the literature search, the research question may need to change or it can be supported by a gap in the literature. More questions to ask about the research question are the following: What is the significance of this problem to nursing education? Is it feasible to study? Do I need to narrow my focus? Which research design is best suited to answer this question?

Once the literature related to the research question is analyzed, there will emerge either gaps or a needed next step to be addressed by this research question. The significance of the problem can be addressed in the aims or objectives of the study. The statement of purpose will summarize the goal(s) of the proposed study. The aims or objectives state the specific ways in which the researcher hopes to conduct the study and answer the research question. The following is an example of a purpose statement, research question, and aims:

- Purpose statement: The purpose of this study is to increase knowledge attainment and retention for pre-licensure nursing students by piloting a new simulation educational experience to supplement a traditional medication administration lecture.

- Research question: Will prelicensure nursing students who participate in a medication administration simulation in addition to traditional lecture have higher medication administration final exam scores than those students who participated in traditional lecture only 4 weeks post lecture/simulation?
- The aim of the study: To assess knowledge attainment and retention by comparing final exam scores of those prelicensure nursing students who received a medication administration simulation in addition to traditional lecture to those who received a traditional lecture only.

Feasibility of the study addresses time, availability of research participants, facilities and equipment, cost, researcher experience and resources, and ethical considerations (Polit & Beck, 2012). For the research question and aims above, there are many factors to consider. How many students do you need to produce generalizable findings, or to power the study? Will you have enough students to participate? How will you recruit? Will you provide incentives? What about the students without the intervention, will it be fair if their scores are lower? How many additional faculty will you need to schedule to conduct the simulations? Do you have the appropriate equipment and space? Do you have buy-in from the faculty and administration? Do you have a validated simulation scenario? It is very important to think through every step and make sure your project is manageable. It is easy to want to solve the world's problems in one study. However, you don't want to end up with a project so big that it is impossible to accomplish. Keep the study manageable by setting concise and simple aims and objectives and focus on those goals. Once the aims are set and feasibility is confirmed, a focus on the appropriate research design for the study is the next step.

Research Design

There are three major research designs: qualitative, quantitative, and mixed methods. The research question will inform which design to use. Quantitative research uses structured methods to gather objective data that can be accurately measured, usually with statistical methods. This method focuses on concepts or variables that are fairly well developed, with an existing body of literature, and have reliable and valid methods of measurement (Creswell & Plano Clark, 2011). An example of a quantitative simulation research project would be to study how simulation learning activities affect test scores in a particular course.

Qualitative research seeks to answer questions about certain phenomena that are not well understood. The underlying assumption of qualitative research is that individuals or groups of individuals socially construct reality. Therefore, the concepts or phenomenon in question require exploration by dialogue or observation in an inductive manner in order to provide a rich meaning

(Creswell & Plano Clark, 2011). Data are usually narrative and subjective and are generally collected in the setting in which the phenomena occur. An example of qualitative simulation research would be to interview students in the simulation lab after participation in a particular scenario to assess their feelings about their experiences.

Mixed methods research rigorously collects both qualitative and quantitative data and integrates, relates, or mixes the data at some stage of the research process (Creswell, Fetters, & Ivankova, 2004). While qualitative methods alone are ideal for exploring previously unknown phenomena, and quantitative methods are ideal for measuring the extensiveness of the phenomena, utilizing both methods combines the strengths and minimizes the weakness of each method in order to more completely answer the research question (Creswell & Plano Clark, 2011). An example of mixed methods simulation research would combine measuring test scores and assessing student feelings after a particular scenario in order to see if the scenario is a valid and satisfactory learning method. Regardless of the design used, the research should have a strong problem statement, robust and replicable methodology, valid scenarios with attention to fidelity (realism), valid and reliable measurement instruments, and attention to protection of human subjects all grounded in theory (Franklin, Leighton, Cantrell, & Rutherford-Hemming, 2015).

Learn what it is like to be asked to be a primary investigator for the largest nursing simulation study ever undertaken by reading Dr. Suzan Kardong-Edgren's Voice of Experience describing the beginning of the National Council of State Boards of Nursing simulation study.

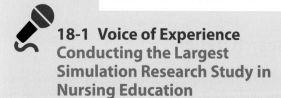

18-1 Voice of Experience
Conducting the Largest Simulation Research Study in Nursing Education

• •

Suzan Kardong-Edgren, PhD, RN, CHSE, FSSH, ANEF, FAAN

• •

The Challenge

When the call came from the NCSBN to consult on the National Simulation Study, I was stunned. Our job was to provide evidence for or against the use of simulation as a substitution for traditional clinical. Thoughts ran through my mind such as "Could we do this idea justice? Did they know how hard a multisite simulation study was to do well? What was our budget? Why did they think I knew anything about simulation? And finally, don't screw this up!" I was delighted to find out I would be working with Pam Jeffries, the original Sim Champion. Jennifer Hayden trusted us to know what to do. When she stepped out of the room at our first meeting, Pam and I looked at each other saying "Can you believe we are doing this?"

Meeting the Challenge

Our first planning meetings were dedicated to devising a multiyear approach to the question. Initially, time was spent in defining terms and gathering preliminary data. Those data were published early and focused on how much simulation was already being used and how faculty were prepared for that use at the time. Based on this, we moved forward with research questions and finding potential sites for the study. We planned and Jennifer guided and executed the plan. Schools were chosen; multiple preparatory training meetings were held. And then, it started at all sites.

Outcome

The study was completed with minimal problems from a research perspective. We experienced one of those ideal outcomes that rarely happens, a study-informed policy. A year after the study was published, the NCSBN called us back to write guidelines for the use of simulation that each US board of nursing could adopt or modify as it so chose. Members of three very active state boards, representatives from the two big nursing accrediting bodies, INACSL, and the NCSBN worked for 2 days to draft the suggested guidelines. These were reviewed by NCSBN committees, edited, and published. The final outcome of those guidelines is not known yet. Arizona used them as a model for their own more stringent simulation guidelines.

Most Valuable Lessons Learned

When you publish, people think you know something. Jennifer found me through my publications. Ask for what you actually need; be bold. We did not know the initial budget for the study, but we knew it was going to be expensive. So we planned as if we had the budget for a study of this size. The NCSBN and Jennifer got us what it took to do the study well.

Inspiration for Simulation Champions

Publish your work. No one can capitalize on what you have done if they do not know about it. Don't be afraid if opportunity knocks. If not you, then who?

Theoretical and Conceptual Models

Theories are sets of interrelated concepts that explain some aspect or view of events or situations by specifying relationships among variables in order to explain and predict the events or situations (Goodson, 2010). Concepts are the integral parts that make up the theory. Theoretical frameworks influence the way questions or problems are identified and studied in that they assist in organizing the concepts or variables, provide a sound description of the events or situations, and predict events or situations.

Theory-based research and interventions are more robust and more effective than research without a theoretical lens (Goodson, 2010). Theories and research are symbiotic in many ways. Theories are created from observations and data obtained from previous research and then tested through further research. The theory then guides ideas for future research intervention development and implementation and development of new theories (Polit & Beck, 2012). To make adequate use of theories, a researcher should apply the theory to guide the research question, data collection, interpretation of results, and recommendations for practice and future research. A review of the literature by Rourke, Schmidt, and Garga (2010) revealed that of 47 nursing simulation research studies, only 10% made adequate use of a theory. Research guided by theoretical or conceptual frameworks is more generalizable, coherent, and robust (Rourke et al., 2010). This is especially important in nursing simulation education research as this area of research has historically lacked in **scientific rigor**. There are no limits on the particular theory that can be used in simulation research. It is only important to choose the theory that will best guide the particular study. Examples of two popular and relevant theories frequently applied to simulation research are self-efficacy theory and the NLN/Jeffries framework, now middle-range theory. For additional discussion on theoretical frameworks, refer to Chapter 16: Theoretical Principles to Effective Simulation.

Self-Efficacy

Self-efficacy is described by Bandura (1977a) as one's belief of being capable of performing tasks in order to achieve particular goals. This is particularly relevant to nursing as students learn basic tasks and progress on to more difficult interventions and critical thinking. Self-efficacy has been linked to success during the undergraduate nursing program, the first year of work experience, and a nurse's general perception of his or her professional role as he or she works from novice nurse to expert nurse. Confidence has been interchanged with self-efficacy, as it is a person's judgement or perception of ability. Historically, this theory has often been applied to clinical research on population health behaviors such as in chronic disease management,

smoking cessation, alcohol use, eating, and exercising (APA.org). There has been a plethora of nursing research related to self-efficacy and confidence in nursing, mostly focusing on clients managing chronic health problems. Recent nursing education research has focused on the self-efficacy of student nurses related to the effectiveness of methods of teaching, in particular, skill acquisition in simulation.

NLN Jeffries Simulation Theory

In 2003, Pamela Jeffries, a leading simulation scientist, developed the first simulation framework at that time, the NLN/Jeffries Simulation Framework. This framework consisted of five constructs: facilitator, participant, educational practices, simulation design characteristics, and outcomes. The purpose of this framework was to provide educators with a consistent and empirically based framework to guide the process of designing, implementing and evaluating simulation in nursing and clarify the roles of the teacher and the student, and to identify best practices in simulation nursing education (Jeffries, 2005). This framework has been used effectively many times in the literature to guide simulation research. A recent systematic review examined simulation studies that used the NLN/Jeffries framework as a guiding lens. Results showed three recurrent themes: simulation provides positive outcomes especially when used in conjunction with traditional teaching strategies, fidelity is an important factor in simulation, and debriefing is a key component for simulation education (Adamson, 2015). To learn more about Dr. Jeffries' thought process as she developed the initial framework, refer to her Voice of Experience in Chapter 1.

This framework recently became the NLN Jeffries Simulation Theory and is considered a midrange theory after extensive synthesis of the literature and discussion among simulation leaders with minor changes within the original concepts (Jeffries, Rogers, & Adamson, 2015). The key concepts of this new theory include context, background, design, simulation experience, facilitator and educational strategies, participant, and outcomes. The contextual factors in the simulation can include circumstances such as the overall purpose of the simulation and the setting or place where the simulation takes place. The background of the simulation includes the specific goals and the theoretical perspective for the simulation experience. These both influence the design of the simulation. The simulation experience occurs in an environment of trust and is experiential, interactive, collaborative, and learner centered. There is a dynamic interaction between the facilitator and the participant in the simulation experience taking into consideration how each one's attributes and characteristics influence the experience. The facilitator responds to the participants' needs by adjusting educational strategies during the simulation such as timing of activities, providing cues during the simulation, and debriefing for feedback after the simulation. The outcomes of the simulation are separated into three areas: participant, patient, and system outcomes, which would equate to improved public health (Jeffries et al., 2015).

Research in Simulation Past, Present, and Future Recommendations

As previously mentioned, it is crucial to search the literature for recent and past literature in order to identify the gaps. Some of the first research in nursing simulation education relates to satisfaction, confidence, and skill attainment. More recent to simulation research is the study of more specific outcomes such as self-efficacy, critical thinking, and transfer of knowledge to the clinical setting. The following is a summary of recent reviews of simulation research.

Satisfaction

Measurement of student and faculty satisfaction in simulation education has been studied fairly extensively over the past years. This is perhaps related to the ease in which satisfaction can be measured both qualitatively and quantitatively with good **reliability** and **validity**. Positive learner satisfaction has been found in most studies. A recent review of the state of the science in prelicensure nursing education described students perceptions related to simulation as beneficial, realistic, enjoyable, and with high satisfaction (Shinnick et al., 2010).

Self-Efficacy/Confidence

Self-efficacy, as mentioned previously, is the belief that one is capable of performing a task or achieving a goal (Franklin & Lee, 2014). It is also frequently referred to in the literature as confidence. Previous research in nursing education has attempted to examine the effects that simulation has on self-efficacy of student or novice nurses. Franklin and Lee's (2014) meta-analysis of 43 studies about the effectiveness of simulation for improvement of the self-efficacy of the novice nurse revealed simulation increased self-efficacy greater than traditional didactic education. Unfortunately, many of these studies have been small in sample size and qualitative, had mainly heterogeneous participants, used unvalidated measurements, and were very focused on specific skills and situations. Of significance, despite studies linking simulation to student confidence in skills, there has not been a significant association between self-efficacy and improved skills or knowledge, which puts to question the value of studying

self-efficacy or confidence gains (Leigh, 2008; Shinnick et al., 2010; Yuan, Williams, & Fang, 2012).

Skill Acquisition and Knowledge

Many studies have looked at simulation's effect on skill acquisition. Systematic reviews of evidence of simulation's effect on improved knowledge and skill acquisition of both nursing and medical students revealed simulation to be associated with enhanced skills and higher scores on knowledge exams (Lapkin, Levett-Jones, Bellchambers, & Fernandez, 2010; Yuan et al., 2012). Objective structured clinical examination (OSCE) assessments are very popular in the literature and are supported by simulation as far as skill gains and improvement. Studies of knowledge gain have yielded mostly insignificant results (Shinnick et al., 2010). Lack of validity and reliability of measurements of both skill acquisition and knowledge plagues most studies.

Critical Thinking/Critical Reasoning

Crucial to a nurse's success and to positive patient outcomes is the ability to build upon prior knowledge and critically think and use proper judgement and decision-making skills when met with an unexpected situation (Lapkin et al., 2010). Results of reviews of the literature of studies measuring the effectiveness of simulation in teaching critical thinking skills are inconclusive given mixed results. This may be because most studies measure more outcomes than just critical thinking in one study, have small sample sizes, and lack measurement tools dedicated to critical reasoning (Fisher & King, 2013; Lapkin et al., 2010; Shinnick et al., 2010).

Safety

One of the most important outcomes nurses strive for is patient safety. A literature review by Shearer (2013) looked at the following safety outcomes in simulation: medication errors, patient identification, communication, knowledge, skills and attitudes, and hygiene. The results of communication studies were inconsistent, and only two studies showed statistically significant improvements on medication errors and patient identifications (Shearer, 2013).

Instrument Development

Reliable and valid instruments are essential in order to adequately evaluate participant performance and measure outcomes in simulation research. As noted in the summary of previous research, the lack of these reliable and valid instruments is frequently mentioned as a limitation in simulation studies. A previous literature review of frequently used instruments in simulation recommended that researchers use existing tools rather than create their own in order to strengthen reliability and validity of those instruments (Kardong-Edgren et al., 2010). This will only add rigor to future research utilizing these instruments. An update of this review in 2015 focusing on four OSCE instruments and other simulation instruments showed that although existing instruments were being used in subsequent research, they were at times not used appropriately, thus negatively affecting their validity and reliability. Also there were new instruments developed since the first review. This updated review again echoed the importance of using existing instruments in future research but with caution that they must be utilized appropriately (Adamson, Kardong-Edgren, & Willhaus, 2013).

Patient Outcomes/Translational Research

Simulation has been studied in a number of settings in the clinical area. A recent review of selected simulation research by Aebersold and Tschannen (2013) revealed how simulation can impact patient outcomes. Settings involved in this review were community hospitals, labor and delivery unit, and pediatric intensive care units. Outcomes included decreased adverse events, increased recognition of deteriorating patients, enhanced teamwork, and improved survival rates in pediatric resuscitations (Adamson, 2015; Aebersold & Tschannen, 2013). A literature review by Fisher and King (2013) showed mixed results of the students' perceived ability to transfer skills into the clinical setting.

McGaghie Draycott, Dunn, Lopez, and Stefanidis (2011) defined translational research in medical education as having three phases to bring the simulation lab to the bedside. The first phase, T1, aims to move from simulation or skills lab to yield improved patient care practices. The second phase, T2, aims to produce evidence of clinical effectiveness at the patient level, leading to improved practice, new guidelines, and policies. The third phase, T3, aims to yield measurable improvement in the health of patients and of society in general (McGaghie et al., 2011). It is of note that although this article referred to simulation in medical education, these outcomes of translational research mirror the outcomes in the NLN Jeffries Simulation Theory (Jeffries et al., 2015). It is critical that we move research in this direction as improved patient outcomes should be a major goal of simulation training in healthcare.

Future Recommendations

Many gaps remain in the literature despite years of simulation research. This is not surprising given small sample sizes, lack of reliable and valid instruments, and a science that is still in early development. Simulation is growing in leaps and bounds, and everyday there is a new question that begs for an answer. The following is a list, albeit not exhaustive, of recommendations for future research as mentioned in the literature.

- Knowledge retainment and transfer in longitudinal study into clinical practice
- Unintended consequences of simulation training
- Cost-effectiveness of simulation training
- Improved measurement practices
- Relationships between confidence/self-efficacy, knowledge gains competence/performance, and patient outcomes
- Debriefing: Which characteristics are most effective for desired outcomes
- Additional simulation frameworks
- Best practices for facilitator training, facilities, equipment and technology
- Prebriefing: Best practices
- Substitution of clinical hours: Further research regarding long-term outcomes and cost
- Team simulation: Instrument development, reliability, and validity for team performance
- In situ simulation outcomes

Developing a Research Program of Excellence

Many leaders in simulation have emerged from less than ideal simulation programs with high-quality research. This was achieved through their sheer determination, perseverance, and desire to advance the science of simulation research. Think of how much more could be produced if the environment was designed to encourage and foster success in research. Developing a simulation research program of excellence is desired by many but obtained by few. Even defining the program may be difficult, yet when certain characteristics are assembled together, the program will have the tools to be successful.

The infrastructure must be in place to support a quality research program. Support from top administrative leadership must be evident in word and action by first selecting a doctorally prepared faculty member who has had formal training and experience in simulation to lead the simulation program. Hiring for this position should not be taken lightly and only someone who is well developed in Kouzes and Posner's (2012) five practices of exemplary leadership should be considered.

The leader of a research program should *Model the Way, Inspire a Shared Vision, Challenge the Process, Enable Others to Act, and Encourage the Heart* in order to serve as a champion and leader for simulation research (Kouzes & Posner, 2012). This leader must:

- Lead by example through developing and growing his/her own **program of research** in simulation
- Collaborate with others within and outside the discipline of nursing to create a team of researchers for future simulation research
- Be able to clearly articulate and inspire stakeholders and colleagues to seize the opportunity to develop a research program of excellence
- Know the current state of the science and where the gaps are in the current simulation literature
- Have the ability to challenge the process in a respectful and professional manner for continual movement toward advancing the science of simulation research
- Support opportunities for faculty development within and outside the institution to empower others to be their best
- Encourage the heart of others through mentoring others to be lifelong learners with the thirst for inquiry, exploring new ideas, and gaining new knowledge through research in simulation.

All of these activities are laying the foundation of success for a simulation research program, and the leader must have protected time to make sure a solid foundation is created and maintained. Anyone can be appointed to direct and/or manage a simulation lab, but it takes a true leader at the helm to develop a simulation research program of excellence and lead a team of simulation researchers.

Personal resources such as research assistants and access to a statistician are invaluable to researchers. Research assistants ease the workload of the researcher by completing tasks that must be done yet do not require the researcher to complete such as performing literature searches, maintaining a reference library, assisting with **grant writing**, and data entry. Collaboration with a statistician when a study is in the planning phase may prevent errors that could not be corrected if the statistician was consulted later in the process. An ideal case would be to have a research assistant and statistician as a member of your research team. Other characteristics that are found within a simulation research program of excellence are that they tend to collaborate with researchers at other simulation programs to conduct multisite studies. This collaboration can also lead to sharing of resources. For example, if you do not have a statistician at your organization, collaborate to conduct research with a nursing program that does.

Dissemination of your research is essential through professional journals and conferences at the local, state, regional, national, and international level. As the authors of simulation review articles have noted, the quality of research design and how outcomes are reported need to be improved in order to better inform our practice. A group of simulation experts developed a steering committee to address the scope of existing reporting guidelines and whether gaps existed related to simulation research (Cheng et al., 2016b). The Consolidated Standards of Reporting Trials (CONSORT) and Strengthening the Reporting of Observational Studies in Epidemiology (STROBE) Statements were identified for potential additions related to simulation research. CONSORT guidelines were developed for randomized trials, while STROBE covers observational studies. A group of consensus panel participants developed simulation-specific extensions to the statements that are meant to guide reporting of research of studies. This work has been published simultaneously by the four largest simulation journals. Using these guidelines when developing your research study, as well as when you document and disseminate the findings, will help to enhance the body of knowledge related to simulation-based learning.

Think broadly when you are disseminating your work. Findings that were nonsignificant may be just as important to publish as results that were significant. Simulation research programs of excellence showcase their work and find innovative ways to assist others through continuing educational programs, fellowship programs, and graduate-level courses specific to simulation.

Finding Funding for Research

It may not be as hard as finding a needle in a haystack, but finding funding for research in simulation can be challenging. The key is to perform a systematic search on a frequent basis. Research funding may be found within your institution, professional organizations, foundations, and government agencies on a state or federal level. If your institution has a grant administrator be sure to introduce yourself and share your interests and program of research. Finding potential funding is one aspect of a grant administrator's job, yet if he/she isn't familiar with your program of research, then opportunities within your area may be missed. If your institution does not have a grant administrator assigned to your school or department, the institution may have a Grant Programs Office or Grant and Contract Office that manages the research portfolios within the institution. Through this office, you should receive support in your search for external funding opportunities by being able to use the Funding Search Database System, which is available to every researcher at the institution. Keywords are used to search the database, and then matching results are revealed to include the funding opportunity number, title, funding agency, posted date, and closing date. A link will be provided to obtain complete information about the grant.

For a novice researcher, you may want to first search for potential funding opportunities within your own institution. These may be classified as research start-up funds, summer stipends, or teaching innovation grants. Often, internal funding covers enough for a pilot project and provides you with an opportunity to showcase your independence as a researcher. No amount of funding should be considered too small or insignificant to apply for. Securing several smaller grants as a novice researcher will lay a solid foundation on which to build a trajectory toward receiving larger funding.

Table 18.1 provides a broad perspective to identify potential funding sources outside of your institution. Simulation may be directly named as the strategy of interest, but more times than not, it will be listed as an optional strategy or may not be listed at all. If you believe the strategy of simulation could meet the desired outcomes of the funding source, then move forward assembling a strong proposal to sell simulation as a solid option. The goal is to find a match between your idea and the funding source's priority. These must be congruent in order to be successful at receiving funding. However, do not wait for grant funding to begin research into your areas of interest. Read the simulation on a shoestring description of how one faculty was successful building a program of research with no outside funding support.

The How-to Guide on Grant Writing

Writing a grant may be perceived by the novice researcher as an insurmountable task or a skill that only a seasoned professor can master, but with dedication, time, and attention to detail, the novice researcher can master the skill like a professional. There are a few preparations that will improve the chances of success. Start by carving out and protecting time in your schedule to dedicate to creative thought and writing. It may work best to reserve one full day per week, 1 hour per day, or a 2-hour block of time on a weekend. The day or time is not important, but what matters is that you are retreating from the world to allow your mind to focus on writing. Reflect on your own workload and schedule to determine what is a realistic time period to dedicate to writing, and then stay firm on the commitment to yourself.

The next step in preparation is to identify a mentor who has had experience and success in grant writing. Ask

Table 18.1	Funding Search Engines and Sources
Agency for Healthcare Research and Quality	http://www.ahrq.gov/funding/index.html
American Association of Colleges of Nursing	http://www.aacn.nche.edu/faculty/funding-opportunities
American Association of Critical-Care Nurses	http://www.aacn.org/wd/practice/content/grant-all.pcms?menu=practice
American Heart Association	http://my.americanheart.org/professional/Research/FundingOpportunities/Funding-Opportunities_UCM_316909_SubHomePage.jsp
Cos Pivot	http://pivot.cos.com/
The Foundation Center	http://foundationcenter.org/
Grants.gov	http://www.grants.gov
International Nursing Association for Clinical Simulation and Learning	http://www.inacsl.org/i4a/pages/index.cfm?pageid=3293
National League for Nursing	http://www.nln.org/professional-development-programs/grants-and-scholarships
National Science Foundation	http://www.nsf.gov
Sigma Theta Tau International Honor Society of Nursing	http://www.nursingsociety.org/advance-elevate/research/research-grants
Society for Simulation in Healthcare	http://www.ssih.org/Membership/Research-Grant
Research	http://www.researchresearch.com/
Robert Wood Johnson Foundation	http://www.rwjf.org/
SPIN Funding Opportunities	http://infoedglobal.com/solutions/grants-contracts/spin-funding-opportunities/
U.S. Department of Health and Human Services, Health Resources and Services Administration (HRSA)	http://www.hrsa.gov/grants/index.html
U.S. Department of Health and Human Services, National Institutes of Health (NIH)	http://www.grants.gov/

Nonfunded Research

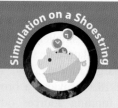

Kim Leighton, PhD, RN, CHSE, CHSOS, ANEF

The Challenge

I was interested in doing research related to simulation-based learning; however, I did not work in a college that conducted research. I had just finished my doctorate and was excited about doing research. The Mission statements revolved around teaching, but leadership did support faculty interested in research and publication; they just didn't fit it into any of the workload formulas. Therefore, research needed to fit into your regular work, and you needed to be willing to do anything more on your own time. We were also a private school with no history of grant funding success; in fact, we had never even applied for a research grant!

I had a lot of burning questions when I started teaching with simulation: Could students actually do CPR after certification? Did they follow BLS guidelines? Does debriefing make a difference? And, my big question: If simulation is going to replace clinical, then isn't it important to know how comparable they are to start with?

Innovative Solutions

To conduct research without funding and time support, the researcher must be passionate about the question and willing to put in some time on their own; however, it's most important to choose a project that is feasible and inexpensive. For the CPR study (Leighton & Scholl, 2009), I created a "treatment scenario" within the software that listed the steps of BLS. As the students provided care, I clicked on the corresponding step when (or if) it occurred. This provided a database that showed length of time between steps and the order they were undertaken. The only cost to this project, which involved a scenario already in the curriculum, was my few minutes to set up the programming. To assess whether debriefing made a difference, students completed the Simulation Effectiveness Tool (Elfrink Cordi, Leighton, Ryan-Wenger, Doyle, & Ravert, 2012) immediately following the scenario and again following debriefing. There were statistically significant gains in the students' perceptions of how well their learning needs were met following debriefing as compared to before debriefing. This tool was already being used in the program so required no additional cost or time. Even the "big question," which was my dissertation, was completed at five sites across the United States at a total cost of $400. As you can see from these examples, it is possible to conduct research on important questions at very little to no cost. Find a topic you are passionate about, consider your resources, and carefully assess feasibility of your project. You don't need large amounts of federal funding to do important work!

the mentor to review your work on a regular basis and then offer suggestions for improvement. Be open to the constructive feedback and learn from it as you move forward. Grant writing is a specific skill set that can be acquired and honed with experience and time. You need the internal motivation and drive to complete your goal of writing a grant, but the mentor provides the experienced guidance toward success. Collaboration with an experienced researcher as a mentor will be essential if applying for a training grant because you may not have any track record of your own.

It is essential that the grant proposal is written to fit the expressed priorities and structured guidelines of the funding source. Begin by grabbing the attention of the reviewer and hold it from start to finish while quickly and efficiently selling the proposal. Keep the sections organized to show detail and logical flow in progression throughout

the proposal much like how a well-developed story is told. The reviewer must be convinced that all the angles have been covered and the proposed plan is realistic, and believe that even a complex proposal can be successfully operationalized to reach the set forth outcomes.

The specific aims of the proposal must be clear, be succinct, and be aligned with a gap in the current knowledge base. Generally, one page is allowed for this section. Provide enough background on the topic that will set the context for the reviewer without overburdening with all of the knowledge about the desired topic. What you decide is a priority, for the background section provides a glimpse as to your thinking on this topic for the reviewer. The significance of the study, as previously mentioned, expresses how and to what extent this study will have an impact. Think of the significance as the "So what? Why is this proposed study so important that I should fund it?" The significance establishes the need for implementation of this study. The background and significance should provide support for the specific aims of the proposal.

Including your study's conceptual or theoretical framework will provide scaffolding on which to build the grant proposal. The framework provides the scientific or conceptual basis and is often included with the review of relevant literature. Describe in detail the relationship and fit between the framework and the grant proposal; it may be best to provide a visual display of this framework in the form of a diagram to support the narrative. It will be important to later link the findings back to this framework and relevant literature.

Up until this point of the grant proposal, the global perspective has been described. Now it is time to describe the details and feasibility of your proposal. This next step in writing a grant proposal will be describing the research approach. This section is often considered the most critical section of the proposal. Identify the specific research questions or hypotheses. Describe the design, sample with inclusion and exclusion criteria, and setting. If relevant, discuss the intervention along with the rationale as to why this intervention was selected and how the intervention differs from standard practice. Report the instruments to measure the dependent variables as well as the reliability and validity of each instrument. The step-by-step data collection plan should be provided followed by the proposed plan for data analysis. It is important for a novice researcher to keep the design and data collection procedures simple and to collaborate with a statistician during the development of the proposal to ensure data are being collected, stored, and analyzed in the appropriate way. Review Adamson and Prion's Voice of Experience to learn how they have used a monthly journal column to mentor researchers in how to manage and analyze data.

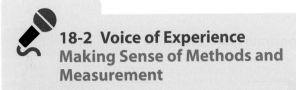

18-2 Voice of Experience
Making Sense of Methods and Measurement

Katie Anne Adamson Haerling, PhD, RN

Susan Prion, EdD, RN, CNE

The Challenge

As early adopters of simulation, we knew from experience that well-run simulation activities provided exceptional learning opportunities. However, we were disappointed by the quality of much of the research about the effectiveness of simulation in nursing education. The early literature in this area relied heavily on author-developed, self-report measures of student satisfaction, confidence, and learning. In order to strengthen the evidence base for simulation practice, we recognized the need for increased rigor in simulation research and resources to assist nurse educators in developing these skills.

Meeting the Challenge

In 2012, at the invitation of Dr. Suzan Kardong-Edgren, editor of *Clinical Simulation in Nursing*, we launched, *Making Sense of Methods and Measurement*, a regular column in the journal. The purpose of the column was to "review a variety of topics directly related to research methodology and both qualitative and quantitative data analysis" (Prion & Adamson, 2012, p. e193). By providing information and guidance related to simulation research methods and data analysis techniques in the column, we hoped to build capacity for improving the evidence base for simulation practice.

Outcome

At the writing of this Voice of Experience piece, over two dozen *Making Sense of Methods and Measurement* columns, including several editions highlighting specific methods by guest author-experts, have appeared in *Clinical Simulation in Nursing*. We continue to receive positive feedback from readers. "Fans" of the column include everyone from struggling graduate students who appreciate the easy-to-understand descriptions of statistical methods to seasoned researchers who see the value of bringing conversations about research methods to the forefront.

Most Valuable Lessons Learned

The most valuable lesson we've learned from this experience is the power of collaboration. While we originally began working together to develop this column, we have leveraged our shared interest in improving the rigor of simulation research to branch out on projects with other methods enthusiasts.

Inspiration for Simulation Champions

Katie: "The most elegant design of a study will not overcome the damage caused by unreliable or imprecise measurements" (Fleiss, 1986, p. 1).

Susan: "Somewhere, something incredible is waiting to be known!" (Begley, 1977, p. 53).

Often, you will be asked to provide a time table for implementation, and a Gantt chart is an excellent way to visually display activities that are planned to occur over time. A quick glance at a Gantt chart will provide information as to what activities are involved, when each activity starts and stops, which activities will overlap, and the length of the overall project from start to finish. A simple Gantt chart is provided in Table 18.2, while a more complex example is found in the Toolkit (18-1). A basic professional Gantt chart may be created in PowerPoint or Excel. Step-by-step instructions may be found on YouTube. Gantt chart software may be purchased for more elaborate project management.

Make certain you understand exactly how much finding is available through the grant and what the funds can or cannot be used for. For example: Can the funds be used to pay salaries, benefits, and/or stipends? Can the funds be used to purchase capital equipment, supplies, and/or food? Can the funds be used for advertisement, recruitment efforts, and/or dissemination of results through travel and conference expenses? With this information, create a realistic budget to include all direct and indirect expenses that are projected to incur during the project. A well-thought-out budget with appropriate justification for all expenses provides evidence of credibility for the researcher.

Formal letters of support should be submitted along with your grant application. A letter may be written by your dean to reconfigure your workload assignment to allow you more time to devote to the project if you are successful at receiving the funding. If you will be collaborating with other institutions in a multisite study, then a letter of intent from each institution would be appropriate to submit with the proposal. Experts who have been consulted on the project may submit a letter of commitment and support for the proposal. A project is rarely designed, implemented, and evaluated all on your own. So seek formal letters of support from all the individuals who will make major contributions to your project and submit these with your proposal.

Once a grant proposal has been completed, seek opportunities for an internal review of your work. You will want to find someone other than your mentor who has been successful at writing grants. Up until this point, you and your mentor have read the proposal many times. You need a fresh set of eyes to review your work to determine if your thoughts are clear and progress logically throughout the proposal. An idea that seemed so clear in your mind may not be so clear to others, which is why it is a good idea for others with experience in grant writing to review your work before it is submitted. Work this internal review into your timeline so that the internal reviewer has plenty of time to provide a quality review of your work and that there will be time for you to make any necessary corrections based on the feedback.

When the time has come to submit the grant proposal, be sure to follow the submission instructions exactly and meet the specified deadline. Verify that you have complied with the requested formatting, page lengths, and number of copies submitted as well as included all of the required signatures. Give yourself time for this final step in the process so that the grant proposal may be submitted with confidence that your best work has been submitted. Institutional review board (IRB) approval is not required prior to the grant proposal submission, but if the proposal is accepted, then IRB approval must be obtained prior to the grant being awarded.

Ethical Considerations

Ethical principles are not an afterthought but instead should be woven throughout the simulation and research experience. Grove, Gray, and Burns (2015) describe three ethical principles to consider: (1) principle of respect for persons, (2) principle of beneficence, and (3) principle of

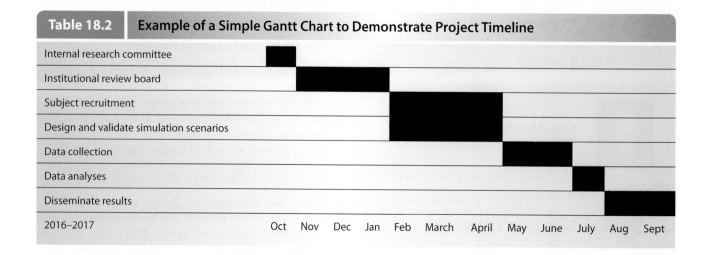

Table 18.2	Example of a Simple Gantt Chart to Demonstrate Project Timeline
Internal research committee	
Institutional review board	
Subject recruitment	
Design and validate simulation scenarios	
Data collection	
Data analyses	
Disseminate results	
2016–2017	Oct Nov Dec Jan Feb March April May June July Aug Sept

justice. All three ethical principles will be discussed in the context of simulation research. Adults who volunteer to participate in research should be perceived as autonomous, therefore having the right to agree or not agree to participate in the research without any repercussions (Grove et al., 2015). This is especially important when your participants are students. They must feel that their participation or decision not to participate will not negatively affect their grades or future status in their program. Proceed carefully with vulnerable populations so that there is no actual or perceived coercion of the participant. Providing full disclosure with no deception is required prior to starting any research. Participants have a right to know if data are being collected, how they are being collected, and how the data will be used. Within the academic setting, participants have a right to know if the simulation experience is graded or not as well as information on whether or not an audio/video recording will be collected. The prebriefing, simulation, and debriefing experience may be required as part of an academic course or training for employment yet be very clear to potential participants that their participation in data collection for research purposes is strictly voluntary.

Beneficence is the belief that the researcher will strive to always do good and avoid doing any harm. The simula-

tion environment must be a psychologically safe environment for the participant to meet Standards of Best Practice: Simulation^{SM} (INACSL Standards Committee, 2016). Participants should have freedom from exploitation. Careful consideration should be made regarding recordings. Just because the simulation center has the ability for audio/video recordings, it doesn't mean it is ethical to obtain the recordings. The following questions should be explored to determine whether or not to record: What are the ethical and legal responsibilities of videotaping? Is a consent specifically for the audio/video recording from each participant signed and on file to document release? What components of the simulation experience will be recorded (prebriefing, simulation, debriefing)? Who will have access to the recording? How long will it be kept? What security measures are in place to protect the recordings? As a researcher, you must never be so focused on acquiring data for a study that you lose sight of the bigger picture, which is to maintain the International Nursing

Association for Clinical Simulation and Learning (INACSL) Standards of Best Practice: Simulation^{SM} and above all do no harm (INACSL Standards Committee, 2016).

Justice occurs when the researcher treats all participants equal and fair in regard to the benefits and risks of the study. The participant selection process as well as the inclusion and exclusion process must exhibit equality

and fairness. As a researcher in simulation, are you using the same group of students for multiple studies out of convenience? It would be better to expand your participant selection process to recruit, which may lead to greater diversity of participants. There should be no difference in how a participant is treated even if the participant decided not to participate in the study. Participants also have a right to privacy meaning they determine whether or not to share private information. Measures need to be put in place for anonymity and confidentiality.

All human subject research including observational studies must be evaluated by the IRB prior to starting the study. The IRB application must include information on how subjects will be protected including specifics on how subjects will be located, recruited, and compensated. Potential risks and anticipated benefits of the study must be clearly stated as well as the informed consent process and specific data collection, management, and security procedures. There are three options for research proposals to be processed through the IRB: exempt (minimal to no risk), expedited (minimal risk), and complete (greater than minimal risk and/or use of vulnerable population). The IRB has the authority to disapprove, approve with modifications, or approve all research proposals. It is your ethical responsibility as a researcher to remain in compliance with institutional and federal regulations as well as educational training required by the IRB. A researcher, no matter what the level of expertise, should be uninhibited at any time to raise ethical questions for discussion to ensure the highest standards are being upheld for human rights.

Summary

It is of great importance that we continue to advance the science of nursing education and nursing practice through simulation research. Not only will simulation research advance nursing science in both clinical and educational practices but also in providing the best care possible for all patients. All it takes is a question or problem and a solid research method to address that question or problem. It is our hope that this chapter will provide you with information to excite and empower you to develop your nursing simulation research project and start your own simulation program of excellence.

Toolkit Resource

Toolkit 18-1: Complex Gantt Chart.

Leading Artistry in Simulation: Moulage and More

Rebekah J. Damazo, Benjamin J. Damazo

 Key Terms

Realism, Fidelity, Fiction Contract, Moulage

 Guiding Questions

1   Is it important to make simulation learning experiences as realistic as possible? Why or why not?

2   What resources are available to simulationists who want to create realism through the use of moulage techniques?

3   What precautions should be taken when choosing and utilizing moulage products?

Theatrical Dimensions of Simulation

The learners participating in a simulated clinical experience may have the same type of experience as if they were part of a theatrical production. The earliest theatrical plays date back to the Greeks in 534 BC and are attributed to Thespis (Buckham, 1830). The first plays were written for one actor, and he interacted with a chorus of people who helped him tell the story. Simulation theater is often the same. There is a primary actor—typically the patient simulator or a standardized patient—and those who interact with the actor to help tell the story. A number of health professionals, as well as scripted family or friends, may work to bring the story of the primary actor/patient to life. In the entertainment theater, the created environment

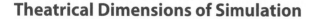

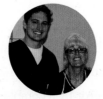

Rebekah J. Damazo, MSN, PNP, RN, CHSE-A
Benjamin J. Damazo, BA

allows the audience to relate to actor, scene, and script. The simulation theater gives learners the opportunity to interact in real time with all theater elements, but they translate to patient, environment, and scenario (Fig. 19.1).

The educator is challenged to develop a workable method to design and implement each element of a simulation-based learning experience. This requires creativity, an understanding of healthcare environments or scenes, and a subset of theatrical skills, which may include staging, costume and prop management, and **moulage** (Smith-Stoner, 2011).

Just as a play poorly written, acted, and staged is difficult to follow and may lead to frustration and dissatisfaction, it is also true that the poorly designed clinical story set in an unrealistic environment without the necessary props or cues can lead to an unsatisfactory learning experience in simulation. Roman Polanski, the famous French Polish film director said: "Cinema should make you forget you are sitting in a theater" (Irving, 2010). Similarly, the simulation scenario should make you forget you are not in a real-world environment. It is the role of the simulation educator to create enough reality to "suspend disbelief" for the participant (Fig. 19.2).

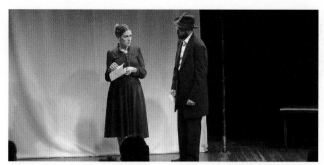

Figure 19.1 Theater Production Showing Minimal Staging to Create the Setting. (Editorial credit: wideweb / Shutterstock.com.)

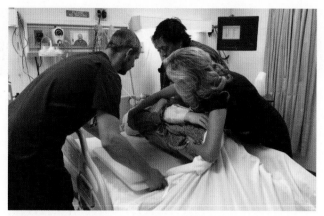

Figure 19.2 Patient Simulation Staging—Creating the Scene by Providing Elements of Reality.

When an individual sits down in a movie theater to watch a story, he or she may become so immersed in the drama that when a shot is fired the moviegoer will jump or even scream at the surprise elements, cry during emotional elements, and laugh out loud when humorous elements are introduced. The same can be true in a well-crafted simulation experience. The better the theatrics and staging, the more likely the learner will "buy in" to the experience and take advantage of the learning opportunity. In a sense, the learner and educator enter into an agreement about what will occur as the learner participates. This agreement is often called a **fiction contract**. Dieckmann, Gaba, and Rall (2007) brought the notion of the fiction contract to simulation in healthcare, borrowing the expression from the famous author Umberto Eco (Whitmarsh & Thompson, 2015). Samuel Coleridge (1817) spoke of "a semblance of truth sufficient to procure for these shadows of imagination that willing suspension of disbelief for the moment, which constitutes poetic faith" (p. 2). Just as the moviegoer decides to become immersed in a screen story, the simulation participant willingly goes on the theatrical journey that will simulate a clinical experience designed for education. The participant must freely accept the experience as real in order to fully experience the educational opportunity.

The effort to create a transparent and believable learning experience falls to the simulation educator or the simulation team. However, the reality of the simulation theater is a partnership between the understanding that the players are not real and the setting may also be artificial. The partners agree that the simulated environment may not exactly represent the learner's typical practice environment. There is an agreement or understanding that the simulation instructor will do all he or she can to create the simulation story as accurately as is reasonable and the learner will buy in to the story without dwelling on small inconsistencies in the setting. Each partner in this relationship has responsibilities. The instructor must develop and maintain an environment with sufficient **realism** that the learner receives appropriate clues to solve the problem presented by the

scenario. The learner's responsibility is to maintain a genuine interest in learning even if the idea of suspending disbelief might become difficult. The learner should also suspend judgement of the realism as a trade-off for the promise of learning new knowledge or skills. This means that the learner won't fixate on the minor details that may not fall in line with his or her understanding of a typical clinical situation and will instead make every effort to understand the clinical case and make appropriate clinical judgements to improve the patient outcomes. A sample fiction contract is located in the Online Toolkit (Toolkit 19-1).

Realism in Simulation

The ability to set the stage for training requires that the simulation instructor consider how to provide the greatest degree of reality for the learning experience. Perception of realism in simulation cases can impact the learner experience and influence learning (Nanji, Baca, & Raemer, 2013). The reality can include information that involves all of the senses including auditory, tactile, visual, and even olfactory. Alfred Hitchcock said: "Always make the audience suffer as much as possible" (Roman, 2009). The Simulation on a Shoestring features in this chapter offer cost-effective methods for increasing realism of the learning environment.

In simulation learning environments, the educator should create enough reality to develop an urgency for treatment and decision-making. Intrinsic motivators in the real-life clinical setting include the risk of patient harm. This fear of harm will naturally motivate the learner to pay attention to the task. Boggs, Mickel, and Holtom (2007) propose that educators "allow the learners to feel some stress" (p. 843). They

Wrapping Walls for Environmental Effect

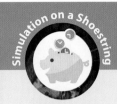

Mark Tuttle, BS, PMD

The Challenge

In the early days, while using simulation, I would place the mannequin in an undisclosed room, and ask the learners what area of patient care they worked in. Then, I created that environment in an effort to help them relax, by feeling they were working in their area of expertise. In 2000, I was one of the first in the United States to create a mobile simulation lab using a motor home, removing the interior structures and placing simulators within. I took the mobile learning lab to various hospital departments, fire departments, and other agencies. I also took the mannequins out and placed them inside an ICU ambulance, and/or an aircraft for training. Still, there are challenges in making the environment seem real.

Innovative Solutions

My program manager at the college asked me if I could wrap some of the walls in the simulation center. I contacted a local photographer and then called the local hospitals to set up time to take photos. All of the hospitals were more than willing to help. I requested a photo shoot of a trauma center, an adult emergency department, a mother–baby unit, and a pediatric scene. I then set out to find a company who could place the wraps on the walls. This meant we had to send the work out to bid. So why did I want to wrap everything? I remember back in the earlier days of simulation, I asked the learner what would make them feel comfortable in simulation. They responded that a simulation environment that portrayed their working environment would place them more at ease. This whole project took about 9 months from start to finish. Figure 19.3 shows the hallway before the

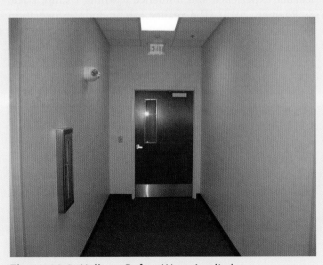

Figure 19.3 Hallway Before Wrap Applied.

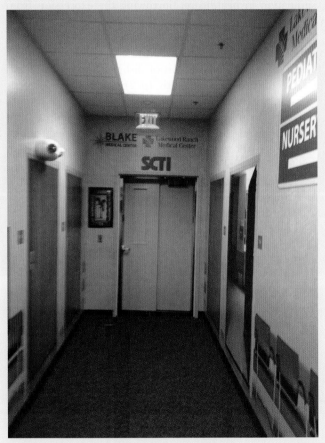

Figure 19.4 Hallway with Wrap Applied.

Wrapping Walls for Environmental Effect (*Continued*)

wrap was applied, and Figure 19.4 is with the wrap applied. A trauma room where only the stretchers with mannequins are

3-dimensional is depicted in Figure 19.5. The infant room is designed in the same manner (Fig. 19.6).

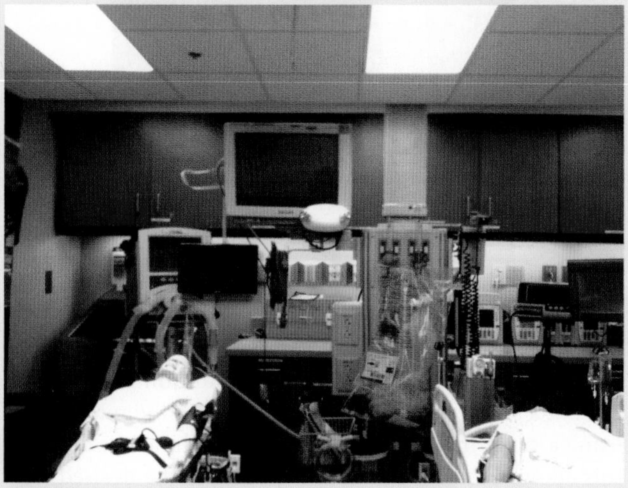

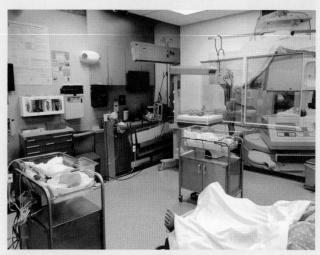

Figure 19.5 Trauma Room with 3D Stretchers with Mannequins and Wrapped Walls.

Figure 19.6 Infant Room with Wrapped Walls.

comment that imposing stress increases the need for quicker action or intervention, thereby leaving less time for the participant to question their performance and become self-conscious. Those observing the simulation also feel an urgency to become involved by wanting to take on the role of a coach or to question the decisions and actions of those caring for the simulated patient. This increased stress may actually improve the level of engagement (Boggs et al., 2007). Additional motivators and attention to realism might be necessary for experiential learning (Sanko, Shekhter, Kyle Jr, De Benedetto, & Birnbach, 2013).

There are variations in what "feels" real for participants. Some learners readily engage in the scenario, while others may be reticent to buy in to the experience (Rudolph, McIntosh, Simon & Raemer, 2015b). Simulation educators guide the social aspects of the simulation learning experience to enhance explicit and implicit motivators, the type of debriefing, and the style of the interactions between the instructors and facilitators. Educators depend on their learner's engagement and can improve that by delivering clear expectations related to roles and the practice of reflection and by building

trust that the educational environment is safe for learning (Dieckmann et al., 2007).

The simulation educator must develop an understanding of the important aspects or components of the simulation scenario to assure there are sufficient and appropriate cues for learner success (Rudolph et al., 2015b). It is also important to know the educational level of the learner and create an experience that provides sufficient reality to move the scenario to its conclusion without providing unnecessary variables that will only serve to confuse the participant.

Determining the appropriate level of realism to achieve the scenario goals is an essential task for the simulation educator. Sometimes, the necessary reality can be achieved simply by increasing the heart rate or decreasing blood pressure. These are clinical cues that are used to determine the state of the patient—real or simulated. However, the learner may benefit from additional cueing that may not be readily apparent using standard patient simulator physiology.

Cues and clues may come in the form of simulated blood, created wounds or burns, or more elaborate moulage. An operating room fire can be simulated with a smoke

Making Simulation Center Rooms More Realistic

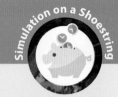

Fran Kamp, MS, RN, CHSE

The Challenge

Getting students to buy into simulation requires environmental **fidelity**. This can be enhanced through very simple and inexpensive solutions, important when starting out and resources, especially funding, are limited. Not having much money to spend, I still wanted equipment to be available for students to see and get used to working with as they would in clinical.

Innovative Solutions

Call bells are an important part of patient care, and I wanted it to be second nature for students to look for them and be sure they were in reach of the patient in all simulations, so that they could then transfer this to clinical. I printed off pictures of call bells and put them on card stock and cut them out in the shape of the call bell. I then attached lanyard to the card stock and tied the other end to the bed's side rail (Fig. 19.7). I did this for all our beds in the lab. I then had the expectation that all students would check for "call bell in reach" every time they entered a simulated patient's room.

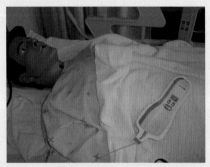

Figure 19.7 Call Bell Created with Card Stock.

My next project was an oxygen flow meter. I did not have working headwalls, yet wanted students to be able to turn the oxygen on. I printed pictures of flow meters, which I then put on card stock, cut out, and utilized double-sided

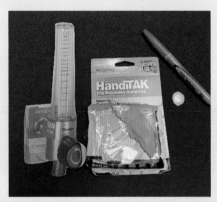

Figure 19.8 Oxygen Flow Meter Created with Card Stock.

tape to hang on the wall. I then took additional card stock, cut out a small circle, and drew a circle in the middle of it using a silver marker. I put ticky-tack behind the dot, and this allowed students to move the dot to the desired oxygen level on the picture of the flow meter (Fig. 19.8). I also used the dot on an actual flow meter that was hung up in the simulated patient's room, but not attached to an oxygen source (Fig. 19.9). Both the call bells and flow meters can be laminated for longer use.

Pulse oximetry is not available for the static mannequins. Creating a wheel allowed me to change the pulse oximetry reading as needed. I cut two circles from card stock. On one of the circles, I cut out a small section. I used a brass fastener to connect the two pieces together so that they would spin

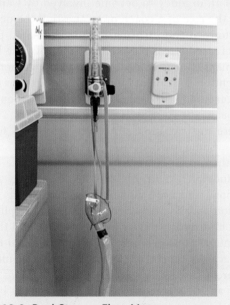

Figure 19.9 Real Oxygen Flow Meter.

Making Simulation Center Rooms More Realistic (*Continued*)

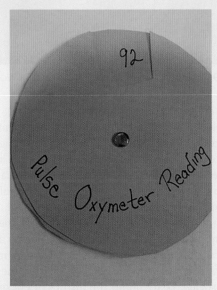

Figure 19.10 Pulse Oximeter Created with Card Stock.

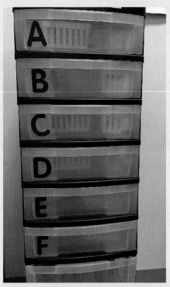

Figure 19.11 Medication Cart.

easily. Then I wrote the numbers of my pulse oximetry readings on the back piece of card stock (Fig. 19.10). You can now dial in the oximetry reading you want.

A med cart was certainly out of the question for me. I purchased a rolling cart with several drawers, labeling each of the drawers with a letter (Fig. 19.11). I placed additional small containers in the drawers, labeling them with numbers. I filled these containers with assorted candies as well as simulation medications. I then created a PowerPoint program with hyperlinks, which allowed students to log in, choose a patient, look up medications, and pull their medications from the appropriate drawer in the medication cart (Fig. 19.12). I also purchased a metal rolling cart with shelves from a home improvement store, stocked it, and used that as our supply room. All of these together helped to enhance the simulation experience for my students.

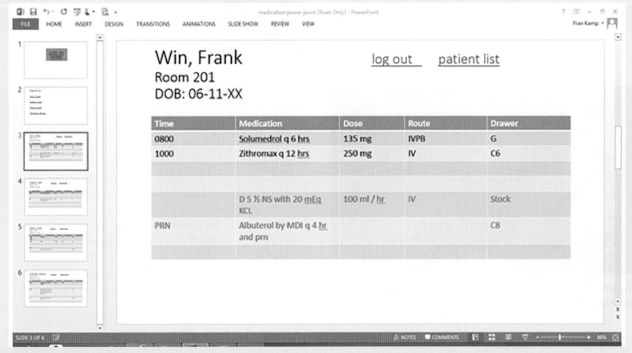

Figure 19.12 Medical Administration PowerPoint.

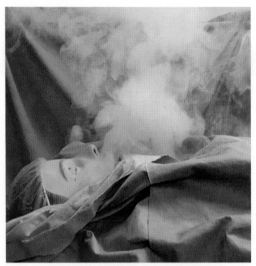

Figure 19.13 Operating Room Fire Simulated with a Smoke Machine. Thanks to Adam Collins, MD for photo staging.

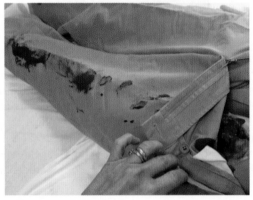

Figure 19.14 Trauma Simulations Wound.

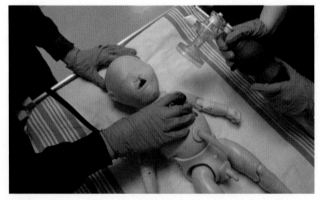

Figure 19.15 Moulaged Cleft Lip Provides Fidelity for Newborn Simulation Scenario.

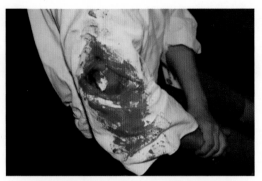

Figure 19.16 Pumping Artificial Blood from a Wound.

machine, creating a sense of urgency (Fig. 19.13), while an actively bleeding wound creates a visual representation of the uncertainty that comes with trauma care (Fig. 19.14). Moulage can be used to create anomalies such as a cleft lip on a newborn simulator (Fig. 19.15). Creating a method to "pump" blood from a bleeding wound simulates the appearance of an arterial bleed, which should lead the learner to act quickly (Fig. 19.16). Signs that the patient needs care and is dependent on the immediate action of the participant create the realism necessary to move the case forward, engage the learner, and assist in the suspension of disbelief. Learn about the history of Pocket Nurse, a leading supplier of simulation supplies, and SimLeggings, an idea that "went viral," using today's terminology.

19-1 Voice of Experience
Creating Pocket Nurse

Anthony J. Battaglia, MS, BSN, RN

The Challenge

I started Pocket Nurse in January 1992 with only one product in my inventory: the Pocket Nurse (Fig. 19.17), a hard plastic case pocket organizer that included gold-plated bandage scissors, hemostat, integrated penlight, and engraved nameplate. While still practicing 7 PM to 7 AM in a Medical ICU I was working during the day in an 8 × 8 room/office adjunct to a medical practice and had the chance to meet with a lot of pharmacy drug representatives. Back in the 1990s, they were still granted the opportunity to hand out generous amounts of giveaways to their customers and that is when I met Nancy who

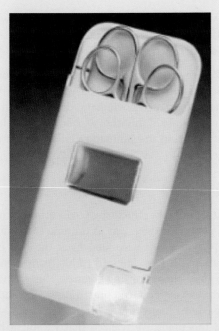

Figure 19.17 Pocket Nurse. (Courtesy of Anthony J. Battaglia, MS, BSN, RN.)

worked for a large pharmaceutical company. Nancy was introduced to the Pocket Nurse and liked it so much that the company purchased 30,000 units in order to promote their drug brand. This initial sale provided me with the necessary funds to get started, and Pocket Nurse began as a promotional company catering to the pharmaceutical market. The sales of the Pocket Nurse allowed us to add more products and eventually offer a 280+ page full color catalog.

Meeting the Challenge

As I realized that no company should rely on only one customer, I started searching for other growth opportunities. I recalled my experience in nursing school and in the "practice" lab when a question hit me: "Where do schools get their supplies?" In order to answer this question, I created a survey, which I sent to local nursing schools. The reply was tremendous, and that gave me the answers I needed to start to sell to colleges and universities. Since that time, the company has expanded its inventory to 8,000 products for healthcare educators and simulation labs worldwide.

Outcome

Pocket Nurse has developed a strong presence in the healthcare education and medical simulation markets since its founding. Throughout its tenure in the marketplace, Pocket Nurse has developed a niche market comprised of Pocket Nurse brand products,

Demo Dose products, Custom Health Totes, and medical supplies and equipment.

Since 1992, Pocket Nurse has expanded its reach within the targeted market by utilizing a variety of marketing vehicles. The goal of the marketing and sales efforts is to provide the customer with "one source, one solution." Additionally, the focus factor "nurse owned and operated" is integrated demonstrating both a collegial and knowledge-based approach.

Pocket Nurse's targeted customers comprise any individual who teaches a healthcare–related course from high school, college, and university programs as well as community-based and governmental programs. The current customer mailing list stands at over 46,000 contacts. To meet the ever-growing needs of the company, a new 122,206 ft² corporate complex was built and opened in 2012.

I also support customer organizations through grants and scholarships, as well as provide product discounts to its membership. I have provided scholarship monies for the following organizations to help their members participate in conferences or programs:

- Pocket Nurse Scholarship through the Pittsburgh Foundation: three academic scholarships are awarded to an allied health, nursing, and nursing faculty student annually.
- Anthony Battaglia Scholarship: INACSL awards this scholarship to eligible applicants to attend the annual conference of simulation directors and educators.
- Pocket Nurse Sim Tech Scholarship: Annual scholarship awarded to eligible applicants to attend the simulation technician conference.
- Pocket Nurse N-OADN Conference Scholarship: Scholarship awarded to nurse educators from community colleges to attend the national conference of Associate Degree Nursing Programs.
- NLN Writing Retreat: Monies given to the National League for Nursing to support research studies on simulation and nursing education topics.

The support of both educators and organizations provides Pocket Nurse with great credibility within our customer market and gives life to the Pocket Nurse focus factor "nurse owned and operated." The past 24 years have been a great success in my life not only from taking a business from virtually nothing to a multimillion dollar company serving the education community worldwide through 100% organic growth and having employed over 80 people to help me take the company to the next level.

Most Valuable Lesson Learned

The American Dream is alive and well, and I am proof of it.

19-2 Voice of Experience
We Wanted Pitting Edema Legs and Ended Up with a Business—The Birth of SimLeggings

Karen Kennedy, MEd, BScN
Colleen Dianne Ward, BSHEc

The Challenge

A student verbally reporting on his/her observations of Mr. Sled, a patient (hi-fidelity simulator) diagnosed with congestive heart failure (CHF):

The patient is in a high Fowler position, hunched over the overbed table. He is diaphoretic with circumoral cyanosis. His respirations are 24/minute, labored and shallow with audible crackles. On his legs are.... sticky notes?!? with the words "Pitting Edema" written on them!

The student saw the sticky notes and could not help but laugh. The seriousness of this patient's condition was lost.

Mannequins are manufactured in what is considered a standard "normal" body type. It is the responsibility and indeed, challenge for simulationists to represent variations of body type and other physical findings in a manner that resembles real life as closely as possible. If we are successful in this endeavor, students will more likely be able to suspend disbelief and immerse themselves in the rich learning from the simulation experience.

Meeting the Challenge

Hi-fidelity mannequins can be programmed to mimic many conditions, but making the legs display a level of pitting edema is not one of them. Unable to find a pitting edema product on the market, I began experimenting with different materials and fasteners. I learned that there were "must haves" in whatever products were to be developed. They must:

- Be able to be put on and taken off quickly as we changed scenarios in a matter of minutes

- Be washable as they would become soiled with all of the students touching them
- Be a tool

With my idea and "must-haves" list, I approached my friend and now business partner, Colleen Ward, who had experience sewing and designing patterns. Within a couple of months, we had a workable prototype to trial in the simulation environment at the college.

Outcome

I can still remember the surprised look and comment of the paramedic who was examining the simulated CHF patient when he pulled back the bed covers to examine his legs. He said to his team members, "Look guys! He has pitting edema!" This was validation from an experienced practitioner who had seen pitting edema many times.

At this point, we realized that we might have a marketable product. We sent a pair of our SimLeggings for evaluation to a nursing colleague who worked in simulation at a nearby university. The response was, "We want this!" With the help of my employer, we were able to apply for a patent just prior to launching our SimLeggings at an international simulation conference. As we expected, our colleagues in simulation were faced with the same challenges as we were. Our SimLeggings were very well received. Based on feedback and requests from colleagues using simulation, we have added a new product every year since we started in business 5 years ago. And yes, we have more ideas!

Most Valuable Lessons Learned

- Develop partnerships with people who have different experiences and skill sets that complement each other. The old adage, two brains are better than one, proved correct again!
- The importance of communication cannot be stressed enough. Share your thoughts with each other regularly and frequently. Jointly decide on the division of responsibilities.
- Seek out resources/mentors who can help you grow your business knowledge. A few examples include web design and management, bookkeeping, long-range planning, legal counsel, liability insurance, and marketing strategies.

Inspiration for Simulation Champions

An idea is only a dream, until you act upon it. Believe in your potential to make a difference.

Morpheus, a character in the Matrix series, poses the question "What is real?" He goes on to state "if real is what you can feel, smell, taste and see, then 'real' is simply electrical signals interpreted by your brain" (Silver, Wachowski, & Wachowski, 1999). The simulation educator's job is to create the "electrical signals" that will provide enough realism to challenge the learners' decision-making.

Simulation Fidelity

When considering the art of simulation and its connection with reality, it is important to understand the interaction of fidelity with realism. Fidelity is defined as:

"The ability to view or represent things as they are to enhance believability. The degree to which a simulated experience approaches reality; as fidelity increases, realism increases. The level of fidelity is determined by the environment, the tools and resources used, and many factors associated with the participants. Fidelity can involve a variety of dimensions: conceptual, physical/environmental, and psychological" (INACSL Standards Committee, 2016, Simulation Glossary, p. S42).

Rudolph et al. (2015b) created a model (Fig. 19.18) that depicts three identified types of fidelity and how they interact to create the perception of realism and subsequent engagement by the learners. Using a fiction contract, as previously discussed, may influence the degree of engagement.

Physical fidelity lies with the believability of the simulation stage: room setup, available equipment, and type of simulator. Patient simulation tools have been classified into low-, medium-, and high-fidelity levels. For an in-depth discussion of fidelity related to simulation equipment, refer to Chapter 6 "The Evolution of Cutting Edge Technology: Today's Simulation Typologies."

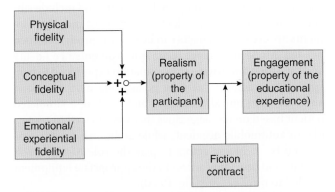

Figure 19.18 Relationship of Fidelity and Realism to Learner Engagement. (From Palaganas, J. C., Maxworthy, J. C., Epps, C. A., & Mancini, M. E. (2015). *Defining excellence in simulation programs* (p. 580). Philadelphia, PA: Wolters Kluwer/Society for Simulation in Healthcare.)

The educator decides on the level of fidelity and realism necessary to set the physical stage for learning. Decisions are made based on the learning objectives for the experience. The simulation educator can enhance the physical fidelity of scenarios with simple embellishments that will establish realism and fidelity. Choosing the right mannequin or actor and the right setting is an essential first step. Allowing learners to progress on simulators of increasing fidelity can lead to superior transfer of a broad range of clinical skills (Brydges, Carnahan, Rose, Rose, & Dubrowski, 2010). Using high-fidelity trainers for simple tasks can create tremendous wear on the sophisticated equipment and may present a diminishing value or educational return for the investment (Norman, Dore, & Grierson, 2012). Conversely, using a low- or medium-fidelity mannequin for complicated problem-solving may not provide the essential physical fidelity to reach learning goals. Munshi, Lababidi, and Alyousef (2015) reported that learning goals and cost ought to determine the level of fidelity, and they propose that both objectives and level of learner should impact the choice of fidelity. Claudius et al. (2015) reported that medical students moulaged as casualty victims provided increased fidelity over that of computerized mannequins. Meurling and team (2014) observed that use of a high-fidelity simulator resulted in a reduction in the frequency of trainer interventions. The group also reports less stress for trainers when high-fidelity mannequins are used. The choice of fidelity and realism must be balanced with cost and degree of desired engagement.

Many simulation educators note the labor-intensive nature of developing scenarios, including planning and implementing the simulation experience. Increasing the physical fidelity and realism of the simulation scenario will add time, expense, and effort for the educator; however, the payout from the time spent developing physical fidelity is improved conceptual and emotional fidelity. Conceptual fidelity refers to the believability of the scenario progression considering the patient's physical condition and responses to intervention, while emotional fidelity is evidenced when realistic emotions are evoked by the experience (Rudolph et al., 2015b). The buy-in, creation of time pressures, and associated stress are created with physical fidelity and lead to emotional fidelity (Rudolph et al., 2015b). Alfred Hitchcock comments "what is drama but life with the dull bits cut out?" (Bell, 2012, p. 82). The difficulty for the educator is to determine the necessary bits to include and which to remove from the scenario.

Holistic Fidelity

The simulation educator is challenged to create fidelity in all areas of patient care. The simulation scenario/theater can be used to immerse students in simulated care situations that require understanding of the developmental, spiritual, psychosocial, and cultural aspects of patient care. There is increased interest in creating scenarios that provide opportunities to address holistic patient care.

Everson and team (2015) designed a three dimensional (3D) immersive simulation experience and reported they were able to positively impact nursing students' empathy in regard to culturally and linguistically diverse patients. The simulation exposed students to an unfolding scene in a hospital ward of a developing country via a 3D video with added smells and tactile stimuli. Students' empathy toward culturally and linguistically diverse patients significantly improved after exposure to the 3D simulation experience.

Scenarios that include the death of a patient, a cultural quandary, or a spiritual dilemma will prepare the student to work in diverse settings and situations. Garrido, Dluglasch, and Grabber (2014) report that when interprofessional education and culture are taught independently, students don't have the opportunity to practice competencies before participating in clinical practice. They used scenario experiences that provided interprofessional practice while simultaneously delivering information about unique cultures. Galbraith, Harder, Macomer, Roe, and Roethlisberger (2014) offer another example where realism was used to give students the opportunity to deliver a death notice. The subject of death and dying can be anxiety provoking. These researchers found that participating in a well-planned, interprofessional, death notification allowed students the opportunity to experience and reflect on their reactions to a stressful situation without the level of anxiety that might be present if the situation were happening in a real clinical setting.

The emphasis here must be on "well planned." Patient death, even when simulated, can be an emotionally traumatic experience. It is impossible for instructors to know or understand every student's background or history. Placing a student who may have recently experienced a similar situation in an emotionally charged simulation may compromise their psychological safety. The instructor must be vigilant when choosing participants—either student or actor—to assure that no emotional damage is created through participation in the scenario. Gaba suggests that facilitators consider ethical and psychological aspects of scenario design before and during the scenario, consider learner vulnerabilities, and provide referrals as needed for untoward effects (Gaba, 2013).

It is important to avoid stereotypical content when developing cultural or spiritual realism for participants. Providing cues or information about a culture or religious group is quite different than putting students in scenarios with stereotypical plots and props that only reinforce negative aspects of either religion or culture. Healthcare professionals have been criticized about impaired holistic care because the spiritual dimension is often overlooked (Baldacchino, 2015). Fink and team (2014) proposed that educators include aspects of diverse religious practices by including environmental and physical props, while avoiding stereotypes by enlisting assistance from religious experts when designing the experience. Persons representative of a culture should be consulted when designing simulation experiences that incorporate a culture other than that of the person or team developing the simulation.

Moulage

Moulage as an adjunct to the high-fidelity mannequin or simulated person is a natural fit with simulation and can provide cost-effective additions to the simulation theater (Damazo & Fox, 2015). Moulage involves various techniques used to simulate characteristics that are important for learners to discover when caring for the simulated patient, thereby increasing fidelity (INACSL Standards Committee, 2016, Simulation Glossary). For centuries, the art of moulage has been used to show illness, disease, and injury (Joshi, D'Costa, & Kura, 2010; Worm, Hadjivassiliou, & Katsambas, 2007). Three-dimensional wax figures were created by the Greeks to teach physicians diagnostic skills (Poulakou-Rebelakou, Karamanou, Rempelakos, & Androutsos, 2012). In an effort to decrease the need for the dissection of human bodies, molds and casts of diseases were created for the study of human anatomy (Damazo & Fox, 2015). Skin manifestations of syphilis and smallpox were created to introduce physicians to the presentation of disease (Joshi et al., 2010; Worm et al., 2007). Many of the wax models have been preserved in museums and galleries and have become of renewed importance as rare diseases are returning due to decreased vaccination rates and supportive environments (Joshi et al., 2010).

Moulage techniques have evolved and now include sophisticated materials that allow multiple uses. Theatrical moulage developed for television and film are now widely used in simulation learning environments and include silicones, gels, and latex products. Castings of moulage elements are created so effects can be easily reproduced when needed. Modern moulage techniques can enhance fidelity and save time, improving the simulation experience to help participants achieve learning goals. Figure 19.19 shows an EMS team quickly assessing and treating a simulated patient based on moulage clues that were placed to resemble an automobile accident, while additional fidelity was created by involving actors to play the role of the child's parents and providing access to the appropriate equipment needed to provide care (Fig. 19.20).

Moulage can be simple or complex. For example, a wig, self-adhesive eye lashes, and stick-on earrings and fingernails will add an element of fidelity when changing mannequins from male to female gender. Effects gel, allowed to dry on a blue pad, with added blood and clots can be used

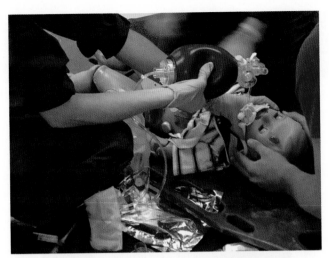

Figure 19.19 Automobile Accident Moulage.

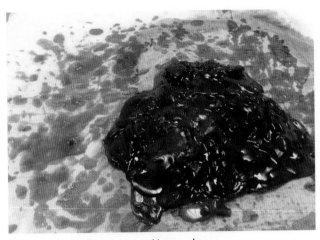

Figure 19.21 Postpartum Hemorrhage.

with a birthing mannequin's bleeding feature for added realism of postpartum hemorrhage (Fig. 19.21), even creating the ability to weigh blood loss (Fig. 19.22). More complex moulage may involve a combination of materials such as effects gels, lubricating jelly, and odor, which were used to create a wound dehiscence (Fig. 19.23).

Early simulationists often placed photographs or transparencies with pictures of wounds or skin diseases on the mannequin in hopes that learners would recognize the injury or dermatological problem. Moulage has since become an important teaching tool, used to create more realistic visuals, particularly in the field of dermatology. While technology has advanced, the ability to appreciate details of a high-resolution, two-dimensional photo does not always correlate to the real-world presentation. Skin lesions are 3D and provide subtle details that

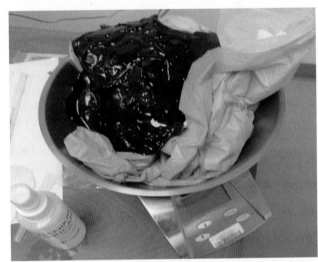

Figure 19.22 Theatrical Effects Create Ability to Weigh Blood Loss.

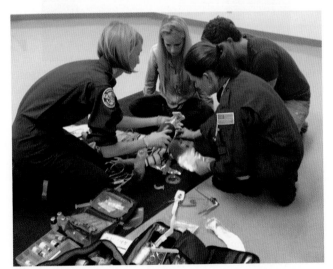

Figure 19.20 Additional Fidelity Created by Actors Portraying Parents and Provision of Appropriate Equipment.

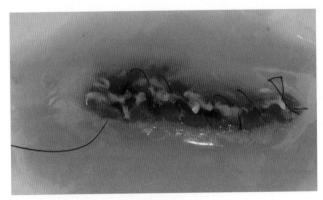

Figure 19.23 Wound Dehiscence.

Creating a Colostomy

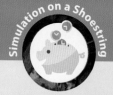

Fran Kamp, MS, RN, CHSE

The Challenge

Taking care of an ostomy, learning how to change an appliance, and assessing an ostomy site were all skills I wanted my students to have practice in, but that opportunity doesn't arise often in clinical.

Innovative Solution

I created an ostomy by cutting a hole in the middle of a wash basin and inserting a stoma (Fig. 19.24). I had many stomas from the abdomens of all the mannequins we had that were not being used. If you don't have a stoma you can use modeling clay to create the appearance of one. I created six setups so a small group of students could work at once. My students were then able to measure and cut a wafer and apply the wafer and skin protectant (I used toothpaste instead of stoma paste since it is so much cheaper). For assessment purposes, I created a stoma with a wafer and an appliance attached. I used a mixture of chocolate syrup and cat litter to create the consistency of the stool inside the bag. I used nail polish to make the area around the stoma red as well as some of the skin where the stoma was "leaking" (Fig. 19.25). Students were able to assess the stoma, characteristics of the drainage, as well as the surrounding skin and document their findings.

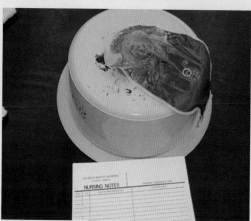

Figure 19.24 Colostomy Created Using Basin and Static Mannequin Ostomy Parts.

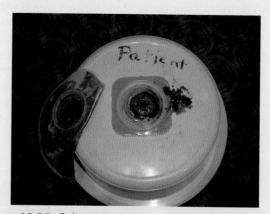

Figure 19.25 Colostomy Prepared for Students to Assess.

may be overlooked when viewing a photograph (Krishna, 2011). Garg, Haley, and Hatem (2010) reported that use of 3D teaching tools for dermatology led to improved outcomes that were sustained. Moulage, using clear effects gel and makeup, was created in only seconds to simulate a rash (Fig. 19.26). Another rash, placed on a patient actor, required 2 to 3 minutes to stage and 30 seconds to remove (Fig. 19.27). Caution must be taken when applying moulage to live actors or standardized patients to ensure that they are not allergic or sensitive to the materials.

Any course level using simulation can benefit from the use of moulage. London's Air Ambulance facilitators found moulage to be an effective way to prepare trainees for an intense and emotionally demanding job (Tariq, Sood, & Goodsman, 2015). They used low-fidelity simulators combined with instructor feedback to stage emergency response training. Figure 19.28 depicts advanced moulage techniques that were used on a real person during a large disaster training drill. A severe hand injury is realistically shown in Figure 19.29. This wound was created with theatrical gels in 15 minutes but is cleaned up in only seconds.

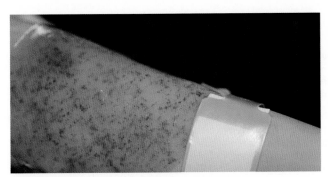

Figure 19.26 Simulated Rash on Mannequin.

The preparation time is offset by the fact that the wound effect can be reused. Claudius et al. (2015) compared training outcomes when using moulaged actors versus computerized mannequins and found increased urgency and improved response time with the use of live actors.

Components of Effective Moulage

Ensuring that the components outlined below are present will make your experience using moulage less time-consuming and ensure increased fidelity of the simulation-based learning experience.

1. A well-planned scenario. A case background and history will help set the learner on the right path. It is important that the moulage provides authenticity to the scenario without taking over the case. Moulage is not the end, but rather the means to the end (Damazo, 2012). Moulage should work with the scenario and not compete or distract from the scenario objectives. "Less is better. This principle should be applied to the entire simulation scenario, including the use of makeup" (Smith-Stoner, 2011, p. 23).

2. Work with the physiology of the mannequin. Modern human patient simulators provide an astonishing level of realism. It is no longer necessary to use makeup to create cyanosis as many mannequins now offer a cyanosis feature that automatically creates cues with a drop in oxygen saturation. Bleeding features trigger a drop in

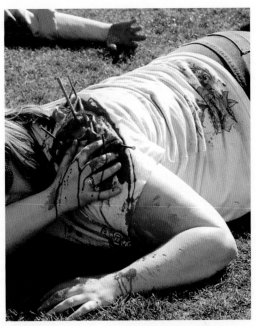

Figure 19.28 Actor Moulaged for Large Disaster Training Drill.

blood pressure to assist in creating a believable scenario. Mannequins sweat, tear, and have trauma limbs—all to increase the fidelity of the scenario. When available, use the full extent of mannequin capabilities.

3. Plan sufficient time for setup and cleanup. Decisions about the use of moulage should be part of the scenario design. It is important to consider time available for setup, cleanup, and time between scenarios. If there is limited time, the moulage should be simple or use theatrical materials that allow for rapid transition between cases.

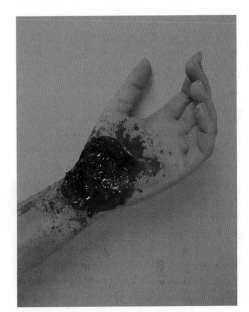

Figure 19.29 Moulaged Hand Injury.

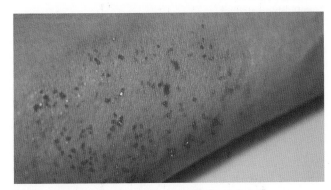

Figure 19.27 Simulated Rash on Patient Actor.

Table 19.1	Instructions for Using Moulage	
Patient Simulators		**Live Actors/Standardized Patients**
Always follow manufacturer's guidelines to avoid the risk of voiding warranty agreements.		When working with older actors, be particularly aware of the potential for thin, sensitive skin.
Test moulage on an inconspicuous area of the simulator that has a similar skin quality. Extra neck skins or old mannequin parts can provide a perfect testing medium.		Provide appropriate makeup removers for products used for simulation. Product removers can be drying so provide lotion to use after the makeup is removed.
Keep a supply of wounds on hand to save time on preparation. Theatrical products are resilient and designed for multiple takes on set. Store products in a cool environment.		Some materials may stain clothing. Warn scenario participants that their clothing may receive permanent stains from the use of some moulage products. Keep a supply of clothing that can be provided to the actor to spare their clothes from damage.
Do not leave moulage or makeup on the mannequins. Because of the increased focus on creating realistic skin on mannequins the skin is now more porous and will absorb ink, colors, and dyes. In addition, the skin is subject to chemical reactions with products that are left on for extended periods. Minimize the risk of damage with prompt and thorough cleanup.		It is important to remember that individuals may be subject to reactions from some theatrical products (Damazo, 2012). Always ask about allergies or sensitivity to products when working with actors. Individuals can also be bothered by smells and sounds used to create simulation reality. Prebriefing actors with the scenario expectations and the makeup required will avoid any potential problems.
Avoid any fluids around the simulators. It seems obvious, but liquids and the electronic simulators don't mix. Use gels with caution as they can melt and seep into the simulation cavity.		

Tips for Implementing Moulage

This chapter has discussed many of the ways in which moulage has been shown to enhance the simulation-based learning experience. There are cautions to consider when using moulage with patient simulators as well as with live actors or standardized patients. Table 19.1 outlines precautions that will help you avoid challenges such as causing an allergic reaction.

A moulage kit is a helpful tool for the simulation educator (Fig. 19.30). By developing a kit, the educator will have all the supplies, materials, and cleaning products in one location. There are many choices in premade moulage kits, but it is possible to easily create an inexpensive kit with materials outlined in Box 19-1 (Damazo, 2012).

Box 19-1	Recommended Supplies for a Moulage Kit

- Makeup, various colors
- Cotton balls
- Gauze pads
- Glycerin
- Palette knife
- Brushes
- Tongue depressors
- Sponges, various sizes and types
- Mixing palette
- Effects gels (blood, clear, flesh-colored)
- Effects gel applicator
- Stage blood
- Scissors
- Utility knife
- Plastic wrap
- Liquid starch
- Pocket comb
- Rubbing alcohol
- Petroleum jelly
- Liquid adhesive and adhesive remover
- Empty mixing bottles
- Flesh putty
- Premade prosthetics (various injuries such as blisters, burnt skin, bone fractures, wounds)

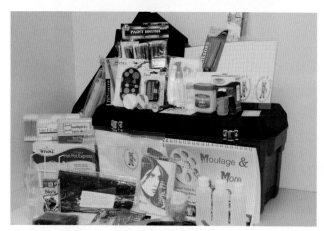

Figure 19.30 Example Moulage Kit.

We have all been amazed at the amount of devastation and damage caused by disaster events. There is renewed interest in disaster preparedness. For disaster scenarios, the moulage can vary from spraying "blood" on victims using gallons of purchased stage blood to specialized wounds such as those that might be created to show the damage caused by a chemical explosion or blast injury (Fig. 19.31). Both the Centers for Disease Control (CDC) and the American Red Cross offer various types of disaster preparedness training that include moulage information via applications accessible through mobile technology.

Moulage Materials

Moulage materials can range from items in the kitchen cabinet to elaborate molding and modeling products using special effects gels, latex, and silicone products. Effects gels come in a variety of colors that can be combined to create the desired effect (Fig. 19.32). The primary colors used in moulage are clear, flesh and blood. The product has a gelatin base and the user must melt the product until it is a liquid consistency. Once the injury is created the product must be stored in a cool place. Washable paint is another material that is very useful in the simulation center. This paint washes off as stated and can prevent staining

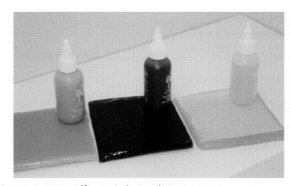

Figure 19.32 Effects Gels Products.

or damage to mannequins. Theatrical supply houses offer a plethora of moulage materials including blood by the gallon, stage makeup and pumps for pulsating blood, and smoke machines.

Silicone molds and casting products are another tool that can be used for simulation. By creating and casting a mold, multiple replications of any created injury can be made. Three-dimensional printing has added a new mechanism to create moulage. One university is even using calf legs created by 3D printing to enhance simulation in a veterinary program (E. Bauman, personal communication, October 30, 2015). This method is being experimented with and may result in a cost-effective way to add to simulation fidelity. The educator interested in exploring advanced moulage techniques could take a course (Fig. 19.33) or try sample products to explore product potential. As with any artistic endeavor, continued study and practice improve performance (Damazo & Fox, 2015). Several examples of moulage recipes are provided to give you ideas! (Table 19.2).

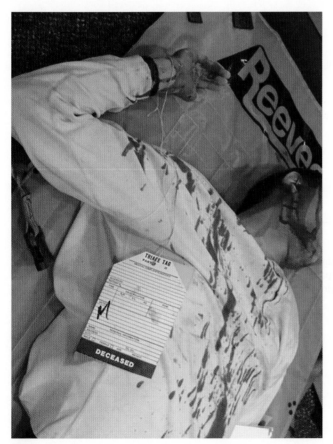

Figure 19.31 Moulaged Actor Triaged at Mass Casualty Drill.

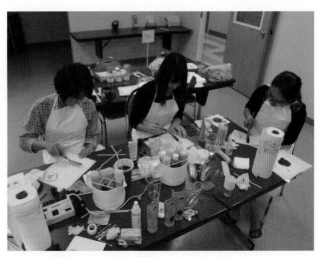

Figure 19.33 Moulage Class.

Table 19.2	Moulage Recipes	
Moulage	**Ingredients**	**Steps for Preparation**
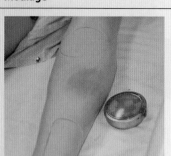 **Figure 19.34** Bruise.	1. Powder makeup in bruise colors: dark and light blues, greens, yellows, and reds 2. Makeup sponge (for application) 3. Face powder 4. Makeup brush	Fresh bruise 1. Start with blush (red/pink) powder makeup to create bruise shape. Very lightly "feather" blue unevenly around the edges using the makeup sponge.
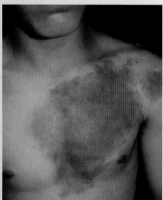 **Figure 19.35** Live Actor Bruise.	1. Ben Nye Bruise Wheels 2. Make up sponge (for application)	Fresh bruise 1. Dab the makeup sponge in several spots on the bruise wheel. Apply the makeup to the actor by dabbing and blotting in the area of the bruise/injury. 2. Layer effects to create the desired age and extent of bruising. The bruise wheel has the appropriate colors and can be applied using a makeup sponge. ● Bruises can be covered with bandages or appear through ripped clothing depending on the scenario.
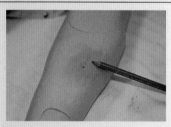 **Figure 19.36** Insect Bite or Sting.	1. Dark red eye liner pencil	1. Use bruising method to create a reddened area. 2. Using the eye liner pencil, place a single dot in the center of the inflamed area. ● For snake bite: the reaction is often very subtle. Use only the dark red eye liner pencil and make two small dots close together. It is helpful to look up a picture of a snake bite using an internet image search tool. ● For Lyme disease: shape the reddened area into a bull's-eye with a darkened center followed by a pale area and a reddened outer circle. Refer to a book or online picture if unsure and match the image to create the effect.
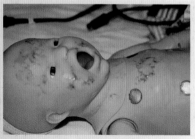 **Figure 19.37** Meconium.	1. Lubricating jelly 2. Petroleum jelly 3. Blue washable finger paint 4. Green washable finger paint 5. Red washable finger paint	1. Mix either lubricating jelly or petroleum jelly with green finger paint. 2. Add blue and a small amount of red to create color desired and a dark tarry, almost black substance. ● Store in container in refrigerator. If you leave the container uncovered for a day or so, it takes on the very sticky, difficult to remove character of meconium. Don't leave uncovered for more than 24 h or the product will become difficult to use.

Table 19.2	Moulage Recipes (*Continued*)

Moulage	Ingredients	Steps for Preparation
Blood	1. A bottle of liquid dish soap 2. Red washable paint 3. Blue washable paint	1. Pour liquid dish soap into a glass container with pouring spout. 2. Add red washable paint and mix thoroughly using a wire whisk. 3. Add a very small amount of blue (dip a toothpick in the paint and add a drop at a time). Mix until it is the desired color and all the paint has dissolved. ● Food color can be substituted for the washable paint if it is to be used on dressings and allowed to dry. **Be cautious! Red can stain the mannequin** if you aren't careful. Use the washable paint in most circumstances. ● Store blood in a bottle (such as an empty dish soap bottle) that can be used to easily dispense the blood.
Urine	1. 1 cup water 2. 1–3 drops yellow food coloring (depending on the desired urine concentration) 3. Ammonia To change urine lab values: ● Hematuria: add a few drops of blood from a *meat package. ● Glucose positive: add a dissolved glucose tablet. ● Protein positive, cloudy urine: add a few drops of *milk. ● Urine sediment: sprinkle with baby powder and stir. ● Urine odor: add ammonia as desired. **Quick Tip:** *Sports drinks and vitamin waters come in a variety of urine colors. Just pour into a catheter bag, bedpan or urinal. The added bonus when using this method is that the urine will test positive for glucose.	1. Mix water and food color together in a clear container. 2. Add a few drops or yellow food coloring to get the look of the desired urine concentration. 3. Add a few drops of ammonia to create desired urine smell. Variations: Add elements to create hematuria, glycosuria, proteinuria, and sediment. 4. Add mix to urinary catheter bag, bedpan, or urinal. ● Absorbent bed pads can also be drenched in urine mix to create incontinence. As with all food color items, allow the drape to dry completely before using with the mannequins.
Sweat	1. Glycerin 2. Water 3. Cold cream or other cream-based barrier 4. Spray bottle	1. Mix 3 parts glycerin with 1 part water. 2. Add mixture to spray bottle. 3. Spritz on the mannequin for desired effect. **Tip:** For longer-lasting effect, add a small amount of cream or similar barrier prior to spritzing on the mannequin. Adding the cream will cause the "sweat" to bubble up to help create the moulage clue. This will help the sweat to last longer. ● If planning to do several scenarios, keep the spray bottle nearby to respritz between cases.

Moulage Cleanup

Our words of advice:

● Think about cleanup before you ever apply any moulage to a mannequin or live actor.
● Plan for the best way to relay necessary clues or change over times between scenarios

● Consider the best way to minimize potential staining or damage to mannequins that might be caused by the moulage application.

Most moulage can be cleaned up with plain soap and water. Wash with a soapy rag and follow with a clean damp rag. Finally, dry and powder the mannequin. For stubborn stains or sticky situations, you might require something a little tougher like an adhesive remover product such as Goo Gone. While this product is amazing at its ability to remove stains and sticky situations, it should be used in moderation. The interaction with the chemicals in the mannequin skin can cause cracking or damage. When this type of product is used, rinse the skin with a damp cloth and then dry and powder the mannequin. Additional tips follow:

- Baby powder can remove the adhesive from tape. Sprinkle mannequin skin with a small amount of powder and rub over the sticky area. The tape will ball up and can be wiped away. Use caution with this method because too much rubbing might remove the skin protection coating applied by the manufacturer.
- Use a barrier. When using any recipe that contains color or dye, we strongly recommend providing a barrier between simulator and moulage. It's amazing how just a small layer of cold cream can decrease cleanup time and protect the mannequin.
- DO NOT use any makeup that is advertised as a "long wearing." Inexpensive makeup that has a short half-life is the best for moulage applications.
- Always use a powder makeup, never a cream-based, liquid, or spray-on makeup. The one exception to this is the white Halloween makeup.
- The simulators consist of both hard and soft plastic skins (the replaceable pieces would be considered soft plastic). Note: The softer plastics will absorb more color and are more susceptible to staining. Think of clean up while you are planning where to place wounds or moulage pieces.
- If you are unsure about whether staining will occur, try the product out on a replaceable simulator neck piece skin first.
- Use caution with live actors who are also susceptible to stained skin. A cream or lotion can assist in clean up and will prevent dry cracked skin that may result from multiple moulage applications.

Summary

Simulation instructors struggle with how much reality matters when including simulation in the curriculum. It is generally understood that enough detail must be provided to allow the student to "suspend disbelief" and enter fully into the simulation experience. However, too many or confusing details that distract from the simulation objectives should be avoided. Moulage is one way to help create a believable reality for students. Everything from bleeding wounds to elaborate 3D theatrical settings can assist students as they work to gain necessary clinical skills.

There are many resources available to simulationists who are striving for simulation reality. Sophisticated high-fidelity mannequins, moulage materials, 3D printing, and environmental settings and staging can be helpful for the design of a believable scenario. The emphasis should always be on the student learning outcomes. Resources are wasted if they do not reinforce the educational purpose.

Precautions should be taken to protect both the mannequin and patient actors using barriers and well-designed theatrical elements. Instructors should also use caution when asking students to embark on the scenarios that may challenge their ethical or emotional limits. Psychological safety should play a prominent role as realism and theatrics are amplified in the simulation setting. "Deception and reality are powerful agents to the uninitiated..." (Nolan, C. *Batman: The Dark Night Rises*, 2012).

Toolkit Resource

Toolkit 19-1: Sample Fiction Contract

20 Curriculum Development in Nursing Simulation Programs

Kim Leighton

Key Terms

Scenario, Debriefing, Confederate (Embedded Actor, Standardized/Simulated Patient, Simulated Person), Coaching, Cue (Prompt), Assessment (Formative, Summative, High Stakes), Fidelity (Conceptual, Environmental, Psychological), Facilitator, Facilitation, Guided Reflection, Interprofessional Education (IPE), Validity, Reliability, Subject Matter Expert, Clinical Reasoning, Critical Thinking, Clinical Judgement, Competence, Prebriefing (Briefing), Script, Simulation-Based Learning Experience (SBLE), Bloom's Taxonomy, Advocacy/Inquiry, Feedback, Reflection-in-Action, Reflection-on-Action

Guiding Questions

1 How does the simulationist integrate simulation into the nursing curriculum?

2 What are the standards of best practice for managing simulation-based education for nurses and nursing students?

3 How do I determine if my teaching is effective when using simulation methods?

Introduction

Where do I start? How do I decide what **scenario** to use? How do I schedule all these learners? How long should a scenario last? And, what about **debriefing**—how long should I plan for that and do I have to use video? These and other questions plague novice simulationists as well as those who have been involved with simulation-based learning for years. The challenge is that there are not

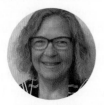

Kim Leighton, PhD, RN, CHSE, CHSOS, ANEF

many answers for us in the literature. One of the reasons is that we all plan, implement, and evaluate our simulation activities differently. That's not necessarily a problem—we are still trying to figure out the "right way"; however, many of the answers to our questions are "it all depends." Simulation-based learning is still a relatively new pedagogy and researchers worldwide are attempting to learn which elements of the experience are most crucial to learning. Fifteen years ago, many of us were likely to not do debriefing if we were running short of time. Research now shows us that this is one of the most valuable features in simulation that promotes learning.

Early efforts to help us better understand how to incorporate simulation into our curriculum were led by Dr. Pam Jeffries and the National League for Nursing (NLN). Details of this work can be reviewed in Chapter 5. Early on, it was recognized that there was interplay between the **facilitator** and participant that was impacted by the way we designed our simulated clinical experiences (and vice versa), which in turn impacted outcomes. We began to question how to best implement design features so that we could achieve best learning outcomes. The literature is replete with examples of how facilitators have implemented simulation but analysis of numerous review articles shows that we haven't yet found those answers.

As a result of extensive analysis of research, specifically in the areas of the constructs of simulation design (see Chapters 3 and 5 for more information about the state-of-the-science project led by the NLN and International Nursing Association for Clinical Simulation and Learning), the INACSL *Standards of Best Practice: Simulation*^{SM} were developed in 2011 and are now in their third revision. These standards were developed to provide guidance on best practices to the simulation community. The standards have found wide acceptance throughout the nursing simulation community, although this is a living document and will be under frequent revision as our ongoing research helps us to better define exactly what the best practices are. There are seven standards, all of which are discussed throughout this chapter: Outcomes and Objectives, Simulation Design, Debriefing, **Facilitation**, Professional Integrity, Participant Evaluation, and Sim-IPE. One new standard is under development: Simulation Operations. The full Standards of Best Practice: Simulation^{SM} are found at http://www.nursingsimulation.org/issue/S1876-1399(16)X0014-X. I encourage you to have them close at hand and review them when making decisions about how you are using simulation with your learners. The standards are also useful as supporting documentation when you are negotiating with faculty and leadership for time, space, supplies, personnel, and other resources. Adhering to the Standards of Best Practice: Simulation^{SM} will help you to be consistent in your approach and help lead to positive learning outcomes.

In addition to offering insight into how to use the INACSL Standards of Best Practice: Simulation^{SM}, this chapter will guide you from start to finish in designing the **simulation-based learning experience** (SBLE). Whether you have just been hired into your simulation position, or were told you are now the simulation coordinator, or even if you've been doing this for years, this chapter will help you to think about why you need to make certain decisions and then help you to implement simulation within the logistical constraints of your environment. Words of wisdom are shared in Voice of Experience features, and cost-effective ways of managing scenario design are discussed in the Simulation on a Shoestring features. Begin by reading Sharon Decker's Voice of Experience where she describes how she initially became involved in simulation and how taking risks informed her career trajectory.

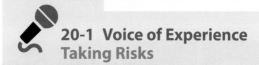

20-1 Voice of Experience
Taking Risks

**Sharon I. Decker,
PhD, RN, ANEF, FAAN**

The Challenge

I've been asked multiple times how I became involved with simulation. My answer: "I was at the right place, at the right time and took the risk." Sounds easy, but opportunities providing the catalyst for a career trajectory do not "just happen." You must be able to recognize the potential of the opportunity and respond appropriately. My response to strategic situations required an awareness of the landscape (both locally and nationally), a continuous immersion in the literature, and an environment that supported innovation and risk taking.

Meeting the Challenge

I was at the right place. I became the Director of Clinical Simulations for the School of Nursing at Texas Tech University (Lubbock campus) in the fall of 1994. With this appointment, I began to explore how the evolving technology could be used as a tool to promote student learning. Over the next several years, grants from local foundations were obtained to purchase then "state-of-the-art" Fuld Institute for Technology in Nursing Education (FITNE) interactive video stations and computer-assisted interactive modules. In the early 2000s, technological advances provided simulators to assist with teaching advanced cardiac life support and pediatric advanced life support. So once again, grants were written to support a project titled "The Enhancement of Teaching Through Simulation." During this time (the mid-1990s through the early 2000s), the healthcare simulation community evolved with the establishment of the Society for Simulation in Healthcare (SSH) and the International Nursing Association for Clinical Simulation and Learning (INACSL), and I was caught in excitement.

It was the right time. An invitation appeared to apply to be a site coordinator for the initial National League for Nursing/Laerdal Industries Multi-site National Simulation Research Study. I applied and was accepted to be a member of this esteemed group led by Drs. Mary Anne Rizzolo and Pam Jeffries. This opportunity occurred at the time I was engaged in doctoral studies. So, I took another risk and asked my advisor, "Instead of aligning my dissertation topic with a faculty at the university, could I explore my passion?" That was and continues to be how simulation (especially the debriefing process) supports the development of **critical thinking/clinical judgement**. After obtaining approval, I was able to use simulation as the focal point for all assignments, discussions, projects, and my research. These two career opportunities evolved and became synergistic. I established collegial relationships with national experts, my knowledge and skill set expanded, and I developed my own expertise and recognition in the simulation community.

Once again *the time was right.* In the mid-2000s as the School of Nursing expanded, enrollment increased, and simulation-based experiences were integrated throughout the curricula, new space was needed. So, once again an opportunity presented itself and *a risk was taken.* I wrote a proposal expanding the proposed new simulation center to be interprofessional and multimodality in focus. Amazingly, it was approved, funding from a wonderful donor was obtained, and in 2003, the F. Marie Hall Sim*Life* Center in Lubbock opened. This 24,500 square foot center served as the template for two additional interprofessional centers at TTUHSC's regional campuses in Abilene and Odessa.

Another risk was coauthoring a Quality Enhancement Proposal (QEP) proposal, Interprofessional Teamwork, that was selected by the President's Executive Council in 2008. As the Director of TTUHSC's QEP from 2008 to 2014, I facilitated the integration of educational opportunities to assist TTUHSC students, residents, staff, and faculty to acquire the knowledge, skills, and attitudes to participate as collegial members of an interprofessional team. This responsibility extended over the TTUHSC system to include six campuses and the Schools of Graduate Biomedical Sciences, Allied Health Sciences, Medicine, Nursing, and Pharmacy.

Outcome

Over the past decade, I've been privileged to assist in the development of the science of simulation influencing healthcare education and delivery by serving on the Board of Directors for INACSL and the SSH. As a member of INACSL's Standards Committee, I assisted in establishing standards of practice for simulation. I was the lead author for the standards on Debriefing and Simulation-Enhanced Interprofessional Education (Sim-IPE) and a member of the interprofessional, international Certification Committee for SSH (currently serve as the Chair of the Certification Committee). Getting involved,

mentoring others, and developing relationships have provided multiple opportunities to be engaged in research projects, presentations, and consultations.

I've been the recipient of multiple awards directly related to my involvement in simulation. For example, the Texas Tech's Chancellor's Council Distinguished Teaching Award; the TTUHSC President's awards for Academic Achievement, Excellence in Teaching, and Outstanding Professor; Distinguished Alumni for the Louise Herrington School of Nursing at Baylor University; and the INACSL Excellence in Academia. Finally, I'm a fellow in the Academy of Nursing Education and American Academy of Nursing. It has been, and continues to be, a wonderful, rewarding journey.

Most Valuable Lesson Learned

"I was at the right place, at the right time and took the risk."

Integrating Simulation into the Curriculum

Many of us became involved in simulation on the day we were told "I need you to implement simulation throughout our curriculum." Some of us were very unfamiliar with simulation—my response was "What is a simulator?" I was promptly sent off to a conference to find out the answer. Learning how to use simulators is only the beginning of the challenge. While a significant focus of simulation is on the use of simulators, we learned in Chapter 6 that there are many types of simulation, and in Chapter 7 we learned that there are a variety of ways in which to use these tools. The challenge is to determine where this all fits into the curriculum.

There is general agreement among most simulationists that simulation should be integrated into the curriculum, rather than having only one or two experiences during a program. One benefit of integration is that learners become more comfortable as they become increasingly familiar with the simulation environment, equipment, and expectations. This may decrease stress and anxiety and may also help them to overcome lack of **fidelity**, enhancing "buy-in." Integrating throughout the curriculum also allows faculty to build on previous learning to promote higher-order thinking. We also know, through our study of learning theory, that practice and repetition impact learning; and hands-on interactive activities impact recall and increase muscle memory. Using simulation throughout the curriculum allows learners to build on prior experiences. Learn how Quality Safety Education for Nurses (QSEN) criteria were integrated throughout one program's simulation curriculum in the following Voice of Experience.

20-2 Voice of Experience
Integrating QSEN into the Simulation Curriculum

Mary Ann Cantrell, PhD, RN, CNE, FAAN

Bette Mariani, PhD, RN

The Challenge

When our school revised its undergraduate curriculum, a major focus was on role formation that included the practice skills of interprofessional collaboration, role transition, scholarly analytical skills, leadership, professional values, accountability, social responsibility, communication, advocacy, collegiality, and a service orientation. Faculty who were responsible for the operationalization of the revised curriculum recognized that an organized simulation program focused on the Quality Safety Education for Nurses (QSEN) competencies to accompany all practice-focused courses across the curriculum was an optimal approach to address professional behaviors among our graduates. Yet, we recognized that faculty's lack of knowledge of simulation as pedagogy and QSEN-identified simulation-based learning activities was a major challenge in achieving our goal.

Meeting the Challenge

To meet our objective and address these known challenges, we attended a QSEN workshop to become immersed in these competencies. We reviewed all of the workshop and published materials by the collaborators and contributors to the QSEN initiative. We then created a template with recommended teaching strategies that intentionally included simulation-based learning activities that would provide opportunities to develop professionalism of our students.

Outcome

There were several positive and negative outcomes from this project. When the template of suggested teaching and simulation-based strategies were introduced to the faculty, several faculty were skeptical and some were wedded to their existing course simulation scenarios; thus, initially, the incorporation of these learning activities into certain courses was minimal.

To be "the voice" of our efforts, we undertook this initiative by developing new scenarios and revising existing scenarios within our own courses being certain to stay true to the outcome goals of our new curriculum, as well as the standards for development of simulation-based learning. One notable positive outcome was the development of a safety-focused scenario, titled Integrating Quality and Safety Education in a Nursing Curriculum through Simulation, within the senior-level nursing leadership and management course. This simulation scenario has now been in use for the past 3 years during which other faculty are exposed to this teaching–learning experience to broaden their knowledge about simulation as pedagogy. This scenario was part of a research study; the findings and simulation scenario were published to share with nurse educators globally to continue the advancement of science for simulation.

Most Valuable Lessons Learned

The most valuable lesson learned was that implementing a structured simulation program across a curriculum must include all stakeholders in the process—administration, faculty, and students. A strong rationale for how and why simulation-based learning experiences can meet the overall program goals must be provided. Promoting simulation as pedagogy grounded in a strong evidence base was the salient message we used for faculty "buy-in" to integrate simulation-based learning experiences across the curriculum.

Inspiration for Simulation Champions

At no other point in nursing education have we experienced such rigorous efforts to provide an evidence base across curricula to educate nursing professionals than we do now through simulation-based education.

Needs Assessment and Gap Analysis of Learners, Environment, Global Concerns

Simulationists often struggle with determining *what* learning experiences can or should be placed in the simulation learning environment. A needs assessment and gap analysis (identifying the difference between actual performance and desired performance) will help to identify opportunities. The Standard of Best Practice: Simulation[SM], Simulation Design supports this analysis, calling it the "foundational evidence" needed to direct us in developing our simulation goals (INACSL Standards Committee, 2016).

We can review learning disparities by evaluating responses to assignments and exams, observing behaviors, analyzing clinical sites, and keeping abreast of global health concerns. Examples of scenarios in response to an analysis of nursing education include the following:

- Review exam item analysis. What concepts do your students struggle to understand? For example, if students do not perform well on exam questions related to management of a patient with schizophrenia, you should consider that they may not have experiences from the traditional clinical environment to draw from and haven't been able to synthesize textbook information. Create a **standardized/simulated patient** experience to enhance learning.
- As a clinical instructor, you are challenged to observe all your students during the day. You realize that you weren't able to observe half your group conducting their physical assessment because you were busy watching others prepare medications. Create simulation experiences using high-fidelity simulators or virtual reality platforms so that you can observe students more closely.
- One of the most common admission diagnoses for hospitalized patients is heart failure; however, we cannot guarantee that every student will care for a patient in heart failure on the clinical unit. Creating a heart failure scenario ensures that all students have the same experience caring for a specific disease process.
- When taking students to clinical, we are faced with random learning opportunities. The patient choices are out of our control; some patients may be too complex for

our level of student. Additionally, many hospitals won't allow students to give certain medications or document in the electronic health record. Create scenarios that allow learners to complete activities expected of them upon graduation but that they don't receive enough practice doing while in school. Table 20.1 provides a comparison of a typical day in the traditional clinical environment versus that in a simulation environment.

- Global health concerns are identified in the media, providing us an opportunity to create scenarios that deal with immediate real-life issues. While many of our simulations focus on care of one patient, we can also create opportunities for community health and leadership courses. For example, the impact of Zika virus reaches beyond a single patient and did not just impact one country but became a global issue due to the Olympics. Create a scenario using various simulation typologies to have community health students demonstrate understanding of disease management across large geographical areas.

In the hospital setting, education needs are driven by analysis of medical error, changes to practice, changes in patient population, new equipment, and regulatory change. Examples of scenarios in response to an analysis of the practice setting include the following:

- Contact risk management to identify the most common causes of error in the hospital. One of the most common is medication error, or errors caused by lack of communication. Create a scenario that involves the medications identified by risk management and include communication. For example, a medication typically ordered in units has been ordered in milliliters. The nurse, during the scenario, needs to contact the healthcare provider to clarify the order. The healthcare provider does not agree that a concern exists so the focus shifts to communication strategies for problem-solving.

Table 20.1	**Comparison of Traditional Clinical Day with Simulation Clinical Day**
Traditional Clinical	**Simulated Clinical**
One patient per student	One patient per group
Instructor time divided among all students	Instructor observes all; opportunity to record sessions
Medications and treatments require most of faculty time.	Collaboration encouraged
Abundant downtime waiting for faculty, when patient sleeping or family visiting, when patient off-unit	Continuous uninterrupted learning; no downtime
Restrictions on administering medications, documenting in electronic health record	Provide all care without restrictions; perform as a nurse
Trajectory of illness difficult to see during time with patient	Can see progression of illness or recovery based on interventions or lack thereof

- A new order set has been distributed that has a new treatment added, and the order of implementation of treatments has changed. A scenario that requires implementation of the new order set can be created to help nurses learn the new process.
- The medical–surgical unit will begin accepting progressive care patients. Scenarios can be created for the most common type of new patient they will begin caring for.
- New equipment has been purchased by the hospital. A scenario can be created that includes use of the new equipment, allowing nurses to familiarize themselves with the functionality and providing for repetition in use.
- Electronic health records are connected to payment systems, a regulatory change that has created a need for nurses to better understand documentation systems and informatics. Including electronic documentation in all scenarios will allow for repetitive practice in this area.

Leveling and Scaffolding to the Learner

The next challenge for the simulationist is to determine *where* to place SBLEs in the curriculum. It is important that we consider the level of the learner when making these decisions. Applying Benner's (1984) novice-to-expert approach as well as Kolb's experiential learning cycle (1984), we know that experiences should be created that build upon prior knowledge and experience. Creating SBLEs that focus on concepts not yet learned will frustrate the learner and facilitator when learning objectives are not met. Carefully consider course placement within the curriculum as well as placement of content within the course.

Another consideration is whether to create SBLE that are unique to each course or that build in repetition of skills and knowledge. The needs assessment and gap analysis will drive this response to a certain degree; however, consider if you want to expose your students to a wide variety of unrelated illnesses and disease processes or whether you want to expose them to increasingly complex scenarios all related to the same concept. There is no specific research to support that one method is better than the other; however, scaffolding on the same concept is supported by several learning theories. If you have the ability to use simulation for a large number of hours, then you may be able to do both. Consider the comparison in Table 20.2. The examples of unique scenarios may represent specific gaps that were discovered in the needs assessment as areas of difficulty for the learners, while the scenarios for increasing complexity demonstrate how curriculum can be designed to build upon prior knowledge. The same thought process is used to develop SBLE for hospital or other organizational education.

Curriculum mapping is one method used to determine best placement for SBLE while ensuring that they are connected to the learning objectives of the course and overall program. Following is an example of how to integrate increasingly complex respiratory content (see Table 20.2) into simulations across a nursing program:

Table 20.2	Integration Comparison	
Curriculum	**Unique Scenarios**	**Increased Complexity (One System)**
Assessment	Abdominal pain	Asthma
Medical–surgical	Deep vein thrombosis	COPD
Pediatrics	Asthma	Cystic fibrosis
Obstetrics	Preeclampsia	Allergic reaction
Mental health	Schizophrenia	Anxiety with hyperventilation
Critical care	Chest pain	Acute heart failure

- Assessment Course: Students have just received their stethoscopes and are learning lung sounds but have not yet learned about patient care. However, most all students are familiar with asthma or allergic reactions as these are frequently encountered personally or with childhood friends. Build a simple scenario that exposes the students to wheezing lung sounds while allowing them to become more comfortable with their stethoscopes. Show an inhaler and answer questions about that. Return simulator lung sounds to normal so students can hear the difference. No interventions are expected.
- Medical–Surgical: Chronic obstructive pulmonary disease (COPD) is frequently encountered in the hospital setting. As this course typically falls early in the curriculum, add basic interventions after assessment, such as oxygen, elevating head of bed, instructing the patient on use of inhaler, or administering a nebulizer treatment.
- Pediatrics: Students now have some experience behind them but are challenged by caring for a child within the context of family. Consider keeping interventions to a minimum while focusing the scenario on communication and education strategies with a child at their level of development.
- Obstetrics: Respiratory issues in the obstetrics setting are often complex and critical. Carefully consider course objectives to determine the desired level of criticality. Using an allergic reaction scenario allows for a great deal of discretion as it can progressive along a continuum.
- Mental Health: While most mental health situations do not have any respiratory component, much of what we teach students in mental health is about communication. An anxious patient who is hyperventilating provides one opportunity to continue the respiratory theme, while also integrating communication strategies.
- Critical Care: Since this course is usually at the end of the program, more license can be taken to increase the critical nature of the scenario. Acute heart failure is an example of a scenario that pulls together all the

interventions learned previously, but with the expectation that the student will recognize problems faster, interpret findings more accurately, look at the situation more holistically, and communicate clearly.

Logistics and Resource Availability

Now that you have completed your needs assessment and gap analysis, and determined how you might best level and scaffold learning for your students, the next step is to consider your resources and logistics. It would be wonderful if we could use SBLE to assist with all of our educational needs, but the reality is that there are only so many hours in a day, and a limited number of physical and human resources available to accomplish your goals. Logistics to consider are space, time, equipment, people, and scheduling.

Space

SBLE can take place in a variety of locations such as a simulation center, a simulation lab, in an area of a skills lab, in situ in a healthcare setting, outside, in a car, in the back of an ambulance...anywhere patient care situations can occur. The simulationist needs to consider the location when determining other resource needs. Is the existing learning space large enough for the activity you are planning? Is the location accessible to multiple groups of learners entering and leaving? If you're planning an outdoor activity, what is your backup plan if it rains that day? If needed, is there electricity available where the training will occur? Do you need permission to use an area other than the simulation lab space? As one example, we were training to provide care in the back of an ambulance but did not have access to an ambulance. We used tape to outline the dimensions on the floor around the stretcher. This visual helped learners to see the space in which they had to work.

Time/Scheduling

When planning for SBLE, the simulationist will need to identify how much time is needed, and not just for the actual scenario. Consideration also needs to be given to the amount of time needed to create a scenario, program the scenario, gather equipment and complete the setup, create associated materials such as preparatory questions and electronic (or paper) health records, do a dry run (sometimes more than one), implement the scenario (including **prebriefing**, debriefing, and evaluation), put equipment and supplies away, clean the simulation equipment, order replacement supplies, analyze the evaluation data, and communicate outcomes to faculty, leadership, or other stakeholders. Even if a scenario is purchased, considerable time is spent on the associated aspects of running SBLE.

As you can see, significant thought needs to go into how time will be managed for each scenario that is developed and implemented. The exact amount of time is quite variable and depends on the complexity of the scenario, associated computer programming, and the skill of the person developing the scenario. It is important to automate routines when possible, for example, creating a database of supplies and equipment so the simulationist knows how many of each item is needed in each scenario (each semester, each year), having predetermined alarms to trigger an order when supplies are low, and automated emails to remind faculty and others of their responsibilities. Additional ideas on how to manage the laboratory functions are found in Chapter 11.

The second aspect of time deals with scheduling the simulation experiences. Numerous ideas have been shared in the literature, but this seems to be very individualized for each location. This is also determined, in part, by whether your state board of nursing allows you to replace traditional clinical with SBLE and if your leadership supports that. You may find that where you work, each course is going to use simulation during a certain week or, perhaps, one course wants to use the lab every Tuesday. At one of the labs I managed, we scheduled differently for every course, while sharing space with a hospital and conducting their simulations as well. Most typologies other than tethered simulators can take place outside the lab; however, laboratory personnel may still be needed to implement. Here are a few ways that SBLE can be scheduled:

- Assessment or skills course has simulation as part of their "skills stations." Students rotate through self-directed learning stations of which facilitated simulation is one.
- Courses (e.g., medical–surgical) use class time for simulation, bringing simulators into the classroom or using virtual reality (VR) or SPs.
- Courses send one group of students to the lab every week during the semester until all have completed simulation.
- Courses schedule all simulation over a 1-week block of time, and all students are complete at the end of the week.
- Make the simulation lab an "official" clinical site. When rotations are scheduled for the semester, student groups are rotated through the simulation lab instead of a hospital unit.
- Combine courses. For example, if mental health and medical–surgical courses are in the same semester, implement a scenario that meets learning objectives for both courses.

One last thought on scheduling and time management for simulation: **interprofessional education**. There is a lot of emphasis on interprofessional education (IPE) using simulation as a platform. While a worthy goal, the simulationist must also consider the time of various other disciplines. What are their course and clinical schedules like? Where is their available time and when are faculty available for scenario development? Further discussion on IPE follows later in this chapter.

Dumpster Diving! Ideas for Obtaining Supplies for Simulation

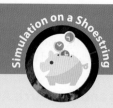

Ruth Braga, MSN, BA, RN

1. I post signs everywhere in the operating room (OR) making staff aware that we need sutures, gowns, gloves, drapes, etc., and then I put a bucket/special garbage can at the front desk or by the decontamination area for them to put them in.

2. I tell the students to speak up when they are in a case and ask the scrub tech if they can take any leftover opened suture.

3. I also tell the student on orientation to watch for anything that gets contaminated and ask to have it—they know where they can dump it for me. This gets them paying better attention to sterility and speaking up for something that is nonthreatening!

4. Get in touch with other hospitals that are not necessarily in your group or where your students/learners are going. They may be happy to have you take expired items off their hands.

5. Every OR has a nurse that is a hoarder—you just have to find them! I have one who stashes for me, and when audit time rolls around, my shelves get filled!

6. I have another nurse hoarder who collects the scissors and needle drivers from the central line kits when they aren't used; these are perfect for training medical students.

7. Become best friends with the people in hospital supply. I get a TON of stuff this way. Sometimes, they have things that they received as samples or were sent by mistake that they can't return.

8. Become best friends with the person who purchases instruments too; sometimes things are tossed because they aren't quite up to par for surgery, but they work for simulation/education.

9. For items that I can never get, such as staplers, I purchase them on eBay, but regulations are getting tougher there and it's difficult to know where they are coming from.

10. Anything that can go back to a vendor for recycling does, of course. "Dumpster diving" puts better use to a product that is paid for and turns it around for educational purposes.

Equipment and Supplies

Fidelity has been addressed elsewhere in this text (see Chapter 19), so this discussion is about logistics. First, what type of SBLE have you decided to conduct and what are the learning objectives? What type of simulation will you use to best meet those learning objectives? If VR is the platform, your equipment needs will consist of computer access with Internet and possibly wearable headgear. While the majority of schools and hospitals have strong Internet connectivity, not every learner does once he or she heads home; therefore, access to computers should be made available to the learner. If mannequin-based simulation is to be used, you will decide the right level of fidelity (see Chapter 6).

Supplies and equipment are needed to make the experience as realistic as possible; however, many budgets are not prepared to cover those needs. The simulationist will need to determine what is feasible from a budget standpoint and logistically possible. For example, a scenario that requires a patient to be on a ventilator will be challenging as most nursing labs do not own a ventilator; however, a hospital your school is affiliated with may be able to loan you one, along with a respiratory therapist who will also help with student learning. Durable medical equipment businesses can rent ventilators for you to use short-term. I've even seen a washing machine box painted to look like a ventilator. The fidelity of the equipment depends on how they need to be used to help meet the learning objectives.

Large hospitals have warehouses where extra supplies and equipment are housed. Ask for a tour! After visiting the warehouse at a hospital I worked at, I had a truckload of supplies and equipment that were outdated or no longer used on its way to my simulation center. Also, let your hospital partners know that you would be happy to take open, but unused, sterile kits (e.g., central line insertion kit) off their hands. Many supplies used in simulation can be used repeatedly. For example, I dried my bloody dressings after use, so I could store them. When I was ready to use, I spritzed them with a water bottle. Using sterile water in a Pleuravac allowed me to use the same system 7 years without mold growth. Reuse of supplies has a major impact on costs. Read about Ruth Braga's experience with "dumpster diving" in the following Simulation on a Shoestring feature.

People

People can be the most logistically challenging of all! No one has extra time in their day, so when they are asked by the simulationist to meet to discuss their scenario, to provide learning objectives, to identify how students will be evaluated, and to schedule run-throughs, you may meet with resistance; however, this collaboration is vital to the success of the SBLE and the impact on learning outcomes. Some ways to gain buy-in from faculty and staff are to invite them to observe simulations involving learners or to create a scenario in which the faculty and staff are the learners. Often, once they have participated, they better understand the potential of working with simulation. Encourage your students to talk to their faculty about the impact SBLE has on their understanding of content and ability to provide better patient care. It is also important that leadership communicates their expectations regarding use of SBLE in the curriculum and provides levels of support that promote success.

Another challenge relates to the role of the facilitator. Is that person ready for their role? Do they have the knowledge, skills, and attitude to be an effective facilitator of SBLE? The

Educator/Facilitator Readiness for Simulation Self-Assessment Survey (Toolkit 20-1) guides the facilitator through questions related to organization- and educator-specific knowledge; simulation resources including standards and guidelines; knowledge, skills, and attitudes about simulation-based teaching and learning; and simulation technological operations. Those who are not prepared to take on the role should seek additional knowledge and skills through reading and participation in webinars and workshops.

Designing a Simulation-Based Learning Experience (SBLE)

Now that you've identified potential topics from your needs assessment and gap analysis, considered how to integrate scenarios into the curriculum, and worked through the logistics of time, space, money, and personnel, it's time to start creating the SBLE. You may also hear the terms scenario, case, or simulated clinical experience (SCE) used to describe this; they are often used interchangeably. Consider the SBLE the big picture—the experience you are creating for your students. The scenario (or case, as this is commonly referred to in medical education) is one part of your larger experience, the SBLE. To promote consistency in terminology use, I will use SBLE in this discussion. As you work through designing and implementing your simulations, refer to the review tool for Evaluating the Design and Implementation of Simulations Using Best

Practices, a checklist created by Jane Page to ensure that the Standards of Best Practice: Simulation[SM] are followed. The review tool is located in the online Toolkit 20-2.

Outcomes and Objectives

The simulationist should consider what the desired end result is following learners' participation in an SBLE, both outcomes and objectives. The INACSL Standards of Best Practice: Simulation[SM], Outcomes and Objectives provide guidance in developing these. Outcomes are broader and consider the overall impact of the SBLE. Desired outcomes may be satisfaction; change in knowledge, skills, or attitude; change in behavior; or improved patient safety, for example. Development of specific learning objectives is driven by the desired outcomes (INACSL Standards Committee, 2016). It is imperative to the success of your students that you clearly identify what the learning objectives are for their SBLE.

Bloom's Taxonomy (1956) is a commonly used framework for developing learning objectives and includes three domains: cognitive, affective, and psychomotor. In 2001, the framework was revised to reflect a more active way of managing learning, resulting in the categories of remembering, understanding, applying, analyzing, evaluating, and creating. Types of knowledge that form the foundation of these categories are factual, **conceptual**, procedural, and metacognitive knowledge (Anderson & Krathwohl, 2001). The model has now become two dimensional, as depicted in Figure 20.1, with the cognitive process dimension correlating with the knowledge dimension. The cognitive process dimension builds from lower-order to higher-order thinking skills. While this may seem confusing, consider the following examples of how to use the table to write learning objectives:

1. I want my students to *remember* the steps of CPR. I can have them demonstrate this knowledge by having them *list* the steps, give them a video and ask them to identify (*recognize*) each step, have them describe to me (*recall*) how they will perform CPR, or have them use mental imaging to *identify* the steps.
2. If I want my students to *analyze* CPR, I can have them *select* between two lists of CPR steps for the right order, *differentiate* between two video examples for the most correct CPR technique, *demonstrate* how they integrated their knowledge by performing correct CPR, or *deconstruct* an IPE code scenario to determine differences in professional roles or culture.

As you can see, the second learning objectives are at a higher level of thinking than the first; however, a learner must perform at the lower level of knowledge gain before they can demonstrate how to use that information. Each

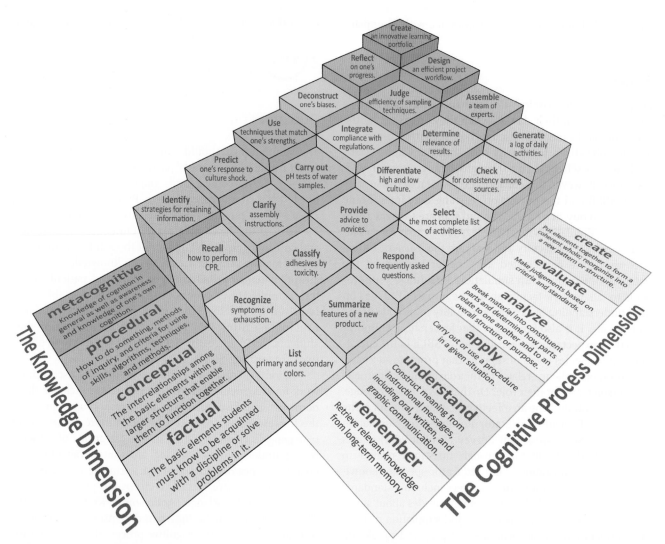

Figure 20.1 Revised Bloom's Taxonomy Model. (Model created by Rex Heer, Iowa State University Center for Excellence in Learning and Teaching, Updated January, 2012. Licensed under a Creative Commons Attribution-NonCommercial-ShareAlike 3.0 Unported License. For additional resources, see www.celt.iastate.edu/teaching/RevisedBlooms1.html. Used with permission.)

of the six steps builds on each other. We can't expect our learners to analyze or evaluate information that they don't understand. This supports the earlier suggestions that learners should be exposed to new information before a SBLE, rather than after. For additional detail about the revision of Bloom's Taxonomy, review Krathwohl's (2002) overview of the revisions, available for download at https://goo.gl/95QdmK. There are numerous resources on the Internet to learn more about writing learning objectives using Bloom's Taxonomy. One of my favorites is the Pedagogy Wheel, now version 4.0, that associates each level of the taxonomy with verbs and then adds learner activities that can be used to help them meet the objectives. The new version includes iPad applications that can be used to complete those assignments. Allan Carrington's work is licensed under Creative Commons and can be found at http://tinyurl.com/padwheelV4. Consider how

your simulation design can fit into these assignments in order to meet your learning objectives. I keep a copy of the model in Figure 20.1 and the Pedagogy Wheel at my fingertips and refer to them often.

Another consideration when writing learning objectives is the format. These are objectives that you want your learners to achieve so should be written from their perspective: "The learner will..." In 1981, the acronym S.M.A.R.T was presented at a conference as a method of writing goals and objectives that were specific, measurable, assignable, realistic, and time related, with the hope that this would improve successful outcomes (Doran, 1981). The Centers for Disease Control (CDC, 2009) adapted the terminology for academia and healthcare, resulting in the terms: specific, measurable, achievable, realistic, and time supported. The Outcomes and Objectives Standard (INACSL Standards Committee, 2016) has listed numerous considerations for the educator to make as they develop specific objectives (p. 17–18). For example, a *specific* objective should have only one action verb; a *measurable* objective requires identification of the reliable and valid tool that will be used for the measurement; an *achievable* objective includes a reasonable time frame; a *realistic* objective is leveled to the learner's abilities and knowledge; and a *time-phased* objective includes an end point by which the learning objective should be met.

Lastly, there is some debate over whether to give the learners the objectives prior to the SBLE. Consideration should be given to the purpose of the experience. If the goal is to conduct **summative** evaluation to determine the learner's ability to demonstrate management of a certain type of patient at semester end, then they should know what type of patient they will be expected to manage. This may be specific or general depending on your purpose. You might choose to tell the learner that the patient will have heart failure, or you might choose to tell them they will care for a patient with a cardiac condition. The learner should know the context within which they will be expected to learn or perform; however, critical action checklists used for evaluation might not be provided (INACSL Standards Committee, 2016). Debate also arises over whether to tell learners what the patient diagnosis is. The response again depends on your purpose. If you are working with undergraduate nursing students to help them learn care of a patient with a deep vein thrombosis, then consider providing that information. Undergraduates are not taught to diagnose. However, running the same SBLE with nurse practitioner students could be done without providing the diagnosis, since assessment leading to diagnosis is part of their role.

Types of Scenarios

Will you create your own scenarios? Will you use purchased scenarios? How do I decide whether to create an experience that encompasses one moment in time or whether to create unfolding cases? And, should I have my nursing students participate in simulation with other disciplines? These are all challenging questions for the simulationist and the answers often go back to some of the earlier questions—How much time do you have? Who can help you? How skilled are you in scenario design? What is your budget?

Create Your Own

Many simulationists create their own scenarios. This requires at least one **subject matter expert (SME)** as well as someone who is competent in scenario design. This might be one person or require several. Often, all faculty

in a course want to be involved in creating the scenarios. It is vital that SMEs use evidence-based current practice to design a SBLE that is realistic and adheres to current practice standards. Benefits of creating unique scenarios for your own courses are that this allows for a great deal of control over how the simulation fits into your curriculum, how learning objectives are met, and the content that is covered. The downside is that, depending on complexity, it can take many hours to create just one scenario. The simulationist, or a designee, will need to program the computer. Fortunately, programming simulators has become easier over the past several years while still maintaining the fidelity of more advanced physiological modeling. I recall programming a scenario about acute coronary syndrome that took over 50 hours because of the complexity. With today's advances, as well as skill developed over time, I would estimate that would now take 4 hours. It can't be overstated though that programming takes a significant amount of time, especially for the novice. Programming can take several forms, including an "on-the-fly" approach, manual progression, or automatic progression. Table 20.3 outlines the advantages and disadvantages of the different types of programming.

Purchased Scenarios

Individual scenarios, scenario bundles, and full simulation curricula are available for purchase through different vendors. The advantage of purchasing these products is that they are designed to be "off-the-shelf" ready-to-use scenarios, allowing the simulationist to enact them quickly without spending the time to start development from scratch. The scenario products typically include all standard elements of good scenario design, including the programming. The inclusion of the programming creates an interesting budget discussion. While the cost of the purchased scenarios may seem high to some, you must consider how many hours it would take you to create the same work based on your level of **competence** and experience. In many cases, it is more expensive to create your own when the cost of your time is factored in. The disadvantage of purchased scenarios is the loss of control over the content. Many, if not most, faculty find something in each purchased scenario that they want to change! It may be that one of the learning objectives doesn't fit your course, or one of the medications is recommended in a dose different than what healthcare providers use in your region. Perhaps the flow of the scenario or the timing doesn't fit your needs. The majority of those problems can be easily resolved by giving your students objectives or healthcare provider orders that supersede those in the purchased scenario. The real challenges are those related to programming. Simulationists with the ability to program will be able to change the scenario flow to meet local needs.

Table 20.3	Advantages and Disadvantages of Programming Types	
Programming	**Advantages**	**Disadvantages**
On the fly	Decreases programming time Use for **formative** SBLE Operator makes changes based on learner action or inaction	Increases variability among learner groups Cannot be used for summative evaluation or research Scenario may last different lengths of time, creating scheduling challenge
Manual progression	Decreases programming time Use for formative SBLE Make changes based on learner response, action, inaction, or predetermined time	Scenario may last different lengths of time, creating scheduling challenge Variability in progression can preclude use in summative evaluation or research Learners receive different experiences
Automatic progression	All experiences last the same length of time, creating ease in scheduling Decisions to move scenario forward is automated; scenario progresses regardless of learner action or inaction Decreases variability for summative evaluation and research	Increased programming time and complexity Scenario may progress at a pace too rapid for learners

Single Case or Unfolding Case

Two ways to design scenarios are single case and unfolding cases. A single-case scenario plays out within the time allotted for the SBLE, while an unfolding case evolves over time, in two or more steps. The time for an unfolding case study could occur in one session or over several. Compare the two examples in Box 20-1. As you can see, the single case is self-limiting and ends within a specific period of time while focusing on resolution of one major problem. The unfolding case study can take place within one time frame or over several visits to the simulation lab. The focus is on an ongoing, evolving problem and allows learners to see progression over time. Recall earlier that you were challenged to identify whether you wanted to have discreet scenarios for each course or whether to have one concept (e.g., respiratory) play out across the curriculum. This is an example of how those decisions can play out in the type of scenario you decide to implement.

Interprofessional Simulation

Review of errors and patient safety reports all point to the need for interprofessional education. Interprofessional education (IPE) includes learners from two or more professions and is designed to "promote collaboration and enhance the quality of care" (Palaganas, Maxworthy, Epps, & Mancini, 2015, p. xxviii). Using simulation as the vehicle for this type of education allows for learners to engage in management of a variety of scenarios in which communication and teamwork are vital to successful outcomes. Scenarios appropriate for simulation-enhanced interprofessional education (Sim-IPE) might include individual patient care (e.g., cardiac arrest), management of a crisis in a particular environment (e.g., operating room), management of a systems issue (e.g., overwhelming influx into ED), environmental changes (e.g., patient movement within a new facility), or management of a community concern (e.g., disaster management), among others.

Box 20-1 Example of Single-Case and Unfolding Case Scenarios

Single Case: The patient has heart failure and has arrived in the emergency department for care. The learners are expected to assess the patient, communicate findings, administer treatments and medications, and give report to the progressive care nurse. This scenario takes place over 30 minutes.

Unfolding Case: The patient has bloody stools and has arrived in the emergency department for care. The learners are expected to assess the patient, communicate findings, administer treatments and medications, and give report to the medical–surgical nurse. The scenario takes place over 30 minutes.

The patient is now 12-hours status post bowel resection with colostomy. He is hypotensive with low urine output. Expectations of the learners are as above, with a treatment focus of resolving fluid volume deficiency.

The patient is now 36-hours post-op and has learned his treatment options. He is anxious and not interested in learning how to manage his colostomy. The expectation of the learner includes the above, but with a focus on relieving anxiety and providing education.

The patient returned to the clinic regularly, and 6 months postdiagnosis, he learns that treatment options have failed. He decides to engage hospice, and learners are now expected to provide end-of-life care to a terminal patient.

Creating Sim-IPE has many advantages including promoting interprofessional competency (Saylor, Vemoony, Selekman, & Cowperthwait, 2016), improved communication (Bolesta & Chmil, 2014), enhanced teamwork (Luctkar-Flude et al., 2013), increased collaboration (Nicely & Farra, 2015), and, anecdotally, a better understanding of the roles and responsibilities of the participants. However, it is not easy to create these SBLE due to competing schedules, different curriculum, and variability in simulators, facilitator strategies, and the types of programs each profession promotes (INACSL Standards Committee, 2016).

The INACSL Standards of Best Practice: Simulation[SM], Simulation-Enhanced Interprofessional Education (Sim-IPE) identify the need to meet the following four criteria:

1. Conduct Sim-IPE based on a theoretical or conceptual framework.
2. Utilize best practices in the design and development of Sim-IPE.

3. Recognize and address potential barriers to Sim-IPE.
4. Devise an appropriate evaluation plan for Sim-IPE (p. 49).

You'll notice that these same criteria are necessary to create discipline-specific SBLE as well; however, it's just more complicated when involving different disciplines! First, there has to be an identified need for the disciplines to work together—what is the problem identified by the needs assessment and gap analysis that you are trying to resolve? What role does each discipline have in the resolution? Identifying the "right" people to work with in other departments can be challenging, and sometimes several attempts need to be made before the right person is located. Those champions may not be in your same building, on the same campus, or even in the same town. It is easy to overlook important stakeholders; early in the process, brainstorm who needs to be at the planning table. Then, it becomes about negotiation: simulationists and SMEs from each discipline will need to come to agreement on the development, implementation, facilitation method, debriefing strategy, and evaluation method that will be used for the SBLE, as well as how the budget and oversight for the experience will be managed. For additional detail on leading interprofessional education, refer to Chapter 26.

Creating the Scenario

Now that you have decided what type of scenario you plan to develop, there are several key components that should be included. If you are using prepackaged scenario products, you will want to review them carefully to ensure that the components meet your needs, and if not, you will need to alter them. Because of the amount of information required for a robust scenario, many simulationists find

Table 20.4	Scenario Design Templates (Free Resources)
Organization	**Link to Template**
National League for Nursing Simulation Innovation Resource Center (NLN SIRC)	https://goo.gl/xxApqJ Sign in to Designing & Developing Simulations Course for free template download
University of Alabama—Birmingham	https://goo.gl/wE3yt9
University of Washington	https://goo.gl/EAU437
QSEN Institute	https://goo.gl/NFCXsF
Laerdal Simulation Users Network (SUN)	https://goo.gl/5Muztq https://goo.gl/LEK385 Sign in to access
Dr. Jeff Taekman, Duke University	https://goo.gl/mrFpJf
MedEdPORTAL	https://goo.gl/INu15o
Hennepin County Medical Center	https://goo.gl/cPbmfq

that a template is useful to prevent overlooking any of the components. There are a variety of templates readily available, or you might create your own if those don't meet your needs. Table 20.4 provides information on some of the free templates available online. As you will see during your review, in most cases, the information requested is the same, but it might be organized differently. Because we all view the process just a little differently from each other, this is not surprising. The key is to get all the information—the order of presentation is not as important. A Master Simulation Design Template and Companion Intake Form are provided in Toolkit 20-3, along with a Completed Master Simulation Design Template, so you can see it in its finished form with all necessary information complete (Toolkit 20-4).

Components

Creating the patient and his or her story is one of the most challenging—and fun—parts of scenario design. This is where your creativity takes over. Below are the patient factors you need to consider when writing your scenario with examples for each. This is not all-inclusive, but will provide you with ideas to use when completing a template.

- Patient Identity: Gender and age
- General Health: Healthy, chronically ill, acutely ill, injured, and end of life

- Psychosocial Factors: Culture, religion, financial resources, and social/family issues
- History/Background: Medical history, medications, allergies, treatment compliance, and what medical history has contributed to the current situation
- Current Situation: Circumstances leading to the patient being where he is now and in his current situation
- Expected Behaviors of Learner: Dependent upon learning objectives; for example, assessment, communication, medication administration, documentation, patient education, family interaction, etc.
- Expected Reaction of the Patient: When the learner behaves as expected, how will the patient respond? If the learner does not behave as expected, how will the patient respond?
- Timeline: Identify the first actions you expect of the learners and how long that should take to occur (it will always take longer than you think!). How long will the patient's response take? What do you expect next of the learner and then the patient? How long will the scenario take to play out?
- Resources: What information does the learner need in order to be successful in their expected behaviors? For example, if the learners are expected to conduct an assessment and then give medication, they will need healthcare provider orders, simulated medications, and a method to document medication administration.
  - Human Resources: **Confederates, simulated persons**, patient family
  - Moulage: Makeup, wax or latex molding, clothing, wig, glasses
  - Equipment: IV pumps, monitor, ventilator, suction, glucose monitor. Read Lu Sweeney's suggestions for providing glucose readings in the Simulation on a Shoestring feature
  - Supplies: Dressings, nasogastric tube, yellow food coloring, urinary catheter bag
  - Electronic Health Record: Documentation forms, results of diagnostic testing, order forms. Read how Margaret Hassler and Cynthia Rubbelke created an electronic medication administration scanning system using QR codes and handheld scanners in the Simulation on a Shoestring feature
  - Medication Administration: Simulated medications, syringes, IV bags, and tubing
  - Holistic Care: Picture frame with family photo, religious icon, get-well cards
  - Information Resources: Pharmacology book, phone applications, computer access
- **Script**: Writing down responses to potential learner questions will help to maintain consistency among learners and groups. Many questions that learners will ask the patient are expected and can be scripted, for example, Describe your pain. How long have you been ill? The simulationist should consider using the voice of the patient to gain additional information

as well. For example, the patient can ask the learner questions like "How long before this medication kicks in?" or "Are there any side effects I should be worried about?" Student responses to these scripted questions help the simulationist to determine their level of comprehension.

- Logistics: A scenario that looks logical on paper may not work when enacted. It is important to do test runs of a planned scenario to determine how much time the scenario will take, where equipment and supplies should be located, how learner movement will occur, and access to electronic resources and, in general, to make sure the scenario runs the way you expect it to.

Another resource for simulation design is to review scenarios that others have already developed. Chapter 23 contains examples of scenario ideas for a variety of courses and patient types. Some of the authors have provided full documentation for their scenarios, and these can be found in the Toolkit for Chapter 23. Standards of Best Practice: Simulation^SM, Scenario Design provides additional ideas and support for the components of a well-designed scenario.

Level of Fidelity

Criterion 3 of the Scenario Design Standard focuses on the format of the SBLE, its purpose and modality. Criterion 5 considers how to use different types of fidelity to enhance realism (INACSL Standards Committee, 2016). To meet the criterions for this standard, you may review information about the typologies of simulation in Chapter 6 and modalities in Chapter 7. Additionally, information about moulage and realism is found in Chapter 19. It is important for the simulationist to create an experience that is engaging to the learner. This helps place the patient care into context and may help to make the connection from learning in the simulation environment to care of human patients. There are three main types of fidelity to consider in scenario design, **environmental, conceptual**, and **psychological** (INACSL Standards Committee, 2016), and examples of each follow:

- Environmental Fidelity: You are conducting an in situ simulation on the obstetrics unit. To ensure environmental fidelity, you will create the SBLE to closely mirror the actual patient care unit, using equipment and supplies that would be used on real patients. The simulator should lie in a hospital bed designed for obstetrics patients surrounded by the furniture and environs of the patient room. The fetal heart monitor and abdominal belts should be the same as those used for real patient care. If the simulator is on a gurney, dressed in street clothes, and has the appearance of a male simulator, it will be harder to get learner buy-in.

Glucometer Readings

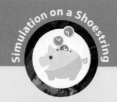

**Natalie Lu Sweeney,
MS, CNS, RNC-NIC**

The Challenge

One of the challenges of implementing scenarios is to decrease "pretending" by increasing fidelity without increasing expense or setup time. Two simple but key procedures, obtaining a blood glucose and taking a temperature, presented difficulties. Complex approaches using glucose test solutions or red glucose solution saturated injectable pads were problematic due to erroneous glucose values and/or loss of learner buy-in because of fumbling with nonintuitive props that were time and labor intensive for staff to set up. Our goal was for students to complete the psychomotor task (obtaining a blood glucose or taking a temperature) and receive a result in a more intuitive way and realistic time than having results phoned into the room or using an unpredictable prop.

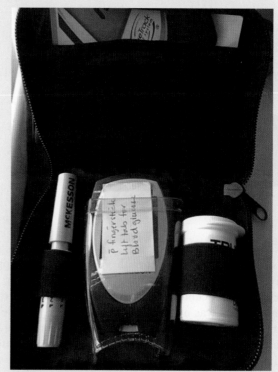

Figure 20.2 Glucometer.

Innovative Solution(s)

Students use a needleless lancet to obtain a "specimen" from a mannequin or standardized patient and, after a few seconds, lift a tab applied to the front of a glucometer (Fig. 20.2) to find the result written on a small sticky note. Multiple values could be layered for use during the same scenario. A similar approach was taken for obtaining a temperature using "temp tabs" (Fig. 20.3). A card stock organizer was created and laminated with clear packing tape to hold dozens of different tabs made from colorful, adhesive plastic folder tabs cut in half with Fahrenheit on one side and Celsius on the other. The desired tabs for the scenario could be slid under a paper "pocket" taped to the front of the digital thermometer and withdrawn after the psychomotor actions were completed. One difficulty noted was distraction from the central objectives of the scenario if students were not familiarized and shown the glucometer and thermometer props with an explanation of how they would provide data during the scenario before *each* scenario.

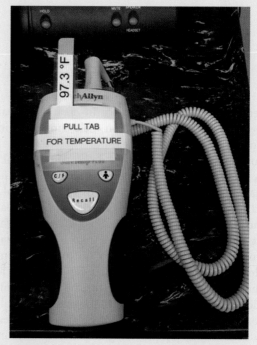

Figure 20.3 Thermometer.

Creating an eMAR Scanning System using QR Codes and Handheld Scanners

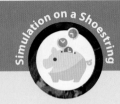

**Cynthia Rubbelke,
MEd, MSN(R), RN**

**Margaret Hassler,
MSN, RN-BC, CHSE**

The Challenge

A simulated electronic health record using Google Drive spreadsheets was being utilized effectively in our simulation center, yet students and faculty felt that some realism was missing because they were unable to administer medications safely using the common practice of a scanning system. Unfortunately, the commercial scanning products offered were cost prohibitive for our laboratory budget. We also could not justify charging students an additional fee to subscribe to another product.

Innovative Solution

For approximately $1,000, we created a functional, realistic medication scanning system comprised of a rolling office cart, a basic laptop computer, and a 2D barcode scanner. The laptop and cart simulate the workstation on wheels that is commonly used in healthcare settings. Using a free QR code generator (https://www.the-qrcode-generator.com/), QR codes were created for each patient's armband and each medication. The QR code on the armband is the URL of the patient eMAR and opens that page within Chrome browser. Once the eMAR is opened, each of the medications can be scanned within a specific cell. Using conditional formatting, font colors, and spreadsheet formulas, the cells are formatted to indicate whether the student scanned the correct medication, incorrect medication, a high-alert medication, or a medication that requires dosage calculation (e.g., the pill needs to be split). Students have commented that the system mimics the scanning systems used in the hospitals and agree that it helps to practice safe medication administration similar to how they will administer medications in their clinical experience. One drawback of this scanning method is lack of time stamping ability for medication administration. Students must still enter the time manually. The file revision feature in Google allows simulation faculty to quickly revert the eMAR to begin another session with new students. The greatly reduced cost outweighs the drawbacks.

Read Sue Thelan's experience in creating a realistic obstetrical overlay for use on male simulators in the Simulation on a Shoestring feature.

- Conceptual Fidelity: You have developed a virtual reality scenario in which the learner enters an online virtual environment and responds to a bus accident. The actions and activities in the scenario need to be realistic and accurate. For example, one would expect orthopedic injuries in an accident. The trauma would result in blood loss and deformities to fractured extremities. Blood loss would lead to hypotension and tachycardia. These are all areas of fidelity for the simulationist to address. If there is no blood, vital signs are normal, and no one is in distress, then it will be hard for the learner to believe they are providing care during a traumatic event.

- Psychological Fidelity: You have developed a cardiac arrest scenario to take place in the simulation lab. The sights and sounds that you create will add to the tension and realism of the situation. A beeping heart monitor or one with alarms going off, the sound of overhead pages, pagers sounding, and the defibrillator charging noise all lead to increased psychological fidelity. Having family members in the room adds to the drama and the realism. However, the simulationist also has to take care not to overdramatize. Often, simulated patients or actors will overdo their efforts. This is seen when students are placed into family roles in situations that they don't have experience with. They tend to overact and the focus shifts from patient care to dealing with an out-of-control person when that wasn't the objective of the scenario.

Changing the Simulator from Male to Female with an Overlay

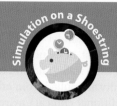

Susan L. Thelen

The Challenge

I am an artist and mother of a nurse educator. My daughter, Lynde Rabine, was teaching at Augustana College in Sioux Falls, SD, when she called saying she needed a way for their male mannequin to be female and made to simulate a pregnancy.

The Innovation

I first designed a "belly" that was made of four layers of foam ovals. I had glued them together, hollowed out the middle and carved the exterior to resemble a pregnant belly. This belly was encased in a stretch fabric and attached with hook and loop tape to a large bra with the cups stuffed with fiberfill. The bra straps and back closure were extended with hook and loop tape to fit the mannequin and make it easier to put on and take off.

This first attempt worked well using a soft-bodied baby doll inserted under the foam. However, when multiple students performed the Leopold method on the belly, the layers began to separate where they had been glued.

The next design worked much better, with a redesigned belly and the same bra. The belly was created by cutting an oval from 1″ foam and cutting out narrow pie-shaped pieces all around the edge. I then used a large needle with a 3′ length of elastic cord and inserted it about ½ in. above the edge all the way around the oval. By tightening the cord, the belly had a perfect mound shape and could be pushed into different sizes of an obese belly or a pregnant belly. The foam was topped with a layer of fleece fabric to imitate a layer of fat. The top of the belly case had a strip of hook tape and the inside bottom of the bra had a loop tape allowing the overlay to be used to simulate a pregnant female or an obese female, or when the belly was removed from the bra, it could be used to simulate an obese male. I also added a boggy and firm uterus made from foam balls shaped so they would stay in place. To simulate the firm uterus, I used a small foam ball, and for the boggy uterus, I used a larger foam ball with the center removed.

This first design of the overlay was so well received that I designed two more overlays including edema overlays for arms and legs, which were made from memory foam glued with a foam glue to stretch fabric and strapped onto the arms and legs with the hook and loop tape, and simulated swollen testicles made from gel balls encased in stretch fabric.

I applied for and received a provisional patent on the design, but the cost of hiring a patent attorney and other costs involved in securing a final patent were prohibitively expensive.

Along with these types of fidelity, I want to make special mention of the holistic aspects of patient simulation. As nurses, we provide holistic patient care, attending to not only the physical aspects of patient care but also the psychosocial, spiritual, developmental, and cultural aspects. We get to know our patients as whole beings, rather than just their illness. It is important for us to build in props, cues, and other information to help our learners provide holistic care. For example, managing a patient with a heart attack is different than managing a 42-year-old construction worker who has a heart attack when you learn he has a wife and four little girls, lacks health insurance, and physically won't be able to return to his job. Focus on holistic aspects of patient care also allows simulationists to create situations that learners often don't know how to handle such as communicating with a young dying patient, a 14-year-old mother,

a lesbian couple experiencing childbirth, or a patient who asks the nurse to pray with them. Experiencing holistic patient care in the simulation lab may lead to greater comfort, less anxiety, and confident patient interaction.

Roles and Responsibilities of the Facilitator

The role of the facilitator encompasses many elements of the SBLE including preparing the learners for the experience, leading prebriefing, managing the scenario, debriefing, and evaluating outcomes. The INACSL Standards of Best Practice: Simulation^{SM}, Scenario Design and Facilitation (INACSL Standards Committee, 2016) provide information as to the necessary

STANDARDS

skills required to facilitate SBLE toward achievement of desired outcomes. The Standards and the NCSBN Guidelines (Alexander et al., 2015) are both clear that facilitators must be educated and trained to function in this role. Historically, and still the case in many organizations, faculty are pulled from other areas such as the skills lab or traditional clinical environment and told that they need to facilitate simulation; however, they are not given the education and training to do so effectively. The need for education and various methods for obtaining that are covered in Chapter 21. In this section, I will talk specifically about the parts of SBLE that the facilitator is responsible for: preparing, prebriefing, facilitating, debriefing, and evaluating.

Preparation

Preparing for the SBLE involves several steps: scheduling, creating learning objectives, planning the activity, determining fidelity, identifying supply and equipment needs, developing preparation requirements, and choosing evaluation methods. Attending to these items early in the process should increase your opportunity for successful implementation of the SBLE as well as learner outcomes.

Scheduling

The facilitator needs to consider the size of the learner group. I am often asked "how many learners should be in a simulation?" The answer, as often spoken related to simulation, is "It all depends." If the simulation is being run for summative evaluation, then you will likely need to run it for each individual learner; however, if you are conducting summative evaluation of a team, then all the members of that team should be involved. If simulation is designed for formative evaluation, then you have more options; however, most simulationists will agree that a small number at the bedside tends to work best. In order for each learner to function in their role, overlap in expectations needs to be eliminated and roles clearly defined. One study showed that learning was equivalent on a posttest (Kaplan, Abraham, & Gary, 2012), reinforcing the opportunity to have a small number of learners at the bedside while others observe the scenario. And, of course, if the simulation is done in VR, or other individualized platform, then group size is less important.

In order to accommodate larger groups, some learners may be given an observer role. They might observe throughout an entire scenario or they may change places with a learner at the bedside at a pre-determined point in time. One method of managing observers is to have half the group provide care for the patient, while the other half observes. The group providing care then gives report to the incoming "shift" and the observers then take over. In order to keep the observing group members engaged, consider asking them each to observe for different aspects of the care, such as opportunities for patient education, holistic considerations, communication opportunities, interaction with family members, and so on. This will help them to contribute to the debriefing as well. Read Sarah Clark's ideas for managing large groups of learners in the Simulation on a Shoestring feature.

I wrote earlier in the chapter about scheduling methods. It is important for the learners to be scheduled in a way that creates an optimal learning experience for them. While you may not have direct responsibility for scheduling the sessions, you must ensure that your groups are on the schedule. While this sounds basic, more times than I can count, I have had groups show up on a day they were not scheduled for, and I have also waited for groups who do not show up on the scheduled day. It is your responsibility to make sure everything is scheduled correctly.

Creating Learning Objectives

Above, I reviewed how to write learning objectives. These objectives should address cognitive, psychomotor, and affective domains. Affective objectives seem more difficult—how do we impact the learner's emotions and help them to appreciate the subtleties of care and its impact on patients? This is where creating fidelity of the holistic aspects of patient care becomes important as this may help learners to see beyond the physical care of their patient and to see them as an entire being. Objectives should be written at the level of the learner, ensuring that they have the knowledge and abilities to be successful while stretching them beyond their comfort level.

Planning the Activity

Make sure that you communicate your learning objectives, scenario, and logistical plan with the simulation laboratory staff. It's not enough to just let them know that you are bringing your students on Wednesday at 3:00 PM. It takes a collaborative effort to ensure that SBLEs go as planned. Test run your scenario with the lab staff to ensure it runs the way you expect, people respond as you desire, and that equipment and supplies are available.

Determining Fidelity

Much has been written already about the fidelity level for SBLE. We tend to use the simulation method that we are most comfortable with; however, we should choose the method that best leads to our desired outcomes. For example, it is unnecessary to use a high-fidelity simulator to teach learners how to insert an IV. This is better accomplished on a task trainer. Many simulationists are instructed to use the high-fidelity mannequin in every course to ensure full curriculum integration. Because there are a variety of types of simulation and various modalities, we have a wide selection of possibilities to meet our fidelity needs and closely replicate the environment of care.

Viewing or Doing

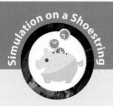

Sarah Clark, MSN, RN, CCRN, CHSE

The Challenge

Our challenge is to provide effective simulation education that keeps large groups engaged in the learning activity with limited space and time. Our simulation center provides education for nurses, paramedics, medical residents, physicians, and interdisciplinary teams. We have large numbers of learners in many simulation activities, a full schedule, one full-time simulation specialist (me), and a handful of part time facilitators.

Innovative Solution

We conduct simulations using facilitators and live video from the bedside into the debriefing room. A series of scenarios are designed to achieve the learning objectives for each session. Participants are divided into teams; each team participates in one scenario and views other teams in their scenarios. After each simulation, all participants come together for a debriefing about the patient care goals.

Three facilitators actively engage all the learners. The bedside facilitator coaches participants in patient care. The mannequin facilitator interacts as the patient and the "voice" of physician, pharmacy, rapid response team, etc. The observation facilitator guides participants viewing the simulation, who record significant patient information on a whiteboard (Fig. 20.4). The whiteboard notes drive the debriefing discussion. Simulations are designed so the actions at the bedside that are recorded by the viewers will reflect the learning objectives. Debriefing is led by the facilitators, using a problem-based learning format. This design employs adult learning principles, encouraging active, self-directed learning.

We conducted a research study with new graduate nurses to compare the self-reported confidence of participants viewing versus participating at the bedside followed by a facilitated debriefing. Participants completed a validated Student Satisfaction and Self-Confidence in Learning tool (NLN, 2005) after each scenario. The findings of this study showed no difference in the self-confidence between viewing and bedside participation. Through the use of multiple facilitators, we have been able to provide effective simulation for large groups, who stay engaged in learning and report gaining self-confidence.

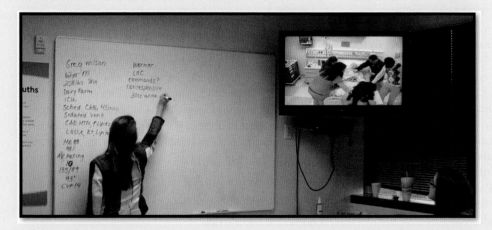

Figure 20.4 Facilitated Observation. Participants view the simulation using video feed. With the facilitator's guidance, viewers record patient information on the whiteboard to be used during debriefing discussions.

Identifying Supply and Equipment Needs

As you develop your scenario, you may be surprised at the amount of supplies and equipment that you need. That is why it is vital to make a list! But, you also need to realistically consider the cost of some items and the logistical ease of access. You want to use materials that enhance the fidelity of your experience but also prioritize their need. For example, a critical care scenario may involve a patient on the ventilator. While it would be great to have an actual ventilator for the experience, consider whether you can use a prop instead. Remember the washing machine box I mentioned earlier? This was designed to appear realistic, and tubing was connected to appropriate areas and then to the endotracheal tube of the simulated patient. The mannequin was set to breath at 10 breaths/minute. The objectives of the scenario focused on management of a critically ill post-op patient—managing breathing, intravenous fluid resuscitation, control of bleeding, and medication administration—so the function of a ventilator was not the focus. If a learning objective was to appropriately manage a ventilator then a real ventilator is important to the cause. Prioritize what is most important to your outcomes.

Developing Preparation Requirements

Many simulationists have their learners complete activities prior to arrival that will help them to be more successful in the SBLE. These activities may include readings in the course text; watching a video; completing a quiz; writing a list of potential nursing diagnoses based on the provided history, physical, and medication list; or creating medication cards, for example. The goal is to help the learner be prepared. Your role is to determine if they are, in fact, prepared. I do not advocate that you have learners hand in assignments that you grade. You will know through responses during prebriefing and actions during the scenario just who is prepared and who is not. Your responsibility is then to determine what that means for the learner. In a traditional clinical unit, unprepared learners pose danger to the patients and may be sent off the hospital unit. Will you ask unprepared learners to leave the simulation? If so, will they be sent home and return later for remediation (increasing your workload!), will you send them to the library to complete a supplemental assignment, or will you mark them as an unexcused absence? These are all philosophical questions to discuss with your course faculty, curriculum committee, and leadership. Anecdotally, rightly or wrongly, it does not take long for word to spread that a student was not allowed to participate because they were unprepared and that often triggers a change in everyone's behaviors.

Choosing Evaluation Methods

Preparing for evaluation is often overlooked. At the start, many simulationists are most interested in whether their learners like coming to simulation. While we prefer that our learners appreciate our efforts and enjoy coming to our class, we also know that not all learning is fun and that there are life and death consequences of how well learners understand material. Editors of simulation journals will tell you to look beyond satisfaction and plan for ways to evaluate effectiveness of the experience, facilitator, learning outcomes, and then consider how this is transferred to practice. It is vital that you choose tools that are validated for use with your learner group and are considered psychometrically sound.

Prebriefing

When learners arrive for the SBLE, especially the first time, they will be anxious and unsure as to what they are to do. For most of them, simulation-based learning is a new experience. They are used to demonstrating knowledge through written tests and demonstrating skills in order of a checklist. In SBLE, we are expecting to observe critical thinking and clinical judgement skills that lead to safe, effective patient care. We need to help our learners understand our expectations. Prebriefing involves several components: setting expectations, reviewing learning objectives, identifying roles, and creating the learning environment. Attending to these items should increase your learner's opportunity for success.

Setting Expectations

The facilitator should explain the purpose of the SBLE and what is expected of the learners, including full participation, respect toward patient and fellow learners, and effort toward realistic response to the simulated experience. Fiction contracts are often used by facilitators to document the agreement of learners to maintain confidentiality, and therefore, integrity of the experience, to not share information about the performance of their peers, and to engage to the best of their ability despite limitations in fidelity. Examples of fiction contracts are in the Toolkit for Chapter 19.

During the prebriefing, the facilitator orients the learners to the environment and what they can expect of the facilitator. Learners should be familiarized with the functions of the simulator, associated equipment and supplies, functionality of the electronic medical record, and any equipment used in the simulation. Learners should not have to wonder what is real and what is not. Discourage the use of the word "pretend" and assure learners that the patient will respond to all attempts to obtain information from or about the patient. If you will be the voice of the patient or provide information (such as lab results) upon request, tell the learner.

Share information about your role with the learners and answer their questions. Let them know how long the scenario will last and that you will facilitate the debriefing session that follows. If the SBLE is a formative experience, let the learners know that it is ok to make mistakes and learn from them. Ensure they know what resources are available to them, including supplies, equipment, electronic resources, and a phone to call the healthcare provider. Make sure the learner has the number to call for healthcare provider assistance, lab results, and other diagnostic findings.

Reviewing Learning Objectives

Review the preparation activities and the learning objectives with the learners, clarify misconceptions and answer questions, or assist them to find answers in their texts or digital resources. Earlier I wrote about the decision to provide learning objectives ahead of time. I'm a firm believer that learners will make every effort to meet learning objectives and perform well—if they know what the objectives and expectations are. Withholding your "plan" may lead to unnecessary anxiety and stress for the learner, and frustration for you when they don't perform as expected. Consider that learners who are unprepared will need you to prepare them when they come. You are now using your valuable simulation time to teach—to teach them information they could have learned on their own ahead of time.

Identifying Roles

Many simulationists have learners take on various roles during the SBLE. These may include professional roles such as primary nurse, medication nurse, documentation nurse, etc. Others assign roles of parent, sibling, chaplain, respiratory therapist, licensed practical nurse, nursing assistant, etc. Consider that assigning professional roles helps the learner to develop their understanding of the responsibilities associated with each role. Assigning roles of other healthcare providers is challenging as the learners do not know and understand those roles until they have worked with these professionals over time. In addition, many of our learners have never been in a hospital environment prior to school so may not have a conceptualization of how a parent or family member might act in the chosen situation. Many are not yet parents or have not experienced death of a close relative, while others may have experienced a traumatic healthcare event.

All assigned roles should come with a detailed description of the associated expectations. Consider providing this information ahead of time, especially to novice learners, so they have time to ask you questions. More expert learners might choose from nametags you have laid out to determine their role. You should also consider assigning specific roles to learners who need more experience in certain areas. For example, the learner who is struggling to take charge could be assigned the role of the primary nurse.

Creating the Learning Environment

The facilitator needs to have an acute awareness of the learning environment, ensuring that learners are not singled out, embarrassed, or made fun of. All learner concerns can be addressed as a group, rather than pointing out one person's lack of understanding. For example, a learner has just asked you the same question about the simulator's capabilities for the third time. You might respond "I know this is a new experience for everyone. Let's review the simulator's capabilities again before we start." Chances are that others have the same questions but are too shy, nervous, or intimidated to ask. During the SBLE, the facilitator needs to monitor the emotions of the learners to make sure they don't interfere with learning. When stress, anxiety, or cognitive load becomes too high, learning may not occur. One strategy is to stop the scenario and conduct a mini-debrief or reflection on action, allowing learners to reflect and discuss the current situation, defusing the tension, and allowing forward movement. The group should also be monitored following the entire SBLE as emotions may not come out until later. This is a potential outcome when the scenario deals with end-of-life issues. Throughout the SBLE, the facilitator needs to role-model positive, encouraging behaviors that promote learning.

Once prebriefing is completed, the scenario can begin. Additional information on how to set the stage during prebriefing for SBLE is found in Criteria 7 of Standards of Best Practice: Simulation^SM, Scenario Design (INACSL Standards Committee, 2016).

Facilitation

Facilitating the simulation experience must be done by a person who is trained to be a facilitator and functions in a way that correlates to the learner's level of learning, experience, and abilities while upholding ethical and professional behaviors. The INACSL Standards of Best Practice: Simulation^SM, Facilitation and Professional Integrity (INACSL Standards Committee, 2016) include guidelines to help the simulationists in their roles. Components of facilitation to consider include focus, guidance, participant engagement, performance, time/length, and evaluate.

Focus

The facilitator needs to place full attention on the learners and closely observe what they are doing, how they are doing it, and what aspects are strengths and areas for improvement. I have seen many facilitators checking email, scrolling through the Internet, and even grading papers while facilitating. This definitely does not meet the standard for professional integrity (INACSL Standards Committee, 2016). The learners deserve your full attention. In addition, you need to be ready to change gears on short notice. While we can predict, to a certain extent, what our learners will do, they often surprise us. They may make one wrong decision that takes them down a path in which they will never meet the learning objectives.

One method that a facilitator might use to return to the desired learning experience is to use cues. **Cues/prompts** are methods used to get learners "back on track" and have also been referred to as "lifesavers." Cues can take many forms such as verbal, written, or digital. Consider a scenario in which you want the learners to recognize that a patient is bleeding internally. They have missed the cues embedded in the assessment such as abdominal tenderness, distention, decreased amplitude of peripheral pulses, tachycardia, and hypotension, and as a result, they believe that their trauma patient's only problem is his fractured tibia. Your learning objective is management of a patient with acute blood loss so it is evident the students have missed this entirely. However, you might use the voice of the patient to complain of light-headedness or to say that you feel like you're in a cold sweat and don't feel well. Or, you could deliver lab results that indicate a low hemoglobin and hematocrit. Pending orders, you may put up a digital radiographic image showing a fractured pelvis. You could also don a lab coat and enter as the charge nurse and ask for a report, then use questions to guide the learners back on track.

Guidance

Closely related to providing cues is providing guidance or coaching. The facilitator needs to decide when it is appropriate to rescue the learner and when it is not. When do we stop mistakes from occurring? Or do we stop them at all? It is my belief that we learn more from the mistakes that we make than when we do everything right. Carefully consider if this might be the case with the error your student will make and how your response will or will not help them to meet the learning objectives for the SBLE. I'd like to offer you two examples to help you process this:

1. On the traditional clinical unit, my student was preparing to administer a medication. I could see that her math was incorrect. Do I stop her or give her time to figure this out on her own? The medication was promethazine 25 mg and she was going to administer 50 mg in error. Because promethazine was a very inexpensive medication, I didn't stop her. She drew up the medication. I had to decide again whether to stop her. I asked her questions about the medication, its side effects, purpose, and dosage, but she still didn't realize her error. I decided to allow her to continue and walked with her to the patient's room. Before we entered, I drew her into an alcove, pulled a notepad from my pocket, and asked her to calculate the dosage again. It was then that she realized her error. We returned a few brief minutes later with the correct dosage of medication. By her own admission, she always had someone double-check calculations from that point forward. In similar situations,

when I stopped students from making an error they responded "I would have figured it out if you'd given me the time."

2. Consider the same scenario using a high-fidelity simulator. I'm in the control room observing the care. The student makes errors in dosage calculation, draws up the medication, and administers twice the ordered dose. I need the mannequin to respond to this as realistically as possible. Because promethazine causes drowsiness, after a few minutes, I close the simulator's eyes and he is sleeping and not responding to the learner's questions. They then problem-solve and critically process why their patient's condition has changed.

In both situations, learning occurred as a result of the error. If I had stopped either of those students, would the impact on their learning been different? While I can't prove it, I'm certain it would have.

Another common topic that stimulates much discussion is "Where should the facilitator be located?" Many believe that the facilitator should be in a control room and out of sight of the learners. The rationale is that the learners should make decisions on their own without interference from the facilitator. However, I also encourage a different viewpoint, one reflective of a novice-to-expert approach.

When learners are new to simulation, they are anxious and afraid of making mistakes or looking foolish. When doing assessment scenarios with new students (who hadn't learned how to use their stethoscopes properly yet), I stayed in the room with them. While the student was listening to lung sounds, I might nudge their stethoscope over a bit so they were closer to the speaker and correct landmark. We would run a scenario but it would be in small pieces while we processed each step together. In the next semester pediatric course, the facilitator was the patient's mother at the bedside. She had a different hat and different personality for each patient. The role-playing allowed the facilitator to ask pointed questions to determine comprehension. When the facilitator felt she must become the instructor, she removed the hat. When I needed to remind her to stop teaching and start facilitating again, I asked her to put the hat back on. In subsequent semesters, I drew further away from the students requiring them to be in charge of their patient care. I would use cues as necessary; however, I was not in the room for immediate help anymore. This method worked well for us. I encourage you to explore options that meet the needs of your learners and your environment. Many of you don't have a control room to work from so will always be in the patient's room. Others may observe the simulation via audiovisual streaming directly to your office or home. There are many ways to facilitate learning.

Learner Engagement

Have you ever run or observed a scenario in which only some of the learners in the room participated? Perhaps one learner stands at the end of the bed, offering no feedback to the team; or one learner always chooses to be the person documenting rather than engaging with the patient. There are also learners from cultures where it is not considered professional to speak up or offer an opinion. The facilitator is challenged to have everyone involved in the learning experience.

Consider the cues discussed above and how you might use them to draw in learners. If using the patient's voice, direct questions specifically to individual people. "Nurse Sarah, why is my blood pressure so low?" or "Nurse Brian, can you tell me about the medication that Nurse Alex just gave me in my IV?" If you are delivering lab results to the room, hand them to the unengaged learner and ask them to review them and share them with the group. The goal is to engage the learner without embarrassing them. If you don't believe the learner is prepared or doesn't know the answer, then deal with that behavior later.

Performance

In addition to level of preparation, you will be observing the learners closely to determine if their performance meets your expectations. Identifying strengths and weaknesses of the learners individually and as a team will provide information to share later in the debriefing and also help to inform evaluation efforts. Take it a step further though—why do you think you are seeing these strengths and weaknesses? Is it because of your program's curriculum design, or the design of your scenario? Are the students unmotivated? Is the group comprised of people who don't like each other? One of your jobs as facilitator is to dig deep and better understand what you are observing. You may find your answers in the debriefing if you ask the right questions. In one program, I facilitated eight groups of students who were graduating in 2 months. The scenario was complex and required the learners to use a nonrebreather mask. None of the groups knew how to use the mask. We wondered how that could be since they were at the end of their program. By asking questions about the observation, we learned that while we had taught them about oxygen delivery devices, we had done so the first week they entered school. After all, isn't oxygen the most important intervention of all? What we had failed to realize is none of the subsequent clinical experiences were in a critical care environment where a nonrebreather mask would be used. The learners had forgotten during the time since they were taught and the time they were to implement. It was our fault they weren't performing to expectation.

Time/Length

How long should a scenario last? What a great question that doesn't have a definitive answer. You should have scheduled enough time to meet the learning objectives based on the trial runs that you did. I encourage you to add about 25% more time to your estimate. It will always take students longer than you think it will. Most programs are restricted by the available hours in the schedule. While you might want 2 hours per group, your reality may be that you have 30 minutes per group. Adjust your learning objectives and expectations accordingly.

What do you do when you're in the middle of facilitating a scenario and it becomes apparent that the students won't finish the scenario in time? The facilitator has several options, the first of which is to continue to the end of the scenario and decrease or eliminate debriefing time. This option should be carefully considered and discouraged. Consider adjusting time within the scenario. For example, rather than waiting for learners to order labs and then ask for results, hand them the results stating "The lab drew your patient's blood and here are the results." A second option is to stop the scenario at the end of the allotted time and move to debriefing. In this situation, you can ensure learning objectives are met within debriefing. For example, during debriefing, you might ask "Right before the scenario ended, you administered furosemide intravenously. How do you think the patient would have responded to that?" As with performance, the facilitator should determine why the scenario ran long and make necessary adjustments.

Evaluate

This is the culmination of the facilitator's role as described above. It's now time to take all the information that you have learned by observing the strengths and weaknesses of your learners and synthesize it to develop a holistic reaction to the scenario that will guide debriefing. You don't want to walk in with a list of everything the learner has done wrong, but instead, have notes as to your general reaction. What did the learners do well and what areas require improvement? If you have used video recording during the scenario, think about the areas you marked for review and how you will use those to guide discussion during debriefing. Spend a few moments to prioritize the most important areas to reflect on with the learners and then move on to debriefing.

Debriefing

Debriefing is often referred to as "the most important part of simulation" as significant learning opportunities exist during that experience. Debriefing facilitators should have formal training in techniques that support learners in reflecting on their performance within the experience (INACSL Standards Committee, 2016). **Guided reflection** is defined as a process that "reinforces the critical aspects of the experience and encourages insightful learning allowing the participant to link theory with practice and research" (Lopreiato et al., 2016). "Debriefing promotes understanding and supports transfer of knowledge, skills, and attitudes with a focus on best practices to promote safe, quality patient care and development of the participant's professional role" (INACSL Standards Committee, 2016, p. 28).

The literature is teeming with research supporting the need for debriefing, and numerous academicians have promoted different methods of conducting debriefing. While there is no research to support one best debriefing model, there is little disagreement that debriefing is a vital part of the SBLE. The INACSL Standards of Best Practice: Simulation^SM, Debriefing outlines criteria necessary to meet this standard (INACSL Standards Committee, 2016).

Debriefing needs to be a "safe" experience. By that, I mean that the students should be reassured that the discussion that occurs will not be shared outside the group. They also need to be assured that they will be treated respectfully and not be made fun of or intimidated when taking part in debriefing. Rudolph, Raemer, and Simon (2014) define this as a safe container where learners are free to be honest without risk of impunity. Most promote conducting debriefing away from the patient room, in a comfortable area where professional respect is a priority. Components of debriefing include model/plan, facilitate reflection, engagement, active listening, performance **feedback**, learning objectives, transfer of learning, and summary.

Model/Plan

There are numerous models promoted for use in debriefing. Each is conceptualized in a way that attempts to fit together the pieces of the debriefing experience and help us to logically assist our learners to reflect. The creators of the models use research findings to help inform their decisions about how to focus efforts on the areas that we believe are most helpful to enable learning to occur. The models all have different names and a different focus area and promote different strategies; however, they are designed for one end goal—to support learners to transfer new knowledge, skills, and attitudes to the traditional practice environment—and as a result, we hope that patient care will improve and impact patient safety in a positive way.

The facilitators should adopt a debriefing model—or two—or more. Many believe that there is no one right model and that we should use whichever model meets the needs of the SBLE and its objectives. Models are typically built on theoretical frameworks and therefore built upon a solid foundation of learning theory. Just as one learning theory does not meet all our needs, neither does one debriefing model. If you are debriefing after an SBLE that focuses heavily on psychomotor skill acquisition, you may choose a debriefing method that is more focused on feedback than on reflection as your objective is for learners to do a task or complete a skill correctly, rather than reflect on how they did the skills, why they made errors, and their plan to do it differently next time. Of course, you might want to consider both of these options and combine debriefing methods. Table 20.5 shows examples of common debriefing methods that you will want to explore further as you practice becoming a better debriefer.

Table 20.5	Examples of Debriefing Models
Model	**Characteristics**
Plus/Delta	● Plus = What was done well ● Delta = What could be done better
GAS	● Gather, analyze, summarize ● Goals and actions (American Heart Association)
Debriefing with Good Judgement	● Process of self-reflection to resolve concerns encountered during simulation ● Uncovers learners' internal frames, helps to reframe assumptions, uses curiosity, and advocacy to learn more about the learner's actions ● Conversation uses advocacy/inquiry approach to combine instructor's judgement with learners' frames to maintain trust between parties while sharing critical evaluation (Rudolph, Simon, Dufresne, & Raemer, 2006)
Debriefing for Meaningful Learning	● Iterative but consistent process that uses Socratic questioning and active learning principles to promote reflective thinking that is used to develop **clinical reasoning** and reflective practice ● Uses reflection in action, reflection on action, and reflection beyond action to develop clinical reasoning ● Six phases: engage, explore, explain, elaborate, evaluate, extend (Dreifuerst, 2015)
3D Model	● Three phases: defusing, discovering, and deepening ● "Description and reaction to experience, analysis of behaviors, and application or synthesis of new knowledge into clinical practice" (Zigmont, Kappus, & Sudikoff, 2011, p. 52)
Promoting Excellence and Reflective Learning in Simulation (PEARLS)	● Integrates learner self-assessment, facilitating focused discussion, and providing directive feedback/teaching (Eppich & Cheng, 2015)

The person who debriefs the SBLE should be formally trained (Hayden, Smiley, Alexander, Kardong-Edgren, & Jeffries, 2014; INACSL Standards Committee, 2016) in using debriefing models and strategies. The session should be planned, consistently approached, and designed with the goal of meeting learning objectives and improving practice. The debriefer must have been actively observing the SBLE in order to effectively debrief the group (INACSL Standards Committee, 2016). Most debriefing models have common foundations, which can be generalized as expression of feelings (reaction), review of the scenario performance with feedback or guided reflection (analysis), and summary with assistance to look toward future practice change. Read about the intricacies of the PEARLS model for debriefing in the Voice of Experience.

20-3 Voice of Experience
PEARLS for Debriefing

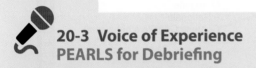

Vincent J. Grant, MD, FRCPC

Although there are several accepted methods for conducting postsimulation debriefing, there are no objective data comparing one method to another (Raemer et al., 2011). Rather than ascribing rigidly to one single method, it is believed that most simulation experts blend various debriefing methods together depending on the context and objectives for each debriefing (Dieckmann, Molin Friis, Lippert, & Ostergaard, 2009; Fanning & Gaba, 2015). The Promoting Excellence and Reflective Learning in Simulation (PEARLS) framework advocates for a multiphase framework for debriefing simulation sessions, including a blending of commonly used debriefing methods (Eppich & Cheng, 2015). The framework includes tools and scripts that provide specific examples of language that can be used in the various phases and methods. These tools have been shown to accelerate the debriefing learning curve (Cheng et al., 2013). Novice debriefers are encouraged to use these tools as they learn and consolidate debriefing skills.

Debriefing Phases

In the PEARLS framework, four main phases are used: (1) reactions, (2) description, (3) analysis, and (4) summary (Fig. 20.5). The reactions phase immediately follows the simulation scenario (Ahmed et al., 2012; Dieckmann, Reddersen, Ieger, & Rall, 2008; Fanning & Gaba, 2007; Rudolph, Simon, Raemer, & Eppich, 2008; Zigmont, Kappus, & Sudikoff, 2011). Learners are asked to share initial emotions and feelings about what they have just experienced. Learners naturally want to talk about their experiences among themselves, so debriefers must be careful not to miss these initial reactions. The reactions typically highlight topics that learners want to review during the debriefing, sometimes referred to as the "learner agenda." The debriefer must pay careful attention to these shared feelings, as they establish a list of items that require discussion in the debriefing. Questions asked in the reactions phase should be open-ended and allow each learner to participate. Paraphrasing what has been said may demonstrate to learners that the debriefer is an active listener and trying to understand their point of view, helping to establish credibility and trust at the onset of debriefing, and allow learners to feel validated for sharing their thoughts.

The next phase of the debriefing is the description phase where the main objectives of the scenario are reviewed or the learners are asked to describe what they felt the scenario was about (Eppich, O'Connor, & Adler, 2013; Steinwachs, 1992). Team members may have different mental models around the scenario and believe the scenario's subject was something different. All team members must "be on the same page," so that discussion leading into the analysis phase is pertinent and makes sense to all the learners. If it is obvious to the debriefer that the team is all on the same page, they could skip this phase; however, if the assumption is incorrect, it may lead to confusion later in the debriefing.

The main part of the debriefing is the analysis phase. During this phase, all performance gaps, positive or negative, should be analyzed and closed. A positive performance gap is present when a team meets or exceeds expectations for a given objective. The debriefer wants to reinforce positive behavior or have learners understand why the positive performance was so important. There are multiple debriefing methods for analyzing and closing performance gaps, which are addressed in greater detail below. Ideally, the analysis phase should begin with the "common agenda," topics for discussion that are shared between the team members and the facilitators. These can be based on scenario objectives, observations from the simulation, and reactions or reflections identified in the reactions phase. Beginning the analysis phase with

(Continued)

20-3 Voice of Experience (*Continued*)

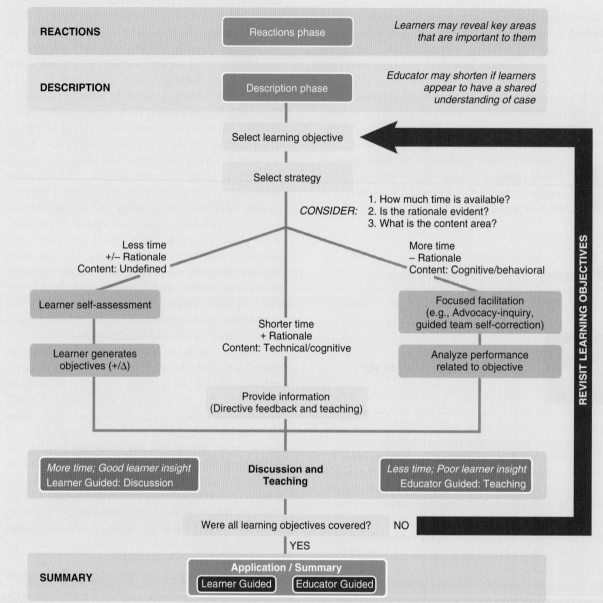

Figure 20.5 PEARLS Debriefing Model. (From Eppich, W., & Cheng, A. (2015). Promoting excellence and reflective learning in simulation (PEARLS). *Simulation in Healthcare, 10,* 106–115.)

the common agenda will help put the learner-centered reactions at the center of the learning process while ensuring that instructor-centered objectives are also met.

Once the items on the learner agenda or the debriefer agenda are analyzed, it is essential that performance gaps are closed. This can be done in a learner-driven manner by asking them to strategize possible solutions for the performance gap, or in an instructor-driven fashion by teaching to the objective, using the debriefer's experience and knowledge of appropriate resources, pathways, and algorithms.

Finally, the debriefing concludes with a summary phase. This is an extremely useful way of finding out what the learners feel they have learned from the session while also providing the debriefer a chance to reiterate key messages or link back to the session objectives. The summary phase can be learner driven, instructor driven, or a combination of both. A blended approach where the learners first provide their summary statements, followed by the instructor filling in any other important gaps that were missed can be a valuable way of concluding the simulation session.

Debriefing Methods

There are several specific methods of debriefing used during the analysis phase of debriefing. The PEARLS framework uses a blended model of debriefing that incorporates the majority of debriefing methods currently used in simulation-based education. They are incorporated into three broad categories: (1) providing information (directive performance feedback and/or focused teaching), (2) learner self-assessment, and (3) focused facilitation to promote critical reflection and deeper understanding of events. The main considerations in choosing which method to use during the analysis phase include (1) available time; (2) clinical or simulation experience; (3) whether performance gap is related to knowledge or clinical reasoning, a technical skill, or a behavioral or teamwork issue; and (4) whether rationale for performance gap is clear (Eppich & Cheng, 2015).

Providing Information (Directive Feedback)

Of all the debriefing methods, directive feedback is the most instructor focused as it represents mostly unidirectional feedback from instructor to learners. It may be the most comfortable for novice debriefers, since it mimics traditional teaching methods. The main advantages are that it is time efficient and rapidly closes performance gaps. However, one of the main disadvantages of the directive feedback method is that assumed rationale may actually be incorrect, and if so, then the proposed solution (the learning) may not close the actual performance gap. Directive feedback is felt to be beneficial for technical skills, pure knowledge gaps, and novice learners. One of the most important elements for effective teaching using this method is that a debriefer must provide rationale for their feedback. This can be as simple as adding a "because" statement following the feedback (Archer, 2010; Dieckmann et al., 2009; Dismukes, Gaba, & Howard, 2006; Hewson & Little, 1998).

Learner Self-Assessment

Learner self-assessment asks learners to reflect on their own performance during the scenario. One common technique is plus/delta, where the plus is a question about "what went well" and the delta is a question about "what would you change for next time." Other versions include asking "and why" to the delta statement, as well as changing the vocabulary slightly to "what was easy" and "what was challenging." The advantage of learner self-assessment is that it rapidly generates a list of topics for discussion. Once the lists are completed, the facilitator can then negotiate with learners which areas require further discussion and reflection, based on available time and session objectives. The main disadvantage of learner self-assessment is that it does not lead to the frame or rationale behind the learner's actions. Learner self-assessment is an easy technique to learn and best used for situations when the debriefer is short on time or unsure of what to debrief about. Finally, it is a technique that is amenable to all learner types from varying levels of experience (Ahmed et al., 2013; Fanning & Gaba, 2007, 2015; Gaba, Howard, Fish, Smith, & Sowb, 2001; Mullan, Wuestner, Kerr, Christopher, & Patel, 2013).

Focused Facilitation

Focused facilitation is a method that allows for full exploration of thought processes, rationale, or frames behind actions and behaviors observed during a scenario, allowing for specific and targeted feedback. The common threads of focused facilitation are being (1) honest with learners, (2) transparent with your thoughts around performance, and (3) curious in understanding rationale behind learners' actions. Of all the methods presented, focused facilitation is the most learner focused, in terms of promoting reflective learning and allowing for better understanding of the learners' frames or rationale and more accurately targeted feedback. Focused facilitation is generally better than the other methods for discussing team dynamics and team behavior. It is also well suited to more experienced groups, either more experienced clinically or more experienced with simulation (Dieckmann, 2012; Dieckmann et al., 2008; Dismukes et al., 2006; Eppich, O'Connor, & Adler, 2013; Fanning & Gaba, 2015; Flanagan, 2008; Lederman, 1992; Rudolph, Simon, Rivard, Dufresne, & Raemer, 2006; Steinwachs, 1992).

The main disadvantage of focused facilitation is that it can be very time-consuming. Since it is a bidirectional discussion that requires input from multiple learners and the debriefer in terms of exploring performance gaps and identifying underlying frames and rationale for observed actions, enough time must be available to allow this discussion to take place, as well as to fill performance gaps. The other disadvantage of focused facilitation is that it can be difficult to learn and master. The PEARLS manuscript provides specific scripts that can be used to help novice debriefers become more comfortable with the vocabulary and flow of focused facilitation. Supplemental digital content that guides the educator through the advocacy–inquiry model of debriefing can be found at http://links.lww.com/SIH/A175 (Eppich & Cheng, 2015).

Facilitate Reflection

In the reaction phase of debriefing, facilitators are encouraged to let the learners talk about how they felt before, during, and after the experience. They need to get this "out of their system" before they can begin to process for learning. My experience is that the learners frequently feel like they performed poorly. Allow them to feel that but then guide them forward by responses such as "Yes, I noticed that didn't go well when you made that decision. Let's talk about that further in a few minutes." Allow expression of feelings but take care not to let it digress into further self-blame, a focus on failure, or blaming the simulator (very common response). Acknowledge the feelings and move on.

The debriefer is responsible for reviewing the scenario and associated activities with the learner, exploring with them the rationale for their decisions. Using an established model will help you to facilitate their reflective process through the questions that you ask. Socratic questioning is a common technique used to learn the rationale for an action. I call it "Why'ing." If the learner reflects that they made a medication error, I ask "Why do you think that happened?" They respond that they made a calculation error. "Why do you think that happened?" I did the math on a paper towel and should have used my calculator. "Why did you do that?" As you can see, each why question forces the learner to reflect on the cause of an action and helps them identify where things went wrong.

Engagement

Just as occurs within a scenario, there are often learners who don't participate in the debriefing. They may be angry, shy, afraid of ridicule, or stubborn, but it is important for everyone to participate in order to enhance learning. Set the expectation for engagement during prebriefing and again when debriefing starts. Remember though that this learning strategy is new for most learners and they don't know what to expect. Remind them of the confidentiality expectations and the reason for debriefing and how their engagement will promote learning for themselves and others. Consider building debriefing sessions in a novice-to-expert way. During the first session, you may need to go around the circle and ask each person a specific question. A couple of sessions later, the expectation is set. There will still be some learners that you need to ask pointed questions of in order to involve them. After a few times guiding the reflection, you will begin to notice that learners will self-reflect. That is a worthy end goal but will likely take some time to reach.

Active Listening

It is hard to sit back and listen. I once participated in a research study in which the debriefing sessions were audio-recorded and transcribed. The debriefers were considered competent in their abilities. However, the transcripts were stunning. On average, three-fourth of each page was filled with the debriefer's words, while the rest was the student responses. More distressing was the fact that most of the student responses were cut off by the debriefer before they were finished talking.

Don't be afraid of silence. Ask your question and be prepared to wait. Learners will often wait for someone else to start before adding their opinion. We often "rescue" our students by answering for them—because silence is awkward. Remember though, they need time to process your questions and determine how they want to respond before doing so. Offer cues, as needed, but don't rush to rescue. Higher-order thinking skills take time.

Performance Feedback

The debriefer must be prepared to provide positive and negative feedback to the learner to affect change. Feedback is defined as constructive information provided back to the learner that addresses specific areas of performance (Lopreiato et al., 2016). We tend to focus our feedback on negative behaviors and performance but also need to provide feedback on good behavior and outcomes. One method of feedback in debriefing is plus/delta. This method focuses on identifying the positive areas of the scenario and the negative, most commonly written on a chart in two columns. The debriefer then helps the learner process why the positive and negative occurrences happened.

Another questioning strategy, called advocacy/inquiry, is helpful. In this method, the debriefer (or another observer) shares what they have observed and insights about the observation and then asks for an explanation from the learner (Rudolph et al., 2007). This strategy is associated with the Debriefing with Good Judgement model and requires some practice to learn how to frame the discussions. Using the medication error example from earlier, an observer who was part of the SBLE might say "When you were trying to figure out your dosage calculation, I noticed that you stopped once to answer the phone, another time to respond to a peer, and a third time to check something in the chart. I believe these interruptions may have led to the error. Can you tell me more about what was happening at that time?" Follow-up questions continue until the learners have reflected on the issue and analyzed the problem.

Learning Objective

During debriefing, it is important to ensure learning objectives are met. They may not have all been met during the scenario itself, which is fine. Remember that much of the learning in simulation occurs during the debriefing, when learners reflect and analyze the scenario. It is your responsibility to ensure the objectives are all addressed in some manner. For example, a simulated patient has a bowel obstruction and one of your objectives is "learner will manage fluid volume deficit." During the scenario, the learners were slow in their assessment and interventions. While there was one liter of gastric fluid in the suction canister, the learners didn't notice that and, therefore, did not follow-up with a call to the healthcare provider for additional orders. In the debriefing, using advocacy/inquiry or Socratic questioning, explore this situation with the learners, asking them how they would respond to the large fluid volume output and what changes they would expect to see if specific orders were received. In other words, walk them through the completion of the scenario in order to meet the objectives.

Transfer of Learning

One of our most important goals for simulation is to transfer what is learned in the simulation activity to real patient care. This is a continuum to assess as learners progress. Many learners don't wash their hands prior to simulated patient care, and we know that most don't wash their hands in real patient care either. If we set an expectation for handwashing in simulation, can we impact it in real life? Can we deliberately practice this until it is etched in muscle memory and no longer an afterthought? And, can we point back to simulation as the turning point? "My students always wash their hands when caring for hospitalized patients (at least when I am observing them) because I make them do that in simulation!" There are so many barriers and variables that conducting this type of research is very challenging; however, many researchers are making strides in this area.

Transfer to practice is our ultimate goal, but we must also understand that negative behaviors can also be transferred to practice. Many times, I have observed facilitators with undergraduate nursing students. When the student makes an assessment that requires intervention, they might implement the intervention without a required order (think night nurse giving patient Maalox for indigestion rather than waking the physician). If we allow that to happen without correction in the lab or during debriefing, we risk the student making the same decision on clinical. Consider the hand-washing example—if we don't hold them accountable in simulation, then they won't believe it to be important enough to do in real-life situations.

Debriefing Summary

Summarizing the scenario either for or with the learners is a valuable way to end the event. Start again with the reactions and summarize the patient care. For example, "Today you cared for an elderly man who presented with new-onset confusion. You felt that you didn't provide care as best you could; however, you did a really good job with his assessment—Sam, remind us of the first step you

took… Sally, you did a nice job of communicating with the physician—what was one thing you learned as result of that conversation?…I noticed that you all struggled with remembering how to obtain a urinalysis from a catheter bag so I want you to come to the skills lab tomorrow and practice that skill." To round off your summary, ask learners what they have learned today that they can use tomorrow when they care for their next patient.

Special Considerations

Many facilitators believe that debriefing should only happen at the end of the scenario; however, many facilitators promote **reflection-in-action**, and **reflection-on-action**. These terms are attributed to Schön, a philosopher who delved deeply into reflective practice. In simplistic terms, reflection-in-action occurs when a learner self-corrects in the middle of a task—"thinking on their feet." For example, the learner is inserting a central line on the task trainer. He is unsuccessful. He steps back, re-evaluates his efforts and realizes that he needs to guide the needle 2 cm to the right. Reflection-on-action occurs after an experience. The learner reflects on their actions and consequences, exploring the situation reflectively. Consider a trauma event that is reviewed by the team after the patient is transferred to the ICU. The practitioners reflect to determine if they did all they could do or if one of their actions worsened the situation. I also encourage you to think about the novice-to-expert approach again and your new learners. Think of them like your children. If your 5-year-old does something wrong and you say "Wait till your Dad gets home," the consequences will occur too late. The 5-year-old won't remember what he or she did wrong 5 hours later. I would suggest that your novice, stressed out learners will be better served if you stop them immediately following an incorrect action (and consequence) and review it then, rather than wait until the full debrief that might not occur for another 30 or more minutes.

Lastly, I'd like to mention the role of video in debriefing. Many simulation labs spend a great deal of money on audiovisual systems with the intent of using video for debriefing. Like other major purchases, ensure that you know what your objectives are for using video and the logistics for how it will be used. While there is little evidence that video improves debriefing outcomes (Cheng et al., 2014), there is no doubt that video can be valuable, and here is an example. I ran a code scenario with students ready to graduate, with my only expectations that they should initiate BLS, call for help, and turn over care to the code team. All learners had been trained in CPR within 3 months. Not one group performed according to protocol—perhaps because they were trained out of context of a real patient environment. One group in particular struggled. They didn't start CPR for 9 minutes. They picked up supplies and equipment that had fallen on the floor, they straightened the simulator's gown, they started (several times) to turn the patient over to see if he was breathing. But, they didn't actually do that for 9 very long minutes. After the scenario ended, I asked them how it went (reaction phase of debriefing). Surprisingly, they all thought they had done a great job! I suggested that we watch the video and they sat in stunned silence for 9 minutes. One student leaned over to me and said, "I never want to be that nurse who doesn't know what he or she is doing. I'm going to rethink how I study and prepare."

This is the only time I have ever used a video in its entirety for debriefing, but it was worth the time, as that is what made the impact. I would recommend that you judiciously use video, marking the places that you want to review—both positive and negative parts to discuss during debriefing. Most A/V products allow you to mark a spot with one click of the mouse. The challenge with video is that many students do not want to be recorded and are concerned about how you will use the video. Some programs ask students to consent to the use of video but then what do you do when some in the group have refused? You've lost the opportunity to use a great teaching tool. The discussion is inherently about trust. One school created a policy—not for what students did with video—but what faculty did. It was the faculty's promise to the students that they would destroy the video immediately following the debriefing and while students were still in the room. That was important to those students because the camera used had a one-button "upload to Facebook" feature. In programs that use simulation for formative evaluation, video may be necessary and nonnegotiable. In that case, clear policies for obtaining, keeping, and securing video need to be in place.

Evaluation

The last consideration for the facilitator is evaluation of the SBLE components. Depending on the learning objectives and desired outcome of the SBLE, the simulationists can choose between formative, summative, and high-stakes evaluation:

- "Formative evaluation of the participants fosters personal and professional development, to assist the participant in progression toward achieving objectives or outcomes.
- Summative evaluation focuses on the measurement of outcomes or achievement of the objectives at a discrete moment in time, often at the end of a program of study.
- **High-stakes** evaluation refers to an **assessment** that has major implications or consequences based on the result or the outcome (such as on merit pay, progression or grades)" (INACSL Standards Committee, 2016, p. 36)

The INACSL Standards of Best Practice: Simulation^SM, Participant Evaluation identifies criterion related to each of these types of evaluation. The criterion reinforces the need for strong design features of the scenarios used for assessment. Additional caveats apply to summative and high-stakes evaluation, pointing to the need to notify learners of the testing situation in advance and ensuring they understand the purposes and desired outcomes of the evaluation and that raters or evaluators are objective and well trained. Establishing interrater reliability is necessary if more than one rater will be evaluating the learner (INACSL Standards Committee, 2016).

Common tools used to evaluate performance include checklists, rubrics, and objective structured clinical examinations (OSCEs). Tools must be evaluated for **reliability** and **validity** prior to use in summative and high-stakes situations. Reliability of a measurement tool is important because we want every individual or group to be evaluated in a consistent manner, over time, and by different people. Each evaluator should be able to use the same tool to evaluate a learner and come up with very similar answers. Reliable tools decrease bias by decreasing subjectivity. The challenge is establishing that interrater reliability and measurement tool developers work hard to ensure the items are as clear and objective as possible.

Validity is also important—does the tool measure what it intends to? Using a tool that measures knowledge when you are really interested in performance won't give you accurate results. An easy example: You are asked to measure someone's waist circumference. You have three valid tools: flexible tape, metal tape measure, and a wooden ruler. These are all accurate (valid) ways to measure distance; however, only one—the flexible tape—can be used accurately by all evaluators (reliability); however, if evaluators do not all measure from the beginning mark on the tape, or if some pull tighter than others when they wrap the tape around the stomach, then there will not be interrater reliability. While the difference in abdominal measurement may not be of critical importance, failing someone on an exam because of lack of reliability, validity, or interrater reliability is not acceptable. One last note on reliability and validity: Just because a tool is reliable and valid for use in a baccalaureate nursing student population does not mean it can appropriately be used for associate degree programs or for practicing nurses or physicians. These properties need to be re-established for the population they are being used for.

There still seems to be a lot of focus on learner satisfaction, though journal editors will tell you that it is time to move on to higher-level evaluation of learning and transfer to practice. Make sure that you have a plan for your data. Many programs collect massive amounts of evaluation data but don't do anything with them! I once had a stack of evaluation forms two feet deep on my desk that covered responses from numerous courses over two semesters. At that time, there weren't electronic methods of data collection so everything was entered manually. I am a big fan of electronic methods of data collection as they are huge time-savers, are more cost-effective, and eliminate data entry errors. One other consideration as you look at evaluation methods is to check the date the tool was developed and review it carefully to see if remains conceptually valid. This is important as simulation practice has grown and changed a lot over the past several years and some tools are now over 10 years old. See Adamson, Kardong-Edgren, and Wilhaus's review of published evaluation instruments (2013). Here are four areas that have tools with established reliability and validity that you may find useful to consider using in your SBLE program for evaluation of the experience, participants, curriculum, and facilitators. Examples of evaluation tools with demonstrated reliability and validity are in Table 20.6.

Experience

Evaluation of the experience includes all aspects of the SBLE, although you may not evaluate all components every session. To go beyond satisfaction, use methods designed to collect data from participants, staff, and faculty about the SBLE. Use the data analysis to better inform future SBLE and lead to continually improved learning outcomes. Existing tools evaluate design features such as fidelity and debriefing or overall effectiveness of the SBLE (Table 20.6).

Table 20.6	Examples of Evaluation Tools	
Area of Evaluation	**Evaluation Instrument**	**Characteristics**
Experience	Debriefing Experience Scale (Reed, 2012)	● 20 items related to debriefing ● Four subscales: analyzing thoughts and feelings, learning and making connections, facilitator skill in conducting the debriefing, appropriate facilitator guidance
	Simulation Effectiveness Tool—Modified (SET-M) (Leighton, Ravert, Mudra, & Macintosh, 2015)	● Updated terminology of original simulation effectiveness tool (Elfrink Cordi, Leighton, Ryan-Wenger, Doyle, & Ravert, 2012) ● 19 items ● Four subscales: prebriefing, confidence, learning, and debriefing
Participants	Creighton Competency Evaluation Instrument (CCEI)* (Hayden, Kardong-Edgren, Keegan, & Smiley, 2011).	● Modified version of the Creighton Simulation Evaluation Instrument (C-SEI) (Todd, Manz, Hawkins, Parsons, & Hercinger, 2008) ● 23 items ● Four subscales: assessment, communication, clinical judgement, and patient safety
	Simulation Thinking Rubric (Doolen, 2015)	● Identifies developmental stages of language and knowing ● Evaluates higher-order thinking
	Lasater Clinical Judgement Rubric (LCJR) (Lasater, 2007a)	● 11 dimensions ● Four behavioral categories: noticing, interpreting, responding, and reflecting
	Spielberger's State-Trait Anxiety Inventory (STAI) (Spielberger, Gorsuch, Lusbene, Vagg, & Jaccobs, 1983)	● State—20 items ● Trait—20 items
Curriculum	Clinical Learning Environment Comparison Survey (CLECS)* (Leighton, 2015)	● Compares learners' perceptions of how well learning needs met in traditional clinical environment versus simulated clinical environment ● Six subscales: teacher–learner dyad, holism, communication, self-efficacy, nursing process, and critical thinking
Facilitators	CLECS* (Leighton, 2015) Debriefing Assessment for Simulation in Healthcare (DASH) Facilitator Competency Rubric (FCR) (Leighton, Mudra, & Gilbert, in development)	● As above ● Six elements addressing various dimensions of debriefer functions ● Novice-to-expert theoretical foundation ● Five subscales: preparation, prebriefing, facilitation, debriefing, and evaluation

*Used in NCSBN National Simulation Study.

Participants

The facilitator should ask for feedback from other faculty or staff who observed or participated in the SBLE and discuss those observations prior to debriefing and evaluation. One challenge with evaluation of learners is to determine if you are evaluating each individual or evaluating the group (or team). Consider that an accurate evaluation of individual learners would require that you considered every item on the instrument for every person involved in providing care to the simulated patient. Many have reported that this is very difficult to do, especially in a summative evaluation. Choose from instruments designed to collect data about the participants and their learning and then use those data to create an action plan to enhance future outcomes (Table 20.6).

Curriculum

Many simulationists don't think about using simulation evaluations to inform curriculum design or change; however, as you've seen in examples throughout this chapter, gaps in learning can become glaringly obvious in simulation and are often due to curriculum design and teaching methods rather than learner lack of motivation or effort. Results from evaluations should be shared with the curriculum team so that you can collaborate to ensure learning needs are met. Choose from instruments designed to collect data beyond that of the experience. One option is the Clinical Learning Environment Comparison Survey (Leighton, 2015), a tool that compares students' perceptions of how well their learning needs were met in the traditional clinical environment and in the simulated clinical environment. Results of this type of instrument will help you to monitor outcomes if you are transitioning hours from traditional clinical to simulation, as supported by the results of the NCSBN study (Hayden et al., 2014).

Facilitators

There is a lot of information in this chapter that points to the need for the facilitator to be educated and trained in simulation pedagogy before they are responsible for managing learning in this environment. However, we have not had a way to measure competency in this area before. It has only been through observation that we gain a sense of whether a facilitator is at a novice, competent, or expert level of practice. Because simulation is still relatively new to many organizations, and the simulationist and simulation operations positions are not yet well developed, many

simulationists are hired into positions that they haven't been adequately trained for. This discussion is covered in detail in Chapter 21. There is now a rubric in development that will help us to objectively evaluate level of competency for our facilitators. The results of this evaluation can then be used to inform faculty development needs and help facilitators to progress along the continuum. Data analysis is under way to evaluate psychometric properties of the Facilitator Competency Rubric (FCR) and to learn more about the correlation between a wide number of demographic variables and the rubric scores; however, the manuscript is still under development and not yet published—though it will be by the time this book is published!

Summary

This chapter was intended to provide simulationists with a broad overview of an SBLE and all of its components, to take you from the first thought of creating a simulation through evaluating outcomes of your efforts. There were many things to consider: needs assessment and gap analysis; creation of learning objectives; designing, scheduling, and implementing scenarios; finding supplies and equipment; preparing and prebriefing learners; and facilitating, debriefing, and evaluating SBLE. My goal was to provide you with numerous ways to consider how you might use simulation in your unique environment and not just tell you the "best" way to do this. As you've learned, there is no one right way or best way. How you introduce and integrate simulation into your program "all depends" on careful consideration of this wide variety of topics. Don't let it overwhelm you—you may find the ability to be creative and think "outside the box" to be one of the most enjoyable aspects of your role.

Toolkit Resources

Toolkit 20-1: Educator/Facilitator Readiness for Simulation: Self-Assessment Survey

Toolkit 20-2: Review Tool for Evaluating the Design and Implementation of Simulations Using Best Practices

Toolkit 20-3: Master Simulation Design Template and Companion Intake Form

Toolkit 20-4: Completed Master Simulation Design Template

21

Developing the Team: Simulation Educators, Technical, and Support Personnel in Simulation

Lori Lioce, Leslie Graham, H. Michael Young

Key Terms

Certified Healthcare Simulation Educator (CHSE), Certified Healthcare Simulation Operations Specialist (CHSOS), Training, Standards of Best Practice, Certification, Accreditation, Facilitator

Guiding Questions

1. What are the roles of various team members in creating and implementing simulation experiences?
2. What guidelines are available for team member development for simulation-based learning?
3. Identify the barriers and facilitators for team members when integrating simulation-based learning.

There are many different roles that are required for simulation programs to run well. In the early days, there was often only one person to manage these roles—and that is often still the case today! A variety of considerations must be made when determining the number of personnel, skill mix, and resources required to maintain a lab or simulation program. Additionally, strategic planning should identify the desired capacity of the program. Will simulation be used for the students in one nursing course? One semester? One program? Or will the program be one that also includes clinicians and their unique simulation needs? There is certainly not a one-size-fits-all answer, as each program should define its own needs. In this chapter, authors discuss the roles of educators, technical personnel, and support personnel in simulation. Keep in mind that there is often significant overlap in the roles so it is not always clear "who is supposed to do what." As such, it was difficult to clearly combine these roles in the discussion. Follow as authors Lioce and Graham discuss the role of the nurse educator, and author Young discusses the role of the **simulation technician** and support personnel.

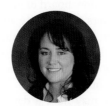

Lori Lioce, DNP, FNP-BC, RN, CHSE, FAANP

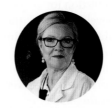

Leslie Graham, MN, RN, CNCC, CHSE

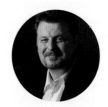

H. Michael Young, BBS, MDiv, CHSE

Traditional Attitudes and Facilitating Role Transition for Educators

Lori Lioce, DNP, FNP-BC, RN, CHSE, FAANP

Leslie Graham, MN, RN, CNCC, CHSE

Simulation-based learning (SBL) experiences are integrated within many nursing programs and gaining broad acceptance as research firmly supports this educational strategy. As a patient safety initiative, the learner is exposed to learning opportunities without risk to the patient. Early SBL experiences for nursing education included practicing injections on an orange or role playing in the skills lab. Integrating simulation into the classroom and the practice domain continues to expand into all aspects of nursing education (Beyer, 2012a). Educator development is essential to ensuring quality, evidence-based education.

Historically, simulation educators evolved from traditional skills laboratory faculty, providing practical instruction in a decontextualized format. Separating theory from practice led to fragmentation of nursing education, which left learners struggling to see the larger picture (Benner, Sutphen, Leonard, & Day, 2010). Educators attempted to minimize the practice–theory gap through linking classroom theory to the skills lab experience. There is a greater impetus to integrate SBL experiences across the curriculum due to access barriers in the clinical setting, increased patient acuity, lack of specialty placements, and changing student/learner needs. Active learning strategies have been implemented in the laboratory and in the classroom setting. The National League for Nursing (NLN) Vision Series provides clear guidance for adopting SBL within the curricula, with prescriptive roles for deans/directors, faculty, and for the NLN (NLN Board of Governors, 2005).

There is greater emphasis on the use of simulation for teaching and learning, yet, faculty and staff development is lagging behind (Waxman & Miller, 2014). Educators are prepared for teaching in the classroom or have a clinical background that prepares them for teaching in the skills laboratory setting, yet few have the theoretical preparation necessary for using SBL. As the current healthcare milieu fosters interprofessional practice, novice healthcare providers require learning opportunities to become proficient at this essential competency. This puts greater demands on the simulation educator to provide interprofessional educational experiences. This chapter discusses educational strategies, standards, and best practices used by simulation experts globally.

Defining the Facilitator's Roles and Responsibilities

One of the biggest challenges in healthcare simulation is transitioning the educator from the "sage on the stage" lecturer to an effective inspiring **facilitator**. The process should begin by defining a clear purpose for the simulation program and should align with the organizational mission and vision (Society for Simulation in Healthcare Council for Accreditation [SSH], 2014a). Special attention to the development of the educator/facilitator's role is crucial and may be greatly influenced by the following four factors as defined by Six Sigma Lean (George, 2005):

1. Purpose—long-term thinking/philosophy
2. People—respect, challenge, and grow
3. Process—eliminate waste
4. Problems—continuous improvement and learning

Purpose

The purpose of facilitation and debriefing **training** is to improve educational outcomes, provide a safe learning environment that promulgates discovery learning, support learner self-reflection, and provide the opportunity to practice peer review (INACSL Standards of Best Practice Committee, n.d.). Hospital-based SBL may address learner remediation, process improvement, team building, performance improvement, orientation, patient safety, knowledge transfer, education updates, and/or competency validation. Academic SBL most typically addresses development of critical thinking, patient safety, competency/mastery, psychomotor skill development, communication and/or interprofessional development.

People (Staffing)

Staffing models for SBL are typically subject to institutional regulations, budgeting, and administrative influence. For instance, the state board of nursing may regulate the number of learners per faculty or the number of simulation hours per course. All simulation educators must understand local and state regulatory requirements. Simulation staffing models may differ in a hospital setting versus an academic center.

A hospital center may have a department for simulation, quality, education, or even a unit-specific nurse educator measuring competencies, simulating high-acuity cases, conducting in situ simulations, and focusing on near misses, or sentinel events. Academic simulation laboratories may employ faculty and staff to execute a more formal simulation environment to prepare and evaluate learners. The staffing model must provide for a standardized consistent method of facilitation and debriefing, decreasing variability of the SBL experience, while controlling extraneous variables that may interfere with measuring educational outcomes (Alexander et al., 2015; Hayden, Smiley, Alexander, Kardong-Edgren, & Jeffries, 2014; INACSL Standards of Best Practice Committee, n.d.). The amount of staff employed will determine the number of simulations that can be run at one particular time, regardless of the number of simulators a lab or center may own.

Other labs or centers may provide technical staff support and training to prepare and support simulation educators in facilitation and debriefing. Each of these models has inherent challenges related to institutional barriers, standardization, staff turnover, budgeting, and ownership of the outcomes. Regardless of which staffing model is used, there are common roles and responsibilities for the educator, technical support, and support personnel. This section will focus on the educator role, with the technical and support personnel discussion to follow later in this chapter.

Process (Accountability/Responsibility)

Intentional and thoughtful planning is required to define roles and responsibilities within a simulation program. Identification of the process is typically a good place to start. Draw a diagram of your simulation process to identify where the accountability resides for each member of the simulation team. In doing so, roles will be clarified to ensure a standardized process. The process should begin with designing a simulation experience. Think about where your process starts. What steps are important to reinforce your simulation program? Who do you contact to schedule a time in the simulation lab? What specific information do you need to have and what do you need to schedule? Which pieces of the process should the educator be aware of or trained on?

Figure 21.1 illustrates elements of a simulation experience, which commonly require faculty development. Most people underestimate the information required to properly schedule simulation activities. Preparatory meetings should occur to develop and identify the simulation learning objectives, performance measures, and a comprehensive scenario design that fulfills the course objectives. Finally, the process must include a continuous quality improvement measure with development of a comprehensive evaluation plan. Each of these elements is an integral part of the simulation program, key in developing quality simulation experiences.

While diagramming, consider the staff you have and what roles are essential to efficiently support and execute this process. Some common roles, regardless of chosen staffing requirements, will include a person responsible

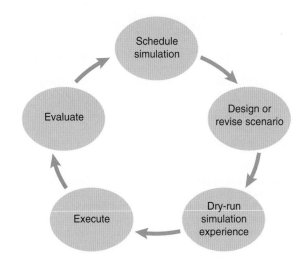

Figure 21.1 Elements of Simulation Design.

for organization, engineering, facilitating, and supporting the simulating. In some cases, these roles may be filled by only one person, whereas larger simulation programs will have more people to take on each responsibility. Table 21.1 further outlines these roles.

Formal role preparation should be provided for all team members, including cross-training in the entire process and roles of the other team members. Small programs may be run by one person. As shown in Figure 21.1, each element may be defined as an individual responsibility or several elements shared among a team. Each element of the process is dependent on the other to be successful, making teamwork and coordination essential to provide a truly immersive experience. The educator plays an important role assuring the overall experience achieves the expected outcomes. Staff and faculty prebriefing and debriefing are recommended with each simulation experience as part of the continuous improvement process.

Challenges

While simulation laboratories use various staffing models and face many barriers, the focus is on preparing the educator as a simulationist, knowledgeable of all the roles that interact in simulation education. Regardless of setting, simulationist preparation requires foundational training on process, framework elements, and best practices (INACSL Standards of Best Practice Committee, n.d.). Many barriers are encountered by educators when implementing SBL. Educators are not often awarded clinical credit time for the additional planning and development required to transition from instructor-led to learner-centered education. Lack of formal onboarding and focused education and training for the new simulation educator may result in a gap in learner satisfaction and outcomes, as well as create discomfort and dissatisfaction for the educator themselves. Because of timelines, dissatisfaction

Table 21.1	Team Member Roles and Responsibilities	
Role (Common Titles)	**Responsibilities**	**Challenge**
Organizer (director, coordinator, staff, administrator, administrative assistant, advisor)	Scheduling, support staffing, budgeting, supplies, and reporting	Details for simulation execution, changes in scheduling
Engineer (simulation technician, operation specialist, coordinator)	Prepares, develops, and executes a simulation experience	Consistency in all paperwork, adding value, detailed setup, and replication for subsequent SBL
Facilitator (campus clinical instructor, staff development, simulation-specific faculty)	Guidance, attainment of objectives, performance evaluator, debriefer	Adequate preparation, theory-based methods, staying learner centered
Supporter (graduate teaching assistants, staff, faculty, educator, technical support)	Voice of patient, embedded actor, audio-video assistance, debriefing room technical support	Multiple room support, technical difficulties, and consistent cueing

and poor outcomes may not be discovered until the end of a semester or program, resulting in repetition of undesired characteristics. Current training may lack development of evidence-based and transparent evaluation criteria, management of generational differences of learners, and integration of active teaching strategies. Furthermore, problems arise when programs fail to formally adopt theoretical frameworks and identify procedural processes vital to achieving a healthy simulation learning environment.

The role of the simulation educator remains relatively new. Considering the above challenges that include lack of faculty development and workload release time, retention of qualified simulation staff is an ongoing leadership challenge, not aided by budgetary limitations. The strategic planning process should clearly identify the need for faculty development, where that support will come from, and how it will be financed. All of these issues contribute to the barriers associated with sustainability a simulation program.

Faculty Development Recommendations

Internationally, healthy debate continues on the educational requirements of simulation staff and educators. Historically, there were no guidelines regarding professional development for healthcare simulation. Simulation educators and staff learned by "trial and error" as the body of evidence grew. As simulation experiences increased, resulting in learner confidence and satisfaction (Jeffries, 2012b), more attention was directed toward the simulation program and equipment development. The rapid expansion in technological capability available to engage the learner spurred early adopters and innovators to integrate discovery learning. The popularity of simulation in healthcare highlighted the need for formal healthcare education for all who facilitate simulation activities. Subsequently, as educational methods changed, debate continued as to whether there was a need for formalized education specific to simulation. As educators were assigned roles in simulation, some believed current preparation was sufficient, while others felt a need for specific simulation-based

knowledge. These debates ultimately resulted in research that supports formal education. Facilitators should be formally educated in facilitation and debriefing methodology (Alexander et al., 2015; Hayden et al., 2014; INACSL Standards of Best Practice Committee, n.d.). Four pivotal formal recommendations for facilitator development currently exist in the literature. These recommendations, set forth by international simulation organizations and regulatory boards, include evidence-based standards, **certification** requirements, simulation program **accreditation** benchmarks, and faculty and program checklists.

Recommendation 1

The International Nursing Association for Clinical Simulation and Learning disseminated the Standards of Best Practice: Simulation^SM (INACSL Standards of Best Practice Committee, n.d.). The educator should receive formal training on all of the Standards in order to be cognizant of pitfalls and become proficient in using simulation as an education method. The simulation program should formally adopt and implement the Standards to aid curricular integration, implementation, and evaluation. The Standards include:

- Professional Integrity
- Outcomes and Objectives
- Facilitation
- Debriefing
- Participant Evaluation
- Simulation-enhanced Interprofessional Education
- Simulation Design

Recommendation 2

The SSH **Certified Healthcare Simulation Educator (CHSE)** certification program provides an exam blueprint (http://www.ssih.org/Certification/CHSE/Exam-Prep) to assist potential candidates to prepare for certification.

Table 21.2	Practice Domains for Certification Examination (SSH, 2016d)	
	Domain	Percentage of Exam Content
1	Educate and Assess Learners Using Simulation	52%
2	Demonstrate Knowledge of Simulation Principles, Practice, and Methodology	34%
3	Manage Overall Simulation Resources and Environments	6%
4	Engage in Scholarly Activities	4%
5	Display Professional Values and Capabilities	4%

The blueprint was developed using a formal process to gain insight from international simulation experts after an extensive practice analysis of SBL in healthcare. This resulted in identification of five major domains that can serve as a guide for educator development (Table 21.2). The five domains are broken down further in the full document. The performance measures in each domain may be used as a self-evaluation tool for educator development.

Recommendation 3

SSH's Council for Accreditation of Healthcare Simulation Programs provides a self-study review, located at http://www.ssih.org/Accreditation/Full-Accreditation, to assist in preparation for accreditation visits. The purpose of accreditation is to establish comparative international benchmarks for simulation programs. The self-study is useful for individual programs to benchmark their program against accepted industry standards, even if not seeking formal accreditation.

The core standards for accreditation are (1) Mission & Governance; (2) Organization and Management; (3) Facilities, Technology, Simulation Modalities, and Human Resources; (4) Evaluation and Improvement; (5) Integrity; (6) Security; and (7) Expanding the Field (Society for Simulation in Healthcare [SSH], 2016d). The focus areas provide specific guidance and a foundation for facilitator development.

The accreditation standards also provide specific areas of focus, one of which is Teaching/Education Standards and Measurement. This focus area is for programs demonstrating that clearly stated objectives are met throughout the simulation program with evidence of ongoing improvement (SSH, 2016d).

The third criterion in this focus area addresses qualified educators and requires programs to demonstrate that they have qualified educators that correspond to the learners' level of study and that there is a process in place for orientation, development, and competence assessment of educators at least once/year (SSH, 2016d). Processes and procedures must support these activities.

Recommendation 4

The National Council of State Boards of Nursing provides Faculty and Program Checklists (Alexander et al., 2015), which are useful in assisting leadership and simulationists to evaluate their program and faculty/staff development efforts. They are useful when developing a program or educator self-evaluation tool and can assist in documentation for program accreditation. These checklists organize evidence-based criteria that should be used to create an educator development plan, guide the development process, and evaluate skill and competencies.

These four recommendations can be blended to create a comprehensive detailed educator orientation agenda, competency checklist, self-evaluation, and/or formal evaluation tool. Two options for assessing educator readiness and self-evaluation are (1) The Educator Readiness for Simulation Self-Assessment tool, developed as a simple to use self-assessment that allows the educator to rate knowledge in simulation and also to track professional growth in using simulation (Chapter 20 Toolkit 20-1); and (2) The University of Alabama Huntsville's Faculty Simulation Self-Assessment Form (Toolkit 21-1).

Online Toolkit

In all settings, administrators must be mindful and adhere to accreditation requirements of their institution or organization. Accreditation standards vary for clinical environments and academic environments in requirements related to SBL and teaching. Consideration should be given to requirements related to educator education, training, preparation, and experience levels. Accreditation standards may also address the process—how the educator is prepared, mentored, or evaluated may need to be reported. The number and type of learning events provided by the organization may need to be documented along with the number of learners who benefitted and how they were evaluated. Internationally, and in different types of organizations, these requirements will vary in their rules and regulations. The Priority List for Building Your Educator Team (Box 21-1) provides a checklist of items to consider as you build your team.

Passion, Authenticity, and Stance

Educators who possess a *passion* to improve, engage, and change educational practices tend to do well in simulation education. The simulation educator is accountable to ensure detailed planning, facilitation, and evaluation so each experience is conducted seamlessly. The passion

---

Box 21-1 **Priority List for Building Your Educator Team**

1. Find innovators/early adopters to create the enthusiasm.
2. Consider workload credit for development of a formal simulation program no matter the size of your lab.
3. Select and share your theoretical framework and process with educators and learners.
4. Select a design or scenario template, evaluation tool, performance measures, and simulation objective map to guide the learning. (See Chapter 20 for additional information and resources.)
5. Collect usage data such as number of scenarios completed and hours of learner time in lab to support increasing resources such as staff and educators.
6. To maintain competency, provide annual facilitation and/or debriefing training, with peer feedback.
7. Require dry runs for new educators or those new to particular scenarios prior to implementation with learners. Strongly consider a dry run each semester, if academic environment or yearly if conducting annual competency evaluation in the hospital.
8. Record and standardize orientation to the environment, simulation, and mannequins.
9. Offer biannual open houses for equipment demonstration and standardization of skill protocols.
10. Annual group facilitator training may not be enough to maintain competency. Facilitators must be fully trained and integrate educational frameworks in day-to-day practice to optimize learning.
11. Deliberate integration of ethical principles in every aspect of SBL.
12. Have job descriptions for the technician, educator, and director roles, with appropriate educational preparation and experience detailed. Each role should work collaboratively and to full scope.
13. Evaluate the facilitator, debriefer, the environment, as well as the participants using valid and reliable tools.
14. Each SBL experience should be evaluated by the participants, with the feedback incorporated for continuous quality improvement.

Adapted from Rutherford-Hemming, T., Lioce, L., Kardong-Edgren, S., Jeffries, P. R., & Sittner, B. (2016). After the National Council of State Boards of Nursing simulation study—Recommendations and next steps. *Clinical Simulation in Nursing, 12*(1), 2–7. http://doi.org/ http://dx.doi.org/10.1016/j.ecns.2015.10.010

---

of the simulation educator is contagious to the staff and learners engaged in SBL.

While the traditional lecture may be easier to deliver in many ways, independent delivery of what the educator determines is important, the *authenticity* of clinical simulation, is more effective in examining the critical thinking of the learner. SBL requires intricate planning and coordination, but the value and worth are evident as the simulation educator witnesses the learner making clinical connections, improving critical thinking, and applying key concepts. In no other setting can on-demand experiences be created that allow educators to see the live interpretation, intervention, and evaluation processes undertaken by learners and then immediately offer feedback to improve the experience without consequence to a patient.

Stance, or the attitude assumed by the educator role in SBL, is a philosophical approach to advance the science of simulation. This may be accomplished through ethical comportment, conducting realistic simulations, adhering to best practices, introducing clinical protocols, and inclusion of evidence-based articles pertinent to the simulated experience. Sharing the educational outcomes and innovations in simulated experiences through scholarly presentations and publications contributes to the advancement and science of simulation education.

Educators should examine their attitude toward simulation education and adhere to a learner-focused approach while role modeling professional behaviors. Share the simulation framework with the learner, including the debriefing method, so they may become better debriefers, implementing debriefing methods into their own practice. The educators' adherence to standards of best practice and integration of them into each simulation is crucial. For instance, scheduling and ensuring full team participation in a dry run of the simulated clinical experience prior to implementation with the learner is important because it will identify potential problems and allow resolution prior to running the scenario with learners. Dry runs are important to repeat when new educators have joined the team or when the learners have changed (e.g., running an anaphylaxis scenario with critical care nurses after doing it last year with medical/surgical nurses).

Educators must demonstrate accountability by being prepared and focused on the learning objectives, stay focused on the learner performance toward those objectives, and not be easily distracted from those objectives. A well-developed facilitator uses simulation objectives as a guiding framework to unfold the scenario, sets up a safe environment in prebriefing, cues only as appropriate and necessary demonstrating patience as the learner struggles so as not to steal their learning moment, utilizes performance measures to objectively guide video annotation (if used) and debriefing to close performance gaps, incorporates peer-to-peer evaluation, and assists the learner to make connections between experiences in the lab and experiences in the clinical environment.

Mitigating Barriers to Simulation-Based Learning

Despite the expansion of SBL, barriers continue to exist in the adoption of simulation as a tool for teaching and learning. These barriers fall into four main themes: learner factors, facilitator influences, simulation design, and environmental issues (Gobbi et al., 2012). With a solution-focused approach, many of these influences may be mitigated or minimized with the goal of improved learner outcomes. Table 21.3 shows the challenges related to each barrier and offers numerous solutions to the challenge.

Table 21.3	Solutions to Enhance Adoption of Simulation-Based Learning	
Barrier	**Challenge**	**Solution**
Learner Factors	Negative experience with SBL	● Begin with formal briefing to create a psychologically safe environment
	Level of preparedness	● Provide scenario and preparatory materials in advance (depending on nature of evaluation)
	Preferred learning style	● Appeal to different learning styles (i.e., program the mannequin to provide directions or briefing verbally for the auditory learner; provide video information in advance for visual or independent learners)
	Willingness to learn	● Engage all learners in the simulation experience, either directly or in an observational role
	Inability to suspend disbelief	● Use alternative methods to enhance realism using the right tools to meet objectives; provide support and time as this is a new way of learning for most participants
Facilitator Influences	Formalized education in simulation pedagogy	● Support formal education in simulation pedagogy (workshops, webinars, graduate, and postgraduate) that provides feedback on competency. Ongoing professional development will provide current practices and ignite creativity
	Expertise in facilitation methods	● Expertise as educator, clinician, and proficiency with SBL
	Expectation of the learner's ability	● Create experiences that challenge the learner to expand their current knowledge, skills, and attitudes
	Perceived enthusiasm	● Enthusiasm conveys positive attitude and sets welcoming environment to foster self-discovery
	Ability to respond in real time to unfolding events	● Be flexible and know that the experiences will not always go as expected; adapt as events unfold
	Facilitator uptake of SBL	● Strengthen facilitator uptake of simulation by mentoring and supporting during the early adoption phase
Simulation Design	Purpose of the scenario	● Arises from curricular or functional needs. Design, conduct, and evaluate SBL experience based on standards of practice (NLN, 2015b)
	Learning objectives	● Well-developed learning objectives are foundational to SBL success as all design decisions are made to support meeting learning objectives
	Complexity of the scenario	● Complexity based on learning objectives and participant level
	Fidelity	● Appropriate moulage of simulator and environment to enhance fidelity or realism to fully engage participant ● Incorporate interprofessional education to prepare for working in effective teams
	Prescenario activities	● Assign learning activities (reading, video) to prepare for engagement ● Orient to environment, simulator, and equipment
	Postscenario activities	● Engages in a structured debriefing using evidence-based method ● Evaluation of participant, facilitator, experience, and the environment, using valid and reliable, appropriately leveled tools
Environmental Issues	Leadership	● Role delineation according to experience and educational preparation ● Foster collegial relationships ● Create healthy work environment ● Decisions are learner centered
	Cost of simulation	● Creative use of simulation resources ● Reuse supplies when possible
	Equipment failure	● Know that technology does fail ● Collaborative relationship with technician or support personnel ● Proactive planning (dry runs), backup plan (substitute equipment, be the "technician" fixing equipment, create distraction by giving or getting report from learners to allow time to correct problem) ● Basic trouble-shooting ability ● Engage in preventative maintenance and operations testing ● Investigate extended warranties
	Technical expertise	● Personnel with expertise in the technology (simulator, audiovisual equipment, virtual environment, other healthcare equipment) ● Ongoing educational development for skill acquisition and maintenance

Professional Development Programs for Educators

Many professional development programs exist as it is important to obtain formal, purposeful education, while mini conferences or workshops can provide continuing education, hands-on training, and immersive development. A list of some of the existing programs are found in Table 21.4.

Competencies for Nurse Educators

Simulation educators require a broad range of skills to conduct quality simulations. Clinical experience is invaluable for the simulation educator in order to replicate the healthcare environment and enhance realism for learning. Experience as an educator will provide the depth and breadth of foundational knowledge for SBL, especially of educational theories. Providing the context for the SBL

Table 21.4	Educational Programs for Using SBL	
Organization	**Description**	**Link**
The Australian Society for Simulation in Healthcare	National Health Education and Training in Simulation	http://www.nhet-sim.edu.au/
Boise State University	Healthcare Simulation Certificate	https://hs.boisestate.edu/nursing/sgcp/
Bryan College of Health Science	Certificate in Simulation Education	http://www.bryanhealthcollege.edu/bcohs/academic-programs/certificate-programs/simulation-certificate/
California Simulation Alliance	Courses, Mentoring	https://www.californiasimulationalliance.org/
Center for Medical Simulation	Courses, Consultation	https://harvardmedsim.org/
Drexel University	Masters of Science in Medical and Healthcare Simulation	http://www.drexel.edu/medicine/Academics/Graduate-School/Medical-and-Healthcare-Simulation/
	Certificate in Simulation	http://drexel.edu/cnhp/academics/continuing-education/Nursing-CE-Programs/Certificate-in-Simulation/
Gordon Center for Research in Medical Educations	Research Fellowship	http://gcrme.med.miami.edu/research_fellowship.php
HealthPartners Clinical Simulation	Courses, Workshops	http://www.hpclinsim.com/
International Nursing Association for Clinical Simulation and Learning	Webinars, Standards of Best Practice Simulation^{SM} INACSL/CAE Simulation Fellowship	http://www.inacsl.org/
Mayo Clinic Multidisciplinary Simulation Center	Instructor Development	http://www.mayo.edu/multidisciplinary-simulation-center/transformative-education/minnesota/instructor-development
National League for Nursing	Leadership Development Program for Simulation Educators	http://www.nln.org/professional-development-programs/leadership-programs/leadership-development-program-for-simulation-educators
National League for Nursing Simulation Innovation Resource Center (SIRC)	Basic and Advanced Courses	http://sirc.nln.org/mod/page/view.php?id=842
New York Institute Technology College of Osteopathic Medicine	Masters of Science in Medical/HealthCare Simulation	http://www.nyit.edu/medicine/academics/icc/
Quality and Safety Education for Nurses Institute	Simulation Education	http://qsen.org/teaching-strategies/simulation/
Robert Morris University	Certificate in Leadership in Simulation Instruction and Management	http://admissions.rmu.edu/online/nursing-and-health-care/simulation-instruction

Table 21.4	Educational Programs for Using SBL (*Continued*)	
Organization	**Description**	**Link**
Royal College of Physicians & Surgeons of Canada	Simulation Educator Trainer Course	http://www.royalcollege.ca/portal/page/portal/rc/resources/ppi/simulation_education_training_course
SimGHOST	Online Videos	http://www.simghosts.org/medical-simulation-videos
Scottish Centre for Simulation & Clinical Human Factors	Facilitator Development	http://scschf.org/faculty-development/
Society for Simulation in Healthcare	Certification, Accreditation, Onsite Preparation Courses	http://www.ssih.org/
United States Department of Veteran Affairs	Simulation Instructor VHA SimLearn	http://www.simlearn.va.gov/SIMLEARN/rsrc_9-how_to_be_a_simulation_instructor.asp
University of Central Missouri	Online Simulation Education Course Series	https://www.ucmo.edu/inquire/?ptype=simulations
University of San Francisco	Master of Science in Healthcare Simulation	https://www.usfca.edu/catalog/graduate/nursing/master-of-science-healthcare-simulation
University of Washington, Center for Health Sciences, Education, Research, and Practice	Online Modules	http://collaborate.uw.edu/faculty-development/teaching-with-simulation/teaching-with-simulation.html-0
WISER	Simulation Training	http://www.wiser.pitt.edu/sites/wiser/training/simTraining.asp

will facilitate learning and knowledge transfer. Experiential learning theorists such as Dewey and Kolb provide guidance in a practical approach to learning experiences (Morrison & Deckers, 2015). [More detailed information on learning theories related to simulation can be found in Chapter 16]. Having in-depth understanding of SBL completes the role of simulation educator. Formalized training in prebriefing, scenario enactment, debriefing, and evaluation will strengthen the simulation educator's role.

Tools for Assessment of Simulation Educators

A standardized approach to facilitator development begins with the educator self-assessment. Through self-assessment, the educator can formulate an individualized plan to develop the necessary simulation competencies. Other tools assist the educator to design learner-centered simulations, evaluate the facilitator conducting the debriefing after the simulation scenario, and provide valuable feedback on delivery of critical elements of SBL. In the Toolkit 21-2, you will find the Educators Advancing Simulation Education Excellence program booklet that will help

you to see how MacEwan University developed a comprehensive simulation education program for its staff. As with all education offerings, an evaluation of the experience should be solicited. Many of these evaluation tools (Table 21.5) provide data that are invaluable when evaluating a program of simulation over time, such as for Joint Commission or accreditation purposes. Additional tools designed to evaluate the experience, the learner, the facilitator, and the curriculum are located in Chapter 20.

Ethics in Simulation

Facilitators

Regulatory bodies provide ethical frameworks to direct the practice of healthcare providers, whether learners, staff, or faculty (American Nurses Association [ANA], 2015). Values such as privacy and confidentiality, maintaining commitments, truthfulness, and fairness (Burkhardt, Nathaniel, & Walton, 2014) are foundational to nursing practice both in academia and in clinical practice. As simulation experiences are considered to be a representation of the clinical environment, ethical values that are the underpinning of clinical practice are the same as those found in simulation experiences. Mutual honesty

Table 21.5	Examples of Evaluation Tools to Assess Simulation Educators
Tool	**Description**
Educator Readiness for Simulation Self-Assessment	*Online Toolkit* There are 4 subscales and 48 items to determine educator readiness for simulation; self-assessment.
Objective Structured Assessment of Debriefing (OSAD) (Imperial College London, n.d.)	A simple, effective tool that can be used by a novice simulation educator to promote high-quality debriefings. A score is provided on eight core elements of debriefing. https://goo.gl/UNbxWr
Debriefing Assessment for Simulation in Healthcare (DASH) (Harvard Medical Simulation, 2009)	This tool rates the debriefing facilitator on six behaviorally rated competencies. Training is required to use this tool effectively. https://goo.gl/N4jbUx
Facilitator Competency Rubric (FCR) (Leighton, Mudra, & Gilbert, manuscript in development)	This rubric allows for observation/evaluation of the facilitator or self-assessment for the purpose of guiding facilitator development. The five concepts include Preparation, Prebriefing, Facilitating, Debriefing, and Evaluation. There are 29 items on the rubric.
The University of Alabama Huntsville Faculty Evaluation (Lioce, 2015)	*Online Toolkit* This evaluation checklist provides feedback to the simulation educator based on the National Council of State Boards of Nursing Faculty Checklist and INACSL's Standards of Best Practice: Simulation[SM].

and trust are integral to simulated experiences, as in clinical practice (ANA, 2015). Fairness and equity during the scenario contribute to learning that occurs during a simulated experience. Ethical practice holds the practitioner accountable for one's own practice (ANA, 2015).

Demonstrating ethical behavior during a simulation experience is necessary to create a safe and positive learning environment (INACSL Standards of Best Practice Committee, n.d.). As educators are held to a higher standard, role modeling expected ethical behavior is necessary for the learner's professional socialization and role clarity (Hill & Zinsmeister, 2012; Wiseman, Haynes, & Hodge, 2013). With such emphasis on the facilitator's role in demonstrating ethical comportment during SBL, tenets such as trustworthiness and transparency impact learning (Oren, Elzas, Smit, & Birta, 2002). Learners need to feel safe in the environment, trusting educators to lead them through a simulated experience that will meet the learning objectives, leveled to their ability and level of experience, and incorporating appropriate fidelity to enhance realism. The facilitator needs to actively neutralize any perceived or actual power disparity between themselves and the participant that can negatively influence the simulation. If the learner feels anxious, it will be difficult to engage in the experience for full benefit of the learning (Gantt, 2013b).

Facilitators demonstrate ethical attributes as a teacher when they have mastery of the content or are subject matter experts (Hill & Zinsmeister, 2012) for the classes they

teach. It would be considered unethical to teach a class with little content expertise, or being unprepared to deliver the lesson. Facilitators need to prepare an environment that is open and welcoming to the learner while diminishing any power disparity, by providing presimulation activities that support the learning objectives, through vigilantly monitoring learner reactions for any distress the scenario may illicit, conducting a thorough prebriefing and debriefing that creates a safe learning environment while diminishing the actual or perceived power differential. Educators demonstrate ethical behaviors when course assessments are fair and align objective measures with course objectives (Caputi, 2010). The learners should be informed in advance of the criteria on which they will be assessed. For fairness and equity, within the simulation context, facilitators need to maintain consistency from one assessor to the next, as well from participant to participant. Using an instrument with established validity and reliability within the environment of the assessment supports fair and equitable assessment for all of the learners.

Importantly, the focus of the ethical educator is on the professionally appropriate relationship. Being sensitive to the vulnerabilities of the learners and having awareness of professional boundaries will maintain an open and transparent relationship. Avoid situations that may lead the learner to perceive the relationship is more than professional. Facilitators should not have the participant engage in personal endeavors such as babysitting children. The ethical educator avoids social networking (e.g., Facebook) for personal interaction with the learner (Hill & Zinsmeister, 2012). Facilitators also need to be attentive to the psychological safety required when conducting SBL experiences. Psychological safety is defined as the feeling experienced during a SBL, where the learner may ask questions, share thoughts, and take risks without fear of embarrassment or retribution (INACSL Standards of Best Practice Committee, n.d.). When there is a high degree of fidelity, the learners can be overwhelmed with emotion throughout the case scenario, and this can create a negative effect on learning (Calhoun, Boone, Miller, & Pian-Smith, 2013). The educator must constantly observe learners for signs of distress and manage emotions before, during, and after the SBL experience. In more extreme cases, psychological assistance may be required.

Learners

Learners also bear responsibility to uphold ethical conduct during a SBL experience. One of the most important ways a learner can demonstrate ethical behavior during a simulation-based experience is by maintaining confidentiality (INACSL Standards of Best Practice Committee, n.d.). Learners are required to attend the simulation lab with presimulation preparatory work completed, mimicking the clinical experience. Learners attending the SBL require the necessary knowledge to participate in a meaningful learning experience (Goldsworthy & Graham, 2012). Academic integrity is maintained by learners in a simulated learning experience by adhering to institutional policies regarding submission of one's own work.

Education-Related Policies and Procedures

The real question facing simulation educators is, how do we operationalize all of the evidence? How do we engage the learners? How do we effectively standardize the simulated experiences enough to accurately measure the outcomes?

Every simulation program must determine policy requirements for facilitator development prior to engaging in simulation with learners. The SSH policy and procedure manual template is available for members. The template has a policy and procedure manual outline with descriptions of what should be placed in each section, saving the educator much development time. Nonmembers might seek assistance in policy development from organizations that have achieved accreditation for their simulation program.

Simulation educators must be intentional in their planning and may need to be advocates for development time and resources. Policies and procedures should be developed with administrative leadership, curriculum committees, and educator teams. These policies include clinical credit time, educator orientation to simulation, theoretical basis for simulation, procedure for simulation education,

educator evaluation, scenario design (INACSL Standards of Best Practice Committee, n.d.), formal job descriptions/roles, and participant evaluation.

Summary/Conclusion

In the past century, there has never been a greater opportunity for educators to shape an emerging technology as there is now with SBL. If one adverse event has been prevented through the use of simulation for teaching and learning, then the educator's goal has been achieved. Through partnership with the simulation team, fostering a culture of learning as scholarship is advanced. SBL is deeply rooted in evidence-based practices supporting formalized education for healthcare educators to gain knowledge, skills, and attitudes for effective, ethical simulation experiences.

Building a simulation program is highly individualized to every setting based on budgets, organizational structure, and learner needs. There are a wealth of resources to assist educators in developing their expertise and designing evidence-based simulation experiences. Self-assessment tools will further support professional development for staff and faculty. Additionally, educators may pursue certification in healthcare simulation to demonstrate the achievement of professional expertise.

Simulation Technicians/Technologists and Support Personnel

H. Michael Young, BBS, MDiv, CHSE

Regardless of a professional's role or expertise, the authenticity, stance, and passion of such individuals help define who they are and how others perceive them. Perception alone does not make a *champion* in any field and the same is true for those working as technicians and technologists. Other parts of this book have explored these three elements (authenticity, stance, and passion) as well, but in this section, I intend to apply them to this integral role among the simulation team. The expertise between those working in simulation operations and simulation education gets very blurry and difficult to distinguish between one role and the other. Smaller simulation programs may have one person who is responsible for education content as well as daily operations. Nevertheless, for the purposes of this chapter, the specialty of *operations* is ideally addressed by any of the technical roles that have emerged over the last decade or more.

Authentication/Authenticity of the Emerging Simulation Operations Specialist

In 2015, the pilot program for the **Certified Healthcare Simulation Operations Specialist (CHSOS)** credential came to an end, and validated roles emerged as Simulation Operations Specialist (SOS) (Bartley, 2016). The SOS represents a general description of anyone, regardless of title, whose professional responsibilities address the day-to-day operations of a simulation program. Table 21.6 shows examples of the numerous titles given this role. New titles continue to emerge.

However, as a consequence of the CHSOS credential, simulation programs have begun to title their technicians as a *Simulation Operations Specialist* (SOS). This was not the intent of the SSH Certification Committee, but is increasingly becoming more common. The idea behind the certification is that it would continue to give simulation programs the freedom to define the operations role to meet program needs. Regardless of the title or background of the role(s), the healthcare simulation community has and will continue to be the beneficiary of a lot of hard work and analysis by SSH and its affiliates. Table 21.7 identifies the five domains covered in the CHSOS exam that address the knowledge, skills, and attributes for the CHSOS certificant.

Note that each domain is very close in weight on the exam, but that *Simulation Modalities and Technologies* represents a full one third the exam. Nevertheless, a candidate must demonstrate competency in ALL of these areas to pass the CHSOS exam or to excel in this operations role. Certification, whether as a CHSE or CHSOS, is a means for demonstrating competency in the field of healthcare simulation. Consideration of professional certification would be wise as some employers are beginning to make certification compulsory for existing employees or prerequisites for candidate employment. For many, the CHSE and CHSOS will remain optional. In either case, the competencies defined are often required to excel in simulation education

Table 21.7	Domains of the CHSOS Exam	
Domain		**Weight**
Concepts in HealthCare and Simulation		19%
Simulation Modalities and Technologies		34%
HealthCare Simulation Program Practices/Processes/Procedures		17%
Professional Role Development		16%
Instructional Design and Theory		14%

From Society for Simulation in Healthcare: Committee for Certification. (2014). SSH certified healthcare simulation operations specialist handbook. Retrieved from http://www.ssih.org/Portals/48/Certification/CHSOS_Docs/CHSOS%20Handbook.pdf, p. 13.

or operations; anyone wanting to excel in healthcare simulation should explore the domains and related resources.

Whether an SOS has the title Simulation Technician, Simulation Specialist, or Technology Specialist or any of the possible titles in this field, the success of such individuals depends very much on their competence and integrity combined. Competence in the field of operations should not be the only goal for these roles. Those who work as an SOS are just as likely to come from a background alien to their current role. While some are RNs or EMTs, others in these roles come from diverse backgrounds, many of which have little to do with healthcare at all (Griffin-Sobel et al., 2010; Young, 2016). What has become clear is that few are entirely prepared when they start working in simulation operations. Those that succeed must be authentic and realize that healthcare simulation has grown, evolved, and matured and likely will always be in a state of flux as continued research and new technologies emerge.

To be authentic, the SOS must be ever curious and never satisfied with what one already knows; there is always more to learn and master. Curiosity should be the stance of the operations staff. While this is true of all professionals, it is especially true of the SOS, because the technology and techniques are always changing. If an SOS does not come from a technical background, and is the only staff member in the program, then it is important that they are curious enough to learn more about technology as they go. Technical expertise is important as one considers that the largest domain in the CHSOS Blueprint is indeed *simulation modalities and technologies*. However, for an SOS coming from a technical background but not from a healthcare field, curiosity and authenticity should drive that person to learn healthcare concepts and terminology. Regardless of the background, the SOS should also have a basic understanding of instructional design concepts and terminology (Patel, 2016). Simulation educators speak this language whether they work in a hospital-based simulation program or in higher education. Consequently, an SOS

Table 21.6	Examples of Titles	
Simulation Technician		Simulation Technologist
Simulation Technology Specialist		Simulation Specialist
Simulation Operations Specialist		Simulation Lab Coordinator
Simulation IT Specialist		Simulation AV Specialist

From Education Advisory Board. (2013). *Considerations for online medical simulation technician training programs.* Retrieved from Education Advisory Board Website: http://www.eab.com/research-and-insights/continuing-and-online-education-forum/custom/2013/12/considerations-for-online-medical-simulation-technician-training-programs

should strive to understand those elements of simulation that concern those who design scenarios and endeavor to integrate simulation into various healthcare–related courses. In essence, an SOS is an "instructional technologist." However, the technologies are unique for simulation-based education.

An SOS should be passionate about their area of expertise and about the expertise of their teammates. This passion drives their curiosity regarding all things simulation and how they can be a part of improving simulation practice. Educators are often quite busy, and the technologies and techniques adopted are very complex. No one person can master it all. The ultimate focus of an SOS' passion must be learners, but at a more practical level, the educator is ultimately responsible for learner curriculum. Thus, the most direct focus of the SOS should be on those tasked with ensuring improved learner outcomes and competency: the educator. The best way to be successful as an SOS is to work to support the success of the educator.

Technology and the Simulation Operations Specialist

The most challenging aspect for any simulation professional is the role that technology plays in the implementation of simulation-based education. This is true regardless of the simulation modality or the discipline (nurse, physician, allied health, etc.). Even the simplest of technologies must be considered carefully or be damaged, misused, underutilized, misapplied, or misunderstood. Maintenance of these technologies is as important as the context in which they are used. Thankfully, many manufacturers of these technologies offer training. The better courses are typically expensive. Some companies offer free training. However, a failed simulator may be far costlier to repair than the cost of a well-developed budget for staff training.

The personal computer has become as ubiquitous as a toothbrush, yet surprisingly few people know how to maintain and repair these systems. Computers are typically the conduit by which an operator controls a simulator, yet when they break down, assistance likely comes from outside the simulation program staffing. In the meantime, the simulator remains dormant. Being a competent SOS doesn't necessarily mean that one has to be a computer "wiz" capable of replacing a hard drive or install software, but it does mean that the SOS should know enough to take appropriate steps for resolution. Swapping out a computer is very intimidating to those who do not do so often. What plugs in where? Is the computer operating system compatible with the simulator software? Solving problems is likely the most important part of an SOS's job. The better at understanding the cause of the problem, the sooner the problem can be resolved.

The typical full-body, programmable simulator utilizes more than one type of platform within the IT spectrum. Aside from the personal computer, control of simulator facilitation occurs over a network, whether that it is a wired or wireless network (Bartley, 2016). The network provides connectivity between the simulator, the personal computer, a server, an audiovisual (AV) system, and other related technologies. Having an understanding of how these different systems comprise the *simulation technology system* is critical to knowing appropriate steps to problem resolution (root cause analysis). Having at least one person on the operations team with an understanding of this broader system will reduce downtime and inspire innovation (Vollmer, Mönk, & Heinrichs, 2008; Young, 2016). However, every SOS should have a basic understanding of those technologies they operate every day (Bartley, 2016).

Audiovisual Concepts and the Simulation Operations Specialist

Audiovisual technologies had originally emerged independent of personal computers. However, in recent years, AV and IT are becoming less distinct of each other (Bartley, 2016). The most common application of audiovisual technology in a simulation program is a video camera viewing and recording system. While there are some detractors in the simulation community regarding the use of video with debriefing, necessity has made AV solutions a staple in most simulation programs.

An SOS must understand, at the very least, the role of audiovisual technologies and how to view, record, retrieve, and play back the video recordings. Whether debriefing does or does not utilize recordings is a choice of the facilitator/educator. A larger simulation center may actually employ a full-time qualified AV specialist as one member of the simulation operations team. As most of the simulation-specific AV systems are quite expensive and costing in excess of $250,000 to $750,000, it is reasonable to consider hiring an SOS with AV technology expertise, just as it is reasonable to consider an IT specialist for the same reasons: reduction of downtime and improved innovation.

Aside from simulation AV systems, integration of other AV-related technologies add value. Many of these technologies have emerged in the IT sector, but are still built around many of the same concepts used in advanced video recording systems. The use of microphones and remote speakers project an operator's voice as the voice of the patient or over speakers used for announcements. Other simulation programs utilize prerecorded audio to emulate ambient sounds consistent with the environment in which the scenario is set. An emergency department mock up benefits from being able to hear a helicopter land nearby, or an ambulance siren screaming as it arrives at the doors of the ED. Codes are announced over a PA speaker. AV technologies are an important part of learners' suspension of disbelief as they immerse themselves into the scenario. An SOS with a basic knowledge of AV can help an educator meet their objectives in improving scenario design and simulation participant outcomes. In essence, the SOS must have a passion to learn (stance) new technologies to support educational objectives.

Academia and the Simulation Operations Specialist

Academia plays an important role in simulation-based education. This is just as applicable in hospital-based simulation settings. The simulation educator has emerged from the academic setting, and the academic setting has influenced professionals directly or indirectly. Instructional design is the primary element that academia relies on for translating ideas to the next generation of learner or trainee. While an engineer or even a nurse may not be aware of the principles that fueled their learning, they are certainly beneficiaries of it. The SOS can be a great asset to an educator by learning the basic concepts and terminology so they can better support the process (Bartley, 2016).

Theater and Performance of the Simulation Operations Specialist

Consider any television program; those that are successful are believable and draw the viewer into the situation as if they are a passive participant. In simulation scenarios, the participants should not be passive, and scenario design can benefit from elements from the entertainment domain. Makeup (moulage), props, and even some semblance of a script increase fidelity (realism). The SOS should commit themselves to learning the various techniques to make the scenario believable to the point that the participants immerse themselves into the "story." Poorly implemented moulage can distract the participant and even mislead them. Moulage, if not done well, can also damage the simulator. If standardized/simulated patients are utilized, they can be injured as well. The same passion that has driven an SOS to learn about the simulation technologies and instructional design should also drive them to be smart about the use of moulage (Bartley, 2016).

Professional Development and the Simulation Operations Specialist

Professional development is a lifelong process. For the SOS, it should include all of the concepts mentioned previously but also other elements that will ultimately improve simulation. This is the difference between being

a good operations team member and being a simulation champion. An SOS who is not improving their skillset and knowledge base will inevitably become obsolete and incompetent. While this is true for just about everyone, an SOS must see their role as equally important as those of physicians and nurses. An SOS helps shape the future of healthcare by helping to shape future practitioners. Future practitioners are at the front lines of patient care outcomes. Learn from Lance Baily's Voice of Experience how he organized a conference for the SOS and turned that into SimGHOSTS.

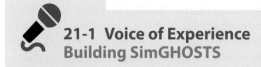

21-1 Voice of Experience
Building SimGHOSTS

Lance Baily, BA, FF1

The Challenge

In 2008, my mother, who worked as the Director of El Camino's Nursing Program, wanted to show me some new "lab technology" that I would "love": a Laerdal SimMan. For the first time, all of my various interests—computer technology, audiovisual systems, robotics, healthcare, and experiential learning—had combined in one place: a simulated human patient mannequin lab. Within minutes, I programmed the mannequin to speak on command and my medical simulation career began.

Shortly thereafter, I attended my first simulation conference. While a wonderful introduction into the unique world of simulation, it did little to quench my thirst for simulation knowledge and I began to attend every simulation conference I could. While providing some discussion regarding operation of simulation technology, in 2009, these events lacked advanced content. Learning on the job and visiting many simulation centers were still the best ways to rapidly improve my technical knowledge. Other Sim Techs shared my frustrations with available resources.

Meeting the Challenge

I was promoted to Director of the newly opened Clinical Simulation Center of Las Vegas (CSCLV). I faced a new challenge: ensuring that our Sim Techs were trained to run a successful multi-institutional multidisciplinary simulation program, even though they had never seen a mannequin, sim lab, or audio-visual system. With 500 students starting in 2 weeks and 80 faculty across three schools scheduled for simulation, it was not clear how we would be able to get our program up and running. Unfortunately, the only way for our new Sim Techs to learn was through stressful trial and error, which took almost a year. I decided there had to be a better way.

I presented my supervisors with the idea: "let's build a simulation technology specialist focused conference so our techs can learn from and support the growing community." The Deans supported the opportunity, and I begun marketing the event at the 2011 INACSL conference and on my free simulation resource website: HealthySimulation.com.

Outcome

The event launched 6 months later in August, and to our surprise over 85 Sim Techs from all over North America attended. Utilizing my Hollywood production background, I created a high-energy, fun, and efficient meeting that offered dynamic courses covering all aspects of running simulation labs. Knowing simulation champions come from different backgrounds like healthcare, A/V, IT, the military, and more, I knew we could all learn more from these unique backgrounds. Pocket Nurse and CAE Healthcare (then METI) sponsored the meeting and provided technical training workshops. Attendees demanded the meeting become an annual event; thus, SimGHOSTS was born.

In 2012, I began running SimGHOSTS.org full time. We became an official 501(c)(3) nonprofit tax-exempt organization and grew to nine board members. Today, SimGHOSTS provides four annual hands-on simulation training events around the world, supports research into the development of our emerging profession, and connects the global community through online resources. Our international team of board members and staff continues to grow, as do our plans to support those operating healthcare simulation technology.

Most Valuable Lessons Learned

With enough passion, anyone can improve the healthcare simulation industry, which is still in an "early-adopter" phase.

Inspiration for Simulation Champions

"If you build it they will come."

Whether or not an SOS comes from a healthcare background, or licensed in a healthcare field, the impact of each member of the simulation team on the future of healthcare is very significant. Consequently, participation/membership with professional organizations such as SSH and INACSL is critical to understanding best practices, if not helping to establish best practices. Additionally, the development of formal education courses and degrees will allow those who want to work in the field of simulation operations to be better prepared for employment and professional certification.

Consider all of the domains identified in the CHSOS blueprint (SSH, 2014b). Bartley envisioned many of the blueprint domains merging to define simulation operations (Fig. 21.2). The likelihood that any one individual will be fully prepared to draw from all of these areas is extremely low. However, the operations team can come together to bring their collective knowledge and expertise into the simulation program (Bartley, 2016). A wise program director will evaluate whether the operations staff has a blending of these skillsets and knowledge base, and seek ways to either fund continuing education opportunities or hire appropriate operations specialists to fill in the gaps. The obvious challenge here is that funding is not always readily available for either. Therefore, a simulation champion, whether administrator, educator, or operations specialist, should actively advocate for appropriate funding. As simulation standards become compulsory by nursing boards and other accreditation bodies, funding must trickle down from a variety of sources to ensure that a simulation program is compliant with accepted standards and employee certification.

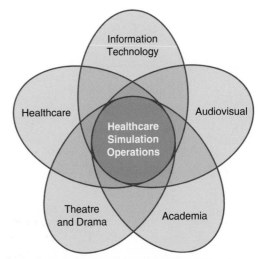

Figure 21.2 Simulation Operations Domains. (From Bartley, E. J. (2016). Foundations for the simulation operations specialist. In L. T. Gantt & H. M. Young (Eds.), *Healthcare simulation: A guide for operations specialists* (pp. 91–112). Hoboken, NJ: Wiley.)

Summary

The SOS should be as much a champion of simulation as any other member of the professional community. An underpaid, underappreciated SOS that is not treated like an integral part of the operations team will eventually seek employment elsewhere. Why should this be any less true than for a clinical educator? The skillset and knowledge base needed for daily operations and technology implementation are quite complex when evaluated. The expectation that busy educators will continue to teach traditional courses and manage a simulation center is unrealistic. A simulation program will not fully benefit from the technological investments until expertise in those domains are represented in the operations staff.

Toolkit Resources

Toolkit 21-1: The University of Alabama Huntsville's Faculty Simulation Self-Assessment Form

Toolkit 21-2: Educators Advancing Simulation Education Excellence Program Booklet

22

Supporting Learners in Simulation
Ashley Franklin

Key Terms

Participant Integrity, Learning Theory, Formative Assessment, Summative Evaluation, Anxiety, Facilitation, Psychological Safety, Peer Learning, Reflection, Reflection-in-Action, Reflection-on-Action, Deliberate Practice, 'Think Like a Nurse', Lifesaver, Debriefing, Safe Container, Clinical Judgement, Clinical Reasoning

Guiding Questions

1 How can I operationalize active simulation roles and observer roles at my institution?

2 Who can be my resources for decreasing learner anxiety and providing psychological support in simulation? What type of training and development does my team need?

3 Will it be more effective to do team-based or individual simulations on my campus?

Introduction

Supporting learners in simulation requires facilitators' expert skills of planning learning activities, anticipating how learners will need support, and responding to unexpected challenges learners experience during simulation and **debriefing**. Because supporting learners in simulation involves a unique combination of teaching strategies and **learning theory** compared to other healthcare education/clinical environments, this chapter starts with an explanation of learning theory and describes how learners fit into several theories that inform simulation. Next, readers will find a discussion of learner **anxiety** in simulation and strategies to mitigate anxiety with expert scenario

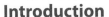

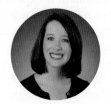

**Ashley Franklin, PhD,
RN, CCRN, CNE, CHSE**

design. Then, the chapter presents a variety of methods to support learners during a scenario. Finally, it concludes with a summary of takeaway messages to help learners apply what they have learned in simulation, feedback, and debriefing to their future independent practice. Interwoven with content related to decreasing learner stress, voices of experience from an expert simulation facilitator pertaining to mitigating anxiety bring chapter content to life. With all of these features, this chapter guides simulation facilitators through many stages of supporting learners in simulation and offers tips for successful simulation implementation.

The Learner Within the Theories

National League for Nursing/Jeffries' Simulation Theory

Though several theories inform simulation teaching, the NLN/Jeffries' Simulation Framework, now Theory (Jeffries, 2015), has been consistently used and frequently tested in education research. The framework was developed based on literature and research from nursing and medicine as well as other healthcare and non–healthcare disciplines (Jeffries & Rogers, 2012). The framework details five conceptual components and a number of variables. Specifically, the participant learning construct informs facilitators on how to support learners in simulation. The participant construct helps us understand that facilitators expect simulation learners to accept responsibility for their own learning, meaning they should be self-directed and motivated (Jeffries & Rogers, 2012). Forthcoming information within this chapter will relate to increasing motivation through learner preparation and setting clear expectations for simulation performance. The self-directed element of simulation participation involves **reflection-in-action** and **reflection-on-action**, which are also described in this chapter. Finally, the participant construct of the NLN/Jeffries' Simulation Framework helps us understand that participant characteristics, such as age, past experience with healthcare, and formal education, influence how learners view simulation.

Simulation Learning Cycle—Kolb

Kolb's (1984) theory of experiential learning explains the simulation learning cycle through four stages of experience: concrete experience, reflective observation, abstract conceptualization, and active experimentation. Kolb explained that learning is "the process whereby knowledge is created through the transformation of experience" (p. 38); transformation happens through many different pathways in simulation. For example, learners who actively participate in simulation have opportunities to apply theoretical knowledge to practice (test hypotheses in new situations), while simulation observers relate what they see in simulation to previous knowledge they bring to a clinical situation (**reflection** and observation). Learners who actively participate in or observe simulation relate their simulation experience to previous knowledge through debriefing (abstraction and generalization), and the global simulation and debriefing experience results in new knowledge (concrete experience). Kolb describes the four stages of learning as cyclical, wherein learning, action, and reflection interact over time (Fig. 22.1) (Dreifuerst, 2009). Further, Kolb's theory points out that good reflection incorporates the multiple perspectives of the active learner, the learner who is observing the experience, and from the variety of roles that may have been assigned to the learners.

Vygotsky's Zone of Proximal Development

Though founded on preschool and primary education research, Vygotsky's (1978a) stages of development in learning help faculty understand that learners' zone of proximal development represent problem-solving abilities that are in various stages of development. Vygotsky's

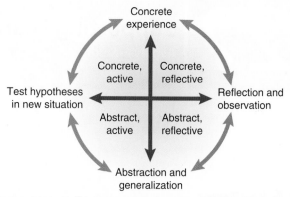

Figure 22.1 Kolb's Experiential Learning Theory. (From Kolb, D.A. (2015). Experiential Learning: Experience as the Source of Learning and Development, 2nd Ed. Reprinted by permission of Pearson Education, Inc., New York, New York.)

proximal development stage represents the buds or flowers on a developing fruit tree, whereas the soon-to-be-mature problem-solving processes represent mature fruit, which is the end product of learning to problem-solve. Zones of proximal development help simulation facilitators understand that some of our learners' problem-solving abilities may be complete (e.g., ability to perform a comprehensive physical assessment on a new postoperative client), while other problem-solving tasks are still in development (e.g., postoperative assessment on a 4-year-old child and explanation of salient assessment findings to family members). In simulation, we are privileged to challenge learners to reach just beyond the comfort zone of the problem-solving tasks they have mastered and help them *test out* the next challenge of thinking like a nurse.

I really appreciate what Vygotsky (1978a) wrote about problem-solving tasks—what our learners *test out* today and complete with assistance will be the same tasks they can complete independently tomorrow. I've had many simulation experiences where learners could not do what I asked them to do by themselves (e.g., prioritize a list of orders that includes medication administration and many other interventions), but I frequently saw the benefits of helping learners prioritize today (or complete any other problem-solving task) so that they could do that task on their own after a few days of **deliberate practice**. This helps reinforce the importance of repetition of structured simulation experiences throughout a curriculum and also helps empower learners to recognize that simulation becomes easier and more meaningful over the course of their nursing school experience because they have more knowledge to apply to clinical problem-solving over time. Vygotsky also wrote about **peer learning** and learning through social development as an aide to "awakening" developmental processes and problem-solving tasks that learners eventually master.

For novice nurses, both active simulation with peer teams and observing peers in simulation help novice nurses' formation of skills, behaviors, attitudes, and knowledge required for independent practice.

Inverted U Theory

Early psychology research also informs the way facilitators approach implementation of simulation activities while aiming to strike a balance between challenging learners to 'think like a nurse' and managing their anxiety in simulation. From the psychology discipline, simulation facilitators understand the relationship between emotional arousal and performance as described by the Yerkes-Dodson Law. Yerkes and Dodson (1908) explain that learners tend to do their best work when they experience the right amount of pressure and perceived stress (Fig. 22.2). Thus, learners who experience moderate pressure tend to achieve peak performance (Sanders & Lushington, 2002; Yerkes & Dodson, 1908). One risk is that learners view simulation as not being a challenge, in which case they would perform nursing care to the simulated patient in a sloppy manner and may miss achieving the learning objectives due to their lack of attention to the problem-solving case at hand. The Inverted U Model helps us understand that learners view challenges in simulation as motivating factors, but that too much of a challenge might make them fall apart under the pressure of simulation performance. Unfortunately, research has yet to uncover characteristics of at-risk learners who may have tremendous simulation-related stress (McKay, Buen, Bohan, & Maye, 2010), but we have identified best practices in simulation **facilitation**, including utilizing specific learning objectives and facilitation methods congruent with expected outcomes to balance learner anxiety in simulation with the challenge to think like a nurse (INACSL Standards Committee, 2016, Facilitation).

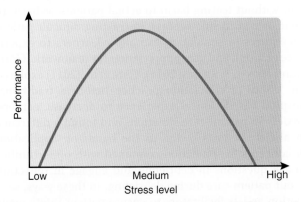

Figure 22.2 Yerkes-Dodson (1908) Inverted U Theory of Stress and Performance. (From Yerkes, R. M., & Dodson, J. M. (1908). The relation of strength of stimulus to rapidity of habit formation. *Journal of Comparative Neurology and Psychology, 18*, 459–482.)

One of my research and teaching interests is facilitating multiple-patient simulations for senior-level novice nurses in academic settings. As an example, learners approach the care of three mannequin patients at change of shift in an acute care medical–surgical setting and have 45 minutes to complete safety checks and focused physical assessments, start to administer morning medications, and delegate appropriately to a trained actor who portrays the role of unlicensed personnel. This simulation-based learning experience is a unique example of the Inverted U Theory (Yerkes & Dodson, 1908) and zones of proximal development (Vygotsky, 1978a), because managing multiple clients and competing challenges is developmentally appropriate for senior-level novice nurses who have previously managed tasks like assessment and medication administration to one patient in an acute care medical–surgical setting, but they have not yet *tested* out the challenge of managing multiple patients concurrently. To decrease their anxiety, I have used standardized learner preparation, prebriefing, and a video orientation to the simulation environment as a way to help learners know what to expect in multiple-patient simulation. Further, I provide many layers of cues from the simulated patients and ancillary services (lab tech calling and charge nurse) and from a trained actor to decrease learners' anxiety in multiple-patient simulation and help them function in the sweet spot of a moderate level of stress where they are able to achieve peak performance.

Cognitive Load Theory

Cognitive load refers to the amount of information that working memory can hold at one time. Because working memory is limited, educators should limit redundancy in content and instructional methods that do not directly contribute to learning (Sweller, 1988). Cognitive Load Theory suggests that using pretraining before a complex learning activity will reduce cognitive load. As such, Cognitive Load Theory helps us with simulation design by supporting use of targeted simulation preparation before complex and/or technically challenging simulations. Importantly, Sweller highlights the importance of leveling learning activities appropriately according to learners' previous experience. Applied to simulation, Cognitive Load Theory helps facilitators identify simulation learning objectives that match participants' experience in previous didactic and clinical courses. Additionally, Sweller identifies cognitive schemas or structures, also called long-term memory, that permit learners to perceive, think, and solve problems rather than memorize a group of facts in rote memory (1988). In simulation, facilitators organize cues so that learners can use long-term memory to bring forward knowledge pertaining to their simulation patient (e.g., signs and symptoms of a condition represented by a mnemonic) as a method to utilize schemas and therefore free-up cognitive space for more advanced thinking processes. In summary, Cognitive Load Theory is an instructional design theory that supports scenario development and implementation to help learners process information in simulation.

Reflection-in-Action, Reflection-on-Action

Reflection is the core of debriefing in simulation, and it is a process of assessing what factors are relevant to a situation and determining the reasons for actions taken during a simulation (National League for Nursing [NLN], 2015d). During simulation, learners have to filter data provided from the facilitator, patient, monitors, and health record in *live* time to implement and potentially reorganize their plan of care. Schön (1983) describes this process as reflection-in-action whereby learners "think on their feet" as they reflect, analyze, and amend their plan of care while participating in a simulation. Facilitators guide reflection-in-action during simulation by offering support through coaching and responding to learners' questions and actions with further cues.

Schön (1983) distinguishes debriefing after a scenario as reflection-on-action and reinforces the importance of formation of new cognitive models during debriefing discussions. Reflection-on-action allows learners to examine a scenario to see the whole of reality (Friere, 1970/2000; NLN, 2015d) as they start to understand why particular actions were taken and the knowledge, assumptions, values, beliefs, and feelings behind action (NLN, 2015d).

Stress in Simulation

Causes of Stress and Anxiety

Regardless of how long ago we learned to think like a nurse, it is important to recognize that practice of any healthcare role imposes stress on the learner (Willhaus, 2013) and that perceptions about a successful or failed performance, combined with physiologic responses to stress, are individually variable (McKay et al., 2010). Simulation experiences can cause learners to report feelings of anxiety, inadequacy, or incompetence (Gantt, 2013a), but there are many facilitation techniques aimed at decreasing learner distress. One technique is to normalize the anxiety by telling learners that I get nervous too (both in simulation and in real-life situations that are not familiar). We have evidence from research that practicing physicians, nurses, and technicians experienced an increased heart rate and salivary cortisol levels before and after a team training simulation despite

their years of independent practice (Bong, Lightdale, Fredette, & Weinstock, 2010). Much of the remainder of this chapter addresses strategies to decrease learner distress and to provide insight into theory that underpins the relationship between stress in simulation and learning.

Helping Learners Perceive Simulation as a Realistic Experience Without Causing Undue Stress

Learners recognize when simulation closely resembles a traditional clinical setting and they appreciate the fidelity offered through room set up, moulage, simulation cues, and the background details that bring a scenario to life. My experience has been that it takes four or five simulation experiences for learners to make a connection between simulation and traditional clinical learning. I've always accredited this to learners requiring time and repetition to build a knowledge base from didactic learning and traditional clinical experiences so they can bring forward knowledge to apply to simulation. Allowing learners with various levels of expertise to have both active and observer roles in simulation may help them see the big picture of how simulation is an effective training method for helping them to think like a nurse in traditional clinical settings. Anecdotally, many learners have reported that they learn more when they are observing peers in simulation, likely owing to decreased nervousness because no one is watching or judging active simulation performance.

Safe Environment

Maintaining a safe environment in simulation means that it is okay for learners to make mistakes in simulation without fearing harm to actual patients or harm to their own academic success. Recreating difficult patient encounters in simulation can allow learners to experience emotion and gain appreciation for teamwork (Gore, Hunt, Parker, & Raines, 2011). Gore et al. (2011) explored the utility of simulation practice before a traditional hospital-based clinical experience to decrease learners' anxiety in patient care situations and found a difference in anxiety reports owing to the hands-on application of concepts in simulation combined with opportunities to ask questions in debriefing and engage in reflection about patient care during debriefing. In these ways, simulation assists facilitators to ensure patient safety while also providing educational opportunities for learners to develop the competencies needed to provide patient care (Decker, 2012).

The Caring Facilitator

The root of caring for learners in simulation is the ability to engage them in all phases of the experience. Expert nurse educators have identified use of humor as an aid to building a relationship with learners as well as the ability to be quiet and allow learners to identify their plan and carry it through in simulation (Parsh, 2010). I have found it effective to model "thinking like a nurse" (Tanner, 2006) during prebriefing and debriefing interactions with simulation learners and pose questions to each group of learners, such as "What did you notice when you walked in the room?" and "Why was ____ important to you, and how did you respond to your concern?" Not only do these types of questions engage learners and promote conversation about their thinking processes, but they also help convey a stance of genuine curiosity that promotes learner engagement during prebriefing and debriefing.

One of the challenges for simulation facilitators is responding to learners who do not engage with simulation. Learners from countries outside of the United States, introverted learners, and those who are too shy to "think like a nurse" require expert facilitation and may benefit from individual attention. I have found it helpful to first use cues during the scenario where the simulation patient or trained actor asks learners direct questions; hopefully, this will help learners overcome their fear of speaking up in simulation. Yet, some learners can't respond in simulation and instead need support during debriefing to share their reactions to simulation and deconstruct the thought frames during the scenario. I will usually make an effort to hear reactions from every simulation participant during the early phase of debriefing, even by calling them by name and asking, "Do you have anything to add?" to open the floor for them to share. If that doesn't work, then I might ask questions in debriefing related to the role that quiet participants assumed, such as "As the medication nurse, what assessment data was important to you?" I have found that these patterns of questioning norm the debriefing experience and help learners know what to expect. Finally, if these strategies are not successful to engage learners in either simulation or debriefing, I would recommend providing individual feedback and offering encouragement either in person or in written feedback (or both) to demonstrate caring to vulnerable simulation learners and convey to them your specific expectations (and rationale) for their engagement in future simulations.

The "goal of simulation is to promote learning" (Willhaus, 2009, p. 220) even when it does not come easily—often because of the intensity of processing abstract and concrete learning within a fast-paced simulation scenario. Simulation taps into cognitive, psychomotor, and affective domains of learning, thereby presenting a more complicated milieu for decision-making practice than other learning activities in nursing education. One goal of a simulation facilitator in debriefing is to advance learners' cognitive, psychomotor, and affective knowledge, which is necessary for their success as independent professional nurses (Dreifuerst & Decker, 2012). Engaging in all phases of simulation allows learners to experience an ambiguous clinical situation and practice recognizing salient elements and filtering out distractors to their decision-making process in a learning environment that is safe for patients and for learners.

At my university, we are beginning three new, dedicated simulation courses and have committed the three semesters prior to course roll-out for simulation faculty development. We talk about what it means to be caring simulation facilitators and how to operationalize caring in the new simulation courses. Our faculty has considered separating simulation faculty from clinical faculty so that learners in simulation would have no fear that mistakes made in simulation might impact the way they are evaluated in traditional clinical coursework. This distinction personifies caring for simulation learners because it protects the **psychological safety**—meaning a simulation environment maintains integrity, trust, and respect for and between learners in a safe environment where there are no consequences to patient care or academic evaluation (INACSL Standards Committee, 2016, Scenario Design). We want simulation learners to value opportunities to make mistakes in simulation so they can learn about their own perceptions and interpretations that influence their **clinical reasoning** and **clinical judgement**. This separation of simulation faculty from clinical faculty might be a unique way of thinking, particularly related to that National Council of State Boards of Nursing suggestion that simulation can replace clinical (Alexander et al., 2015). Many nursing programs are moving toward a model of "sameness" of clinical faculty rather than being different (especially with evaluation); however, my university has found that the extensive requirements for faculty preparation in simulation, combined with an exclusive focus on **formative assessment** for our learners, support the distinction of simulation from clinical faculty wherever possible.

One of the challenges I encountered as a novice simulation facilitator was balancing learners' emotions before and after a simulation. For me, compassion toward learners comes fairly naturally, but my desire for learners to be high achievers sometimes made me overlook the fact that they could be paralyzed by fear of what would happen in simulation and if they would know how to respond. I've learned to use phrases like "Tell me more about that" in prebriefing and debriefing to explore learners' feelings. This reminds me to avoid making the assumption that I know how they feel and how I might be able to "fix them." Simulation mentors reinforced the importance of drawing out the learners' emotions and mental frames that underpin their thoughts and clinical judgements.

22-1 Voice of Experience
Important Responsibilities to Support Learners

Mary Cato, EdD, RN, CHSE

The Challenge

In over 10 years of teaching nursing students through the use of simulation, I have developed ideas and techniques of facilitation that have helped create positive environments for learning.

Meeting the Challenge

We have responsibilities as faculty to do several things to support our learners in simulation, and I think the most important are these:

1. Role-model kindness. It may be easier to base a debriefing only on what was done well and what could be improved, but doing so would deprive learners of the opportunity to dialogue about the patient, what they think was happening, and why they chose the assessments and interventions that they did. Learners will only feel empowered to have these conversations if we accept and encourage their thoughts and ideas. We must be open to their explanations and their questions, and seriously consider the validity of their decisions. Learners have changed my mind about some of my ideas in the past, and they have also had inaccurate ideas and conclusions that needed thoughtful discussion and correction. My job as their facilitator is to create the open and accepting atmosphere in which they can feel encouraged to be their real and vulnerable selves. I hope that by thoughtfully leading these dialogues, learners will realize how much they can gain for themselves, their colleagues, and their patients by accepting and treating others with kindness.

2. Understand that anxiety happens, and sometimes prevails, as a response to simulation. Our simulation hours are a required part of clinical hours, and therefore, attendance is mandatory. There is no separate grade for simulation: there is no A, B, or C, no satisfactory or unsatisfactory, no points allotted, not even a pass or a fail. While in theory this would seem to lower the stakes and relieve

some of the anxiety, that is not always the case. My doctoral work was focused on anxiety, and how it affects learning in simulation. I learned that while too much anxiety (which is the learner's response to stress) was debilitating and no anxiety at all could decrease investment in the learning, there is an optimal level that motivates the learner to prepare and engage in simulation activities. Palethorpe and Wilson (2011) developed what they call the "comfort–stretch–panic" model, in which they identified this optimal level of stress as the "stretch" zone. Learners in the stretch zone are motivated to optimal performance, and learning here is maximized. This model is readily applied to simulation activities and can impact our expectations and interactions with learners.

Outcome

By role-modeling kindness and considering the effect of anxiety on learning, we can create safe spaces where our learners grow and develop into expert nurses.

Most Valuable Lesson Learned

I believe that our role in teaching nursing through simulation is challenging, and our responsibility is great.

Decreasing Stress When Designing Scenarios

It is impossible to overestimate the importance of having a well-developed plan to support learners in simulation. As a critical care nurse, my motto was to always have a code cart ready near my patient's room, because it would warn off bad spirits of an impending cardiac arrest. I have the same philosophy when planning for how to support learners in simulation.

Preparing the Learner

My experience in teaching and simulation research has been that learners are most nervous about that which is unknown in simulation and traditional clinical learning activities. Surely, no one likes to feel like they have no control over their future. A recent descriptive survey of nursing students ($n = 10$) confirmed this belief that learners feel stress when they don't know what to expect in simulation (Ganley & Linnard-Palmer, 2012) and when they lack the knowledge or skills to respond appropriately to simulation cues (Willhaus, 2013). Thus, it is important to be intentional about choosing simulation preparation activities to assist learners to anticipate how the simulation will unfold. Assigning simulation preparation is a standard practice (INACSL Standards Committee, 2016, Scenario Design), and simulation facilitators should not fear they are "giving away the answers" by having learners come prepared to a simulation-based experience (Willhaus, 2009). In fact, we know that learners in simulation most often need several repetitions of a scenario to master the content and decision-making at the heart of the learning objectives. Preparation materials may focus on skills, medications, pathophysiology, patient teaching, or cultural/age-related considerations of the simulated patient. Preparation sheets or focused information from an electronic health record are helpful to promote the

best possible outcome for participants to successfully address the simulation objectives (INACSL Standards Committee, 2016, Scenario Design; see Box 22-1).

Box 22-1   Example of a Preparation Sheet

● Postpartum Hemorrhage Simulation Prep Sheet

Objectives

1. The student will be able to identify and respond to signs and symptoms of postpartum bleeding emergencies.
2. The student will be able to demonstrate therapeutic communication techniques.
3. The student will be able to communicate effectively with members of the healthcare team.

Jenny Smith is a 28-year-old patient of Dr. Meyers who delivered a viable male infant weighing 4.450 kg 90 minutes ago. Jenny has just been transferred to your care on the postpartum unit. She has an IV in her left forearm with an infusion of lactated ringers with 10 units of pitocin added running at 75 mL/hr. Jenny is married to an Air Force officer who is currently deployed in Afghanistan. She is accompanied by a friend from their military family support unit. She nursed the baby for 20 minutes shortly after delivery. Her last assessment revealed a BP 115/70, pulse 80, resp. 18, temp. 98.6. Her fundus was firm at the umbilicus and she had a moderate rubra vaginal discharge. She had no perineal repair. She has required no pain medication and reports her pain at 2/10. Her epidural is beginning to wear off, but she is still unable to walk to the bathroom to void. Her bladder was emptied by straight catheterization upon delivery.

Skills to practive: Postpartum assessment, catheterization, IV fluid management, medication administration, therapeutic communication, SBAR (Situation-Background-Assessment-Recommendation) communication, fundal massage.

Medications to study: Analgesics, narcotics, medications used to control bleeding in the childbearing setting.

From Willhaus (2009, p. 222 Box 17.1).

Prebriefing

Prebriefing is also an important part of preparation wherein facilitators orient learners to the simulation lab and simulation patient. During prebriefing, learners should have time for hands-on practice with the specific features of the simulator (e.g., locating speakers where heart and lung sounds are best heard) and locating equipment in the simulation lab. Facilitators should clarify roles that learners will assume during simulation as well as encourage learners to verbalize their plan for providing care. Facilitators should use guided questions to help learners anticipate what they might see or experience during the simulation. Guided questions assist learners to develop patterns of *noticing* that gives them a grasp of the larger clinical situation (*noticing* as an element of clinical judgement identified by Tanner, 2006).

Scripting and Cues

Cues can be provided directly from the facilitator or through the voice of the patient or trained actor. It is important that cues are scripted in advance and vetted through a "dry run" scenario practice so facilitators have confidence that cues portray the intended message. Primary cues are delivered to all simulation learners, while secondary cues are available as needed, depending on the learner's actions or questions. As an example, reporting a subjective pain scale would be a primary cue in a postoperative scenario, whereas reviewing symptom analysis using the OLDCART framework (onset, location, duration, characteristics, aggravating or relieving factors, and treatment) would be a secondary cue that is only provided if learners actually ask the related questions to their patient. In this way, secondary cues reward learners for expanding their plan of care while "thinking on their feet" by providing additional cues to guide decision-making. The combination of primary and secondary cues may help learners filter out salient data during the scenario.

Expert cue giving allows simulation facilitators to respond to learners who experience maximum stress. As an example, I may choose to call in to the scenario and offer some direction from the charge nurse or provider perspective to direct their decision-making and/or reassure them that they are on the right problem-solving path. I've found that calling in to simulation and speaking with the primary nurse (while I maintain character of a logical provider interested in care of the simulation patient) is an effective way to offer psychological support and support learners' reflection-in-action. Such cues tend to increase learners' confidence and motivate them to continue working their plan of care delivery instead of caving in to their perceived stress and abandoning the simulation objectives.

Simulation "**lifesavers**" are plans made before simulation and interventions during simulation that allow learners to achieve the objectives for a simulation scenario by adapting the content and form (Dieckmann, Lippert, Glavin, & Rall, 2010). These "lifesavers" frequently emerge during simulation "dry runs" or conversations with faculty colleagues before and after simulation. I have learned to write "if and then" scripts to plan potential scenarios that may arise and how I will respond. As an example, I can send a nursing assistant (read: simulation technician) to help learners problem-solve how to take their patient's vital signs or I can send a pharmacy tech (read: simulation technician) to troubleshoot the electronic medication cart or deliver a medication from the central pharmacy (read: extra medication kept in the control room). All of these interventions have helped me to decrease learner anxiety successfully by meeting their unexpected needs while still maintaining the integrity of the scenario. Remember, no one likes to feel like they have no control over their future in simulation; so, I use "if and then" scripts and offer human resources as support, I've been successful giving control back to simulation learners.

Simulation "lifesavers" help me adapt a scenario when learners are travelling down a path that is a valid interpretation of presented cues—even when it isn't the path I had originally planned. My goal is to always have options to dial scenarios either up or down in terms of complexity to accommodate for learner responses to the simulation scenario. As an example from a trained actor scenario where the patient is on a medical–surgical unit following a suicide attempt, I can cue the patient to cover her head with the blankets or pillow (cue through a walkie-talkie earbud) if learners are asking questions in a rapid-fire manner or being too casual and therefore insensitive to the patient's perspective. Having these plans to adjust scenario complexity in advance helps me to respond more consistently to large cohorts of learners who may experience simulation over a period of several weeks. I always have a plan of scripted cues including comments made by the simulation patient/mannequin, standardized patient actors, or family members who provide cues to learners. Other potential sources of cues include a change in vital signs or sending in ancillary personnel as "lifesavers" (e.g., send the charge nurse to check on a patient whose telemetry alarms have been sounding at the nurse's station and prompt a drop-in visit). Such a repertoire of simulation "lifesavers" enables me to respond to learners and help them achieve the predetermined learning objectives at the same time.

Planning to Repeat Scenarios

An option for decreasing learners' distress is to repeat a simulation scenario after debriefing; there is a potential decrease in both psychological and physical stress when learners repeat scenarios and therefore have no surprises about how the scenario will unfold (Willhaus, 2013). I have found that repeating scenarios is particularly helpful to reinforce major concepts (e.g., performing safety checks or a focused physical assessment) that learners can apply to many different types of patient care settings. However, one downside to repeating scenarios is the potential lost time that has to be accounted for in the simulation schedule. To mitigate this, my university uses parallel cases that revolve around the same concept; we use four simulation cases within a 4-hour simulation experience. Thus, items learned in the first case are applicable to the remaining three so that learners have many opportunities to put their learning into action and have a concrete experience that will solidify their knowledge and skills practice to aide transfer to future clinical settings. As an example, if perfusion were the primary concept for a simulation experience, then simulation cases would address diagnoses like anaphylaxis, sepsis, postpartum hemorrhage, and electrolyte imbalance causing dysrhythmias. Learning related to intravenous fluid boluses would carry over throughout the simulation experience, while the nuances of administering a fluid bolus to a specific population (e.g., a pediatric patient with an allergic reaction to medication administration versus an elderly patient with congestive heart failure and sepsis) would provide concrete experience to solidify learning and decrease learner anxiety as the simulation experience progressed.

Dry Runs to Assist With Scenario Implementation Success

A critical step in decreasing learner stress and developing a plan for psychological support is to schedule a "dry run" of the scenario where other faculty portray the role of learners and also help me to plan how to support learners during prebriefing, simulation, and debriefing. I schedule dry runs at least 1 week before the simulation activity with learners. Dry runs help me to be more familiar with scenario content and cues, so that more of my cognitive load is available to respond to learners when it counts. When I am more familiar with the simulation case and nuances of operating the mannequin, microphones, telephones, and audiovisual system, I can more effectively read the cues from learners who may be telling or showing me that they have reached their maximum level of tolerated stress.

Upholding Participant Integrity

 One of the goals that underpins simulation pedagogy is mutual respect between learners and facilitators, recognizing that this impacts the willingness of both learners and facilitators to engage in simulation (INACSL Standards Committee, 2016, Professional Integrity). Facilitators should clearly outline expectations for appropriate attitudes and behaviors, such as speaking directly to simulation patients, performing hand hygiene and safe medication practices in simulation, and using point-of-care equipment like a pulse oximeter

| Box 22-2 | **Example of a Simulation Contract** |

Simulation Contract

1. Assume "goodwill" of other simulation learners and facilitators.
2. Stay in character during simulation.
3. Treat the mannequins and standardized patient actors as real patients.
4. Use patient care equipment like you are in a real hospital (e.g., wash your hands, and wear gloves).
5. Call for help when needed!
6. Call a team huddle to take a time out.

From Health Professions Learning Center, Texas Christian University, Harris College of Nursing and Health Sciences, with permission.

and intravenous pump just like they are used in traditional hospital-based clinical environments.

It is important to convey the necessity of confidentiality of the simulation experience, which I frequently describe as "What happens in sim stays in sim." Maintaining confidentiality is important because it preserves learning experiences for large cohorts and those learners who come at the end of a simulation cycle (which may be weeks after the first learners). One strategy for upholding **participant integrity** is to review a "simulation contract" at the beginning of each course (see Box 22-2). A simulation contract is a simple contract to clearly explain facilitator expectations for simulation performance and confidentiality. When using a simulation contract, facilitators should plan in advance for consequences that will take place if learners break the contract (e.g., learners will earn an unsatisfactory for the learning activity and be required to write a reflection about the importance of confidentiality in academic and patient care environments). I've adopted the practice of posting the simulation contract in the simulation lab, control rooms, and debriefing rooms to serve as a consistent reminder of confidentiality and expected behaviors in simulation.

Supporting Learners During a Scenario

Basic Assumption

One of the principles that guides simulation facilitation is the assumption of good will of learners in their statements and interventions. Even as an experienced nurse, when I participate in simulation, feelings of anxiety while being watched (judged) by my peers impacts my performance; so, I have found that assuming good will of learners in simulation helps me approach simulation pedagogy from a caring worldview. Simulation experts who have participated in the Center for Medical Simulation Instructor Training Course are encouraged to adopt a basic assumption of

simulation learners, which reads "We believe that everyone who comes to simulation is intelligent, well-trained, cares about doing their best, and wants to improve the way they care for patients" (Center for Medical Simulation, 2015). Facilitators are challenged to clearly communicate detailed feedback to simulation learners and hold them to high performance standards (Parsh, 2010); posting this basic assumption statement in the control room, debriefing room, and simulation lab helps remind me to treat simulation learners with respect in all of my interactions even when I am delivering potentially bad news along with my constructive feedback.

Learner Satisfaction and Early Simulation Research

We have anecdotal and research evidence that demonstrates learners are generally satisfied with simulation and agree that simulation helps to increase their self-confidence. The satisfaction reports are helpful to reward faculty's time and effort in planning and implementing simulation and to give recognition to administration teams and funders who provide state-of-the-art simulation laboratories in schools and hospitals around the country. Many of us have used the National League for Nursing's *Student Satisfaction and Self-Confidence in Learning* scale (Jeffries & Rizzolo, 2006a) as a teaching evaluation to provide evidence of simulation satisfaction to stakeholders. But, it is important to recognize that empirical evaluation of learner satisfaction as a stand-alone outcome is no longer needed in the simulation literature (Franklin, Leighton, Cantrell, & Rutherford-Hemming, 2015). Early research in simulation centered on learner satisfaction, but the current call for simulation research is to use experimental methods and evaluate the effect of simulation on competence-based performance outcomes alongside other subjective measures of simulation success (Franklin & Lee, 2014).

Peer Learning

It could be that opportunities for peer learning are what make simulation so successful in the eyes of learners. Peer learning is reciprocal learning, wherein participants share knowledge, ideas, and experience with each other (Boud, Cohen, & Sampson, 2014). This may assist learners to be intentional reflective practitioners, to develop coping strategies when they make mistakes, and to strengthen their in depth understanding of concepts central to nursing practice (Valler-Jones, 2014). Peer learning in simulation allows learners to take responsibility for their own learning, without relying on faculty or facilitators to input knowledge. Learners report their simulation experience is meaningful when it builds upon concepts that were introduced earlier in the curriculum (Valler-Jones, 2014) and when simulation provides opportunities for learning with, from, and about the experiences, clinical reasoning and clinical judgements of their peers.

I have used peer learning as formative assessment in simulation. Previously in this chapter, I described organization of simulation with 12 novice nurses and four simulation cases in a 4-hour simulation experience. My goal is for learners to work together in teams of three to provide care to simulation patients. Peer learning in this fashion promotes teamwork and communication that is characteristic of modern nursing practice. I tend to designate roles of primary nurse (responsible for seeing the "big picture," calling a team huddle, and communicating with providers over the telephone), assessment nurse (responsible for vital signs and other physical/emotional assessments), and medication/skills nurse (responsible for medication administration and other skills during the scenario). It is important that simulation learners know that I intend the roles to be guidelines that are not restrictive; as such, transition of roles and leadership during the scenario is allowed in order to meet relevant problem-solving tasks. Informal and formal transition of roles usually brings forward a meaningful conversation in debriefing about role clarity. I record which learners have filled the various roles in simulation so that roles rotate during the academic semester. I am very open with simulation learners about the rationale for rotating roles and the responsibility each learner has to assume the leader role during the semester. Sharing the primary nurse role and accountability of leadership in the simulation contributes to learning, even when novice nurses may not think of themselves as natural leaders.

Having Fun in Simulation

Learners tend to think simulation is more fun when they have more practice experience in simulation environments. My teaching experience in simulation has been that learners may not verbalize their enjoyment until the fifth or sixth time they come to simulation because it takes that long to feel comfortable performing in front of peers and thinking on the spot in ways they may not routinely do in traditional clinical settings. I started out using simulation as an active participation-only experience, and I found that learners reported they were having more fun and also learning from their peers when they also had regular opportunities to observe their peers providing care in simulation. As a result, my preference for facilitating simulation now is to have four simulated cases within a 4-hour time period which all revolve around a common conceptual theme. Out of a group of 10 to 12 learners, everyone gets an opportunity to be an active participant in one scenario and an observer in the remaining three scenarios. Whether learners have active or observer roles in simulation, my goal is to create an environment

where learners feel safe enough to take interpersonal risk (Rudolph, Raemer, & Simon, 2014) and also to recognize that interpersonal risk occurs both during active simulation and by offering your own misperceptions or misinterpretations during debriefing and reflection-on-action. When learners are more mature in their curriculum and have developed a sense of camaraderie, I've found they tend to have more fun in simulation and taking risks with their peers.

Expanded Resources for Crisis Management

When anticipating learners' needs for psychological support, I have found it helpful to confer with my faculty colleagues to help me anticipate how learners might respond to simulation cues (either based on their personal history or class/clinical content) and how they might break down in simulation. It is important to talk with clinical faculty about the scenario objectives and expected learner behaviors, because they can relate experiences from clinical (great discussion topics for prebriefing and debriefing) or learners' personal history with the scenario content that might affect simulation flow. In some cases, I've elected to assign a learner to an observer role in a scenario, because the topic was too close to home in their personal life, based on conversations with faculty colleagues. As an example, I have found scenarios involving hospice caregiving experiences and/or planned simulator death to be particularly critical related to learner support. Faculty colleagues who have closer relationships with learners than I have been particularly helpful to brief learners individually and talk with them about how past personal experiences with death of family members informs their nursing worldview surrounding end of life care. Only in one instance that I can remember did we elect to excuse a learner from a simulation death scenario because she wasn't emotionally ready for the experience; in this situation, having foresight and support from faculty colleagues to provide anticipatory support for crisis management in simulation was critical to helping all simulation learners achieve the scenario objectives.

Option for Team Huddle

I want learners to call a time out during simulation so they can consult with their peers about priority setting and how to proceed. Though I facilitate prebriefing and make sure learners have a plan of care in place when they begin a scenario, there are many occasions when unexpected findings make learners feel uncertain, and they want to seek cognitive or task support. Team huddle is a concept introduced in TeamSTEPPS training (Agency for Healthcare Research and Quality, 2015b), used with learners at my university during their senior year. Calling a team huddle is a norm I create in simulation by introducing the concept at the beginning of simulation each semester and norming the team huddle on my university's simulation contract (see Box 22-2). I try to reinforce that any member of the simulation team (e.g., primary nurse or any team members) can call the team huddle and also model the importance of team huddle in terms of sharing new orders received over the telephone as a result of a call to the provider to report a change in patient condition. By their fourth or fifth simulation experiences, learners gain appreciation for the team huddle/time out to redirect their active simulation, and frequently debriefing conversations turn to simulation elements that active participants noticed that triggered their decision to call a team huddle. On these occasions, it is easy for learners to draw connections between calling a team huddle during simulation and calling the charge nurse for a consult in a traditional clinical setting. Therefore, using team huddles in simulation is another method to help learners draw connections between simulation and independent practice.

Supporting Learners Following a Scenario

Debriefing and Safe Container

Debriefing is a structured time for reflection that should occur soon after simulation where a facilitator guides learners to revisit their simulation experience to reflect, review what occurred, discuss with peers, correct errors in practice, and solidify learning concepts that learners can apply to future clinical situations (Dreifuerst & Decker, 2012; Shinnick, Woo, Horwich, & Steadman, 2011). The goal of debriefing is to facilitate learners' self-reflection on their own mental models (Fey, Scrandis, Daniels, & Haut, 2014) and correct any errors in thinking processes that occurred as a result of misperceptions or misinterpretations of the simulation experience. Structured debriefing provides intentional, systematic inquiry to support learning (INACSL Standards Committee, 2016, Debriefing), encourage reflective thinking, and uncover potential errors in thinking that informed decision-making during the simulation (Dreifuerst & Decker; Shinnick et al.).

Simulation leaders from the Center for Medical Simulation in Boston have described the importance of a **safe container**, also referred to as an environment where learners face meaningful challenges and are held to high standards in a way that engages them but without impending humiliation or intimidation (Rudolph et al., 2014). Creating this safe container in simulation and in debriefing increases learners' motivation for risk-taking wherein learners feel safe enough to embrace feeling uncomfortable, recognizing that all feelings of interpersonal risk probably have not been taken away. By establishing a safe container in simulation, facilitators create a setting for learners to practice new or familiar skills without a fear that they will be shamed, humiliated, or belittled (Rudolph et al.). In debriefing, I have found it effective to use a standard structure for debriefing, which normalizes the debriefing conversation and helps learners know what to expect. Other strategies to create a safe container include explicitly acknowledging interpersonal risk, confidentiality, and the importance of learning through debriefing. Posting a simulation contract, as previously described, and referring to it in debriefing as well as prebriefing and simulation orientation also conveys the message of a safe container for learners.

Other Ways to Support Learners

Healthy Competition: SimWars

SimWars is a friendly competition where teams demonstrate knowledge, behaviors, and attitudes related to teamwork while providing patient care in simulation and competing for a prize. Most of my exposure to SimWars involves teams of practicing healthcare professionals designing a scenario and presenting it in the form of a talent competition at professional meetings. It's really a lot of fun to watch! Frequently, simulation center teams (faculty, simulation technicians, and debriefing specialists) compete in a game of skill, creativity, and educational best practices. The Society of Simulation in Healthcare operationalizes SimWars as a live simulation competition on the main stage on the conference hall where simulation teams develop and perform their best simulation and debriefing within about 5 hours of receiving the scenario prompt and a list of required elements of simulation—such as the case background, props, goals, and objectives. Audience members rate each sim center team based on their effectiveness to accomplish learning objectives and on their overall innovation. Competing teams are provided the same set of resources and props, and each team is allowed to bring one carry-on sized bag of additional props to the competition.

The SimWars competition is catching on for professional meetings like emergency medicine and critical care nursing where simulation is a common pedagogy used for team training. Some groups have provided expert simulation mentors/coaches to help simulation center teams to think creatively, and other groups leverage a celebrity judges' panel to draw attention to the healthy competition. It is not unheard of to have simulation center teams submit a 5-minute video entry of a scenario along a given theme (e.g., rapid sequence intubation in critical care settings) to qualify for SimWars. One group from Australia even added a twist with extra points awarded for variations on a Star Wars theme integrated into the simulation experience. Broadly, SimWars competitions are a fun way to demonstrate educational best practices and use the creative sides of our simulation brains.

Graduate Learners Writing and Implementing Scenarios in Informal Competitions

I have been involved with graduate learners who wrote simulation cases as informal competitions as well. In a postmaster's certificate program for nurse educators, graduate learners complete a summer course in simulation pedagogy and gain a foundation of didactic knowledge related to simulation best practices, learning objectives, and basic simulation operations in terms of mannequin capabilities and medical equipment frequently used in simulation (e.g., how do we take a capillary blood glucose on a mannequin patient). The informal competition took place during a week-long face-to-face intensive experience where learners worked in teams to write, practice, and implement scenarios for their peers over the course of 3 days. While this is a lot of fun, it is also very labor intensive from a simulation operations perspective. Because these graduate learners were visitors to the simulation lab, they weren't familiar with the capabilities of the audiovisual system or mannequins. We found it most helpful to embed a simulation technician into each team of learners to guide them through the process of scenario development from an operations perspective. One of the fun parts about this experience was the camaraderie that existed between the teams and the way they wrote scripts for standardized patient actors who were funny at times and still maintained the character of practicing nurses. Writing and implementing scenarios in our informal competition was a meaningful way for graduate learners to apply their knowledge of simulation theory and get hands-on experience implementing simulation cases in a safe environment.

Team Versus Individual Learning in Simulation

Most of my experience in simulation involves team training with groups of learners working together to provide patient care and problem-solve for a simulated patient. Though critics point out that most patients do not have multiple nurses at the same time in practice, teamwork in simulation accomplishes the goals of reducing the cognitive load, alleviating distress, and providing an opportunity for intentional practice of teamwork behaviors. From our colleagues in medical education, many simulation facilitators have adopted the concept of "shared mind"

wherein two or more individuals share their cognitive and affective schemas and are able to process complex information that would otherwise overwhelm an individual (Epstein, 2013). My goal is to remember that in real life and in simulation, most of our important decisions emerge from interactions between groups of interprofessional providers and patients. Therefore, social interactions with other interprofessional providers in simulation enhance both our individual and relational autonomy as nurses (Epstein, 2013).

Teamwork in simulation may help learners avoid premature closure of their clinical judgement processes (e.g., stop *noticing* and move to *interpretation* too quickly) through interaction with other learners in simulation. Teamwork allows healthcare providers access to multiple ways of knowing—that is, using both logic and intuition as decision-making models—and offers opportunities to clarify values or assumptions made in the context of patient care with other trusted individuals (Epstein, 2013). Thus, deliberation between team members (e.g., team huddle) is a social process, which promotes collective decision-making as a more effective alternative to potentially biased individual decision-making.

Deliberate Practice in Simulation Teamwork

One of the most consistent accolades I receive from learners in simulation is how much they appreciate the debriefing conversation as a time for intentional learning and reflection, where an important element of feedback comes from simulation facilitators drawing attention to performance gaps and helping learners brainstorm alternative strategies to approach clinical problem-solving. Ericsson (2007) wrote that the availability of valid immediate feedback is fundamental for performance improvement through practice. When I receive this feedback from learners, I ask them a question in return, "Where is there a better place to practice teamwork and problem-solving than in simulation?" Ericsson describes deliberate practice as activities designed to provide opportunities to improve particular aspects of performance in an environment that allows gradual refinement after problem-solving and repeated variations with immediate feedback (McGahie, Issenberg, Petrussa, & Scalese, 2006). Deliberate practice increases the argument for allowing learners to repeat simulation scenarios after participating in a debriefing session where simulation facilitators unpack learners' cognitive frames and correct performance gaps through guided reflection. Deliberate practice of teamwork and other simulation skills may increase the learning and reflection our learners both need and desire.

Deliberate practice offers a path to skill improvement and expertise (Clapper & Kardong-Edgren, 2012), but it is important to recognize that there are several important elements to deliberate practice. First, *critical reflection* happens in debriefing when learners realize they need more skill practice or practice applying a specific concept in the context of patient care delivery. Second, *ongoing reflection* is an iterative process of internal performance evaluation against a set standard; ongoing reflection may start in debriefing and continue for days or weeks after when learners have opportunities to put the pieces of a clinical puzzle together within their own cognitive schema. A third characteristic of deliberate practice is that *learners frame why a task was performed and the way it relates to improving patient care* in order to fully understand the steps of skill performance and acquire a deeper understanding of the task. Finally, the goal of deliberate practice is *mastery of the task* and mastery of cognitive knowledge to anticipate problems or next steps (Ericsson, 2006).

Simulation Remediation

My preference for simulation teaching is emphasizing the learning that comes from immersion in clinical problem-solving in a safe environment. Applying the deliberate practice framework to simulation can be a solution to the common need of learner remediation and enhancing performance outcomes for learners who struggle. The deliberate practice framework helps simulation facilitators and learners to agree upon a mutual purpose for remediation while keeping in mind the mutual respect that is a critical element of participant integrity in simulation. Once a mutual purpose is established, facilitators can adapt scenarios and objectives to challenge learners' problem-solving abilities related to the task at hand, objectives, skill set, and learning needs (Benner, Sutphen, Leonard, & Day, 2010; Hamilton & Morris, 2012). Careful facilitation promotes learner motivation to improve their own performance, especially through use of a rubric and specific feedback to guide future practice (Evans & Harder, 2013). Rubrics may augment debriefing and provide specific objectives for shared reflection between the simulation facilitator, clinical faculty, and learner. Rubrics also provide the learner with an artifact to use for goal setting in their future clinical practice. Use of these best educational practices in simulation remediation further promotes learning and improved performance.

Many times, simulation remediation is a one-on-one experience, but it continues to utilize essential simulation characteristics including learner preparation, reflection-in-action, and reflection-on-action. Two unique characteristics of simulation remediation may be direct feedback to the referring faculty member who initiated simulation remediation and a journal or written reflection from the learner after simulation to provide evidence of knowledge gained and goals for the future. Success of simulation remediation may be measured by qualitative feedback in the reflection (Evans & Harder, 2013) or by performance observations when the learner returns to a traditional clinical setting.

It is important that simulation pedagogy and technology allow for remediation beyond psychomotor skills to include realistic scenarios that support critical thinking (Lisko & O'Dell, 2010) and clinical judgement (Evans & Harder, 2013). I have used simulation remediation for learners whom clinical faculty identify as at-risk based on performance in clinical or team simulation. I have had more success with problem-solving scenarios where learners receive a handoff report, identify a plan of care, and implement their plan to include physical assessment, medication administration, communication with other providers, patient teaching, and some psychomotor skills as relevant to the simulation case. Utilizing these options for creating learning objectives in simulation remediation provides for a much more robust experience than psychomotor skills practice alone, which may be well suited for practice lab and task trainers. As an example, instead of doing a short scenario involving a urinary catheter insertion, a simulation remediation case might involve an elderly patient with congestive heart failure who complains of shortness of breath and swelling in her feet. In remediation, learners could identify a plan for physical assessment, medication administration with intravenous furosemide, patient teaching related to the medication, reporting an abnormal lab value to a provider over the telephone, titrating oxygen administration, and inserting a urinary catheter for precise measurement of intake and output. Not only does this type of problem-solving scenario provide more opportunities for learning, but it also potentially uncovers hidden performance gaps and objectives for further remediation.

Simulation facilitators from the University of Maryland use a more prescriptive remediation approach that assists, instills, and reinforces confidence within learners, while at the same time ensuring competence with clinical skills and safe care (Lynn & Twigg, 2011). There are four steps in their remediation program, including identifying the learning needs, developing an individualized simulation lesson plan, completing the lesson plan, and completing clinical readiness testing with a clinical remediation grading rubric to determine options for future simulation remediation. Clinical readiness testing is a simulation of the first hour of a clinical day when learners tend to make errors in clinical judgement that impact their holistic nursing performance. A unique feature of this remediation program is the use of graduate nurse teaching assistants (with at least 18 months of practice experience) who assist with the first two steps of the remediation program and help with skills practice in a nonthreatening environment. At the University of Maryland, learners in simulation remediation are not allowed to attend activities in the hospital or community setting until they complete the simulation remediation lesson plan, which may help to deescalate their performance stress about clinical expertise. Overall, the simulation remediation activities on this campus have positively impacted learners' knowledge and growth (Lynn & Twigg).

Application to Future Practice

Debriefing Questions to Connect the Dots

Some simulation learners easily visualize how scenarios apply to their future practice, while others require facilitators to connect the dots between a scenario and real-life practice during debriefing. Simulation is most helpful when experienced following content delivery in a didactic setting so that simulation builds on knowledge acquired in course lectures (Kirkman, 2013). Even in cases where simulation may introduce new content to learners, debriefing can serve as a meaningful introduction when it's bolstered by clinical stories from real practice and/or videos or handouts that appeal to different learning style preferences. Debriefing sessions should include discussions by the learners about the takeaway points they will apply to their own practice, offering an opportunity to demonstrate retention and actualization of scenario content. Research evidence points to transfer of knowledge and skills from simulation to future traditional clinical experiences among samples of novice nurses (Kirkman, 2013). Transfer of knowledge and skills from simulation increases when debriefing involves sharing of insights between learners and their facilitator using standards of best practice (INACSL Standards Committee, 2016, Debriefing).

Formative Assessment: Assessment for Learning Versus Learning for Assessment

 Formative assessment fosters "progress toward goal attainment" (INACSL Standards Committee, 2016, Simulation Glossary, p. S41) by using a scenario to ask learners,— "How are you doing?"—and allowing them time in the curriculum to improve their performance (McDonald, 2013). The intended outcome of formative assessment is improvement of learners' performance after simulation and debriefing to unveil the rationale that informed the way they provided patient care. In simulation, learners frequently need to focus on anticipating what may happen with their patient, plan how to respond, and reflect-in-action to alter their plan of care as needed. Because formative assessment is appropriate for learners getting used to the culture of simulation, it is natural for them to need improvement related to thinking in their professional role and implementing patient care during simulation. Constructive feedback from peers and simulation facilitators is an important element of formative assessment. The

Simulation on a Shoestring feature describes a cost-effective method for gathering data to help facilitators better respond to learner needs.

Summative Evaluation in Simulation

 Summative evaluation provides feedback on meeting outcomes or determining competence (INACSL Standards Committee, 2016, Simulation Glossary) by using a scenario to ask learners, "How did you do?" (McDonald, 2013)—in order to assess the degree to which learners achieved desired outcomes and to document a specific competency level. Intended outcomes may be a course grade, promotion, certification, or competency achievement; thus, the importance of using valid and reliable evaluation tools and measuring interrater reliability is important with summative evaluation (Bensfield, Olech, & Horsley, 2012). Evaluators should share the rubric for summative evaluation with learners and explain the evaluation process prior to the simulation experience (INACSL Standards Committee, 2016, Participant Evaluation). For learners, the consequence of summative simulation may include the potential to fail a course or program on the basis of simulation performance (Kardong-Edgren, Hanberg, Keenan, Ackerman, & Chambers, 2012). Summative evaluation requires that participants are well acquainted with simulation practice in order to provide fair evaluation and make sure participants' performance is not negatively impacted by their anxiety about simulation in general. A hallmark of summative simulation is the focus on evaluating outcomes without providing participants with opportunities for debriefing; instead of debriefing, facilitators provide structured feedback on participants' performance compared to a benchmark or rubric/checklist.

Transitioning the Learner to a New Way of Learning

The Institute of Medicine (2011) suggested that simulation will play a more important role in health professions education in the future. Through use of simulation best practices presented here, facilitators inform the simulation culture that best supports learning for novice nurses and other health professions learners. I've previously mentioned the importance of learning how to simulate both to decrease learner stress and to help them have fun in simulation. But, an additional reality of learning to simulate is that learners will be more likely to transfer their simulation learning to actual independent practice when they can anticipate what will happen in simulation and both think and act in their professional roles by responding effectively (Benner et al., 2010). Through intentional simulation experiences carefully threaded throughout

PALS Form as Formative Assessment

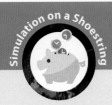

Mary Cato, EdD, RN, CHSE

Ashley Franklin, PhD, RN, CCRN, CNE, CHSE

Participation and Learning in Simulation

The purpose of this form is to provide learner feedback about participation and learning in simulation. The form will be completed by simulation participants after each simulation session and be provided to simulation faculty for further comments. The completed form will be returned to learners using the learning management system.

Learners must complete the PALS form by the **24 hour deadline after simulation**. For example, if your simulation finished Monday at 12 Noon, then PALS submissions are due by Tuesday at 12 Noon.

1. Provide your simulation patient's name.

2. Your preparation and contributions to group learning are an important part of simulation. These are 5 elements of participation that are meaningful to simulation learning.

   1. Thoughtful communication that reflects preparation
   2. Concise and clear presentation of ideas
   3. Avoids inappropriate use of personal experiences/interpretations
   4. Demonstrates critical analysis of nursing care in the simulation and in debriefing
   5. Uses resources to contribute to patient outcomes and to debriefing discussion.

Using the criteria above, rate your own preparation and contribution to group learning in terms of how frequently you demonstrated the behaviors above.
   ____   Never
   ____   Occasionally
   ____   Often

3. Inquiry and reflection are an important part of debriefing. These behaviors demonstrate inquiry and reflection:

   1. Initiates responses and questions and debriefing
   2. Seeks information, knowledge, and feedback in simulation and debriefing discussion
   3. Asks pertinent and relevant questions
   4. Considers opinions, views, and ideas expressed by other participants.

Using the criteria above, rate your own inquiry and reflection in terms of how frequently you demonstrated the behaviors above.

   ____   Never
   ____   Occasionally
   ____   Often

4. Reflect on your "takeaways" or "aha moments" in simulation today. Write about things you learned related to your role in simulation, your patient, working with a team, communication, or your own nursing judgement.

5. What was difficult for you today? Write about your teamwork, communication, or clinical judgement.

Figure 22.3 Participation and Learning in Simulation (PALS) Form. (Used with permission from Ashley Franklin and Mary Cato [personal communication 2015])

(Continued)

PALS Form as Formative Assessment (*Continued*)

The Challenge

Implementing a formative assessment activity after each simulation experience with our undergraduate learners in a meaningful way to promote additional reflection-on-action and provide constructive feedback on specific behaviors that might not have been appropriate for large group discussion.

Innovative Solutions

We implemented the Participation and Learning in Simulation (PALS) form using our learning management system's quizzes and test feature with no added cost to our budget but a large reward in terms of learning. Using the PALS form helped simulation faculty respond to individual learner needs and also infused the language of clinical judgement intentionally into learner feedback. Learners completed the PALS form in approximately 5 minutes and could use their laptops or the computer lab to complete

their part of the formative assessment before leaving the simulation center. Anecdotally, we heard that learners very much appreciated the intentional feedback on their individual simulation performance (see Fig. 22.3).

An unintended outcome of the PALS form provided additional evidence of simulation learning for the learners' professional portfolios and reflections about their clinical judgement development during annual benchmark essays. PALS feedback from simulation faculty identified specific areas of concern, such as potential assumptions made about simulation patients, alternative patient education methods, and elements of team communication to consider for future practice. Facilitators took specific notes during simulation, including the way learners worded questions and patient education, to enable individualized PALS feedback. In essence, the PALS form helped us create action plans for future simulations, which helped learners be more intentional about their patterns of behavior during future simulations.

---

health professions' curricula, learners have opportunities for practice improvement. For example, novice nurses cite substandard practice in their clinical experiences as a major ethical concern during school (Benner et al., 2010), but the controlled nature of simulation learning can curb exposure to poor quality practice and instead replace it with more active learning opportunities that really do change the face of health professions education.

It is important to recognize the role of simulation from the perspective of education experts related to transformation of education. Simulation is an opportunity for powerful learning experiences that integrate clinical and classroom teaching, which Benner et al. (2010) recognize as one of three important findings in the seminal Carnegie study report. Simulation is a place to practice communication between nurses and interprofessional providers, which is of ultimate importance given the current climate of healthcare where "*doctor's orders* are not specific directions but instead are guidelines and parameters for nurses to judiciously adjust therapies according to patient responses" (Benner et al., 2010, p. 22). Finally, simulation is a place for learners to develop relational skills by practicing patient education and delivering patient care in a team setting that is characteristic of modern healthcare delivery. Surely, the transformation of health professions education is upon us.

I appreciate that simulation is a safe place for learning where facilitators observe and provide feedback, using

what Lave and Wenger (1991) called "legitimate peripheral participation" as a way to teach learners about high-risk situations before they are ready to actually perform in them with real patients. In simulation, we are privileged to create situations where a patient's conditions changes on demand and therefore provides an opportunity for novice nurses to detect the changes, respond effectively, and alert other providers about the change in condition (Benner et al., 2010); through debriefing or using scripted cues to clue learners in to the change, simulation facilitators can guide the way learners approach an unstable patient, notice salient cues, and respond. Thus, the "legitimate peripheral participation" encourages learners to take a risk in their own clinical judgement, make decisions, and implement a plan of care in a safe simulation environment. Simulation facilitators should help learners recognize that their risks in simulation translate directly to application to future practice following in real patient care settings.

We have empirical evidence to support transfer of learning from simulation to traditional clinical settings from nursing and other health disciplines; the evidence supports a continued transformation of health professions education and supports the use of more simulation in our curricula. Kirkman (2013) evaluated transfer to practice in a time series repeated measures design study where didactic faculty introduced content in lecture during week one, learners applied content related to respiratory assessment in hospitalized adults during week two, learners participated in an asthma simulation during week three, and trained raters observed learners' respiratory assessments in the traditional clinical setting during week four of an academic semester. Similar to findings from other simulation research, Kirkman found that simulation increased the knowledge learners were able to demonstrate in a traditional clinical setting and that performance assessment scores documented the effectiveness of simulation pedagogy. Such evidence helps me understand the importance of utilizing simulation best practices and talking with learners about the rationale for simulation practice to both reinforce prior knowledge and practice newly learned skills.

Summary

This chapter presented theory and application related to supporting learners during various stages of simulation. Integrating best practices for learner support should enhance the overall quality of learning and transfer of knowledge into actual practice following simulation experiences. Supporting learners in simulation requires careful planning, anticipating how learners will need support, and responding to unexpected challenges learners experience during simulation and debriefing. After considering best practices presented in this chapter, readers should be able to describe how simulation learners fit into several learning theories. Specifically, readers should be able to describe contributors to learner anxiety in simulation and strategies to mitigate anxiety using strategies for scenario design and facilitation such as prebriefing, standardized cues, and creating a safe container during debriefing. Finally, readers should be able to apply their increased understanding of formative assessment and summative evaluation in simulation to consider which type of simulation fits best with their own curriculum and program outcomes.

23

Simulation Examples for Nursing Practice and Clinical Specialties

Kim Leighton

Key Terms

Distributed Learning, Second Life, Leadership, Delegation, Blog, Broadcast Simulation

Guiding Questions

1 I've been asked to create a scenario to use with a high school group of learners. What have others done?

2 How do I create a simulation experience for a group of over 70 students?

3 What methods have other simulationists used to evaluate the effectiveness of their simulation?

Introduction

When faced with the task of integrating simulation experiences throughout an entire curriculum, it can be daunting to know where to begin. Chapter 20 outlined the steps to take when deciding what topics might meet the learning objectives you have identified; however, we thought that it would be helpful for you to read about some of the unique experiences that other simulationists have created, implemented, and evaluated—some ideas to help get your own creative juices flowing! The examples in this chapter can be adapted to both academic and clinical learning environments.

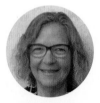

Kim Leighton,
PhD, RN, CHSE, CHSOS, ANEF

These examples are not meant to be perfect exemplars, and use of the INACSL Standards of Best Practice: Simulation[SM] may not always be evident; however, the goal of this chapter is to provide you with ideas, rather than off-the-shelf, ready-to-implement scenarios. These examples, provided by numerous simulationists, have all been run with learners and the authors share with you the rationale for why the scenario was created, how they prepared for the experience, and their outcomes—both the good outcomes and the lessons they learned along the way. Use these experiences as a springboard to developing your own experiences. As you read through the examples, think to yourself, "Could this work with my students?" "Would this work in my hospital?" or "This is an interesting idea. How can I adapt it for the needs of my learners?"

Many years ago, I worked for a vendor and project managed the development of the first vendor-produced set of simulation scenarios. We wanted the product to be one that educators could just take off the shelf and use. Over 125 masters and doctorally prepared educators contributed to the project, which included, at that time, 90 scenarios that crossed the continuum of a baccalaureate degree nursing program. What I learned during that project is that no two educators saw scenario design the same way! Some preferred a different format, others preferred a different order, while others thought there was too little or too much information provided to the students! And this variation wasn't just with the authors—I also heard this from the customers. There were also variances in practice that occurred in different regions of the country, and in countries outside the United States, that became issues of debate. The moral of my story? There may not be a "perfect" scenario! However, I believe that you will learn from these examples how others have conceptualized and implemented simulation, which will further inform your own practice.

The template that was used for these contributions include scenario title, learner population, the performance gap that was identified, learning objectives, performance assessment plan, scenario synopsis, preparation for learner and educator, event flow data, debriefing strategies, evaluation of the event, and lessons learned. It is my hope that you can adapt some of these scenarios to your own environment. A quote that you will often hear related to simulation is "Let's not recreate the wheel."

This chapter is organized into the following sections:

- *Nursing Care Specialties:* Medical/Surgical, Preoperative Education, Obstetrical Care, Mental Health, Pediatrics, Gerontology
- *Critical Care:* Intensive Care, Trauma/Emergency, Neonatal Intensive Care, Distributed Learning for Practicing Nurses
- *Graduate Studies:* Nurse Practitioner Simulation With Second Life
- *Leadership/Management:* Leadership, Delegation
- *Community:* Poverty, High School, Public Health/ Veteran Care
- *End of Program Evaluation:* Case Management 1:1
- *Unique Experiences:* Lauren's Blog, the 12-Hour Night Shift, Broadcast Simulation

Nursing Care Specialties

Medical/Surgical: Mock Hospital Unit Simulation as Initial Clinical Experience

Teresa Gore, PhD, DNP, FNP-BC, NP-C, CHSE-A

Caralise W. Hunt, PhD, RN

Karol C. Renfroe, MSN, RN

Population

First clinical semester baccalaureate nursing students.

Performance Gap

Faculty realized the nursing students' anxiety levels were too high on the initial inpatient clinical day, hindering the transition of learning from the classroom and lab into the patient care setting. The teachers believed the cause of the anxiety was because students did not know what to expect or have an opportunity to "put it all together" until the initial inpatient clinical day. The simulation was designed to give the students an opportunity to be in a simulated clinical day at the hospital.

Learning Objectives

1. Provide total patient care in a safe environment.
2. Use personal data assistant (PDA) for bedside medication administration.
3. Detect and correct a specific problem with the assigned simulated patient.
4. Develop, implement, and evaluate plan of care for the assigned simulated patient including documentation.

Performance Assessment

This simulation was a formative assessment. Students were expected to come to the simulation/clinical lab at the university as if attending an inpatient clinical day with uniform, resources, and equipment needed to complete a clinical day. This simulation was graded using a satisfactory/unsatisfactory rating. An existing evaluation tool was modified to incorporate Quality and Safety Education for Nurses (QSEN) competencies and critical thinking.

Scenario Synopsis

Synopsis of the Patient Background

Four patients were selected for this simulation: (1) a congestive heart failure (CHF) patient admitted with an acute exacerbation with multiple chronic diagnosis with wrong intravenous (IV) medication hanging; (2) a chronic obstructive pulmonary disease (COPD) patient with acute exacerbation who has accidentally become disconnected from the oxygen; (3) a trauma patient third day post-op with nasogastric (NGT) and chest tube (CT) and one has become disconnected from the wall suction; and (4) an abdominal surgery patient who has an antibiotic ordered for which she has an allergy.

Modality/Typology Selection and Rationale

Low- and medium-level fidelity mannequins were used (Fig. 23.1) because this was a pilot study to determine the feasibility of conducting this experience with a large number of students.

Fidelity Achievement

Using actual equipment that would be used in the hospital setting: IV pumps, suction, oxygen (O_2) tubing, CT, NGT, medication cart in a designated medication area, and patient charts at the bedside.

Preparation

Learner Preparation

Read about assigned diagnosis. Key briefing points on day of simulation included ethical considerations, discussion of formative versus summative evaluation, and creation of a safe environment.

Educator Preparation

Three facilitators participated in this simulation. Each facilitator assisted with the design, development, and preparation and planned for how to interact with the students.

Event Flow Data

The total group size was 79 students enrolled in the class. During each simulation session, two students were

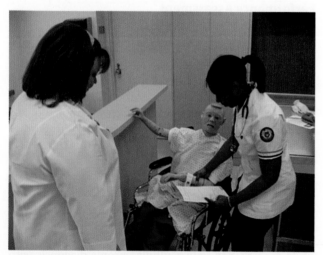

Figure 23.1 Mock Hospital Patient Care. (Courtesy of Auburn University School of Nursing, with permission.)

assigned to each of the four patients. Students were given a report on their patient, reviewed the chart, used PDAs to obtain information, discussed the patient with the clinical instructor, prioritized interventions, and assumed care. A problem was built into each scenario to assist in the development of clinical judgement/critical thinking along with spontaneous problems in response to student action or nonaction. At the end of the simulation, each student gave a report and discussed the events of the day. The students were debriefed on the scenarios.

Debriefing

The facilitator asked at least one question from each section of our debriefing tool—aesthetic, personal, empirical, and ethical—followed by review of the care plan, diagnoses, and interventions performed during the simulation.

Evaluation of Event

The Spielberger State–Trait Anxiety Inventory (STAI) was used as a self-report measure of the students' anxiety level on their first inpatient clinical day. The control group completed the STAI on the morning of their initial inpatient clinical experience. The experimental group participated in the simulation as their initial clinical experience and completed the STAI the next day prior to their initial inpatient clinical day. The anxiety scores of the experimental group ($n = 47$) were statistically significantly lower than the control group. The Simulation Effectiveness Tool (METI/CAE) data showed that the experience was beneficial for students.

Lessons Learned

Simulation is instructor/facilitator time intensive. The experience included the use of an electronic medical record whenever possible. It was difficult remembering to change out the chart between students. Another lesson learned is to keep the first simulation simple. Chest tubes were identified as a gap in the student learning but that scenario may have been too complicated for these students. After the school had students purchase a simulation scenario with electronic medical record product, the scenarios were changed to commonly occurring diagnoses and clinical issues.

Preoperative Education: Veterans Receive High-Fidelity Simulation Preoperatively

Bonnie Haupt, DNP, RN, CNL, CHSE

Population

Patients undergoing coronary artery bypass graft (CABG) surgeries.

Performance Gap

There is a lack of diverse educational methods in healthcare utilized for patient education. Traditionally, most patient teaching experiences involve face-to-face education with printed materials. This form of education is lacking and does not meet different learner needs. My personal experiences working in the surgical intensive care unit (ICU) caring for postoperative CABG patients confirmed a gap in patient understandings of expectations of care, increasing postoperative anxiety.

Learning Objectives

1. Participate in a high-fidelity simulation experience mimicking the ICU environment after CABG surgery and postoperative plan of care activities.
2. Describe ICU and postoperative devices, equipment, sounds, and expectations for care in the postoperative period.
3. Apply increased knowledge of postoperative expectations to reduce anxiety and increase learner satisfaction.

Performance Assessment

This scenario was conducted as part of a study. To assess knowledge and patient understanding, the CABG pre–post quiz was developed by the researcher to measure understanding of key topics provided in the education experience and usual pre- and postoperative teachings. Length of stay (LOS) data were collected. Patient satisfaction data were obtained after the educational experiences and anxiety was measured using the State–Trait Anxiety Inventory (STAI) (Spielberger, 1970).

Scenario Synopsis

Synopsis of the Patient Background

The case stem was variable due to different patient ages, genders, and unique health histories. The general age range was 60 to 80 years old, male/female gender with a history of heart disease status post CABG surgery.

Modality/Typology Selection and Rationale

To increase patient understanding of the CABG postoperative period, high-fidelity simulation was incorporated into the educational experience.

- The control group received usual CABG preoperative VA-established education, which included a one-to-one, face-to-face session that lasted no longer than 1 hour.

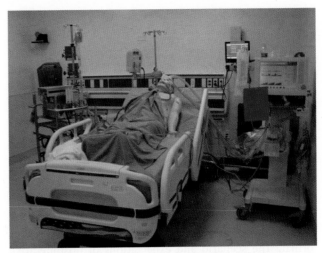

Figure 23.2 Preoperative Staging for Preop Patient Education Class.

- The simulation intervention group education included a high-fidelity simulation experience, with a mannequin in an educational setting resembling an ICU environment in place of the usual education (Fig. 23.2).

Fidelity Achievement

The 1-hour session immersed participants into the simulated ICU environment with the high-fidelity simulator in an ICU bed with arterial line, catheter, chest tube, compression boots, dressings, endotracheal tube, IVs, IV pumps, monitor, sternal and leg incisions, pacemaker, restraints, SWAN catheter, and ventilator in place. Sounds were introduced during the experience to educate participants to usual ICU noises and alarms, and included use of the call light and bed, compression boots, coughing and deep breathing exercises along with trial of the incentive spirometer, pain scale, splinting and restraints, and tactile experience of any equipment of interest.

Preparation

Learner Preparation

There is no learner preparation for the class. The learners signed an informed consent for the study and completed the pretest for knowledge and State–Trait Anxiety instruments prior to education.

Educator Preparation

Familiarity with CABG pre-, intra-, and postoperative and discharge plans of care. Postoperative devices and equipment. Set up the simulation room to mimic the ICU environment post CABG surgery.

Event Flow Data

The study groups consisted of 10 patients in the simulation intervention and 10 patients in the control group. In each educational session, one patient was present, but some had a family member or caregiver as well. The time allotted for the educational sessions was up to 1 hour; however, the sessions lasted an average of about 30 minutes.

Debriefing

After completion of the posttest for knowledge, state anxiety, and satisfaction evaluation, the patients and family participated in an informal debrief of the simulation education intervention utilizing the advocacy and inquiry format. The scenario and expectations of postoperative care were reviewed with the patients. Statements such as "I observed" and "How did you feel" were used in the debrief process. Participants were also encouraged to identify the plus/delta elements of the simulation scenario.

Evaluation of Event

The post-knowledge scores were higher for the high-fidelity learner group, and they reported higher satisfaction. State anxiety was reduced more for the intervention group, and unsolicited follow-up communication revealed additional positive remarks. There was no difference in LOS.

Lessons Learned

The outcomes suggest use of high-fidelity simulation as an educational tool as a means for meeting patients' individual learning needs. A great opportunity exists through the use of simulation education to improve patient and family understanding of their specific healthcare plan. There is also the potential to reduce psychological and physical postoperative complications.

Obstetrical Care: High-Risk Obstetrical Scenario: Putting It All Together

Barbara Sittner, PhD, APRN-CNS, RN, ANEF

Population

Undergraduate Bachelor of Science in Nursing junior-level students completing their obstetrical clinical rotation.

Performance Gap

Nursing students have limited opportunities to provide care for high-risk obstetrical patients from the time of admission throughout the four stages of labor.

Learning Objectives

1. Assess risk factors contributing to a high-risk pregnancy.
2. Provide care throughout the four stages of labor.
3. Prioritize care based on clinical manifestations.
4. Effective communication with healthcare team based on patient condition.

Performance Assessment

Faculty summative evaluation on student clinical evaluation. Simulation is a clinical day and students are to come to the Simulation Center prepared (read assignments and completed medication worksheet). Student satisfaction using the Simulation Experience Questionnaire (SEQ; Sittner, Hertzog, & Ofe, 2013) that has QSEN competencies threaded throughout is used as an evaluation tool. The SEQ can be found in Toolkit 23-1.

Scenario Synopsis

 The scenario for "Putting It All Together" can be found in Toolkit 23-2.

Synopsis of the Patient Background

The scenario was designed to capture risk factors associated with preeclampsia: history of preeclampsia with a previous pregnancy, African American ethnicity, and family history of preeclampsia (her mother).

Modality/Typology Selection and Rationale

High-fidelity birthing mannequin with a wireless tablet PC with a variety of options that the educator can change as the scenario evolves. Changes made from the tablet PC are shown in real time on the virtual monitor (Fig. 23.3).

Fidelity Achievement

Labor and delivery (L&D) equipment: L&D bed, electronic fetal monitoring (EFM) equipment (tocotransducer, ultrasound, belts), and fetal heart rate and contraction changes shown on virtual monitor in patient room.

Preparation

Learner Preparation

Review textbook reading assignments, including prenatal history assessment, vaginal birth, hypertensive disorders

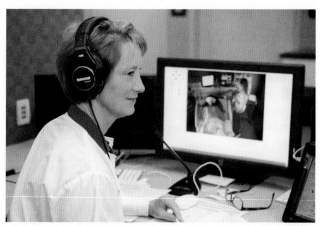

Figure 23.3 Monitoring the Simulation With Audiovisual Equipment. (From Bryan Medical Center, Lincoln, Nebraska, with permission.)

of pregnancy, postpartum assessment, and hemorrhage. Review the Hypertension in Pregnancy Executive Summary (ACOG, 2013a) and Postpartum Hemorrhage from Vaginal Delivery Patient Safety Checklist (ACOG, 2013b). Complete Postpartum Hemorrhage Medication Worksheet. Key briefing points including ethical considerations on the day of the simulation are for everyone to come prepared, work as a team, and not to share information on the activity with other classmates.

Educator Preparation

Schedule dates and times for the student's simulation experience at the Simulation Center. Include the simulation schedule for student simulation groups in the syllabus and learning management system. Discuss expectations of the simulation experience with students on the first day of orientation.

Event Flow Data

A total of eight clinical groups, each with six students, participated in 4-hour simulations. Students "draw" their assigned role for the simulation activity. For my simulation activities, there was a Part I and Part II of an unfolding simulation experience. There were three students who provided care and three students who observed. At the completion of Part I, there was a "handoff" to the next shift. Those who observed were now the care providers, and those who had been the care providers now had new roles.

Debriefing

Methods used included guided reflection, reflective thinking, and constructive peer feedback using the Quality and Safety Education for Nurses (QSEN) competencies as a guide.

Evaluation of Event

Overall, this has been a positive learning experience for the students. They know what to expect and arrive at the Simulation Center prepared. Here is one comment that captures the essence of the experience: "I enjoyed this sim. It was nice to have a scenario where a patient has major complications before/during/after labor. This didn't occur for me during the OB rotation, so it was nice to use the info I have learned in class."

Lessons Learned

Organization is imperative. Critical elements include beginning with an identified need; utilizing the International Nursing Association for Clinical Simulation and Learning Standards of Best Practice: Simulation^{SM} (INACSL Standards Committee, 2016), as guides to design, implement, and evaluate experiences; creativity; communication; and being prepared for the unexpected—have extra supplies available. Another key point is work as a team—that means setup and teardown. Oftentimes, I have been thanked for helping stock and assist in putting the simulation room back in order. Always seems strange to me not to help. Lastly, have fun with this teaching strategy...the possibilities of simulation are endless!

Mental Health: Bipolar Disorder, Weight Gain, and Fatigue: An Interprofessional Standardized Patient Simulation

Kirstyn M. Kameg, DNP, PMHNP-BC

Population

Doctoral-level psychiatric mental health nurse practitioner (PMHNP) students and medical residents/students.

Performance Gap

Primary care is frequently referred to as the *de facto* mental health system in the United States. Primary care clinicians are facing the burden of an ever-increasing number of patients presenting with major mental illness. Failure to recognize and appropriately treat mental health conditions has a significant impact on health outcomes and costs leading to recommendations for integration of psychiatry in the primary care setting. Furthermore, the Institute of Medicine has recommended that interprofessional education competencies be integrated into health professionals' curricula in order to improve healthcare quality. In response, we developed, implemented, and evaluated a standardized patient simulation depicting a patient with a history of bipolar II disorder presenting to the primary care setting with the chief complaint of recent weight gain and fatigue.

Learning Objectives

1. Perform history and physical exam.
2. Assess the patient's mental status.
3. Order appropriate labs.
4. Establish list of differential diagnoses.
5. Formulate treatment plan based on most likely diagnosis(es).
6. Educate patient on selected treatment plan emphasizing both pharmacologic and nonpharmacologic treatments.

Performance Assessment

The pre-/post-knowledge test (23-3) and performance checklist (23-4) are located in the Toolkit.

Scenario Synopsis

Synopsis of the Patient Background

The patient is a 35-year-old administrative assistant working at a local high school. Over the past 4 months, she has gained weight, almost 20 lb, reaching her highest weight of 170 lb. She also reports that she has been feeling more fatigued lately. She has a history of bipolar II disorder and was hospitalized 2 years ago for depression and a suicide attempt by overdose. At that time, she was started on Prozac, which precipitated a hypomanic episode. Most recently, she has been following on an outpatient basis with a psychiatrist and was started on quetiapine (Seroquel) 300 mg every night 3 months ago. She is presenting to the primary care setting with concerns regarding this recent weight gain.

Modality/Typology Selection and Rationale

A standardized patient (SP) was used for this scenario to enhance fidelity and to meet one of the learning objectives, which was to assess the patient's mental status.

Fidelity Achievement

Creating a primary care office setting.

Preparation

Learner Preparation

Because of the focus on interprofessional collaboration and the fact that the PMHNP students and the medical residents/students had not worked together prior to this simulation activity, the experience began with a team-building exercise. Participants completed a 10-item pretest to assess knowledge related to the simulation objectives. Participants were provided with the patient's past history, current medications, vital signs, weight and BMI, and chief complaint. Ethical considerations regarding confidentiality, respect, and professional behaviors were reviewed.

Educator Preparation

The PMHNP faculty is doctorally prepared and nationally certified. She has had experience facilitating prior simulations. Additionally, a primary care physician assisted with the development of the SP script and with the content debriefing.

Preparation of Others

The SP used in this scenario had time to review the script prior to the simulation and also had the opportunity to come in for training and to have any questions answered prior to the simulation.

Event Flow Data

The total group size was 20 students. During each simulation, there was one medical resident or student and a PMHNP student participating. Three simulations ran simultaneously in different rooms and were observed by students not participating at the time. Each scenario lasted 20 minutes followed by 30 minutes of debriefing.

Debriefing

The model used was the Promoting Excellence and Reflective Learning in Simulation (PEARLS) debriefing method (Eppich & Cheng, 2015). The four phases of this debriefing process include reaction, description, analysis, and summary. Guiding reflective questions and key content questions guided the discussion.

Evaluation of Event

Participants completed an Attitudes Toward Healthcare Teams Scale (ATHCTS) to evaluate perceptions of the interprofessional team and a Simulation Evaluation Survey to evaluate the simulation itself. The T-TPQ is divided into the following five domains: team building, leadership, situational monitoring, mutual support, and communication. Mean scores in each of the domains for both the medical residents and PMHNP students were four or greater indicating that the participants strongly agreed/agreed that the simulation experience assisted in meeting those domains. Results of the Simulation Evaluation Survey indicated that they were satisfied with the experience. Results from the pre- and post-tests did not reveal a significant increase in knowledge following the simulation, nor was there a significant different between the PMHNP students' and medical residents/students' knowledge.

Lessons Learned

It was difficult to coordinate schedules for an interprofessional simulation, requiring advance planning. Because we ran three rooms simultaneously, there was inconsistency in debriefing, which may have impacted knowledge gain on the post-test. In the future we will include a training day for debriefers.

The participants were apprehensive so we included an ice-breaker activity involving team-building skills prior to the simulation. Team members lacked knowledge about the role of the PMHNP. We provided an overview of the role prior to the simulation. It is also important to note that simulations with a focus on mental health may trigger participant anxiety/other emotional responses. Include a debriefing question that addresses whether or not the scenario evoked an emotional response.

Pediatrics: Ruptured Appendix

Teresa W. Atz, PhD, RN, CHSE

Population

Undergraduate nursing students in their third or fourth semester of an accelerated BSN program, pediatric nursing course.

Performance Gap

Pain and comfort measures, SBAR report (Situation–Background–Assessment–Recommendation) to physician, prioritization, nasogastric tube (NGT) insertion, and communication with an anxious mother.

Learning Objectives

1. Evaluate patient assessment information including vital signs, focused abdominal, and pain assessment.
2. Recognize need for intervention related to constant nausea/vomiting and pain.
3. Communicate therapeutically and calmly to family who is refusing anesthesia and communicate effectively to healthcare team.
4. Demonstrate safe and appropriate insertion of NGT.

Performance Assessment

Grading criteria are preprogrammed. Each critical event that the students must achieve is given a score of 1. There are a total of 15 critical events in this scenario.

Scenario Synopsis

The scenario can be found in Toolkit 23-5.

Synopsis of the Patient Background

An 8-year-old boy is brought to the emergency department (ED) by his parents and diagnosed with acute appendicitis. While awaiting surgery the next morning, his mother becomes anxious and does not want to sign the surgical consent. The student is expected to care for the physical needs of the child and psychosocial needs of the mother.

Modality/Typology Selection and Rationale

SimJunior high-fidelity mannequin for ability to mimic real-life vital sign changes and ability for students to insert NGT.

Fidelity Achievement

Through preprogrammed voices and vital signs. The room was set as a patient room. SimJunior mimics the child's age and a prerecorded child's voice is used. Also used are prerecorded voices for the mother and the physician.

Preparation

Learner Preparation

Mosby skills for NGT placement are reviewed before the simulation day as an assignment, the instructor gives a demonstration, and students practice before the scenario begins.

Educator Preparation

The instructor reviews the Mosby skills and sets up the room with all supplies and equipment needed for the scenario.

Event Flow Data

The overall group size is 4 to 6 fourth semester senior nursing students. Two students participate in the scenario with one in the primary nurse role and the other as the secondary nurse. There are a total of 65 students in the course; each scenario lasts approximately 20 minutes.

Debriefing

Standardized plan for this patient includes open-ended questions, review of learning objectives, and performance. Performance includes knowledge, skills, and attitude items.

Evaluation of Event

The author observed this scenario and evaluated outcomes. As this was the first time the scenario was run, no formal grade was given to the students. The scenario ran very smoothly, and the students performed most of the critical events. Students generally became flustered with the constant retching and vomiting but are able to work through this distraction and critically think through the scenario.

Lessons Learned

It is great to have preprogrammed voices so that the instructor can focus on the scenario. However, students often ask questions that may not have appropriate responses recorded. They also have trouble talking to someone who isn't there; perhaps having a mother there with a script is better than the preprogrammed voice of the mother. The students were usually unsure how to handle the mother's refusal to sign the consent. Few want to call the surgeon. Prebriefing for better understanding of the surgical consent process is warranted.

Gerontology: Advancing Care Excellence for Alzheimer's Patients: George Palo

● ●

Susan Gross Forneris, PhD, RN, CNE, CHSE-A

● ●

Population

Prelicensure students as well as nurses in practice needing to enhance their skills/knowledge on care of the older adult with Alzheimer disease.

Performance Gap

This is a simulation scenario that is designed as an unfolding case. There are three scenarios that unfold to address knowledge gaps in the use of appropriate tools to assess cognition, depression, and physical and functional assessments. The scenarios also enhance communication and education skills to provide emotional and family support.

Learning Objectives

1. Assess and interpret the patient's physical and functional status, individual aging pattern, and emotional and cognitive status using the appropriate assessment tools (i.e., Confusion Assessment Method [CAM],

Mini-Cog, Brief Evaluation of Executive Dysfunction, Geriatric Depression Scale, and Katz).
2. Use updated Beers criteria to assess medications ordered for the patient.
3. Discuss appropriate criteria and resources to support maintaining patient independence.
4. Implement appropriate communication techniques and nursing interventions that meet patient safety needs and patient-centered care.

Performance Assessment

Each scenario has a detailed list of expected interventions and nursing behaviors that the student needs to demonstrate as evidence of achievement of the scenario-specific learning outcomes. As an example, in scenario 1, the student is to assess and interpret the patient's cognitive status. There are five expected interventions that are evaluated.

Scenario Synopsis

Synopsis of Patient Background and Case Stem

George Palo is a 90-year-old male who has been diagnosed with early-stage dementia. George's wife died 2 years ago, and one of his five children lives nearby. He resides in an independent living setting that allows him to keep his dog. His only health problem is medication-controlled high blood pressure. His family is supportive but concerned about his safety. He is stubborn, passionate about remaining independent, and adamant about never going to a nursing home. As George relates his story, he is unaware that he is getting more forgetful and often repeats himself.

Modality/Typology Selection and Rationale

The modality most used is the standardized patient. Mannequins can also be used. These unfolding cases require George to demonstrate both cognitive and functional deficits.

Fidelity Achievement

The medical record and props contain George's actual responses to the assessment to assist in the fidelity. These unfolding cases combine the power of storytelling with the experiential nature of simulation scenarios. Audiotaped monologue of George's story also accompanies this scenario.

Preparation

Learner Preparation

Orientation to program's home visit protocols; head-to-toe assessment. Become familiar with typical services provided in retirement housing facilities and other resources for older adults in the community. Read textbook and lecture notes on dementia, Alzheimer disease, and cognitive changes in older adults. Tools in the *Try This:®* and *How to Try This* Series are available on ConsultGeriRN.org (http://consultgerirn.org/resources). Specific tools recommended for this scenario are Confusion Assessment Method (CAM), Brief Evaluation of Executive Dysfunction tool, and SBAR or other standardized communication tool.

Educator Preparation

The ACE.Z educator toolkit provides additional ideas on how to use the monologue effectively as well as other strategies to prepare for engaging students in conversation on care of the older adult with Alzheimer disease (http://www.nln.org/professional-development-programs/teaching-resources/aging/ace-z/unfolding-cases/george-palo). Embedded in each scenario template are direct links to resources to assist faculty to enhance their knowledge base.

Event Flow Data

Approximately six to eight students participate per group. Two students can play the role of the nurse and secondary nurse. There are also the roles of George's daughter as well as the community health nurse. The remaining students can play the role of observers assessing whether QSEN competencies such as safety, patient-centered care, etc. are addressed and how during the scenario. The simulation runs for 20 minutes with at least a 45-minute debriefing session.

Debriefing

The debriefing questions are presented in two parts. There is a series of questions that were designed to discuss the simulation run in general with more specific guided questions for the facilitator/debriefer to cover the essential knowledge domains of care of the older adult. Debriefing questions (using ACES precepts) consider the following: assess function and expectations, coordinate and manage care, use evolving knowledge, and make situational decisions.

Evaluation of Event

These scenarios were piloted across the country to assure that the scenarios were realistic and easily implemented. The pilot results indicated that scenarios were engaging and realistic with valuable learning resources. The ACE Seniors scenarios have been used with students in a multisite study to determine whether the theory-based debriefing method—Debriefing for Meaningful Learning—would improve clinical reasoning skills (Forneris et al., 2015).

Lessons Learned

These series of unfolding cases and teaching strategies are designed to help the student become more proficient in understanding Alzheimer dementia as a disease process and the care management implications. Faculty and students who engaged in pilots of these simulations have found them engaging and a meaningful way to better educate our future nurses to care for a complex population.

● The Advancing Care Excellence series of simulations can be obtained at http://www.nln.org/centers-for-nursing-education/nln-center-for-excellence-in-the-care-of-vulnerable-populations.
● The ACE.Z simulation scenario specifically George Palo can be obtained at http://www.nln.org/professional-development-programs/teaching-resources/aging/ace-z/unfolding-cases/george-palo.

Critical Care

Intensive Care: Sepsis Patient with PEA Arrest

Penni I. Watts, PhD, RN

Jason L. Morris, MD, FACP

Summer Langston Powers, DNP, CRNP, ACNP-BC, AACC

Population

Prelicensure nursing students (can be interprofessional).

Performance Gap

Upper-level prelicensure students may not have the opportunity to care for an acutely declining patient in a busy critical care unit during their clinical rotations. Making quick decisions and working with the healthcare team to care for critically ill patients requires more than just technical skills; this simulation allows learners to apply what they have learned to a lifelike situation.

Learning Objectives

1. Collaborate with team members to manage care of complex clinical situation.
2. Describe strategies for dealing with a difficult team member.
3. Implement standards of practice for caring for a sepsis patient.

Performance Assessment

Expected to defuse team member conflict. Apply systemic inflammatory response syndrome (SIRS) protocol according to hospital policy.

Scenario Synopsis

Synopsis of the Patient Background
Ms. Barbara Walker was admitted 2 days ago from home with a 3-day history of worsening weakness and confusion.

Modality/Typology Selection and Rationale
Mannequin-based simulation due to skills involved and potential resuscitation measures needed (Fig. 23.4).

Fidelity Achievement
Use of a high-fidelity patient simulator

Preparation

Learner Preparation
There are no preparation activities as students come with what they know. Key briefing points included the following: general objectives of the experience (manage care of a critically ill patient); confidentiality of cases and performance of other learners; act as a newly licensed registered nurse; the embedded simulated participant (ESP) nurse will help verify mannequin responses and provide a link to diagnostic and laboratory results; and every learner comes to the simulation experience with the goal of providing better patient care.

Educator Preparation
Will have attended the institution's simulation courses and have attended a prebriefing and preparation session for the simulation. The ESP nurse will have been instructed on the case flow and level of learners. With senior-level nursing students, minimal support is needed except for environmental orientation, and delivery of diagnostic and laboratory test results.

Event Flow Data
Seventy to one hundred nursing students participate in this simulation that is part of a larger ICU interprofessional (IP) simulation. There are six simulated patients with approximately 12 assigned nurses (one is assigned a charge nurse role, another a float nurse role). Typically, this patient has two nurses assigned. Other participants may include a medical student and two residents or other professionals including respiratory therapy, physical therapy, nuclear medicine, laboratory, or physician assistant. The scenario lasts 15 minutes followed by a 45-minute debriefing.

Debriefing
Debriefing with good judgement and use of structured debriefing are used. Components include (1) reactions, (2) facts of the case, (3) preview of objectives, (4) analysis and investigating learners' frames, and (5) summary and wrap up.

Evaluation of Event
A general evaluation of the simulation was used to evaluate the event. Educator outcomes were to discover curricular areas that needed improvement related to critical thinking and crisis management as well as communicating within teams.

Lessons Learned
While many thought the mock ICU was too much for learners, they stepped up to the challenge. It is necessary to raise the complexity for our learners so they experience the stress and chaos of an ICU prior to real clinical practice. Also, with complex cases, details become more important to the realism. Ensure medical records, lab values, timing of events, physical assessment findings, and previous viral signs are accurate. Advanced learners expect these details when caring for complex patient situations.

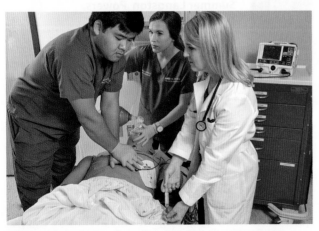

Figure 23.4 Caring for a Septic Patient in ICU. (From University of Alabama at Birmingham School of Nursing, with permission.)

Trauma/Emergency: Primary and Secondary Survey in the ER: The Importance of Assessment, Prioritization, and Clinical Management of the Trauma Patient

Catherine Bowman, MN, RN

Population

Fourth year nursing students in a senior nursing elective titled *Perspectives of Trauma and Injury* and postgraduate students or registered nurses participating in orientating to new clinical areas such as the emergency department.

Performance Gap

Many Canadians who survive traumatic injuries suffer long-term disability that impacts them physically, emotionally, socially, and economically. Rapid assessment and treatment of the trauma patient ensures that injuries are not missed and morbidity and mortality decreased.

Learning Objectives

1. Perform a primary survey and correctly identify all life-threatening conditions.
2. Perform a secondary survey and identify all underlying injuries sustained by the trauma patient.
3. Identify and demonstrate the application of clinical interventions necessary to treat life-threatening and non–life-threatening conditions.
4. Enact essential team management competencies within the scenario.

Performance Assessment

The criteria was created based on the Emergency Nurses Association Trauma Nursing Core Course resource (ENA, 2014) and includes universal precautions, general impression, safety, primary survey, secondary survey, reassessment, organization and delegation, verbal and written communication, and professionalism. The Trauma Performance Checklist is available in Toolkit 23-6.

Scenario Synopsis

Synopsis of the Patient Background

A 30-year-old male presents to the emergency department with right arm pain after falling from an all-terrain vehicle (ATV) 2 days ago. He has experienced increasing swelling and pain to his right upper extremity with some trouble breathing. His temperature, heart rate, and respiratory rate are elevated; his blood pressure and oxygen saturation are low.

Modality/Typology Selection and Rationale

A high-fidelity mannequin is used to heighten realism for this scenario, as it allows for students to perform a primary and secondary survey and identify specific assessment findings while allowing us to depict a progressively deteriorating patient.

Fidelity Achievement

Mannequin programming that can change depending on assessment and prioritization. Moulage of obviously deformed arm and pink frothy sputum. All necessary equipment that would be found in the emergency department.

Preparation

Learner Preparation

Classroom content and activities related to trauma management and musculoskeletal trauma.

Educator Preparation

This acute care scenario can quickly lead to systemic decompensation of the patient if the students fail to recognize key findings. The earlier the students can recognize and treat this patient, the less hemodynamically unstable he becomes. Therefore, it is vital that the educator have a solid understanding of assessment findings and underlying pathophysiology. An educator needs to be aware of key interventions that may result in improvement or further deterioration of the patient.

Event Flow Data

A team of three students, each with assigned roles with specific responsibilities. The initial primary and secondary surveys, including interventions, are run over 15 minutes. Reevaluation of assessment and interventions are done in the last 5 minutes for a total running time of 20 minutes. Debriefing is 40 minutes. Afterwards, a second run-through occurs, with the student's assigned different roles.

Debriefing

The Plus Delta Gamma debriefing model (Decker & Anderson, 2013), as well as Advocacy Inquiry (Rudolph, Simon, Rivard, Dufresne, & Raemer, 2007), was used to uncover the learners' perspectives about what went well, what could be enhanced next time around, and to identify what to base their plan for change on. Debriefing and teaching points include the following:

1. Which signs and symptoms were you most concerned about and why?
2. What laboratory and diagnostic procedures will help the trauma team determine a clinical diagnosis for this patient?
3. What clinical interventions will the patient require based on the patient's presentation?
4. Describe essential team management competencies that contribute to improved health outcomes for the patient.

Evaluation of Event

The first time the trauma scenario ran, the students were only given 2 minutes to complete the primary survey; however, they needed more exposure to this type of clinical scenario to complete the primary survey effectively. Subsequently, students were given 5 minutes, which was more appropriate for fourth year undergraduate nursing students.

Debriefing revealed many areas of student growth, specifically their ability to put clinical pieces together and begin to see the patient holistically, versus by separate body systems. They were able to connect assessment findings with the patients' clinical presentation, anticipate, and advocate for nursing and medical interventions with sound rationale. Watching confidence grow during subsequent running of the simulation, after they had identified their learning needs during debriefing, was empowering to witness as a faculty member.

Lessons Learned

High-fidelity simulation is a very stressful event for students and instructors alike. Ensuring students have adequate preparation for simulation is key in reducing their anxiety. However, when the synthesis of knowledge, skills, and attitudes is required in an unstable acutely ill patient scenario, it is very common for students to regress in their learning and perform somewhat unremarkably at first. Allowing them to debrief, reflect, and then repeat the scenario increases confidence, competence, and overall satisfaction with their performance.

Neonatal Intensive Care: Using Simulation as a Methodology for Implementing Bedside Report

Nikki Wiggins, MSN, RN, CCRN

Leslie Allen, MA

Note: Exemplar simulation designed as a result of Oregon Health and Sciences University's work on improving patient safety, affiliated with the Vermont Oxford Network.

Population

All neonatal intensive care unit RN and MD staff.

Performance Gap

We were required to implement bedside report and to incorporate family members who were present. RN staff had no experience giving report with families present as the unit had been closed during shift change. Staff frequently have to deliver or disclose information to families that can be uncomfortable or not routine. This can be confounded by family dynamics, and a heightened stress response due to the nature of having a baby in the NICU. There is no training specific to neonatal care that is available for staff regarding role-play and evaluation of delivery of information based on specific measurable criteria.

Learning Objectives

1. Simulate bedside report that is inclusive of parents using a standardized work format established by the institution.
2. Effectively use Family Conversation Simulation and Simulation Measurement tool during bedside report simulations.
3. Demonstrate empathetic listening, verbal and nonverbal communication as measured by the Simulation Measurement tool.
4. Reflect on performance based on measurement tool and feedback from family graduate standardized parent and educator.

Performance Assessment

Evaluate empathetic listening and verbal and nonverbal communication. Individual and group feedback from parent participants. Results of Simulation Measurement Tool (based on the Behavioral Assessment Tool) to assess performance of standardized bedside report of ICU patient. The Simulation Measurement Tool is within the Family Conversation Scenario Design Tool for Simulations (Toolkit 23-7).

Scenario Synopsis

Synopsis of the Patient Background

The scenarios were based on patients that the nurses had cared for in the previous 2 weeks.

Modality/Typology Selection and Rationale

Standardized parents were used as the focus on communication strategies and listening skills. The standardized parents provided feedback.

Fidelity Achievement

High fidelity was achieved through the use of standardized parents communicating about patients that the nurses had actually cared for. EPIC computers and charts were made available during simulations. Nurses participated in their regular role.

Preparation

Learner Preparation

Review of bedside report standard work description; recall of a recent patient. The Family Conversation Scenario Design Tool for Simulation is included in the Toolkit 23-7.

Educator Preparation

Special training regarding standardized workflow for bedside report from the institution prior to simulations.

Other Participant Preparation

Standardized parents become familiar with the demographics and variables specific to the family of the patient being reported upon. Careful consideration was given to use only graduate family members who had been out of the NICU for greater than 1 year. Additionally, families were asked about their comfort level with each scenario in recognition that there may be an emotional response if the situation was similar to their own experience.

Event Flow Data

One-hundred-and-twenty-two RNs participated in giving and receiving bedside report from one another. The simulations were completed in pairs with one or two standardized family members present and lasted approximately 10 minutes each.

Debriefing

Debriefing was completed after both RNs had given report to one another using a reaction, understanding, and summary debriefing model. Participants discussed their initial reactions to including families in bedside report, as well as their understanding of the standardized workflow, their scoring on the Simulation Measurement Tool, and how they would apply this learning to their practice when implementing bedside report in the NICU. Family participants gave feedback specifically about strategies for including families and specific ways to discuss difficult topics.

Evaluation of Event

Evaluations of the simulations were completed using a handwritten evaluation tool to score the effectiveness of the simulation and how applicable it was to each RN's practice. Specific areas for comments were made available. Evaluations and verbal feedback were overwhelmingly positive and indicated that realism was achieved. Staff had an increased level of comfort for implementing the bedside report process in the NICU following the simulations. Feedback from the graduate families proved to be invaluable.

Lessons Learned

Staff was initially skeptical and downplayed the value of simulating something nonclinical like bedside report. There was also concern about graduate family participants in the role of the standardized parent and worry that the simulations would be uncomfortable because of that. Furthermore, some staff speculated that realism would not be achieved in this nonclinical simulation. The biggest lesson learned was that you can simulate anything. Simulations should not just be limited to codes or the clinical setting.

Distributed Learning for Practicing Nurses: Care of the Critically Ill Patient Experiencing Liver Failure

Sandra Goldsworthy, PhD, RN, CCNCC(C), CMSN(C)

Population

Registered nurses enrolled in a critical care program. This scenario is targeted at nurses who are new and transitioning into critical care units. We have also had many experienced critical care nurses participate.

Performance Gap

Scenarios were designed to address foundational competencies required of nurses working in the intensive care unit (ICU). The scenarios are delivered with minor critical care cases (i.e., myocardial infarction) initially, leading to more complex major case scenarios such as septic shock and cardiogenic shock to allow for scaffolding of learning and mastery through repetition of each scenario.

Learning Objectives

1. Perform a focused assessment based on the patient's presenting status or change in the patient condition.
2. Recognize abnormal lab values related to liver failure.
3. Recognize and manage complications associated with liver failure.

A complete list of learning objectives can be found in Goldsworthy and Graham (2013).

Performance Assessment

Demonstrates safe management of pharmacologic agents, ability to accurately interpret arrhythmias and quickly recognize and prioritize the patient's deteriorating condition. Able to suggest anticipated ventilator changes based on arterial blood gas interpretation. The complete checklist can be found in Goldsworthy and Graham (2013).

Scenario Synopsis

Synopsis of the Patient Background
A 54-year-old disoriented male patient was admitted to the ICU 3 days ago experiencing loss of appetite, diarrhea, nausea, and vomiting. He has a 15-year history of alcoholism, 10-year history of chronic liver failure, and depression. He is hypotensive and hypoxic, with a markedly distended abdomen, scleral icterus, muscle weakness and tenderness, and palmar erythema.

Modality/Typology Selection and Rationale
High-fidelity patient simulator for realistic physiological portrayal of condition.

Fidelity Achievement
Use of ICU equipment including radial arterial line, triple lumen central line, and Foley catheter draining small amounts of light brown urine

Preparation

Learner Preparation
Provided with pretest questions prior to scenario

Educator Preparation
Standardized template is applied to all critical care scenarios (Goldsworthy & Graham, 2013).

Event Flow Data

Class size varied from 10 to 42 students. Scenarios were run in groups of three to five students per one to two instructors. The prebrief lasted 15 minutes, scenario 20 minutes, and debriefing 30 minutes. The final testing station groups consisted of two students and were 20 minutes in duration with no debriefing period. Feedback was provided at the end of the simulation module.

Debriefing

Combination of a number of established debriefing frameworks. Each debriefer had predeveloped posttest simulation questions and guided debriefing questions (with expected answers) to standardize the process and content of debriefing for each scenario. Debriefing and posttest simulation questions were intentionally linked to the learning objectives for the scenario.

Evaluation of Event

The critical care simulation program is evaluated by several measures. A critical care self-efficacy scale was developed and validated among critical care nurses participating in our simulation program (Goldsworthy, 2015). Other measures that were used included the Transfer of Learning Scale (Facteau, Dobbins, Russell, Ladd, & Kudisch, 1995).

Lessons Learned

Faculty development and direct "side-by-side" mentorship are critical to the standardized delivery of scenarios. Nine partner simulation labs deliver our program in their own communities. The educators traveled to our simulation lab to be mentored and to build their competence and confidence in the preparation, delivery, and debriefing of these complex scenarios. Ongoing communication between our "hub" sim center and the nine partner labs continues. Also, repetition of scenarios is important. When participants had the opportunity to repeat each scenario, they reported that this increased their confidence and gave them an opportunity to improve their performance and master the beginning-level critical care competencies. Building or scaffolding the learning by including critical care skills stations was also reported by the students to be very helpful in building their confidence. Beginning with minor cases and advancing to complex scenarios also built confidence.

Graduate Studies

Nurse Practitioner Simulation: The EBOLA Pandemic: A Virtual Mentored Practice Experience

Linda C. Carl, EdD, MSN, RN

Dee McGonigle, PhD, RN, CNE, FAAN, ANEF

Debra L. Duncan, BS, MLS

Paul Woodcock

Population

Students enrolled in the informatics, executive, education, and public policy Master of Science in nursing program specialty tracks, faculty mentors, and virtual world designers.

Performance Gap

The 2014 Ebola pandemic demonstrated a performance gap in managing communicable disease transmission and elevated the need for a protected virtual learning environment (VLE).

Learning Objectives

1. Script a virtual interprofessional pandemic disaster practice scenario.
2. Create self-regulated student debriefing evaluation criteria.

3. Analyze a pandemic disaster practice experience using the DIKW (data, information, knowledge, wisdom) virtual, clinical education model.
4. Describe any effect a virtual pandemic disaster practice scenario has on interprofessional team learning outcomes.

Performance Assessment

The following performance assessment strategies are used for formative and summative assessment: prospective, direct observation by faculty mentor; retrospective, scripted simulation video reviews; self-regulated student evaluation; student-led weekly planning and evaluation meetings with mentor and team; student-led postsimulation clinical debriefing; and one-to-one faculty–student virtual communication feedback meetings at the beginning, middle, and end of the practice experience.

Scenario Synopsis

Synopsis of the Patient Background

The Ebola Treatment, Teaching, and Learning Center provides a protected, interactive environment where students, faculty, and virtual world designers create, build, script, simulate, and demonstrate real-world public policy, best practices, and protocols, in real-world time (Fig. 23.5).

Modality/Typology Selection and Rationale

A VLE provides realistic, real-time, real-world practice experiences that can be simulated at the time a disaster or crisis occurs. Students are in a safe, controlled, intentional learning environment.

Fidelity Achievement

The experience uses 3D scripted avatars in a simulated Ebola pandemic VLE. The pandemic scripted simulation is driven by daily and current events so that the simulation mimics clinical practice as a team in the real world. The experience is designed to include the panic, chaos, disruption, and ethical issues that occur in practice in spite of standards and best practices.

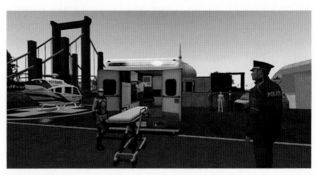

Figure 23.5 Ebola Prehospital Care Design in Second Life.

Preparation

Learner Preparation

Participate in VLE orientation to practice the art of avatar puppeteering skills, establish weekly meetings, appoint a student project manager, and create a scripted, pandemic scenario and project proposal with realistic milestones and timeline. The simulation script is studied and followed during the videotaped simulation.

Educator Preparation

Mentors participate in orientation as well. Student and faculty watch multiple news broadcasts and Internet searches of current events to prepare for daily disruptive changes to incorporate.

Event Flow Data

A faculty mentor, two to four students with scripted roles, and one to two VLE support personnel are in a group. This multiplies if students from different program tracks are also involved. Complex experiences may require more support personnel if new infrastructure is required. Interprofessional simulations may involve 8 to 10 students with four faculty; numbers vary based on the design of the experience. There is a 10-minute prebrief, followed by a 30-minute scripted scenario, ending with critical debriefing for 60 minutes.

Debriefing

Student-led debriefings of the video and learning experiences occur weekly, using a self-regulated student evaluation model, and reported to the mentor during each meeting. Verbal evaluation data are used to drive change in teaching and student-learning strategies implemented the next day.

Evaluation of Event

Debriefing is the core of the evaluation process used to drive change in learning objectives and to redirect student learning during the practice experience. Evaluation data can be collected by administering weekly meeting and simulation debriefing surveys to engage formative assessment and then analyzed as a faculty–student team. Individualized learning is assessed by the faculty mentor through direct observation during the experience and at the start, midterm, and end of the practice experience using virtual communication modalities.

Lessons Learned

3D virtual simulation can be successfully used to engage students in higher-order thinking; in global, cultural competence; and in public health and public policy health mandates. A VLE can build trust and topic expert confidence; teach real-world, real-time change in clinical standards and best practices; and deliver complex content

that can be assessed using a competency-based education model in a safe robust, fun, and effective learning environment that can be accessed globally.

Leadership/Management

Prioritization and Delegation Utilizing vSim

Sarah Lynn-Sells Lambert, MEd, BSN, RN

Population

Prelicensure nursing students.

Performance Gap

Challenges exist in providing clinical opportunities to nursing students for the development of the leadership skills of prioritizing and delegating patient care.

Learning Objectives

In prelicensure nursing students:

1. Enhance the knowledge, skills, and attitudes of prioritization and delegation in delivering safe patient care.
2. Enable autonomous action in the decision-making process of prioritizing, delegating, and delivering safe patient care with multiple virtual adult medical–surgical patients.

Performance Assessment

Participation in 100% of the 4-hour simulation experience, evaluated satisfactory or unsatisfactory; individual submission of the DocuCare assignment postsimulation; and individual response submission to "You are the only RN caring for the three patients, how would you prioritize the care?" and "You have an unlicensed assistive person (UAP) working with you; what would you delegate to the UAP?"

Scenario Synopsis

Synopsis of the Patient Background
All adult medical–surgical patients available on vSim.

Modality/Typology Selection and Rationale
Virtual patients chosen to broaden opportunity to make decisions related to prioritization and delegation; low and medium fidelity for interventions and procedures (Fig. 23.6).

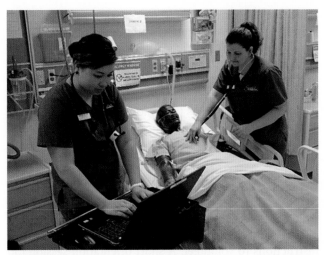

Figure 23.6 Hybrid Simulation Using vSim and Mannequins. (Courtesy of Sandhills Community College, with permission.)

Fidelity Achievement

Virtual via individual laptops, IV arm task trainers for any IV activity, medium-fidelity simulators for medication administration (other than IV), blood glucose check, urinary catheterization, oxygen application, tracheostomy suctioning/care, dressing change, and NGT insertion.

Preparation

Learner Preparation

Each student was asked to bring a laptop capable of accessing vSim. Students were paired and could decide what professional resources and texts to have available during the simulation. Three patients were randomly drawn from those available on the vSim program.

Educator Preparation

The schedule of activities was written on a flip chart. Expectations, objectives, location of supplies, and room setup were all provided. Students were informed that all scenarios would be launched simultaneously. "Pause" activities were written on a flip chart for each pair of students to view throughout the simulation. Each completed the adult medical–surgical vSim patient scenario and prepared Student Information sheet for using vSim. A third laptop was available for each pair of students to access the third patient.

Event Flow Data

Twelve students were in the group. Each pair of students worked with three vSim patients over a 4-hour time frame.

Debriefing

Dreifuerst's Debriefing for Meaningful Learning (Dreifuerst, 2011) and Tanner's Clinical Judgement Model (Tanner, 2006) informed the debriefing.

Evaluation of Event

The pilot group of students who had access to vSim for two semesters achieved a higher raw mean score on the HESI exam than their counterparts who had no or limited access (0.5 semester), but the difference was not statistically significant. Every student in the pilot group was positive in postactivity comments, and each one expressed a desire to have another opportunity to participate in a follow-up simulation utilizing vSim.

Lessons Learned

Plan for additional time to use the vSim tutorial. Consider using one of the adult vSim medical–surgical patients as the practice patient for each pair of students to become accustomed to the program and where to locate the nursing actions under the specific tabs. Although the Student Information sheet had this information, most of the students forgot to use the sheet. Remind the students that communication with the vSim patient is based on the program's preloaded questions.

Community

Missouri Community Action Poverty Simulation©

Teresa Boese, DNP, RN

Marion Donohoe, DNP, APRN, CPNP-PC

Population

Community leaders, advocates, policy makers, students, and organizations. The following discussion focuses on the use of this simulation with nursing and healthcare professionals.

Performance Gap

Caring for persons living with limited resources is a challenge for undergraduate nursing and other health professional students in part because of a lack of awareness, understanding, and experience of patients' daily struggles. Developing trust and probing gently to learn a person's concerns and vulnerabilities requires an awareness of the world in which one lives.

Learning Objectives

1. Become aware of everyday realities facing low-income people.
2. Comprehend what living in a low-income family may be like.
3. Demonstrate patient-centered communication in the course of collaboration with people living in poverty.

Performance Assessment

Pre–/post–self-assessment for participants focused on attitudes toward people with low income. This assessment tool that measures change is provided as part of the purchased Poverty Simulation Kit.

Scenario Synopsis

Synopsis of the Patient Background

Participants role-play a month in the life of low-income families, from single parents trying to care for their children to senior citizens trying to maintain their self-sufficiency on Social Security.

Modality/Typology Selection and Rationale

Volunteers (faculty and community members) play the roles of staff workers at various resources, which are businesses and agencies found in any community such as a food store, a bank, a utility company, a daycare, a school, and an employment agency (Fig. 23.7). Role-play promotes personal communication. There are no mannequins or standardized patients.

Fidelity Achievement

This is a low-fidelity simulation. While the stories of the low-income families are based on real cases, the environment in which the simulation is run represents the actual setting where low-income people live.

Preparation

Learner Preparation

No special preparation is necessary on the part of the learner.

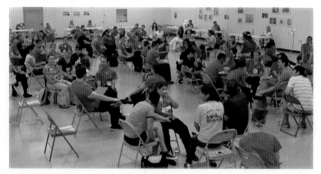

Figure 23.7 Poverty Simulation Scope of Simulation Activity.

Educator Preparation

Attend the facilitator training provided by the Missouri Association for Community Action if possible. This provides an opportunity for the educator to participate in the simulation and become familiar with all aspects of both participation and management of this simulation. The Poverty Simulation Kit comes with all props (play money, signs, name badges, etc.) and packets of materials needed. A DVD with files of all materials that might need to be replaced comes in the kit.

Preparation of Others

Depending on number of participants, 18 to 20 volunteers are needed to staff the resource tables. These volunteers need to be recruited (may be faculty or community volunteers) and trained in their roles. Assign roles and send instructions to volunteer. A short orientation session (30 to 40 minutes) before the simulation will serve to familiarize the volunteers and answer any questions.

Event Flow Data

The minimum number of participants is 25; the maximum is 88. All participants are active in the simulation at the same time. A room that has approximately 3,000 square feet is needed to accommodate all participants and resources. Timing is important for this simulation. Every 10 minutes, an overview is provided. Students read a packet of family information and receive instructions. A whistle is used to keep time and begins each 15-minute week, which is followed by 2-minute weekends for 4 weeks. During the week, participants use their money and resources to manage their family needs. Following this, a debriefing occurs.

Debriefing

Debriefing gives participants time to reflect and then share their experiences and emotions related to their month living in poverty. Numerous questions are suggested by MACA and focus on feelings, attitude change, function of families and meeting their needs, mutual help, child's perspective, and insight into how to change perception of low-income people.

Evaluation of Event

No formal evaluation tool is provided by MACA. However, it is important to gather data from participants related to the educational and behavioral strengths and weaknesses of the simulation event. Query participants via written or electronic means. A formal evaluation tool for the simulation has been developed according to INACSL guidelines.

Lessons Learned

The Community Action Poverty Simulation is a time- and labor-intensive event to manage. It is helpful to have a dedicated team (five or more) to organize and direct the simulation. It takes 8 hours for one faculty to review and prepare the kit before an event. Ten persons are needed for 1 hour to prepare the room for the event, and it takes four people 2 hours to repackage the kit after a simulation.

High School/Summer Camper Health and Dietary Considerations

Desiree A. Díaz, PhD, RN-BC, CNE, CHSE-A

Robin June Miller, PhD, RN, CNE

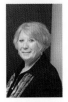

E. Carol Polifroni, EdD, RN, CNE, NEA-BC, ANEF

Population

Undergraduate and accelerated second-degree students during a pediatric rotation mentoring prenursing high school students. The scenario takes place during the university-hosted summer soccer camp program when approximately 330 campers per week are on the campus.

Performance Gap

The performance gap that is addressed in the simulation is similar to mock code blue in the hospitals. Students have been trained on emergency procedure; however, they are never able to practice without prior knowledge of an event or until something actually happens.

Learning Objectives

1. Recognize immediate signs of anaphylaxis.
2. Initiate safety protocols such as 911 activation and assessment of camper and scene (e.g., nut or potential allergy on camper meal tray).
3. Effectively communicate with the camper, interdisciplinary team, and head nurse.
4. Recognize proper protocols and chain of command while communicating effectively in a TeamSTEPPS approach and conducting handoffs using SBAR.

Performance Assessment

Performance assessment included the initial treatment only. The main focus was in the recognition of the life-threatening situation of anaphylaxis of a camper in a defined population that the learners were responsible for. A faculty member observes the scenario, which is being recorded.

Scenario Synopsis

Synopsis of the Patient Background

Nursing students are responsible for documenting and communicating food allergies, possession of EpiPens, diabetic diagnoses and insulin needs, and special dietary needs of the campers. During a meal in the Student Union food court, surrounded by members of the university community (not involved in the simulation), a standardized patient (SP) portrays an anaphylactic reaction to a known nut allergy (Fig. 23.8). The scripted SP role is performed by a high school prenursing student.

Modality/Typology Selection and Rationale

The SP's ability to act increases the high-stakes nature of the experience.

Fidelity Achievement

Placing the simulation in a common area of the university during normal daily activities promoted realism and allowed for involvement of dietary aides and other diners. All were aware that a simulation was in progress.

Preparation

Learner Preparation

CPR for the professional rescuer, community health scenarios, and preparation with emergent situations in school health and community settings. Standing orders, laws pertaining to allergies in the school setting, and American Academy of Pediatrics' recommendations for nut allergies were reviewed.

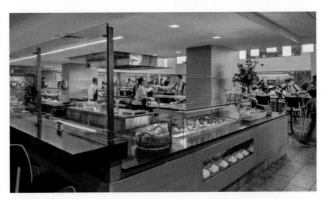

Figure 23.8 Site of Anaphylactic Reaction to Food Item.

Educator Preparation

Faculty are all CPR for healthcare provider trained. Preparation regarding emergent treatment for anaphylaxis reaction reviewed with standing orders and Academy of Pediatrics' recommendations.

Preparation of Others

Discussion with observers prior to the event with an explanation that a training activity would ensue much like that of lifeguard training. SP preparation for the high school students includes basic knowledge of CPR, allergic reactions, and signs of a beginning allergic reaction.

Event Flow Data

An entire clinical group of 10 students participated in the simulation. The group was eating lunch with the five high school students when the scenario occurred. The scenario is completed in real time providing resources based on crisis resource management (CRM) principles. The simulation lasted 15 minutes with the debrief lasting approximately 45 minutes.

Debriefing

Debriefing for Meaningful Learning (DML) (Dreifuerst, 2011) was used to explore actions within the scenario as well as what is appropriate in other situations. Students are asked to reflect on their actions from the simulation. The dietary aides, the servers, the cashiers, and the community members who just happened to be in the Student Union at the time of the simulation all spoke of bearing witness to feeling scared, not sure what do, but also comforted by the action of the nursing students and knowing it was a simulation.

Evaluation of Event

High school students with an interest in healthcare experience the patient role and see the nursing role from a patient's viewpoint. The community partners are active in the student learning process and also educated on the potential for anaphylactic reaction in daily life. Based on 2 years of evaluations, all individuals value the opportunity. The students learn that critical thinking is based on knowledge but also common sense. They learn that they are the nursing student in all settings not just when they "are on duty." There is a reasonable expectation to act, and this expectation is tested when students are not thinking they are in a school or educational situation.

Lessons Learned

It is important to have realism, with the public watching the event, but also to protect the learner. Conducting the simulation when there are fewer people in the union would minimize the observers and decrease the risk of someone calling 911 inadvertently. The faculty member is critical to the simulation, knowing when to intervene or let the experience evolve. The videographer needs to maintain calm and distance throughout, as the video is a critically important aspect of the debriefing.

Advancing Care Excellence for Veterans (ACE-V) Simulated Clinical Day Replacement

Maureen Tremel, MSN, ARNP, CNE, CHSE-A, ANEF

Sharon Saidi, MSN, RN, CNE

Rita Swanson, BSN, RN

Marguerite Abel, MSN, RN

Note: Maureen Tremel passed away on August 6, 2016, after a distinguished career in nursing. Maureen was a Nursing Professor and faculty member at Seminole State College of Florida, Altamonte Springs, Florida, since 1986. She was recognized as an amazing role model and mentor for innovation in teaching and learning. She was a tireless advocate for simulation at local, national, and international levels. She helped to establish the Florida Healthcare Simulation Alliance, participated in the NLN Advancing Care Excellence for Veterans simulations pilot, and led innumerable other simulation initiatives. Maureen made a sustained and significant contribution to nursing simulation through her creative vision and her quest for excellence. The many people that knew, loved, and admired her will miss her and we are pleased to have honored Maureen through her contribution to this book.

This work was supported by a Florida Blue Foundation Grant.

Population

Basic medical–surgical nursing course in prelicensure Associate Degree nursing program.

Performance Gap

Florida, as well as the rest of the United States, has an increasing problem with homelessness, particularly with the veteran population. The ACE-V unfolding cases were developed by the National League for Nursing (NLN) to support the White House Joining Forces Project. The NLN ACE-V Butch Sampson case provides an effective replacement for a traditional clinical day. The entire simulation toolkit is available free of charge on the NLN website (NLN, 2015c).

Learning Objectives

1. Demonstrate knowledge of disease process and patient care needs for type 2 diabetes mellitus (DM) and connection to military service.
2. Deliver prescribed medications and treatments to veteran hospitalized for complications of type 2 DM.
3. Employ therapeutic communication skills, which take into consideration the military culture.
4. Consider individual needs of homeless veteran when planning discharge teaching and follow-up home care.

Performance Assessment

Several presimulation assessments were completed including the Military Cultural Self-Assessment, the Student Preconception of Simulated Clinical Day survey, Presimulation Planning Record, and a Simulation Pretest. Postsimulation assessments included a Simulation Posttest, Postsimulation Reflections, Postsimulation Student Perception Survey.

Scenario Synopsis

Synopsis of the Patient Background

A chronically homeless Vietnam veteran with type 2 diabetes, related to Agent Orange exposure, has a wound on his foot that he has examined at a free clinic (Fig. 23.9). He provides his history and story to the student nurse at the clinic. He is assessed, referred to a local hospital for treatment, and provided with discharge education and resources including a place to stay; however, he is having a difficult time complying with treatment regimens and restrictions regarding smoking and alcohol expected of houseguests.

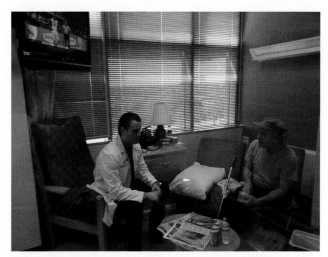

Figure 23.9 Interaction with Standardized Actor Portraying a Veteran.

Modality/Typology Selection and Rationale

Hybrid simulation using trained standardized patients (SP) combined with task trainers and props was chosen to achieve the desired fidelity.

Fidelity Achievement

Two SPs with varied acting experience, who were actually Vietnam veterans about the same age as Butch, were hired and trained.

Preparation

Learner Preparation

Students were given links to various web resources, documents, and videos regarding veterans' issues, homelessness, and DM. They synthesized the information by completing the Presimulation Planning Worksheet. Prebriefing was conducted.

Educator Preparation

Experienced simulationists provided clinical lab staff with directions for setup and conducted an orientation session with clinical faculty to review skill practice sessions, the flow of scenarios, student assignments, and basic principles of debriefing method. A facilitator's guidebook was compiled. Clinical faculty participated in a run-through of all scenarios.

Standardized Patient Preparation

Reviewed storyboard and expected student performance. The SPs collaborated on character development, their roles, and responsibility for delivery of monologue. They participated in a run-through of scenarios.

Event Flow Data

There were 7 to 10 students per group. The educator team consisted of two nurse simulationists and four clinical instructors. Students reviewed skills specific to the scenarios in a structured skills practice session. Patient care for each of the three scenarios was divided into three to four individual student assignments (15 minutes). Clinical faculty observed the performance but allowed students autonomy in decision-making. Students not assigned to active roles in a scenario watched their peers via a webcast projected to a conference room and recorded observations on an observer worksheet.

Debriefing

The three dimensions of Element 3 of the Debriefing Assessment for Simulation in Healthcare (DASH) (Rudolph, Raemer, & Simon, 2014) tool served as the framework for the debriefing plan. Students were asked to express their reactions to the simulation, followed by a review of scenario objectives and analysis of students' performance. Clinical instructors used the advocacy inquiry approach promoted in the Debriefing with Good Judgement method to elicit students' mental models and rationales for actions through each patient care assignment (Rudolph et al., 2007). Each session concluded with a summary and projected application of learning.

Evaluation of Event

Postsimulation surveys indicated clinical objectives were met; overall, second semester students did not want to decrease the time they spent in the hospital. Students felt the use of a live patient actor increased the realism of simulation and the ACE-V case enhanced their understanding of challenges facing the veteran population. Pre- and posttests showed improvement but scores were lower than desired. Written post-simulation reflections revealed personal insight toward development of cultural competence caring for military veterans and the homeless.

Lessons Learned

Online links to resources provide a wealth of information but may be difficult for novice students to navigate and recall the most important information. A reading guide or narrated presentation to use while visiting websites would help direct attention to the critical information. Space may be a concern. Conducting the on-campus clinical on the weekend posed no scheduling problems; however, scheduling during busier weekdays will require advance planning.

End of Program Evaluation

Case Management 1:1

Kathy Carver, MN, RN

Rochelle Quinn, MSN, RN, CHSE

Mindy Ritter, MS, RN, CEN

Timothy J. Laughlin, BA, CHSOS

Population

Undergraduate, last semester.

Performance Gap

This simulation evaluates program outcomes by comparing simulation-based performance to clinical-based performance. Students are not evaluated as part of their course criteria. The intent of this final simulation was to provide additional data that students had achieved end of program objectives. These scenarios were not intended to grade or evaluate individual students but to look at the class statistics as a group.

Learning Objectives

1. Assessment: With proficiency, systematically collect and evaluate significance of data pertinent to the patient's health or situation.
2. Implementation: Independently deliver safe and efficient care, based on changing patient needs.
3. Therapeutic Communication: Compassionately perform therapeutic communication skills during an emergent patient care change.
4. Professional/Team Role: Report information accurately using appropriate terminology in SBAR format.

Performance Assessment

Data from each student are scored using a 20-point Case Management Rubric (Toolkit 23-8) focusing on both assessment and interventions performed during the scenario, but we added the postsimulation verbalization of their thought process. We asked three questions to illicit their clinical reasoning. Additional data that could be analyzed: video of each simulation and debriefing, SBAR documentation included during simulation, clinical evaluation, and final exam and ATI NCLEX predictor score.

Scenario Synopsis

Synopsis of the Patient Background

Four different patient problems were used; hypoglycemic event with IV insulin administration, new onset of chest pain postoperatively, sepsis with pneumonia, and alcohol withdrawal seizure. Scenario details are located in Toolkit 23-9.

Modality/Typology Selection and Rationale

All patients were mannequin-based for consistency.

Fidelity Achievement

Realistic setup, medication, and nursing orders.

Preparation

Learner Preparation

Student orientation details for Case Management include the timeline, type of mannequin, objectives, and details of the simulation. Patient information is not provided prior to the simulation. All prior scenarios have preparation required. Since this simulation was to assess for level of critical thinking and performance, students had to rely of previously learned information and skills.

Educator Preparation

Scenario details, setup, report, and all patient information provided for instructors are located in the Toolkit 23-9.

Event Flow Data

Students have completed similar simulation scenarios during the previous semesters. Each student is randomly assigned one of four possible patient scenarios and will complete this 1:1 with a facilitator. The scenario lasts 1 hour including review of simulation details (5 minutes), chart review, report, and MAR review (10 minutes), patient care (10 minutes), complete SBAR on chart (5 minutes), and debrief (15 minutes).

Debriefing

During the debrief, all students were asked the same three questions to elicit perception and understanding: priority concerns, why is the problem occurring, and what needs to be done. Debriefing reflection contributes to the overall evaluation of clinical judgement. The 1:1 debriefing was completed with an informal format that included one video clip. Students overwhelmingly preferred this type of debrief with the instructor compared to clinical group size debriefings. Comments centered on the individualized learning, and they requested to repeat this type of simulation format and to do it sooner in the curriculum.

Evaluation of Event

Students evaluate simulation using a Likert scale, with additional comment options. The scenario evaluation form is found in Toolkit 23-10. Not one student wanted to delete this simulation scenario and format. Students express anxiety prior to the experience so these evaluations were a surprise outcome. A review of student performance data supported our intuitive conclusions that we were seeing a difference in student performance and clinical judgement. The mean score and variance of student performance demonstrated achievement of program outcomes. We are encouraged by the fact that 90% the students were performing consistently at the same level—and did not have students struggling to assume the RN role as reflected by the tight variance.

Lessons Learned

Faculty were evaluating if this format should continue. Students were 100% in favor of this format and 1:1 debriefing; however, faculty were ready to let go of the scenario. The time is exhaustive for faculty. To accommodate 72 students, five total faculty are involved for a total of 24 hours. Training additional faculty would be advisable. Timing of this needs to be carefully considered and should be in the last semester. Students know that they are not graded but are still anxious about completing the scenario. It is also vital to pilot the scenario with all involved faculty for validity.

Unique Experiences

Lauren's Blog

Cynthia M. Thomas, EdD, MS, BSN, RNC

Population

Lauren's Blog is an interactive, narrative-based online simulation used as an independent teaching/learning strategy for prelicensure undergraduate nursing students in a baccalaureate program. Lauren is a "virtual new graduate nurse" that blogs about her clinical experiences. This nontraditional simulation approach requires that students engage and respond in blog form to Lauren's personal narratives throughout an entire semester.

Performance Gap

Newly licensed registered nurses experience difficulty transitioning from student to professional nurse role. New nurses often experience difficulty working within a team, using critical thinking and problem-solving strategies, communicating with other team members including physicians, and seeing the "big picture."

Learning Objectives

1. Cultivate quality and safety strategies by expanding critical thinking skills.
2. Improve problem-solving and prioritizing skills.
3. Develop better communication strategies and foster the value of working within a team concept.

Performance Assessment

The intent of the simulation is to help students transition to the professional registered nurse role. Specific questions based on each blog topic are presented. Students are required to thoughtfully respond to other student's postings. All 18 blogs must be completed for a passing grade of 100 points. If faculty believe the students do not understand a specific concept being addressed, they respond to the post or further address in class.

Scenario Synopsis

Synopsis of the Patient Background
Lauren is a 24-year-old new registered nurse embarking on her first career opportunity. Students receive information about her family, living situation, personality, and relationships.

Modality/Typology Selection and Rationale
Blogging is a common method of communicating electronically. Using this method provides a way for learners to communicate and learn more about the transition to practicing nurse in a way they wouldn't while using traditional teaching strategies such as interviewing a nurse.

Fidelity Achievement
The blog is comprised of topics directly related to the activities, thoughts, and feelings that a new nurse might have.

Sample Blog Portion: Friday
This was not a good day. I was supposed to work with Karen who has been an RN for 5 years, but Karen called in sick so I was placed with Alice. Alice has been there for 30 years. Can you believe that? She has been in the same hospital for 30 years. I heard that she is stuck in the 1900s, avoids the computer, and is always the last person to accept changes. Alice watches my every move. She's driving me crazy already. I realize I am a new nurse, but I believe I am well prepared to accept the challenges. Anyway, I just got so tired of her checking on me so I told her that I really didn't need this much help, and I would come and get her if I needed anything. I started out with three patients this morning, and I was supposed to get the first admit—Mrs. Brock, a breast cancer patient. I got the room ready then everything started to fall apart. One of my other patients started vomiting. While I was cleaning her up, Mrs. Brock arrived on the unit. The transporter just put her in the room and didn't tell me. How was I supposed to know that she was there? Well, to make a long story short, she fell on the floor trying to get to the bathroom because she was having diarrhea. Alice helped me complete the incident report, assess the patient, and I hate to admit this, but Alice apologized to the husband and took the blame herself. She actually defended me. Can you believe that, after the way I treated her this morning, she still defended me. Maybe I have misjudged Alice. I cried all the way home. I just feel awful.

Questions
How could this incident have been avoided? What could Lauren have done differently? What do you think about Alice's approach to the incident?

Preparation

Learner Preparation
Faculty lecture on blog topics in the classroom prior to each blog assignment. Students are expected to read textbook chapters that correspond to the blog topics and review online and in class lecture notes prior to completing each blog assignment.

Educator Preparation
The course faculty continually update the blog based on current research and trends in nursing and healthcare.

Event Flow Data

Average class size varies from 47 to 100. Students are provided a specific date for assignment completion on the course calendar. On average, it may take 30 minutes to

1 hour for a student to complete the assigned set of blogs for the week.

Debriefing

Since Lauren's Blog is an online independent simulation, debriefing is accomplished through individual and group responses by the course faculty. The intent of the faculty response is to reinforce correct or appropriate thinking and to correct any misinterpretation of a concept presented in the blog. If faculty identify that a large percent of the students do not understand a concept, faculty will do an additional lecture on the topic.

Evaluation of Event

The evaluation is ongoing for the faculty to make appropriate updates to the blog and to ensure students understand specific concepts being presented. Students complete a final evaluation at the end of the blog assignment.

Lessons Learned

We learned very early on that students do not like to read common slang language, as if Lauren was actually talking to them. The blog was written from the perspective of a young 24-year-old new registered nurse so we intentionally did not use correct grammar and punctuation. However, we had complaints from the students and eventually had to go back and make the corrections. Older students do not always identify with a 24-year-old new nurse but understand that they may be working with one; therefore, older students may respond to the questions from that perspective.

A 12-Hour Night Shift Simulation Event

Holldrid Odreman, PhD, MScN-Ed, RN

Population

Student nurses from different levels in the nursing program; medical students.

Performance Gap

Current clinical placements do not offer 12-hour night shift experiences, so learners do not know how they will function emotionally, cognitively, and physically for that period of time.

Learning Objectives

1. Witness mentors engage in meaningful communication with simulated patients, peers, and medical students.
2. Experience increased learning and self-efficacy when providing nursing care.
3. Prioritize patient needs.
4. Verbalize the experience of professional and personal self-discovery.

Performance Assessment

The goal was practice of clinical skills and use of knowledge without fear of evaluation, to be allowed to make mistakes and learn from them, and to increase confidence in knowledge and skills without pressure or stress of performance.

Scenario Synopsis

Synopsis of the Patient Background

Type A businessman, reluctant to comply 2 days following appendectomy; several patients with minor or no health issues; a critically ill patient that required transfer to the ICU.

Modality/Typology Selection and Rationale

Two high-fidelity mannequins so that changes in condition can be controlled. Two standardized patients (SP) to enhance communication and family support. Volunteer patients for communication opportunities.

Fidelity Achievement

Props and decorations to furnish the lab as a real hospital medical–surgical ward (Fig. 23.10).

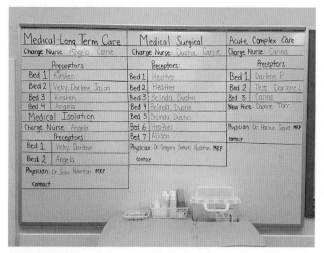

Figure 23.10 Assignment board reflecting assignments for the shift-long simulation activity.

Preparation

Learner Preparation

Before the experience, nursing and medical students are given information about their simulated patient assignments, including medical history and 12 hours of prior nursing documentation. They are also given a list of expected clinical skills for the night shift routine to review.

Educator Preparation

The simulationist guides the experience by providing cues to the actors and medical students to guide their responses.

Preparation of Others

Support staff, standardized patient actors, and volunteers have 1:1 meetings to review expectations for their role and to learn the overall idea of the simulation, objectives, and goals.

Event Flow Data

Eleven practical nursing students had roles of consolidation (capstone experience) or preceptored student nurses; four support staff played the role of nurse preceptors. Two medical students portrayed medical residents. Two standardized patient actors and 10 additional volunteers played the role of ward patients. Midway through the 12-hour event, a 1-hour debriefing was held (3 AM) and again at the end of the simulation shift when a report was given to the person portraying the day shift charge nurse.

Debriefing

All participants in the event participated as a group to share experiences and feelings based on their interactions with one another. The questions focused on what went well and what did not, importance of observing mentors perform skills and respond to difficult situations, to what degree communication skills have improved, and the potential of this experience to inform future practice.

Evaluation of Event

A survey asked what students had learned about night shift work, the greatest concerns night nurses have, how they physically felt, strategies they used to stay awake, and how well pre-identified goals were met. Surveys showed that the simulation event and the simulation environment were well received. Furthermore, surveys showed an increase in students' perception of self-confidence after the simulation experience while the interaction with nurse preceptors, patient actors, volunteers, and the use of high-fidelity mannequins enhanced the overall learning of each student nurse. Nurse preceptors expressed a sense of pride to witness the growth in confidence of learners from the time

that the simulation event started to the time of the structured debriefing. Finally, all participants expressed a sense of transformation in their experience, attributed to the numerous times of meaningful communication between learners and nurse preceptors, nursing students and medical students, and learners and simulation patients.

Lessons Learned

Due to the positive feedback from each participant, a similar simulation event involving more students from different healthcare programs was planned for the following academic year. The goal is to continue to provide meaningful simulation events that inform the practice of nursing and allied healthcare students so that they are equipped with the academic and professional skills to effect positive social changes within healthcare.

Live Broadcasting Simulation in the Classroom

Dustin Chan, BScN, RN

Brandi Pawliuk, MN(MH), BScN, RN, CPMHN(C)

Jillian Thomas, BScN, RN, CPMHN(C)

Population

Undergraduate nursing students enrolled in a psychiatric nursing theory block.

Performance Gap

Created a high-fidelity classroom broadcasting simulation experience to augment existing theory and traditional and simulation lab experiences (Fig. 23.11).

Learning Objectives

1. Formulate and implement a plan of care for four clients with diverse medical–surgical needs.

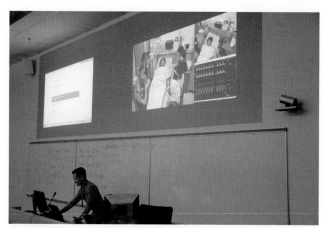

Figure 23.11 Broadcasting the Simulation Suite into the Classroom.

2. Identify the possible causes of respiratory dysfunction in four patient scenarios.
3. Manage the nursing care of the patient with respiratory distress secondary to chest tube dysfunction, asthma, and COPD.
4. Employ therapeutic communication strategies in the care of the psychiatric patient.

Performance Assessment

The students were expected to carry forward therapeutic communication from a previous mental health course and apply that in this simulation. Formative assessment of their prior knowledge and review of mental health disorders used in this simulation was expected.

Scenario Synopsis

Synopsis of the Patient Background

Two patients involve surgical trauma patients with chest tubes, while the other two are medical patients with lung disease. All scenarios begin with a decline in respiratory status. Each patient is also experiencing a mental health issue.

Modality/Typology Selection and Rationale

High-fidelity simulators were chosen to best exemplify the physiological changes that occur with patient deterioration.

Fidelity Achievement

High-fidelity mannequins were used to allow for hands-on nursing interventions and corresponding physiological responses. The high-fidelity mannequin experience provided a voice for nurse–patient interaction, allowing students to employ therapeutic communication strategies for the patient.

Preparation

Learner Preparation

One week in advance, students are assigned to teams which are then assigned to prepare for one of the four scenarios, using preparation questions to review pathophysiology, pharmacology, and health assessment.

Educator Preparation

Scripting and training for the voice actors. Complete scenarios were designed and tested and included a list of standardized guided reflection questions for the facilitator within the large group debrief.

Event Flow Data

Web-based broadcasting technology recorded live-streaming action from the Clinical Simulation Centre (CSC) to the classroom. Small teams provide care in the CSC while peers in the classroom watched in real time. Participants included 40 to 45 learners, two faculty to facilitate lab and classroom activities, and two volunteer faculty for mannequin voices. Prebriefing (15 minutes) described the event flow and scenario overview to participants. The assigned groups were further divided into observer and doer groups. The simulation lasted 10 minutes followed by a 15-minute individual team debriefing. This process was repeated the following week where teams switched roles to enact observation and simulation experiences.

Debriefing

A Plus, Delta, Gamma approach was used. In the classroom, students from observer groups made notes for large group debrief and participated in an instructor-facilitated feedback session, using GoSoapBox (GSB) (http://www.gosoapbox.com/), a web-based clicker tool used to encourage student engagement, deeper thinking, and self-reflection by having them provide online, up-to-the-minute feedback during the event. The classroom facilitator used thought-provoking critical thinking questions to promote discussion.

Evaluation of Event

GSB allowed the student feedback to remain anonymous. Student and faculty evaluation of the event stated that the GSB methods of reflection contributed to effective discussion and learning of key concepts.

Lessons Learned

Positive student feedback affirmed the demand for more broadcast simulation. Students shared an appreciation for this delivery method, finding it especially useful prior to clinical practice. They self-reported increased confidence

Table 23.1	Free Scenario Ideas
Organization	**Link to Resources**
American Association of Medical Colleges MedEdPORTAL	https://www.mededportal.org/collections/
University of Washington Center for Health Science Interprofessional Education, Research and Practice	http://collaborate.uw.edu/tools-and-curricula/scenario-building-and-library.html
Geriatric Clinical Simulation at the University of North Carolina at Chapel Hill	http://geroclinsim.org/
QSEN Institute	http://qsen.org/teaching-strategies/strategy-search/advanced-search-results/?strat_type=Simulation%20Exercises
Massachusetts Nursing Initiative	http://www.mass.edu/currentinit/Nursing/Sim/Scenarios.asp
Montgomery Community College	http://cms.montgomerycollege.edu/nursingsims/
Minnesota Healthcare Simulation Library	http://www.healthforceminnesota.org/simulation/m-shep-simulation-library-2/
NLN Advancing Care Excellence Series (ACE.S, ACE.Z)	http://www.nln.org/professional-development-programs/teaching-resources/aging
thesimtech	http://thesimtech.com/scenarios/

while validating cumulative knowledge and communication skill. The teaching team is currently reviewing the use of valid and reliable tools for assessment. The Creighton Competency Evaluation Instrument holds promise for improved performance assessment in this context (Hayden, Keegan, Kardong-Edgren, & Smiley, 2014).

Summary

A variety of scenario ideas have been shared across a wide continuum of learners, from the novice to the advanced, from academia to practice settings, within the hospital and outside of it and using technology that ranged from the physical mannequin to virtual tools. As you develop your own scenarios, refer back to these ideas. At different times over your development, you may find that scenarios that didn't "speak to you" now may later.

While the chapter provides a plethora of ideas, it also highlights the need for standardization of terminology and adherence to the INACSL Standards of Best Practice: Simulation. Using standardized templates (more in Chapter 20) will also help simulationists to communicate their work more clearly to others. There are many other resources for scenario ideas and I encourage you to explore them all. Table 23.1 provides a list of some of the freely available resources. Don't limit yourself to only reviewing

nursing-specific scenarios as most healthcare scenarios can be adapted to other disciplines. Building a repertoire of simulated clinical experiences is important, but not the end goal. As we move simulation forward as an art and science, it is also vital that we assess the reliability and validity of the learning experience, particularly when scenarios are used for assessment purposes and most importantly when they are used for high-stakes testing.

Toolkit Resources

Toolkit 23-1: Simulation Experience Questionnaire

Toolkit 23-2: High-Risk Obstetrical Scenario: Putting it All Together

Toolkit 23-3: Pre/Post Knowledge Test

Toolkit 23-4: Performance Checklist

Toolkit 23-5: Scenario Pediatric Acute Appendicitis

Toolkit 23-6: Trauma Performance Checklist

Toolkit 23-7: Family Conversation Scenario Design Tool

Toolkit 23-8: Case Management Rubric

Toolkit 23-9: End of Program Scenarios

Toolkit 23-10: End of Program Scenario Evaluation Form

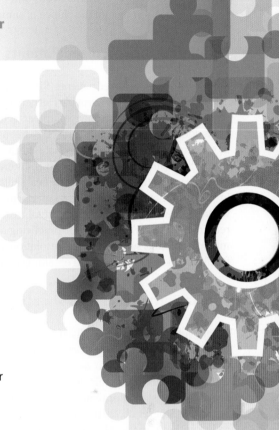

24

Simulation in Medicine

Purnima Rao, Meghan Andrews, Amy Fraser

Key Terms

Medical Simulation, Interprofessional Team Training, Assessment, Competency-Based Education, Fellowships, Accreditation, Global Health

Guiding Questions

1   What types of simulation do physicians and other healthcare professionals use in their training and assessment programs?

2   What role will simulation play in the future of medical education?

3   How are medical simulation educators trained and credentialed?

4   How are simulation programs accredited?

5   How will simulation help diverse healthcare professions work better together?

Introduction

Now more than ever, simulation-based education and assessment are an integral part of medical education. Across healthcare professions, medical educators and practitioners are using simulation to accelerate and maintain skill acquisition, reduce risk to patients, expose trainees to rare or critical events, and even reduce training time (Sonnadara, Mui, McQueen, Mironova, Nousiainen, et al., 2014). Formal programs of simulation-based training for physicians and other healthcare professionals will very likely become universal in the near future. This chapter will explore the efforts of pioneers in medical simulation, the current types and uses of simulation for medical healthcare professionals, and the future of medical simulation for learner assessment and competency-based training.

Simulation Modality and Typology Use in Medical Education

Medical simulation involves a variety of teaching techniques (modalities) and associated types of simulation tools (typologies) to replicate aspects of real patient care. Simulation typologies range from low-fidelity simulators,

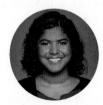

Purnima Rao, MD, BSc(Hon), FRCPC

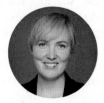

Meghan Andrews, MD, BSc, FRCP(C)

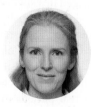

Amy Fraser, MD, MSc, BScH, FRCP(C), MHPE

such as part task trainers, to high-fidelity simulators, such as fully equipped mock operating theaters with mechanized mannequins that speak, breathe, and even bleed. Relying exclusively on the use of high-fidelity trainers would be cost-prohibitive, therefore, learners' needs and best evidence in medical education dictate the choice of simulator typology.

Simulated/Standardized Patients

Simulated or standardized patients (SPs) are paid or volunteer actors who are trained to provide learners with a predefined clinical scenario. Commonly, volunteer actors are termed embedded actors or volunteers. SPs are used extensively in undergraduate and postgraduate healthcare programs to simulate clinic or wardlike settings. Interacting with SPs allows learners to develop nontechnical skills while engaged in medical history taking or to perform clinical exams where no invasive procedures or actual treatment would be required. They are also ideal for practicing additional communication skills such as conflict resolution, interacting with family, breaking bad news, and obtaining consent.

Part Task Trainers

Often, specific technical skills are taught without the participation of a patient. In these circumstances, part task trainers (also referred to as task trainers or partial task trainers) are used to train learners in key elements of a procedure or skill (Lopreiato, Downing, Gammon, Lioce, Sittner, & Slot, et al., 2016). These learning tools are typically synthetic-material models made to mimic the look and feel of specific parts of the human body (e.g., an arm, leg, or chest). Sometimes, part task trainers also contain mechanical or electronic interfaces that provide augmented interactivity and feedback for learners (Lopreiato et al.). Examples of part task trainers include those used for learning airway management, vascular access, cardiopulmonary resuscitation, suturing, ultrasound, lumbar puncture, pelvic procedures, and even basic laparoscopic skills. Part task trainers can be purchased as ready-made synthetic models from vendors or can also be homegrown innovations such as the example you see depicted in Figure 24.1. This homemade part task trainer is made from a combination of synthetic materials and live animal tissue (an approach known as hybrid or blended simulation) to create an open fracture for practicing suturing (see Fig. 24.1). Learners engaged in a single scenario can use multiple part task trainers simultaneously. Part task trainers may also be used in conjunction with standardized patients to increase realism. For example, an obstetrician in training may be required to deliver a fetal mannequin from a pelvic floor model that has been attached to a standardized patient mimicking a real patient in labor. This would allow the learner to practice the technical skill of delivery and the nontechnical skill of patient communication.

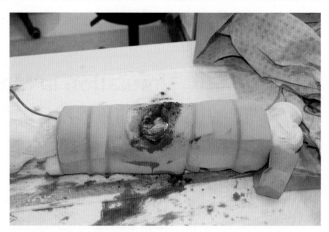

Figure 24.1 Hybrid Simulation Model. This model designed to practice suturing skills may be applied to a standardized patient in order to increase realism. (Photo courtesy of the University of Ottawa Skills and Simulation Centre; used with permission.)

Computer-Based Simulation: Gaming and Virtual Reality

Virtual reality simulation occurs when the learner interacts solely within "a computer-generated three-dimensional environment that gives an immersion effect" (Lopreiato et al., 2016, p. 40). Information is typically fed to the learner via auditory, visual, and tactile means—where the learner is otherwise isolated from their environment. This simulated/synthetic learning modality is particularly useful in teaching complex medical procedures such as laparoscopic, endoscopic, and endovascular procedures because the execution of these procedures in real life requires interaction with video screens and tools or instruments that are controlled by fine motor movements. The advent of newer promising technologies includes the use of holographic augmented reality simulation where trainees can interact with holographic representations of humans while using real equipment. One such example is the medical simulation software by SimX, creator of augmented reality platforms for medical training (https://twitter.com/simxar).

Cadaveric Simulation

Originally used to teach anatomy, cadavers are also used extensively for procedural skills training. As opposed to using replicated synthetic tissues, as is the case in part task trainers, practicing procedural skills using cadaveric tissues provides trainees with sensory feedback that more closely resembles live human tissues. One such example is the Clinical Cadaver Program, at Dalhousie University in Nova Scotia, Canada. This program uses a new embalming technique that produces tissue that looks, feels, and reacts in almost the same way as a live patient's body. This process allows surgical residents to practice procedural skills—

without the risk of harming patients (https://medicine.dal. ca/departments/department-sites/emergency/education/ Simulation-BasedMedicalEducation.html). Despite being the gold standard for procedural surgical training (Aydin, Ahmed, Khan, Dasgupta, & McCabe, 2015), cadavers' prohibitive cost and limited availability have required the development of more sustainable training modalities.

High-Fidelity Mannequin Simulators

High-fidelity mannequin simulators (also termed fully computerized human patient mannequins) allow healthcare providers to care for realistic "patients" in a representative physical clinical environment. The "patients" are typically expensive computer-controlled mechanical mannequins housed in a simulation lab and surrounded by real clinical equipment, such as resuscitation supplies. Often, embedded actors or role-players will act as additional healthcare team members to increase the fidelity, or believability of a simulation-based learning situation. Participants are allowed to care for the simulated patient during a critical event, after which they undergo a formal debriefing in order to discuss technical and nontechnical skills used during the simulation. The simulators are typically equipped with video and audio recording devices that allow for review of events during the debriefing. These simulators are particularly well suited to teaching and evaluating how teams work in crisis situations (Kim, Neilipovitz, Cardinal, Chiu, & Clinch, 2006).

High-Fidelity/Cadaveric Hybrids

The mechanized and artificial nature of high-fidelity mannequins makes it difficult to use them to simulate realistic surgical pathology. This has resulted in the development of high-fidelity mannequin–cadaveric hybrids. For example, human or animal organs can be arranged inside a box to simulate a particular body cavity. This box can then be placed on or near the high-fidelity mannequin. The mannequin and box can then be draped or covered to make it appear as if they are both part of a single patient. This allows for a surgical trainee to "operate" on the mannequin, encountering real organs and pathology, while the computer-driven vital signs can be changed from a nearby control room. This results in a much more realistic clinical scenario.

3D Printing

The advent of 3D printing technology has opened the door to numerous applications to the field of medical simulation, in particular tissue fabrication for anatomical models. This technique may even negate the need for human and animal cadaveric models in the future. 3D printing has been used to created replica heart valves, allowing surgical trainees to practice a variety of cardiac surgical procedures,

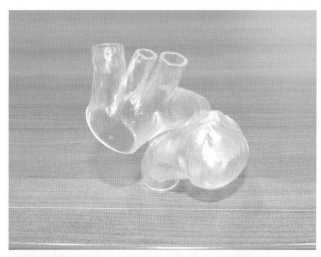

Figure 24.2 3D Sim Model Made with a Printer in Preparation for a Real Case. Photo courtesy of Dr. Bin Zheng, University of Alberta. Used with Permission.

ranging from simple valve replacements to complex valve repairs (Royal College: 3D printers, innovating medical education, 2014). Surgeons can also use CT scan and MRI information to create 3D-printed models of a specific patient's anatomy to better help them plan for complex surgical procedures. Figure 24.2 depicts a 3D model that assists surgeons in practicing and preparing to perform complex surgical procedures (http://www.3dsystems.com/ solutions/healthcare).

The Integration of Crisis Resource Management into Medical Simulation

The value of simulation in medicine is found not only in the opportunity to practice and perfect technical skills but also in the opportunity to learn and apply nontechnical skills, such as communication, decision making, and leadership. These skills are essential in the delivery of safe and efficient patient care within complex, ever-changing team dynamics. High-fidelity simulators provide the ideal vehicle for healthcare providers to practice these skills in a supportive and safe environment.

To that end, the term "crisis resource management" (CRM) began to appear in the patient safety literature in the early 1990s, thanks to the pioneering work of Dr. David Gaba and his collaborators (Gaba, 2010). Originating in the aviation industry, CRM refers to the "principles of individual and crew behaviour in ordinary and crisis situations that focuses on skills of dynamic decision making, interpersonal behaviour, and team management" (Helmreich & Foushee, 1993). The application of CRM principles is intended to ensure the "avoidance, trapping, and mitigation of risk" that could lead to adverse patient outcome (Eisen & Savel, 2009).

Within the healthcare field, there are numerous training programs based on CRM principles. These include the

Anesthesia Crisis Resource Management Course (ACRM) (Gaba, 2010), MedTeams (Small et al., 1999), TeamSTEPPS (Clancy & Tornberg, 2007), and the Acute Critical Events Course administered by the Royal College of Physicians and Surgeons of Canada (RCPSC) (Neilipovitz, 2005). All of these use high-fidelity simulation to teach and reinforce various CRM principles in a multidisciplinary context.

The Pioneers of Medical Simulation

Anesthesiologists were among the first physician specialty groups to realize the potential of high-fidelity simulation (Gaba, Howard, Fish, Smith, & Sowb, 2001). Anesthesiologists have a unique role in healthcare: they are not considered to be the patient's "primary physician" until a crisis occurs. At that time, the anesthesiologist must collaborate with and lead the operating room team to provide lifesaving care to the critically ill patient. However, such crises occur rarely, and the opportunity to practice leading the team in managing a crisis is not often available to anesthesia trainees. Through simulation, we can create opportunities for medical trainees to practice CRM while diagnosing and managing unanticipated critical illness.

Because anesthesiologists were among the earliest adopters and pioneers of high-fidelity simulation, they also created, refined, and disseminated early simulation-based training materials. Anesthesiologists also became established researchers in the field of high-fidelity simulation. More recently, anesthesiologists have established groundbreaking collaborations in **interprofessional team training** initiatives with surgeons, emergency medicine specialists, nurses, respiratory therapists (RTs), and anesthesia assistants (AAs).

A "typical" anesthesia simulation scenario might take place in a mock operating room, using a patient simulator mannequin and realistic equipment, personnel, information, and supplies. A real anesthesia machine is often used for ventilation and vital signs monitoring. The scenario has been prewritten, detailing what happens in the mock OR as the patient becomes critically ill, is treated, and possibly begins to recover. Preplanned events in the scenario include aspects of the patient's illness, such as changes in vital signs and availability of new laboratory results. These events also can include aspects of team functioning that can add to the degree of difficulty of the simulation, such as an incompetent colleague. Following the scenario, the trainee(s) and instructors take part in a debriefing session, during which they discuss both the medical events and the functioning of the team during the crisis (see Fig. 24.3).

Obstetricians were also early adopters of simulation. Obstetrical emergencies are high-pressure, time-sensitive situations requiring interprofessional (physicians,

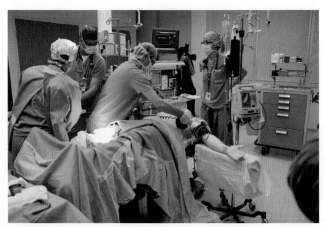

Figure 24.3 Public Demonstration of Anesthesia Crisis Resource Management Skills using a High-Fidelity Simulator. (Photo courtesy of the University of Ottawa Skills and Simulation Centre; used with permission.)

nurses, and midwives) and interdisciplinary (obstetrics, anesthesia, and neonatology) teamwork. Elements of good team functioning include communication with the patient and her family, excellent technical performance, and ethical decision making to ensure the safety of the mother and fetus. Simulation is a technique that is used to teach, practice, and improve all of these skills to better patient outcomes. For example, an obstetric simulation might focus on a healthy patient under the care of a midwife, who develops a massive postpartum hemorrhage requiring surgical intervention. This simulated scenario would require all members of the medical team to practice their own unique tasks as well as team-based tasks. The midwife would recognize the medical emergency, perform initial resuscitation, and call for the rest of the medical team. The obstetricians would continue resuscitation, recognize the need for surgical management, and practice surgical skills. The nurses would prepare the patient and operating room for an emergency procedure and assist in management of postpartum hemorrhage. The anesthesiologist would manage an unstable postpartum patient requiring emergency surgery. All members of the team would also practice leadership, followership, closed-loop communication, and other CRM skills.

To increase scenario complexity, healthcare educators can consider inserting an embedded actor to play the role of a distressed family member. For example, the addition might require a team member(s) to communicate a poor outcome to the family. The presence of the actor allows participants to practice disclosure of adverse events and other difficult conversations.

General surgeons are also well represented in simulation-based medical education (SBME), likely because of their early efforts to use simulation to improve laparoscopic skill acquisition (Derossis et al., 1998) for both residents and staff surgeons.

Today, the use of medical simulation is diverse with evidence of increasing depth and breadth of use across most medical specialties. Examples of such specialties and/or subspecialties include noninvasive cardiology, cardiothoracic surgery, emergency medicine, family medicine, gastroenterology, genitourinary surgery, internal medicine, neurosurgery, obstetrics and gynecology, ophthalmology, orthopedic surgery, otolaryngology, palliative care, pediatrics, psychiatry, respirology, critical care, radiology, and diagnostics, as well as military and battlefield medicine (Levine, DeMaria, Schwartz, & Sim, 2014).

Respiratory Therapists and Anesthesia Assistants

As members of the Code Blue team in many hospitals, Respiratory Therapists (RTs) are often present during critical patient care events, as part of a multidisciplinary patient care team. In some jurisdictions, including Canada, RTs can become AAs after pursuing extra training. AAs are often invaluable members of OR teams during management of critical events. For these reasons, simulation has been identified as a highly useful complement to training for both RTs and AAs. Simulation facilities are becoming increasingly available to trainees in RT and AA programs. Interprofessional team training initiatives (Direnna, Boet, & Crooks, 2012) have also included RT/AAs as key members of the crisis response team. Training programs for RTs and AAs incorporate various types of simulation, including low-fidelity part-task trainers for airway management skills and high-fidelity simulators for team training exercises.

Interprofessional Simulation

Simulation was initially developed to teach technical skills such as cardiac physical examination, central line placement, delivery of a baby, and resuscitation. Its use as a medical education tool leads to improved performance of medical students and residents in both nonclinical and clinical environments (Okuda et al., 2009; Willems, Waxman, Bacon, Smith, & Kitto, 2013). However, teamwork skills including communication, leadership, followership, and knowledge of other professionals' roles are just as important as technical skills in contributing to patient safety and outcomes (Yule, Flin, Paterson-Brown, & Maran, 2006). A systematic review by Fung et al. found that simulation-based CRM training was associated with significant improvements in CRM skill acquisition with some studies showing improved workplace team behav-

iors and reductions in adverse patient outcomes (Fung et al., 2015). A variety of crises may be simulated in order to challenge the whole team, or focus on specific members of a team (Tan, Pena, Altree, & Maddern, 2014). Examples have included the death of a pediatric patient in critical care (Youngblood, Zinkan, Tofil, & White, 2012), patient demise during a massive transfusion in the operating room, or even a multipatient trauma in the emergency department (ED). These situations will involve the entire team of healthcare providers: physicians, nurses, hospital aides, ward clerks, respiratory and radiation technologists, pharmacists, spiritual care professionals, and many others depending on the resources and creativity of the simulation instructors.

In situ simulation (simulation that occurs within a healthcare worker's own clinical environment) allows participants to train and learn within their own interprofessional team, in a familiar environment, and with the resources normally available to them. If well executed, the potential benefits of simulation training are improved realism and better "buy in" from the participants (Kalaniti, 2014). High impact simulation training has also been found to lessen the time spent away from clinical responsibilities, lower care costs (Lois, Pospiech, Van Dyck, Kahn, & De Kock, 2014), bring wider accessibility to rural and remote areas, and aid in the identification of latent safety threats (Yajamanyam & Sohi, 2015). As with all simulation sessions, the complexity of the cases can range from management of a relatively uncomplicated patient in a low-acuity setting to coordination of a hospital-wide response to a large-scale disaster such as a train derailment or industrial fire (Fig. 24.4) (see Box 24-1).

Simulation-Based Assessment and Competency-Based Medical Education

The emergence of **competency-based medical education** (CBME) has revolutionized the approach to the assessment of medical trainees (Hamstra, 2012). Simulation offers great potential as a solution to assessment challenges in medical training programs, most importantly the capacity to assess complex, team-based competencies.

One example of such a competency might be the ability to lead a cardiac arrest or "Code Blue" team. The building blocks of this competency (e.g., knowledge of ACLS protocols) are easily identified and can often be assessed through written tests or clinical observation. However, leading a Code Blue team incorporates not only basic knowledge but also the ability to set priorities, sort important from unimportant information, generate hypotheses, balance competing issues, communicate

Box 24-1 **Education Exemplar: Interprofessional Team Training with a Hybrid Simulator**

Dr. Meghan Andrews, Anesthesiologist, Department of Anesthesiology, The Ottawa Hospital, The University of Ottawa

Dr. Maher Matar, General Surgeon, Department of General Surgery, The Ottawa Hospital, The University of Ottawa

Dr. Purnima Rao, Anesthesiologist, Department of Anesthesiology, The Ottawa Hospital, The University of Ottawa

Ms. Melissa Waggot, Nurse Educator, Emergency Department, The Ottawa Hospital

Dr. Simone Crooks, Anesthesiologist, Department of Anesthesiology, The Ottawa Hospital, The University of Ottawa

Dr. Jacinthe Lampron, General Surgeon, Department of General Surgery, The Ottawa Hospital, The University of Ottawa

Scenario Title

Interprofessional Trauma Code

Population

Postgraduate trainees in Anesthesiology and General Surgery, Practicing Emergency Department Nurses

Performance Gap

Assessment and management of an unstable patient with multiple injuries, communication between team members with conflicting priorities.

Learning Objectives

● To manage the elements of interdisciplinary teamwork in a crisis: communication skills, leadership, collaboration, and resource allocation.
● To apply the principles of ATLS management of a trauma patient, resulting in identification of a tension pneumothorax and insertion of a chest tube and performance of a FAST and interpretation of the results.

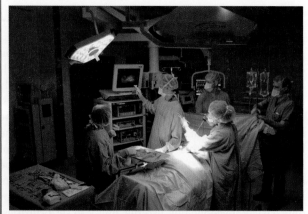

Figure 24.4 Interdisciplinary High-Fidelity Simulation Session Involving General Surgery and Anesthesia Participants. (Photo courtesy of the University of Ottawa Skills and Simulation Centre; used with permission.)

● To generate and execute a management plan for an unstable trauma patient with a potentially difficult airway and an intrathoracic injury.

Performance Assessment

● Adherence to ATLS protocol including early resuscitation goals
● Chest tube insertion technique
● FAST interpretation
● Anesthesia nontechnical skills scale

Scenario Synopsis and Case Stem

A motor vehicle collision trauma patient has been delivered to the ED trauma bay. The patient presents as follows: features concerning for a potentially difficult airway, clinical signs and symptoms of a hemopneumothorax, and a positive abdominal FAST.

A trauma code has been called, resulting in the arrival of an ED nurse, a senior surgical resident, and an anesthesiologist, followed by the staff surgeon. The team must manage the patient according to ATLS guidelines.

A high-fidelity mannequin with a chest tube box applied to the chest and an ultrasound apron applied to the abdomen was created for this scenario. This technique was chosen as it allowed the team to assess the patient, perform appropriate diagnostic and therapeutic procedures, and respond to changes in the patient's status.

Fidelity was achieved by recreating the setup and equipment of the local ED. A combination of synthetic and animal parts was used to create the chest tube box, allowing a realistic sensation during chest tube insertion. The high-fidelity mannequin was programmed to achieve features of a difficult airway.

Preparation: Describe Key Preparation Considerations

● Learners received an orientation (prebriefing) document 2 weeks prior to their scheduled session outlining the nontechnical objectives and the formative nature of the session.
● Educators were familiar with all objectives and content of the scenario and were prepared to play the role of confederates within the scenario.

Event Flow Data

● Five learners participated in each event: two General Surgery residents, two Anesthesiology residents, one Emergency Department Nurse
● Two confederate actors were required for each event: one ED physician and one ED nurse
● Duration of 15 minutes

Debriefing Topics

● Role clarity during a trauma code
  o Trauma team leader
  o Charge nurse

Box 24-1 **Education Exemplar: Interprofessional Team Training with a Hybrid Simulator (*Continued*)**

- Communication within the team and with the operating room staff
- Early and late resuscitation goals in trauma
- Prioritizing management steps in a patient with multiple injuries

Evaluation of Event

This was a formative session and was evaluated using the University of Ottawa Skills and Simulation Centre Multidisciplinary Evaluation form. Participant feedback was collected regarding the fidelity of the scenario, the application to clinical practice, and individual lessons learned.

Lessons Learned

When implementing this scenario in your own institution, we suggest early involvement of educators from all fields to ensure that all elements—learning objectives, environmental and physical fidelity, and participant roles—are relevant to your own learners.

---

with a team, and integrate the demands of a compressed timeline (Wilkinson & Harris, 2002). These multifaceted competencies are challenging to measure using the above methods.

There is a lack of opportunity in medical education to assess complex skills. This reality is especially unfortunate considering that many medical trainees struggle acquire skills that require logical, sequential, and time-sensitive patient evaluation (Boulet & Murray, 2010). According to Boulet and Murray (2010), "the 'borderline' resident often struggles with setting priorities, managing time effectively, and recognizing when to call for help. In clinical practice, residents with serious skill deficits in these essential domains are often not recognized until multiple questionable judgements and skills deficits are observed in a crisis setting" (p. 1044).

It is vitally important for medical educators to develop novel ways to assess competency attainment, so that we can give trainees opportunities to demonstrate mastery in areas that we have conventionally claimed to value, but for which we have found few methods of assessment (Costa & Kallick, 1995).

The assessment of competencies that are complex, team-based, or based on uncommon clinical events can be accomplished using simulation. Simulation is especially powerful as a way to provide "cognitive fidelity"—that is, it can trigger the same thinking processes used in a real patient care setting (Weaver, Lyons, Diazgranados, Rosen, Salas, et al., 2012). In fact, a simulation may be the best way to assess skills such as decision making and communication (Boulet & Murray, 2010). The capacity of simulation to produce realistic, responsive, and reproducible experiences lends itself to the development of good quality assessment tools (Boulet, 2008; Boulet & Murray, 2010). Simulation has been listed as a recommended assessment method by at least one ACGME milestones task force (Green et al., 2009) to date. Some national anesthesia societies are already using high-fidelity simulation for high-stakes certification examinations (Berkenstadt, Ziv, Gafni, & Sidi, 2006), and the ACGME Advisory Committee on Educational Outcome Assessment has recommended that programs be encouraged to develop and use simulation for assessment (Swing, 2002).

24-1 Voice of Experience
The Canadian National Anesthesia Simulation Curriculum (CanNASC) Collaboration

Michelle Chiu, MD, FRCP(C)

The Challenge

Anesthesia simulation programs across Canada did not share a universal vision or standardized curriculum. There was an opportunity to create a nationwide program to address teaching and assessment of critical anesthesia learning objectives.

Meeting the Challenge

In 2013, Dr. Michelle Chiu founded the Canadian National Anesthesia Simulation Curriculum (CanNASC) Collaboration. CanNASC uses simulation to standardize anesthesia training by delivering critically needed simulation-based education to anesthesia residents. A panel of anesthesia simulation leaders from across Canada selected 13 clinical scenarios that included both common and rare events. Together, these scenarios comprise a core set of anesthesia skills essential to safe practice.

Outcome

Two years later, piloting of scenarios began. The scenarios are now being used as a resource both for training and assessing senior anesthesia residents. Before CanNASC, simulation was not widely used in the assessment of anesthesia residents. This groundbreaking initiative will help to establish simulation-based assessment of critical skill sets in anesthesia residents.

Fellowships in Medical Simulation

The use of simulation for teaching and assessment in medical education has expanded significantly over the past decade. The introduction has resulted in a drive to formally train experts in SBME through specialized education programs, including continuing professional development courses, fellowship programs, and master's degree programs. A number of institutions in the United States and Canada offer 3- to 5-day simulation instructor courses.

- The Royal College of Physicians and Surgeons of Canada (RCPSC), *Simulation Educator Course* (Royal College: Simulation Educator Training Course, 2015)
- Harvard University's Center for Medical Simulation: *Comprehensive Instructor Workshop* ("Simulation Instructor Training | Institute for Medical Simulation (IMS)—Center for Medical Simulation," n.d.)
- The Mayo Clinic's Multidisciplinary Simulation Centre *Simulation Instructor Development, Comprehensive Course*

The increased role of simulation in medical education has also prompted the expansion of formal postresidency **fellowships**. Fellowship training programs are primarily designed for physicians and are typically 1 to 2 years in duration. The literature highlights a few attempts at cataloguing fellowship programs. An abstract submitted to *Simulation in Healthcare* by An-Grogan, Jansson, Park, Salzman, and Vozenilek (2014) identified 34 fellowship training programs in the United States and Canada. A 2015 survey by Kotal and colleagues (Kotal, Sivertson, Wolfe, Lammers, & Overton, 2015) identified 17 fellowship programs in the United States. At the time of publication, two of these programs accepted nonphysician medical professionals.

Such training programs also exist in Europe, Asia, and Australia/New Zealand. As is the case for Canada and the United States, information about individual programs is not centralized, but can be accessed by contacting individual academic institutions, simulation centers, or professional associations. The Society for Simulation in Healthcare maintains a list of accredited simulation centers worldwide.

Accreditation of Medical Simulation Programs

Critical advances in the quality of medical education have historically been attributed to the impact of the Flexner Report in 1910 (Flexner, 1910a). One of Abraham Flexner's key recommendations was the adoption of a centralized **accreditation** process for medical residency programs. Before this report, medical training programs had largely operated on an independent basis with little oversight, resulting in a highly variable quality of education.

Parallels between the histories of medical education and medical simulation can be drawn with respect to the rise of accreditation. Although some simulation modalities were described in the medical literature more than 50 years ago, widespread uptake of simulation as a medical education tool did not take place until the late 1990s (Fernandez, Wang, Vozenilek, Hayden, McLaughlin, et al., 2010; Rosen, 2008). At that time, medical simulation programs typically operated in isolation, developing most of their own materials and engaging in limited collaboration with other centers. Although large simulation interest groups formed, such as the Society for Simulation in Healthcare (SSH, 2016e), these groups initially promoted education and collaboration, rather than offering oversight and accreditation (SSH, 2016d).

Since approximately 2005, simulation interest groups and medical specialty organizations have begun to advocate for accreditation of both simulation educators and medical simulation programs (Fernandez et al., 2010; SSH, 2016e). The purpose of accreditation is twofold: to set benchmarks for quality and to promote evidence-based best practices in the delivery of SBME (Fernandez et al., 2010).

Currently, multiple national and international organizations offer centralized quality assurance through accreditation of both simulation providers and programs. In North America, the three most prominent groups offering accreditation are the RCPSC, the SSH, and the American College of Surgeons (ACS, 2015). However, there are substantial variations in the conceptualization of accreditation between these three groups. For example, while the RCPSC offers oversight of simulation programs, the SSH program into different accreditation standards and associated criteria, listed as Core, Assessment, Research, Teaching/Education, and Systems Integration (SSH, 2016d).

In general, accreditation is achieved through peer review of the quality of a simulation center's facilities, its educators, and its learning activities. Facilities are expected to be up to date and in compliance with safety and confidentiality standards. Educators must have appropriate and current expertise and may be required to have leadership skills and maintain active collaboration with leaders at other simulation centers. Educational experiences are expected to be developed in accordance with best practices and have demonstrable positive impact on patient safety and quality care (Royal College of Physicians and Surgeons of Canada, 2015 [http://www.royalcollege.ca/rcsite/cpd/accreditation-simulation-programs-e]; Society for Simulation in Healthcare, 2016 [http://www.ssih.org/Accreditation/

Full-Accreditation]). Accreditation status is typically renewable every few years.

In Canada, the RCPSC offers accreditation for healthcare simulation programs run by and for health provider professions, including nursing, medicine, and others. Often, simulation centers are certified on the basis of the provision of services to multiple health provider types.

Internationally, the SSH has been able to establish a significant presence as an accreditor of simulation programs. As of January 2016, SSH reports having accredited 65 programs, with 10 more programs having achieved provisional accreditation status (See Chapter 4). Its definition of "simulation programs" is wide, encompassing universities, hospitals, medical associations, and stand-alone facilities. The SSH also offers credentialing programs for both simulation educators and simulation operators.

The ACS offers to certify "Accredited Educational Institutes" for surgical simulation programs that encompass physician and nonphysician members of the surgical team (www.facs.org). To date, this certification has been limited to universities and their associated hospitals. The RCPSC also offers training programs and simulation center accreditation to programs throughout the world (http://www.royalcollege.ca/rcsite/cpd/accreditation-simulation-programs-e).

Simulation in Low- and Middle-Income Countries

Affordable, low-fidelity simulation tools and education programs have the potential to transform patient care in places where there is minimal access to continuing education programs. Despite this, there are few groups specifically dedicated to simulation education in low- and middle-income countries.

One example of affordable simulation-based education is the *Helping Babies Breathe* Initiative. *Helping Babies Breathe*, is a collaboration between the American Academy of Pediatrics, the World Health Organization, the U.S. Agency for International Development, the charity organization Save The Children, the National Institute of Child Health and Development, and several other **global health** organizations. This program is an evidence-based educational program to teach neonatal resuscitation

techniques in resource-limited areas (Helping Babies Breathe, 2015). With the ongoing development of healthcare simulation education in North America and Europe, perhaps more of these programs will arise.

Disaster Management

Simulation has also been used to replicate large-scale disasters, pandemics, and humanitarian crises. In particular, these allow for the identification of gaps in existing emergency response systems (Gaba, 2014; Kobayashi, Shapiro, Suner, & Williams, 2003).

Military

Because of their unique exposure to large-scale trauma and involvement with disaster relief and chemical, biological, and nuclear weapons, military forces worldwide have long used simulation for training personnel (Bradley, 2006; Leitch, Moses, & Magee, 2002).

Summary

In summary, simulation has become a vital component of all healthcare professionals' training and assessment programs. There is a wide variety of simulation modalities and typologies available and their use will vary depending on the learner and the skills being taught. Standardized/simulated patients, part task trainers, computer-based simulation, and high-fidelity simulators can be used alone or as part of a hybrid simulation in the instruction and assessment of technical and nontechnical skills. Simulation is expanding at all stages of medical education, from its use as teaching and assessment modality for students to its role in continuing medical education for practicing healthcare professionals. To meet this growing need, universities, medical schools, and accrediting bodies will need to establish their own simulation programs with formally trained staff and educators. These programs will enable healthcare professionals from different fields to learn together and from each other in an effort to improve patient care and safety.

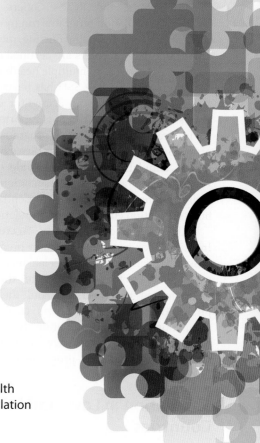

25 Simulation in Allied Health
Norbert Werner

 Key Terms

Allied Health Professionals, Simulation-based Training (SBT),
In Situ Simulation, High-Acuity Low Occurrence (HALO) Clinical
Events, Soft Skills, Crisis Resource Management, Objective
Structured Clinical Examination (OSCE), Multimodal, Simulated/
Standardized Patients, Hybrid Simulations, Virtual Patients,
Interprofessional Education (IPE), Interprofessional Collaborative
Practice, Debriefing, Formative and Summative Assessment/
Evaluation

 Guiding Questions

1 Are you able to identify and describe *allied health professions*?
2 What does the use of simulation look like in allied health discipline
   education compared to nursing education? What is unique to allied health
   simulation? How is it similar and different to nursing and medicine simulation
   programming? Alternatively, is it the same?

Introduction

The use of simulation exists in almost every facet of
healthcare education today as a result of relatively
recent and significant uptake of this powerful teaching and learning strategy. *Allied health* is no exception
to this rule and has also continued to expand its use of
simulation within curricula. Although simulation-based
teaching and learning is an accepted evidence-based
educational methodology in nursing and medicine,
the literature has been sparse in allied health academics (McAllister, 2015). Nevertheless, many allied health
prelicensure programs are adopting and translating the

tenets of simulation-based education (SBE) to their
teaching contexts for similar purposes and outcomes as
in medicine and nursing. This chapter provides a brief
introduction to the use of simulation in the context of
allied health education followed by an exemplar demonstrating the championing of simulation in various
applications within the Northern Alberta Institute of
Technology (NAIT) School of Health and Life Sciences
(SHLS) in Edmonton, Alberta, Canada.

What Is Allied Health?

The majority of the health workforce still consists of the
primary groups of nursing, medicine, and midwifery;
however, the broader health workforce has become
extensive and includes a diverse and broad range of
highly skilled professionals educated in varying universities, colleges, and polytechnic institutes (Brownie,
2015). So, what exactly constitutes an allied health
professional?

The Association of Schools of Allied Health Professions
(ASAHP) defines **allied health professionals** in the following manner:

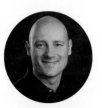

Norbert Werner,
MEd, ACP

Allied Health professionals are involved with the delivery of health or related services pertaining to the identification, evaluation, and prevention of diseases and disorders; dietary and nutrition services; rehabilitation and health systems management, among others. Allied health professionals, to name a few, include dental hygienists, diagnostic medical sonographers, dietitians, medical technologists, occupational therapists, physical therapists, radiographers, respiratory therapists, and speech language pathologists. (http://www.asahp.org/about-us/what-is-allied-health/)

Allied Health Professions Australia (AHPA) provides further insight into the field of allied health:

The allied health sub-set of the Australian health professions does not include medical, nursing or dental professionals, [and] there is no universally accepted definition of allied health professions. Instead, a range of definitions are used in various sectors. (http://www.ahpa.com.au/Home/DefinitionofAlliedHealth.aspx).

The Canadian Association of Allied Health Programs (CAAHP) is "an affiliation group for Colleges and Institutions across Canada offering programs of study in the 'allied health' fields. These fields encompass all professions in healthcare with the exception of Medicine and Nursing" (http://www.caahp.ca/about-us/). Moreover, the definition of allied health can differ depending on where one lives, works, or resides and from province to province, from state to state, and from one country to the next. Allied health, although somewhat ill defined, is, for the most part, understood to include all healthcare disciplines and professions beyond the traditional medicine and nursing role. Whatever the case, allied health education and professionals play a critical role in the complex and technical healthcare system that exists today. As a result, the allied health community has embraced high-quality education delivery methods including the use of various modes of simulation to ensure competent, highly trained, and safe practitioners.

Simulation in the Context of Allied Health Education

Not unlike the nursing and medicine professions, allied health has many similar opportunities to champion and apply simulation-based instructional methods in curricula and for many of the same reasons. Theoretical underpinnings and justification for the use of simulation-based teaching and learning in both traditional and allied healthcare education are plentiful in the current literature. **Simulation-based training** (SBT) continues to grow within the current body of knowledge and research community with many positive outcomes and evidence-based teaching and learning benefits in healthcare education. Rosen, Salas, Silvestri, Wu, and Lazzara (2008) describe several benefits to SBT in healthcare education (see Box 25-1) that augment allied health education, curricula, and programming at the prelicensure level.

Situated learning is also a common instructional model within the literature that closely resembles and supports *scenario-based* or *context-based* SBT. Situated learning characteristics include the following:

- Learning is situated in the activity in which it takes place and implies doing
- Design effectiveness and realism—(Murdoch, Bushell, & Johnson, 2012)
- Meaningful learning will only take place if it is embedded in the cultural, social, and physical context within which it will be used
- Knowledge is situated, being in part a product of the activity, context, and culture in which it is developed and used; and
- Learning methods embedded in authentic situations are highly meaningful for the learner (Brown et al., 2000, as cited in Kommers, 2012, p. 379).

The tenets of simulation described above are increasingly becoming commonplace in every healthcare professional's education experience, including allied health.

Box 25-1	**Benefits to Simulation-Based Training (SBT) in Healthcare Education (Rosen et al., 2008)**

- Accelerates the acquisition of expertise through the provision of structured learning experiences that represent certain aspects of the real-world setting and its complexity.
- Exposure to a simulated environment that closely resembles real life and enhances transfer of learning to the workplace.
- SBT is a safe place to practice and is tolerant of errors compared to real patient care settings.
- SBT provides an opportunity for immediate and thorough feedback on the learners' performance due to no other competing priorities in the clinical environment, allowing for rich debriefing post-SBT.

- SBT provides further control regarding the content of experiences, standardizing the experiences for all learners with predetermined scenarios as opposed to unpredictable events in the real clinical setting.
- Use of structured observation protocols during SBT assists in guiding feedback and performance measurement as well as decreasing variability in student experiences in receiving variable feedback from differing clinicians and educators.
- All simulation technologies have a common goal of providing practice activities for the learner.

NAIT: An Allied Health Polytechnic Exemplar

To further illustrate the successful adoption, integration, and the various applications of simulation-based training and instructional methods in allied health, we will highlight a School of Health and Life Sciences (SHLS) in a Canadian Polytechnic Institute, namely, NAIT in Edmonton, Alberta, Canada. We will briefly explore the greater vision and strategies for creating a new simulation movement across the SHLS followed by a few examples from some of their allied health programs. Each allied health program example will feature similar uses and applications for simulation-based education for the purpose of reinforcement as well as include some unique applications to their respective discipline. I encourage you to actively read the following exemplars by using a pencil or highlighter to underline or circle each of the key terms, the various concepts, and themes as they emerge and resonate with you. Focus on the similarities and/or unique features in the adoption and application of simulation in allied health education.

The Greater Vision for Simulation at NAIT SHLS

NAIT, being a polytechnic, is well known since its inception for its "hands-on" training and use of experiential learning tools such as task trainers and other simulators. Nevertheless, a new movement of simulation emerged in healthcare in the early 2000s creating a paradigm shift in the understanding and use of simulation-based teaching and learning in both pre- and post-licensure education. NAIT SHLS spent significant time reflecting on the current state of simulation in the curricula including the continued use of "tried, tested, and true" techniques, as well as defining a greater vision for simulation in allied health education within the SHLS based on this new movement. Box 25-2 summarizes this greater vision and its guiding principles used in the pursuit of a new era and chapter of simulation-based education at the NAIT SHLS.

Box 25-2	**The *Greater Vision* for Simulation in the NAIT SHLS (Created and Adopted in 2009)**

- Patient Safety
- Immersive Learning
- Optimized Clinical Performance
- Interprofessional Education (IPE) via Simulation
- Learner-Centered Education
- Comprehensive Simulation Integration

Core Pillars of Activity and Strategic Directions for Simulation

In alignment with NAIT's academic model and strategic plan, the SHLS collaboratively defined four key pillars of activity and 10 strategic goals or outcomes to drive their greater vision for simulation. These strategies continue to evolve each year due to ongoing evaluation, organizational climate change, and an attitude of reflexivity and responsiveness from the leadership team, faculty, and staff. Box 25-3 features the 2009–2014 SHLS core pillars of activity and strategic goals devised to drive simulation forward within the allied health school. The following program-specific examples of simulation adoption and integration are a result of this greater vision and strategic plan.

Allied Health Program Examples of Simulation Integration

Advanced Care Paramedic Program

Williams and Edwards (2015) discuss the use of simulation in paramedic clinical education, suggesting that "simulation training allows paramedic students to practice and consolidate their clinical problem-solving skills, practical and assessment skills, and 'nontechnical skills' such as empathy

---

Box 25-3	**Four Pillars of Activity and 10 Simulation Outcomes Pursued over 3 to 5 Years within the NAIT School of Health Sciences to Guide the Vision in Enhancing the Use of Simulation in Allied Health Education**

Pillars

A. Build Capacity and Access for Clinical Simulation
B. Promote Intelligent Use of Simulation Application
C. Develop Strategic Partnerships
D. Advocate Applied Research in Simulation

Simulation Outcomes

1. Simulation Integration Alignment with Outcomes-Based Education (OBE) Curriculum Renewal
2. Faculty Development and Competency in the Use of Simulation Methodology
3. Dedicated Simulation Center Space for SHLS
4. IPE Simulation Activities Embedded Within IPE Curriculum
5. Online Simulation Knowledge Management, Learning Community, and Resource Center for the SHLS
6. A Defined and Focused Simulation Research Program
7. Strong Partnerships in the Simulation Community
8. A Multimodal Approach to Simulation in the SHLS
9. A Robust Communication Plan for Simulation
10. A Comprehensive and Sustainable Simulation Integration Team/Committee

and communication in a controlled and safe environment" (p. 441). The NAIT Advanced Care Paramedic program has no doubt embraced the powerful teaching and learning technique of simulation as an allied health program. The use of simulation has expanded beyond task trainers and technical training in recent years by adding realistic and immersive simulations across the paramedic curricula. Now, learners can practice individual technical skill proficiency in such areas as prehospital assessment, triage, harm reduction, and crisis resource management (St. Pierre, Hofinger, Buerschaper, & Simon, 2011). **Crisis resource management** (CRM) is an approach to healthcare that "aims to coordinate, utilize and apply all available resources to optimize patient safety and outcomes" (Rall & Dieckmann, 2005, p. 107). Nontechnical skills or *soft skills* such as *professionalism* and the skill of delivery of bad news to patients are critical to positive outcomes in patient care. **Soft skills** may focus on areas of team communication, leadership, situational awareness, and interpersonal exchange and are crucial to facilitate the best achievable results during critical situations (Von Wyl, Zuercher, Amsler, Walter & Ummenhoffer, 2008). Using simulations to assess the students' readiness to practice before clinical practicums and rotations, as well as enhancing their clinical competence and confidence is also a primary purpose and outcome of the expanded use of simulation in this program. The enhanced realism and relevance of the simulations, as well as the enhanced formative feedback through rich **debriefing**, self-reflection, and peer assessment opportunities has resulted in greater student satisfaction with simulation activities and improved student success Early on, NAIT adopted Debriefing with Good Judgement (DWGJ) as the primary approach to debriefing in the curriculum (Rudolph, Simon, Dufresne, & Raemer, 2006). **In situ** simulation is used extensively in the advanced care paramedic program to replicate "the workplace" that paramedic students will be expected to work in upon graduation. These in situ settings occur across campus such as at swimming pools, racquetball courts, administrative offices, hockey arenas, automotive shops, and the washroom, as well as off-site locations such as the inner-city homeless shelter and the local seniors lodge (Fig. 25.1). **Simulated/standardized patients (SPs)**, "high-tech" *human patient simulators*, and a combination thereof, known as **hybrid simulations**, augment paramedic simulations. Also, prospective paramedic students (i.e., EMT students) volunteer their time as *confederates* and are embedded participants/actors (sometimes referred to as confederates) into each simulation for further realism and authenticity of each case. Additionally, the paramedic program incorporates the use of local junior high school drama students from the seventh to ninth grade as junior SPs. Simulations utilizing junior SPs provide paramedic students with valuable exposure to "pediatric populations" and afford them the opportunity to engage and interact with this subgroup of patients. Meanwhile, the drama students have an opportunity to apply their drama skills to challenging clinical situations.

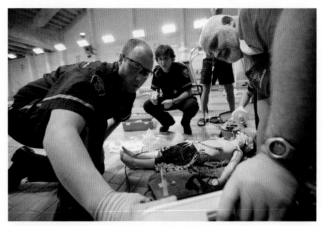

Figure 25.1 Paramedic Students Completing an Interprofessional In Situ Simulation on Deck at the NAIT Swimming Pool of a 6-Year-Old Cardiac Arrest. Courtesy of NAIT, with permission.

Respiratory Therapist Program

The respiratory therapist (RT) program offers another example of simulation adoption and enhancement in recent years at NAIT. In 2008, the RT program received provincial funding to address clinical capacity issues (the inability for clinical placement sites to meet learning needs and numbers of learners) in the hospital practicum setting, approving the SCORE (Simulation for Clinical Optimization of Respiratory Education) Project. The 3-year funded project explored the use of simulation for both enhancing and replacing several weeks of the clinical component of the program. With assistance from clinical preceptors, 72 clinical simulation scenarios were developed to populate several weeks of simulation that was embedded within the RT students' clinical education experience. In the third year of the project, preceptors from clinical sites were hired to assist NAIT RT clinical faculty in the delivery and debriefing of these simulation scenarios. The simulations primarily target skills and situations that allow our students to be more prepared and capable in the first few shifts in clinical rotations. Through capital project funds, the RT program has purchased five high-fidelity mannequins, two test lungs with spontaneous breathing modules, as well as other simulation, respiratory, and storage equipment to enhance realism and assist in the delivery of these simulation scenarios. The project outcomes (1) resulted in the *replacement* of several weeks of clinical time throughout the duration of the 3-year program, (2) provided increased capacity and decreased pressure on the clinical sites as well as on the clinical instructors with "reduced preceptor burnout," (3) provided an opportunity to address *experiential learning* gaps with simulation, (4) enhanced student preparedness for each of their clinical rotations, and (5) improved student–preceptor relations. This project has become a permanent and sustainable addition to the delivery of the RT curricula and continues to be refined even further each year to ensure quality in the clinical education of RT students.

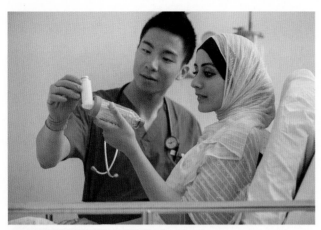

Figure 25.2 Respiratory Therapy Students are Participating in an Immersive Simulation, Assessing and Treating a Short of Breath, Asthmatic Patient with an Emphasis on Cultural Diversity (Utilizing SPs). Courtesy of NAIT, with permission.

The RT program has also integrated a **multimodal** approach to the adoption of various types of simulation beyond computerized full-body simulators, including the use of SPs (see Fig. 25.2) and web-based **virtual patients** in the curricula. These learning experiences provide further opportunities for self-directed learning, clinical decision-making, and enhanced experiential learning.

Diagnostic Medical Sonography

Several diagnostic imaging programs at NAIT have also embraced simulation-based education including the allied health discipline of sonography (ultrasound). Feedback from industry partners revealed that diagnostic medical sonography (DMS) students lacked history-taking and professionalism skills. Simulations using SPs were developed and integrated in 2010 to address this gap, including scenarios related to geriatrics, trauma, multiculturalism, auditory/visual impairment, grief, anger, anxiousness, and cardiac arrest.

The National Competency Profile for Sonography Canada requires that two major competencies be taught and assessed in a simulated environment. These include (1) recognizing and responding to emergency situations and (2) providing support in emergency situations. The Clinical Sonographer course addresses this requirement by using immersive medical emergency simulations as part of the curriculum. These simulations use mannequins and SPs to portray various signs and symptoms of a disease or reaction that result in a medical emergency. Learning in these simulations employs both **formative and summative assessment/evaluation**.

With the demand and growth of the DMS profession, increased class sizes resulted in an insufficient number of clinical placements to accommodate 60 DMS students at one time. Therefore, a 2-week clinical simulation course was created to allow second-year students to return to

NAIT from clinical rotations and avoid clinical overlap with other first-year students who also require access to the clinical sites (a similar clinical capacity issue to the RT program above). The course includes more than 32 hours of simulation to optimize the students' clinical learning while at the same time replacing clinical practicum time. This course exposes students to a variety of activities and contexts that simulate the workplace. Simulation scenarios engage the students in activities such as reporting exam findings to a radiologist and performing various core competencies. Other simulations focus on professionalism, collaborative practice, and body mechanics. Every simulation includes a facilitated debriefing to ensure rich feedback and conversation specific to the learning objectives, behavior modification, and closure of any knowledge, skill, or attitudinal gaps. One of the NAIT DMS students expressed her appreciation for the enhanced feedback and debriefing from this course, saying: "I really liked the debriefing at the end of each where we could actually talk about how we felt because we finally got an opportunity to express the stress and frustrations we experienced as students during different difficult clinical situations." Some of the DMS program lessons learned from using simulation for enhancing clinical rotations as well as replacing clinical time are featured in Box 25-4.

Combined Laboratory and X-Ray Technology

Another allied health program example at NAIT includes the discipline of combined laboratory and x-ray technology (CLXT). In addition to traditional labs and experiential learning activities, the CLXT incorporated a "Simulation Day" near the end of the program as a capstone event. This "Sim Day" offers a full day of 12 different simulation scenarios that immerse students in realistic clinical situations, allowing the application of their knowledge,

---

Box 25-4   Lessons Learned from DMS

- Through a series of simulated scenarios, the students had the ability to practice skills and interactions allowing them an opportunity to improve their abilities before attending practicum.
- These workplace simulations offered students the chance to encounter situations in a learning environment without the fear of jeopardizing patient safety.
- Time to discuss an exam or professional interaction is not always available while in a practicum, incorporating the time to debrief an activity or situation as part of a simulation helps to solidify the learning and work together as a team to problem solve.
- Developing multiple simulations that offer a unique and valuable learning experience can be difficult.
- Designing the simulations to encourage student buy-in can be challenging.
- Scheduling 32 hours of simulation labs in a 2-week block can present challenges; this 40-hour course equates to 264 hours of instructor time.

skills, and attitudes. The students rotate through each of the 12 different simulation scenarios (utilizing SPs and other volunteer actors) that provide an opportunity to practice and develop the following skills:

- Communication and professionalism skills
- Taking a blood sample and perform an ECG on a sweaty, short of breath patient
- Transfer of a patient with a broken hip onto the x-ray table using a slider board
- Identify and respond to a medical emergency (fainting patient) before performing a blood collection
- Professionally interact with patient that is intoxicated and behaving flirtatiously with healthcare providers while performing a hand x-ray
- Performing blood collection while managing the emotional stress reaction of an injured, pregnant female patient that has been in a car accident and recently discovered that her husband died in the collision

The simulations throughout the day become increasingly more complex and stressful, building on each of the previous simulations. The "boot camp" simulation modality provides our CLXT students an opportunity to experience a "full work day in the real world" and practice critical skills in a context-specific setting. Each simulation is designed to ensure relevancy and authenticity. To accomplish this, we base our simulations on real events and situations that our students may or may not experience within the hospital setting during their clinical training experiences. This approach addresses both core competencies as well as **high-acuity, low-occurrence (HALO) clinical events** for our students.

Magnetic Radiographic Technology (MRT)

Radiography education has been known to use simulated-based teaching and learning instructional methods such as anatomical models, SPs, and computer-generated systems that replicate clinical scenarios for the purpose of clinical skill development (Ng, 2015). The magnetic radiographic technology (MRT) program at NAIT is no exception and has used various forms of simulation in the curricula, ranging from traditional skills and lab education to highly contextual Simulated Clinical Immersion experiences with an emphasis on rich debriefing. The MRT program has also addressed clinical capacity issues at their clinical sites by incorporating several days of simulation-based education to replace some clinical time and to enhance the clinical learning experience for the students. Students return to NAIT from their clinical sites, thus alleviating the pressures on clinical partners while allowing increased access to these sites for other MRT students. Box 25-5 further highlights this simulation initiative in the MRT program.

Diagnostic Laboratory Programs

The Medical Laboratory Assisting (MLA) and Medical Laboratory Technology (MLT) allied health disciplines were

Box 25-5	**Optimizing Clinical Rotations and Enhancing Capacity with Simulation in the MRT Program**

- The simulations are intended to fill the experiential learning gaps and HALO events during the clinical practicum.
- All simulations were grounded in a comprehensive needs assessment and gap analysis that included input from students, industry partners, clinical partners, and advisory committees (i.e., the need for enhanced communication skills).
- To maximize fidelity and realism, the simulations in the MRT program accommodate 1 to 2 students that participate in a high-intensity simulation while being observed remotely from an observation/debriefing room by other students and the facilitator. All students and the facilitator participate in the debriefing of each scenario. Students are allowed to make mistakes in this safe/controlled environment and are ensured to learn from that experience. Simulations were developed and scripted by NAIT MRT staff members and based are on past real-life experiences.
- Each simulation reflects current industry practices and potential incidents.
- Each student can participate in a scenario that they may have not yet experienced but could potentially experience during their clinical practice as a student or future employee.
- MRT simulations unfold in the NAIT MRT lab space, or a simulation center, using SPs, human patient simulators (high-fidelity mannequins), moulage/makeup (for enhanced realism), and both paid actors and staff members in the embedded actor role.

early adopters of the "new world" simulation movement to supplement their existing simulated lab activities. The program has developed and integrated more than ten realistic simulations using SPs various types of human patient simulators, task trainers, and hybrid simulations into courses to address common themes and needs. Simulations encompass enhanced communication and professionalism soft skill development to supplement clinical exposure and experience during practicums. Simulations involved situations with patients from various age groups that experienced intoxication, grieving, and fainting, or demonstrated flirtatious behavior. The simulations also provide opportunities for promoting collaborative practice with other professions while challenging the traditional medical laboratory scope of practice.

The MLT/MLA programs have also enhanced their teaching and learning methods with the development and integration of computer-based simulations to help students further enhance their confidence in concepts that, at one time, could only be practiced in the lab. Some examples of developed computer-based simulations include (1) data entry and patient demographics, (2) microscope use, (3) phlebotomy practice, and (4) analyzer maintenance/troubleshooting. One area for improvement in these individual, self-directed

Box 25-6	Lessons Learned from Simulation Integration in the MLT/MLA Programs

- The difficulty with incorporating traditional lab testing with the use of simulation (analyzers, specimens processing, handling, and testing) without the high cost presents unique challenges.
- There is a need to include more opportunities for med lab simulation-based education to help with clinical placement gaps
- Debriefing sessions post-simulation are incredibly powerful learning moments. It is crucial to leverage these transformational moments even further by having skilled facilitators (as debriefers). Skilled facilitators guide meaningful learning through conversations that cover learning objectives while allowing the students to "get there" on their own as much as possible without defaulting to directed learning or teaching methods

learning computer-based simulations is the gap and need for richer feedback to be provided to the learner after the simulation. This facilitative approach requires greater complexity in computer programming and development, yet is a critical element to ensuring that learning has occurred and errors are corrected prior to real patient care.

The MLT/MLA programs report positive outcomes from the use of SPs, stating that they have been beneficial to student learning by adding a "real human" experience that is more authentic and effective compared to role-play by the students. Student testimonials repeatedly indicate that SP-based simulations have been incredibly valuable in providing a "complete clinical picture" and in addressing learning gaps that cannot be taught in the classroom and labs alone.

Additional lessons learned from the MLT/MLA programs specific to the use of simulation are described in Box 25-6.

Denturist Programs

Although some definitions of allied health exclude dental education, NAIT SHLS includes three highly successful dental programs, namely, dental assisting, denturist, and dental technology. Each of these dental allied health programs uses various types of simulation in their delivery methods. Task trainers, real dental equipment, and cases based on real patients are used to simulate various dental procedures and skills. In addition, the denturist program added the combined use of Simulated/Standardized Patients and **Objective Structured Clinical Examinations** (*OSCEs*) within their simulation curricula for added consistency and validity in their assessments. OSCEs, as a clinical skills evaluative approach "have been used by many health professions to test the development of skills" (MacLellan, 2015, p. 495). The NAIT Denturist program, working closely

with the licensing/regulatory body in Alberta for the last 8 years, has developed, piloted, and integrated more than 12 OSCEs in dental education curricula for enhanced formative and summative assessment/evaluation. The partnership has also resulted in enhanced educational experiences at NAIT. In addition to curricular improvement, the collaborative efforts have produced more than 30 OSCE scenarios to reform the current provincial licensing examination. The change has standardized and improved the validity and reliability in high-stakes testing processes, once again, in reponse to industry and regulatory feedback. Additionally, in collaboration with NAITs Digital Media and Information Technology program students, we have developed a computer-based simulation for teaching clinical decision-making and partial denture competencies.

Animal Health Technology and Veterinary Medical Assistant Programs

Similar to the use of simulation for teaching crisis resource management for anesthesia in the human world (Gaba, 2004), the Animal Health Technology (AHT) program developed several simulations staged in the operating room for our "furry friends" from the feline and canine populations. Through the use of human **embedded actors/**

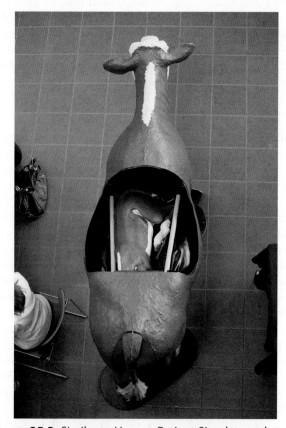

Figure 25.3 Similar to Human Patient Simulators, the Animal Health Technology Program at NAIT Utilizes True-to-Life Simulators Including Feline, Canine, Bovine, and Equine Simulators. Courtesy of NAIT, with permission.

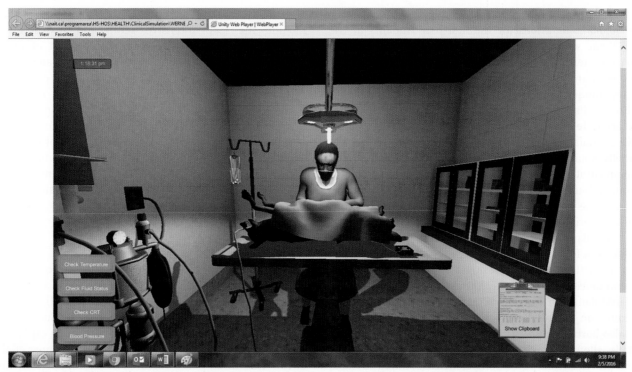

Figure 25.4 An AHT Desktop Simulation Allowing Students to Practice the Care and Monitoring of an Anesthetized Patient (German Shepherd). Courtesy of NAIT, with permission.

participants as clients, and **animal patient simulators** (see Fig. 25.3), realistic simulated clinical immersions have been developed and integrated into the AHT program to enhance experience and confidence in AHT students. Simulations allow students to manage intraoperative patients with all of the associated technical and nontechnical dynamics inherent in this high-risk context. Some examples of anesthesia-related simulations include the following:

● An immersive introductory simulation to demonstrate the setup of an anesthetic machine and perform a low-pressure leak (LPL) test and trace oxygen flow, allowing them to "get their feet wet" in this setting
● The induction of a feline or canine patient to practice general anesthesia skills and the placement of an endotracheal tube
● Simulations to focus on the care of the patient during the maintenance phase of anesthesia in the operating room
● Emergency anesthesia situations and critical events

Dr. Greg Woodard, AHT instructor at NAIT and veterinarian describes the following positive outcome:

One thing that I have seen since we have been adding more simulation in the Anesthesiology course is how much better prepared the students are for the anesthetist rotations in 2nd year. The students also appear to be able to handle better the unexpected and stressful situations and seem more accepting of constructive criticism during other rotations, in part due to greater use of debriefing and feedback in simulations.

The AHT program also developed a computer-based desktop simulation (see Fig. 25.4) to further support anesthesia training and better prepare their students before arrival at the lab. Students complete a staged learning process by completing e-simulations, followed by the face-to-face simulation, and, finally, practicing and applying their skills in a real anesthesia setting with live animals, seen in Figure 25.5.

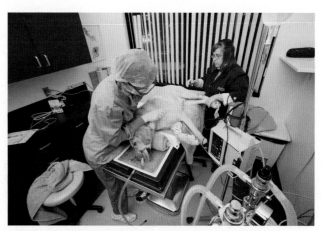

Figure 25.5 An AHT Student Participates in a Real Anesthesia Monitoring Case, but not Before the Completion of Computer-Based and Mannequin-Based Simulations to Ensure Safe Practice, Competency, and Confidence in the Learner. Courtesy of NAIT, with permission.

The program has also developed *history-taking telephone simulations* for the first-year students in the AHT and veterinary medical assistant (VMA) programs to promote clinical questioning and the practice of engaging with and managing clients in a professional manner. These unique simulations require that students field telephone calls from simulated/standardized clients, gather an accurate history, and multitask to manage a busy office. We stimulate all of the students' senses with the real smells, sounds, and sights of a real clinic. Students must demonstrate professional communication, conflict resolution, and effective office management skills, then receive immediate peer and instructor feedback in the post-simulation debriefings.

Simulation has become popular among healthcare educators for delivering IPE activities with several studies reporting short-term impacts such as improved communication within healthcare teams (Kenaszchuk, MacMillan, Van Soeren, & Reeves, 2011). Not only is simulation potentially effective for skills development, it is also particularly well suited for team training and soft skills, allowing participants to interact with one another and practice team-based competencies (Fanning & Gaba, as cited in Rogers et al., 2012). This is evident at NAIT as emergency simulations are also integrated into the AHT/VMA curricula to provide **interprofessional education (IPE)** and **interprofessional collaborative practice** opportunities between the roles of AHT, VMA, and Doctor of Veterinary Medicine (DVM). Students have a chance to practice the skills and competencies of emergency management and care of the animal patients and their upset owners with an emphasis of interprofessional competencies in these predetermined emergency situations created by instructional program staff.

Personal Fitness Trainer Program

The NAIT SHLS has a reputation for their highly successful 2-year Personal Fitness Trainer (PFT) diploma program. The PFT program, included in the broader allied health realm and definition at NAIT with the focus on prevention of illness and injury, uses various simulation-based teaching and learning methods using task trainers and scenario-based simulations. For example, PFT students utilize blood pressure task trainers for learning this core skill before practicing blood pressure readings with real clients in pre- and post-exercise assessments. Grounded in formative assessment, students also engage with standardized clients that represent geriatric populations to gain experience and receive feedback in aerobic monitoring, client assessment, and information gathering skills. Simulations have proven to be more effective and realistic than the previous practice of student role-play.

The major challenges as described by PFT staff include the labor-intensive setup and instructional design time required before the deployment of these simulations. These challenges have often been an impediment to the integration of simulations in the curricula. In some cases, the barriers have resulted in reverting to past, more *instructor-time-friendly* learning activities that are less demanding. This reality is concerning because the PFT program found the quality of learning experiences to be exponentially greater with simulation. It is important to find ways to allocate more time within instructor workloads to develop and deploy simulation further.

Research in Allied Health Simulation

Several of the program examples above have also included formal research to evaluate the effectiveness and drive best practice in the use of simulation. NAIT SHLS was an active participant in a Simulation-Enhanced Curriculum Research Study, a Canadian allied health study exploring the use of simulation within the curricula (Gropper et al., 2010). This three-phase research study investigated the question: Does simulation-enhanced curriculum reduce "time to competency"? The competencies selected for the study included four patient interaction competencies from the radiological national (Canada) entry-level competency profile. Student participants were recruited from six different allied health disciplines including these NAIT programs: diagnostic medical sonography, medical radiological technology, magnetic resonance, combined laboratory and x-ray technology, radiation therapy, and medical laboratory.

Phase one resulted in the development of a tool to evaluate student performance. Results in phase two indicated improved OSCE performance in the interventional group. Phase three results indicated a reduced "time to competency," specifically, students who had received prior simulation training achieved patient interaction competency 4 weeks earlier than the control group students. In response to the research question: "Does simulation-enhanced curriculum reduce time to competency?" this study indicates that yes, it does, in all four identified patient interaction competencies. Limitations of the study included a smaller sample size than preferred. The research investigators recommend continued exploration of the research question utilizing (1) different competencies such as technical and/or other nontechnical competencies, (2) competencies from similar or different allied health science professions, and (3) a larger sample size. This study is just one example of exciting research and evidence-based practice that continues to grow in the field of allied health simulation.

Common Themes in Allied Health and Nursing Simulation

So....what key terms related to simulation did you underline or highlight when reading the examples above? What reoccurring themes stood out from your perspective between allied health and nursing? Were you able to identify similarities as well as unique issues and features of simulation in allied health education? Compare your notes and highlighted words and phrases with some of the highlighted themes in Box 25-7.

Moving Forward...A New Interprofessional Allied Health Simulation Center

NAIT SHLS has much to celebrate about simulation integration after several years of hard work and commitment. To this day, we continue to grow the allied health simulation movement. Enhancing teaching, learning, and assessment/evaluation through simulation continue to be the focus for

the SHLS. See Toolkit 25-1 for a copy of the floor plan. NAIT's future includes increased physical capacity for simulation growth with the new SHLS Simulation Center designed and developed to serve all of the allied health programs at NAIT as well as other internal and external partners and users. This dynamic learning space will encourage and support both single-discipline and interprofessional simulation activities. The center includes a welcoming multi-purpose foyer, nine flexible simulation theaters four elevated and four nonelevated control rooms, five dedicated observation/debrief rooms, office space, a simulation technician workshop, and ample storage (see Chapter 27, workbooks two and three). Program-specific simulation labs adjacent to the Simulation Center include Paramedic (ambulance simulator included; see Fig. 25.6), Respiratory Therapy, and Diagnostic Medical Sonography, creating an impressive collective space to further champion simulation-based education at NAIT SHLS.

Box 25-7	Key Themes and Examples for the Use of Simulation in the Allied Health Exemplar

- Patient safety
- Experiential learning
- Predetermined simulations such as high-acuity, low occurrence (HALO) events
- Creation of an immersive clinical context in simulation scenarios including the use of in situ simulation
- OSCE simulations for summative and high-stakes evaluation
- Multimodal use of simulation that incorporates the use of including task trainers, SPs, hybrid simulations, high-tech human patient simulators, and virtual patients
- IPE and collaborative practice via simulation
- Evidence-based augmentation and replacement of some clinical practicum time to address not only clinical capacity issues but also the need to enhance and optimize clinical learning such as "time to competency" in allied health students
- A greater emphasis on rich feedback, debriefing, and formative assessment/evaluation post–simulation-based learning activities.
- Growing research in the use of simulation in allied health education.
- Not just for the technical, hard skills…. Please give us soft skills! A significant portion of new simulation scenarios in the curriculum now address the nontechnical, or soft skills of relationality in patient care, professionalism, and team dynamics, to complement existing emphasis on clinical skills competency.
- Partnerships, both internal and external, provide further support and opportunity for simulation enhancement.

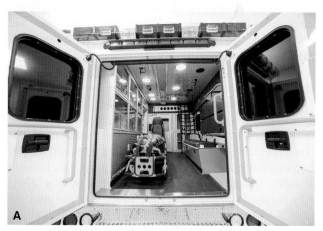

A

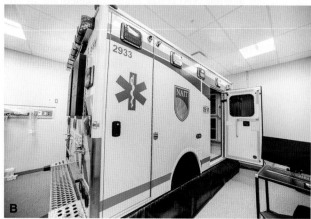

B

Figure 25.6 NAIT Created an Industry-Standard Ambulance Box with a Motion Platform and Monitors in lieu of Windows that Project Recorded Video of Edmonton Streets and Roadways Synchronized with the Movement of the Ambulance, Offering Paramedic Students an Immersive Opportunity to Practice Safe Patient Care During Transport. Courtesy of NAIT, with permission.

Opening in August 2016, the SHLS leadership team has created a simple, yet vital *operational readiness* strategic plan to ensure that the simulation center will be fully functional and deployable on opening day. Box 25-8 highlights the seven key deliverables and outcomes of the operational readiness plan. Each Chair of the leadership team has accepted the challenge to lead the charge of one of these deliverables along with the support of a subcommittee team to ensure the completion of the action plans and deliverables to ensure that their assigned strategy comes to fruition. This collective and collaborative approach across the leadership team is a testament to the continued dedication and commitment to simulation in the SHLS.

Summary

Revisiting the opening guiding questions at the start of this chapter, it is apparent that there are few differences between allied health simulation and other groups such as nursing and medicine. In fact, we utilize and apply the same grounding theory and simulation modalities and typologies found within other healthcare education curricula. We are much more alike than we are different. What is unique to our discipline, however, may simply be the size and type of the simulator!

After several years of change leadership and management, and a commitment to continuous adoption and integration of simulation within the allied health curricula, positive outcomes have emerged, and the proposed simulation outcomes from previous strategic plans have become a reality (including the examples shared in Box 25-8). As a result of collaboration, early adopters at the program level, and support from both "top-down" and "bottom-up" change agents, NAIT has much to celebrate in the enhanced use of simulation in allied health education in the School of Health Sciences.

Allied health is becoming a leader in the use of simulation in prelicensure education. This chapter explored the definition of allied health, the basic benefits, and tenets of SBE and provided an exemplar of the adoption and use of simulation in allied health prelicensure programming and curricula. It is imperative that all stakeholders continue to embrace and harness the potential of SBE in allied health education and beyond. We trust that some of the examples shared in this chapter will act as a catalyst for creativity and innovation as well as further support your role as a Simulation Champion in your organization.

Box 25-8	**Seven Strategies of the *Operational Readiness* Plan for NAIT's Allied Health Simulation Center**

1. A defined HR Model for the simulation center
2. An Equipment and Storage Plan
3. A Scheduling Plan
4. A defined Budget for the simulation center
5. An Operations Plan and execution of the plan for day-to-day activities within the simulation center
6. An Educational Plan and execution of the plan to support staff end-users of the new learning space
7. A Communication and Marketing Plan and execution of the plan to all stakeholders of the simulation center

Toolkit Resource

Toolkit 25-1: Floor Plan of the NAIT SHLS Simulation Centre. NAIT is pleased to share the floor plan of our Simulation Centre, opened in August 2016. Assorted pictures featuring many innovative design ideas are located in the Chapter 27 online toolkit, Companion Image Collection of Simulation Centres and General Nursing Skills Labs.

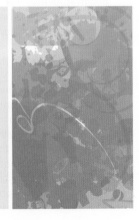

Reflection Activity 25-1
Similarities and Differences Between Allied Health and Nursing Education

Having read the various applications of simulation-based learning in allied health education, which examples resonate most with you? What examples or adoption strategies from *simulation in allied health* resonate most with you? How might you be able to apply and champion these applications and strategies for simulation growth in your organization?

26

Leading Interprofessional Education: Shaping Tomorrow's Healthcare

Sharla King, L. Dawn Ansell

"If healthcare providers are expected to work together and share expertise in a team environment, it makes sense that their education and training should prepare them for this type of working arrangement." (Sando, Coggins, & Romanow, 2002, p. 109).

Key Terms

Interprofessional Education (IPE), Interprofessional Collaboration (IPC), Interdisciplinary, Simulation-Enhanced IPE (SIM-IPE), Leadership, Hidden Curriculum

Guiding Questions

1 What models exist to increase collaboration and enhance patient safety?

2 What is Sim-IPE and what healthcare issues can you best address by using Sim-IPE?

3 What about IPE attracts learners?

4 Where would you be able to host IPE? What other institutions exist in your local area that you can partner with to develop and implement Sim-IPE?

5 How can you create sustainability in developing and offering Sim-IPE experiences?

Our Story—The Interdisciplinary Health Education Partnership

In 2008, the Alberta provincial government in Canada had a call for proposals from academic institutions to create innovative educational opportunities for a broad range of learners. Rather than compete for funding dollars, health science programs from four postsecondary institutions and the provincial health provider decided to partner to explore simulation-enhanced interprofessional education (Sim-IPE) opportunities across our organizations. Each postsecondary institution had different levels of expertise related to simulation and IPE. By also partnering with a health provider, we ensured a strong connection to the practice setting. Thus was created the Interdisciplinary Health Education Partnership (IHEP). The goals of the project included "developing, implementing and evaluating three simulation-based education modules targeting gaps/inadequacies in healthcare practitioner's competencies, especially as they relate to patient safety and interprofessional healthcare teams" (IHEP, 2012).

This chapter will outline the practical strategies and approaches our partnership developed and implemented to ensure that our students had access to high-quality simulation-enhanced interprofessional education. We draw on examples from our experiences and resources we developed and utilized. However, we also refer to the

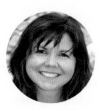

Sharla King, PhD

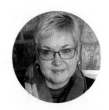

L. Dawn Ansell, BN

evidence in the literature to support our actions and highlight additional resources others may find helpful. Before we get started, a quick note about **interdisciplinary** versus interprofessional language. In the literature, there are strong advocates for a clear distinction between "interprofessional" and "interdisciplinary" (Gilbert, 2005). However, additional voices are highlighting the similarities between the two (e.g., the challenges with the silo mentality in both) (Smith & Clouder, 2010). At the time that we created IHEP, the word "interdisciplinary" was more reflective of the current thinking of all partners. As the project evolved, we shifted our language to "interprofessional" with the intent of being inclusive of all health team providers, regardless of credentials. Therefore, throughout this chapter, we will use the word "interprofessional" with the same intent for inclusivity.

Brief Background of Interprofessional Education (IPE)

Interprofessional education "occurs when two or more professions learn with, from and about each other to improve collaboration and the quality of care" (CAIPE, 2002). IPE is viewed as a means to enhance collaborative practice (WHO, 2010b). Optimizing interprofessional collaborative teams can help improve patient outcomes and make the healthcare system more sustainable (Dinh, Stonebridge, & Theriault, 2014; Reeves, Boet, Zierler, & Kitto, 2015). Support for and interest in IPE and collaborative practice are increasing on a global scale (Frenk et al., 2010; IOM, 1999; Reeves, Tassone, Parker, Wagner, & Simmons, 2012; Sando et al., 2002; WHO, 2010b). As such, healthcare professionals should have opportunities to develop **interprofessional collaboration (IPC)** competencies (Dinh et al., 2014).

Global Interprofessional Networks

Across the globe, eight interprofessional networks represent each major geographic region featured in Table 26.1. These networks are also members of the World Coordinating Committee established in 2013 to facilitate resource sharing between the networks and establish relationships with other organizations.

Competency Frameworks and Guides to Support IPE

Before the development of interprofessional competency frameworks, educators used frameworks focused on patient safety highlighting teamwork and communication competencies (King et al., 2013). For example, the Canadian Patient Safety Institute's Safety Competencies has two domains focusing on effective communication and teamwork (2009) providing a useful structure for educators.

World Health Organization's Patient Safety Curriculum Guide: Multi-professional Edition (WHO, 2011a) synthesized frameworks from Canada and Australia to develop a guide to assist academic institutions with capacity building in the area of patient safety education. The guide clearly highlights the critical need for students to understand teamwork, team dynamics, and effective communication across professions, not just within their profession.

There now exist specific interprofessional competency frameworks with the Canadian Interprofessional Health Collaborative Competency Framework (2010) and the Interprofessional Education Collaborative Competency Framework (2011) in Canada and the United States respectively. In Australia and the United Kingdom, postsecondary institutions have created Interprofessional Capability Frameworks (CUILU, 2004; Curtin University, 2010). These documents guide the development of educational initiatives ensuring that the skills, knowledge, and attitudes necessary for collaborative practice are intentionally built into learning experiences. The specific language used to describe the competencies across these documents may vary; however, the concepts are similar. Table 26.2 features varied interprofessional competencies and featured terminology.

Also, IPE is integrated into the accreditation standards for six health professions in Canada (medicine, nursing, occupational therapy, pharmacy, physical therapy, and social work) (AIPHE, 2009). This document outlines principles to guide and support the integration of IPE into curricula to meet accreditation standards. The WHO (2010b) created a document providing a framework for IPE and collaborative practice to guide the development of initiatives around the globe.

TeamSTEPPS is an evidence-based teamwork system and training program developed jointly by the United States Department of Defense and the Agency for Healthcare Research and Quality. It is focused on optimizing patient care by improving communication and teamwork skills among healthcare professionals. The TeamSTEPPS website houses a comprehensive set of ready-to-use resources (checklists, videos) and a training curriculum to successfully integrate teamwork principles into a variety of care settings. Although the TeamSTEPPS curriculum targets practicing professionals, many of the resources are easy to incorporate into health professional curricula for students (AHRQ, 2015c; Baker & Fowler Durham, 2014).

Common Barriers to Implementing IPE

Anyone involved in health professional education understands that despite a belief in IPE, often the barriers to bringing students from other disciplines together are challenging, especially when integrating the learning experience into the curriculum. Some of these challenges include the unique culture of practice of each discipline; disciplines that work together in practice are often not educated at the same

Table 26.1	Global Interprofessional Networks	
AIHC	The American Interprofessional Health Collaborative https://aihc-us.org/	Transcends boundaries to transform learning, policies, practices, and scholarship toward an improved system of health and wellness for individual patients, communities, and populations
AIPPEN	The Australasian Interprofessional Practice and Education Network http://www.aippen.net/	Brings together individuals, groups, institutions, and organizations committed to promoting and supporting interprofessional learning and improving collaborative practice, with the ultimate goal of achieving quality patient-centered care
CAIPE	The Centre for the Advancement of Interprofessional Education https://www.caipe.org/	Formed in 1987, this *think tank* comprises individuals, corporate, and student members who work with organizations in the United Kingdom and overseas to "improve collaborative practice and thereby the quality of care by professions learning and working together."
CIHC	The Canadian Interprofessional Health Collaborative http://www.cihc.ca/	The CIHC is the hub for interprofessional activity in Canada, and it works at the edges and interfaces of health, education, and the professions to discover and share promising practices to promote interprofessional education and collaboration in areas that will enhance patient care.
EIPEN	European Interprofessional Education Network http://www.eipen.eu/	Develops and shares effective IP training programs, methods, and materials for improving collaborative practice in health and social care in Europe.
JAIPE	The Japan Association of Interprofessional Education https://www.jaipe.net/	Launched in 2008, the role of the association is to implement IPE, to conduct research, and to train health professionals to collaborate.
JIPWEN	Japan Interprofessional Working and Education Network http://jipwen.dept.showa.gunma-u.ac.jp/	Established in 2008 by 10 Japanese universities engaged in health professions education. The network aims to discuss critical issues of IPE and to present plural models so that institutions who are interested in the IPE programs can adapt the models to their academic and social settings. Nowadays, more and more institutions intend to start IPE activities.
NIPNET	The Nordic Interprofessional Network http://nipnet.org/	Created in 2001 in Norway, network members collaborate in designing, delivering, and evaluating interprofessional education programs by sharing experiences and addressing underlying theoretical issues.

Table 26.2	Comparing Interprofessional Competencies and Terms		
CIHC Competencies (2010)	**IPEC Competencies (2011)**	**The Combined Universities Interprofessional Learning Unit (2004)**	**University of Curtin IPE Capabilities (2010)**
Interprofessional Communication and Patient-, Client-, Family, and Community-Centered Care 1. Role clarification 2. Collaborative leadership 3. Team functioning 4. Interprofessional conflict resolution	Values/Ethics for interprofessional Practice 1. Roles/responsibilities 2. Interprofessional communication 3. Teams and teamwork	Domains: 1. Knowledge in practice 2. Ethical practice 3. Interprofessional working 4. Reflection (learning)	Core elements: 1. Client-centered service 2. Client safety and quality 3. Collaborative practice Core elements are underpinned by five collaborative practice capabilities: 1. Communication 2. Team function 3. Role clarification 4. Conflict resolution 5. Reflection

institution, and even when they are, timetabling, logistics, physical location, and traditionally defined curriculum are barriers and issues such as workload, reward systems, research and teaching objectives vary within and across institutions for faculty members (Thibault, 2011). Even when an interinstitutional collaboration is possible, the different terminal credentials (certificate, diploma, degree) may be perceived as a limitation, yet in certain environments, the disciplines work together in the practice setting, regardless of the terminal credentials. Additionally, faculty may be unprepared to facilitate in an interprofessional environment, adding another layer of complexity (Dinh, 2012).

To help overcome some of these challenges, IPE "best practice" models have been proposed, such as didactic programming (team building and knowledge of interprofessional practice), community-based practice, and interprofessional simulation (Bridges, Davidson, Soule Odegard, Maki, & Tomkowiak, 2011; INACSL Standards Committee, 2016). To operationalize these best practice models, it is often essential to (1) develop cross-institutional relationships, because only a small percentage of schools offer a diverse range of programs (Thibault, 2011), and (2) create relevant interprofessional experiences that mirror students' future practice (Jeffries & Rizzolo, 2006b). Faculty preparedness must be addressed through faculty development sessions. If there is an office of IPE at your institution, they may be able to assist in preparing faculty or clinical/community educators to facilitate in an interprofessional environment. Attending IPE conferences, such as Collaborating Across Borders, a conference jointly planned by the CIHC and AIHC and held in alternating years either in Canada or in the United States, can provide further knowledge and exposure to instructors new to IPE. More formal training is available through a program called Educating Health Professionals in Interprofessional Care (http://ehpic.ca/).

Our partnership overcame many of these barriers by remaining focused on the key objective—preparing our students for collaborative practice. We searched for creative strategies to address challenges, which often meant taking a few risks. Additionally, we started with cocurricular learning experiences to pilot ideas and scenarios, rather than focusing on integrating the learning into curriculum immediately. We harnessed our local expertise and developed our own faculty development workshops for interprofessional simulation.

Why Simulation-Enhanced IPE?

Healthcare simulation primarily evolved from issues in patient safety (Palaganas, Epps, & Raemer, 2014). Additionally, the introduction of human factors research into crisis resource management simulations (Gaba, 1997) resulted in a focus on areas such as IP relationships and hierarchy, communication, and organizational cultures in high-stress, high-risk environments. The Institute of Medicine's (1999) report *To Err is Human* initiated a surge in team training with health professionals (Salas, Burke, & Cannon-Bowers, 2000). Thus began the era of IPE in simulation. Simulation provides an environment to explore issues of power imbalances, gender, hierarchy, status, and professional divisions; sociohistorical factors often ignored in the IPE literature (Palaganas et al., 2014; Reeves, Kitto, Alexanian, & Grant, 2016). The siloed approach to health professional education has nurtured a culture of ineffective collaboration (WHO, 2010b), as is evident in the statistics reported in hospital, patient safety, and risk management studies. Simulation-enhanced IPE provides the opportunity to address this culture of ineffective collaboration and the theory-to-practice gap in most health professional programs (Bridges et al., 2011; Greenstock, Brooks, & Bingham, 2011; Sharma, Boet, Kitto, & Reeves, 2011).

Why is there a natural merging of simulation and IPE? Simulation-enhanced IPE allows for a closer resemblance to actual clinical practice with more relevant feedback provided (Palaganas et al., 2014). The simulation learning experiences can be designed to address the learning needs of different levels of learners. Students can observe the simulation and then participate in the debrief—a critical aspect of simulation. Additionally, issues such as social hierarchy, and diversity can be examined through the debrief. Reflection and discussion during the debrief may reveal cognitive frames related to these social issues and provides a safe environment to explore them.

Research in **Simulation-Enhanced Interprofessional Education** (Sim-IPE) has shown improved team communication (Kenaszchuk, MacMillan, Van Soeren, & Reeves, 2011) and augmented team performance and knowledge (Capella et al., 2010). Sim-IPE "enables participants from different professions to engage in a simulation-based experience to achieve shared or linked objectives and outcomes" (INACSL Standards Committee, 2016 - Sim-IPE, p. S34). Simulation has been identified as an effective interactive platform for interprofessional education (Reeves et al., 2012) and a strategy that provides for a more authentic replication of the workplace in which learners can participate (Failla & Macauley, 2014).

Why did we start Sim-IPE? We realized that collectively, we had expertise in multimodal simulation using SPs, mannequin-based simulation, and virtual simulation and we had expertise in IPE. We decided to bring our experience, knowledge, and skill in simulation and healthcare education together to create authentic interprofessional learning experiences for disciplines from each of the institutions. We also held the belief that even if a discipline did not have a perfect fit within a given simulation, the learner could still develop an appreciation for and exposure to others' work and the patient experience. Moreover, we understood that including those "nonperfect fit" learners in the debriefing sessions is valuable. Regardless of the students' roles, we knew that we could create Sim-IPE to engage and excite the learner.

26-1 Voice of Experience
Sociological Fidelity in Interprofessional Learning: The Need for Critical Thinking

Scott Reeves, PhD, MSc, PGCE

The Challenge

In simulation, fidelity refers to the degree to which a simulated learning activity can accurately reproduce environmental and behavioral elements of the real world. Indeed, there are many forms of fidelity, including physical fidelity (degree of visual and spatial accuracy), psychological fidelity (degree of perceived realism), and task fidelity (the degree to which tasks are realistic). Collectively, these different types of fidelity help us understand the complexity related to attempting to recreate faithful versions of the real world. However, educators often fail to look beyond these standard forms of fidelity to explicitly incorporate key social factors (e.g., professional power differentials, gender imbalances) into their interprofessional simulation designs. As a result, interprofessional simulation activities lack a true degree of realism, which can compromise the effectiveness of this type of education.

Meeting the Challenge

With colleagues, I developed the notion of sociological fidelity—an approach that can allow educators to increase the realism of the learning and that in turn can enhance the transferability of skills and behaviors gained from the simulation. To achieve this, one needs to combine sociologically real simulations with appropriate postsimulation debriefing, an approach that can support effective interprofessional learning.

Facilitation of the debriefing session is of vital importance. Facilitators need to model interprofessional collaborative practice and create safe spaces where participants can focus on collaboration and communication skills to help tease out issues of conflict/friction. Skilled facilitation also helps the different groups verbalize the benefits they gained from their colleagues. Issues surrounding hierarchy,

leadership, followership, and professional identity need to be explored honestly and openly. (For further information about this form of fidelity, see Libby and Reeves [2011].)

The Outcome

The outcome of introducing this term has been positive as a number of colleagues involved in developing and delivering simulation activities are now employing sociological fidelity to enhance and enrich the quality of their interprofessional simulated learning.

Most Valuable Lesson Learned

Most valuable lesson learned is to think critically about education—consider the nature of a learning activity and problematize it. Such an approach can lead to the development of new concepts and methodologies that can ultimately enhance the learning experiences for students.

Inspiration for Simulation Champions

A critique does not consist in saying that things aren't good the way they are. It consists in seeing on just what type of assumptions, of familiar notions, of established and unexamined ways of thinking the accepted practices are based…To do criticism is to make harder those acts which are now too easy.—

Michel Foucault

Getting Started: Building an IPE Education Team

The next sections of this chapter tell the story of a Canadian inter-institutional partnership called the Interdisciplinary Healthcare Education Partnership (IHEP) that collaborated to build a context relevant IPE curriculum for prelicensure students from healthcare programs across Edmonton, Alberta to advocate for, and promote grassroots changes in healthcare culture. IHEPs flagship IPE event is called *HELP! Save Stan.*

IHEP received funding in 2009, and the real work began. It was time to roll up our sleeves and dig in. The task before us was considerable and at times seemed overwhelmingly impossible. We asked ourselves, "How do four postsecondary institutions and a health authority start the work of developing Sim-IPE for such a diverse group of learners?" The following sections outline building context relevant curriculum, developing and supporting faculty for Sim-IPE, assessing and evaluating the experiences, and changing the culture.

Building and Implementing Context Relevant Simulation-Enhanced IPE Curriculum

Developing curriculum in nursing can be viewed as the holistic mix of educational philosophies that explain the knowledge, skills, and judgement that make up the authentic practice based experience that is nursing (Paige & Daley, 2009). Dynamic and collaborative curriculum development in nursing is informed by evidence, context, and connections (Iwasiw & Goldenberg, 2014). The evolution of all healthcare disciplines followed a similar process with professional programs emerging in silos. The blending of discipline-specific curricula to create Interprofessional education is complex and difficult to achieve. IHEP employed two key supporting documents published after IHEP's work began, the INACSL Standards of Best Practice: Simulation^{SM} - Standard VIII (Decker et al., 2015) and 12 Tips for Successful Interprofessinal Team-Based High Fidelity Simulation (Boet, Bould, Burn and Reeves, 2014). The 12 tips (Box 26-1), and the the INACSL Standard of Best Practice: Standard VIII (now INACSL Standards Committee, 2016, Sim-IPE) were used to frame our curriculum development work.

The Simulation Enhanced Interprofessional Education (Sim-IPE) Standard was first introduced in June of 2015, and has since been updated (INACSL Standards Committee, 2016) to include the following criteria:

1. Conduct Sim-IPE based on a theoretical or a conceptual framework.
2. Utilize best practices in the design and development of Sim-IPE.
3. Recognize and address potential barriers to Sim-IPE.
4. Devise an appropriate evaluation plan for Sim-IPE (p . S34).

The Sim-IPE standards link team collaboration to patient safety and align well with interprofessional competencies as identified by the Canadian Interprofessional Health Collaborative (CIHC) in the National Interprofessional Competency Framework (2010) and by the Interprofessional Education Collaborative (IPEC) document on Core Competencies for Interprofessional Collaborative Practice (2011).

The INACSL Sim-IPE criteria are summarized in the sections that follow with examples of IHEP's application of each criterion. At the time, IHEP program development was based on the 2015 Sim-IPE Standard (Decker et al.), therefore the next section will feature work related to that version.

Box 26-1 **12 Tips for Developing Sim-IPE**

1. *Focus on the "interprofessional"*—Learning objectives must focus on enhancing interprofessional knowledge, behaviors, and attitudes (Zwarenstein et al., 2009); use competency frameworks to guide the learning.
2. *Anticipate complex logistical challenges,* such as scheduling, financing, and human resources.
3. *Find your interprofessional Simulation "Champions."*
4. *Balance diversity with equity*—This means no profession is privileged in the scenario or debriefing (Hammick, Freeth, Koppel, Reeves, & Barr, 2007); balance of professions (not 4 medical students to 1 nurse); optimal size of group of learners is determined by objectives.
5. *Develop scenarios that are relevant to all professions*—All professions have a significant and balanced role.
6. *Be mindful of sociological fidelity*—Consider cultural and sociological issues that could arise (Reeves & Pryce, 1998; Sharma et al., 2011); power and hierarchical considerations need to be thought through; does the simulation reproduce the same hierarchy and power relations found in a clinical environment and that can be a barrier to good teamwork?
7. *Put all the professions on the same page—The importance of prebriefing*—set the "ground rules"—social acceptance of feedback from all peers, despite any real or perceived authoritative positions; helps prevent any complications during interprofessional debriefing (Husebø, Friberg, Soreide, Rystedt, & Nestel, 2012; Rudolph, Raemer, & Simon, 2014).
8. *Beware of interprofessional debriefing challenges*—May be challenging to maintain emotional and psychological safety with interprofessional learners as they reflect upon the sim experience; Lindqvist and Reeves (2007) state that IP debriefings are often challenging and demanding; no gold standard with interprofessional debriefing, although codebriefing is often adopted.
9. *Use simulation to add value within the broader interprofessional curriculum*—interprofessional sim needs to be embedded within a wider mandate for IPE and Interprofessional Practice (IPP).
10. *Focus the assessment on the team*—Consider both quantitative and qualitative methods when designing a team assessment.
11. *Support the interprofessional simulation educators*—Train the trainer courses help debriefers (van Soeren et al., 2011) to ensure that they don't miss any "teachable" moments.
12. *Interprofessional-simulated learning is underresearched*—use teaching opportunities to foster research.

Adapted from Boet, S., Bould, M., Burn, C. & Reeves, S. (2014). Twelve tips for a successful interprofessional team-based high-fidelity simulation education session. *Med Teach, 36*(10): 853–857.

Applying Criterion 1: Simulation-Enhanced Interprofessional Education Should Be Based on Theory

To create the highest interprofessional learning experience, the "use of theories (educational, organizational and/or management), frameworks, standards and competencies to guide the development and implementation of Sim-IPE" is critical (Decker et al., 2015, p. 294). In the 2016 version of the Sim-IPE Standard, criterion one has expanded to include the need for Sim-IPE to be based on *theoretical and conceptual frameworks.* The remaining three 2015 criteria headings are unchanged. Adult learning theories, social learning theory, interprofessional competency frameworks, and crisis resource management frameworks are all excellent resources to guide the development of the learning experience. Curriculum mapping is helpful to ensuring sustainability and appropriate integration of the experience. See Toolkit 26-1 for a list of applicable theories, frameworks, and resources.

The Sim-IPE curriculum developed for IHEP and the HELP! Save Stan event is based on a combination of theories, competency frameworks, and standards. Initially, the learning objectives for each scenario were based on the Canadian Patient Safety Institutes' Safety Competencies (Frank & Brien, 2009), specifically Domain Two (Work in teams for patient safety) and Domain Three (Communicate effectively for patient safety).

One year later, the CIHC-Interprofessional Competency Framework (2010) was published, and we revised our learning objectives and followed this competency framework to ensure the scenarios retained an interprofessional focus.

Applying Criterion 2: Follow Best Practices in Simulation-Based and Interprofessional Education

The second INACSL Criterion for Standard VIII calls for integrating best practices in simulation and IPE, including promoting interprofessional communication and collaboration and team-based structured debriefing. The scenarios used in HELP! Save Stan were written and vetted by subject matter experts and faculty experienced with simulation. We had to design the scenarios to be flexible enough to accommodate a range of undergraduate/graduate, diploma, and certificate learners, mimicking the realities of the healthcare workplace in each situation. Authors of the simulation scenarios drew from their experience in both academic and practice environments to inform their simulations. Therefore, in keeping with the project's overall objectives to be inclusive of all types of team members, the scenarios fell into two overall categories: either dynamic (complex care) or routine.

The use of IPE and simulation in the education of undergraduate health professionals is well documented within the dynamic realm. However, the use of simulation and IPE within the routine domain and with certificate and diploma level populations is less well documented.

Dynamic urgent care simulation scenarios tended to focus on skills, algorithms, and **leadership** consisting of clinical teams that form for short periods to manage an emergent care situation (King et al., 2014; Manser, 2009). Routine scenarios that take place in geriatrics, rehabilitation environments (Sheehan, Robertson, & Ormond, 2007), and continuing care such as transitioning to home care (King et al., 2014) are grounded in foundational interprofessional competencies such as communication, collaboration, and relationship building (Kenaszchuk et al., 2011).

HELP! Save Stan offers learners a supportive, learner-centered, environment and a safe psychological learning place. Students are encouraged to take part in formative self-evaluation and peer evaluation of the IPE competencies as they relate to their program, learning, and expectations. The overall objective is to develop reflective practitioners and team players in healthcare by challenging them through Sim-IPE scenarios that are relevant to their education and practice. Sim-IPE offers opportunities to develop synergy as learners share goals with team members and participate in shared decision-making. The overarching goal of the simulations is the attainment of core IPE competencies and promoting patient safety through effective team behaviors such as (1) communication particularly in patient care transitions; (2) collaboration by offering opportunities to discover differences and overlaps in their roles; and (3) opportunities to discuss these situations as they debrief and make sense of their experiences.

Applying Criterion 3: Address Institutional and Local Issues

New or emerging IPE initiatives have often lacked a strong sustainability plan, thereby dissolving after a few years. Sim-IPE is no different. We now know that creating simulations to address institutional and local issues in addition to educational goals have a greater chance of success.

The HELP! Save Stan scenarios reflect current issues that real clinical practice environments face every day. The simulations replicate authentic situations that would highlight IPE competencies and offer learners opportunities for working together in teams. In many cases, we adapted existing unidisciplinary scenarios, modifying them to have an IPE focus. Subject matter experts that originally wrote or reviewed these scenarios then identified which disciplines could realistically participate in the interprofessional version. We devised specific roles for each level of learner, and in some cases, several iterations of the scenario had to be written to ensure fidelity. This strategy was critical because learners participating in HELP! Save Stan come from a variety of backgrounds, educational levels, experiences, cultures, and differing levels of professional socialization. The unique blend of students forced the scenario authors to anticipate what each participant would bring to the scenario and to think with intentionality about which circumstances, equipment, or components would be necessary to make the scenario relevant for each level and/or discipline.

An interprofessional cofacilitation model is used for HELP! Save Stan to ensure an interprofessional perspective throughout the event. We found it most helpful to have facilitators from backgrounds other than the participants to keep the focus of debriefing squarely on the acquisition of team competencies.

Our first Sim-IPE pilot run experiences took place in the evenings and weekends in simulation centers on campus, and we enlisted volunteer students and faculty. We called these early events "Bootcamps" and invited small numbers of learners to participate in either a mannequin-based or a standardized patient-based simulation as relevant to their actual working environments. We developed this approach as a "proof of concept" to work through scenario details and begin to evaluate the value of these experiences. Initially offering extracurricular opportunities to participate in IPE may have mitigated some of the problems with scheduling; however, we ran the risk of learners viewing IPE as "optional" rather than as essential.

In these initial events, lessons learned included the following:

- Learners opting to participate in IPE are engaged learners who elect to involve themselves in such opportunities. This extracurricular approach may attract self-selected high achievers and perhaps contribute to lower attendance by students who need to work or have families.
- Learners were more likely to commit and to attend the event if they received recognition or marks for attendance. We needed to increase the value of these experiences from their perspectives.
- Learners or faculty had misunderstandings or stereotypes about other disciplines. When it happened that one student did not show up for a scenario, other students or faculty keenly jumped in to replace the missing student. For example, a nurse might interpret the role of a respiratory therapist based on past experiences. The substitution of non–discipline-specific participants to fill other disciplines' roles (even for faculty engaged in role-playing) did not produce the authentic learning we had planned for, and we did not continue that practice.

While watching the scenarios unfold, volunteer faculty members prepared for debriefing by writing down their observations and listing events to discuss with the students in debriefing. Many struggled with the transition to focusing on debriefing IPE competencies. The educators came to the realization that we collectively needed to better understand the IPE competencies. As we engaged in discussions and team learning about collaborative practice, we evolved to become a learning community. Many synergies resulted from team learning, including the development of new dimensions in our simulations such

as power differentials to increase "sociological fidelity" (Sharma et al., 2011).

If At First You Don't Succeed....

We discussed the strengths and shortcomings of the Bootcamp approach and felt there might be efficiencies in consolidating our efforts in a 1-day event instead of small evening simulations. We introduced the idea of a full-day simulation blitz on the weekend. The first HELP! Save Stan was held March 12, 2011. That first event offered ten multimodal simulations to learners (Box 26-2) from certificate, diploma, undergraduate, and graduate degree health-based programs from the four postsecondary educational institutions. Table 26.3 lists the original interprofessional simulation scenarios offered at HELP! Save Stan in 2011. The initial HELP! Save Stan event was branded with the slogan, "The scenario is simulated, the team experience is real!" Simulation scenarios were designed to cover the full spectrum of the healthcare continuum and addressed patient care in primary, secondary, and tertiary care settings.

Since that time, we have developed more simulations and learning activities, all focused on interprofessional competencies. Faculty observers from other institutions have attended, including the University of Calgary, St. Francis Xavier, Dalhousie University, and Brandon Community College. Some are preparing to host a HELP! Save Stan within their institutions!

One of the many challenges with IPE that also impacts sustainability is the logistics of managing large numbers of students, particularly the task of balancing large numbers of nurses and practical nurses while having smaller numbers from other healthcare programs. Interestingly, this balancing act mirrored the composition of today's workforce teams and, hence, formed the basis of the ratios we used to determine the number of participants from each discipline per scenario. As interest in HELP! Save Stan increased and numbers grew, we chose to formalize an observer role. This approach was particularly useful for disciplines not typically involved in a scenario, but for whom the experience was helpful. The observer role also proved helpful for faculty who were inexperienced with simulation and initially preferred to watch.

Box 26-2	**The HELP! Save Stan Experience— Who Are the Learners?**

Learners included in HELP! Save Stan were from: emergency medical responder, emergency medical technician, healthcare aide, med-lab technology, med-lab assistant programs, medicine, mental health rehabilitation, nursing, nutrition, occupational therapy, paramedic, pharmacist, pharmacy technician, physical therapy, practical nursing, recreational therapist respiratory therapy, social work, speech–language pathology therapy assistant, ultrasonography, and x-ray tech.

Table 26.3	2011 Original HELP! Save Stan Simulations
2011 HELP! Save Stan Simulations	Simulation Typology Used For Simulated Clinical Immersion
"Postoperative teamwork and communication"	Mannequin
"Hospital to homecare" (parts 1 and 2)	Standardized patient
Paramedic hand-off to ER staff	Virtual world-Avatar
"ER mashup"	Hybrid (mannequin and SP)
"Giving bad news"	Standardized patient
"Balancing priorities"	Role-playing
"Palliative care"	Hybrid (mannequin and SP)
"Team interviews"	Standardized patient
"Help my baby!"	Hybrid (mannequin and SP)
Inner city youth	Standardized patient

Applying Criterion 4: Include an Evaluation Plan

The final INACSL criterion highlights the importance of thinking about evaluation from the beginning of the development of the learning experience. Evaluation plans need to include valid and reliable measures, examine how participating in the Sim-IPE improves learner and patient outcomes, and measure how the experience helps change the culture. The issue of evaluation will be explored in more detail in the following section.

Assessing Students and Evaluating the Experiences

Perhaps the area for greatest growth in Sim-IPE is in the domains of assessment and evaluation. An evaluation plan needs to be developed concurrently with the development of the learning experience (Decker et al., 2015; Palaganas et al., 2014; Reeves et al., 2015; Seymour et al., 2013). As highlighted by Reeves et al. (2015), the evaluation of IPE experiences is increasing; however, the quality of the empirical studies has room for improvement. For example, the evidence directly linking IPE and Sim-IPE to patient and population outcomes is lacking (Brashers et al., 2005); however, the direct cause–effect relationship of any health professional education intervention to the patient, population, and system outcomes is limited (Brashers et al., 2005). Existing research with Sim-IPE includes inconsistencies in study designs and methods and the lack of full reporting

on study methods thereby limiting the applicability and generalizability of findings (Brashers et al., 2005). A realist approach or qualitative design captures contextual issues or variables—moving beyond just the quantitative approach capturing "what occurred." It is also necessary to capture "the how or why" outcomes by employing a mixed methods design. Other challenges with the current research are that changes in behavior are often self-reported by participants (Reeves, Lewin, Espin, & Zwarenstein, 2010), and there are few longitudinal studies that follow students through the continuum of learning. Details are often lacking on how students were assessed on interprofessional competencies with many studies mentioning that teamwork and collaboration and communication were observed/improved (Luctkar-Flude et al., 2014). In the simulation literature, a link has been made between simulation education and patient outcomes (Barsuk et al., 2014; Zerdejas, Brydges, Wang, & Cook, 2013). Similar work in Sim-IPE is necessary.

Based on Reeves et al. (2015) and the National Academy of Practice's (NAP) document, Measuring the Impact of IPE on Collaborative Practice and Patient Outcomes (2015), the following points should be considered when evaluating Sim-IPE experiences:

- Think about evaluation early
- Be clear about the purpose the evaluation
- Consider learning outcomes
- Include theory
- Employ an evaluation model
- Select an evaluation design

The NAP (2015) identified areas in IPE where research is necessary. These same areas would apply to Sim-IPE and include the following:

- Construct well-designed mixed methods studies that utilize robust qualitative data, as well as validated tools for evaluating IPE outcomes.
- Develop a consistent framework for reporting the methodological details of IPE studies.
- Examine the cost and cost-effectiveness of IPE interventions.
- Link IPE with changes in collaborative practice behavior.

We mapped out our plan for evaluation early and executed it with minor modifications as we went along. We used the University of West England Interprofessional Questionnaire (Pollard, Miers, & Gilchrist, 2004) and the Readiness for Interprofessional Learning Scale (McFadyen et al., 2005), both considered reliable and valid at that time (Thannhauser, Russell-Mayhew, & Scott, 2010). We documented student responses to the innovations, and we modified our approach according to their responses. We evaluated the experience immediately after the event and then contacted students several months later to ask them what they remembered. The debriefing at HELP! Save Stan was for formative purposes, only. The event was co-curricular therefore, no summative evaluation of learners occurred. We wanted the students to relax, have fun, and learn without the worry of grades.

A key lesson for us was the need to "check in" with students. We asked "What do you think you learned?" and then compared that to what we wanted them to learn (Greidanus, King, LoVerso, & Ansell, 2013). By recording simulations and debriefings, we observed what occurred during both components and heard from students what they experienced. We could then compare to the scenario's learning objectives and make adjustments to the experience, if necessary. This process was lengthy, yet critical to validate the learning experience. Learners acquire knowledge individually based on what they know, who they are, and the connections they make with the other learners (Paige & Daley 2009; Wyrostok, Hoffart, Kelly, & Ryba, 2014). Therefore, it was critical to determine what the learners felt they learned in the simulation scenarios.

Changing Healthcare Culture by Building Team Excellence

Cultural influences are ubiquitous impacting us on many levels. Professional cultures commonly build on history and tradition and demonstrate long-standing features of hierarchical teams and competitive members. As such, professional socialization into healthcare culture may be more focused on interactions with each other (health professionals) than with the patient (Failla & Macauley, 2014). Successful professional socialization and transformations of professional culture may depend on exposure to situations that contradict cultural understandings and the professional's response to the situation.

Professional Culture and the Hidden Curriculum

Healthcare professionals have traditionally learned, practiced, and socialized within their own "silos" and subcultures (Palaganas et al., 2014). Classically, this approach to healthcare provider education has too often been associated with ineffective collaboration and communication-associated patient errors (WHO, 2010b). Interprofessional simulation builds on Failla's description of collaboration to change healthcare culture by building team excellence (Box 26-3; 2014).

Student experiences are heavily influenced by factors existing outside the formal curriculum. Hafferty and Franks first highlighted the concept of the **hidden curriculum** in the medical education literature in 1994. The hidden curriculum comprises what students learn in the hallways, in lecture theaters after class, and in the cafeteria and even includes such factors as architecture and the physical layout of the learning space (O'Donnell, 2014). O'Donnell (2014) outlined four types of curricula at work in an educational setting:

Box 26-3	The HELP! Save Stan Experience—The Hidden Curriculum Finds a Life of Its Own!

A postgrad student from the University of Alberta and a long-standing member of IHEP were facilitating an interprofessional simulation scenario at one of the Bootcamps. The students were from two different institutions and programs. They were communicating and collaborating beyond our expectations. My observant colleague noted that the students did not need to have us pass on our current culture to them; she said: "they are busy building their own culture."

IHEP Faculty

1. The *intended curriculum*, or the planned and formal curriculum
2. The *actual curriculum*, or the informal learning, role-modeling, and interpersonal dynamics in the learning environment that happens outside of the formal classroom
3. The *hidden curricular space* and professional, cultural subtexts that exist at the level of the organizational culture and is where students learn "how things work around here"
4. The *null curriculum*, what is not taught or not attended to within a program

Educators tasked with socializing learners to professions model their personal perspectives and stereotypes in an informal and hidden curriculum rather than overt features of a current cultural paradigm. Additionally, learners engaged in the apprenticeship model of learning may assimilate some of their preceptor's perspectives, stereotypes, and misunderstandings about other team roles. Passing on out-dated and inaccurate understandings or personal perspectives reinforces the hidden curriculum and negatively impacts the culture of the workplace. Educators need to be aware of the hidden curriculum when working with students in the classroom, simulation space, clinical environment, or hallway and attend to issues within their institution.

Success in interprofessional teams is dependent on mindful self-awareness about personal beliefs and behaviors, the current healthcare culture, as well as a clear picture of the collaborative culture and community we want our learners to embrace. Kelly and Hager (2015) encourages the use of informal, affective, and contextual learning in simulation situations that facilitate professional socialization as learners engage "in the process of becoming a healthcare professional" (Kelly & Hager, 2015, pp. 376–377).

Professional socialization intersects largely in communication, collaboration, and leadership (King et al., 2013). Interestingly, these areas represent some of the major performance gaps in patient safety. Learners who take part in Sim-IPE report being more confident in communicating and collaborating with team members. Their ability to

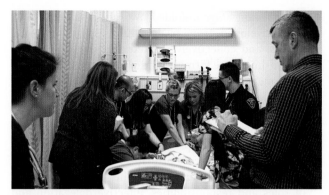

Figure 26.1 The Team Experience—ER Mash Up, Child Accompanied by Mother with Acute Asthmatic Episode. Image taken during HELP! Save Stan 2014, used with permission.

present their opinion in a new working group improved in simulations based in acute and nonacute settings. Exposure to workplace relevant simulation scenarios based on a common patient-centered approach empowered all of the members of the healthcare team (King et al., 2014). In the HELP! Save Stan simulations, the IHEP team educators used simulation to build bridges between existing and desired cultural communities (Fig. 26.1).

Using a Change Model to Change Culture

Over the past 9 years, the IHEP project has become a successful and internationally recognized interprofessional partnership. We can outline a retrospective analysis of how we were able to facilitate successful shifts in organizational and professional culture to include the basic tenets of both interprofessional education and collaboration by using Kotter's 8 Step Change Model (Kotter, 2015). Refer to Chapter 9 for a detailed review of Kotter's Model. We apply Kotter's eight steps to the IHEP initiative in the following sections.

Step One—Create a Sense of Urgency

Once IHEP was awarded the funding from the provincial government in 2009, the initial working group shared a great sense of urgency to achieve the proposed objectives. The specific outcomes of proposed project included the following:

- The development of an interinstitutional, interprofessional community of educators from healthcare professions
- Opportunities for instructors to facilitate interprofessional learning using simulation
- Evidence-based standardized interprofessional curriculum across the education sectors
- Opportunities for students to develop interprofessional collaboration competency through facilitated experiences

- Creating interprofessional learning opportunities for groups of learners with low access to other health team members. These low access groups often care for at-risk populations (e.g., immigrant, aboriginal, or low-income populations) (King et al., 2014).

To enhance the transformative nature of this iterative project, the working group decided that learning and feedback/debriefing after scenarios would be based on the attainment of IPE core competencies rather than on discipline-specific clinical performance competencies. Developing trained facilitators to lead the debriefing was critical (King et al., 2013).

Step Two—Build a Guiding Coalition

The next step was to create organizational structures to support the project and ensure that we achieved our objectives. The initial working group became the IHEP Steering Committee whose members included senior executive leaders from the participating institutions. The leading participants in the IHEP group consisted of change agents, and innovators: people who were excited by change and who were willing to be members of the guiding coalition. Retrospectively, it is now clear that the leading participants of the IHEP project were a powerful combination of innovators, early adopters, and pragmatists—as featured in the Theory of Diffusion of Innovation (Kaminsky, 2011).

Step Three—Form Strategic Vision and Initiatives

The vision of the IHEP Steering Committee was to create a transformative interprofessional learning community of educators to enhance health science practitioner's readiness for practice. Initially, the Steering Committee guided decisions and provided stewardship over the funds. Each of the IHEP partners had an equal seat at the table regardless of institutional size, credentials, the number of students, or the educational qualifications of faculty/staff; everyone was welcome (King et al., 2013).

Next steps involved forming a Curriculum Committee with representation from each of the partners to establish core competencies for the team members in both simulation and IPE. Subcommittees were formed with content experts from a variety of practice settings to discuss and develop specific modules, identify needed resources, and write scenarios.

Simulation as a learning strategy and IPE, in general, were relatively new concepts for some partners. For example, many partners lacked experience with certain simulation modalities such as Virtual Simulation. Figure 26.2 depicts the online interprofessional virtual learning module that was developed in Second Life. Consequently, the most experienced simulationists and IPE specialists led scenario development initially. It was apparent that before we could increase capacity in our students and impact the healthcare system, we had to increase capacity in our educators. We then formed a Faculty Development Committee, consisting

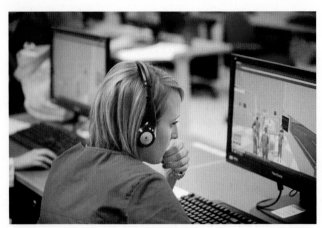

Figure 26.2 Virtual Sim-IPE in Second Life. (Developed for *HELP! Save Stan* 2014, used with permission).

of Simulation Champions, IPE experts, educators, content experts, and researchers from each partner group, and went to work. It was not long before we built capacity in the team and less experienced committee members were assuming leadership roles.

The evolution and growth of the IHEP team mirrored Tuckman's Stages of Small Group Development; forming, storming, norming, performing, and adjourning (Tuckman & Jensen, 1977). The newly appointed members of the group had a big picture idea of the tasks ahead. They were honored to represent their institutions and programs and excited at the potential that lay before them.

We did not start out as friends. For many, we had been long-standing competitors that at times in other forums had fiercely defended our students, programs, and processes. Nursing programs, in particular, had a history of competing for students in undergraduate programs. Other challenges included shifting scopes of practice and a lack of shared understanding of roles of team members.

● During the *forming stage*, team members started getting to know each other and to discern member roles on the team. There was an unearthing of preconceived notions and assumptions about our professions, about IPE, and about simulation. Differences surfaced in our use of terminology and theory, our understanding of essential components of simulation-based learning and scenario development, and our assessment and evaluation practices and tools. We worked to build trust in one another and to address issues as they arose, keeping our focus on the project outcomes.

● The *storming stage* played out, and tensions grew as members established themselves and their credibility. Early in the process, some members questioned the project's likelihood of success and chose to bow out. This reality allowed others to bring their passion to the table, and the group forged on. One of many positives that surfaced was our willingness as a team to explore differing approaches and to focus on personal and professional strengths.

● The *norming stage* unfolded over about a year as our team developed strong relationships, established group norms, and collectively worked past our differences. Friendships were forming, and we realized that each of us brought unique richness in skills and knowledge to the table. As we came to realize how much we had to learn with, from, and about each other, it became easier to establish project norms, goals, and a team identity. The group was developing into a high-performing team. We were living the core principles of Interprofessional Practice (IPP): understanding the team, knowledge of roles and responsibilities, effective delegation and follow-up, regular and crisis communication, conflict management, and continuous learning (UCSF, 2014) (https://interprofessional.ucsf.edu/framework-competencies). In fact, we became the team that we wanted to model for our students.

● During the *performing stage*, the membership of the committee and our approach changed several times. We had developed a strong sense of team identity, roles, and shared goals, making it easier to integrate others quickly. The main team performance was the first IHEP HELP! Save Stan that took place on March 12, 2011, at MacEwan University. Each institution turned to their content experts to create more scenarios to ensure we could meet the demand for growing student interest. Since then, we have planned and successfully hosted five HELP! Save Stan events, alternating between hosts; the University of Alberta and MacEwan University. Approximately 800 students and 300 faculty and staff volunteers have participated over the last 5 years. On March 11th of 2017, IHEP will offer 7th Annual HELP! Save Stan event with both institutions hosting over 1000 students, faculty, and staff. There are plans afoot to expand to even more sites as IHEP partners open new simulation facilities. Following their participation at HELP! Save Stan, other Canadian institutions have followed suit to host, or are working to host their own HELP! Save Stan event. Informally, we have welcomed the participation of external academic stakeholders as observers and have trained facilitators from colleges, institutes, and universities in several Canadian provinces.

● The opportunity for the *adjourning stage* came in 2012 with the end of the project funds. Collectively, we refused to lose the momentum and relationships we had worked so hard to develop. We elected to continue to build on our successes.

Step Four—Enlist a Volunteer Army

To be successful, IHEP had to enlist a massive army of passionate volunteers. As we offered IPE debriefing and simulation development workshops, the pool of simulation and IPE champions grew in our community. According to Kotter, we succeeded in engaging the minds and hearts of people and capably moved them to action (Box 26-4).

Box 26-4	A Word to Inspire

"Innovation is less about generating new ideas and more about knocking down barriers to making those ideas a reality."

—*John Kotter Accelerate*

Step Five—Enable Action by Removing Barriers

There are some significant barriers to IPE and collaboration including practice-academe, resources, and logistical type challenges. *Practice-academe barriers* can include culture, attitudes, weak leadership, history, stereotypes, content, curriculum, disciplinary jargon, levels of evidence, accreditation, regulation, competencies and outcomes. *Resource barriers* stem from funding, faculty workload, education and training, IPE event staffing, and equipment. Whereas, *logistical barriers* are tied to infrastructure, delivery models, institutional calendars, time, distance, practice schedules, course credit systems, and credit for clinical practice hours (Reeves et al., 2016; Sunguya, Hinthong, Jimba, & Yasuoka, 2014).

Resource issues about funding and financing models for IPE continue to be an ongoing barrier to IPE. With IHEP, the varying value placed on IPE and simulation at times resulted in competing or conflicting priorities for allocating funds and human resources. Also, variations in organizational size between the IHEP partners presented challenges related to human and physical capacity. We continue to seek funding and increased resources.

Logistics including academic schedules, timetables, and norms as well as employee contracts and schedules are often the reason for a lack of interaction between learner groups. Conducting the IPE events in an extracurricular manner reduced scheduling barriers. Institutional and individual valuing of IPE and simulation as service, teaching or scholarship resulted in varying work assignments and often related to the faculty and staff expectations and experience in IPE and simulation (King et al., 2013).

A lack of dialogue and the power status associated with individuals and professions can lead to a lack of team cohesion or success (Lichtenstein, Alexander, McCarthy, & Wells, 2004). Other factors include frequent transitions between team members increasing the need for communication, unbounded teams with a lack of coordination (Wageman, Hackman, & Lehman, 2005), and the complexities of dealing with personalities and relationships (Steiner, 1972) (Box 26-5).

IHEP was changing healthcare culture by intentionally removing existing barriers and building team excellence. We developed egalitarian infrastructure and governance processes that supported an interprofessional community focused on collaborative learning, patient safety, research, cross-institutional relationships, and a vision for simulation-based IPE based on common goals. We built a platform on which educators and administrators could base socialization and networking to overcome common barriers and collaborate on efficiencies (King et al., 2013).

Box 26-5	The HELP! Save Stan Experience: I Don't Mean to Mow Your Grass...

In one of our very first Bootcamps, students from a registered nursing program, a practical nursing program, and the medical program were debriefing after a scenario in which the mannequin patient incurred postsurgical complications. In the discussion about their performance in the scenario, the practical nurse student said to the med student: "Hey, I don't want to mow your grass, but I thought maybe Benadryl might have been a good idea." To which the medical student replied: "Great idea—wish I would have thought of it".

—IHEP Faculty Narrative

The IHEP team members' ability to address and mitigate barriers and our passion for collaboration and Sim-IPE were the drivers that often had us all working off the sides of our desks so that we could participate.

Step Six—Generate Short-Term Wins

The IHEP team members collected, communicated, and celebrated every move forward, every accomplishment, and every success. We announced when we met our project outcomes and our successes with sustainability to postsecondary education, our original funders, simulation education, and IPE. With every event, we captured the learning in pictures, videos, interviews, and a graffiti board for student comments (Fig. 26.3). We collected testimonials about the transformational impact of participation and circulated them to our institutional leaders and volunteers (King et al., 2014). We talked about HELP! Save Stan as we toured potential funders, community leaders, and corporate visitors in our institutions. We used the successes to demonstrate to our volunteers and students, as well as to our Steering Committee and funders that we were moving in the right direction.

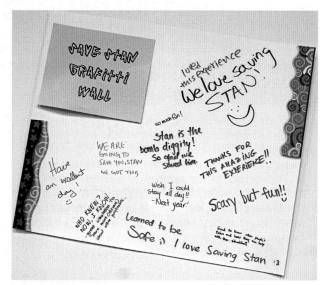

Figure 26.3 HELP! Save Stan Graffiti Wall. An Annual Tradition, used with permission.

Our research demonstrated successes as students reported that they learned about each other; about differing scopes of practice and roles, and about the views and perspectives of other health team members. They learned about communication, teamwork and leadership. They learned how to work together, about leadership and team dynamics. They told us they learned about themselves, about their role in the healthcare team, and interprofessional learning and how ready they were to participate in collaborative practice (King et al., 2014).

Following IHEP events, particularly during and after HELP! Save Stan events, all participants reported a subjective flush of pride in participation and accomplishment. At the end of the activities, we literally had to tell the students there were no more events for the day. Participants reported feeling part of a membership and a community of learners (Box 26-6). Learners were learning informally and professionally in the affective domain. Affective learning can impact motivation, commitment, appreciation, and valuation of learning (Huitt, 2011; Kelly & Hager, 2015).

Step Seven—Sustain Acceleration

The IHEP team developed three interprofessional modules, HELP! Save Stan, Facilitating Interprofessional Debriefing, SimETC, Digital Storytelling, and databases of processes, curriculum, and an inventory of the products and processes of the partners. In addition to tangible deliverables, the IHEP team was also associated with building Sim-IPE capacity in our institutions, faculty, staff, students, and workplaces. IHEP successes with interprofessional communication, collaboration, and teamwork supported efficiencies in institutional interprofessional activities such as a well-established workshop for workplace preceptors, a long-standing interprofessional course on team development, a series of video learning objects for interprofessional team curriculum, adoption of the nonconfrontational style of communication offered by the Advocacy Inquiry approach to debriefing in the workplace, and infusion into a long-standing simulation educational series. The diffusion of interprofessional

---

Box 26-6	The HELP! Save Stan Experience: Feeling Right at Home

At a Post HELP! Save Stan IHEP meeting, a representative from MacEwan University disclosed that she had received a call from a student in the practical nurse program at NorQuest College asking to book some practice time in their nursing skills practice lab. The MacEwan faculty member was quite taken aback, yet thrilled that the student felt comfortable to call and ask. When I called the student to follow up, she said, "Even though times were open at NorQuest, I knew you guys worked together, so I thought I might be able to practice there." This student showed us what shared resources in the future might look like.

—IHEP Faculty Story

Box 26-7	The HELP! Save Stan Experience: I Broke my Paramedic Brain!

A paramedic student in his last year arrived at the Palliative Care scenario with a first year paramedic student whom he was mentoring. He had participated in the Palliative Care scenario at the last HELP! Save Stan and had demonstrated an exceedingly high level of compassionate and collaborative care in the scenario. He explained that he wanted his mentee to take part in the scenario. He spoke of the important role this scenario played in his development by changing deeply ingrained patterns of thinking, saying of his experience in this scenario that "It broke my paramedic brain."

—IHEP Faculty Narrative

---

successes was taking place on numerous levels from student to student, from faculty to faculty, and from institution to institution. As we translated what we learned locally, nationally, and internationally in academic articles, media, and at conferences, workshops, and meetings, we established our community of practice. Colleagues, institutions, and other groups approached us wanting to attend events, workshops, and courses. We grew daily, forever changed by availing the opportunities we were afforded. We were transformed.

Step Eight—Institute Change

We had forever altered the landscape of the professional culture of Sim-IPE. For the fifth anniversary of HELP! Save Stan, we celebrated with a party, an updated marketing package, and an international award. In 2015, IHEP was awarded the Sigma Theta Tau International Practice-Academe Innovation Collaboration Award. This award was affirming and reflected the extent to which we had truly succeeded at changing our healthcare culture by building team excellence (Box 26-7).

Developing and Supporting Faculty for Simulation-Enhanced IPE (Sim-IPE)

We recognized the need to support faculty and staff as we worked toward building the capacity of our community of Sim-IPE Champions. The IHEP Faculty Development Committee developed two workshops: the Facilitating Interprofessional Debriefing Workshop and the Simulation Educators Interdisciplinary Training Course (SimETC). In keeping with the vision of IHEP, both of these workshops were developed by a cross-institutional team with an interprofessional approach and based on experiential learning. We based our approach on evidence from established experts in the simulation and IPE fields. Some of our IHEP members had taken courses that highlighted interprofessional education (http://ehpic.ca/), the Harvard Center for Medical Simulation https://harvardmedsim.org/ or the Mayo Clinic

Simulation Center (http://www.mayo.edu/multidisciplinary-simulation-center). These courses, combined with the experience of more experienced IHEP members, allowed us to acquire the perspective to develop the faculty development we thought the facilitators of the IHEP project would need.

Faculty development would have to be efficient and focused, as well as prepare the faculty and staff team for collaboration and Sim-IPE. We also acknowledged that reflection played an essential role in experiential learning (Rudolph, Simon, Rivard, Dufresne, & Raemer, 2007), and we wanted to build in reflective practice opportunities as part of faculty development.

Facilitating Interprofessional Debriefing Workshop

Best practice in simulation includes a planned and facilitated debriefing that guides learners in reflective thinking on the events of the simulation with a goal of making sense of the experience with reference to their previous understandings: in other words, learning from the experience (Decker et al., 2013). Reflective thinking is best taught and learned in the context of active learning (Decker et al.).

Debriefing describes a facilitated discussion wherein learners think reflectively reflect on a situation in order to learn from the event (Darling, Parry, & Moore, 2005; Dreifuerst, 2009; Fanning & Gaba, 2007; Salem-Schatz, Ordin, & Mittman, 2010). Facilitated debriefing is valued, may be less threatening, may be framed in a more relevant way, and may enhance collaboration (Fey, Scrandis, Daniels, & Haut, 2014; Kim-Godwin et al., 2013; Pastor, Cunningham, & Kuiper, 2015).

The Debriefing with Good Judgement method of debriefing (Rudolph, Simon, Dufresne, & Raemer, 2006; Rudolph et al., 2007) offers a balanced, good judgement approach to debriefing that supports reflective practice and offers the opportunity to collaboratively address performance. This approach identifies three elements: (1) learner "cognitive frames"—"knowledge, assumptions, and feelings that drive (their) actions" (Rudolph et al., 2006, p. 49); (2) an authentic and genuine curiosity about the frames, actions and consequences; and (3) a conversational technique called Advocacy Inquiry. The IHEP team felt that this model was consistent with our project goals and adopted it as our primary debriefing model.

We developed a 4-hour workshop titled, Facilitating Interprofessional Debriefing. Although the short workshop would necessitate continued faculty practice in the workplace, we hoped that the introductory offering would ignite an interest in continuing development in our passionate faculty volunteers. Ice breaking, sharing, and breaks would take an hour; didactic introducing simulation, IPE, and the debriefing model would take an hour; and the final 2 hours would include two simulation scenarios including prebriefing, participation, practice debriefing of the participants,

Box 26-8   **The HELP! Save Stan Experience—Faculty Debriefing Workshops: Learning from our Mistakes**

A group of very experienced nurse educators offered to participate in the first Facilitating Debriefing Workshop at my institution. In that inexperience, we presented a dynamic simulation scenario and in debriefing defaulted to a discussion on clinical competencies involved in the patient's deterioration. Several of those educators were very put off and never took part in simulation again. They expressed feeling put on the spot and vulnerable. We learned, albeit the hard way, the importance offering educators a simulation experience in which they could feel safe and experience some success.

and feedback to the debriefers all using the Debriefing with Good Judgement model. A unique feature of the HELP! Save Stan event that increased capacity and experience with debriefing included more experienced debriefers providing feedback to the less experienced debriefers (Box 26-8).

Initially, we offered faculty the same clinical simulation scenarios we offered the students. We discovered that learners often defaulted to their comfort level—debriefing discipline-specific clinical competencies, instead of addressing the IPE objectives particularly if the scenarios are clinical situations. We also discovered that in the faculty development, volunteers were asked to perform in situations that were no longer familiar reducing the safety of the learning environment and leaving them feeling somewhat vulnerable. The safe containers that we capably learned to build for student groups became even more important to create for groups of faculty.

Simulation Educators Interprofessional Training Course SimETC

To further increase capacity for simulation and Sim-IPE in our community, we designed the Simulation Educators Interprofessional Training Course—SimETC. We collaborated on the course objectives and content, and we each adopted areas to champion. We used an evidence-informed approach to support our content. SimETC became a 3-day workshop that offered participants the opportunity to hear some of the original IHEP committee participants share their knowledge and experience on Sim-IPE. The 2011 SimETC modules addressed

1. Simulation from 25,000 ft—An Overview
2. Simulation Technology and Modalities
3. Theater 101—The Art and Design of a Simulation Experience
4. Interprofessional Education and Simulation—A Happy Marriage
5. Assessment Considerations
6. What Happens Now? Debriefing Simulation
7. Considering Simulation? Consider Research
8. Lights, Camera, Action

During the 3-day experience, participants spent the first 2 days moving from presentations to small group work to apply the didactic and create a scenario with the guidance of the workshop leaders. Each working group wrote an interprofessional simulation scenario in which another working group participated. The third day was almost entirely devoted to Sim-IPE and debriefing. The author group debriefed the participants of the scenario they designed and were provided feedback on their debriefing by the leaders of the course and a group of experienced graduate students. Learners used the Debriefing with Good Judgement model to debrief IPE objectives.

On retrospect, our faculty development efforts met the objectives we had outlined for them. We built capacity in simulation, IPE, and Sim-IPE.

The Debriefing with Good Judgement method of debriefing remains the introductory model supported by the IHEP project. Faculty volunteers either attend or facilitate the Facilitating Interprofessional Debriefing workshop annually, just like CPR certification. Resources including debriefing resources have been sourced, created, and shared in Virtual Interprofessional Educator Resource (VIPER) on the University of Alberta website (http://www.hserc.ualberta.ca/TeachingandLearning/VIPER.aspx).

It is critical to remember that debriefing methods or approaches do vary. The IPE experience, learning, and perspective change that take place as a function of reflection in the debriefing are the critical factors in making sense of Sim-IPE.

Sim-IPE is also being deployed in clinical practice contexts with postlicensure groups. Dr. Bin Zheng describes a perioperative course designed to enhance healthcare team performance in the OR.

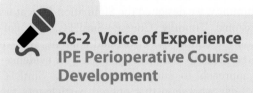

26-2 Voice of Experience
IPE Perioperative Course Development

●●●

Bin Zheng, MD, PhD

●●●

The Challenge

Surgical care requires a team of healthcare providers with a variety of skills and expertise. Nurses are core team members in the operating room who share critical responsibilities with surgeons and anesthesiologists for patients in need. Thus, it is important to establish an interprofessional education (IPE) opportunity for the nursing and medicine trainees to work collaboratively to develop the team skills and cognition for better patient care.

Meeting the Challenge

To meet the demand for a stronger collaborative team practice, we designed a simulation-based IPE course that allows learners from medicine and nursing to be trained together during the perioperative care.

Outcome

The IPE perioperative course incorporates various simulation models (standardized patients, high-fidelity mannequins, and specific task trainers) at different phases of perioperative care. Individual and team performance (communication, collaboration, leadership, and team awareness) are evaluated by multiple means, including knowledge tests, standardized patients' comments, and behavior patterns recorded through video. Excellent education outcomes have been reported from the self-administered survey from our trainees. Education leaders in both faculties of medicine and nursing are motivated by the outcomes and are considering the development of a joint curriculum to enforce the interprofessional education between faculties.

Most Valuable Lessons Learned

A shared vision among the educators from different faculties is imperative for the success of any IPE attempt. Throughout the course development, principal educators in nursing and medicine frequently meet to share our thoughts on educational objectives and challenges in achieving these objectives. A collective goal and keen collaboration allows us to find solutions to the challenges and conquer barriers in the development of an IPE course. Another takeaway from our work thus far is to maintain research priority while developing the perioperative IPE course. Strong research property enables us to obtain sufficient funds to evaluate education outcome and facilitate course implementation.

Inspiration for Simulation Champions

"Talent wins games, but teamwork and intelligence win championships."

—*Michael Jordan*

Telling Our Stories: Digital Storytelling for IPE

Storytelling is a traditional way of passing on knowledge and traditions in many cultures. Offering a narrative on one's personal experience as a story offers the author of the story the opportunity to reflect on the experience and to frame that experience for others in a story format. Narrative pedagogy is a term used to describe an approach to nursing education that includes the use of sharing stories of lived experiences to enhance understanding of each other, of experiences, and of emotions. This approach is a perspective that acknowledges faculty and student as colearner, encouraging thinking in seeking to understand lived experiences (Ironside, 2013).

When educators provide opportunities for students and themselves to develop relationships, understanding, and trust, demonstrating respect for each other in safe psychological learning spaces, they support engagement and learning (Kelly & Hager, 2015). Moreover, using respectful and nonconfrontational communication techniques encourages the development of relationships (Rudolph et al., 2014). Relationship building includes listening to stories about the background and culture of students and faculty members with the intent to understand how these have impacted perspectives. "The students and I would engage in conversations, uncovering frames that pertained to topics ranging from Ramadan to the Easter Bunny, from raising teenagers to understanding folk traditions, and from the lived experience of being one of many wives to professional scopes of practice..." (Foisy-Doll, 2013).

Sharing involves personal integration or framing of an experience and can take place face to face, in writing such as in wikis (Beyer, 2012), or in alternate formats such as digital stories (Gazarian, 2010). One of the means by which the IHEP project sought to extend the affective learning experience was to offer volunteers an opportunity to develop a digital story about their HELP! Save Stan experience (https://sites.google.com/site/ihepsavestan/about-save-stan/digital-stories).

Summary

The increasing complexity of patient care and healthcare environments demands a more collaborative and inclusive approach to healthcare provider education. A more inclusive approach means creating interprofessional learning experiences for early learners throughout the duration of their programs to ensure that a culture of collaboration and team excellence can be translated into practice. Sim-IPE has been found to be one of the most relevant and realistic ways to create meaningful learning experiences for learners and impact downstream positive outcomes (Palaganas et al., 2014). Simulationists are naturals as Sim-IPE champions. Using their skills in providing immersive, high-context learning within educational institutions and clinical practice contexts, they are well positioned to foster a new culture of collaboration. As Simulation Champions in all healthcare environments, we need to embrace new ways of delivering healthcare education, starting with changing how we educate new generations of healthcare providers. Collectively, we must lead and manage change toward a new healthcare culture of collaboration and team excellence to deliver the highest quality, patient-centered care. Currently, we have at our disposal a host of amazing tools and resources to ensure that all learners and practicing healthcare providers acquire interprofessional core competencies to meaningfully transform the professional practice of future health providers. We send out a plea to each one of you to join the cause!

Toolkit Resource

Toolkit 26-1: Resources for Simulation, IPE, and Sim-IPE

27

Space Planning, Design, and Construction for Simulation: A 10-Step Process and Companion Workbooks

Damian A. Henri, Susan Morhart

Note: Damian is a Senior Associate and Simulation-Based Learning Environment Design Leader and has created innovative and modern simulation learning spaces. Susan serves as a Simulation Administrator at the Northern Ontario School of Medicine in Ontario, Canada. This chapter and the online companion workbooks were a collaborative effort by both authors. Damian was the primary author on the chapter while Susan was the primary author on the companion online workbooks.

 Key Terms

Building Program, Design-Build, Simulation-Based Learning Environment, Simulation Learning Spaces, Program (Functional Program)

 Guiding Questions

1 You have just been asked to take on the task of working on a project team to design and build a new simulation center. Would you know where to begin?

2 How can your knowledge as an educator contribute to the success of the project?

3 With whom will you be working, and how do you help select your project team?

4 What kinds of spaces will you include as part of your new facility?

5 What do you need to know about architecture and engineering to lead and participate effectively in this process?

Introduction

The dean of a nursing program once held up a picture of patient beds lined up against a wall in a nursing skills lab and said, "You see this? I don't want this." In setting forth

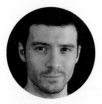

Damian A. Henri, RA, LEED AP

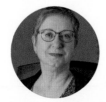

Susan Morhart, RN (Retired)

this mandate, she immediately communicated that she was seeking a learning environment that defied conventional understanding of what nursing students needed to learn. Why is this important? The learning environment influences the learning, and this particular dean recognized that (Fig. 27.1).

Educators, especially, are poised to make crucial contributions to the process of designing and building simulation learning environments. Your experience and knowledge in teaching and learning within a skills laboratory setting puts you in an excellent position to know what it is you want, as well as what you don't want in a new learning space. As a matter of fact, it has been our experience that educators in healthcare spend quite a bit of time envisaging how to improve or replace existing

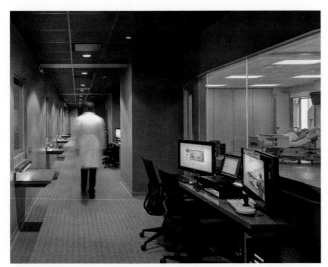

Figure 27.1 Simulation Lab Hallway, Standardized/ Simulated Patient (SP) Suite Stations on the Left, with Open Concept Monitoring Station and Simulation Lab Viewing Window on the Right. (Photo credit ©Brad Feinknopf Photography, 2012.)

teaching spaces and as a result are brimming with great ideas. Don't ever underestimate the pivotal role you play as an equal partner in creating spaces that inspire learning for students and enhance teaching for faculty. It is interesting to note that in an analysis of simulation resources, needs and plans completed by 185 hospital administrators and deans of schools of nursing (SON) in Florida (Sole, Guimond, & Amidei, 2013), "less than half of SON/hospitals (41.8%) had laboratory space designated specifically for simulation activities (dedicated space) and/or a dedicated debriefing room (44.4%)" (p. e268). Of those programs that had simulation spaces, the average space size was 1,916 square feet (178 m²). Those without dedicated space transported simulators to classrooms, lab spaces, and other learning areas.

Can simulation happen "anywhere?" Certainly, but simulation labs can be high fidelity, too! Consider the potential educational benefits that a few clinically accurate learning environments could provide to those who are taking on some of the most challenging and rewarding careers in our society. Any learning space should be explicitly designed from its initial conception to support pedagogy and key educational objectives and provide maximum realism.

What follows is a cursory explanation of the design and construction process that goes into creating **Simulation-Based Learning Environments** and, ultimately, a simulation center. What is unique about this chapter is that it is written from the first-hand experiences of an architect who has been specializing in simulation and a simulation operations manager, each with over 15 years of experience. This chapter and the associated online companion workbooks (See Toolkit 27-1 through 27-10) will guide you through an intricate process using the 10 steps to

design and construction. We break each step down in a clear and substantive way. Also access the Companion Image Catalogue of Simulation Centres and General Nursing Skills Labs (Toolkit 27-11). The *10-Step Companion Workbooks* are rich with amazing tools, photos, and additional content to facilitate your design build journey. **Design-build** refers to one option of many project delivery models whereby there is "One entity, one contract, one unified flow of work from initial concept through completion [for both design and construction]"(Design Build Institute of America, 2014, p. 1). Other project delivery approaches feature separate contracts for design and construction. Although different aspects of design are presented as "steps" in this chapter and the companion workbooks, do not be deceived into thinking that planning a building or learning space is, by any measure, a linear process. As you move through your design, you will find yourself shifting focus among these interdependent steps on a regular basis. Others also have determined incremental approaches to simulation design and building projects, such as, a seven-phase approach articulated by Kuiper and Zabriskie (2012) and Seropian et al. (2015). Kutzin (2016) highlights many helpful design elements that can add to the flow and functionality of simulation spaces that must be though through carefully with your simulation design team.

Given the sizable scope and inherent complexity of building design, we advise that you assemble a team of simulation champions from among your colleagues, so you don't have to make this journey through the quagmire of design and construction complexities all alone.

Please remember this: The purpose of this chapter is *not* to make you an expert in architectural design, engineering, or construction. The majority of the responsibility for carrying out the work related to those disciplines will be borne by others. At the same time, your leadership and participation in that process will be vital to positive outcomes, and the better prepared you will feel to engage knowledgeably in the deliberations surrounding design and construction decisions, the more confident you will feel about the direction of the project, and the more satisfied you will be with the outcomes. You can consider the chapter and companion workbooks as combined Voices of Experience from many our many years in practice and involvement in numerous simulation projects. If you are about to embark on a design build project, this is no doubt an exciting time for you. While there are specific considerations for space development for mobile, distributed, in situ (Horley, 2008; Miller, Riley, Davis, & Hansen, 2008; Tang, Kyaw Tun, & Kneebone, 2013; Thorkelson, 2015), and virtual learning programs (Aebersold, Tschannen, Stephens, Anderson, & Lei, 2016; Bauman, 2010; Kapralos, Hogan, Pribetic, & Dubrowski, 2011; Shelton & Pierce, 2011), this chapter focuses primarily on designing and building simulation centers. Context will also inform your space needs, for example, when simulation occurs on the battlefield,

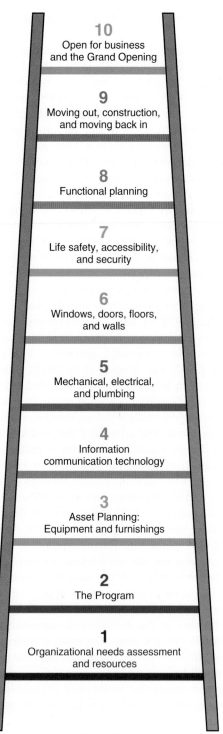

Figure 27.2 Simulation Champions: Ten Steps to Designing a Simulation Center.

disaster zone or in a simulated helicopter or ambulance (Alfes & Manacci, 2014). So grab a cup of your favorite beverage, a sharpened pencil, some paper, and your laptop and settle in with us to begin the process of designing and building. The 10 steps to designing a simulation center are featured in Figure 27.2.

Step 1: Organizational Needs Assessment and Resources

Before you do anything else, make sure you have a capable and committed team from within your institution to take on collectively what will be an exciting and monumental transformation. Using simulation not only changes where teaching and learning takes place, but also how teaching and learning transpires. As you will see throughout the book, adopting change leadership and management practices are key to positive outcomes. This premise holds true for creating simulation-learning environments.

Who's In?

The individuals on your designing and building team can be hard workers, creative thinkers, efficient organizers, decisive managers, or fearless leaders, but it is most important that they have enthusiasm. While this may seem trite, it is, in fact, the single most critical characteristic for achieving buy-in to the endeavor and harnessing the best output from the varied skills of all team members. At first, your team may include only those within your department who have an interest in simulation. As momentum grows, your team may expand to include a broader representation of departmental faculty and leadership, design and construction personnel from your institution, and outside consultants from the fields of architecture, engineering, construction, and simulation. All of these experts will bring diverse and complementary skill sets to the table, some of them daunting and seemingly arcane. Remember that you, too, are an expert who is contributing to this team and bringing valuable insight and perspective to the project. Sprehe and Haley (2012) described how naming the interdisciplinary development team, the STREET team (Simulation Training Resource Education Experts) helped give them a team identify and create a formal presence within the partnering organizations.

Getting Started

You don't need to be an architect or engineer to start designing a simulation center; you just need a list or two, or three. Get your core champions together, and write down all the simulation activities you currently incorporate into the curriculum. Then, make a list of all the things you'd *like* to see happen. Take an account of all faculty and staff who are involved in simulation, even tangentially at first. List the specific courses and the numbers of students in each. Make an inventory of the various tools, devices, and equipment you use to teach. By simply assessing the information you already know about your institution and the ways it uses simulation, you are establishing the necessary foundational data upon which any design effort must build. For this reason, you don't need to be a design expert. You're already an expert in your field! Refer to Toolkit 27-1 for the Step 1 Workbook. We also recommend that you complete the Simulation Culture Organizational Readiness Survey (SCORS). To download a copy of the tool and guidebook, follow this link or go to Toolkit item 9-1 (https://sites.google.com/site/scorsfile/).

All great projects begin with a comprehensive needs assessment that includes identifying benchmarks. We recommend that teams ground new space development in current simulation best practices by learning from the evidence. For example, INACSL Standards of Best Practice: Simulation^SM serve as an excellent starting point in the needs assessment phase. To uphold the INACSL Standards, simulation programs should attend to space requirements for simulation events and the briefing and debriefing of participants.

 Moreover, the Society for Simulation in Healthcare's core accreditation standards (2016) require that Programs have "appropriate physical areas for activities such as education, technology storage, and debriefing, as appropriate with the mission of the Program" (Core Criterion 3. b, p. 3). They also request floor plans, blueprints, and/or photographs of primary simulation facilities or for plans to enlarge or enhance spaces, and at a minimum, a narrative description of in situ simulation facilities (SSH, 2016a). Most recently, the NCSBN Simulation Guidelines for Prelicensure Nursing Programs (Alexander et al., 2015) denote the need for Programs to have appropriate facilities to conduction simulation, including storage areas, staging areas, a place for debriefing, and spaces to house technological resources and store simulation equipment. Physical space development, however, is only one piece of the equation. More precisely, successful simulation integration comes from pairing adequate space development with sufficient program and faculty preparation. From a regulatory standpoint, many jurisdictions now allow the substitution of clinical hours in a traditional practice setting with simulation. This finding is further supported by Jansen, Johnson, Larson, Berry, and Brenner (2009) who cited the top seven obstacles for nurse educators in simulation as, time, training, attitude, lack of space and equipment and scheduling of the lab, funding, staffing, and engaging all students while a few are involved in simulations.

For many, compliance with regulatory standards also involves providing evidence of adherence to best practices in simulation teaching and learning and also the provision of adequate physical spaces and equipment (e.g., Arizona State Boards of Nursing Use of Simulation in Approved RN/LPN Programs (2015) (https://www.azbn.gov/Documents/advisory_opinion/AO%20Use%20of%20Simulation%20in%20Pre-Licensure%20Programs.pdf). Dozens of conference presenters, as well as several book authors and simulation consultants, have addressed simulation space development providing valuable advice from their own lived

experiences (Alinier, Bello, Kalbag, & Kneebone, 2015; Baily, Bar-on, Yucha, & Snyder, 2013; Bar-on, Yucha, & Kinsey, 2013; Horley, 2008; Kuiper & Zabriskie, 2012; Kutzin, 2016; Kyle & Murray, 2008; Nelson, 2013; Seropian & Lavey, 2010; Seropian et al., 2015; Young & Scherwitz, 2015); however, there is little to be found in the literature on best practices in designing and building simulation centers (Rothgeb, 2008; Seropian et al., 2015). The lack of standardized approaches may in part be due to the many variables that exist between health disciplines, programs, and institutions. It is difficult to create standards that fit everyone's space design needs, although Kutzin (2016) suggests that hospital design standards are applicable to simulation environment design; however, allowances for unusual simulation operational and educational requirements exist. What we can offer you is our collective knowledge from designing multiple simulation learning spaces, coupled with many years of healthcare and architectural experience.

Alone, stellar learning spaces are insufficient for the magic of simulation to transpire. Refer to Chapter 3 for information on the INACSL Standards of Best Practice: Simulation^SM (http://www.nursingsimulation.org/issue/S1876-1399(13) X0013-1), Chapter 4 for Simulation Program accreditation, Chapter 11 for Simulation Program management, Chapter 20 for curriculum development, and Chapters 10 and 21 for pointers on simulation team development. Sole, Guimond, and Amedei, (2013) cited that beyond obtaining funding for simulation, the greatest challenges faced by nursing programs were the lack of faculty knowledge, lack of time to implement simulation, lack of equipment, lack of technical support, and lack of buy-in. Therefore, programs must start by conducting a needs assessment followed by creating a plan optimize learning outcomes by strategically tackling each of these challenges prior to or at least in tandem with building simulation learning spaces (Alexander et al., 2015; Meakim, 2007; Rothgeb, 2008; Seropian, Brown, Gavilanes, & Driggers, 2004a, 2004b). Seropian et al. (2004a) offer a sample project timeline that incorporates all of the elements involved in Simulation Program development, including the designing and building of new **simulation-learning spaces** (spaces that are purpose-built for simulated learning experiences) (see Fig. 27.3).

If you're feeling especially daring, go ahead and make a list of the rooms you would want in your simulation center. That is how conceptualizing a new facility starts, and this chapter presents that in greater detail in the next section. When determining what types of spaces should be part of your simulation center, site visits to peer institutions can often be quite helpful. Learning directly from those who actively instruct through simulation and have possibly gone through their own design and construction process can aid you in identifying an approach you should take, components you should include, and especially pitfalls you should avoid. Gathering the best ideas from other facilities can help give you confidence that you're in line with accepted standards

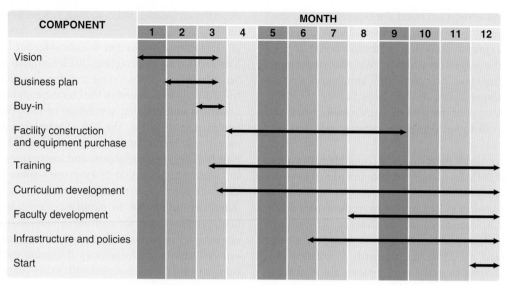

Figure 27.3 Time Line for Components Involved in the Development of a Simulation Program. (From Seropian, M. A., Brown, K., Gavilanes, J. S., & Driggers, B. (2004a). An approach to simulation program development. *Journal of Nursing Education, 43*, 170–174, used with permission.)

of practice and even inspire you to innovate with your own design. While site visits are an excellent source of inspiration and ideas, the lists of spaces and characteristics you are developing should clearly embody the essence of *your* school. They should enumerate goals that reflect *your* institution's vision, mission, and values. You will also need to establish a unique vision for the simulation program: a step that is crucial to positive outcomes in building simulation learning spaces. Seropian et al. (2004b, 2015) remind us that vision development ultimately informs the final size of the space, the scope of the project, the extent to which you choose to collaborate with other disciplines, the budget, the populations you serve, the simulation modalities and simulation typologies you choose to employ (See Chapter 6 and 7 for more information), and the structure of Program governance. Therefore, clearly articulating your *why* provides boundaries that prove essential when making key decisions.

If your lists don't seem to be quite accomplishing this yet, tweak them little by little until they do. By starting with this approach in mind, the result will have a higher chance of success in the evolution of student learning and the facilities that support it. These lists then give simulation champions an early centerpiece around which to discuss how simulation-based learning fits into the institution.

As might be imagined, simply generating lists does not necessarily address the feasibility of implementing any of the ideas they contain. Rather, such lists help set targets through which plans can be scrutinized and perhaps re-aligned as you work through the process (see Box 27-1). Most of these issues are difficult to answer without input from internal facilities managers or external design consultants like architects and engineers. Nonetheless, understanding some of the questions to ask—even if answers are still elusive—is a significant step in recognizing all the factors that will influence your project.

Don't let any early doses of reality douse your dreams when you're in this ideating phase. Although there are inevitable outside influences that will mould and shape your project, anticipation and fear of those realities should not get in the way of honing an idealized concept for your simulation center. Once your team feels confident in understanding its aspirations for your new center, it is time to take the next steps. Those next steps can vary, depending on the nature of your institution, and it will require at least some investigation on the part of the simulation champions. Make sure these ideas are supported by the leadership in your Program, department, or school and then reach out to those in your organization who are responsible for capital improvements, facilities management, or design and construction. Without the strong support of your executive sponsor and department heads, you will have an uphill battle. You may also need to seek input from the overall leadership of your college, university, hospital, or medical center. Again, this requires investigation, understanding, and collaboration on the part of simulation champions.

As more individuals buy in and get on board with your project, those at your institution who internally manage

Box 27-1	Initial Questions to Ask in Context

- How much funding is available?
- Will it be sufficient to renovate your current facilities or will you have to look to expand your footprint?
- How much space is available in existing buildings?
- How much space and funding is available to construct new buildings?
- How much time and effort to allocate to completing the project?
- How much support is there for faculty, staff, departmental administration, and institutional leadership?

construction projects will be able to answer many of your difficult questions. Suddenly issues of building schedule, cost, and existing infrastructure gain clarity and begin to refine or even whittle down some of the ideas you generated by way of your initial lists. It is important that you keep discussions moving forward in the realm of all possible ideas. You'll soon find that you have a loose outline that addresses room types, their functions, and capacities. Not only that but the impacts of the budget, schedule, and the reality of what is possible to create at your institution will inform your team. The answers, to a great extent, are thanks to the input of your new team members who oversee capital improvements. This outline is the beginning of what is known variously as a **building program**, program of required spaces, functional program, or program of functional requirements. For the purpose of this chapter, we call it the Program. Throughout all stages of development, communication between team members and internal and external stakeholders is key to positive outcomes. People really do want to know what is happening and want to have a say in plans (Kuiper & Zabriskie, 2012).

Step 2: The Program

Before drawing any walls, doors, or windows, most building projects start with a **Program**. In its simplest form, it is the initially written summary of what spaces and features go into a building. You may even have already started down the programming road through one of the lists you've already made with your team of champions. If so, review that list to make sure that what you itemized will be an enabler of your current or future curriculum, as well as the curriculum of other programs for which you are planning. The curriculum is the initial generator of the recipe for your facility, and in many ways, the Program is analogous to a list of ingredients for that complicated recipe. See Box 27-2 for the major headings commonly contained in a Program. Once you have read through this section, access Toolkit 27-2 for the online Step 2 Companion Workbook. There you will find a step-by-step guide to describing the Program for your project.

The Project Scope

In construction and building projects, the scope is expressed as a written statement that is used to specify project outcomes and help keep decision-making during the project on point. A *project scope* generally entails the project objective, deliverables, milestones, technical requirements, and any limitations or exclusions. A sample scope objective might read: We will build a high-quality, state-of-the-art simulation center in 18 months that is not to exceed $ 8M dollars. The building will include a 10,300-square-feet facility with four basic simulation rooms, four simulated patient

---

> **Box 27-2   The Program Outline**
>
>   I. Overview, purpose, and description of program
> II. Room Overview
>   **a.** Quantity
>   **b.** Floor area (SF or m²)
>   **c.** Occupancy level
>   **d.** Priority level
>   **e.** Description of use and unique requirements
> III. Room detail (room data sheets)
>   **a.** Critical adjacencies and separations
>   **b.** Hours of usage
>   **c.** Use by specific faculty or students
>   **d.** Interior finish descriptions
>   **e.** Door and windows requirements
>   **f.** Special construction (acoustic walls, lead-lined walls, raised floors, etc.)
>   **g.** Mechanical needs (HVAC, plumbing, medical gas, fire suppression, etc.)
>   **h.** Electrical needs (power, lighting, fire alarm, etc.)
>   **i.** Audiovisual needs (cameras, microphones, monitoring, sim software, etc.)
>   **j.** Information technology needs (computers, network infrastructure, etc.)
>   **k.** Special furniture needs
>   **l.** Special equipment needs

---

rooms with adjoining monitoring rooms, one SP lounge, one operating room theatre, associated control/monitoring rooms, one lecture theatre, six briefing/debriefing rooms, one 24-station eLearning pod, a café area to accommodate 40 people, two breakouts gathering spaces, one procedural skills training room equipped with 12 virtual haptic learning stations, and a clear entrance and exit. Technical requirements speak to things like LEED Certification, building codes, energy ratings, and capacity will include a web-based integrated IT/AV system for recording and storing simulation events and accommodations for full body computerized simulators. *Milestones* can include statements regarding stages of permit approvals, key building stages (e.g., pouring concrete, building enclosure), or final inspection and move-in date. It is important to clearly state that what is in and what is out of the project. You don't want any nasty surprises like, "What do you mean refrigerators are not part of kitchen appliance packages?" Be clear on what the builder, subcontractor, and owner are providing. The budget ultimately affects the scope of the project.

Programming for Buildings

As with the ingredient list in a recipe, a building program includes the types of components that will make up the final product and also the quantities of each, their sizes, and descriptions of unique characteristics that are fundamental in defining those spaces. Additionally, it may be helpful to identify the number of occupants expected for each space, key location relationships with other spaces, and likely final location within the finished building—basement versus top floor, the perimeter versus the center of the building. Any relevant detail that you can summarize with a numerical value or brief written description is worth considering for inclusion in the Program. Note that some of these spaces are required by accreditation or regulatory bodies as previously stated, so you are wise to verify and comply with requirements that apply to your organization.

Once assembled, a summary of all this information may be a one- or two-page spreadsheet that reduces a complex structure to a series of numerically defined, easily understood line items. As the Program develops, each of those line items is isolated or expanded on, within their own page. In this way, you can give even more detail and description of the room or space, still without drawing or designing anything. While you cannot confirm all the specifics of each space in their entirety before completing the full building design, you can use programming tools to define a substantial portion of those attributes that will characterize each room.

As you go through the exercise of programming your project, remember that there is no neutral space. It is either helping or hindering your mission in some way. Given that understanding of the Program, what types of spaces should be included? Of course, the answer to this question will vary, depending on your needs. Terminology for naming and describing these may also vary, depending on geographical region and institutional culture, but here are some simple descriptions of the primary constituent space types of most simulation centers. Additional detail and considerations for these spaces will follow later in this chapter. As well, the workbook exercises and fill in tables will drill down deeper into your specific needs.

Simulation Lab

There are as many different types of simulation labs as there are clinical specialties. Broadly speaking, a simulation lab is any space dedicated to simulation-based learning through the use of individual or team-based scenarios. Also included are simulation spaces that recreate vehicle environments for EMTs and flight nurses, exam rooms for simulated/standardized patient interaction, and even nonclinical environments to recreate scenarios in locations other than medical facilities. A simulation lab will often replicate to some degree of detail the characteristics of specific clinical settings unless it is a lab intended to be more flexible. In that case, the lab may pull attributes from a variety of clinical realities to broaden the utilization of available space.

Control or Monitor Room

Today, given the commonplace use of sophisticated patient simulators and integrated AV/IT capture

systems, there are definitely specialized design needs. Simulation operating systems and equipment require designated spaces, even for the most modest of simulation centers. The approach to creating control locations can vary vastly, from single, large, centralized rooms that serve an entire center to multiple, smaller control rooms with proprietary, direct views to each simulation lab. Those views may be via windows and/or flat panel displays. In all cases, these spaces will provide multiple seating locations for technicians and instructors to use computer workstations, which often have multiple monitors to view video feeds, live data from mannequins, and scenario-related documents like scripts, checklists, and fictional patient records.

Prebriefing and Debriefing Room

The prebriefing/debriefing room is where students prepare for, and consolidate learning in simulation. Until students have the opportunity to discuss and analyze their performance in a simulation scenario, the full cycle of learning has not been completed. While it is possible to debrief in the simulation lab, a classroom, or other impromptu location, a dedicated debriefing room can be configured to optimize postsimulation discussions. In particular, integration of audiovisual playback systems allows a debriefing team to review and discuss footage from the scenario in an environment specifically tailored to this style of interaction.

Nursing Skills Laboratory

The nursing skills laboratory (aka skills lab) has been a common component of nursing and health science education that long predates modern simulation technologies, and as its name indicates, is the location where students can learn and practice tasks and psychomotor skills in a low-stakes environment (see Fig. 27.4A, B). For nursing programs, this space usually includes an array of patient bed stations that allow a large class of learners to break up into small groups to practice and discuss skills and patient care modalities in a low-stakes environment. In this setting, low-fidelity static mannequins are generally the surrogates for an actual patient, as opposed to the more advanced patient simulators used in dedicated simulation labs. A skills lab may also be a location to work with task trainers or virtual reality surgical simulators. In all cases, a skills lab should provide an opportunity for active learning and engagement with faculty. Skills labs can also be environments that support the acquisition of specific procedural skills, as with procedural skills labs that house things like task trainers or virtual workbenches.

Storage and Supply (Including Lockers)

The need for storage space in a simulation center is chronically underestimated and is usually the first to be sacrificed

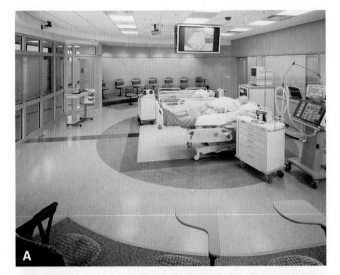

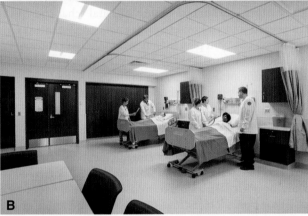

Figure 27.4 Examples of Nursing Skills Labs. **A.** Division of Nursing Facility at Cuyahoga Community College's Metro Campus. (Architectural Photography by Barney Taxel, Cleveland OH.) **B.** Lorain County Community College's Nursing Program (LCCC) Health Science. (Todd Williams, Shooting Star Architectural Photography)

when additional space is needed for other purposes. This double hit leaves most simulation centers wanting for storage space, often resulting in the largest and most ungainly pieces of equipment being shunted aside in corridors or, worse yet, tucked away in learning spaces, thus hampering the primary purpose of the simulation center. Be sure to allocate sufficient storage area within the Program. While there is no definitive ratio of storage space to simulation space, make a reasonable initial estimate based on what you will need to store and how much of it there will be, both now and in the future. Keep in mind that storage needs are greater for a multidisciplinary center with each additional discipline introducing storage needs that are specific to its profession. Remember to include locations for consumable supplies, especially those that require being secured in a limited access setting. Consider whether or not to plan for lockers for simulation participants to store personal belongings while participating in simulation activities and debriefings.

Reception/Check-in (If Necessary)

For many simulation centers, a front desk area can serve many roles, depending on the location and layout of the center. Generally speaking, in a solely academic setting where the simulation participants are students, this reception area may not be a critical component but could take on a dual-purpose form to simulate a nurse station or a monitoring location for faculty or staff overseeing a large skills lab. It may also be strategically located to provide faculty with oversight of most of the spaces in the simulation center.

For facilities that are serving learners from outside the institution or providing continuing education for practicing professionals, such a reception area almost always requires a full-time equivalent staff member. This kind of "front door" does help provide not just a welcome but also orientation to the site, directions and information, a mechanism for tracking schedules and attendance, and even a measure of security at the entrance to the facility. Consider in the design idea phase whether you currently have the funding to support this position or if it is feasible and desirable to seek funding for it in the future.

Administrative Support

Any simulation center needs administrators, faculty, technicians, and other dedicated staff to perform the day-to-day duties of operating the center and teaching students. If these individuals are not already accommodated in offices elsewhere, they will likely need a workstation somewhere within or nearby the simulation center. This reality is particularly the case for new staff whose role is to provide technical skills, guidance, and support to those using the simulation center. Additionally, it may be useful to provide conference space, project worktable areas, and room for a copier or other office equipment if they are not otherwise existing in the building and available for use. While office environments may not seem highly relevant to a discussion regarding the design of a simulation facility, it is critical to account for the square footage used by these rooms in the Program to have a complete picture of your overall space needs.

Other (Classrooms, Meeting Space, Lounge Space, etc.)

Many space types don't fit well into distinct categories but nonetheless perform particular functions in a simulation center that are worth describing. For example, given the ubiquity of computer workstations and the increasing emphasis on using sophisticated simulators with highly technical attributes, the technicians you may have on staff might require a small workshop dedicated to the maintenance and repair of your equipment. If your simulation center is to include facilities dedicated to simulated/ standardized patient (SP) interaction, it may be advisable to provide clothes changing spaces and lockers, prebriefing rooms, and even a lounge where actors can wait during a day of structured examinations. You may also want to explore whether faculty or simulation participants may benefit from having a lounge space of their own. Also, consider the need to provide a location for amenities that would support meal breaks. Of course, given that a simulation center is an educational facility, consider the need for didactic learning space—that is, classrooms—to supplement the practical learning environments as the heart of your center.

 Refer to Toolkit 27-2 in the online Step 2 Companion Workbook for examples of Program summary spreadsheets and room data sheets. As mentioned before, room data sheets contain a higher resolution of descriptive information than the overall program summary when it comes to defining the needs of individual spaces. The following sections in this chapter help educate you on the necessary design understanding you will need to better establish the needs of each room and fill out a room data sheet.

Step 3: Asset Planning: Equipment and Furnishings

A reflection of modern healthcare delivery, simulation-based education in health sciences is dependent on regular usage of tools and devices of varying degrees of complexity. This equipment plays a significant role in defining how the design of each space will take shape. It is not uncommon to use a major piece like a hospital bed as a basis on which to plan a basic work and learning area module. By planning around equipment elements that often have sizes and requirements predetermined by manufacturers, you can be sure that you will have the *dimensional clearances* and *building utilities* you will need to support productive use of the equipment and, by extension, support the learning experience. As an educator, your primary role related to this area is to understand what equipment you plan to use and to inform your team how you use it in a teaching setting. Once you have read through this section, access Toolkit 27-3 the online Step 3 Companion Workbook. There you will find a step-by-step guide to planning for equipment and furniture for your project.

Generally speaking, the three major categories of equipment are *simulators, medical devices,* and *audiovisual and information* technology. This section of the chapter focuses on the first two of those topics and how they inform the design of your center, focusing especially on storage strategies. Audiovisual and information technology are addressed in the section following this one.

Simulators

The term "simulator" can be used to describe a wide range of teaching tools that reproduce physiological realities for

the purpose of providing low-risk training for learners. When selecting what simulation technology you want to incorporate in your center, again start with your curriculum to help ensure that the devices you choose will possess the appropriate features that are best aligned to fulfill the learning objectives you have devised for your students. The simulators that you plan to use will need to be apportioned space in your simulation center, both in the labs or classrooms where they will be used, and when they are not in use, in the location where you will store them. Your simulators may also have electrical, technology, or medical gas requirements for which your team needs to plan.

Perhaps no simulation technology has influenced health science education in the past two decades more than patient simulator mannequins. While instructional mannequins have long been in use for medical and nursing education, the advent of simulators that can be programmed to exhibit a series of vital characteristics, symptoms, and responses to care and treatment has an impact on how you plan for a new simulation center.

Each simulator you have or plan on acquiring will have specific utility needs, even if it's as simple as a location where it gets plugged in when it needs to be charged. While this seems straightforward, do inform the design team where that charging location should be—while the mannequin is in the bed or gurney in the simulation lab or while it is in a dedicated storage location. It may not occur to the design team to provide outlets dedicated to charging devices in a storage area. Peripheral devices such as laptops and tablets that control the operation of the mannequins generally accompany programmable patient simulators. Decide whether these control stations will be mobile or have a dedicated workstation in a control room, for example. This will help your team understand the number and locations of power outlets and data connections.

Simulators also transmit data, either wirelessly or through hard-wired connection. Again, all of these issues can be handled and accommodated in the design by the architects and engineers with whom you will be working. While you as the educator should be aware of these requirements, it is more important that you communicate to your team how you intend to take full advantage of the features of your simulator. If you want patient data to display on a bedside monitor, it may require special data, audio, and video connections in the wall to permit the display of this data. If you would like to capture patient data from the simulator in parallel with video and audio feeds during the simulation, the design will need to incorporate yet another set of these connections.

Although the latest efforts in mannequin design have strived to make these simulators as untethered as possible, respiratory gas exchange provided with some of the most sophisticated patient simulators is often enabled by an accompanying rack of equipment that comes as part of that simulator's included components. If you intend to use a tethered simulator in your facility, you should be aware of how much floor space the rack(s) take up and how the length of the umbilical connecting the rack to the mannequin limits the distance separating those two pieces of the system. If these limitations dictate that the rack is in the same room as the mannequin, it may become an obstacle to having reasonable clearances to move around the patient or to simultaneously use actual medical equipment like ventilators, crash carts, and the like. Furthermore, these equipment racks must often be supplied with nitrogen, oxygen, and carbon dioxide for the mannequin's gas exchange to function properly. This application may require the introduction of a dedicated closet for medical gases or even to have gas cylinders located within the teaching area, further impinging on the available space for students to learn.

In many centers, a patient simulator may enjoy the luxury of lazily reclining on a dedicated bed or gurney in a simulation room for the majority of its lifetime. On the other hand, if a mannequin needs to be stored elsewhere, a specific storage solution will be required to efficiently and safely stow this expensive piece of equipment. In general, when considering storage, it is best to consider design tactics that maximize the density of storage, allowing you to keep the maximum amount of content in the smallest amount of floor area—think compact and think vertical. If you roll the gurney and simulator wholesale into a storage room where there is enough floor space to accommodate it, plan on lowering the gurney to its lowest height so that you leave the potential to introduce shelving or cabinets above it for storing other items.

Another option for storing a patient simulator mannequin is in a customized cabinetry solution. A large cabinet with shelves that glide out can allow for the transfer of a mannequin to a bed or gurney using the same methods typically used for safe patient transfer. Such cabinetry solutions will require heavy duty hardware to support the weight of the simulators and invariably large cabinet doors. This kind of solution has the potential to house multiple mannequins on stacked tiers of shelves, resulting in a highly efficient use of a small area.

The important lesson, here, is not so much that you are fully versed in the technical ins and outs of all your simulators and every impact they will have on your project's design but more that you are judicious and deliberate in the selection of your simulation equipment. It is also important that you are as thorough as possible in communicating to those designing your space how you intend to use that equipment and what you want to get out of it.

Task Trainers

A subset of the simulator category, task trainers (also referred to as part- or partial task trainers) come in many forms—for example, a forearm and hand model used to practice IV insertion, a torso "phantom" to help hone ultrasound scanning skills, or a surgeon's laparoscopy training kit that often bears no resemblance to any portion of human anatomy. All task trainers generally have one thing in common in that they are each specially designed to allow students to gain aptitude in a specific skill or modality.

Because of this, task trainers are uncomplicated in contrast to full body, patient simulators and commensurately less expensive, allowing institutions to purchase them en masse to support larger group training sessions. Due to the variety of task trainers and the fact that they involve volume purchasing, their greatest influence on the design of the facility is in formulating an appropriate furniture solution for their use during class and lab sessions and in designing a place for their storage when not in use. Unlike mannequin simulators, which often reside on a semipermanent basis in a bed or on a gurney, task trainers usually need to be set up on a table or countertop when students are learning on them, and put away after their use in a class session is concluded. Like the full body simulators, some task trainers require electrical power or to be plugged in as a peripheral device to a computer workstation in order to take most complete advantage of their full range of features. Be sure that, in the location where you intend to use any device, you have the work surface, physical clearances, and access to utilities that you will need to use it. Use the design of your facility as an opportunity to locate the resources your students will need to achieve the learning objectives set forth through your curriculum.

Major Medical Equipment

In many ways, the use of hospital beds, crash carts, and preengineered headwalls will introduce to a simulation center the greatest degree of clinical realism because they are the actual products that are found in hospitals and other healthcare settings. There is little more to be said about considerations for medical equipment that hasn't already been stated for patient simulators and task trainers. Ask yourself what are the physical space, electrical power, data network, and daily usage requirements for each piece of equipment? What differentiates major medical equipment from other equipment types is the impact it has on defining the size and layout of each space. A simple patient bed, and not the mannequin that resides there, becomes the kernel of an educational workstation module. This module includes a bed and a zone of open floor area around the bed for students and instructors to work and circulate. When configuring a series of these patient bed modules in a skills lab, for example, the overall size and shape of the room begin to take form.

It is easy to imagine then, how the instructional environment for x-ray technology or a simulated operating room will involve a combination of medical equipment and teacher/learner workspace. As the largest items in the room, medical devices are predominant when making initial estimates of room sizes and when planning out each space as the design process proceeds.

Medical Consumables and Supplies

Medical supply purchases will likely be from an operations budget, rather than a major capital improvement budget. Either way, their presence and use in a simulation center should have an influence on the building design. You will need to think about any possible impacts their use may have on the center, and how the design might need to respond to those possibilities. In one interpretation of such impacts, the use of a substance like Betadine might require the selection of stain resistant material for countertops, cabinetry, and flooring. This example features a particular product, however, with all supplies the key consideration is how consumable products of any kind will be stored, secured, distributed to students when it's time to learn, and disposed of when they are no longer usable.

Thinking about designing around your equipment is important, but if you are not able to acquire the new equipment you need, the exercise of developing a design strategy around it is moot. Like most other aspects of your project, equipment comes at a price. How high that price is, depends on how diligent and creative your team is in pursuing the best opportunities available for maximizing the value of your equipment purchase. The first and most often overlooked opportunity is the availability of reduced pricing, if not outright donations of new or used medical equipment. While you should address this possibility with all equipment manufacturers and vendors representatives, however, companies that are in the business of selling major medical equipment are most likely to work with educational institutions toward the goal of minimizing the cost of everything from beds to medical gas booms to clinical grade cabinetry.

Should negotiations for attractively priced new equipment not yield everything you might need for your center, another option for securing equipment at a reduced price is through companies that refurbish previously owned items and sell them at a discount. This approach does not guarantee the most current models of what you'll need, but in many cases, it does not matter for equipment where core functionality has not changed significantly over time.

If you're not the primary person responsible for procuring equipment, be sure that the individual who holds that responsibility is well aware of cost-saving opportunities. It can potentially add up to thousands of dollars in savings that can then be applied to benefit other areas in your simulation center project. For this reason, it is never too soon to begin these discussions. If your team waits too long to explore these options, you may miss out on opportunities to maximize the distance your project budget can go. Another consideration is that large purchases (capital expenses—generally speaking, those exceeding $1,000.00) require time for procurement processes. For example, institutional tendering procurement processes to ensure fairness to competitors can take up to several weeks or months to complete.

Furnishings

The last category of what might be considered equipment is simple furniture: tables, chairs, and any other furnishing that is not built in with the construction of your facility. By that definition, furnishings as a category do not include cabinetry and countertops. Fixed built-ins are also called millwork.

It may seem that there is not much to say about the topic. However, furniture purchases can impact the functionality and flexibility of spaces and their usability. Because of this, furniture is sometimes overlooked until the last moment, so be sure to keep tabs on all your furniture needs for offices, debriefing rooms, control rooms, and any other instances where someone will need a place to sit or do work. Consider buying flexible, collapsible, stackable, lightweight, durable, portable, and mobile furniture. Nesting chairs and tables, for example, can impact your ability to take quickly down or reset a room independently. Spend time thinking about each piece of furniture or equipment and how it will affect program delivery. Discussions could revolve around the selection of a family caregiver chair in a patient room or furniture for a simulated domestic setting—most of these decisions would appear to be self-evident, however, can significantly affect day-to-day functionality.

As with most of the building materials in your project, you should especially consider durability when it comes to furniture, especially if you are reconfiguring rooms on a regular basis. With more movement comes more opportunity for incidental damage. Aside from these practical concerns, ask which design needs require a furniture solution as opposed to using built-in work surfaces or seating. It is desirable whenever possible to eliminate the need for built-ins as they are costly to install and remove and can impede space flexibility. The rationale for making such decisions is rooted in the degree of flexibility you desire, your institutional standards, and sometimes, mere preference.

Step 4: Information and Communication

The use of information and audiovisual technology is pervasive in all learning environments, and education for nursing, medicine, and other health sciences is no exception. For simulation-based learning in these disciplines, this kind of technology plays a critical role in capturing and archiving the simulation activities of students, allowing them to review and learn from their experiences in a more objective way than firsthand involvement can provide on its own. Please refer to Toolkit 27-4, for the online Step 4 Companion Workbook information and communication.

Whether they are in offices, classrooms, control rooms, or on a bedside cart in a simulation space, the ubiquity of computers applies just as much, if not more, to the simulation center as it does other, more traditional learning environments. Because they're so commonplace, it's easy to overlook them when considering how a room will be furnished. The most common uses of simulation-specific computers are for simulator mannequin control and for the software that helps manage video, audio, and data captures from simulation events. You will also require computers for simulated medical records, simulation through a virtual reality interface, or as a workstation for computer-based, interactive task trainers, such as haptic devices. Be sure that your team identifies all the computers you will use—yet another list that your team should make.

Once you have identified all of the potential usage of fixed computer workstations, mobile workstations on wheels, laptops, tablets, and even personal mobile devices, you will need to work with your design team to designate locations for each of these uses. For example, most advanced patient simulator packages include a laptop or tablet holding the software that provides control and monitoring of the simulator. This computer could be in a control room, in the simulation lab itself, or stored in a locked location when not in use. Of course, those faculty and staff with offices will have a natural, dedicated home for their computer usage.

In addition to computers that have dedicated locations, your faculty, staff, and students will bring their own laptops, tablets, and other devices and expect to be able to use them *wherever* they are in your facility. It's hard to imagine the individual who would enter any educational facility without one, two, or even more personal devices of some kind. You and your team will need to figure out how to prioritize the assignment of space for people to work independently. Whether they are distinct lounges or small niches carved into a corridor wall, this kind of incidental space will be competing for a slot in your building program alongside other support areas, such as the ever-important equipment and supply storage.

Wherever there are computers, there will be the need for network connectivity. One of the most important reasons for identifying computer usage locations in your facility is that it tells the architects and engineers where they need to provide network access. Much of this access is wireless, but until security and bandwidth improve on Wi-Fi, you will likely also have wired network connections that manifest as data jacks on the walls of your labs, control rooms, and offices.

Perhaps the most frustrating part of planning for information technology is the obligation to set aside a not insignificant amount of space for server closets and network rooms. Your design team should make sure that these are included and sized and ventilated appropriately in your design. Just know that those rooms will forever be staring back at you from the floor plan as essential square footage that you and your team will rarely visit.

Audiovisual

The ability to capture video and audio recordings of a simulation scenario is highly desirable where possible to achieve full effectiveness in simulation-based learning. During active participation in a simulation activity, students are not able to apply an analytical perspective to their performance because they are actively focusing on the tasks and objectives of the scenario. Even the sharpest minds will encounter difficulty in attempting to recall with accuracy a sequence of events that may have transpired in a high-stress and possibly chaotic setting. By following the simulation activity with a review of a recording of their work in a calm, conversational, and collaborative context like a debriefing room, students are able to assume a more objective viewpoint of their performance and maximize what they learn from the experience. Well-conceived audiovisual equipment integration, along with the software to manage that equipment, will provide such advantages to your students.

If you intend to make the capture of video, audio, and simulators' vital signs a part of your simulation center, you will need to explore the variety of options on the market for simulation software. Such software packages cover a wide range of capabilities and costs, and it would benefit your team to research the available product choices as much as possible. Depending on the software and the features you elect to incorporate, not only you can simultaneously capture multiple, synchronized streams of data from different cameras, microphones, instruments, and monitors but you may also be able to type and attach comments that are bookmarked to a specific time in the video as a scenario is being recorded, embedding performance feedback for students that becomes part of the digital file. Some simulation software might include a scheduling tool, allowing you to plan and coordinate your resources for simulation events. Many software packages extend beyond simple multimedia recording and playback platforms, and they can now be used to manage an entire simulation center. Be sure to couple your research with the knowledge brought to the table by your design team, especially if your team includes an AV specialist with a deep background in simulation.

While you and your team of champions do not need to understand the technical intricacies of video cameras and microphones, it is important to know what they can contribute to the learning experience and how you should be prepared to discuss this with the design team experts. When it comes to video cameras, consider the variety of views you may want to capture of the activity in a simulation lab. More accurately, determine what action you would like to capture from a variety of different simulation scenarios based on what will be most useful in aiding students to learn from their experiences. This content may vary from a wide view of all the activity in the room to a close-up look from directly over the patient—or even a certain part of the patient's body. Cameras can allow you to consider perspectives from almost any direction and with any degree of detail, keeping in mind that the greater the versatility of the camera or the higher its definition, the more expensive it will be. Figure 27.5 demonstrates the

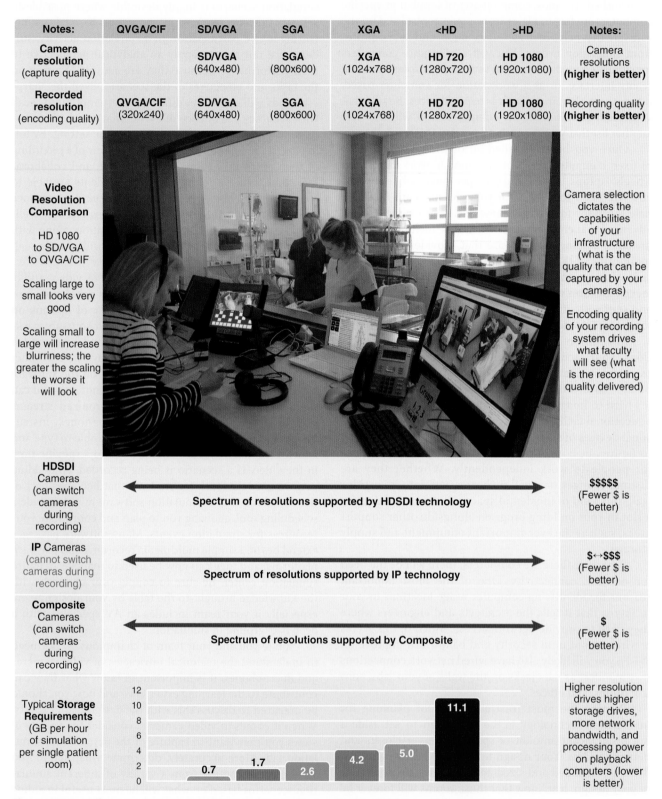

Notes:	QVGA/CIF	SD/VGA	SGA	XGA	<HD	>HD	Notes:
Camera resolution (capture quality)		SD/VGA (640x480)	SGA (800x600)	XGA (1024x768)	HD 720 (1280x720)	HD 1080 (1920x1080)	Camera resolutions **(higher is better)**
Recorded resolution (encoding quality)	QVGA/CIF (320x240)	SD/VGA (640x480)	SGA (800x600)	XGA (1024x768)	HD 720 (1280x720)	HD 1080 (1920x1080)	Recording quality **(higher is better)**

Video Resolution Comparison

HD 1080 to SD/VGA to QVGA/CIF

Scaling large to small looks very good

Scaling small to large will increase blurriness; the greater the scaling the worse it will look

Camera selection dictates the capabilities of your infrastructure (what is the quality that can be captured by your cameras)

Encoding quality of your recording system drives what faculty will see (what is the recording quality delivered)

HDSDI Cameras (can switch cameras during recording)

Spectrum of resolutions supported by HDSDI technology

$$$$$ (Fewer $ is better)

IP Cameras (cannot switch cameras during recording)

Spectrum of resolutions supported by IP technology

$↔$$$ (Fewer $ is better)

Composite Cameras (can switch cameras during recording)

Spectrum of resolutions supported by Composite

$ (Fewer $ is better)

Typical **Storage Requirements** (GB per hour of simulation per single patient room)

0.7   1.7   2.6   4.2   5.0   11.1

Higher resolution drives higher storage drives, more network bandwidth, and processing power on playback computers (lower is better)

Figure 27.5 Differences between the Various Camera Technologies. (Table credit Lucas Huang, 2016, with permission. Image credit, MacEwan University Clinical Simulation Centre, 2014. Used with Permission.)

vast array of options and technological considerations for camera capture. Through your involvement in the design process, you will become well versed in technical language if you are not already.

When you convey these objectives to the design professionals, they will advise on the right types of cameras and the optimal locations for those cameras. Depending on the comprehensiveness of video capture that you are striving to achieve, a single simulation room or site may have several cameras. Outside of simulated patient care areas, cameras have also been installed in skills labs to capture students' work at the bedside or their technique on an IV practice arm. Cameras could be located in corridors to capture patient transport that is part of a multiroom simulation scenario, or they could be located in debriefing rooms, so teachers can hone their skills through review of debriefing procedure and technique.

Microphones follow many of the same design rules as cameras, though of course their function is to capture the sounds of a simulation. Given the emphasis on strong communication skills in simulation-based team training, be sure to advocate for well-integrated microphone design for the project. As with cameras, you will likely need to include multiple microphones for each simulation area. Some of these may be mounted to a headwall or in the ceiling above a bed and able to pick up sound from a wide area. This approach can be a budget-friendly way to mix one or two microphones into the capture feed, but sound quality may be unreliable as participants move in and out of range of the microphones and excessive collateral noise makes picking out individual voices challenging during debriefs and other review sessions.

A more expensive, but more dependable alternative for capturing sound is the use of an individual lavaliere-style microphone for each simulation participant and confederate. When strategically used, this manner of capturing sound will provide the most consistently intelligible audio output. Aside from the increased cost associated with purchasing and maintaining several microphones, transmitters, and receivers, the major drawback of this model is that it often does not capture incidental sounds from the simulation area—for example, equipment sounds—that can fill the audio capture with an important additional layer of sound information.

Because of these oppositional advantages, most audio capture solutions involve both approaches—one "area" microphone to record the general atmosphere of sound in the simulation and a number of personal "close" microphones that capture individual voices. Often, having three to five personal microphones should cover most simulation situations. For those scenarios that involve more principal participants, you can often fall back on the ceiling or headwall-mounted area microphone to capture those without personal devices. As always, make these

decisions in the context of what you and your champions know about your curriculum, the scenarios you plan to run, and the depth of information you want to generate for debriefing. Given those considerations, you may only consistently need two personal microphones or you may need six or more.

While cameras and microphones fulfill the need for recording input, flat panel monitors, and speakers provide playback output. It is commonplace to equip debriefing rooms and smaller classrooms with flat panel displays and ceiling or wall-mounted speakers. Sometimes, more than one monitor is needed to display more content or enable distance learning and teleconferencing functionality. Aside from these more obvious uses, think of how these devices can contribute more directly to simulation activities. They are essential in simulating telemedicine-based scenarios. Additionally, speakers coupled with a microphone in the control room can introduce opportunities for voice over intercom style announcements for paging, codes, and alarms. In a surgical setting, monitors can display not only patient data and vitals but also simulated views from laparoscopic devices.

Finally, to store all the data, you will be recording, you will need file servers—those large computers that sit in a tall rack somewhere in a room you rarely visit. Like the IT network closet, the room where these servers live is a "necessary evil," taking up valuable floor space but also indispensable in a modern and fully equipped simulation center. In many cases, this room will be separate from the IT network closet because two different groups of personnel manage them. Even so, when space is at a premium, it pays to ask whether or not to combine these spaces in the name of efficiency.

Also found within the technology and IT/AV category are health informatics and patient care technologies. These systems of course include the electronic healthcare record (EHR). Hanberg and Madden (2011) underscore the importance of providing learners with hands on, immersive, contextual experiences that integrate patient care situations for optimize learning information learning outcomes. There is also evidence to support that the integration of EHR systems into high-fidelity simulation produces increases in a student's speed and accuracy of use (George, Drahnak, Schroeder, & Katrancha, 2016). Greenawalt (2014) warns educators that advance planning is essential to mitigate the many challenges inherent in teaching and learning about healthcare informatics systems and their use in simulation.

Simulation labs can either create internal simulated EHRs, purchase them ready made from vendors, or tap into existing health authority systems. Each of these options will require detailed consideration. For example, many labs will include either fixed computer stations or alternately use computers on wheels (COWs) for access to the EHR.

Step 5: Mechanical, Electrical, and Plumbing

When you think of the MEP (mechanical, electrical, and plumbing) systems in a building, it may be difficult to envision what they are and what they do. There is a good reason for this since designers will hide these components behind walls, above ceilings, and under floors. The umbrella category of building MEP encompasses a broad variety of utilities and functionality including HVAC (heating, ventilation, and air conditioning), electrical power, and plumbing for both water and medical gasses. While the design engineers on your project team will bear the responsibility of understanding the technical details for each of these, it is important that you comprehend how they may have an impact on your simulation center and the experience of the learners. Refer to Toolkit Workbook 27-5 after reading this chapter section to begin your planning for MEP.

Mechanical Systems

You will often hear the HVAC components of a design referred to as the mechanical systems because, in part, a mechanical engineer typically designs them. While it is rare that direct interaction with HVAC becomes part of the simulated experience, it is important that this engineer has experience designing simulation centers or, barring that, is at least well versed in design for healthcare facilities. For example, while your center may not end up providing low-temperature, laminar flow air in its simulated operating room, you may want the ceiling diffusers to have the right look that suggests laminar air supply. Details like this affect the perception, if not the operation, of the environment, and it takes a well-informed designer to pick up on those details and incorporate them.

On the other hand, you may be seeking to create some unique learning environments for which you will want to explore unique HVAC designs. A simulation lab that is intended to emulate various outside conditions could have a broad range of variability in air speed and temperature control and would therefore need separate heating and cooling as well as additional wall insulation between it and adjacent spaces. A simulated home care setting may incorporate an old style radiator, baseboard heaters, or other residential grade components that would otherwise be foreign to new or renovated buildings at an educational institution.

In all cases, the design of mechanical systems must account for enough cooling power to offset the heat given off by medical equipment, simulators, and the computers that accompany them. Again, this reinforces the need for you to help the design team ensure that the equipment list is comprehensive and well understood by each team member.

Nurse Call and Code Call Systems

This chapter is not intended to apply to in situ simulation, and given that simulation centers are mostly in educational settings, and in no way ever provide real patient care, nurse call systems are permitted and incorporated for use in simulation scenarios. As always, consider how nurse call functions can play a part in your simulations. The question of how far you go with the available features may be both a question of practicality and cost. Most nursing schools with active simulation programs almost certainly include scenarios for simulating code events, so installing a code button—even a mock one—in a patient bed area is advisable. Other features like patient call buttons or intercoms can also be useful, especially if your simulation involves a standardized patient or other confederate participant acting as a family member or an affiliated medical professional.

Building Security

As much as it can be dismaying and even uncomfortable topic to address, well-conceived building security measures are an essential part of keeping staff, students, and the expensive tools they use safe and out of the reach of any who might bear ill intent. There are two components to building security. The first is "Defensible Design," a design philosophy detailed in Oscar Newman's (1972) book *Design Guidelines for Creating Defensible Space*, through which a building's inherent design characteristics serve to passively and naturally serve as controls for building access and even deterrents to crime. While some attributes like adequate lighting levels or a well-positioned reception desk are common sense measures, there are others that might not as immediately be evident. For example, maximizing the number and size of exterior windows and interior windows between spaces promotes a secure environment by providing for natural surveillance through expanded visibility. Be sure to discuss these ideas with your champions, administration, and design team if security is of particular concern to you.

Electrical

Most people don't think twice when plugging something into an electrical outlet, and it is easy to take for granted continuous power to so many of the devices used to care for patient care, sometimes on a round-the-clock basis. Those outlets, along with light fixtures and the occasional electrical panel, are the only visible evidence of the extensive, hidden system of conduits and junction boxes that route electricity throughout buildings.

Every room in your center will require power provided through electrical outlets. Control rooms will require them for computers and monitors. Simulation labs will have them arrayed around every patient care area. Storage rooms may require them for anything that needs recharging when not in use. Your task here is to work with the designers on what needs power and when and where it is needed. For example, the headwall of a typical patient bed is home to a host of outlets that provide power to everything from ventilators to pumps to the bed itself. The number of receptacles is often augmented to include additional red emergency outlets that, in a clinical setting, would be fed by a generator or an uninterruptable power source. When designing your simulated patient care areas, use standards derived from the healthcare settings you are modeling as a starting point to determine the outlet count. We recommend that you confirm these standards against your anticipated power use in your most equipment-intensive scenarios. If you decide to incorporate "emergency" outlets—albeit, not connected to an auxiliary power source—it will likely for code purposes be necessary to post a sign indicating that those outlets do not, in fact, supply emergency power.

The type and location of an outlet should be governed based on its usage. Given the frequency with which equipment is plugged in and unplugged, it is wise to mount outlets higher up on a wall for accessibility and to save wear and tear on students, staff, and faculty by minimizing the need to bend over or crouch. For a patient bed or anything else that is rarely unplugged, a lower, more conventional mounting height is appropriate. It is also advisable to locate outlets to either side of the bed head rather than directly above it, both due to the ergonomic advantage for caregivers, but also to avoid power cords being accidentally draped over a patient, if even temporarily. Other details like the length of the power cord on a device, the device location, and whether or not it would need to move while plugged in, will also help the design team locate outlets.

When deciding on the type of power outlet, a push toward efficiency or cost savings may tempt you to install "quad" outlets with space to plug in four items at a time. While these may certainly be useful in some instances, they could cause frustration that first time you plug in something that has a large plug head, finding that it blocks off the other three outlets. Instead, use two duplex outlets and separate them with just enough distance to offset any potential plug head interferences.

You will also need to understand specific issues when it comes to the other half of electrical systems: lighting. While sufficient light levels to conduct learning activities are essential in any educational environment, clinical education often demands specialized and often higher output lighting design solutions. A good example of this difference arises when recreating various inpatient rooms, where you may want to simulate as many as three levels of lighting: low-power night-lights mounted low on the walls, general room lights, and a higher-intensity exam light directly over the patient bed. Exam lights of adequate brightness are essential for any simulations requiring students to engage in finer detail work like wound care or IV insertion. Lighting considerations, like so much of the design of your center, force you to scrutinize care settings—so often treated as no more than a backdrop—as a way of understanding how you will teach your students.

If you include a simulated OR environment, then make decisions about the level of general illumination of the surgical field as well as the degree to which you may use boom-mounted surgical lamps. For control rooms using one-way viewing glass, you may want to consider dimmable lighting that offers lower light levels in the monitoring space relative to the simulation space while still allowing technicians and faculty to see what they are doing. You should also consider any above-counter wall cabinets and the need for undermounted cabinet task lights to illuminate the counter surface. Lighting issues range from the highly detailed to the seemingly mundane, but you should certainly give some thought to lighting needs in all spaces.

Plumbing

The "P" of MEP—plumbing—will also require you to deliberate on a number of important decisions, especially due to the specialized nature of plumbing systems in healthcare environments. When thinking about plumbing, most will immediately zero in on those fixtures that deliver domestic water service at sinks, showers, and toilets. Most skills labs will either have several hand-washing sinks distributed throughout the room or a dedicated hand-washing area where small lab groups can work with an instructor on proper washing technique. However, you approach it, hand-washing sinks should be present in any skills or simulation area to help condition students toward a habit of hand washing before and after interacting with any patient. If you are simulating an operating room, a surgical scrub sink should be located immediately outside the OR in a prep area or at least in a dedicated alcove in the corridor. Finally, a large-basin utility sink with a sprayer hose attachment should be installed in the space where you intend to provide maintenance and repair of equipment. Coupled with adjacent counter space for drying, this is an invaluable amenity for cleaning reusable equipment, including mannequins.

Simulated inpatient rooms of all kinds will often include an adjoining private restroom, critical for training on patient transfer modalities, infection control, and general patient care skills. Because of their universal usefulness, sinks in these bathrooms should nearly always be operable while showers and baths can have unplumbed, mock fixtures for reasons of safety and general cleanliness.

Water closets have occasionally fallen into an inconvenient and often unfortunate middle ground, especially in challenging renovations where new plumbing piping is expensive and disruptive to install. While a toilet may not be *intended* for use, it is probably best where possible to connect it to a water supply and sanitary waste lines, just in case someone decides to avail him or herself of the amenity—despite the presence of prohibitive signage and other deterrents. Should you choose to use unplumbed toilets, clearly mark them as nonfunctional.

The other subset of plumbing considerations involves medical gasses, and given their necessity for patient care, you and your team should be very intentional about their design into your center and their eventual use. First and foremost, think about the safety requirements for any real gasses you intend to use, particularly with an inexperienced student population. Pressurized gas cylinders are large and heavy, so unless there is a secure closet in which to store them, they could pose a risk in more heavily occupied rooms. Pure oxygen, in the presence of heat and anything remotely flammable, constitutes a hazard such that building codes require special construction measures to accommodate it. Your safety-related line of inquiry may lead you to move away from including live gasses and instead to rely on dummy outlets for the purpose of simulating connecting and disconnecting equipment. However, if you intend to take advantage of the full features of certain high-performance simulators, ensure that you prompt the design team to incorporate gas supply infrastructure for oxygen, nitrogen, and carbon dioxide—with a reminder for you to identify and share all the requirements for any equipment you will use in the center.

Regardless of whether medical gas outlets will be functioning or simulated, you will need to make decisions about the types and quantities of outlets. At the patient bedside, it is typical to have medical grade air, oxygen, and vacuum/slide with one of each outlet on either side of the bed. While it is possible to locate gas outlets inboard of electrical outlets (within), for practical and safety reasons, the design should nonetheless avoid placing outlet locations on the wall above a patient's head.

There are also some more specialized applications for medical gas including carbon dioxide for cavity insufflation, nitrogen for some surgical tools, and nitrous oxide and gas waste disposal when anesthesia use is to be simulated. In an operating room or other procedure space where these gasses are most commonly found, medical booms provide maximum flexibility in getting gas outlets wherever they need to be around the surgical area. These booms are also highly customizable, enabling even greater flexibility. The use of booms or any of these medical gasses will, of course, depend on the programming of these spaces and the degree of fidelity you want to bring to more specialized environments.

Step 6: Windows, Doors, Floors, and Walls

The preceding two sections of this chapter have dealt with building systems that, although essential, are mostly hidden from view to the casual observer and even the everyday occupant. Occupants of the center will largely form an impression of and remember physical spaces based on the following five things: windows, doors, walls, ceilings, and floors. These components define the size and shape of enclosed space, allow seeing into it, and grant passage to enter and leave it. The finish materials applied to these surfaces provide visual, tactile, and even acoustic impressions, allowing occupants to perceive and comprehend the room at a fundamental level. While this chapter not delve into the aesthetics of finish selection, be aware that the colors and patterns your team selects will have a significant and highly subjective impact on how any one individual feels about being in the space. Because of this elemental role that walls, floors, and doors play, it is

 easy to take them for granted, but they require no less design attention than any other aspect of the center. See Toolkit 27.6 for the corresponding workbook.

Doors

Since doors are the first thing with which anyone would come into contact upon arrival at your center, let's talk doors. They certainly seem uncomplicated enough, but if you think of how much you interact with doors, if only in passing, it becomes easy to see that there are opportunities for maximizing their functional contribution. They also serve as a surface on which to locate signage to aid in room identification and way finding. Nowhere might this purpose be better exemplified than at the main entrance to your center, where the doors and the design of the building in the immediate vicinity give the first impression of your simulation program. Be deliberate in your consideration of the entry and how it will shape what students and visitors experience upon their arrival.

On the other hand, if not specifically designed for their purpose, doors can be the bane of day-to-day operations for a simulation center. While this may seem an overstatement, consider this: a standard door opening is only 35 in. wide. Most standard patient beds are now at least 36 in. wide, requiring an oversized or double-door opening. While this incompatibility may seem an obvious condition to avoid in designing any healthcare environment, simulated or not, an inexperienced or inattentive project team can easily miss these kinds of details that make or break the success of a design. This detail-focused approach applies to a variety of characteristics. Simply adding a window in a door can allow someone to determine whether a room is in use without entering and can also enhance safety by providing a view of anyone who might be coming at you through a door you are about to open. Applied stainless steel kick plates on the lower half of heavily used doors will help them endure repeated collisions with carts and beds moved in and out of storage rooms or patient bedrooms on a daily basis.

Aside from such modifications to conventional doors, healthcare facilities are replete with door types that are largely unique to clinical settings. A sliding or breakout ICU door poses an entirely different type of interaction from a conventional swing door, especially when students are moving a cart or patient bed in or out of the room. An automated OR door can become an integral part of teaching proper sterile technique after scrubbing in to take part in a procedure. Incorporating specialized doors like these can contribute to a thorough and high-fidelity simulation experience and allow students to become comfortable with basic modalities so that they are second nature by the time they fully enter into their chosen professions.

Windows

Nearly everyone appreciates the natural daylight and views to the outside world that windows provide, especially when the majority of waking hours are spent inside the walls a building. While exterior windows are considered a considerable asset, the building exterior is not the only location where glass, also known as glazing, can be incorporated to admit light. Among the details listed on each room data sheet should be a note as to whether a space should feature transparency to other rooms or the outside.

Generally speaking, everyone will make a case to get access to exterior windows—for an office, classroom, lab, reception area, or any room where someone will spend an appreciable portion of her or his day. What is intuitive to most people has been studied and repeatedly proven: access to daylight and views can boost morale, reduce absenteeism, and increase productivity (Figueiro, Rea, Rea, & Stevens, 2002; Heschong, Wright, & Okura, 2001; Leslie, 2003). The reasons for wanting windows, however, may be less concrete and run more deeply, more subtly. Some projects present finite opportunities for windows, and simulation centers contain numerous spaces that perform better when they *do not* have daylight access. A control room that has a direct view into a simulation lab should eschew all excess light, including daylight, to remain relatively darkened compared to the lab. Simulation spaces themselves can benefit from a window, but so often the goal is to build as much into a single lab as possible. Therefore, there is precious little wall space left after incorporating control room windows, patient monitors, headwall utilities, crash cart alcoves, and equipment such as sphygmomanometers. With all the storage capacity requirements, ensure that no wall in a storage room is interrupted by a window that otherwise deprives you of prime real estate for shelving or wall hooks. Save the exterior windows for offices, workshops, debrief and conference rooms, and you minimize any infighting over getting that window, if not altogether eliminate it.

As mentioned before, windows aren't just for looking out at the trees and sky. The strategic use of interior glazing can imbue your center with a greater feeling of openness, modernity, and welcoming while also granting significant functional advantages. In the vein of functionality, simulation center design immediately calls to mind one of the single most important windows: the control room window. If your team elects to have a control room or rooms from which you can directly view into one or more simulation spaces, it is advisable that the viewing windows employ one-way viewing glass. These windows also referred to as mirrored glass, a one-way mirror, or, inexplicably at times, a two-way mirror. Most people are familiar with the advantages they provide in concealing activity. You will find a more detailed discussion in the workbook should you want to learn more about the pros and cons of viewing windows. Additionally, these window units can also be built to have acoustic isolation properties to prevent sound transmission. The best performance of the one-way window is heavily dependent on the relative light levels of the control and simulation rooms, respectively. Specifically, light levels should be considerably dimmer on the control monitoring side than on the simulation activity side, and wall and work surface finishes should be dark in color to prevent highlights and silhouetting. Given the elevated level of illumination in most simulated environments, this is generally not a problem. You may, however, encounter difficulties when conducting OR simulations where the concentration of light over the procedure area is greatest and the remainder of the chamber may be minimally lit or even fully dimmed. In this case, the complete darkening of a control room may be necessary. If you are striving for an elevated level of immersion for the students participating in the simulation, it is important that they not be distracted by the control room activities of faculty and staff. A window like this helps to prevent this from occurring.

Important roles for interior glazing can certainly be found elsewhere. As mentioned before, a window in a door—a door lite—or built into the door frame adjacent to a door—a side lite—allows someone to easily determine whether a room is currently in use without opening the door and disturbing those inside. Windows that enclose a reception area open up lines of sight for the reception staff while providing a measure of security. If you would like to allow daylight to pass through a room at the perimeter of your building into a corridor or adjacent space that would otherwise not have daylight access, part or all of the wall separating those two spaces could be glass—a borrowed light. Finally, you may want to create transparent teaching spaces that feature students' learning through the glass. Usually, privacy and confidentiality are paramount, so this application is not the norm. Having said this, windows into your labs and classrooms can showcase and promote your important work to anyone who visits your center.

Walls

Despite the importance of doors and windows, they would serve little function at all were it not for the walls that are home to them all. Walls enclose and define space, provide visual and acoustic privacy, can be a place to hang equipment, and generally establish the character of the room. Interior partitions are those walls that separate one room from another. Movable interior partitions are generally folding or accordion-style panelized walls that can be deployed to divide a room or stowed in a wall-based cavity or even above the ceiling. When correctly designed and regularly used, they can add significant flexibility to a space. They are briefly addressed later in Section 8 of this chapter, under the "Flexibility" heading.

In simulation centers, walls and partitions are subjected to an elevated level of use and abuse and should be designed accordingly. As has been evident in this chapter so far, the walls in your simulation spaces could be covered with power and gas outlets, bed locators, microphones and cameras, patient monitors, otoscopes, and blood pressure cuffs. As crowded as the walls will be, it is important to review how they are laid out with your faculty colleagues and discuss with them the functional and ergonomic implications as well as you can anticipate them based on the design drawings. Furthermore, coordinate the locations of all these items with the architects so that they can be sure to design concealed wood or metal blocking in the wall construction, thus providing adequate purchase for heavier items to be screwed in.

Healthcare settings are notorious for subjecting walls to enough daily stress to rival the heavy commercial and industrial world. With carts, beds and gurneys, IV poles, and all manner of mobile equipment being indiscriminately shoved in and out of place on a regular basis, you may find yourself looking through a hole in the wall into the next room over if you don't plan proper wall protection. Some of this protection is imperceptible, like spacing wall studs more closely to create sturdier construction and using high-impact gypsum wall board (aka GWB or drywall). Other wall protection is more obvious like plastic or metal corner guards, bumper rails, chair rails, and sheet wall protection. While these measures may not needed everywhere in your facility, include wall protection wherever you will be regularly moving equipment. To that end, your simulation spaces and storage rooms should incorporate sheet wall protection on the lower 4 or 5 ft of every wall surface. Along the entire length of major corridors, you may install continuous bumper rails roughly 3 feet above the floor. Aside from protecting your walls, all of these products are standard in healthcare environments

and therefore augment the clinical realism of your simulation center.

In both medical and educational facilities, acoustic privacy and noise distraction mitigation is an important and often overlooked aspect of design. Interior partitions are the primary building components that accomplish this separation, and while conventional wall construction cannot fully eliminate all unwanted sound transmission, proper design and construction techniques will reduce it to manageable levels. With few exceptions, interior partitions should always be built fully to the underside of the building structure, whether it is the underside of the roof or the floor slab above. This prevents sound from transmitting up through the ceiling over the top of a partial height wall and into the next room. Adding sound attenuation insulation inside a partition or applying additional layers of drywall to the wall are other reasonable ways to increase acoustic absorption. Advise the design team about specific locations that might be more acoustically sensitive, and they can propose additional methods for enhancing acoustic separation of spaces.

Floors

While it may be possible to carefully avoid colliding a cart into a wall, there's no getting around the punishment that floors take—and dole out—because we literally walk all over them. The selection of flooring materials is something you must consider in a bidirectional manner. For example, a terrazzo floor may be handsome and the most durable—and most expensive flooring option you might consider, but its unyielding nature also accelerates the fatigue of those who continually walk those floors on a daily basis. With that in mind, there are less expensive options that can offer some of the same durability characteristics as terrazzo while also exhibiting greater resiliency and cushion. Your flooring selection will vary based on which room you are considering. Offices and debriefing rooms will likely feature carpet. Storage rooms may be simple vinyl composition tile or even sealed concrete. Your architect will likely put numerous options in front of you to consider for each space. Ask plenty of questions about the options, price, physical characteristics, and expected longevity for each product, and weigh the answers against what you can reasonably project about the traffic and usage patterns each room will experience.

As you select materials, pay attention to where the transitions between different flooring types will occur in your center. These changes of material are sometimes accompanied by a small bump when two materials of differing thicknesses meet or the transition is covered using a transition strip. This has the potential to become an aggravating detail every time you or one of your colleagues rolls a cart or bed over it, so look for these transitions along those routes used for transporting your wheeled equipment. Floor color changes using the same material, on the other hand, can be useful for indicating different zones in a simulated patient bedroom, a sterile procedure area around an OR table, designated pathways through your center, or different simulated clinical departments. Though flooring serves an uncomplicated purpose, don't sell it short when it comes to innovative ways that it can improve the function of your space.

Ceilings

Given how little day-to-day interaction we have with them, ceilings are largely underappreciated for everything they do to improve every environmental quality of a space. They provide a place for lighting and air distribution fixtures. Projectors, projection screens, cameras, microphones, and speakers are all often installed in ceilings. Smoke detectors and sprinkler heads can be located there. Ceilings are most likely to provide the majority of acoustically absorptive surfaces through the use of acoustic panel ceilings. They accommodate all of these disparate functions while organizing them in a deliberate, systematic, and aesthetically calm way. Where some of this environmental organization and control is less needed—storage spaces, utility closets, and AV and IT server rooms—ceilings are sometimes eschewed altogether, exposing the building structure, ductwork, and piping that you may prefer not to see in the more regularly populated areas of your center.

In healthcare settings, there are specialized ceilings that are primarily incorporated for their infection control or pressure stabilization properties. Given that these are not concerns in an educational environment, the use of these substantially more expensive products in a simulation-based learning environment is not recommended. The design of the ceiling will place lower demands for your attention, except where it concerns the locations of lights, cameras, and the other devices already addressed in previous sections of this chapter.

Step 7: Life Safety, Accessibility, and Security

If you ever ask an architect what the primary responsibility of the profession is, the knowledgeable and responsible designer will tell you that it is the health, safety, and welfare of the building occupants. As with many of the other topics covered in this chapter, it isn't necessary for you and your team of simulation champions to have intimate knowledge of the technical requirements of building and life safety codes. You should be aware that they exist and will have an inevitable influence on your facility's design. Refer to Toolkit 27-7 for planning windows, doors, floors, walls, and furniture.

If architects, engineers, and those in the medical profession have anything in common, it is that they uphold a code to preserve life. They simply do it in different ways. Architects and engineers follow building codes whose primary purpose is to help preserve life and secondary purpose is to preserve property. Ironically, building codes accomplish this by *first* protecting the building in order that building occupants might safely leave a building in the event of an emergency.

Building Egress

Multiple sections of most building codes are dedicated to the technical requirements of designing a way out of a building. Having multiple doors out of a large room, planning redundant hallways that give options when exiting, eliminating dead end corridors, and having clearly visible exit signage are just a few of the many ways that building codes help promote safe options in the face of a potential disaster. These parts of the code will affect the design of corridors, stairways, and doors, so be prepared to have some of the floor plan ideas that your team discusses modified—if not outright thwarted—by the egress criteria of the applicable building code.

One classic example is the issue of fire-rated wall construction, which is exactly what it sounds like—walls or partitions that are designated with a time rating to indicate their resistance to burning and failing in the event of a fire. All stairways, elevators, and other shafts that move vertically through a building require fire-rated construction. Additionally, if your facility is not equipped with a sprinkler system throughout the building (see section later on "Fire Suppression"), all corridors used for exiting a floor must also be rated. Once an interior wall or partition has been designated with a rating, its cost, and the cost to penetrate it with an air duct, a door, a window, or anything else goes up. So, if you have hopes of looking through an expansive window from the corridor into a lab that you really want to see into, and your building doesn't have sprinklers, that window will need to be rated and consequently entail a cost four or five times the amount it would cost if it was not rated. Life safety issues like this will prompt questions in your design discussions about the value of such a window as well as questions about the merits of adding full building fire suppression to reduce rated construction costs and enable more design freedom.

Accessibility

Designing a building that is universally accessible by all who visit your facility is not only legally required of your architect, it is simply good and responsible design. It is imperative that you source out accessibility guidelines for your institution, as well as context-relevant legislation and regulatory requirements. Regardless of background or disability, any person should be able to reasonably navigate the public areas of your simulation center and feel welcome doing so. When thinking of accessibility in this sense, your most immediate consideration may be for disabilities of persons using wheelchairs. While wheelchair access is a major determinant of accessibility requirements, you should keep in mind that these requirements are also shaped by other mobility impairments involving the use of assistive devices like canes, crutches, or braces. Being professionals in the area of patient care, you will naturally be familiar with all of these, even if you may have never considered them as influencing the design of the built environment. The current concept of accessible or universal design goes several steps further, accommodating those with vision and hearing impairments, learning or literacy difficulties, and diverse social, economic, and cultural backgrounds.

When this concept is applied to physical structures, it manifests as ramps and railings to negotiate floor elevations changes; countertops, light switches, and drinking fountains at appropriate heights to allow use by all; room signs with Braille letters and pictographs; fire alarms with both visible and audible components; and perhaps lactation rooms, prayer rooms, and gender-neutral restrooms, depending on the demographics of the community being served. Everyone on your extended team of champions—educators, technicians, administrators, and designers—should examine each decision through the lens of universal accessibility and allow that ideal to shape your design as much as any other influence so that everyone feels there is a place for them at your institution.

Fire Suppression

Commonly referred to as sprinkler systems, fully automated fire suppression has become prevalent in new construction around the world and has contributed to dramatic declines in deaths and casualties related to building fires. Despite this beneficial impact, many college and university campus buildings were still being designed and built without such systems as recently as the 1970s. Globally, many life safety codes still do not require them for certain types of buildings, including higher education facilities. Should your project be protected by a fire suppression system, you should know a few key points ahead of time.

Not all fire suppression systems are the same, and some aren't even water based. In environments where there is an appreciable amount of expensive electrical equipment, certain dry chemical agents are often used in place of water. These agents will both cool and smother a fire while leaving sensitive and costly gear largely

unharmed. Due to their cost, the decision to include such a system is usually limited to those areas where it can provide the largest potential benefit—for example, the audiovisual server room where all of your scenario recordings will be stored. There are some sprinkler systems whose pipes are constantly filled with water, ready to extinguish at a moment's notice. There are other systems whose pipes remain dry and only fill with water once the system is activated. In any case, should your design team not bring up the topic, be sure to ask whether or not there should be any special considerations given to the design of the fire suppression system in your facility.

Believe it or not, there have been simulation champions at some institutions that have inquired about the feasibility of activating a live sprinkler system during a simulation scenario. While there will certainly be occasions in nurses' and doctors' careers when they are providing care to a patient under emergency conditions, there are simply some situations that are too impractical, difficult, messy, or unsafe to simulate. If you want to simulate anything having to do with life safety systems, find a way that will communicate this to the simulation participants in a way that is unambiguously part of the scenario protocol. Your faculty, staff, and students should never be in a situation where they are uncertain about a potentially life-threatening situation.

Fire Alarm Systems

The other major life safety system present in every built structure is the fire alarm. Because building and life safety codes require smoke and fire detection that work in concert with audible and visual alarms, you will see familiar components like pull stations, annunciator horns, and flashing strobes regularly located throughout your facility. The rules for locating these devices are fairly strict, but most designers are skilled at coordinating their inclusion so as not to be an eyesore or interfere with other building components.

As with fire suppression systems, you will not be able to interact with your building's fire alarm system as part of a simulation nor will you be able to create a second simulated fire alarm for educational purposes. Despite this, you can still conceive ways to conduct training in a simulated fire emergency through the use of voice announcements over a public address system internal to your center. As always, these announcements should be unambiguous about the alarm being part of the simulation.

The other half of building security is an actual security system—a network of devices dedicated to controlling access, detecting entry, and recording video in your facility. Sometimes, security may be as simple as a door lock. Your institution might also have a standard for card swipes or proximity readers to gain entry to those spaces in most critical need of close monitoring. What you should think about for the building and each room is how and which staff, students, and visitors you want to come and go from each space. Main entries to your facility, whether they are doors into your simulation suite or into a building you share with others, are important control points that should be monitored, either by reception staff or cameras for off-hours surveillance. Once inside, each room type—office, classroom, laboratory—may have different security characteristics, and the design team will be relying on you and the security personnel from your institution to help define those. Because of their low occupancy function and need to protect property, storage rooms are often locked from the outside such that the door will always be secure when it closes behind anyone retrieving anything there. You may have a computer lab for which you want to monitor usage by staff and students. In this case, a networked card reader at the door can track ID badges that are used to enter the room. This kind of access control, along with strategically placed security cameras, will not always deter an individual who is intent perpetrating harm, but it will keep life and property safe in the vast majority of cases.

Step 8: Functional Planning

Up until this point, this chapter has been sharing with you some of the easy-to-define characteristics that come in the form of equipment, fixtures on the walls, and even the walls themselves—hard, tangible aspects of the design process. As suggested before, these are all possible ingredients of a simulation center. The specific configuration in which they will be combined is akin to a recipe. This recipe comes in the form of design documents. Floor plans, wall sections, interior and exterior elevations, details, and specifications are all terms used to describe documents that convey how the various components of a building fit together. The majority of your interaction with the design professionals who become part of your team will revolve around the design decisions that will ultimately inform these documents. The decisions are myriad and varied and sometimes hard to define using all the pieces and parts this chapter has introduced thus far. What follows are a few examples of some of the design characteristics that might fall outside more easily definable categories and have an impact on how your center will look, feel, and operate. Though this chapter is introducing these concepts late in the narrative, your discussions about these topics should

commence at the very beginning of your project and continue through to the end, becoming progressively more detailed and refined along the way. Refer to Workbook 27.8 for the online Step 8 Companion Workbook.

Flow

The topic of "flow" may find its way into your team's design conversations. Unless you are discussing plumbing or electricity, it likely refers to how an individual might enter, traverse, use, and depart your facility. This topic becomes an especially important point of deliberation for simulation centers because there is a pedagogically reinforced sequence of learner activities. These student activities often then relate to the use of prescribed space types. Additionally, the placement of rooms relative to one another and the design of the circulation spaces that connect those rooms must support the workflows of faculty and staff. Depending on their purpose for being at your facility, consider how various individuals might use the center.

Let's start at the entry to your facility. It may be that anyone arriving at the simulation center will use the same entrance and that is perfectly acceptable and even a predominant model. If the program of spaces for your simulation center includes multiple and diverse components—a variety of simulation labs; standardized patient interaction, faculty office and support areas, etc.—it may be wise and even necessary to consider multiple entrances, if only due to the sheer size of your center. Besides size, another reason to consider multiple entrances is directly related to the quality of learning, itself. So much of the success of simulation-based learning is dependent on the degree of realism that is perceived by the learners. A perception of realism equates to a perception of risk, and a lived experience that supports improved retention. With that in mind, much of the students' learning can be heightened by enhancing the authenticity of their experience from the time to enter the facility right up until they debrief after their simulation. If their arrival takes them by the sim lab control rooms or has them encountering the standardized patient actors with whom they will be interacting later in their day, it compromises the benefits of suspending disbelief in simulation-based learning. A dedicated separate entrance for learners and sequence of governed access through the center is part of shaping their learning beyond the boundaries of the lab and classroom. Are there practical limits to this approach? Certainly, but adopting a general premise of sustained credibility can be a strong guiding principle in the planning of your center. In the spirit of a comprehensively conceived curriculum, it seems natural to strengthen the contribution that the built environment brings to learning outcomes wherever possible.

There is an even more pragmatic side to flow. Simply put, you will need to manage the throughput of your center. Logically choreographing the movement from space to space helps regulate and optimize utilization. For example, consider this standard list of sequenced tasks that a student might need to complete: check in, change clothes, stow belongings, preliminary briefing/didactic session, simulation activity, debrief, change clothes, check out. Now, consider that same set of tasks with several groups of 8, 12, or 20 students starting at staggered times. The building plan should organize the rooms associated with each of those tasks in a way that reflects the actual physical movement associated with the enactment of the curriculum. The alternative is a sense of chaos or a reduction in your capacity to offer your students a quality learning experience.

Finally, and just as importantly, the strategic planning of adjacency—which rooms are placed next to which—will figure largely into how efficiently and productively faculty and staff are able to function in their place of work. Poor understanding of critical adjacencies can lead to difficulties in foot traffic safety, property security, and employee fatigue. These conditions arise when paths of travel that should not intersect are caused to cross one another. Just imagine the implications of positioning storage or supply rooms that serve simulation labs on the opposite side of a heavily used student corridor. Conveying equipment or supplies between those two rooms could lead to ineffective operations, damage, theft, or even injury. Much as for those who work in a hospital setting, simulation center staff are on their feet for much of the day. Through thoughtful design, regularly traversed routes can be shortened to minimize the impact of fatigue and wear on the people who are the lifeblood of your operation. The workflow and daily routines of your center's employees should inform the shape of your facility at least as much as the circulation patterns of the students.

Flexibility

There are few concepts being emphasized in building design for higher education more than flexibility. Due to increasing pressures being exerted on and by educational institutions to maximize use of existing spaces and to accomplish as much of the curriculum as possible with those spaces, educators and designers are coming up with increasingly creative ways to build as much function into each room as is conceivable. Depending on the design strategies employed, an individual space can serve a few different roles, provide several furniture and equipment layouts, or accommodate a variety of class sizes. The opportunities for flexibility will vary from project to project, and while your team should imagine at an early stage, which approaches best align with your needs and goals, you should also urge your architectural team members to propose ideas for flexible room usage.

Overlaying multiple purposes for a single space may be obvious. Debriefing rooms can also serve as conference, seminar, or group workrooms. Some combination uses may be less apparent. For example, one might envision a setup that would allow a simulation control room to double as a simulated nurse station so that it could be used to teach charting and floor management skills when it's not being used to run a simulation. Exploring options for flexibility within a simulation lab is fairly commonplace and is generally achieved by using one space to provide educational settings that replicate multiple types of clinical environments. In many cases, this can be simply achieved by reconfiguring the equipment in the room. Keep in mind that this is not simply a case of rearranging the furniture, and the room must be designed to accommodate such changes in usage. Even simply moving a patient bed from one wall to a different one, you will need to be sure that you have the electrical power outlets and medical gas connections, whether real or simulated, that you will need to conduct your simulation.

Designing for multiple patient positions in a flexible simulation lab is advisable, and it doesn't need to be restricted to wall-based locations. With their rising use in hospital environments other than operating rooms, small-scale medical gas booms are a flexible and realistic way of providing services in the center of a room. Another method of accomplishing flexibility in your teaching spaces is with the use of floor box–based service access. A floor box is simply a method of recessing power outlets and other services into the floor, rather than a wall. If you're building a brand new building, floor boxes are easy to design and install. If your project is a renovation, introducing floor boxes becomes more of a challenge, requiring invasive modification of existing floor slab structure—not to mention potentially invoking the ire of any building occupants on the floor below who might be disrupted by construction work in the ceiling above them.

For this reason, raised access floor systems have risen in popularity over the past several years to simplify the retrofit of new floor-based utilities and to provide more space flexibility, even in entirely new buildings. A manufactured raised access floor is a modular, grid-based system that is installed directly on top of a building's floor structure, effectively raising the finished floor surface and creating an underfloor cavity through which everything from electrical power to data connectivity to conditioned air can be delivered to building occupants. Finish materials like carpet or interlocking tile can then be installed over the access floor. Because these are modular systems, the locations of power outlets, data jacks, or any other utility devices can be reconfigured to better suit the changing use of a room. Especially relevant in a simulated medical environment, any fluids spilled on a raised floor will quickly find their way through the copious seams in the flooring, allowing the spill to collect down in the cavity and making for challenging cleanup.

Additional flexibility can be accomplished by subdividing a room using one or more mobile partitions. For example, a 600-square-feet simulated operating room can be bisected by a movable partition in order to create two 300-square-feet intensive care unit rooms. Having this modification as an option to you can help you cut down on the number of spaces you may need to fulfill your curricular needs or, conversely, allow you to get the most use out of the space you have been allotted. It can also bolster your educational offerings by giving you more tools to expose your students to as many varied experiences as possible. Just keep in mind that while a mobile partition introduces new capabilities to a room, it also limits your ability to permanently mount any equipment to it or to have live power and gas outlets.

Fidelity

You and your fellow champions will be the best judges of best to balance your needs for fidelity and flexibility. As you are making that judgement, you should be aware of the inverse relationship that the flexibility of a space has with its perceived fidelity. Consider this: when a space is designed to flexibly convert from portraying an intensive care unit to an OR to a labor and delivery room, it is likely not able to portray any single one of those with a high degree of clinical realism. Conversely, if you have designed a high-fidelity emergency room trauma bay nearly indistinguishable from its real-life counterpart, its ability to also serve as some other clinical setting is, at best, significantly compromised by inaccuracy, potentially to the detriment and confusion of learners. Exact replications, however, are not essential for many scenarios and your team will need to consider which elements are necessary to create the highest levels of fidelity. Today, there are also many props such as wallpaper, movable screens, or curtains that can transform spaces and enhance fidelity.

Given this relationship, you will work with your team to find the balance of flexibility and fidelity for each space. For most educators, it is easiest to address this from the fidelity side. In other words, you are asking the question, "What characteristics and functions from actual clinical environments will it be important to incorporate in this space?" In some ways, this chapter has been touching on that question from the beginning by addressing this issue as it pertains to gases, medical equipment, finishes, and MEP infrastructure details. As always, the answer to this question will come down to what supports your curriculum and the best learning outcomes for your students.

The rest of this section touches on specific design decision points relevant to a few of the spaces that might be part of your simulation center.

Prebriefing and Debriefing Rooms

The spaces where you review with simulation participants their performance during a scenario should be designed to foster productive discourse between students and instructors. For this reason, many debriefing rooms are nothing more than a conference room for 6 to 12 people with the requisite audiovisual resources for reviewing the simulation capture. However, the conference format is certainly not required. If you want an environment that better promotes dialogue as part of the debriefing process, you can establish a more relaxed atmosphere by using lounge seating with built-in writing surfaces informally gathered around the instructor and audiovisual display. On the other hand, if you are debriefing larger groups, a conference or lounge style space might be undersized. A debriefing room set up like a classroom could also work, provided that your team gives special attention to making sure the room is suitable for conversation-based learning. Additionally, a debriefing room in the style of a classroom makes available an additional didactic teaching space for your facility.

When determining the number of debriefing rooms required for your new center, a good rule of thumb is to match that quantity to the number of simulations that you would typically be running simultaneously. That way, if all the simulations conclude at around the same time, each scenario group has a place to go to continue their learning. On those rare occasions when you are conducting more simulations than usual, it's always good to have a spare classroom or conference room available to stand in as a debriefing room so that you don't have teams waiting too long to review their work. Your debriefing spaces can be grouped together in one area of your simulation center or distributed and more closely coupled with your simulation space. This decision goes back to the question of flow and how you want your students and faculty to move through the center.

For simulation centers with audiovisual capture systems, debriefing rooms are the ideal location to provide an interface for accessing and reviewing simulation footage that is saved on your servers. This will likely require a resident computer—that is, one that permanently stays in the debriefing room—and a flat panel display large enough for the entire room to easily view. There is no question that these technology aids contribute immense value to the learning process, but they are not absolutely essential to the objectives of simulation-based learning. For that matter, neither is the debriefing room. The postsimulation conversation can even happen right in the simulation room. If you desire video playback, any private space that has a computer will also have access to streamed video or cloud storage. Also, the use of portable devices like tablets makes it easy to view video content anywhere. As long as the students can assess their performance with the help of an objective observer, the cycle of learning can continue so they can apply what they've learned to their next educational challenge.

Control Rooms

There is possibly no more contentious design topic in the realm of simulation centers than the best way to design a control room, also known as a monitor room. Depending on the circumstances of any given project, such spaces are sometimes seen as a luxury, and for others, they may be a nonnegotiable necessity. It is not rare that you have two champions, presumably on the same team, digging in their heels on opposing sides of the issue. It may be that, in the absence of audiovisual capture or high-fidelity patient simulators, there isn't as much need for a control or monitor room. When this technology is incorporated, however, the computers controlling it all must have a home somewhere and that is where a space like this starts to make sense.

Without a dedicated room, it is possible to configure a control station right in the simulation space itself. This reduces the formality of simulation events and can put learners in a position where they are tempted to glance over at a faculty member for some guidance during a particularly challenging sequence. There are mobile one-way viewing screens that can help to counteract this potential for distraction. When the control station is planned to be in the room, set aside enough floor space for a desk or small workstation that won't risk encroaching on the area where students will be working.

When simulation control and monitoring is accommodated in a separate room, one of the most hotly contested debates arises: direct view versus remote view. On one hand, some assert that a control room should be immediately adjacent to a simulation lab with the ability to view a scenario through a window. Some users attest that directly viewing a scenario offers the best opportunity to catch as much action and detail as possible, rendering greater benefit when it comes time to debriefing. This vantage point offers viewers quick access to the entire room without camera delays. The opposing stance counters with the argument that, because a simulation center will already have numerous cameras and microphones recording the action, there is no need to take up additional floor space with dedicated control rooms and expensive one-way viewing windows for each simulation lab. Some say that all you need is a single, consolidated control room with great cameras located anywhere in your facility and from which a smaller staff of faculty and technicians can monitor all of your simulation events on large monitors. Sometimes, those in different camps reach a compromise when the conditions of the project limit space for additional rooms. One option features a long linear control room with windows into simulation spaces on either side.

A similar approach that takes the concept a step or two further situates the control room in the middle of a horseshoe configuration or an entire circle of simulation labs, more fully surrounding the control location. The goal of each of these options is to reduce the amount floor space required for monitoring purposes. One of the primary drawbacks of multisided control rooms is that windows opposite from on another can backlight those working from the control room, compromising the effectiveness of one-way viewing windows. The noise in open configurations can also pose a challenge. To mitigate this problem, use sound-attenuating headsets.

For control rooms from which you can directly view the simulation through a window, having an elevated view can provide a line of sight advantage, especially when faculty and other observers are trying to watch the activities of a group of students gathered around a bed. A raised access floor system in a control room allows for this superior viewing angle while also creating a floor cavity that can conceal the innumerable data and audiovisual cables connecting all the control room technology and thereby decrease clutter underneath the control workstations. The disadvantage of differing floor levels between control and the simulation room is that the design will need to incorporate a ramp for access between the two. According to most accessibility guidelines, ramps cannot exceed a 1:12 scope, meaning that even a 6-in. height difference would require you to accommodate a 5-foot-long ramp with railings. See Figure 27.6 for an overall summary and relationships of audiovisual equipment.

Storage

If the issues surrounding control rooms come nearest to the classification of "most contentious," then the final topic in this section, storage, easily instills the most anxiety in those charged with running a simulation center. This is because the determination of how much storage will be needed is an inexact science, to say the least. The best that the following paragraphs will be able to do is offer a few guiding principles that will help you maximize storage with the space you have available and get you to a reasonable understanding of what you will actually need.

Elementary though it may seem, the first task is to assess what you are storing today and decide whether it will all need to move to your new facility. It is common that a not insignificant amount of housecleaning may need to occur before an exact needs assessment can begin. Make sure you also account for those items that have overflowed from your current storage and are currently improperly stored in inappropriate locations, like a corridor, office, classroom, or lab. Once you have made an initial assessment of your stored materials, make a loose determination of how efficient current storage is and whether you can store it in a smaller or larger footprint than you are currently using. Comparing to your current condition and including projected purchases will give you and the entire project team a rough idea of how much space you will require to store needed materials and equipment.

The next decision involves determining what you will store and where. You will undoubtedly find a need for a dedicated storage room, and you will also want to consider distributed storage within other rooms in your center. Centralized storage can be for larger or less frequently used items and if need be, may be less conveniently located due to its size and less regular usage. Consider the centralized storage area the least often accessed space. Some, however, prefer to have centralized storage be front and center as a hub space with easy access. Centralized storage areas often do double duty as with a technician's workspace, therefore, might include

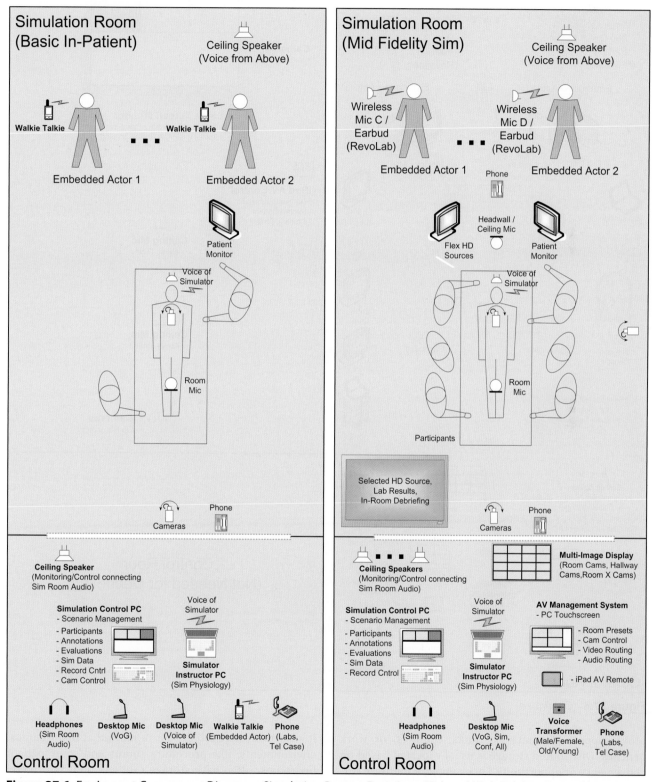

Figure 27.6 Equipment Component Diagrams: Simulation Rooms: Basic Low, Mid, and High Fidelity; Control Room; and Debriefing Room. (Image credit, Lucas Huang, with permission.)

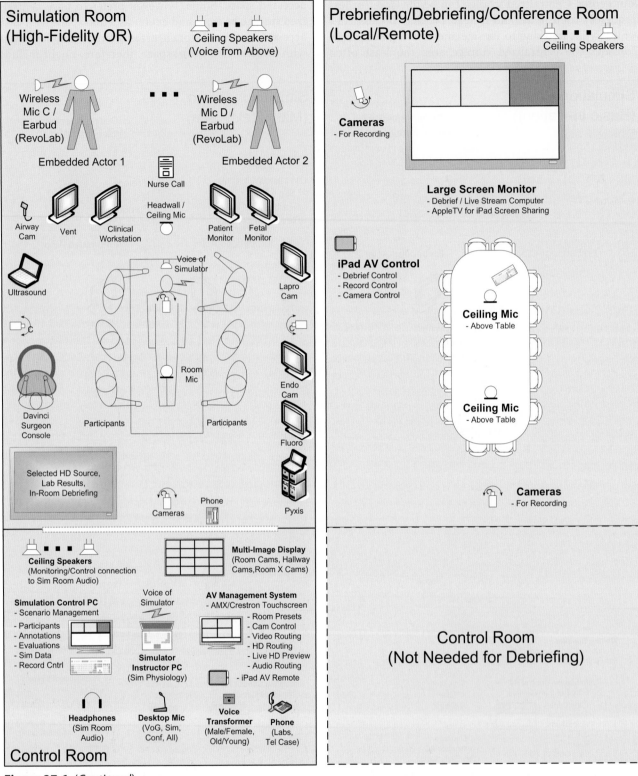

Figure 27.6 (*Continued*)

other support elements like sinks, counters, or work benches. Distributed storage is usually located based on convenience or opportunity. For example, if there are student supplies regularly in use during sessions in the skills lab, a small bedside cabinet is preferable to keep those

items readily accessible. Bear in mind that many clinical environments, like procedure rooms and some patient bedrooms, often have storage cabinets built into them. Including similar storage in your simulation labs is not only practical but it will also make them more realistic.

When a project team is reluctant to dedicate square footage to storage at the expense of additional learning space, designing built-in, lockable cabinets along corridors adds capacity without sacrificing significant square footage. To find often-overlooked storage areas, stop and look above, below, and around you.

The design of the storage system itself is your opportunity to maximize capacity through compactness and efficiency. Built-in casework (or millwork) is a common and effective way to stock and organize supplies in cabinets, drawers, and on countertops, particularly when it will be in more publicly visible areas. In your storage rooms, allocate enough open floor space for the storage of carts, stretchers, IV poles, patient beds, or any other equipment that won't fit on a shelf or in a drawer. Remember to plan for the electrical requirements of all the equipment housed in your storage areas. Don't pass up the chance to use the full height of your storage room if some of these items, like beds and carts, allow for wall cabinets or shelving to be installed above them. Locate these more open floor areas close to the entrance of the room and reserve the more remote portions of your closets for full-height shelving systems. Perhaps the most efficient form of shelving is a high-density system that allows you change where the aisle between shelving units occurs by sliding or rolling individual units from side to side. Instead of an aisle between every pair of shelves, high-density systems stack mobile shelving units against one another, permitting only one aisle to be opened at a time at the location where you need to access the shelves.

Step 9: Moving Out, Construction, and Moving Back In

Whether you are renovating your existing space, expanding on it, or moving to a wholly new facility, there will be a point when you will need to coordinate the arrival of newly purchased equipment and supplies into your new facility and ready them for that first day of operation. If you are relocating to a new space from your current home, you will also likely need to take inventory of and pack up those items already part of your program that will be transferred to your new location. On the other hand, if the facility you are currently using is going to be renovated in place, not only do you have develop and implement an approach to relocation, you will probably have to do it *twice*, assuming that you will be maintaining some semblance of your daily educational operations in an alternate location—known as "swing" space—

before moving back after a lengthy construction period. Refer to Toolkit 27-9 online Step 9 Companion Workbook for information on moving out, construction, and moving back in.

In some ways, this part of the process can be the most daunting because, aside from the actual physical transport of your belongings, you and your fellow faculty and staff will be primarily and possibly solely responsible for strategizing, organizing, and executing this effort. If you outsource this duty, there is a strong chance that it will not be conducted with the same degree of care, thoughtfulness, and specificity with which you and your team would be likely to do it. So, identify those on your team whose natural organizational skills would be best applied to the task. The workbook provides a great starting point with detailed information and immediately usable worksheets to help track and pack your supplies and equipment with maximum organization and efficiency during a hectic relocation process. If you and your champions are able to develop your own strategy or adapt one from an example in the workbook, don't hesitate to do so. What is most important is that, whatever system you use, it makes sense to you and does the most to alleviate some of the stress associated with moving.

Finally, as anyone who has ever moved before knows, a relocation is an opportunity for cleaning house. Be deliberate and honest about what in your current facility will be worthwhile to move. Ask when was the last time something was used and whether it is likely to be regularly used going forward. Take advantage of resale, surplus, and donation opportunities. Keep in mind that anything you bring over needs to be stored somewhere, and why take up space in your new center with something that you'll never use?

Construction

Once the design is complete and your project enters into the construction phase, the site of your simulation center, whether it's a new building or a renovation of an existing one, will be taken over by the construction team. You will no longer own that space or have free access to it. Depending on how your institution decides to execute your project, some of the contractors who are responsible for the physical construction of the project may have already been onboard with the team even during the design phase. In other cases, the builders may not be selected until after design is fully completed. In either situation, your team's responsibilities relative to helping guide the project's design are concluded at this point in the project but that doesn't mean you shouldn't maintain your involvement in the process through periodic visits to the construction site. Construction sites can often seem intimidating to those who have not visited many in their lifetime, but you should let any sense of trepidation stand between you and your understanding of how work is progressing. You may even be called upon to interact with contractors to provide them with additional guidance as they build your new simulation home.

Any time you wish to visit the site first keep in mind that the contractor is responsible for just about everything that transpires onsite during the construction period, and good contractors take this responsibility seriously. Through your institution's project manager or the architect, contact the construction team ahead of time and coordinate your schedules for the visit. In other words, a surprise visit is almost never a good idea, if only from a safety standpoint. When it comes to safety apparel, you will likely need to wear a hardhat, protective eyewear, appropriate footwear, and possibly hearing protection on a noisy day.

While there may not be much to look at if you visit early in construction, it pays to visit nonetheless. Take photos—lots of them—all along the way. Document the progress of construction so you can share it with others as well as continue the creation of a record that memorializes your progress from idea to reality. When the picture looks like this beautiful space, it is exceedingly rewarding (see Fig. 27.7). Also, ask questions—lots of them. At first, these queries may just be about where certain rooms will be built or some of the early utility work that needs to be performed before walls start appearing. As time goes on, your questions can become more detailed about the spaces you will use every day. Asking questions does two things: firstly, it keeps you and the contractors mutually informed; secondly, it serves to expose potential differences in understanding or interpretation about the design intent. Design and construction of something as sophisticated, as a simulation center is a complicated process, and the potential for legitimate confusion about the design is high, especially if the construction team members are not brought in until after design is completed. The discussions spurred by your good questions can help avoid missteps during construction that may compromise your team's vision. Do not underestimate your ability to contribute to the process.

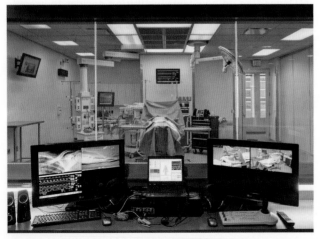

Figure 27.7 Control Room View of a Simulation Lab. (Photo credit, © Brad Feinknopf Photography, 2012.)

Step 10: Open for Business and the Grand Opening

The process has been long, the wait for the final result, seemingly even longer. Once you have finally arrived at the completion of the construction of your new simulation center, once you have moved in, once you have trained your staff, but may be before those first students walk through the door, you should give you and your entire team permission to recognize the occasion. Depending on the course your project has charted, this may be a grand, formal celebration to which you invite all who you feel may want to celebrate with you or to whom you want to show off what you have accomplished. If you go this route, be as inclusive as possible. When your team of champions slows down to think of all the individuals who have touched your project in some way, you will undoubtedly find that the list is long. The occasion may, on the other hand, call for a deliberately more modest event that simply allows those whose contributions have led the effort to step back, take a breath, and share with colleagues an acknowledgment of the team's success before immersing themselves in the task of educating the learners who will

come to the center. However it takes shape, do something! Pull out Toolkit 27-10 for the Step 10 online Companion Workbook to start planning how to open your new learning space and a grand opening.

Even before construction has finished—or may be even before it has started—promote the event both internally to your institution and externally to your city or region. You will certainly want your colleagues from other parts of the campus to be aware that your team has just brought a new learning resource to the school. Additionally, a simulation center is often seen as newsworthy in the local community and that kind of exposure can provide an outstanding portrayal of your academic programs and the facilities you have to support them. Publicity like that can be pivotal in attracting students, staff, and faculty to your institution for all the right reasons.

Given that many architectural design firms now use sophisticated 3D Building Information Modeling software, it is relatively commonplace to create attractive 3D sketch renderings at a relatively reasonable cost. Photo-realistic images require significantly more effort and cost much more than their sketchy counterparts, but an ultra-real depiction may be just what you need to attract not only students or faculty but also new donors to your program. These images can be used over and over again for mass emails, print advertising, websites, and other promotional purposes, including getting people to your grand opening.

So, what happens at these events? Aside from the camaraderie and vegetable trays, it is a time to recognize the major contributors—of time, effort, money, and goods. Pick a few key players to make short speeches. Have the entire gathering gratefully acknowledge the donors, institutional leadership, designers, contractors, and, of course, you and your team of champions! The occasion may call for a dedication or naming ceremony for that one donor who really made the project possible. More than anything else, give tours of your new center that show off the facility *and* what you do there. Simulation-based learning is a pedagogy to which very few have been exposed, and while the physical environments may themselves be impressive, witnessing simulation activities firsthand will make a lasting impact on your guests and remind them why your project is so important to nursing and medical education.

Summary

While a broad swath of content has been addressed in this chapter and the accompanying online companion workbooks, it is intended to focus your attention on specific topics or attributes of design. The goal is to strengthen your understanding and resultant contributions to the design effort so that the project outcome most closely aligns with what you require to effectively teach your students. Work as a team with your fellow champions, your institution's administration, the architects and engineers, and the contractors on the day-to-day progress of the project. As a team, explore innovative and atypical directions that the design could take and don't be afraid to discuss ideas that may, at the outset, seem impractical or unrealistic. Indeed,

refer to both this chapter and the workbooks regularly as you make your way through your own design journey, and if you ever feel confused or unsure, ask yourself, "How will this better help my students learn or my simulation team function?" In fact, that question should be asked by your entire simulation project team when the decision-making becomes challenging. In the end, how well your students learn will be the single most important criterion by which you will evaluate the project's success. We wish your simulation champion teams every success in the process of dreaming, building, and innovating within your new simulation learning spaces.

Toolkit Resources

Step One: Organizational Needs Assessment and Resources
Step Two: The Program
Step Three: Asset Planning: Equipment and Furnishings
Step Four: Information Communication Technology
Step Five: Mechanical, Electrical, and Plumbing
Step Six: Windows, Doors, Floors and Walls
Step Seven: Life Safety, Accessibility, and Security
Step Eight: Functional Planning
Step Nine: Moving Out, Construction, and Moving In
Step Ten: Open for Business and Grand Opening
Toolkit 27-11: Companion Image Catalogue of Simulation Centres and General Nursing Skills Labs

28 Simulation Champions: Visionaries of the Future

Colette Foisy-Doll, Kim Leighton

Key Terms

Health EdTech, Virtual Reality (VR), Augmented Reality (AR), Mixed Reality (MR), Disruptive Innovation Theory, e-Patients, Health Hackers, Time-Based Program, Competency-Based Program, Smart Glasses, Head-Mounted Displays (HMD), Virtual Conferences, Touch-Sensitive Interactive Glass Display Systems, Flexible Glass, Photovoltaic Glass, Just Culture

Guiding Questions

1 What changes have characterized the past 35 years in nursing education?

2 If you had a crystal ball that could tell the future, what would it foretell about simulation in the next 10, 15, or 20 years? What is on the horizon for healthcare education? What will the simulation lab and related technologies look like then?

3 How will the road we chart as simulationists and healthcare educators living and working in a globalized world shape the social forces that will inform system change, educational and healthcare policy, regulatory standards and guidelines, safer patient care, quality improvement, and culture?

4 As technology continues to advance at a gallop, how will tomorrow's simulation teaching practices, simulation delivery modalities, and simulation typologies change? How can the digital immigrant keep up with the pace of technological change to ensure the best use of technology in healthcare education? As technology advances and the lines of technology and humanity become increasingly blurred, what ethical and moral imperatives will healthcare educators be facing?

5 What is an e-patient and how are patients themselves impacting the future of healthcare and healthcare education?

6 What will you bring to the simulation practice community as a Simulation Champion leader, follower, and manager?

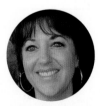

Colette Foisy-Doll,
MSN, RN, CHSE

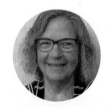

Kim Leighton,
PhD, RN, CHSE, CHSOS, ANEF

To begin telling this great story, you could simply place the now 150-year-old stethoscope and 135-year-old blood pressure cuff beside an augmented reality virtual patient that is interacting with a trainee in a fully immersive virtual space (The Medical Futurist, 2016). The stark contrast between these two realities defies anything we could have imagined 20 years ago. The cyber world has arrived and now provides "beam-me-up-type" healthcare learning experiences for the next generation of healthcare providers. We are living in a time of unprecedented and astonishing change. Technology is galloping forward at breakneck speed, and we are simply no longer able to predict what life will look like for the next generation of learners. For example, if we ask you to describe what a university will look like 30 years from now, how would you answer? Most would say, "I'm not sure, but I know it won't be anything like the university of today." We are going to explore that question in this last chapter of the Simulation Champions book.

We begin this chapter with a salute to the past and then move on to taking a glimpse at today and a look to the future. Over a few short decades, we have realized incredible advances in teaching and learning and in the use of disruptive innovations for learning in healthcare. **Disruptive innovation theory** is the theory that explains the "phenomenon by which an innovation transforms an existing market or sector by introducing simplicity, convenience, accessibility, and affordability where complication and high cost are the status quo" (Christenson Institute, 2016, para. 2). For example, the major disruptive innovation of our time is the personal computer. Although we cannot fully conceptualize what the future of healthcare education will look like, we can envision that it will be nothing like what we have today. What will become of the full-body computerized mannequin? What of task trainers, and screen-based computer learning modules? What of simulation centers? We invite you on a journey to explore what might be possible. Whatever comes, Simulation Champions will be challenged to keep up-to-date with emerging technologies and to establish new best practices to meet the needs of a new generation of healthcare professionals, the next users of the next disruptive innovations. Let's begin by taking a quick look back.

A Salute to Yesterday

As we reflected on our journey in nursing and nursing education over the past 35 years, we were able to pinpoint milestones in the evolution of nursing education over the past quarter century. Pedagogically speaking, there has been a distinct shift from the use of behaviorist-centric approaches to more constructivist-centric and socio-centric learning theory and associated teaching and learning methodologies. Ortiz posits that we must foster advancement toward more transdisciplinary "personalized, holistic, and research-based pedagogy" (Launchship.com, 2016, para. 2). In contrast, current trends in psychomotor skills acquisition are grounded in diverse learning theory, such as deliberate practice, cognitive load theory, situated cognition, and mastery learning among many others. The advent and use of such learning paradigms are complemented by the evolution and availability of incredible new educational technologies.

Whereas the vast majority of nursing programs used to offer a diploma in nursing, today most programs offer degrees requisite for entry to practice. Venues and facilities for delivering nursing programs differ vastly from yesteryear.

Whereas nursing programs between the 1960s and 1980s unfolded in hospital- and college-based locales, today they unfold in sophisticated, technology-rich replications of clinical environments that are housed in educational institutions or virtual worlds. Back in the day, training programs used the apprenticeship model. In this model, most psychomotor skills were learned on the patient while working in the hospital using the "see one, do one, teach one" approach. Students were lucky if they had one skills practice room furnished with a few old beds and maybe an IV pole and a static mannequin or two. Times have certainly changed.

What of Today's Healthcare Education Technologies?

Healthcare educational technology (Health EdTech) is "the study and ethical practice of facilitating learning and improving performance [in healthcare] by creating, using, and managing appropriate technological processes and resources" (Robinson, Molenda, & Rezabek, 2008, p. 15). In the space of 30 short years, Health EdTech has moved from a reliance on such technologies as reel-to-reel film, slide projectors, microfiche, and computer-based learning modules, to the use of disruptive innovations like simulation using **virtual reality (VR)**, **augmented reality (AR)**, **mixed reality (MR)**, and cloud computing platforms. These are the revolutionary products that are now fueling the educational technologies market (Murray, 2016). Technavio.com (2016) reports that these technologies, plus the introduction of simulation in e-learning, have the potential to increase the compound annual growth rate in Health EdTech by 18% through 2020. The total revenue for VR and AR is projected to increase from $5.2 billion in 2016 to over $162 billion by 2020 (International Data Corporation [IDC], 2016). Universities are also undergoing threat from low-cost or no-cost courses like massive open online courses (MOOCs), Coursera, and edX (Murray, 2016). As such, educational institutions are challenged to develop innovative digital offerings or run the risk of being undercut by lower-cost options that are adopted by millions of people around the globe. Watcher (2015), however, tells us that amid this technological explosion, healthcare has remained seemingly immune to computerization. He states that "until recently, in many communities, the high school was more wired than the local hospital" (p. xiii). The truth is that the vast majority of hospitals and educational instructions remain sorely under resourced. Simulation programs must take heed and pay attention to the cost of Health EdTech and yet be forward thinking when developing on- and off-campus offerings. Educators should plan to incorporate contemporary simulation design, such as the inclusion of games and the use of VR, AR, and MR environments. Innovators who are embracing the integration of disruptive technologies in healthcare education curricula lead cutting-edge schools.

As was discussed in Chapter 1, there has been a tremendous swing in the social forces that have shaped new realities in healthcare and healthcare education. Among them are the following:

- Globalization and global mandates for more equitable access to education by working to develop sustainable, ethical, and responsible education on the global platform
- Current "superdiversity" migration patterns creating the need for culturally and linguistically competent care providers that embrace diversity by enacting the professional practices of cultural humility and culturally safety
- The call to disrupt, reshape, and transform nursing and other healthcare education programs that includes access to quality experiential learning to better bridge between theory and today's complex and dynamic professional practice settings
- The need for quality research toward critical examination of current practices and to inform future changes in education and healthcare
- The cry for deep, pervasive, and sustainable organizational culture change in healthcare to shift from a culture rooted in blame, shame, hierarchy, and power distance to a **Just Culture** and a culture of safety
- The need to break down silos between healthcare professions and educational and healthcare institutions to shape a new team culture that places patients and their families as central participants on the healthcare team
- Increasing interprofessional collaboration (IPC), interprofessional education (IPE), and team training to achieve safer patient care
- The need for increased intersectoral partnering to promulgate innovation and then to enact best practices in the use of such innovations in teaching, learning, and clinical practice
- The need for sustainable practices in a world whose resources are finite and for which we must be responsible ambassadors and stewards
- The need for skilled leaders, followers, and managers to create high-reliability organizations through the use of systems approaches to effect change in complex adaptive systems
- The need to keep abreast of advancements in technology as well as the impact it has on human existence - and to honor the ethical imperative we all have to play our part in shaping the future.

As simulationists, we are called to continue our efforts in attending to these key drivers and to commit to best practices in all facets of simulation-based education. It is a large mandate, but we have clearly demonstrated as a simulation community of practice that we are up for the challenge. Areas of focus to date have included the following:

- Translational research in simulation, including both research studies on simulation and research that uses simulation

- A commitment to the ongoing creation, dissemination, and adherence to Standards of Best Practice: Simulation^SM (INACSL Standards Committee, 2016) and other established benchmarks for simulation success
- Striving for pervasive culture change within educational organizations and healthcare systems
- Embedding cortical concepts into simulation-based curricula, including such concepts and constructs as values-based and complexity leadership, relationality, human factors, patient safety, patient- and family-centered care, interprofessional teams, culture and diversity, systems approaches, advocacy, social responsibility, distributive justice, Just Culture, global citizenship, and theory-based learning

Futuristic Healthcare Programs— Where Are We Going?

The information age has fundamentally changed the way humans behave and interact on the planet (Carroll, Bruno, & vonTschudi, 2016). Social, economic, and environmental structures are forever changed by technology. It is fascinating, for example, that today we can hold the collective knowledge of all of human existence in the palm of our hand, available within seconds on any smart device. It is in this context that we had a great discussion about the universities of the future. At one point in our conversation, someone mentioned the need for more interprofessional education (IPE) within existing curricula, when the other blurted out, "No, you are thinking too small. If I had to build this from scratch, I would build an IPE University where all disciplines learned core healthcare content together from day one!" We went on to talk about a hypothetical Virtual Interprofessional University (VIP-U) (see Fig. 28.1 for a depiction of the VIP-U Crest and Motto). As off the wall as it may seem, we share our vision for VIP-U. Let's check in again in 5-10 years or so to see how far off the mark we were.

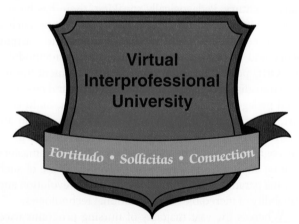

Figure 28.1 Hypothetical Virtual Interprofessional University—VIP-U Crest and Motto (*Fortitudo-Sollicitas, Connection* (Latin for) Courage, Caring, and Connection).

The VIP-U and the IPE Program Delivery

Dr. Christina Ortiz, former Dean at MIT, professes that the university of the future will have "no classrooms, no scheduled lectures, and lots of technology" (Launchship. com, 2016, para. 1). If you think this is unlikely, think again. As you read, she is busy "building a radical non-profit research institution focused on the intersection of technology and humanity, to increase college access for underprivileged students" (para. 1). This initiative is not the first of its kind. Dr. Hubert Rampersad just spear-headed the opening of the *Innovation University of Silicon Valley*, using mostly online learning to reach a target audience of talented students from Africa and Asia who could never afford the costs of studying at traditional universities (http://www.iusv.university/). Unlike traditional universities with campuses, buildings, staff, onsite students, and lots of "stuff," VIP-U will be a borderless university that is unbound by time, physical spaces, and the need to access local people and house key learning resources. VIP-U will admit learners from anywhere in the world.

The VIP-U Program

VIP-U will exist within a conglomerate of learning entities as partners in IPE excellence around the world. Christenson

(2013) believes "consumers will ultimately adopt the [online education] disruption, and a host of struggling colleges and universities—the bottom 25% of every tier, will disappear or merge in the next 10 to 15 years" (para. 6). As such, IPE programs will be delivered using blended learning strategies that unfold in a virtual environment. Learners at VIP-U will move through their studies in a nonlinear fashion through four phases of learning: experiential learning, concept exploration, meaning making, and demonstration and application (see Fig. 28.2). VIP-U will unfold in VR, AR, and MR supported learning spaces in combination with in-person practical experiences. VIP-U virtual capabilities will provide teachers and learners with shared learning spaces so realistic that they won't actually miss physically sitting beside their peers in a classroom. Human interaction in future virtual worlds will feel exceptionally real—including provisions for exchanging the sensory data needed to create a fully immersive human interactive experience from anywhere in the world. You will literally feel like other people are sitting right next to you and be able to feel their presence.

Additionally, affective computing will play an increased role in education. Affective computing, studied particularly at MIT since the 1990s has been defined as "the ability of humans to program machines to recognize, interpret, process and simulate the range of emotions" (Johnson et al., 2016, p. 44). Using affective computing to create virtualized persons possessing emotional intelligence can replace some

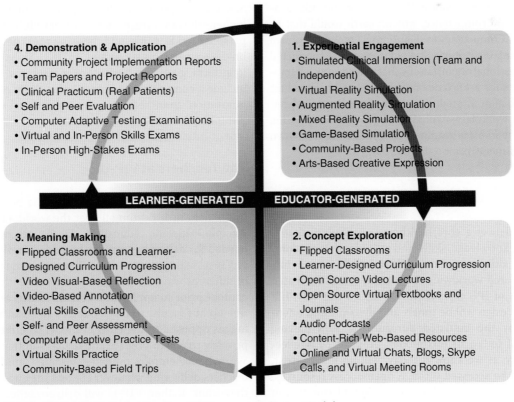

Figure 28.2 VIP-U: An Innovative IPE Program Delivery Model.

dimensions of human-to-human coaching and tutoring for learning. The British Columbia Institute of Technology has developed a technology-based solution to facilitate virtual deliberate practice coaching using an iPad fixed to a mobile rod. Using the iPad FaceTime feature, learners can call from any location for person-to-person coaching anytime during independent practice.

The use of innovative approaches allows programs to shift from the use of on campus **time-based program** delivery models to the use of an off campus **competency-based** delivery model. The time-based programs we employ today require that learners be physically present in a classroom or skills lab for preestablished periods of time on task or topic to become competent (e.g., 120 hours of lecture, 60 hours skills labs, 100 hours practicum) (Gruppen, Mangrukar, & Kolars, 2012). In time-based educational delivery models, curriculum drives courses that are traditionally offered in dedicated classroom spaces equipped with desks, chairs, and walls. Learners in time-based programs, for the most part, must be physically present for the entire duration of the program in order to successfully complete the course. In contrast, VIP-U will build on already existing virtual competency-based programs to create the opportunity for students to use bite-sized, self-regulated learning and to move through the curriculum at their own pace from anywhere in the world. Competency-based outcomes and the attainment of competency-based learning objectives through the use of competency-based learning strategies will drive the curriculum at VIP-U. If students can complete their course work in half the time and still capably demonstrate competence, why on earth would that be discouraged? Competency evaluations will move away from siloed teaching institutions and will instead be conducted by interprofessional organizations that will administer standardized tests for proficiency in IPE. This will help reduce the hyperinflation of grades to meet university mandates. Professional workplaces will also take a role in assessing learners for workplace readiness by conducting their own learner assessments prior to hiring.

The VIP-U Curriculum

VIP-U will deliver a core healthcare curriculum that is grounded in knowledge, skills, and attitudes that are common to all health professionals. VIP-U will deliver a living, breathing shared worldwide curriculum that is cocreated by hundreds of IPE experts worldwide. In this way, IPE curriculum design will be timely and dynamic and unencumbered by the outdated bureaucratic slow-moving structures of today. In this model, proprietary intellectual property, as we know it today, will no longer exist. Content will be accessed through open-access resources, no cost (or low-cost) scalable cloud-based platforms, not unlike today's massive open online courses (MOOCs).

As such, the cost of getting an education at VIP-U will plummet. VIP-U will therefore realize a program cost reduction of at least 75%, as compared to conventional university tuition. Most courses will be offered through global third-party service providers that deliver low-cost courses to the world. To contribute to global development and global equity in education, the program will be delivered at no cost to underserved or low-resource parts of the world.

Core content related to healthcare concepts common to all disciplines will be taught to the entire group of learners regardless of discipline, after which time, learners will branch off into unidisciplinary program tracks to acquire discipline-specific knowledge and competencies. Debriefing will be a core competency that is threaded throughout the entire curriculum and practiced in virtual teams and during actual patient care (National League for Nursing, 2015). At regular points throughout the program, VIP-U learners will come back together to share and learn with and from each other—using a true IPE model. On-site, in-person learning (which may or may not be campus based) will involve clinical groups composed of a blend of core disciplines, instead of the current siloed discipline-specific clinical groups. There will also be accommodations for individualized learning to meet individual student needs: a need that is currently not fully met. In today's programs, learners are saddled with juggling many balls in the air and fall behind, or fail to meet course requirements within the prescribed timelines. Despite the demand, Skiba (2016), points out that there are a "limited number of higher-education institutions that have fully implemented personalized learning, and there is a great need for faculty buy-in to make this successful" (p. 183). Skiba foresees that long-term goals for healthcare institutions will need to include a commitment to creating a culture of change and innovation, to increasing cross-institutional work, and to rethinking how institutions work.

The Teachers at VIP-U

VIP-U will draw on faculty that are the best of the best in the field of IPE from all over the world and top-notch discipline-specific educators. Fewer teachers will be needed for delivering content-based lectures. Classrooms at VIP-U will be flipped and will promote the use of a host of different ways for learners to interact with and absorb content prior to application activities. This approach will free up our faculty to be facilitators and coaches of learning, as opposed to the current model where the teacher's primary role is to prepare and deliver content in lectures. We will not employ outdated teaching models that see teachers delivering whatever content they want, whenever they want. Rather, VIP-U will deliver content created by experts, using a wide variety of technology-based teaching modalities that unfold in virtual spaces. Faculty at VIP-U will become codesigners of learning experiences and facilitators and coaches of both in-person and virtual learning.

The Students of VIP-U

Learners from all health disciplines will learn together in one program with one glaring difference. They won't be sitting in chairs in a classroom that has four walls. Learners will not have to leave home to attend class. The traditional campus residence will be a thing of the past, as learners will engage in both independent and team learning in the virtual environment through smart devices. They will practice skills in virtual simulation centers and skills laboratories, using VR, AR, and MR technology with the use of **head-mounted displays (HMD)** and **smart glasses** (see Fig. 28.3A, B) although that technology will also evolve in coming years. Consider how different Oculus Rift is now, compared to when Mark Zuckerberg purchased the technology in 2014. We first heard of its potential for immersing ourselves in gaming applications; however, it wasn't long before the virtual reality world entered other realms, including healthcare education. Numerous companies continue to strive to enhance this technology for use in managing global issues such as lack of access to technology, education, and healthcare.

Learners will also be given the opportunity to engage in application of knowledge, skills, and attitudes within their own communities, where course projects will unfold within the context of local needs and realities. Hands-on patient care will unfold in actual practice settings accompanied by coaching for competency attainment with the aid of such technologies as See What I See headgear to connect learners and teachers (see Figure 28-6). Evaluation of learner competency and corresponding learner assessments will transpire in both virtual and in-person spaces. Students at VIP-U will be free to learn at their own pace.

Using self-regulated learning will enable them to take classes anytime, anywhere, and be the designers of their own program.

That is our VIP-U vision. Perhaps this is a pie-in-the-sky dream, but the more we talked it through, the more it made sense. We honestly think it is just a matter of time before someone takes the ball and runs with it taking virtual IPE to the next level. One thing is for certain; if we don't dream it, we will never realize it and IPC is vital to improving the healthcare outcomes of future generations.

New Vistas: Disruptive Innovations in Healthcare Education

"Any sufficiently advanced technology is indistinguishable from magic."

—*Arthur C. Clarke (1962)*

Simulation was once touted as disruptive innovation in health education technology and is now described by Bauman (2016) as "a vetted, standard educational practice for nursing and clinical education at all levels" (p. 109). Today, a wide assortment of simulation delivery modalities are enacted using a myriad of simulation typologies and have become ubiquitous in many healthcare learning environments, especially in urban centers. Bauman also reports that game-based learning, mobile applications (otherwise known as apps), and virtual reality are now on track to useful ubiquity, following an expansion pathway similar to that of mannequin-based simulation. In fact, there are currently an estimated 10,000 plus healthcare apps on the market (MedData Group, 2014). While mannequin-based simulation remains quite costly, virtual simulation holds promise as a viable, lower-cost, scalable learning modality (Bauman, 2016). Other predictions include an increase in the use of game-based simulation, mobile apps, learning

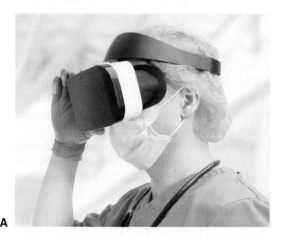
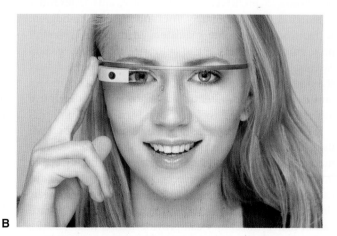

Figure 28.3   A. Surgeon wearing virtual reality glasses (courtesy of Shutterstock.com). **B.** Google Glass (Editorial credit: Peppinuzzo/Shutterstock.com.)

in virtual worlds and environments using computers, and wearable gear to support digital–human interfacing within those worlds. Some nursing programs are already experimenting with AR platforms.

Disruptive innovations, such as simulation, impact many stakeholder groups ranging from administrators, faculty, students, and staff in education and healthcare institutions to industry partners, regulators, policy and lawmakers, and even patients and their families. For example, in today's digital era, everyone has access to information about their genetic composition and even their DNA ancestry information (https://dna.ancestry.ca/). In this day and age, our lives interface with technology to the extent that we have fashion items housing pieces of technology that adorn our bodies and, in some cases, technology that is embedded within the human body. These digital devices provide us with all kinds of information such as how well we sleep, how many steps we take, our vital signs, and other similar health parameters. We are connected to others and to ourselves through technology in ways that were previously unthinkable. Even the need to push the sync button has even been replaced with wireless Bluetooth capabilities for data transfer.

Simulation is a disruptive technology that has grown by leaps and bounds in the past 10 years. Simulation capabilities run the gamut from surgical simulators that allow practice of minimally invasive procedures; to 3D imaging, printing, and photocopying; to virtual reality tools and applications for healthcare professionals and patients alike (Alec, 2016; The Medical Futurist, 2016). As much as there are advantages to disruptive innovations, there are number of significant challenges in the interfacing of Health EdTech and those who use them: educators, administrators, and key stakeholders, such as regulatory bodies, have often not kept up with the times and put up barriers to advancement. For example, in the face of irrefutable high-quality evidence that proves that under the right conditions, simulation can replace up to 50% of traditional clinical practice hours in prelicensure nursing programs (Alexander et al., 2015; Hayden, Smiley, Alexander, Kardong-Edgren, & Jeffries, 2014), some regulators of nursing education programs remain reticent to authorize this practice. It is essential that those responsible for approval of regulatory standards and compliance seek out a balanced perspective on the benefits and potential adverse effects of disruptive innovations.

Educators themselves are often inclined to continue using outdated teaching methodologies, often void of technological innovation. As we embark with lightning speed into a new digital world, it has become apparent that educational institutions are broken in so many ways. Seely Brown stated that "We currently have the very best education that 17th century can provide" (CBC Radio, 2012). Ortiz reaffirms this, saying that "Technology is accelerating, and modernization and expansion of the higher education system is desperately needed…our higher education system is still stuck in the Middle Ages" (Launchship.com, para. 1). Many contemporary postsecondary learning institutions continue to offer learning environments that are similar to the classrooms of centuries long ago. Today; however, emerging technologies and their application to the learning process are challenging outdated pedagogical models. Consider the following questions:

- Do conventional learning models that continue to be characterized by single discipline silos do a good job of teaching healthcare providers how to be effective in teams?
- Is information delivered to passive recipients (our learners) sitting in lecture halls creating the type of thinker we need in this new digital information age?
- Are learners literate and skilled in the use of disruptive innovations for effective learning?
- Are learners empowered by learning critical thinking processes to manage and sift through the myriad of information that is available to them? (Seely Brown & Adler, 2008)

Technological capability alone is simply not enough and educators also must "stimulate intellectual capacity for transforming tacit pedagogical knowledge into commonly usable and visible knowledge" (Seely Brown, 2008). It is, therefore, imperative that a new generation of educators rebuilds how we teach, learn, and share knowledge in the use of disruptive innovations. Globally, the collective efforts of many are in play as new *collaborative learning models* that are enabled by technology and digital world capabilities are being co-developed. Not all simulation educators, for example, are innovators and early adopters, and in fact, most are digital immigrants who struggle to keep abreast of emerging Health EdTech and implement their use in teaching (Prensky, 2010).

Emerging learning models, like simulation-based learning, also spawn the need for leaders who are well versed in transformational, discovery-driven, collaborative learning. Simulation leaders fill multiple complex roles that entail abilities to lead organizational change, manage programs and resources, implement technology-based innovation, and integrate sound curriculum. There is much work to be done to achieve an optimal blend of formal and informal learning through co-creating, experimenting, reflecting, sharing, and reusing accumulated ideas and knowledge about teaching and learning. Technological advances do produce opportunities for the development of new pathways to knowledge acquisition and simulation offers an environment where students learn together with a hands-on, interactive, experiential approach instead of learning alone, memorizing a textbook.

"The most innovative technologies will extend the curriculum beyond the confines of the traditional classroom by creating digital spaces to promote the suspension of disbelief and produce sufficient authenticity or environmental fidelity to allow for deep meaning making" (Bauman, 2016, p. 111).

Introducing innovative technologies in education necessitates capable, knowledgeable, and skilled leaders that inspire action in followers around a united vision for change. Simulationists are called to be transformational leaders that know how to engage a new generation of technosavvy learners as much as the traditionalist educator (Kouzes & Posner, 2014; Prensky, 2013). Additionally, those working as regulators in the health professions, or serving on accrediting bodies, as well as those working in health policy development must be well versed in best practices in simulation. We are at a critical juncture in simulation "with massive advances springing up every week, and there's simply no time to stick to established methods of regulation" (The Medical Futurist, 2016, para. 5). Standards and approvals for simulation programs and their sound use of simulation design, deployment, and evaluation must be established across all health programs and disciplines.

The Virtual Reality Explosion

Once reserved for techies and gamers, VR is surfacing as the next big thing in healthcare (Scher, 2016). Although VR is ubiquitous in gaming, video entertainment, and military, engineering, and flight training, it is certainly not yet commonplace in healthcare. However, due to decreasing costs and the scalability of virtual products, we are seeing the increased application of VR in healthcare education and inpatient care (Ridley, 2013). In Box 28-1, Scher (2016) features five ways that VR will impact healthcare.

Other innovations in Health EdTech include the use of See What I Can See integrated smartphone video capabilities and VR headgear to provide real-time telepresence solutions in healthcare settings (e.g., AMA Xpert Eye http://www.amaxperteye.com/). Figure 28.4 provides an example of using Eyes in the Field technology in nursing. Additionally, surgeons can use 3D-enhanced MRI and CT images to "view and navigate around healthy and damaged tissue, tumors, and blood vessels in order to create a precise plan for surgery that minimizes the risk of complications" (Teo, 2016, para. 5). VR applications also play a role in patient rehabilitation through immersion in virtual environments that stimulate the brain to refocus attention and enhance relearning (Teo, 2016). Patients can use products like Applied VR (http://appliedvr.io/) and Deep Stream VR (http://www.deepstreamvr.com/) to produce deep levels of relaxation.

In healthcare education, the release of virtual learning products is increasing. Examples of virtual reality environments in healthcare include V-Sim, Shadow Health, iHuman Patient, and SimIQ-IPE. Another innovation is the use of QR code readers or scanners on smartphone or tablet apps. These apps are programmed to read QR codes that can literally be embedded into any surface, even on a static man-

---

Box 28-1 **Five Ways That Virtual Reality Will Impact Healthcare in the Future**

Scher (2016) identifies five major ways that VR has the potential to create impact and meaningful changes in healthcare in the coming years:

1. The ability to provide highly realistic educational hands-on learning experiences for students and for faculty development to increase health literacy language and skill development, including critical relational abilities
2. The ability to shorten the learning curve and time needed to train on real patients using virtual workbenches, and the ability to integrate the use of VR into live patient care (e.g., having a patient wear a VR headset to allow for mapping of brain activity to facilitate the removal of a brain tumor [https://www.engadget.com/2016/02/17/patient-wears-vr-headset-during-brain-surgery/])
3. The ability to make available critical tools and information from patient e-records on mobile devices for patient education
4. For therapeutic patient care intervention (e.g., to promote relaxation or for pain management)
5. To use 3D capabilities that bring unbelievable levels of accuracy to ultrasound, CT scan, and MR images (e.g., EchoPixel through its True 3D system, allows healthcare providers to see multidimensional images of human anatomy [http://motherboard.vice.com/read/this-interactive-system-lets-doctors-see-your-guts-in-virtual-reality])

---

nequin or task trainer. Sheffield Hallam University in the United Kingdom uses QR code technology to prompt a video to play when the student points their smart device at various locations on static mannequins. For example, they can point an iPad at the patient's head and a video sequence pops up that allows the student to have an AR experience with a static mannequin. The same technique can be used to bring body parts, wounds, or other aspects of patient assessment to life (https://youtu.be/Sbh2PRrLSZ8). To amp it up, AR can include interactivity where learners can manipulate, pinch, and grab 3D images. As you see, the opportunities for VR expansion in healthcare and healthcare education realms are staggering. When coupled with the potential that VR has for enhancing management of healthcare costs, improving quality, and enhancing the patient experience, Teo posits that the stage is set for an interesting intersection (Teo, 2016).

Virtual Reality—What Do All Those Terms Mean?

Virtual reality terminology can be very confusing for many Table 28.1 provides a summary of the main virtual technology terms and definitions to help you make sense of it all.

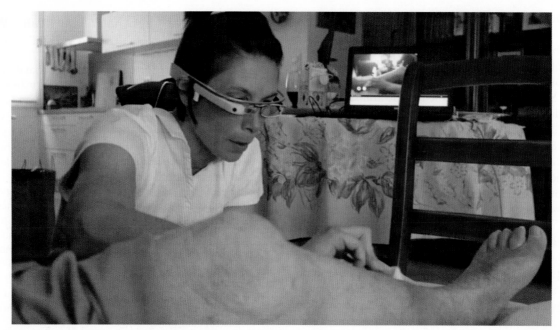

Figure 28.4 Nurse Using *Eyes in the Field* VR Glasses to Capture and Transmit What She Is Seeing to Other Healthcare Providers. (Image courtesy of AMA Xpert Eye Inc., Cambridge, MA.)

Simulation Champions: Leaders Shaping the Future

Blanford (2016) states that despite the advancements in measures taken to improve patient safety, a recent study by Makary and Daniel (2016) reported that medical error persists and is now positioned as the third leading cause of death in the United States. Technology has been proven to lower risks of procedural errors in healthcare, reduce cost of healthcare delivery, better inform patients and families, and improve patient outcomes.

A Look Through the Crystal Ball: Key Advancements in Health EdTech by 2020

We envision that the future of technology in healthcare and healthcare education will bring continued progress in the following areas:

- Steady and continuous waves of *technological innovation* across all healthcare disciplines, such as the progression from wearable glasses and headsets to contact lenses or the 3D printing of almost anything (Meskó, 2014).
- The emergence of *new technology trends* that do not exist today. We suggest that you follow the blogs and writings of healthcare and medical futurists such as Bertalan Meskó (http://medicalfuturist.com/). Stay connected, learn about new healthcare technologies, and then engage in meaningful discussion about best practices for their use. We need to critically think and question technological innovations and their application to healthcare.
- Expanded applications for glass including **touch-sensitive interactive display systems** in all sizes and shapes, even as **flexible glass** you can roll up and carry, and **photovoltaic glass** that can produce electricity through the window itself by converting light into a power source. Corning provides great examples of futuristic glass applications in their video "The Future: A Day of Glass" (https://youtu.be/Hr1ZI9qbgSE). Medical educational equipment is expanding the use of interactive glass workbenches. Body Interact (http://bodyinteract.com/product/) and Anatomage Medical (http://www.anatomage.com/table/) are two such examples.
- More *research to accelerate system change* and advancements in healthcare educational policy. Increasingly, simulation will be recognized as a legitimate and viable learning pedagogy and, in many instances, will trump traditional clinical learning practices.
- Increases in simulationists as **health hackers** participate in Hacking Health on an unprecedented global scale, where "healthcare professionals with designers, developers, innovators and entrepreneurs [can] build realistic, human-centric solutions to front-line healthcare problems" (Hacking Health, 2016).
- Increased emergence of **e-patients**: individuals that are "equipped, enabled, empowered and engaged in their health and healthcare decisions… within an equal partnership between e-patients and health professionals and systems that support them" (E-patients.net, 2016).

Table 28.1	Virtual Reality Terminology and Expanded Definitions
Virtual Imaging	"The images created by an optical display system that in turn creates a larger screen than is physically presented to the user. These optical display systems are used in head-mounted displays (HMD) or goggles" (Ridley, 2013, para. 6).
Head-Mounted Displays (HMD) or Virtual Reality Headsets or Headgear	Gear that is worn on the head that is fed imagery data provided by a camera, computer, or video source. Various makers include Oculus Rift, Sony PlayStation VR, HTC-Vive, Samsung Gear VR, FOVE, and Google Glasses or Daydream Headset. These products create the virtual experience with the help of (1) a desktop computer or smartphone needed to run an app or specific software and (2) a headset, with input from head tracking, eye tracking, and hand tracking devices, and sometimes with voice activation, handheld controllers, smart gloves, or buttons on devices or trackpads. The advent of low-latency motion tracking technology is making these devices much more friendly by minimizing the lag or delay effect that is experienced between the movement of the wearer and the virtual image being displayed (Charara, 2016).
Smart Glasses (also referred to as Data Glasses or Virtual Reality Glasses)	A pair of glasses that look like ordinary glasses but contain specialized polarized lenses that allow the wearer to see two images, one per each eye, giving the illusion of depth (Charara, 2016)
Virtual Reality (VR)	An artificial environment, which is experienced through sensory stimuli (as sights and sounds) provided by a computer and in which one's actions partially determine what happens in the environment (Merriam-webster.com). VR places the user within a fully immersive computer-simulated environment that gives the user the feeling of being in that environment instead of the one they are actually in (Mashable Explains, 2014). VR takes you into an entirely new world and does not interface with your actual world. It involves wearing specialized headgear that suspends a computer-generated screen within the lenses. Computers, gaming consoles, or smartphones equipped with special software or apps and sensors make what you see seem like reality. It can also be accompanied by 3D surround sound effects. Sometimes, controllers are used allowing you to interact with virtual artifacts like avatars or other images (Charara, 2016). When we can move around and interact with virtual environments, our brains are fooled into believing it is real (https://youtu.be/HBNH8tzsfVM).
Hand Controllers	Wireless hand devices that make you feel like you are using your hands in the virtual environment. For example, such devices might make you feel like you are actually using scissors to cut. They can also provide sensory data to the user to enhance the realism of the entire experience (Charara, 2016).
Augmented Vision (AV)	AV involves the visualization process used to realize AR that overlays the viewer's vision with data that are "see-through" so they appear to float in the user's view (where the real world is not occluded to any great extent). In AV, you need to wear something on your head, like specialized glasses that use beam-splitter optics to combine the normal vision path with images provided by a microdisplay. These floating images are usually mounted above or to the side of the optical lens so as not to obstruct the viewer's vision. It is best for use during task focused, simple procedures and allows hands-free experiences (Ridley, 2013). Another example of AV is Augmented Virtuality, which is a mostly virtual world to which real objects are added (with cameras, or by scanning them with lasers, for example).
Augmented Reality (AR)	The key thing that distinguishes VR from AR is that it does not provide the full immersion experience of VR. AR can overlay virtual images on top of the user's actual physical world. With AR we have a world that's mostly real, to which we are adding some virtual objects. Both VR and AR applications move synchronously with the head/body, and both have a wide range of motion, especially for room-sized VR. Quality of the image and latency are purely a function of the hardware, which is often shared between both applications of the technology. Because an AR application doesn't have to render the entire world, it can be less hardware-intensive. AR also has the ability to allow the user complete mobility in the real world while experiencing created content. These features mean that AR is often useful for seamlessly integrating data from the Internet with our world, providing us with restaurant reviews, bus schedules, narrations about pieces of art in a museum, or similar applications." (Chris Ozeroff, Virtual Product Designer, personal communication, Feb, 2017). See https://youtu.be/09vxKN1zLNI for an explanation. One of the first applications was the heads up display used to embed instruments and gauges into the real viewing field of pilots.
Mixed Reality (MR)	MR is the most flexible of the virtual products. In mixed reality, there is a blend of virtual and augmented reality where real objects can be used to view many dimensions of the virtual world, such as a wall or tabletop surface used to display virtual imagery (Ridley, 2013). "I personally think the "divide" between AR and VR is mostly imaginary. They are really just the same thing, with the slider just moved around a bit. Almost all VR things have some grounding in reality, or they would be difficult to relate with. And all AR has at least some virtual objects, or there would be no point to it. They are really two sides of the same coin, and I think the term Mixed Reality is trying to express that. Many of the technologies that are not as new and sexy as VR and AR also play with mixed reality; after all, when I sit in front of a computer and play a video game, I am (usually) playing in a virtual world, so in that sense, it is a mixed reality device as well.... MR unfolds across a spectrum. On one end, there is the pure Real World, and on the other is a purely Virtual World" (Chris Ozeroff, personal communication, Feb, 2017).

- The increased use of *organized social media* for health-care purposes, such as groups of patients and families using Twitter, Facebook, YouTube, and blogs (Carroll et al., 2016).
- The expansion of *shared web-based learning spaces* for faculty development such as Clinical Playground (http://clinicalplayground.com/), Healthy Simulation (http://healthysimulation.com/), the NLN Simulation Innovation Resources Center (SIRC) online modules (http://sirc.nln.org/), and a host of simulation practice community webinars.
- Expanded virtual conferencing that allows for 100% virtual conference attendance. For example, in the past 2 years, the Canadian Patient Safety Conference has been offered as either a full virtual experience or in-person experience. The days of having to take trains, planes, and automobiles to travel the globe for conferences are changing as part of the global mandate for sustainability.
- Continued advancement in the sophistication of educational platforms to deliver simulation will see expansion in *simulation delivery modalities, as well as in simulation typologies* used to enact these modalities (see Table 28.2).
- The *expanded role of e-patients* as equal members of healthcare teams to codiagnose and then cocreate treatment plans and outcomes verification; they will also expand on existing patient online support groups to include more virtual meetings (Meskó, 2014; Trotter & Uhlman, 2013).
- New *apps with advanced analytics* for e-patient and healthcare provider access to information for health tracking and health management (MedData, 2014; Trotter & Uhlman, 2013).

- Use games and AR to assist patients in following health regimes that are often so tough to follow (Fabella, 2016a). For example, we have seen kids jump of the couch and become super physically active because of Pokémon Go and not because they were prescribed 30 minutes a day of exercise. Another healthcare application for computer-based games is to stave off the onset of Alzheimer disease (e.g., Luminosity.com) or AR games to treat conditions like phobias, phantom limb syndrome, posttraumatic stress syndrome, and autism (Fabella, 2016b).
- The practice of coalescing data from multiple apps to create superanalytic capabilities called *Big Data Analytics*.
- The use of *geolocation-sensitive learning* using mobile apps. Imagine how much fun it would be to have learners use location-aware devices to interview virtual characters in various locations and then gather simulated patient assessment data to uncover the source of illness from a hypothetical toxic spill (Educause Learning Initiative, 2009).
- Build on the *creative uses of VR and AR*, such as those from medicine that include AR-assisted skills training, AR-assisted patient diagnosing, AR-assisted procedural design and procedural planning for minimally invasive surgery on hard and soft tissues, thus enabling advance practice runs, the ability to consult specialists, and cut down on time.
- Enhancing simulator functions (both static and computerized) using apps that contain *QR reader technology* to augment reality.
- The use of *robotics* to increase realistic movement in simulators.

Table 28.2	Expansion in Simulation Delivery Modalities and Typologies
Link	**Description**
https://youtu.be/QGZvOrWzV-I https://youtu.be/86wmhfQEQIQ	SimX (2017) uses AR for medical trainees to assess and treat holographic patients in virtual worlds. Using AR gear and real medical equipment, this technology brings scalable, realistic, and relevant learning to the masses at a relatively low cost. For comparison, the cost of a single simulator can run $25,000–150,000 USD depending on the level of sophistication, while AR gear runs $300–$3,000 per pair.
https://youtu.be/SKpKlh1-en0	Case Western University is using Microsoft HoloLens technology to bring high-realism digital anatomy into the classroom.
https://www.cyber-anatomy.com/	Cyber-Anatomy's Cyber-Science 3D fully immersive, interactive holographic human anatomy models are delivered in virtual reality learning spaces.
http://medicalfuturist.com/top-10-virtual-medical-sites-in-second-life/	Second Life is showing great promise; a recent blog post listed the top 10 sites in healthcare in Second Life.
https://youtu.be/saGGNLbU4tl	Surgical training applications using highly sophisticated educational 3D-printed heart valve surgery simulators, like the ones developed and adopted at Maastricht University Hospital (Alec, 2016). These 3D printer–integrated simulation systems allow for three-dimensional reconstruction of patient-specific anatomy for rehearsal of complex cases (Sardari Nia et al., 2016).

- Enhancing simulated clinical immersion to include AR, VR, and MR to *mimic their use in real-world applications* (e.g., patient education to teach about and enable visualization of prosthetics [e.g., iLimb systems] or patient disease self-regulation and access to diagnostic results).

- Creating *better skills training products* that incorporate virtual environments and game-based learning (e.g., the nursing program at Boise State University in Idaho used Oculus Rift to create a virtual catheterization trainer). This approach was found to eliminate the cost of the expensive simulators while providing participants with performance tracking data, such as skeletal positioning to ensure correct hand placement and positioning (Woods, 2015). The additional data provided from AR technology is not currently generated from simulators, nor from task trainers, or low-cost home-made devices. Comparisons in educational outcomes when using different typologies has yet to be studied in depth, however, AR holds great promise as a scalable, more diverse, lower-cost solution (SimX, 2017).

- *Augmenting human capabilities* through technology (e.g., exoskeletons that allow people living with paralysis to walk again, embedded technology to improve health parameter awareness and control, or for remote communication with healthcare providers [MedData, 2014]). Futurists and Health IT specialists speak of *the quantified-self* reality that is emerging through the use of wearable technology and embedded computer chips that make available diverse health data parameters (Meskó, 2014; Trotter & Uhlman, 2013).

- The *hospital of the future* will be connected and extended into patients' homes. There is a proliferation of physicians asking patients to use smart devices to diagnose or management illness. Imagine the limitless utility of the smartphone-driven EEG or ECG (Fabella, 2016b; MedData, 2014; Meskó, 2014).

- The emergence of collaborative e-patient healthcare provider (HCP) data collection, monitoring, and storage in *Cloud-based shared storage spaces*. HCPs can respond and intervene remotely (MedData, 2014). There will be expanded applications of devices like the Fitbit or HexCare. These devices have the potential to offer a fully integrated personal, social, and medical device. The aggregation of data from these apps will be used for research and to inform local, national, or worldwide health initiatives (MedData). Imagine the potential. What if all post-op patients went home with wearable devices that linked health measures back to a data collection and notification system?

- Continued expansion in the *ecosystem of stakeholders* such as health services, government agencies looking out for the public, patients and the public, and industry vendors of health product technologies. What if your health insurance company gave you incentives or reduced rates based on data from a wearable device that was endorsed by your physician? Car insurance carriers already do this.

- Blurring of lines between technology and humanity as we enter a transhumanistic period (a time when humanity can evolve beyond its current physical and mental limitations by modifying itself via all emerging sciences, including genetic engineering, digital technology, and bioengineering) (LaGrandeur, 2014; Locsin, 2005).

- Living in a world populated by post humans (a condition in which humans and intelligent technology overlap and become increasingly intertwined – to the point where the human body may actually be viewed as excess baggage): these beings of the future have been described as technosapiens, neomorts, and cyborgs (LaGrandeur, 2014; Locsin, 2005).

- Facing the challenges inherent in a trans human and post human era, where nurses and other healthcare providers are challenged to define personhood as we once knew it. For example, at what point, if any, does the human body so filled with technology, ever stop being a person? Would the implanting of an artificial intelligence program into the human brain change the personhood of a human being? What is the cost of furthering humanity and science and when do we cross ethical and moral boundaries that ought not be crossed?

- The broadening scope of genetics and genomics in healthcare and the inability of the health professions to keep up with standards of practice for these rapidly emerging screening, diagnostic, and therapeutic interventions.

Technology Related Challenges and Barriers to Advancement

Virtual learning and advanced technologies come with challenges. For example, AR devices are expensive and need more robustness to perform better. Internet-based technology requires ubiquitous network connectivity; therefore, rendering such technologies inaccessible in many places in the world. Even in high-resource countries, connectivity can create performance and reliability issues. There are also device-to-device connectivity issues that can result in poor system-to-system integration. Some of these are examples of why the mandate for widespread use of electronic health records has not yet been realized. Computer-based systems like EHRs also cost time and money to implement, input data and maintain while paper and pen continue to be a practical, efficient, and very convenient alternative (Trotter & Uhlman, 2013). Meanwhile, this thwarts our efforts to streamline patient records to improve patient safety and health outcomes.

Financial concerns are very real, although many will argue that VR and AR learning technologies are much more scalable and affordable than some current simulation technologies. More research comparing the costs and benefits of disruptive innovations is needed. Simulation programs will need to adopt business models and practices to support sustainability for the ongoing costs of simulation, including things like equipment replacement, insurance, and maintenance.

Best practices in technology usage are not yet fully developed as technology is moving faster than educational standards can be created. For example, we still need to learn a great deal about AR and doing so means we need established standards and metrics for evaluation. Research into the use of HMDs will reveal best practices for design based on the tracking of latency, weight, power, heat, and comfort issues. Regulatory standards and the mechanisms to enforce compliance have yet to be developed.

Summary

In conclusion, disruptive healthcare innovations, such as advancements not yet realized in simulation, have the potential to improve healthcare training and education for the next generations of healthcare providers. As such, courses in simulation pedagogy and technological literacy should become the golden standard in faculty development for simulation-based learning. Simulationists also need to educate learners so that they make the most of new technologies and maximize self-regulated learning. Learners need to develop both digital literacy and fluency. Nursing programs of the future will benefit from the complete overhauling of current pedagogical frameworks, teaching and learning methodologies, and the use of new disruptive innovations for experiential learning. There is urgency for healthcare agencies and regulators to understand the coming changes better—both the dangers and the value that can be gained from using technological innovations. Together, we need to strike a healthy balance between the use of nascent technological innovations for transformative learning and the ethical challenges that accompany them.

We took great enjoyment envisioning VIP-U and, in doing so, acknowledge the dire need for change in our sometimes antiquated educational and healthcare institutions.

We are dreamers, but we are also doers. It takes both people that believe in the power of innovation and those willing to dive in and give it a try. One thing we do know for sure is that our healthcare schools and institutions need to be places that set our learners' hearts on fire with a passion for being the best healthcare providers they can be. To make meaningful learning happen for students, simulationists everywhere must uncover what their learners care deeply about and want most to achieve. As educators and healthcare providers, our common point of unification is and always has been the patient and their family. As we forge head on into healthcare in this millennium, we need to remember what unites us—"keeping the patient at the centre of this redefinition gives us a profound sense of optimism about what changes can bring in terms of patient and health economic outcomes, truly innovative health and healthcare approaches, and fundamentally improved economics for the health system, companies, families, and individuals" (Elton & O'Riordan, 2016, pp. 196–197). Together, we can create powerful simulated clinically immersive learning opportunities to pursue the requisite knowledge, skills, and value sets needed to attain our collective goals.

We are now at a remarkable point of convergence in healthcare education—the place where we are letting go of old teaching pedagogy and methodologies to adopt new approaches that will disrupt and shake us up like never before. In the years ahead, we will shape a new reality for healthcare education. Long ago, we came to the realization that although simulation tools are powerfully disruptive technologies, the true revolution that has unfolded has been the transformation of educational practices. Simulation-based education is the catalyst that has deposed the sage on the stage to make way for relationship-, mastery-, and transformational-based learning. As a Simulation Champion, in which ways do you feel called to action? Right here and now, at this point in history, we are poised to impact and imprint the next generation of healthcare providers and systems like never before. We know that your chosen mission and vocation will bring you to a place where no man or woman has ever gone before!

To quote a famous futurist: "To infinity... and beyond!"—Buzz Lightyear

Glossary

We are pleased to be able to include a glossary with this book. We worked toward providing a cohesive taxonomy but were challenged to find a perfect fit between each term used in this book and the comprehensive resources provided by the *INACSL Standards of Best Practice: Simulation*^{SM} Glossary (INACSL Standards Committee, 2016) and the *Healthcare Simulation Dictionary* maintained by SSH (Lopreiato et al., 2016). We have, therefore, provided definitions of the terms that seemed most valuable to have on hand for quick reference and have referred the reader to these other resources when necessary. Both the INACSL Standards Glossary and the Healthcare Simulation Dictionary are available online and are living documents, so the reader would be well served to consult the most current version available:

- INACSL Glossary: INACSL Standards Committee. (2016). Standards of best practice: Simulation^{SM}: Simulation glossary. *Clinical Simulation in Nursing, 12*(S), S39–S47. Retrieved from http://www.nursingsimulation.org/issue/S1876-1399 (16)X0014-X
- SSH Dictionary: Lopreiato, J. O. (Ed.), Downing, D., Gammon, W., Lioce, L., Sittner, B., Slot, V., & Spain, A. E. (Associate Eds.); and the Terminology & Concepts Working Group. (2016). *Healthcare simulation dictionary*. Retrieved from http://www.ssih.org/dictionary

A

Accreditation Standards Established ideal or set of guidelines and associated criteria established by a professional accrediting agency, association, or other entity against which simulation and healthcare programs must demonstrate compliance (Accreditation Commission for Healthcare, n.d.; SSH, 2016).

Administration Administration involves determinative functions such as making key decisions, delegating authority, creating positions for people, creating objectives for transformation, and formulating crucial policies and enforcement of the same, for an organization or entity (Hartherly, 2011).

Adult Learning Theory Learning theory based on the andragogical learning principles of self-concept, learner experience, readiness to learn, orientation to learning, and motivation to learn (Knowles, 1984).

Advocacy/Inquiry See SSH Dictionary.

Allied Health (Professions) "Allied Health professionals are involved with the delivery of health or related services pertaining to the identification, evaluation and prevention of diseases and disorders; dietary and nutrition services; rehabilitation and health systems management" and may include dental hygienists, dietitians, medical technologists, occupational therapists, physical therapists, radiographers, respiratory therapists, and speech language pathologists (Association of Schools of Allied Health Professions, 2017, para. 1).

Anatomical Models Noninteractive, static anatomical parts of the body or the whole body that is used for education (e.g., heart model) (Centre of Excellence for Simulation Education and Innovation, 2016, para. 10).

Andragogy "Expands on pedagogy and refers to active, learner-focused education for people of all ages. It is based on learning principles that involve problem solving that is relevant to the learner's everyday experiences" (Meakim et al., 2013, p. S4).

Anxiety "A fear or nervousness about what might happen" (Merriam-Webster, 2016).

Applicability "One of several aspects of critical appraisal in research that evaluates the study subjects in comparison with the population to whom the evidence will be applied" (Melnyk & Fineout-Overholt, 2011, p. 107).

Assessment "Assessment is the process of obtaining information to use for making educational decisions" (Oermann, 2017, p. 4), and occurs at various points along a trajectory toward an established educational goal using various strategies to collect information about a given entity (E.g. learner, program, curriculum). See Evaluation; see INACSL Glossary.

Assessment, Formative See INACSL Glossary; see also Evaluation: Formative Evaluation.

Assessment, Summative See INACSL Glossary; see also Evaluation: Summative Evaluation.

Augmented Reality See SSH Dictionary.

Association Management Company "A firm of professionals who have expertise and specialized training in providing administrative services to trade associations, professional societies and educational foundation" (IMI Association Executives, 2016, para. 1).

Avatar See INACSL Glossary; see SSH Dictionary.

Aviation Safety Management Systems "A systematic approach to managing safety, including the necessary organizational structures, accountabilities, policies, and procedures" (International Civil Aviation Organization (CA), 2013, p. xii).

B

Benchmark(ing) "Process of seeking out and implementing best practices at best cost" (Ettorchi-Tardy, Levif, & Michel, 2012, 102).

Blog "A website containing a writer's or group of writers' own experiences, observations, opinions, etc., and often having images and links to other websites" (Dictionary.com, 2016).

Bloom's Taxonomy Set of three hierarchical models used to classify educational learning objectives into levels of complexity and specificity (Bloom, Englehart, Furst, Hill, & Krathwohl, 1956).

Boot Camp Approach to learning similar to military basic training that includes tasks designed to improve skills (Aebersold, 2017).

Bounded Team Teams composed of individuals in stable positions working independently with clearly defined rules and established boundaries, having well-defined tasks and a clear and solid presence within an organization (Hackman, 2011).

Briefing See Prebriefing; see SSH Dictionary.

Broadcast Simulation Use of telehealth links and two-way interactive video (e.g., Skype) to provide simulation experiences (Manhas, 2017).

Building Program Programs that describe the sequence in which tasks must be carried out so that a project (or part of a project) can be completed on time (Designing Buildings Wiki, 2016).

C

Call-Outs "Strategy used to communicate important or critical information in healthcare teams" (AHRQ, 2013, p. 10).

Certification The process through which an organization endorses an individual who meets certain established criteria and eligibility requirements (Australian Society for Simulation in Healthcare Simulation, 2012, p. 2).

Certified Healthcare Simulation Educator (CHSE, CHSE-Advanced) A specialist in the theory and practice of simulation education who has the responsibility for developing, managing, and/or implementing educational activities who has achieved certification designation through the Society for Simulation in Healthcare (SSH, 2017). An individual who has demonstrated expertise in simulation education, curriculum design, implementation, and evaluation through qualifications and years of experience. An expert is regarded in the community as an expert in simulation through years of experience or research expertise and often acts as a consultant or mentor for other individuals in the community (ASSH, 2012).

Certified Healthcare Simulation Operations Specialist (CHSOS) Formal professional recognition of specialized knowledge, skills, abilities, and accomplishments in simulation operations (SSH Committee on Certification, 2014).

Change Leadership Change leadership is a necessary solution for sustainable change that change management alone fails to accomplish (Wild & Foisy-Doll, 2017).

Change Management The continuous process of aligning an organization with its marketplace and processes—and aims to do so more responsively and efficiently than do its competitors (Kotter International, 2015).

Change Model A theoretical conceptual approach to understanding process and sustainability in transforming people, organizations, policy, practices, and knowledge/learning that can be created and recreated by employment of the selected model or approach.

Check-Backs "Using closed-loop communication to ensure that information conveyed by the sender is understood by the receiver as intended" (AHRQ, 2013, p. 11).

Classroom Simulation Use of various simulation typologies in the classroom (mannequins, standardized patients, actors or role-players, avatars, holograms, virtual reality) (Milner, 2017).

Clinical Judgement See INACSL Glossary.

Clinical Reasoning See INACSL Glossary.

Closed-Loop Communication "A type of communication in teams that ensures that information conveyed by the sender is understood by the receiver as intended" (AHRQ, 2013, p. 11).

Coaching See INACSL Glossary; see SSH Dictionary.

Cognitive Load Theory A theory that uses instructional design to reduce the total amount of mental effort being used in the working memory (Sweller, 1988).

Cognitive Overload Providing more information than the brain can process in short-term memory.

Complex Adaptive Systems A new worldview that is based on "new science" and strives to make sense in organizations out of chaos. Sense-making is about learning and adapting, and CASs are building blocks that become embedded and form a larger CAS (Wild & Foisy-Doll, 2017).

Competence See INACSL Glossary.

Competency-Based Education "System of instruction, assessment, grading, and academic reporting" that is "based on students demonstrating that they have learned the knowledge and skills they are expected to learn as they progress through their education through the use of learning standards to determine academic expectations and define 'competency' or 'proficiency' in a given course, subject area, or level [of learning]" (Great Schools Partnership, 2014, para. 1. (Also referred to as Competency-Based Learning)).

Competency-Based Program A program of study grounded in competency-based education. See Competency-Based Education.

Complexity Science Complexity science is the study of complex systems and their characteristics: how they are sustained and self-organized and how outcomes emerge. As complexity increases, predictability decreases (Wild & Foisy-Doll, 2017).

Computer-Based Simulation See INACSL Glossary; see SSH Dictionary.

Conceptual Fidelity See Fidelity, Conceptual; see SSH Dictionary.

Confederate See Embedded Actor; see Simulated Person; see SSH Dictionary (Wild & Foisy-Doll, 2017).

Conflict Resolution "The process of limiting the negative aspects of conflict while increasing the positive aspects of conflict… with an aim to enhance learning and group outcomes, including effectiveness or performance in organizational setting" (Afzalur Rahim, 2001, p. 208).

Constructivism See INACSL Glossary.

Crisis Resource Management A safety-oriented training approach to managing challenging situations in a healthcare setting. In CRM style training, the emphasis is on crisis resource management behaviors, such as developing effective teamwork skills including communication and effective management of available resources, rather than on medical/technical knowledge and/or skill (ASSH, 2012, p. 4).

Critical Thinking See INACSL Glossary.

Cue(ing) See Prompt; see SSH Dictionary.

Culture "The totality of socially transmitted behavioral patterns, arts, beliefs, values, and customs, life ways, and all other products of human work and thought characteristics of a population of people that guide their worldview and decision making… patterns are shared by most (but not all) members of a culture… is largely unconscious and has powerful influences on health and illness" (Giger et al., 2007, pp. 6–7).

Culture Bubbles Choosing to socialize with others from a similar or familiar background (Cleary, Walter, Siegfried, & Jackson, 2014).

Culture of Blame A culture where individuals are blamed that is still dominant and traditionally found in healthcare and that undoubtedly impairs the advancement of a culture of safety and ultimately diminishes patient safety (Khatri, Brown, & Hicks, 2009, see Secretive Culture).

Cultural Brokering "A healthcare intervention through which the professional increasingly uses cultural and health science knowledge and skills to negotiate with the client and the healthcare system for an effective, beneficial healthcare plan" (Wenger, 1995, as cited in Bronheim, 2011, p. 3).

Cultural Competence Cultural competence involves the nurse's focus on acquiring the requisite knowledge, skills, and attitudes to provide care to diverse populations to eliminate health disparities. It also involves the ongoing process of respecting differences, actively acquiring new knowledge and skills to fill gaps, and the understanding that others' personal beliefs and worldviews may differ from our own (Leininger, 2007).

Culture-Focused Simulation A simulation-based learning event created through the strategic integration of cultural experiences at all levels of the simulation curriculum so that students can gain comfort and acquire the requisite skills needed to interact capably with diverse patients and colleagues (Foronda, Swoboda, Bahreman, & Foisy-Doll, 2017).

Cultural Diversity "The differences in ethnic or racial classification and self-identification, tribal or clan affiliation, nationality, language, age, gender, sexual orientation, gender identity or expression, socioeconomic status, education, religion, spirituality, physical and intellectual abilities, personal appearance, and other factors that distinguish one group or individual from another" (Goode & Jackson, 2013a, p. 9).

Cultural Humility Cultural humility incorporates a lifelong commitment to self-evaluation and critique, to redressing the power imbalances in the physician–patient dynamic, and to developing mutually beneficial and nonpaternalistic partnerships with communities on behalf of individuals and defined populations (Tervalon & Murray-Garcia, 2013, p. 123).

Cultural Safety A standard in healthcare that first emerged in the late 1980s in New Zealand and has since been refined and embedded as a standard in healthcare education in the region and throughout the world. Unlike cultural competence, awareness, and sensitivity, "cultural safety is not about cultural practices of the nurse, but it is about engaging in a recognition of the social, economic, and political position of certain groups within society" (Nursing Council of New Zealand, 2005, p. 152).

Cultural Sensitivity Employing one's knowledge, consideration, understanding, respect, and tailoring after realizing awareness of self and others and encountering a diverse group or individual (Foronda, 2008).

Cultural Sensibility "A deliberate, proactive behavior by healthcare providers to examine cultural situations through thoughtful reasoning, responsiveness, and discreet actions" (Ellis Fletcher, 2015, p. 3).

Cynefin Model Decision-making, analytic framework, and a sense-making model comparing four system types (or domains) being: simple, complicated, complex, and chaotic. This model recognizes the causal differences that exist between different types of systems, providing agility to move between systems and to choose a decision method that is most appropriate for each system type (Cognitive Edge, 2015).

D

Debrief(ing) See SSH Dictionary.

Delegation The act of delegating or handing off a clear and well-documented process when both the delegator and the delegate acknowledge and adhere to their respective responsibilities (Nursing Management, 2011).

Deliberate Practice See SSH Dictionary.

Design Build Design build, or D-B, is a project-based method of designing and building used in the construction industry. Within D-B, all design and construction services are delivered by one contractor, known as a design-build contractor who serves as a single point of contact for the entire project, to minimize risks and deliver projects on time (Design-Build Institute of America, 2016).

Disclosure of Error Error disclosure involves being honest about what happened, explicitly stating that an error occurred, and explaining to the patient any specific information that might be helpful in terms of necessary follow-up (Kalra, 2011).

Disruptive Innovation Theory "A theory that explains the phenomenon by which an innovation transforms an existing market or sector by introducing simplicity, convenience, accessibility, and affordability where complication and high cost are the status quo, for example the personal computer" (Christenson Institute, 2016, para. 2).

Distributed Learning (Simulation) See In Situ; see SSH Dictionary.

Distributed/Dispersed or Virtual Team Teams that are not in the same geographical location, do not need to engage in real time, nor need to coact simultaneously (Daft, 2012).

Distributive Justice "The apportionment of privileges, duties, and goods in consonance… with the merits of the individual and in the best interest of society [the global society]" (Merriam-Webster Dictionary, n.d.).

Drama Triangle A model depicting complex human interactions and entanglements that unfold in conflict situations that represents the "all-too-familiar three-sided way we sabotage relationships" (Karpman, 2014, p. 15).

E

e-Patient "individuals who are equipped, enabled, empowered and engaged in their health and healthcare decisions… as part of an equal partnership between the e-patient and health professionals and systems that support them" (ePatients.net., 2014, para. 1).

Early Adopter Person who adopts an innovation after a varying degree of time that is significantly longer than the innovators (Rogers, 1962).

Emotional Intelligence A group of competencies that influence our ability to respond to others and manage our own feelings (Goleman, 2006).

Embedded Actor (Participant) See Confederate; see Simulated Person; see SSH Dictionary.

Equity "The absence of avoidable or remediable differences among groups of people, whether those groups are defined socially, economically, demographically, or geographically" (World Health Organization, 2015, para 1).

Error Tracking A systematic integrated process whereby medical errors or healthcare incidents are recorded, tracked, and analyzed. Reports generated from error tracking can show trending and be a source of improved patient safety (AHRQ, 2016).

Ethical Workspace A work environment where coworkers make a commitment to supportive colleagueship, and refuse to get caught up in workplace negativism (Turnbull, 2003).

Executive Sponsorship An individual or team of individuals that possess a solid understanding of simulation-based education and that work to make things happen. These individuals will go to bat for you at board meetings, influence agendas at top levels, secure funding, engage other institutions, and have your back by supporting the simulation project at every opportunity (Wild & Foisy-Doll, 2017).

Expertise Special skill or knowledge in a particular field (Merriam-Webster, 2016).

Expert Modeling "A technique by which an expert demonstrates the procedure in its entirety and then may break down the procedure into its components" (Cheng & Grant, 2016, p. 13).

Evaluation Evaluation is the process of making a judgement as to overall value, merit, and worth of a given entity based on the assessment information collected. "While assessment is the process of obtaining information, when judgements are made about value and worth, the process has extended to evaluation" (Oermann, 2017, p. 4). See Assessment; see INACSL Glossary.

Evaluation, Formative See Assessment, Formative; see INACSL Glossary Formative Evaluation.

Evaluation, High-Stakes See Assessment, High-Stakes; see INACSL Glossary.

Evaluation, Summative See Assessment, Summative; see INACSL Glossary.

Event Flow Event flow is a sequential account and schedule (and often visual depiction) of a simulation event that features the flow of participants through the various stages of the simulation. It usually comprises the number of rooms, number of students, total length of time, breakdown of timing, repetition of the simulation, length of prebriefing, simulation event, debriefing and turnaround time between events.

Evidence-Based Practice Evidence-based practice (EBP) is a problem-solving approach to the delivery of healthcare that integrates the best evidence from studies and patient care data with clinician expertise and patient preferences and values. When

delivered in a context of caring and in a supportive organizational culture, the highest quality of care and best patient outcomes can be achieved (Melnyk & Fineout-Overholt, 2015).

F

Facilitation See INACSL Glossary.

Facilitator See INACSL Glossary; see SSH Dictionary.

Faculty Development Systematic effort to improve faculty skills in the following areas: "(1) educational skills, (2) leadership skills, (3) skills necessary to engage in scholarly activities, (4) personal development, and (5) skills in designing and implementing a professional development plan" (Florida State University, 2016, para 1).

Family-Centered Care "Patient- and family-centered care is an approach to the planning, delivery, and evaluation of healthcare that is grounded in mutually beneficial partnerships among healthcare providers, patients, and families" (The Institute for Patient- and Family-Centered Care, 2010, para 1).

Fellowship "Short-term opportunities lasting from a few months to several years that focus on the professional development of the fellows and are sponsored by a specific association or organization seeking to expand leadership in their field" (Berkley Career Center, 2016, para 1).

Fiction Contract See INACSL Glossary; see SSH Dictionary.

Fidelity See Realism; see INACSL Glossary; see SSH Dictionary (Fidelity, Low-Fidelity, High-Fidelity Simulator, High-Fidelity Simulation, Simulation Fidelity).

Fidelity, Conceptual See INACSL Glossary; see SSH Dictionary Conceptual Fidelity.

Fidelity, Environmental See INACSL Glossary; see SSH Dictionary Environmental Fidelity.

Fidelity, Physical See INACSL Glossary; see SSH Dictionary Physical Fidelity.

Fidelity, Psychological See INACSL Glossary; see SSH Dictionary Psychological Fidelity.

Fee Schedule "A pricing schedule [in a Simulation Program] that shows the dollar amounts charged for various course, workshops, and other activities" (Jamal, Walling, & Arnold, 2015, p. 293).

Flexible Glass "Bendable glass that's thinner than a human hair" (Bourzac, 2016, para. 1).

Fellowship An academic scholarly endeavor that furthers knowledge, skills, and attitudes in a particular field of study, for example, INACSL Fellowship. Fellowships can be specific academic positions that focus on postgraduate research work.

Followership Is the deliberate understanding of styles, behaviors, and characteristics that create understanding about the relationship among followers and leaders. As a new modern theory, it challenges the thinking and the importance of the relationship between leader and follower roles and the human potential in organizations and relationships (Hurwitz & Hurwitz, 2015; Kellerman, 2008, 2014; Kelly, 2008).

Functional Program Articulates client philosophy, vision and mission, and goals, services provided/desired, activities, workloads, people and staff, major equipment, space relationships, grouping of spaces, space requirements, details room specs, and sometimes a delivery schedule, financial projections, budgets, project delivery methods, and site evaluation Also known as design briefs, facilities programs, architectural programs, space programs, space needs analysis, owner's statement of requirements, or output specifications (Saly, 2010).

G

Games (Serious) See SSH Dictionary.

General Operations Pertaining to the logistics of managing the day-in and day-out functions that exist within simulation programs (Foisy-Doll, 2017).

Global Citizen(ship) Responsibility of world citizens that goes beyond the local and national arena, given that some actions impact the planet as a whole, thus creating demand for global responsibility (Mill, Astle, Ogilvie, & Gastaldo, 2010).

Global Health "An area for study, research, and practice that places a priority on improving health and achieving equity in health for all people worldwide" (Koplan et al., 1995).

Globalization(-ism) The worldwide integration of economic and financial sectors, which was made possible by three crucial developments: technical progress, geopolitical changes, and the dominant ideology of regulation of the market (Hiershfield, 2008).

Grant Writing Grant writing involves completion of a proposal designed to fit the priorities and structured guidelines of the funding source (see Chapter 18).

Group A collection of "individuals who happen to be taking up the same space but each going in his or her own direction and working relatively independently of one another with little collaboration" (Bendaly & Bendaly, 2012, p. 14).

Guidelines, Simulation See SSH Dictionary.

Guided Reflection See SSH Dictionary.

H

Haptics (Device) See INACSL Glossary; see SSH Dictionary.

Health Hackers "Groups of amateurs and citizen scientists, using the Internet to connect with other patients, run experiments, and conduct clinical trials on their own diseases" (Bottles, 2013, p. 88).

Hacking Health Communities Organized groups that aim to transform healthcare by connecting healthcare professionals with designers, developers, innovators, and entrepreneurs to build realistic, human-centric solutions to frontline healthcare problems. We believe that innovation is fueled by diverse minds and perspectives (Hacking Health, n.d., para. 1).

Hardware The space, equipment, and other physical resources like simulators, computers and related components, integrated AV/IT systems, medical equipment, consumable supplies, etc., needed to operationalize a simulation program (Cornele & Leland, 2010).

Head-Mounted Display (HMD) Gear that is worn on the head that is fed imagery data provided by a camera, computer, or video source (Charara, 2016).

Health Disparities "A particular type of health difference that is closely linked with social or economic disadvantage and adversely affect groups of people who have systematically experienced greater social or economic obstacles to health" based on any factors or characteristics "historically linked to discrimination or exclusion" (The Secretary's Advisory Committee on National Health Promotion and Disease Prevention, 2008, p. 28).

Health Education Technologies (Health EdTech) "The study and ethical practice of facilitating learning and improving performance [in healthcare] by creating, using, and managing appropriate technological processes and resources" (Robinson, Molenda, & Rezabek, 2008, p. 15).

Healthcare Simulation See SSH Dictionary.

Hidden Curriculum What students learn in the hallways, in lecture theaters after class, in the cafeteria, and even includes such factors as architecture and the physical layout of the learning space (O'Donnell, 2014).

High-Acuity Low-Occurrence Clinical Events (HALO) Situations in healthcare that arise infrequently but still require a high level of cognitive and technical competency as well as mental preparedness (Mileder, Urlesberger, Szyld, Roehr, & Schmölzer, 2014, p. 263).

High-Fidelity Simulation See SSH Dictionary.

High-Fidelity Simulator See SSH Dictionary.

High-Performing Team A team marked by strong cohesion, open communication, and flexibility to change that is heavily invested in cocreating a healthy team climate through interdependence, shared leadership, and a unified commitment to goals (Bendaly et al., 2012).

High-Risk Industry Business or other organization that carries the potential for catastrophic events causing multiple fatalities. Healthcare and healthcare organizations carry "high risk with high numbers of employees, high degree of interdependence, complex technology, and extensive regulations are very complex" (Healthcare Insurance Reciprocal of Canada (HIROC), 2014, p. 3).

Hologram "A three-dimensional image reproduced from a pattern of interference produced by a split coherent beam of radiation (as a laser)" (Merriamwebster.com, 2017).

Human Capital Management Attracting and engaging highly talented people, developing global leaders, improving and sharing new skills, and keeping people aligned and working together in a highly connected way (Bersin, 2013).

Hybrid Simulation See INACSL Glossary; see SSH Dictionary.

I

Impact Factor Measures how often an "average article" in a journal was cited during a given year or period. "The annual Journal Citation Report impact factor is a ratio between citations and recent citable items published. Thus, the impact factor of a journal is calculated by dividing the number of current year citations to the source items published in that journal during the previous two years" (Clarivate Analytics, Reuters, 1994 as cited in Clarivate Analytics, 2017, para. 3).

Imposter Syndrome When surrounded by professional peers, the feeling that one doesn't belong (not at comparable level or skill).

Income (Low, Low-Mid, Mid, High) High-income countries has have an annual per capita income of >= $12,475 USD, mid-income $4,036-12,475 USD, and lower-middle income between $1,026-4,035 USD, and low income <= 1,025 USD (World Bank, 2017).

In Situ Simulation See INACSL Glossary; see SSH Dictionary.

Innovator The group that is the first to try new ideas, processes, foods, and services (Rogers, 2003).

I PASS the Baton *(also referred to as IPASS)* Strategy designed to enhance information exchange during transitions in care that delivers information for introductions, patients, assessments, situation, safety concerns, background, actions, timing, ownership, and next actions (AHRQ, 2013, p. 13).

Intercultural Interaction between two or more different cultures.

Integrated Data Management "A strategic initiative to deliver an integrated, yet modular, data management environment to design, develop, deploy, operate, optimize and govern data, databases, and data-driven applications throughout the entire data management lifecycle" (Hayes, 2010, para. 1).

Interprofessional Collaboration (IPC) "The process of developing and maintaining effective interprofessional working relationships with learners, practitioners, patients/clients/ families and communities to enable optimal health outcomes. Elements of collaboration include respect, trust, shared decision making, and partnerships" (Canadian Interprofessional Health Collaborative National Competency Framework (CIHC), 2010, p. 8).

Interprofessional Education (IPE) See Simulation-Enhanced Interprofessional Education; see INACSL Glossary; see SSH Dictionary.

Interprofessional Team Training In simulation, educational training programs where teams from across varied healthcare practice disciplines collaborate to provide care to simulated patients.

Introspection One's ability to look inside oneself and one's experiences (Kouzes & Posner, 2012).

Inventory Management Activities employed in maintaining the optimum number or amount of each inventory item to provide uninterrupted production, sales, and/or customer service at a minimum cost (Businessdictionary.com).

J

Just Culture A culture in which underlying behavioral patterns and causes of error are examined as opposed to only looking at the consequences of error for the purpose of promoting system change, rather than focusing on penalizing individuals (Reason, 2000).

Just in Time Training See SSH Dictionary.

K

Kirkpatrick's Educational Outcomes Four-step evaluation framework including reaction, learning, behavior, and results (Kirkpatrick, 1994). Commonly used to evaluate learning, behavior change, and implications for clinical practice change.

Kolb's Experiential Learning Theory See Experiential Learning Theory.

L

Leader A person that influences followers, produces a vision and commitment, and contributes to self and others and planetary health (Grossman & Valiga, 2009; Kouzes & Pozner, 2014).

Leadership Complex multifaceted learned intentional phenomenon engaged in by a leader to influence followers, produce a vision and commitment, and contribute to self, others, and planetary health (Grossman & Valiga, 2009; Kouzes & Posner, 2014).

Leadership Development The act of expanding the capacity of individuals to perform in leadership roles. To facilitate the learning of leadership competencies in others to be able to "influence followers, produce a vision and commitment; and contribute to self, others and planetary health" (Grossman & Valiga, 2009; Kouzes & Posner, 2014).

Learning Paradigm Learning theories are grounded in varying paradigms or frameworks containing basic assumptions on the process of learning. The most common are behaviorism, cognitivism, humanism, constructivism, and connectivism, all of which can be related simulation-based learning (Learning Paradigms, 2013; http://www.learning-theories.org/doku.php?id=learning_paradigms).

Learning Resource Center Also called Skills Resource Center. A facility within a school that houses learning resources. In healthcare, this facility commonly mimics acute care hospital environments for training purposes.

Learning Theory Interrelated concepts that represent a phenomenon (Powers & Knapp, 2011) and convey meaning. The concepts form a framework that can then be used to study and explain behaviors and phenomenon, such as learning.

Lifesaver See INACSL Glossary: Life Saver.

Linguistic Competence An organization's capacity, based on "its policy, structures, practices, procedures" and its personnel, "to communicate effectively, and convey information in a manner that is easily understood by diverse groups including persons of limited English proficiency, those who have low literacy skills or are not literate, [and] individuals with disabilities" (Goode and Jones, 2009).

Low-Fidelity Simulators "usually provide for simple, gross movements without joint movement... Best used for the instruction of psychomotor skills" (Nehring, Ellis, & Lashley, 2001, p. 15).

M

Management Is the science of organizationally understanding the operational needs of a work unit to produce desired outcomes characterized traditionally by the functions of planning, organizing, commanding, controlling, and coordinating and by a sixth function of leading (Marquis & Huston, 2012, p. 8).

Manager Those charged with executing the plans of administrators by implementing these plans and frameworks at various levels within the organization.

Mannequin (Manikin) See SSH Dictionary.

Mannequin (Manikin)-Based Simulation See SSH Dictionary.

Mastery Learning See SSH Dictionary.

Medical Error An act of commission (doing something wrong) or omission (failing to do the right thing) [by healthcare providers] that leads to an undesirable outcome or significant potential for such an outcome (AHRQ, 2016, para. 5).

Metrics "The standards of measurement by which efficiency, performance, progress, or quality of a plan, process, or product can be assessed" (http://www.businessdictionary.com/definition/metrics.html).

Mid-Fidelity Simulators Moderate (midlevel) fidelity experiences that are more technologically sophisticated, such as computer-based, self-directed learning systems simulations in which the participant relies on a two-dimensional focused experience to problem-solve, perform a skill, and make decisions or the use of more realistic manikins having breath sounds, heart sounds, and/or pulses (also called intermediate fidelity; NLN-SIRC, 2017).

Mission Mission statements focus on the present, offering a snapshot of today. In a nutshell, a mission statement describes the core purpose of the organization, or what it does, and then how they do it, why they do it, and those who are served by the organization (Businessdictionary.com, 2017, para. 1).

Mixed Reality A blend of virtual and augmented reality where real objects can be used to view many dimensions of the virtual world, such as a wall or tabletop surface used to display virtual imagery (Ridley, 2013).

Mobile Simulation See SSH Dictionary.

Modality Delivery model used to implement various typologies of simulation, chosen to best support learning objectives while using available resources; see INACSL Glossary; see SSH Dictionary.

Moral Courage "The bridge between talking ethics and doing ethics" (Kidder, 2005, p. 6).

Motivation (Intrinsic and Extrinsic) Internal (intrinsic) and external (extrinsic) factors that stimulate desire and energy in people to be continually interested and committed to a job, role or subject, or to make an effort to attain a goal (Businessdictionary. com).

Moulage See INACSL Glossary; see SSH Dictionary.

Multidisciplinary See SSH Dictionary.

N

Networking Developing and using contacts for business purposes beyond the initial reason for contact, that is, networking with colleagues you meet at a conference or online.

New Science of Leadership A phrase that refers to concepts used in forming relationships and connections with others that challenge "old ways of doing things." Margaret Wheatley (2006) interprets quantum physics, biology, and chaos theory as organizing constructs to create a paradigm shift or new worldview of an emerging global understanding within the 21st century for leadership (Wild & Foisy-Doll, 2017).

Neocolonialism "All forms of control of prior colonies or populations, such as Indigenous people who continue to live under conditions of internal colonialism" (Reimer, Kirkham, & Brown, 2006, p. 334).

NLN/Jeffries Simulation Theory Theory evolved from the original simulation framework; includes the constructs of context, background, design, simulation experience, and outcomes (Jeffries, 2015).

O

Operating Budget "Combination of known expenses, expected future costs, and forecasted income over the course of a year. Operating budgets are completed in advance of the accounting period, which is why they require estimated expenses and revenues" (Bradford, 2017, para. 1).

Organizational Chart "Visual representation of how a firm intends authority, responsibility, and information to flow within its formal organizational structure" (Businessdictionary.com, para. 1).

Organizational Climate The feeling or social atmosphere within a group (Schein, 2010; Schneider & Barbera, 2014).

Organizational Culture "Both a here and now dynamic phenomenon in organizations that is constantly enacted and reenacted, created by our interactions with others and shaped by our own behavior" (Schein, 2009, p. 3). It is difficult to articulate, is difficult to pin down and lurks in hidden places like in the "mindsets and frames" [of employees]… "and are powerful in their impact but invisible, and to a considerable degree unconscious" (Schein, 2010, p. 14).

Objective Structured Clinical Examination (OSCE) See SSH Dictionary.

Outrospection The ability to look outside yourself and your experiences (Kouzes & Posner, 2012).

P

Participant See INACSL Glossary; see SSH Dictionary.

Participant Integrity Upholding professional integrity when working with simulation participants, including "confidentiality, compassion, honesty, commitment, collaboration, mutual respect, and engagement in the learning process" (INACSL Standards Committee, 2016, Professional Integrity, p. S30).

Patient Safety "A discipline in the healthcare professions that applies safety science methods toward the goal of achieving a trustworthy system of healthcare delivery." Can also be "an attribute of healthcare systems that minimizes the incidence and impact of adverse events and maximizes recovery from such events" (Emanuel et al., 2008, p. 1).

Patient Volunteers Use of students, alumna, and others who volunteer to be trained to perform a role in a simulation experience.

Peer Learning Learning occurs through interaction with those a person considers to be of equal skill or ability.

Perseverance The day-to-day decision to not give up. It is about committing to see things as they are, as they could be, and working with focused intention to make them what they should be (Wheatley, 2010).

Person-Centered Care Patient- and family-centered care is an approach to the planning, delivery, and evaluation of healthcare that is grounded in mutually beneficial partnerships among healthcare providers, patients, and families (The Institute for Patient- and Family-Centered Care, 2010, para. 1).

Photovoltaic Glass "A technology that enables the conversion of light into electricity through glass that incorporates transparent semiconductor-based photovoltaic cells that are sandwiched between two sheets of glass" (Whatis.com., 2016, para. 1–2).

PICOT Question A method of questioning within the PICOT model used to develop a specific clinical research question structured around (P) patient population, (I) intervention or issue of interest, (C) comparison, (O) outcome, and (T) time.

Plastinate Dissected bodies undergo a lengthy process called plastination that preserves the body in its current position and hardens it so that it can be touched or observed in its motion. Individual organs, bones, and tissues can also undergo plastination so that numerous students can handle the material without it deteriorating (Von Hagens Plastination, 2016).

Policy A course or principle of action adopted or proposed (Oxford Concise Dictionary).

Postcolonialism The period that followed the Colonial Era specifically took root in the late 14th century during an age when Europeans set sail to conquer and build settlements in other worlds. These voyages by explorers and merchants involved the deliberative process of shaping the belief of Indigenous peoples to one that saw white Europeans as superior to themselves (Ertan, Putterman, & Fiszbein, 2012).

Prebrief(ing) See INACSL Glossary; see SSH Dictionary.

Procedure The processes that are needed to comply with a given policy.

Procedural Simulation See INACSL Glossary; see SSH Dictionary.

Professional Integrity See INACSL Glossary.

Program Evaluation "A process used to create information for planning, designing, implementing and assessing the results of our efforts to address and solve problems " (McDavid, Huse, and Hawthorn, 2013, p. 3).

Program of Research Planned progression of study in a researcher's area of interest that builds from prior or current work.

Programmatic Assessment "An integral approach to the design of an assessment program with the intent to optimize its learning function, its decision-making function and its curriculum quality-assurance function" (Van Der Vleuten, Schuwirth, Driessen, Govaerts, & Heeneman, 2015, p. 641).

Project Management A staged process of engaging, planning, implementing, monitoring, and sustaining a desired change or strategy through work tasks and groups to accomplish an immediate desired task or goal or outcome.

Prompt See Cue; see INACSL Glossary.

Psychological Safety See SSH Dictionary.

R

Realism See Fidelity; see SSH Dictionary.

Reconciliation A multistage, delicate, and intricate process that aims to consolidate peace and centers around an acknowledgment and acceptance of past wounds and wrongs with a dedication to renewed peaceful coexistence (Truth and Reconciliation Commission of Canada, 2015).

Reflection See INACSL Glossary; see SSH Dictionary Reflective Thinking.

Reflection in Action Learners assess their actions in real time, adjusting their plan of care concurrently.

Reflection on Action Occurs during debriefing following a scenario; reinforces formation of new cognitive models. Allows learners to examine a scenario as a whole to understand why actions were taken and the knowledge, assumptions, values, beliefs, and feelings behind the actions (Friere, 2000; NLN, 2015).

Reflexivity A domain of knowing where the influence of past experience on the present is made known and further understood (Johns, 2013). Reflexivity is related to deep mindfulness where assumptions and values and beliefs are challenged/transformed and more clearly understood within a present situation and the past is made more intentionally clear. It is about critical reflection (Horton-Deuthsch & Sherwood, 2012; Sherwood & Horton-Deutsch, 2015) and the intentional use of critical thinking and critical reflection for critical action that is required in learning organizations for safety and risk management and for lifelong learning.

Reliability See INACSL Glossary; see SSH Dictionary Simulation Reliability.

Reports (in Simulation Programs) All required documented information used to chart progress status and outcomes and to inform decisions about general operations, educational operations, technical operations, and human capital management.

Research Funding Money, typically in the form of grants or scholarships, that supports research studies.

Return on Investment (ROI) A measure that demonstrates investment outcomes within an organization (Rundio, 2016).

Return on Expectations (ROE) The practitioner's approach to creating and demonstrating the organizational value of training and the degree to which their expectations have been satisfied (Kirkpatrick Partners, 2016, para. 1; Kirkpatrick & Kirkpatrick, 2010).

S

Safe Container An environment that allows learners to face professionally meaningful challenges where they are held to high standards in a way that engages them but does not intimidate or humiliate them (Rudolph, Simon, & Raemer, 2015).

SBAR (Situation, Background, Assessment, Recommendation) A technique for communicating critical information that requires immediate attention and action concerning a patient's condition (AHRQ, 2013, p. 9).

Scenario See INACSL Glossary; see SSH Dictionary.

Scientific Rigor Degree of adherence to the rules and expectations required when designing, implementing, and evaluating outcomes of research.

Script See SSH Dictionary.

Second Life Virtual teaching/learning environment where participants interact using avatars.

Secretive Culture A culture where trust at all levels of the organization is low and when mistakes or latent failures are known but remain hidden or not verbalized and where evaluation of events relies exclusively on data from operational reports and punishment for mistakes follows swiftly (Patankar, Brown, Sabin, & Bigda-Peyton, 2012).

Self-Managed Team A team of between 5 and 20 highly motivated and skilled individuals that ideally do not require a manager and take responsibility for decision-making, expending dollars, adding new members, monitoring performance, problem-solving, adapting to change, and working toward goal attainment as they deem appropriate (Daft, 2012).

SimOps (Specialist) See Simulator Technician; See SSH Dictionary: Operations Specialist.

Simulated Patient See Standardized Patient; see INACSL Glossary; see SSH Dictionary.

Simulated Person See Confederate; see Embedded Actor; see SSH Dictionary.

Simulation See INACSL Glossary; see SSH Dictionary.

Simulation-Based Learning (Training) Experience See INACSL Glossary Simulation-Based Experience(s); see SSH Dictionary: Simulated-Based Learning Experience.

Simulation-Based Learning Environment See Simulation Learning Spaces; see SSH Dictionary.

Simulation Centre (or Center) A physical purpose-build space, created in an actual building, mobile unit, or virtual world in which simulation-based learning is enacted.

Simulation Champions All past, present, and future courageous, caring, and connected leaders, followers, and managers that come together from many backgrounds, disciplines, and industries to drive the advancement of simulation around the world.

Simulation-Enhanced-IPE (Sim-IPE) See Interprofessional Education; see INACSL Glossary; see SSH Dictionary.

Simulated Clinical Immersion See INACSL Glossary; see SSH Dictionary Immersive Simulation.

Simulation Learning Spaces See Simulation-Based Learning Environment.

Simulation Program "An organization or group with dedicated resources (personnel and equipment) whose mission is specifically targeted toward improving patient safety and outcomes through assessment, research, advocacy, and education using simulation technologies and methodologies" (SSH Accreditation Process, 2014, p. 5).

Simulation Research Systematic investigation into various features of simulation to determine overall effectiveness in education and practice environments.

Simulation Researcher A person that conducts and implements a research strategy.... the researcher plans and conducts experiments to increase the body of scientific knowledge on simulation related topics. They may also aim to develop or improve existing processes in simulation or provide a new body of evidence for different aspects of simulation (ASSH, 2012, p. 14).

Simulator See SSH Dictionary.

Simulator Technician See SimOps; see SSH Dictionary: Operations Specialist.

Simulation Delivery Team Team of individuals possessing the educational and operational competencies required to design, deploy, and evaluate quality, evidence-based simulation-based learning.

Simulationist See SSH Dictionary.

Situational Awareness/Monitoring See SSH Dictionary: Situational Awareness.

Smart Glasses A pair of glasses that look like ordinary glasses but contain specialized polarized lenses that allow the wearer to see two images, one per each eye, giving the illusion of depth (Charara, 2016).

SOAR (Strengths, Opportunities, Aspirations, and Results) A systematic approach to conducting a needs assessment that examines an organization's strengths, opportunities, aspirations, and results (Stavros & Hinrichs, 2007).

Social Responsibility "Responsibility that is extended from individuals to groups and communities, but also from private to public institutions and corporations, inasmuch as the latter share the same scope of activities and produce effects that are potentially beneficial or harmful for workers, suppliers, customers, other concerned persons or the environment" (UNESCO, 2010, p. 19).

Soft Skills Also referred to as nontechnical skills. Core cognitive and behavioral factors in healthcare, categorized as situational awareness, decision-making, communications skills, teamwork, stress management, fatigue management, and leadership (Karate, Ross, Anderson, & Flin, 2012).

Software The intangible components of computer systems or operations systems like a computer operating system (Gantt & Young, 2016) and management products and procedures (Cornele & Leland, 2010).

Standards of Best Practice A set of established levels of quality developed through rigorous methodology that provide individuals with terminology, rationale, outcomes, criteria, and guidelines based on evidence-based best practices (Rutherford-Hemming Lioce, & Durham, 2015); see SSH Dictionary Simulation Standard.

Standardized Patient See Simulated Patient; see SSH Dictionary.

Static Mannequin Passive full-body mannequin that represents different stages of the lifespan and has exchangeable parts (e.g., wounds, genitalia).

Strategic Plan(ning) A document that is the end result of strategic planning, which is a long-range organizational planning process that is "deliberate, premeditated, and intentional" ...and focuses on "purpose, mission, philosophy, and goals related to the external environment" (Marquis & Huston, 2012, p.101).

Subject Matter Expert (SME) A person with extensive experience and knowledge in a particular subject area, who acts as a consultant and content expert during development of a course (ASSH, 2012, p. 16).

Superdiversity A term intended to capture a level and kind of complexity surpassing anything many migrant-receiving countries have ever experienced in the history of the world (Vertovec, 2010).

SWOT (Strengths, Weaknesses, Opportunities, Threats) A systematic approach to conducting a needs assessment that examines an organization's strengths, weaknesses, opportunities, and threats.

Systems Approach A method of problem solving that "seeks to identify situations or factors likely to give rise to human error, and change the underlying systems of care in order to reduce the occurrence of errors or minimize their impact on patients" (AHRQ, 2015, para. 2). See Systems Integration; See SSH Dictionary.

T

Task Trainer See SSH Dictionary.

Team "A unit of two or more people who interact and coordinate their work to accomplish a common goal to which they are committed and themselves mutually accountable" (Daft, 2012, p. 597).

Team Assessment Observations of team progress related to knowledge, skills, and attitudes related to context, composition, competencies, and change management practices used to improve future team outcomes (Dyer, Dyer, & Dyer, 2013).

Technical Operations Technical operations involves managing a host of informational technology (IT) and audio visual (AV) systems with the program (Gantt & Young, 2016).

Time-Based Program Educational programs that require that learners be physically present in a classroom or skills lab for pre-established periods of time on task or topic to become competent (e.g., 120 hours of lecture, 60 hours skills labs, 100 hours practicum) (Gruppen, Rajesh, Mangrulkar, & Kolars, 2012).

Telesimulation See Broadcast Simulation.

Think Like a Nurse Using clinical reasoning, diagnostic reasoning, critical thinking, nursing process, evidence-based practice, ethical reasoning, and systems thinking to make judgements as a nurse and not as a student (Tanner, 2006).

Total Quality Improvement The extent to which discipline has been ingrained as a way of life through a core commitment to continuous improvement in organizations (Rampersad & El Homsi, 2007).

Touch-Sensitive Interactive Glass Display Systems A computer-based display screen that is also an input device and is sensitive to pressure from a user's touch (WhatsIt.com, 2017).

Transactional Leadership A leadership style or theory first defined by Burns in 1978 that considers an exchange between leader and follower often with an inherent reward/punishment component. Transactional is synonymous with managerial functions as opposed to what Burns defined/described as transforming or appealing to higher order values or motives (Wild & Foisy-Doll, 2017).

Transcendent Leadership A leadership theory for the 21st century that encompasses leadership of self, others, and the world or planet (Crossan & Mazutis, 2008) with a strong focus on both stewardship and transformation (Gardiner, 2009). Transcendent leadership encompasses the foundational value-based principles of servant and transformational leadership theories in response to a social change or healthy world agenda (Wild & Foisy-Doll, 2017).

Transcultural (Nursing) How the nursing profession interacts with the concept of culture. Relating to or involving more than one culture; cross-cultural.

Transformational Leadership A leadership theory and style developed by Bernard Bass (1995) and characterized by how the leader transforms or changes subordinates or followers by focusing followers on task importance and value; on organizational versus personal goals; and on their higher-order needs. Transformational leadership eventually was termed authentic transformational leadership theory (Bass, 1999) based on four components of idealized influence; intellectual stimulation, inspirational motivation and individualized consideration, plus the moral character and ethical values displayed by the leader, and the morality of the collective process (Bass, 1995). Today Kouzes and Posner (2007, 2014) describe five exemplary practices of transformational leadership and leaders that describe what leaders are doing when they are at their best. The critical features of transformational over the preceding leadership theories are the focus on morality and ethical value-based actions and beliefs.

Transformational Change A transformation that occurs over time with iterative [impactful] changes being sustained and spread across the organization (Lucas et al., 2007), and that become embedded in organizational culture and climate (Schein, 2009).

Transition Shock A rocky period in adaptation, can often occur after the excitement of relocation wanes (Clearly et al., 2014). Foreign workers suffering intense homesickness and feelings of isolation.

Typology Classification of simulation methods (e.g., mannequins, virtual reality); not to be confused with modality, the way in which the typologies are used. See SSH Dictionary.

U

Ubuntu An African philosophical expression and worldview that when translated means "I am because you are." "In essence, you can't be human all by yourself, and when you have this quality—Ubuntu—you are known for your generosity" (Tutu Foundation, 2015, para. 1).

Unbounded Team Teams that are characterized by fluid boundaries and members, such as with shift workers in healthcare teams (Hackman, 2011).

V

Validity See INACSL Glossary; see SSH Dictionary: Simulation Validity.

Value Based A term used to define the ethical principles and beliefs that govern a group or individuals in practice and decision-making. Ethical behavior is of a higher order and distinct from moral behavior (Knights & O'Leary, 2006). The term value-based leadership refers to the highest standards of ethical behavior in leaders and in leadership.

Virtual Conference A conference that is delivered using virtual platforms, for which attendees do not have to travel to fixed destinations and can be full virtual participants.

Virtual Learning Environment See SSH Dictionary.

Virtual Reality See INACSL Glossary; see SSH Dictionary: Virtual Reality, Virtual Reality Simulation, Virtual Simulation.

Virtual Patient See SSH Dictionary.

Vision A look to the future that corresponds to a vision statement in organizations providing a description of what an organization, person, technology, etc., hopes to become.

W

Wearable Technology Computers that are worn virtually anywhere on the body (phones, watches, rings, glasses, etc.). They contain smart sensors, and make use of a web connection, usually using Bluetooth to connect wirelessly to a smartphone app. (Digital Trends, 2017). In simulation, wearable glasses are used for augmented reality (http://www.digitaltrends.com/wearables/).

References

Abdellah, F. (1960). *Patient-centered approaches to nursing.* New York, NY: Macmillan Company.

Aboriginal Healing Foundation. (2002). *The healing has begun.* Retrieved from http://www.ahf.ca/downloads/the-healing-has-begun.pdf

Accreditation Commission for Healthcare (ACHC). (n.d.). *ACHA accreditation standards: Accreditation guide to success workbook.* Retrieved from http://achc.org/docs/default-document-library/achc_accredguidetosuccessworkbook_sample_pharmacy.pdf?sfvrsn=2

Accreditation of Interprofessional Health Education (AIPHE). (2007). *Principles and practices for integrating interprofessional education into the accreditation standards for six health professions in Canada.* Retrieved from http://www.afmc.ca/aiphe-afiss/documents/AIPHE_Principles_and_Implementation_Guide_EN.pdf

Accreditation of Interprofessional Health Education (AIPHE). (2009). *Principles and practices for integrating interprofessional education into the accreditation standards for six health professions in canada.* Retrieved from http://casn.ca/wp-content/uploads/2014/12/AIPHEPrinciplesandPracticesGuidev2EN.pdf

Accreditation of Interprofessional Health Education (AIPHE). (2016). About *AIPHE.* Retrieved from http://www.cihc.ca/aiphe/about

Adams, D. L. (1995). *Health for women of color: A cultural diversity health perspective.* Thousand Oaks, CA: SAGE Publications.

Adams, L. (2015). *Workplace mental health: Manual for nurse managers.* New York, NY: Springer Publishing Company.

Adamson, K. (2010). Integrating human patient simulation into associate degree nursing curricula: Faculty experiences, barriers, and facilitators. *Clinical Simulation in Nursing, 6*(1), e75–e81. Retrieved from http://dx. doi:10.1016/j.ecsns.2010.06.002

Adamson, K. (2015). A systematic review of the literature related to the NLN/Jeffries simulation framework. *Nursing Education Perspectives, 36*(5), 281–291. doi:10.5480/15-1655

Adamson, K. A., Kardong-Edgren, S., & Willhaus, J. (2013). An updated review of published simulation evaluation instruments. *Clinical Simulation in Nursing, 9*(9), e393–e400. doi:http://dx.doi.org/10.1016/j.ecns.2012.09.004

Adamson, K. A., & Prion, S. (2015). Making sense of methods and measurement: Simulation program evaluation. *Clinical Simulation in Nursing, 11,* 505–506. doi:http://dx.doi.org/10.1016/j.ecns.2015.10.007

Adamson, K., & Rodgers, B. (2016). Systematic review of the literature for the NLN Jeffries simulation framework: Discussion, summary, and research findings. In P. R. Jeffries (Ed.), *The NLN Jeffries simulation theory.* Washington, DC: National League for Nursing.

Adelman, L. (Executive Producer), Fortier, J. M., Smith, L. M., Stange, E., & Strain, T. H. (Directors). (2008). *Unnatural causes: Is inequality making us sick?* [DVD]. Retrieved from http://www.unnaturalcauses.org/

Aebersold, M. (2017). Developing psychomotor skills using a "boot camp" approach to training. In C. Foisy-Doll & K. Leighton (Eds.), *Simulation champions: Fostering courage, caring, and connection* (p. 5). Philadelphia, PA: Wolters Kluwer, Inc.

Aebersold, M., & Tschannen, D. (2013). Simulation in nursing practice: The impact on patient care. *Online Journal of Issues in Nursing, 18*(2), 1–13. doi:10.3912/OJIN.Vol18No02Man06

Aebersold, M., Tschannen, D., Stephens, M., Anderson, P., & Lei, X. (2012). Second Life®: A new strategy in educating nursing students. *Clinical Simulation in Nursing, 8*(9), e469–e475. doi:10.1016/j.ecns.2011.05.002

Afzalur Rahim, M., Antonioni, D., & Psenicka, C. (2001). A structural equations model of leader power, subordinates' styles of handling conflict, and job performance. *International Journal of Conflict Management, 12*(3), 191–211. http://doi.org/10.1108/eb022855

Agency for Healthcare Research and Quality (AHRQ). (2011). *TeamSTEPPS curriculum tools and materials.* Retrieved from http://teamstepps.ahrq.gov/abouttoolsmaterials.htm

Agency for Healthcare Research and Quality (AHRQ). (2013). *Pocket guide: TeamSTEPPS.* AHRQ Pub. No. 14-0001-2. Retrieved from https://www.ahrq.gov/teamstepps/instructor/essentials/pocketguide.html

Agency for Healthcare Research and Quality (AHRQ). (2013, May). *Module 14: Creating quality improvement teams and QI plans.* Rockville, MD: Author. Retrieved from http://www.ahrq.gov/professionals/prevention-chronic-care/improve/system/pfhandbook/mod14.html

Agency for Healthcare Research and Quality (AHRQ). (2014a, October). *Facilitator's notes.* Rockville, MD: Author. Retrieved from http://www.ahrq.gov/professionals/education/curriculum-tools/teamstepps/simulation/traininggd.html#intro

Agency for Healthcare Research and Quality (AHRQ). (2014b). *TeamSTEPPS pocket guide* (website). Retrieved from http://www.ahrq.gov/professionals/education/curriculum-tools/teamstepps/instructor/essentials/pocketguide.html

Agency for Healthcare Research and Quality (AHRQ). (2015a). 2014 national healthcare quality and disparities report. Retrieved from http://www.ahrq.gov/sites/default/files/wysiwyg/research/findings/nhqrdr/nhqdr14/2014nhqdr.pdf

Agency for Healthcare Research and Quality (AHRQ). (2015b). Systems approach. Retrieved from https://psnet.ahrq.gov/primers/primer/21/systems-approach

Agency for Healthcare Research and Quality (AHRQ). (2015b). Systems approach Curriculum tools. Retrieved from Retrieved from https://psnet.ahrq.gov/primers/primer/21/systems-approach

Agency for Healthcare Research and Quality. (2015c). *TeamSTEPPS*. Retrieved from http://www.ahrq.gov/professionals/education/curriculum-tools/teamstepps/index.html

Ahmed, M., Arora, S., Russ, S., Darzi, A., Vincent, C., & Sevdalis, N. (2013). Operation debrief: A SHARP improvement in performance feedback in the operating room. *Annals of Surgery, 258*(6), 958–963. doi:10.1097/SLA.0b013e31828c88fc

Ahmed, M., Sevdalis, N., Paige, J., Paragi-Gururaja, R., Nestel, D., & Arora, S. (2012). Identifying best practice guidelines for debriefing in surgery: A tri-continental study. *American Journal of Surgery, 203*(4), 523–529. doi:10.1016/j.amjsurg.2011.09.024

Aiken, L. H., Clarke, S. P., Sloane, D. M., Lake, E. T., & Cheney, T. (2008). Effects of hospital care environment on patient mortality and nurse outcomes. *Journal of Nursing Administration, 38*(5), 223–229. doi:10.1097/01.NNA.0000312773.42352.d7

Aiken, L., Sloane, D., Bruyneel, L., Van Den Heede, K., Griffiths, P., Busse, R., …, Sermeus, W.; RN4CAST Consortium. (2014). Nurse staffing and education and hospital mortality in nine European countries: A retrospective observational study. *Lancet Early, 383*(9931), 1824–1830. Retrieved from http://www.thelancet.com/journals/lancet/article/PIIS0140-6736(13)62631-8/abstract

Akhtar-Danesh, N., Baxter, P., Valaitis, R., Stanyon, W., & Sproul, S. (2010). Nurse faculty perceptions of simulation use in nursing education. *Western Journal of Nursing Research, 31*(3), 312–329. doi:10.1177/0193945908328264

Alberta, A. J., & Wood, A. H. (2008). A practical skills model for effectively engaging clients in multicultural settings. *The Counseling Psychologist, 37*(4), 564–579. http://doi.org/10.1177/0011000008326231

Aldridge, J., Kilgo, J. L., & Christensen, L. M. (2014). Turning culture upside down: The role of transcultural education. *Social Studies Research and Practice, 9*(2), 107–119.

Alec. (2014, Oct). *Educational 3D printed heart valve surgery simulator adopted at Maastricht University Hospital.* Retrieved from https://tinyurl.com/h9gc6ha

Alexander, M. (2014). NCSBN national simulation study. *Dean's Notes, 36*(1), 1–2.

Alexander, M., Durham, C. F., Hooper, J. I., Jeffries, P. R., Goldman, N., Kardong-Edgren, S., … Tillman, C. (2015). NCSBN simulation guidelines for prelicensure nursing programs. *Journal of Nursing Regulation, 6*(3), 39–42. doi:10.1016/S2155-8256(15)30783-3

Alfes, C. M. (2008). Setting the stage for clinical simulation: Developing an introductory video. *Clinical Simulation in Nursing, 4*(3). doi:10.1016/j.ecns.2008.08.005

Alfes, C. M., & Manacci, C. F. (2014). Taking simulation to new heights: Designing a flight simulation center. *Clinical Simulation in Nursing, 10*(9), 442–445. http://dx.doi.org/10.1016/j.ecns.2014.05.006

Alinier, G. (2007). A typology of educationally focused medical simulation tools. *Medical Teacher, 29*(8), e243–e250. doi:10.1080/01421590701551185

Alinier, G., Bello, F., Kalbag, A. A., & Kneebone, R. (2015). Space: Potential to conduct full-scale simulation-based education.

In J. C. Palaganas, J. C. Maxworthy, C. A. Epps & M. E. Mancini (Eds.), *Defining excellence in simulation programs* (pp. 455–472). Philadelphia, PA: Wolters Kluwer.

Alinier, G., Hunt, B., Gordon, R., & Harwood, C. (2006). Effectiveness of intermediate-fidelity simulation training technology in undergraduate nursing education. *Journal of Advanced Nursing, 54*, 359–369. Retrieved from http://dx.doi.org/10.1111/j.1365–2648.2006.03810.x

American Association of Colleges of Nursing (AACN). (2002). Using strategic partnerships to expand nursing education programs. *AACN Issue Bulletin.* Retrieved from http://www.aacn.nche.edu/publications/issues/oct02.htm

American Association of Colleges of Nursing (AACN). (2006). *The essentials of doctoral education and advanced nursing practice.* Retrieved from http://www.aacn.nche.edu/publications/position-statements

American Association of Colleges of Nursing (AACN). (2008a). *Cultural competency in baccalaureate nursing education.* Retrieved from http://www.aacn.nche.edu/leading-initiatives/education-resources/competency.pdf

American Association of Colleges of Nursing (AACN). (2008b). *The essentials of baccalaureate education for professional nursing practice.* Retrieved from http://www.aacn.nche.edu/education-resources/BaccEssentials08.pdf

American Association of Colleges of Nursing (AACN). (2010). *Tri-Council for Nursing issues new consensus policy statement.* Retrieved from http://www.aacn.nche.edu/news/articles/2010/tri-council-educational-statement

American Association of Colleges of Nursing (AACN). (2011). *The essentials of master's education in nursing.* Retrieved from http://www.aacn.nche.edu/publications/position-statements

American Association of Colleges of Nursing (AACN). (2013). *Hallmarks of the professional nursing practice environment.* Retrieved from http://aacn.nche.edu/publications/white-papers/hallmarks-practice-environment

American Association of University Professors. (2015). Academic freedom. Retrieved from http://www.aaup.org/our-work/protecting-academic-freedom

American College of Obstetricians and Gynecologists (ACOG). (2013a). Executive summary: Hypertension in pregnancy. *Obstetrics and Gynecology, 122*(5), 1122–1131. doi:10.1097/01.AOG.0000437382.03963.88

American College of Obstetricians and Gynecologists (ACOG). (2013b). Patient safety checklist: Postpartum hemorrhage from vaginal delivery. *Obstetrics and Gynecology, 122*(5), 1151–1152. doi:10.1097/01.AOG.0000429662. 16341.48

American College of Surgeons. (2015). *Accredited education institutes.* Retrieved from https://www.facs.org/education/accreditation/aei

American Institutes for Research. (2011). *Training guide: Using simulation in TeamSTEPPS® training.* Rockville, MD: Agency for Healthcare Research and Quality. AHRQ Publication No. 11-0041EF.

American Nurses Association (ANA). (2015). *Code of ethics with interpretative statements.* Retrieved from http://nursingworld.org/MainMenuCategories/EthicsStandards/CodeofEthicsforNurses/Code-of-Ethics-For-Nurses.html

American Society of Anesthesiologists. (2015). *MOCA 2.0.* Retrieved from https://education.asahq.org/totara/asa/core/drupal.php?name=Simulation-Education

Amory, D. (2011). *Life coaching: Essential knowledge for personal coaching and self-coaching.* Belgium: CreateSpace Publishing.

Anderson, C. (2013). What's the purpose of a procedure manual? Retrieved from https://www.bizmanualz.com/writing-procedure-manuals/what-is-a-policies-and-procedures-manual.html

Anderson, J. (2015). *Educational effectiveness in healthcare simulation: Improving performance, improving patient outcomes* (endnote conference presentation). International Nursing Association for Clinical Simulation and Learning, 14th Annual INACSL Conference, Atlanta, GA.

Anderson, J. M., & Warren, J. B. (2011). Using simulation to enhance the acquisition and retention of clinical skills in neonatology. *Seminars in Perinatology, 35*(2), 59–67. doi:10.1053/j.semperi.2011.01.004

Anderson, L. W., & Krathwohl, D. (Eds.), (2001). *A taxonomy for learning, teaching, and assessing: A revision of Bloom's taxonomy of educational objectives.* New York, NY: Longman Group.

Anderson, M., & Decker, S. (2013). *SIRC: Beyond basic debriefing module.* New York, NY: National League for Nursing. Retrieved from http://sirc.nln.org/mod/resource/view.php?id=746

Anderson, M., Holmes, T. L., LeFlore, J. L., Nelson, K. A., & Jenkins, T. (2010). Standardized patients in educating student nurses: One school's experience. *Clinical Simulation in Nursing, 6*(2), e61–e66. doi:10.1016/j.ecns.2009.08.001

Anderson, M., LeFlore, J. L., & Anderson, J. M. (2013). Evaluating videotaped role-modeling to teach crisis resource management principles. *Clinical Simulation in Nursing, 9*(9), e343–e354. http://dx.doi.org/10.1016/j.ecns.2012.05.007

Andrews, M. M., & Boyle, J. S. (2012a). Theoretical foundations of transcultural nursing. In M. M. Andrews & J. S. Boyle (Eds.), *Transcultural concepts in nursing care* (6th ed.). Philadelphia, PA: Wolters Kluwer/Lippincott Williams & Wilkins.

Andrews, M. M., & Boyle, J. S. (2012b). *Transcultural concepts in nursing care* (6th ed.). Philadelphia, PA: Wolters Kluwer, Lippincott Williams & Wilkins.

An-Grogan, Y., Jansson, P., Park, C., Salzman, D., & Vozenilek, J. (2014). Board #104—Research abstract the growth of simulation fellowships (Submission #9902). *Simulation in Healthcare, 9*(6), 397. http://doi.org/10.1097/01.SIH.0000459274.00761.c1

Archer, J. C. (2010). State of the science in health professional education: Effective feedback. *Medical Education, 44*(1), 101–108. doi:10.1111/j.1365-2923.2009.03546

Arenas, A., León-Pérez, J., Munduate, L., & Medina, F. (2015). Workplace bullying and interpersonal conflicts: The moderation effect of supervisor's power. *International Journal of Social Psychology, 3*(2), 295–322. doi:10.1080/21711976.2015.1016753

Argyris, C., & Schön, D. A. (1978). *Organizational learning: A theory in action perspective.* New York, NY: Addison-Wesley.

Argyris, C., & Schön, D. A. (1992). *Theory in practice: Increasing professional effectiveness* (Reprint ed.). San Francisco, CA: Jossey-Bass.

Armstrong, C. (2012). *Global distributive justice.* New York, NY: Cambridge University Press.

Aronson, B., Glynn, B., & Squires, T. (2013). Effectiveness of a role-modeling intervention on student nurse simulation competency. *Clinical Simulation in Nursing, 9*(4), e121–e126. doi:10.1016/j.ecns.2011.11.005

Arthur, C., Kable, A., & Levett-Jones, T. (2011). Human patient simulation manikins and information communication technology use in Australian schools of nursing: A cross-sectional survey. *Clinical Simulation in Nursing, 7*(6), e219–e227. doi:10.1016/j.ecns.2010.03.002

Arthur, C., Levett-Jones, T., & Kable, A. (2013). Quality indicators for the design and implementation of simulation experiences: A Delphi study. *Nurse Education Today, 33*(11), 1357–1361. doi:10.1016/j.nedt.2012.07.012

Asia for Educators. (2013). *Asia for Educators,* Retrieved from http://afe.easia.columbia.edu/

Asociación Chilena de Educación en Enfermería (Chilean Association of Education in Nursing) (ACHIEEN). (2015). *Discurso por celebración de los 100 años de la Escuela de Enfermería de U. de Chile 2006.* Retrieved from http://www.achieen.cl/index.php/documentos

Asociación Latinoamericana de Simulación Clínica (ALASIC). (2015). *Latin American Association of Clinical Simulation.* Retrieved from www.alasic.org

Association for Simulated Practice in Healthcare (ASPiH). (2015). *Welcome to ASPiH.* Retrieved from http://www.aspih.org.uk

Association of Schools of Allied Health Professions (ASAHP). (2017). *What is allied health?* Retrieved from http://www.asahp.org/about-us/what-is-allied-health/

Association of Standardized Patient Educators (ASPE). (2017) *Virtual library.* Retrieved from http://www.aspeducators.org/virtual-library

Auerbach, A. D., Sehgal, N. L., Blegen, M. A., Maselli, J., Alldredge, B. K., Vittinghoff, E., … Wachter, R. M. (2012). Effects of a multicenter teamwork and communication programme on patient outcomes: Results from the Triad for Optimal Patient Safety (TOPS) project. *BMJ Quality & Safety, 21,* 118–126. doi:10.1136/bmjqs-2011-000311

Auerbach, J. A., & Hoffenberg P. H. (Eds.) (2016). *Britain, the empire and the world at the great exhibition of 1851.* Abingdon, OX: Routledge.

Australian Society for Simulation in Healthcare Simulation (ASSH). (2012, June). *Australian society for simulation in healthcare simulation: Directory data dictionary.* Retrieved from http://www.simulationaustralasia.com/communities/simulation-learning-programs

Ausland, A. (2010). Staying for tea: Five principles for the community service volunteer. *The Global Citizen: A Journal for Young Adults Engaging the World through Service, 2.* Retrieved from www.kirstafoundation.org

Austin, W., Bergum, V., Nuttgens, S., & Peternelj-Taylor, C. (2006). A re-visioning of boundaries in professional helping relationships: Exploring other metaphors. *Ethics & Behavior, 16*(2), 77–94. http://doi.org/10.1207/s15327019eb1602_1

Australasian Interprofessional Practice and Education Network (AIPPEN). (2011). *Curtin University Interprofessional Capability Network. Interprofessional Capabilities, Competencies, and Frameworks.* Retrieved from http://www.aippen.net/criehcapabilitiesandframeworks

Australian Government Department of Education and Training. (2011). *Tertiary education quality standards agency.* Retrieved from http://www.teqsa.gov.au/

Australian Government Department of Foreign Affairs and Trade. (2017). *About Australia.* Retrieved from http://dfat.gov.au/about-australia/Pages/about-australia.aspx

Australian Health Practitioner Regulation Agency. (2010). *Regulating Australia's health practitioners in partnership with the national boards.* Retrieved from https://www.ahpra.gov.au/

Australian Institute of Health and Welfare. (2015). *National health priority areas.* Retrieved from http://www.aihw.gov.au/national-health-priority-areas/

Australian Society for Simulation in Healthcare (ASSH). (2012). *Simulation directory data dictionary.* Retrieved from http://www.tcen.com.au/sites/newtcen/files/files/SLE/assh_hwa_data_dictionary.pdf

Australian Society for Simulation in Healthcare (ASSH). (2015). *The story of ASSH.* Retrieved from http://www.simulationaustralasia.com/divisions/assh-history

Aydin, A., Ahmed, K., Khan, M. S., Dasgupta, P., & McCabe, J. (2015). The role of human cadaveric procedural simulation in urology training. *Journal of Urology, 193*(S), e273. http://doi.org/10.1016/j.juro.2015.02.1259

Bachen, C. M., Hernandez-Ramos, P. F., & Raphael, C. (2012). Simulating REAL LIVES: Promoting global empathy and interest in learning through simulation games. *Simulation & Gaming, 43*(4), 437–460. doi:10.1177/1046878111432108

Baig, L. B., Beran, T. N., Vallevand, A., Zarrukh, A. B., & Monroy-Cuadros, M. (2014). Accuracy of portrayal by standardized patients: Results from four OSCE stations conducted for high stakes examinations. *BMC Medical Education, 14*(97), 2–8. Retrieved from http://www.biomedcentral.com/1472-6920/14/97

Bailey, J., & Axelrod, R. H. (2001). Leadership lessons from Mount Rushmore: An interview with James McGregor Burns. *The Leadership Quarterly, 12*(1), 113–127. Retrieved from http://www.journals.elsevier.com/the-leadership-quarterly/

Baily, L., Bar-on, M., Yucha, C., & Snyder, S. J. (2013). Six challenges encountered in the opening of a multi-institutional, interprofessional simulation center. *Clinical Simulation in Nursing, 9*(6), e219–e223. doi:10.1016/j.ecns.2011.12.002

Bainbridge, L., Nasmith, L., Orchard, C., & Wood, V. (2010). Competencies for interprofessional collaboration. *Journal of Physical Therapy Education, 24*(1), 6–11.

Baker, E. W., Slott, P. A., Terracio, L., & Cunningham, E. P. (2013). An innovative method for teaching anatomy in the predoctoral dental curriculum. *Journal of Dental Education, 77*(11), 1498–1507.

Baker, G. R., Norton, P. G., Flintoft, V., Blasi, R., Brown, A., Cox, J., & Tamblyn, R. (2004). The Canadian adverse events study: The incidence of adverse events among hospitalized patients in Canada. *Canadian Medical Association Journal, 170*(11), 1678–1686. doi:10.1053/cmaj.1040498

Baker, M., & Fowler Durham, C. (2014). Interprofessional education: A survey of students' collaborative competency outcomes. *Journal of Nursing Education, 52*(12), 713–718. doi:10.3928/01484834-20131118-04

Baldacchino, D. (2015). Spiritual care education of healthcare professionals. Conference report. *Religions, 6*(2), 594–613. doi:10.3390/43l6020594

Bale, H. (n.d.). *Global economic symposium.* Retrieved from http://www.global-economic-symposium.org/knowledgebase/the-global-society/financing-health-care-for-the-poor/proposals/improving-access-to-health-care-for-the-poor-especially-in-developing-countries

Ball, T. (1994). New faces of power. In T. Wartenberg (Ed.), *Rethinking power.* Albany, NY: SUNY Press.

Bandura, A. (1977a). Self-efficacy: Toward a unifying theory of behavioral change. *Psychological Review, 84*(2), 191–215.

Bandura, A. (1977b). *Social learning theory.* Englewood Cliffs, NJ: Prentice Hall.

Barbeito, A., Bonifacio, A., Holtschneider, M., Segall, N., Schroeder, R., & Mark, J. (2015). In situ simulated cardiac arrest exercises to detect system vulnerability. *Simulation in Healthcare, 10*(3), 154–162. doi:10.1097.SIH.0000000000000087

Barnes, C., Blake, H., & Pinder, D. (2009). *Creating and delivering your value proposition: Managing customer experience for profit.* Philadelphia, PA: Kogan Page, Ltd.

Bar-on, M., Yucha, C. B., & Kinsey, J. (2013). Funding a collaborative simulation center: First step in interprofessional education. *Clinical Simulation in Nursing, 9*(11), e531–e534. http://dx.doi.org/10.1016/j.ecns.2013.04.014

Barrows, H. S. (1987) *Simulated (standardized) patients and other human simulations.* Chapel Hill, NC: Health Sciences Consortium.

Barrows, H. (1993). An overview of the uses of standardized patients for teaching and evaluating clinical skills. *Academic Medicine, 68*(6), 443–451.

Barrows, H. S. (1999). *Training standardized patients to have physical findings.* Springfield, IL: Southern Illinois University School of Medicine, Department of Medical Education.

Barrows, H., & Abrahamason, S. (1964). The programmed patient: A technique for appraising student performance in clinical neurology. *Journal of Medical Education, 39*(8), 802–805.

Barsuk, J. H., Cohen, E. R., Feinglass, J., Kozmic, S. E., McGaghie, W. C., Ganger D., & Wayne, D. B. (2014). Cost savings of performing paracentesis procedures at the bedside after simulation-based education. *Simulation in Healthcare, 9*(5), 312–318. doi:10.1097/SIH.0000000000000040

Bartley, E. J. (2016). Foundations for the simulation operations specialist. In L. T. Gantt & H. M. Young (Eds.), *Healthcare simulation: A guide for operations specialists* (1st ed., pp. 91–112). Hoboken, NJ: Wiley.

Bass, B. M. (1995). Theory of transformational leadership redux. *The Leadership Quarterly, 6*(4), 463–478. Retrieved from http://www.journals.elsevier.com/the-leadership-quarterly/

Bass, B. M. (1998). The inspirational processes of leadership. *Journal of Management Development, 7*(5), 21–31. doi:10.1108/eb051688

Bass, B. M., & Steidlmeier, P. (1999). Ethics, character, and authentic transformational leadership behavior. *The Leadership Quarterly, 10*(2), 181–217. Retrieved from http://www.journals.elsevier.com/the-leadership-quarterly/

Bassendowski, S. (2013). Holograms in health care. *Canadian Journal of Nursing Informatics, 8*(3–4).

Battista, A. B., & Antonis, M. S. (2015). *Comparative analysis of how skills-based and scenario-based simulations support learning.* Unpublished manuscript.

Battista, A., & Sheridan, K. (2014, January). Examining learning-in action: A descriptive analysis of what is learned within complex scenario-based simulations. Presented at the International Meeting on Simulation in Healthcare. San Diego, CA.

Bauman, E. (2007). High fidelity simulation in healthcare. (Doctoral dissertation), Dissertations & Theses @ CIC Institutions database (Publication no. AAT 3294196 ISBN: 9780549383109 ProQuest document ID: 1453230861)

Bauman, E. (2010). Virtual reality and game-based clinical education. In K. B. Gaberson & M. H. Oermann (Eds.), *Clinical teaching strategies in nursing education* (3rd ed.). New York, NY: Springer Publishing Company.

Bauman, E. B. (2012). *Game-based teaching and simulation in nursing & healthcare.* New York, NY: Springer Publishing Company.

Bauman, E. B. (2016). Games, virtual environments, mobile applications and a futurist's crystal ball. *Clinical Simulation in Nursing, 12,* 109–114. doi:10.1016/j.ecns.2016.02.002

Bauman, E. B., & Ralston-Berg, P. (2014). Serious gaming using simulations. In P. Jeffries (Ed.), *Clinical simulations in nursing: Advanced concepts, trends, and opportunities.* Philadelphia, PA: Wolters Kluwer.

Bauman, E. B., & Ralston-Berg, P. (2015). Virtual simulation. In J. C. Palaganas, J. C. Maxworthy, C. A. Epps & M. E. Mancini (Eds.), *Defining excellence in simulation programs* (pp. 241–251). Philadelphia, PA: Wolters Kluwer.

Beaubien, J. M. & Baker, D. P. (2004). The use of simulation for training teamwork skills in health care: How low can you go? *Quality & Safety in Health Care, 13*(Suppl. 1), i51–i56. doi:10.1136/qshc.2004.009845

Begley, S. (1977). Seeking other worlds (Profile of Carl Sagan), *Newsweek, 90,* 53.

Beischel, K. P., Hart, J., Turkelson, S., & Churchill, J. (2013). Using a standardized patient to teach fall safety. *Clinical Simulation in Nursing, 10*(4), e183–e190. doi:10.1016/j.ecns.2013.11.007

Bell, J. S. (2012). *Elements of fiction writing: Conflict and suspense.* Blue Ash, OH: Writer's Digest Books.

Bell, M. (2008). Toward a definition of virtual worlds. *Journal of Virtual Worlds Research, 1*(1), 1–5. http://dx.doi.org/10.4101/jvwr.v1i1.283

Bendaly, L., & Bendaly, N. (2012). *Improving healthcare team performance: The 7 requirements for excellence in patient care.* Toronto, ON: Jossey-Bass.

Benner, P. (1982). From novice to expert. *The American Journal of Nursing, 82*(3), 402–407.

Benner, P. (1984). *From novice to expert: Excellence and power in clinical nursing practice.* Menlo Park, CA: Addison-Wesley.

Benner, P., Sutphen, M. Leonard, V., & Day, L. (2010). *Educating nurses: A call for radical transformation.* San Francisco, CA: Jossey-Bass.

Benner, P., Tanner, C., & Chesla, C. (2009). *Expertise in nursing practice.* New York, NY: Springer Publishing Co.

Bennis, W., & Goldsmith, J. (2010). *Learning to LEAD: A workbook on becoming a LEADER* (4th ed.). Philadelphia, PA: Basic Books.

Bennis, W., Goleman, D., O'Toole, J., & Ward Biederman, P. (2008). *Transparency: How leaders create a culture of candor.* San Francisco, CA: Jossey-Bass.

Bensfield, L. A., Olech, M. J., & Horsley, T. L. (2012). Simulation for high-stakes evaluation in nursing. *Nurse Educator, 37*(2), 71–74. doi:10.1097/NNE.0b013e3182461b8c

Benson, J. A. (1991). Certification and recertification: One approach to professional accountability. *American Board of Internal Medicine, 114*(3), 238–242. doi:10.7326/0003-4819-114-3-238

Bergum, V. (2012). Relational ethics for nursing. In J. Storch, P. Rodney & R. Starzomski (Eds.), *Toward a moral horizon: Nursing ethics for leadership and practice* (pp. 127–142). Toronto, ON: Pearson Education Canada.

Bergum, V., & Dossetor, J. (2005). *Relational ethics: The full meaning of respect.* Hagerstown, MD: University Publishing Group.

Berkenstadt, H., Ziv, A., Gafni, N., & Sidi, A. (2006). Incorporating simulation-based structured clinical examination into the Israeli board examination in anesthesiology. *Anesthesia and Analgesia, 102,* 853–858. doi:10.1243/01.ane.0000194934.34552.ab

Berkley, University of California Career Center. (2017). *Fellowships.* Retrieved from https://career.berkeley.edu/InfoLab/Fellow

Berro, E. A., & Knoesel, M. A. (2016). An innovative approach to staffing a simulation center in a college of health professions. *Journal of Nursing Education, 55*(1), doi:10.3928/01484834-20151214-13

Bersin, J. (2013a). *Building a smarter workforce in today's global economy.* Deloitte Development, LLC. Retrieved from http://www.bersin.com/Practice/Detail.aspx?docid=16682&mode=search&p=Human-Resources

Berwick, D. M. (2009). What 'patient-centered' should mean: Confessions of an extremist. *Health Affairs, 28*(4), w555–w565. doi:10.1377/hlthaff.28.4.w555

Beyer, D. A. (2012). Effectiveness of human patient simulator as a classroom teaching strategy. *Clinical Simulation in Nursing, 8*(7), e301–e305. doi.org/10.1016/j.ecns.2011.01.005

Beyer, D. A. (2012, February). Enhancing critical reflection on simulation through wikis. *Clinical Simulation in Nursing, 8*(2), e67–e70. doi:10.1016/j.ecns.2010

BizManualz.com (2016). Policy and procedure template. Retrieved from https://www.bizmanualz.com/

Black, J. S., & Gregersen, H. (2014). *It starts with one: Changing individuals changes organizations* (3rd ed.). Upper Saddle River, NJ: Pearson Education, Inc.

Blackstock, F. C., Watson, K. M., Morris, N. R., Jones, A., Wright, A., McMeeken, J. M., … Jull, G. A. (2013). Simulation can contribute a part of cardiorespiratory physiotherapy clinical education: Two randomized trials. *Simulation in Healthcare, 8*(1), 32–42. doi:10.1097/SIH.0b013e318273101a

Blake, R., & Mouton, J. (1985). *The managerial grid III: The key to leadership excellence.* Houston, TX: Gulf Publishing Co.

Blanchet Garneau, A. (2016). Critical reflection in cultural competence development: A framework for undergraduate nursing education. *Journal of Nursing Education, 55*(3), 125–132. doi:10.3928/01484834-20160216-02

Blanchet Garneau, A., & Pepin, J. (2015). A constructivist theoretical proposition for cultural competence development in nursing. *Nurse Education Today, 35*(11), 1062–1068. doi:10.1016/j.nedt.2015.05.019

Bland, A. J., Topping, A., & Wood, B. (2011). A concept analysis of simulation as a learning strategy in the education of undergraduate nursing students. *Nurse Education Today, 31,* 664–670. http://dx.doi.org/10.1016/j.nedt.2010.10.013

Blanford, R. (2016, May). *A culture of patient safety: Reducing medical errors with simulation.* Retrieved from http://www.meti.com/eng/blog/patient-safety-healthcare-simulation-training-lucian-leape-institute

Bloom, B. S. (1956). *Taxonomy of educational objectives: Cognitive and affective domains.* New York, NY: David McKay Company, Inc.

Bloom, B. S. (1968). Learning for mastery. *Evaluation Comment, 1*(2), 1–12 (ERIC Document Reproduction No. ED053419).

Bloom, B., Engelhart, M., Furst, E., Hill, W., & Krathwohl, D. (1956). *Taxonomy of educational objectives: The classification of educational goals. Handbook I: Cognitive domain.* New York, NY: Longmans, Green, & Co.

Blum, R. H., Raemer, D. B., Carroll, J. S., Sunder, N., Felstein, D. M., & Cooper, J. B. (2004). Crisis resource management training for an anaesthesia faculty: A new approach to continuing education. *Medical Education, 38*(1), 45–55. http://doi.org/10.1111/j.1365-2923.2004.01696.x

Bodek, N. (1988). *Taiichi Ohno. Toyota production system: Beyond large-scale production.* Portland, OR: Productivity Press, Inc.

Boese, T., Cato, M., Gonzales, L., Jones, A., Kennedy, K., Reese, C., … Borum, J. C. (2013). Standards of best practice: Simulation Standard V: Facilitator. *Clinical Simulation in Nursing, 9*(6S), S22–S25. doi:10.1016/j.ecns.2013.04.010

Boet, S., Bould, M., Burn, C., & Reeves, S. (2014). Twelve tips for a successful interprofessional team-based high-fidelity simulation education session. *Medical Teacher, 36*(10), 853–857. doi:10.3109/0142159X.2014.923558

Boggs, J., Mickel, A., & Holtom, B. (2007). Experiential learning through interactive drama: An alternative to student role plays. *Journal of Management Education, 31*(6), 832–858. doi:10.1177/1052562906294952

Bogossian, F., McKenna, L., Higgins, M., Benefer, C., Brady, S., Fox-Young, S., & Cooper, S. (2012). Simulation based learning in Australian midwifery curricula: Results of a national electronic survey. *Women and Birth, 25*(2), 86–97. doi:10.1016/j.wombi.2011.02.001

Bolesta, S., & Chmil, J. V. (2014). Interprofessional education among student health professionals using human patient simulation, *American Journal of Pharmaceutical Education, 78*(5), 1–9, Article 94. doi:10.5688/ajpe78594

Bolton, S. C. (2004). A simple matter of control? NHS hospital nurses and new management. *Journal of Management Studies, 41*(2), 317–333.

Bong, C. L., Lightdale, J. R., Fredette, M. F., & Weinstock, P. (2010). Effects of simulation versus traditional tutorial-based training on physiologic stress and among clinicians: A pilot study. *Simulation in Healthcare, 5*(5), 272–278. doi:10.1097/SIH.0b013e3181e98b29

Bornais, J., Foisy-Doll, C., & Wyrostok, L. (2014). Transforming nursing education using simulation. In D. Gregory, C. Raymond-Seniuk & L. Patrick (Eds.), *Fundamentals: Perspectives on the art and science of Canadian nursing* (pp. 290–313). Lippincott Williams & Wilkins, Inc.

Bottles, K. (2013, January/February). Health hackers and citizen scientists shake up medical research. *Physician Executive, 39*(1), 88–90.

Boud, D., Cohen, R., & Sampson, J. (2014). *Peer learning in higher education: Learning from and with each other.* London, UK: Routledge.

Boulet, J. R. (2008). Summative assessment in medicine: The promise of simulation for high-stakes evaluation. *Academic Emergency Medicine, 15*(11), 1017–1024. doi:10.1111/j.1553-2712.2008.00228.x

Boulet, J. R., & Errichetti, A. (2008). Training and assessment with standardized patients. In Riley, R. H. (Ed.), *Manual of simulation in healthcare.* New York, NY: Oxford University Press.

Boulet, J. R., & Murray, D. J. (2010). Simulation-based assessment in anesthesiology requirements for practical implementation. *Anesthesiology, 112*(4), 1041–1052. doi:10.1097/ALN.0b013e3181cea265

Bourzac, K. (2016, February). *Flexible glass could bring back the flip phone.* MIT Technology Review. Retrieved from https://www.technologyreview.com/s/600894/flexible-glass-could-bring-back-the-flip-phone/

Boutain, D. (2005). Social justice as a framework for professional nursing. *Journal of Nursing Education, 44*(9), 404–408.

Boyd, K. B., & Salameh, J. R. (2006). Surgical residents' perception of simulation training. *American Surgeon, 72*(6), 521–524.

Bradford, C. (2017). *What is an operating budget?* Retrieved from http://smallbusiness.chron.com/operating-budget-61475.html

Bradley, P. (2006). The history of simulation in medical education and possible future directions. *Medical Education, 40,* 254–262. doi:10.1111/j.1365-2929.2006.02394.x

Bransford, J. D., Brown, A. L., & Cocking, R. R. (2000). *How people learn: Brain, mind, experience, and school.* Washington, DC: National Academy Press.

Brashers, V., Phillips, E., Malpass, J., & Owen, J. (2005). Review: Measuring the impact of interprofessional education (IPE) on collaborative practice and patient outcomes. Paper commissioned by the Committee on Measuring the Impact of Interprofessional Education (IPE) on Collaborative Practice and Patient Outcomes, Institute of Medicine. In *Measuring the Impact of Interprofessional Education (IPE) on Collaborative Practice and Patient Outcomes* (Appendix A). Washington, DC: National Academies Press.

Braskamp, L. A. (2008). Developing global citizens. *Journal of College and Character, 10,* 1. doi:10.2202/1940-1639.105810(1)

Braskamp, L. A., Calian Trautvetter, L., & Ward, K. (2008). Putting students first: Promoting lives of purpose and meaning. *About Campus, 13*(1), 26–32.

Bremner, M. N., Aduddell, K., Bennett, D. N., & VanGeest, J. B. (2006). The use of human patient simulators: Best practices with novice nursing students. *Nurse Educator, 31*(4), 170–174.

Brewer, E. P. (2011). Successful techniques for using human patient simulation in nursing education. *Journal of Nursing Scholarship, 43,* 311–317. Retrieved from http://dx.doi.org/10.1111/j.1547-5069.2011.01405.x

Bridges, D. R., Davidson, R. A., Soule Odegard, P., Maki, I. V., & Tomkowiak, J. (2011). Interprofessional collaboration: Three best practice models of interprofessional education. *Medical Education Online, 16*(10), 3e. doi:10.3402/meo.v16i0.6035

Bridges, W. (2009). *Managing transitions: Making the most of change* (3rd ed.). Boston, MA: Da Capo Lifelong Books.

Brock, T. R., & Holtschneider, M. (2016). Simulation operations, curriculum integration, and performance improvement. In L. T. Gantt & M. H. Young (Eds.), *Healthcare simulation: A guide for operations specialists.* Hoboken, NJ: John Wiley & Sons, Inc.

Bronheim, S. (2011). *Promising practices: Cultural brokers help families and providers bridge the cultural gap.* Washington, DC: National Center for Cultural Competence, Georgetown University Center for Child and Human Development.

Bronheim, S., & Goode T. (2013a). *Applying cultural and linguistic competence to a framework for creating learning spaces for the enhancement of experiential learning.* Washington,

DC: National Center for Cultural Competence, Georgetown University Center for Child and Human Development. Retrieved from https://nccc.georgetown.edu/documents/NCCC_PP_Cultural%20Brokers.pdf

Bronheim, S., & Goode, T. (2013b). *Climate of the learning environment: Cultural and linguistic competence checklist for MCH training programs.* Washington, DC: National Center for Cultural Competence, Georgetown University Center for Child and Human Development. Retrieved from https://nccc.georgetown.edu/training/NCCC_Climate_Checklist.pdf

Brookfield, S. D. (1995). *Becoming a critically reflective teacher.* San Francisco, CA: Jossey-Bass.

Brooks, J., & Brooks, M. (1993). *The case for the constructivist classrooms.* Alexandria, VA: ASCD.

Brooks, J., & Brooks, M. (2001). *In search of understanding: The case for constructivist classrooms.* Upper Saddle River, NJ: Pearson/Prentice Hall.

Brown, S., & Kingston, C. J. (2009). Nursing resource centers: Tracking utilization and outcome data. *Clinical Simulation in Nursing, 5*(3), S3–S4. http://doi.org/10.1016/j.ecns.2009.03.141

Brown, T. H. (2005). Beyond constructivism: Exploring future learning paradigms. *Education Today, 2*, 1–11.

Browne, A., Varcoe, C., Smye, V., Reimer-Kirkham, S., Lynam, M. J., & Wong, S. (2009). Cultural safety and the challenges of translating critically oriented knowledge in practice. *Nursing Philosophy, 10*, 167–179. doi:10.1111/j.1466-769X.2009.00406.x

Brownie, S. (2015). Programme accreditation and professional competencies in health profession education. In T. Brown & B. Williams (Eds.), *Evidence-based education in the health professions: Promoting best practice in the learning and teaching of students* (pp. 123–139). London, UK: Radcliffe Publishing Ltd.

Brun, J. P., & Dugas, N. (2008). An analysis of employee recognition: Perspectives on human resources practices. *The International Journal of Human Resource Management, 19*(4), 716–730. doi:10.1080/0958519080195372

Bruner, J. S. (1961). The act of discovery. *Harvard Educational Review, 31*, 21–32.

Brydges, R., Carnahan, H., Rose, D., Rose, L., & Dubrowski A. (2010). Coordinating progressive levels of simulation fidelity to maximize educational benefit. *Academic Medicine, 85*(5), 806–812. doi:10.1097/ACM.0b013e3181d7aabd

Bryson, J. M. (2011). *Strategic planning for public and nonprofit organizations: A guide to strengthening and sustaining organizational achievement.* Hoboken, NJ: John Wiley & Sons, Inc.

Buckham, P. W. (1830). *The theatre of the Greeks* (3rd ed.). Cambridge, UK: J. Smith, Printer.

Buckley, S., Hensman, M., Thomas, S., Dudley, R., Nevin, G., & Coleman, J. (2012). Developing interprofessional simulation in the undergraduate setting: Experience with five different professional groups. *Journal of Interprofessional Care, 26*(5), 362–369. doi:10.3109/13561820.2012.685993

Burgess, G. J. (2013). Leadership thresholds. In L. R. Melina, G. J. Burgess, L. L. Falkman & A. Marturano (Eds.), *The embodiment of leadership* (pp. 1–22). San Francisco, CA: Jossey-Bass.

Burkhardt, M., Nathaniel, A., & Walton, N. (2014). *Ethics and issues in contemporary nursing* (2nd ed.). Toronto, ON: Nelson.

Burns, J. M. (1978). *Leadership.* New York, NY: Harper & Row.

Burns, J. P. (2001). Complexity science and leadership in healthcare. *Journal of Nursing Administration, 31*(10), 474–482. Retrieved from http://www.nursingcenter.com

Businessdictionary.com. (2016a). *Inventory management.* Retrieved from http://www.businessdictionary.com/definition/inventory-management.html

Businessdictionary.com. (2016b). *Metrics.* Retrieved from http://www.businessdictionary.com/definition/metrics.html

Businessdictionary.com. (2016c). *Mission.* Retrieved from http://www.businessdictionary.com/definition/mission.html

Businessdictionary.com. (2016d). *Motivation: Intrinsic.* Retrieved from http://www.businessdictionary.com/definition/intrinsic-motivation.html

Businessdictionary.com. (2016e). *Motivation: Extrinsic.* Retrieved from http://www.businessdictionary.com/definition/extrinsic-motivation.html

Businessdictionary.com. (2016f). *Organizational chart.* Retrieved from http://www.businessdictionary.com/definition/organizational-chart.html

Butteris, S. M., Gladding, S. P., Eppich, W., Hagen, S. A., & Pitt, M. B. (2014). Simulation use for global away rotations (SUGAR): Preparing residents for emotional challenges abroad: A multicenter study. *Academic Pediatrics, 14*(5), 533–541. doi:10.1016/j.acap.2014.05.004

Buykx, P., Cooper, S., Kinsman, L., Endacott, R., Scholes, J., McConnell-Henry, T., & Cant, R. (2012). Patient deterioration simulation experiences: Impact on teaching and learning. *Collegian, 19*(3), 125–129. doi:10.1016/j.colegn.2012.03.011

Caldwell, J. (2012). *A framework for board oversight of enterprise risk.* Toronto, ON: Canadian Institute of Chartered Accountants.

Calhoun, A., Boone, M., Miller, K., & Pian-Smith, M. (2013). Using simulation to address hierarchy issues during medical crises. *Simulation in Healthcare, 8*(13), 14–21. doi:10.1097/SIH.0b013e318280b202

Campinha-Bacote, J. (1998). *The process of cultural competence in the delivery healthcare services: A culturally competent model of care* (3rd ed.). Cincinnati, OH: Transcultural C.A.R.E. Associates. Retrieved from www.transculturalcare.net

Campinha-Bacote, J. (2002). The process of cultural competence in the delivery of healthcare services: A model of care. *Journal of Transcultural Nursing, 13*(3), 181–184. doi:full/10.1177/10459602013003003

Canadian Institutes of Health Research. (2015). *Guide to knowledge translation planning and CIHR: Integrated and end-of-grant approaches.* Retrieved from http://www.cihr-irsc.gc.ca/e/45321.html#a4

Canadian Interprofessional Health Collaborative (CIHC). (2010a). *A national interprofessional competency framework.* Retrieved from on https://www.cihc.ca/library/handle/10296/436 and http://www.cihc.ca/files/CIHC_IPCompetencies_Feb1210.pdf

Canadian Interprofessional Healthcare Collaborative (CIHC). (2010b). *Canadian interprofessional health collaborative national competency framework.* Retrieved from http://www.cihc.ca/files/CIHC_IPCompetencies_Feb1210.pdf

Canadian Nurses Association (CNA). (2001). *Quality professional practice environments for registered nurses: Position statement.* Ottawa, ON: Author.

Canadian Nurses Association (CNA). (2003). *Ethical distress in health care environments. Ethics in practice for registered nurses.* Retrieved from http://www.cna-nurses.ca/cna/practice/ethics/inpractice/default_e.aspx

Canadian Nurses Association (CNA). (2005). Nursing leadership in a changing world. *Nursing Now, Issues and Trends in Canadian Nursing, 18*(1). Retrieved from http://www.cna-nurses.ca/cna/

Canadian Nurses Association (CNA). (2008). *Code of ethics for registered nurses.* Ottawa: Author.

Canadian Nurses Association (CNA). (2009). *Position statement: Nursing leadership.* Retrieved from http://www.cnaaiic.ca/CNA/documents/pdf/publications/PS110_Leadership_2009_e.pdf

Canadian Nurses Association (CNA). (2010). *Position Statement: Promoting cultural competence in nursing.* Ottawa, ON: Canadian Nurses Association.

Canadian Nurses Association (CNA). (2011a). *Position statement: Interprofessional collaboration.* Retrieved from https://www.cna-aiic.ca/~/media/cna/page-content/pdf-en/inter-proffessional-collaboration_position-statement.pdf?la=en

Canadian Nurses Association (CNA). (2011b). *The client, the nurse, and the environment.* Retrieved from http://www.cno.org/Global/docs/prac/41062.pdf

Canadian Nurses Association (CNA). (2012). *A nursing call to action: The health of our nation, the future of our health system.* Retrieved from http://www.cna-aiic.ca/~/media/cna/files/en/nec_report_e.pdf

Canadian Nurses Association (CNA) (2014, December 31). *About CNA: History.* Retrieved from https://www.cna-aiic.ca/en/about-cna/history

Canadian Nurses Association (CNA). (2015, May). *Workplace violence and bullying.* Retrieved from https://www.cna-aiic.ca/~/media/cna/page-content/pdf-en/workplace-violence-and-bullying_joint-position-statement.pdf?la=en

Canadian Patient Safety Institute (CPSI). (2006). *Special interest group on simulation: Final Report.* Retrieved on January 24, 2016 from http://www.patientsafetyinstitute.ca/en/education/simulation/Documents/Final%20Report-Simulation%20Special%20Interest%20Group.pdf

Canadian Patient Safety Institute (CPSI). (2008, May). *Patient simulation needs assessment.* Retrieved from http://www.patientsafetyinstitute.ca/en/education/simulation/Documents/Patient Simulation Needs Assessment - May 2008.pdf

Canadian Patient Safety Institute (CPSI). (2009). *Royal College of Physicians and Surgeons of Canada: Safety competencies framework* (1st ed.). Retrieved from http://www.patientsafetyinstitute.ca/en/toolsResources/safetyCompetencies/Documents/Safety Competencies.pdf

Canadian Patient Safety Institute (CPSI). (2012). *Patient and family stories* (website). Retrieved from http://www.patientsafetyinstitute.ca/en/toolsResources/Member-Videos-and-Stories/Pages/default.aspx

Canadian Patient Safety Institute (CPSI). (2016b). *Patient Safety Education Program* [PSEP]. Retrieved from http://www.patientsafetyinstitute.ca/en/education/PatientSafetyEducationProgram/Pages/default.aspx

Canadian Standards Association (CSA). (2011). Implementation guide to CAN/CSA-ISO 3100, risk management—Principles and guidelines. Retrieved from http://www.iso.org/iso/pub100080.pdf

Canever, B. P., Prado, M. L., Backes, V. M. S., & Gomes, D. C. (2012). Production of knowledge about the training of nurses in Latin America. *Revista Gaúcha de Enfermagem, 33*(4), 211–220.

Canillas, E. N. (2010). *The use of cognitive task analysis for identifying the critical information omitted when experts describe surgical procedures* (Unpublished Ed.D Dissertation). University of Southern California, Los Angeles, CA.

Cant, R. P., & Cooper, S. J. (2010). Simulation-based learning in nurse education: Systematic review. *Journal of Advanced Nursing, 66*(1), 3–15. doi:10.1111/j.1365-2648.2009.05240.x

Cant, R. P., & Cooper, S. J. (2011). The benefits of debriefing as formative feedback in nurse education. *Australian Journal of Advanced Nursing, 29*(1), 37–47.

Cant, R. P., & Cooper, S. J. (2014). Simulation in the Internet age: The place of web-based simulation in nursing education. An integrated review. *Nurse Education Today, 34*(12), 1435–1442. doi:10.1016/j.nedt.2014.08.001

Capella, J., Smith, S., Putnam, P., Gilbert C., Harvey, E., Wright, A., …, Remine, S. (2010). Teamwork training improves the clinical care of trauma patients. *Journal of Surgical Education, 67*(6), 439–443. doi:10.1016/Jsurg.2010.06.006

Caputi, L. (2010). *Teaching nursing: The art and science* (2nd ed). Glen Ellyn, IL: College of DuPage Press.

Carpenter-Song, E. A., Nordquiest Schwallie M., & Jonghofer, J. (2007). Cultural competence reexamined: Critique and directions for the future. *Psychiatric Services, 58*(10), 1362–1365. doi:10.1176/ps.2007.58.10.1362

Carroll, C. L., Bruno, K., & vonTschudi, M. (2016). Social media and free open access medical education: The future of medical and nursing education? *American Journal of Critical Care, 25*(1), 93–96. doi:10.4037/ajcc2016622

Carson, M. L., Gilbert, G. E., Schmoll, H. H., Dolinar, S. M., Anderson, J., Nickles, B. M., … Schaefer, J. J. (2015). Cooperative learning using simulation to achieve mastery of nasogastric tube insertion. *Journal of Nursing Education, 54*(3 Suppl), S47–S51. doi:10.3928/01484834-20150218-09

Carsten, M. K., Uhl-Bien, M., West, B. J., Patera, J. L., & McGregor, R. (2010). Exploring social constructions of followership: A qualitative study. *The Leadership Quarterly, 21*, 543–562. doi:10.1016/j.leaqua.2010.03.015

Carteret, M. (2011). Traditional Asian health beliefs & healing practices. Retrieved from http://www.dimensionsofculture.com/2010/10/traditional-asian-health-beliefs-healing-practices/

Castree, N., Kitchin, R., & Rogers, A. (2013). *A dictionary of human geography.* Oxford, UK: Oxford Press.

CBC Radio. (2012, January). *Recivilization: (Episode two) Open source knowledge.* Retrieved from http://www.cbc.ca/recivilization/episode/2012/01/24/episode-two-open-source-knowledge/

CEB Blogs. (2014, April). *The 12 skills CIOs and their teams must have.* Retrieved from https://www.cebglobal.com/blogs/12-competencies-that-drive-high-performance-in-it/?business_line=information-technology

Center for Disease Control and Prevention (CDC). (2009). *Evaluation briefs: Writing SMART objectives.* Retrieved from http://www.cdc.gov/healthyyouth/evaluation/pdf/brief3b.pdf

Center for Medical Simulation. (2016). *Debriefing assessment for simulation in healthcare (DASH)*©. Retrieved from https://www.harvardmedsim.org/debriefing-assesment-simulation-healthcare.php

Central Intelligence Agency (CIA). (2015, July). *The world fact book: East and southeast Asia China*. Retrieved from https://www.cia.gov/library/publications/the-world-factbook/geos/ch.html

Central Intelligence Agency (CIA). (2015a). *CIA world factbook, Rwanda*. Retrieved from https://www.cia.gov/library/publications/the-world-factbook/geos/rw.html

Central Intelligence Agency (CIA). (2015b). *The world factbook: United States*. Retrieved from https://www.cia.gov/library/publications/the-world-factbook/geos/us.html

Centre for the Advancement of Interprofessional Education (CAIPE). (2002). *Defining IPE—Interprofessional Education*. Retrieved from http://www.caipe.org.uk/about-us/defining-ipe/

Centre of Excellence for Simulation Education and Innovation. *Glossary*. Retrieved from http://cesei.org/global_assessment/

Chadwick, M. M. (2010). Creating order out of chaos: A leadership approach. *AORN Journal, 91*(1), 154–170. Retrieved from http://dx.doi.org/10.1016/j.aorn.2009.06.029

Chaffee, M. W., & McNeill, M. M. (2007). A model of nursing as a complex adaptive system. *Nursing Outlook, 55*(5), 232–241. doi:10.1016/j.outlook.2007.04.003

Chaleff, I. (2009). *The courageous follower: Standing up to and for our leaders* (3rd ed.). San Francisco, CA: Berrett-Koehler.

Charara, S. (2016, October). *Explained: How does VR actually work?* Retrieved from http://www.wareable.com/vr/how-does-vr-work-explained

Chatalalsingh, C., & Reeves, S. (2014). Leading team learning: What makes interprofessional teams learn to work well? *Journal of Interprofessional Care, 28*(6), 513–518. http://doi.org/10.3109/13561820.2014.900001

Chen, L. C., & Berlinguer, G. (2001). Health equity in a globalizing world. In T. Evans, M. Whitehead, F. Diderichsen, F. Bhuiya & M. Wirth (Eds.), *Challenging inequities in health: From ethics to action* (pp. 35–44). New York, NY: Oxford University Press.

Cheney, C., & Josey, K. (2014). Defining roles and building a career in simulation. In B. Ulrich & B. Mancini (Eds.), *Mastering simulation: A handbook for success*. Indianapolis, IN: Sigma Theta Tau International.

Cheng, A., Eppich, W., Grant, V., Sherbino, J., Zendejas, B., & Cook, D. A. (2014). Debriefing for technology-enhanced simulation: A systematic review and meta-analysis. *Medical Educator, 48*(7), 657–666. doi:10.1111/medu.12432

Cheng, A., Hunt, E. A., Donoghue, A., Nelson-McMillan, K., Nishisaki, A., Leflore, J., … Nadkami, V. W. (2013). Examining pediatric resuscitation education using simulation and scripted debriefing: A multicenter randomized trial. *JAMA Pediatrics, 167*(6), 528–536. doi:10.1001/jamapediatrics.2013.1389

Cheng, A., Kessler, D., Mackinnon, R., Change, T. P., Nadkarni, V. M., Hunt, E. A., …, Auerbach, M. (2016). Reporting guidelines for health care simulation research: Extensions to the CONSORT and STROBE statements. *Clinical Simulation in Nursing, 12*(3), A3–A13. doi:10.1016/j.ecns.2016.04.008

Chin, P. (2005). Chinese. In J. Lipson, & S. Dibble (Eds.), *Culture and clinical care*. San Francisco, CA: UCSF Nursing Press.

Chiniara, C., Cole, G., Brisbin, K., Huffman, D., Cragg, B., Lamacchia, M. … Canadian Network for Simulation in Healthcare, Guidelines Working Group. (2013). Simulation in healthcare: A taxonomy and a conceptual framework for instructional design and media selection. *Medical Teacher, 35*(8), e1380–e1395. Retrieved from http://dx.doi.org/10.3109/0142159X.2012.733451

Chow, G. (2004). Economic reform and growth in China. *Annals of Economics and Finance, 5*(5), 127–152. Retrieved from http://aeconf.com/Articles/May2004/aef050107.pdf

Christenson, C. (2013, November). Innovation imperative: Change everything. *The New York Times*. Retrieved from http://www.nytimes.com/2013/11/03/education/edlife/online-education-as-an-agent-of-transformation.html?_r=0

Christenson Institute. (2016). *Disruptive innovation*. Retrieved from http://www.christenseninstitute.org/key-concepts/disruptive-innovation-2/

Churchouse, C., & McCafferty, C. (2012). Standardized patients versus simulated patients: Is there a difference. *Clinical Simulation in Nursing, 8*(8), e363–e365. doi:10.1016/j.ecns.2011.04.008

Clancy, C. M., & Tornberg, D. N. (2007). TeamSTEPPS: Assuring optimal teamwork in clinical settings. *American Journal of Medical Quality, 22*(3), 244–247. http://doi.org/10.1177/1062860607300616

Clapper, T. C. (2009). Moving away from teaching and becoming a facilitator of learning. Professionals Against Improperly Labeling Active Learners, *2*(2). Retrieved from http://www.academia.edu/1180001/Moving_away_from_teaching_and_becoming_a_facilitator_of_learning

Clapper, T. C. (2010a). Beyond Knowles: What those conducting simulation need to know about adult learning theory. *Clinical Simulation in Nursing, 6*(1), e7–e14. doi:10.1016/j.ecns.2009.07.003

Clapper, T. C. (2010b). Creating the safe learning environment. Professionals Against Improperly Labeling Active Learners, *3*(2), 1–6. Retrieved from http://www.academia.edu/1180264/Creating_the_safe_learning_environment

Clapper, T. C. (2011a). *The effect of differentiated instruction on JROTC leadership training* (Doctoral dissertation). Retrieved from Dissertations & Theses: Full Text (Publication No. AAT 3440244).

Clapper, T. C. (2011b). Interference in learning: What curriculum developers need to know. *Clinical Simulation in Nursing, 7*(3), e77–e80. doi:10.1016/j.ecns.2010.08.001

Clapper, T. C. (2012). Development of a hybrid simulation course to reduce central line infections. *Journal of Continuing Education in Nursing, 43*(5), 218–224. doi:10.3928/00220124-20111101-06

Clapper, T. C. (2013a). In situ and mobile simulation: Lessons learned… Authentic and resource intensive. *Clinical Simulation in Nursing, 9*(11), e551–e557. doi:10.1016/j.ecns.2012.12.005

Clapper, T. C. (2013b). Saturation in training. *Patient Safety InSight*. Retrieved from http://magazine.nationalpatientsafetyfoundation.org/magazine/spring2013-saturation-in-training/

Clapper, T. C. (2014a). Situational interest and instructional design: A guide for simulation facilitators. *Simulation & Gaming, 45*(2), 167–182. doi:10.1177/1046878113518482

Clapper, T. C. (2014b). Next steps in TeamSTEPPS®: Creating a just culture with observation and simulation. *Simulation & Gaming, 45*(3), 306–317. doi:10.1177/1046878114543638

Clapper, T. C. (2015a). Theory to practice in simulation. *Simulation & Gaming, 46*(2), 131–136. doi:10.1177/1046878115599615

Clapper, T. C. (2015b). Cooperative-based learning and the zone of proximal development. *Simulation & Gaming, 46*(2), 148–158. doi:10.1177/1046878115569044

Clapper, T. C., & Kardong-Edgren, S. (2012). Using deliberate practice and simulation to improve nursing skills. *Clinical Simulation in Nursing, 8*(3), e109–e133. doi:10.1016/j.ecns.2010.12.001

Clarivate Analytics. (2017). *The Thompson Reuters impact factor.* Retrieved from http://wokinfo.com/essays/impact-factor/

Clark, C. M. (2013). *Creating & sustaining civility in nursing education.* Indianapolis, IN: Sigma Theta Tau International.

Clark, C. M. (2015). Conversations to inspire and promote a more civil workplaces. *American Nurse Today, 10*(11).

Clark, R. E., Pugh, C. M., Yates, K. A., & Sullivan, M. (2008). *The use of cognitive task analysis and simulators for after review of medical events in Iraq.* Technical Report 5-21-2008 developed for the Center for Cognitive Technology. Rossier School of Ed, University of Southern California.

Clarke, A. C. (1962). Hazards of prophecy. In A. C. Clarke (Ed.), *Profiles of the future.* Boston, MA: H.M.H. Publishing Co.

Classen, D. C., Resar, R., Griffin, F., Federico, F., Frankel, T., Kimmel, N., … James, B. C. (2011). Global Trigger Tool shows that adverse events in hospitals may be ten times greater than previously measured. *Health Affairs, 30*(4), 581–589. doi:10.1377/hlthaff.2011.0190

Claudius, I., Kaji, A., Santillanes, G., Cicero, M., Donofrio, J., Gausche-Hill, M., … Chang, T. (2015). Comparison of computerized patients versus live moulaged actors for a mass-casualty drill. *Prehospital and Disaster Medicine, 30*(5), 438–442. doi:10.1017/S1049023X15004963

Cleary, M., Walter, G., Siegfried, N., & Jackson, D. (2014). Contemplating an expatriate health care position? Key factors to consider. *Issues in Mental Health Nursing, 35*(5), 406–409. Retrieved from http://doi.org/10.3109/01612840.2014.899301

Cleland, J. A., Abe, K., & Rethans, J. J. (2009). The use of simulated patients in medical education: AMEE Guide No. 42. *Medical Teacher, 31*(6), 477–486. http://doi.org/10.1080/01421590903002821

Cognitive Edge. (2015). *Introduction to Cynefin framework.* Retrieved from http://cognitive-edge.com/videos/cynefin-framework-introduction/

Cognitive Edge.com. (2016). *Cynefin framework.* Retrieved from http://cognitive-edge.com/

Cohen, E. R., Barsuk, J. H., Moazed, F., Caprio, T., Didwania, A., MGhaghie, W. C., & Wayne, D. B. (2013). Making July safe: Simulation-based mastery learning during intern boot camp. *Academic Medicine, 88*(2), 233–239. doi:10.1097/ACM.0b013e31827bfc0a

Coleridge, S. T. (1817). *Biographia literaria or biographical sketches of my literary life and opinions* (Vol. II). London, UK: S. Curtis, Printer.

Combined Universities Interprofessional Learning Unit (CUILU). (2004). *Interprofessional Capability Framework. A framework containing capabilities and learning levels leading to interprofessional capability.* Retrieved from http://caipe.org.uk/silo/files/cuilupdf.pdf

Commission on Collegiate Nursing Education. (2013). *Standards for accreditation of baccalaureate and graduate nursing programs.* Retrieved from http://www.aacn.nche.edu/ccne-accreditation/Standards-Amended-2013.pdf

Commission on Social Determinants of Health (CSDH). (2008). *Closing the gap in a generation: Health equity through action on the social determinants of health.* Final Report of the Commission on Social Determinants of Health, Geneva.

Connor, J. B., & Miller, A. M. (2014). Occupational stress and adaptation of immigrant nurses from the Philippines. *Journal of Research in Nursing, 19*(6), 504–515. doi:10.1177/1744987114536570

Conrad, M. A., Guhde, J., Brown, D., Chronister, C., & Ross-Alaolmolki, K. (2011). Trans-formational leadership: Instituting a nursing simulation program. *Clinical Simulation in Nursing, 7*(5), e189–e195. doi:10.1016/j.ecns.2010.02.007

Consejo de Rectores de las Universidades Chilenas (Council of Rectors of Chilean Universities), CRUCH. (2015). *Home page.* Retrieved from http://www.consejoderectores.cl

Consortium for Research on Emotional Intelligence Organizations. (2015). *Emotional intelligence measures.* Retrieved from http://www.eiconsortium.org/measures/measures.html

Cook, D., Hatala, R., Brydges, R., Szostek, J., Wang, A., Erwin, P., & Hamstra, S. (2011). Technology-enhanced simulation for health professional's education—A systematic review and meta-analysis. *JAMA, 306*(9), 978–988. doi:10.1001/jama.2011.1234

Cooper, S., Beauchamp, A., Bogossian, F., Bucknall, T., Cant, R., DeVries, B., … Young, S. (2012). Managing patient deterioration: A protocol for enhancing undergraduate nursing students' competence through web-based simulation and feedback techniques. *BMC Nursing, 11*(18). doi:10.1186/1472-6955-11-18

Cooper, S., Kinsman, L., Buykx, P., McConnell-Henry, T., Endacott, R., & Scholes, J. (2010). Managing the deteriorating patient in a simulated environment: Nursing students' knowledge, skill and situation awareness. *Journal of Clinical Nursing, 19*(15–16), 2309–2318. doi:10.1111/j.1365-2702.2009.03164.x

Cooperrider, D. L., & Whitney, D. (2005). *Appreciative inquiry: A positive revolution in change.* San Francisco, CA: Berrett-Koehler.

Corbett, S., & Fikkert, B. (2009). *When helping hurts; how to alleviate poverty without hurting the poor and yourself.* Chicago, IL: Moody Press.

Cornele, J., & Rockstraw, L. J. (2010). Managing a simulation center: People, resources, equipment, and technology. *Clinical Simulation in Nursing, 6*(3), e111. http://doi.org/10.1016/j.ecns.2010.03.019

Corvetto, M., Bravo, M. P., Montaña, R., Utili, F., Escudero, E., Boza, C., …, Dagnino, J. (2013). Simulación en educación médica, una sinopsis. *Revista Medica Chile, 141*, 70–79.

Costa, A. L., & Kallick, B. (1995). *Assessment in the learning organization: Shifting the paradigm.* Alexandria, VA: Association for Supervision and Curriculum Development.

Creative Spirits. (2015). Aboriginal culture. Retrieved from http://www.creativespirits.info/#axzz3oo3KWy00

Cregan, P., & Watterson, L. (2005). High stakes assessment using simulation—An Australian experience. *Studies in Health Technology & Informatics, 111*, 99–104.

Cremin, L. A. (1957). *The republic and the school: Horace Mann on the education of free men.* New York, NY: Teachers College.

Creswell, J. W., Fetters, M. D., & Ivankova, N. V. (2004). Designing a mixed methods study in primary care. *Annals of Family Medicine, 2*(1), 7–12. doi:10.1370/afm.104

Creswell, J. W., & Plano Clark, L. (2011). *Designing and conducting mixed methods research.* Thousand Oaks, CA: SAGE Publications, Inc.

Crispen, P. D. (2010). *Identifying the point of diminishing marginal utility for cognitive task analysis: Surgical subject matter expert interviews* (Doctoral dissertation). University of Southern California. ProQuest Dissertations and Theses (UMI Number: 3403725).

Crossan, M., & Mazutis, D. (2008). Transcendent leadership. *Business Horizons, 51*(2), 131–139. doi:10.1016/j.bushor.2007.11.004

Cueva, M., Kuhnley, R., Revels, L., Cueva, K., Dignan, M., & Lanier, A. (2013). Bridging storytelling traditions with digital technology. *International Journal of Circumpolar Health, 72.* doi:10.3402/ijch.v72i0.20717

Cueva, M., Kuhnley, R., Revels, L., Schoenberg, N., & Dignan, M. (2015). Digital storytelling: A tool for health promotion and cancer awareness in rural Alaskan communities. *International Journal of Circumpolar Health, 74.* doi:10.3402/ijch.v74.28781

Cummings, G. G., MacGregor, T., Davey, M., Lee, H., Wong, C. A., Lo, E., ... Stafford, E. (2010). Leadership styles and outcome patterns for the nursing workforce and work environment: A systematic review. *International Journal of Nursing Studies, 47,* 363–385. doi:10.1016/j.ijnurstu.2009.08.006

Curran, V. R., Heath, O., Kearney, A., & Button, P. (2010). Evaluation of an interprofessional collaboration workshop for post-graduate residents, nursing and allied health professionals. *Journal of Interprofessional Care, 24*(3), 315–318. doi:10.3109/13561820903163827

Daft, R. L. (2010). *Management* (9th ed.). Mason, OH: South Western Cengage Learning.

Daft, R. L. (2012). *Management* (10th ed.). Mason, OH: Cengage Learning.

Daft, R. L. (2014). *Management* (11th ed.). Mason, OH: South Western Cengage Learning.

Damazo, R. (2012). *Moulage and more: Theatrical tricks and amazing tools to create simulation reality.* Chicaco, CA: California State University.

Damazo, R., & Fox, S. (2015). Moulage: The art of providing physical cues for simulation reality. In J. C. Palaganas, J. Maxworth, C. A. Epps & M. E. Mancini (Eds.), *Defining excellence in simulation programs.* Philadelphia, PA: Wolters Kluwer Lippincott Williams & Wilkins.

Darling, M., Parry, C., & Moore, J. (2005, July–August). Learning in the thick of it. *Harvard Business Review, 83*(7), 84–92, 192.

Dauphinee, D. W., & Reznick, R. (2011). Framework for designing, implementing, and sustaining a national simulation network. Building incentive-based network structures and iterative processes for long-term success: The case of the Medical Council of Canada's qualifying examination, part II. *Simulation in Healthcare, 6,* 94–100. doi:10.1097/SIH.0b013e31820695e8

Davies, J., & Alinier, G. (2010). *The emergence of simulation-based clinical training outside of the western world. The growing trend of simulation as a form of clinical education. A global perspective.* Retrieved from http://uhra.herts.ac.uk/bitstream/handle/2299/7614/904558.pdf?sequence=1

Day-Black, C., & Watties-Daniels, A. D. (2006). Cutting edge technology to enhance nursing classroom instruction at Coppin State University. *ABNF Journal, 17,* 103–106.

Decker, S. I. (2012). Simulations: Education and ethics. In P. R. Jeffries (Ed.), *Simulation in nursing education: From conceptualization to evaluation* (2nd ed., pp. 13–23). New York, NY: National League for Nursing.

Decker, S., & Anderson, M. (2013). *SIRC: Beyond basic debriefing module.* New York, NY: National League for Nursing, Retrieved from http://sirc.nln.org/mod/resource/view.php?id=746

Decker, S. I., Anderson, M., Boese, T., Epps, C., McCarthy, J., Motola, I. ... Lioce, L. (2015). Standards of best practice: Simulation standard VIII: Simulation-enhanced interprofessional education (sim-IPE). *Clinical Simulation in Nursing, 11*(6), 293–297. doi:http://dx.doi.org/10.1016/j.ecns.2015.03.010

Decker, S., Fey, M., Sideras, S., Caballero, S., Rockstraw, L. (R.), Boese, T., ..., Borum, J. C. (2013). Standards of best practice: Simulation standard VI: The debriefing process. *Clinical Simulation in Nursing, 9*(6S), S27–S29. http://dx.doi.org/10.1016/j.ecns.2013.04.008

Decker, S., Sportsman, S., Puetz, L., & Billings, L. (2008). The evolution of simulation and its contribution to competency. *The Journal of Continuing Education in Nursing, 39*(2), 74–80.

Delors, J., Al Mufti, I., Amagi, I., Carneiro, R., Chung, F., Geremek, B., . . . Nanzhao, Z. (1996). *Learning: the treasure within.* Paris, France: United Nations Educational, Scientific and Cultural Organization.

Denning, S. M., Jewett Johnson, C. M., Johnson, D., Loen, M., Patow, C., & Brannen, C. K. (2010). Partners in simulation: Public academic-private health care collaboration. In Richard R. Kyle, Jr. & W. Bosseau Murray (Eds.), *Clinical simulation: Operations, engineering, and management.* San Diego, CA: Elsevier, Inc.

Department of Health. (2003). *Guidance on implementing the European working time directive for doctors in training, HSC 2003/001.* London, UK: The Stationary Office

Department of Veteran's Affairs (DVA) and Board of Studies Teaching and Educational Standars (BOSTES) NSW. (2015). Gallipoli and the ANZACS. Retrieved from http://www.gallipoli.gov.au/

Derossis, A. M., Fried, G. M., Abrahamowicz, M., Sigman, H. H., Barkun, J. S., & Meakin, J. L. (1998). Development of model for training and evaluation of laparoscopic skills. *The American Journal of Surgery, 175,* 482–487.

Design-Build Institute of America. (2014). *What is design build? A design-build done right primer.* Retrieved from http://www.dbia.org/resource-center/Documents/what_is_design_build_primer.pdf

Deterding, S., Dixon, D., Khaled, R., & Nacke, L. (2011, September). From game design elements to gamefulness: Defining gamification. In *Proceedings of the 15th International Academic MindTrek Conference: Envisioning Future Media Environments* (pp. 9–15). ACM.

Dewey, J. (1913). *Interest and effort in education.* Boston, MA: Houghton Mifflin.

Dewey, J. (1938). *Experience and education.* New York, NY: Macmillan.

Dictionary.com. (2016). *Blog*. Retrieved from http://www.dictionary.com/browse/blog

Dieckmann, P. (2012). Debriefing olympics: A workshop concept to stimulate the adaptation of debriefings to learning contexts. *Simulation in Healthcare, 7*(3), 176–182. doi:10.1097/SIH.0b013e31824888b8

Dieckmann, P., Gaba, D., & Rall, M. (2007). Deepening the theoretical foundations of patient simulation as social practice. *Simulation in Healthcare, 2*(3), 183–193. doi:10.1097/SIH.0b013e3180f637f5

Dieckmann, P., Lippert, A., Glavin, R., & Rall, M. (2010). When things do not go as expected: Scenario life savers. *Simulation in Healthcare, 5*(4), 219–225. doi:10.1097/SIH.0b013e3181e77f74

Dieckmann, P., Molin Friis, S., Lippert, A., & Ostergaard, D. (2009). The art and science of debriefing in simulation: Ideal and practice. *Medical Teacher, 31*(7), e287–e294.

Dieckmann, P., Reddersen, S., Zieger, J., & Rall, M. (2008). Video-assisted debriefing in simulation-based training of crisis resource management. In R. R. Kyle & W. B. Murray (Eds.), *Clinical simulation: Operations, engineering, and management* (pp. 667–676). Burlington, VT: Academic Press.

Digital Trends. (2017). *Wearables*. Retrieved from http://www.digitaltrends.com/wearables/

Dillon, P. M., Noble, K. A., & Kaplan, W. (2009). Simulation as a means to foster collaborative interdisciplinary education. *Nursing Education Perspectives, 30*(2), 87–90.

Dinh, T. (2012). *Improving primary health care through collaboration: Briefing-barriers to successful interprofessional teams*. The Conference Board of Canada. Retrieved from www.wrha.mb.ca/professionals/collaborativecare/files/CBCBriefing22012.pdf

Dinh, T., Stonebridge, C., & Theriault, L. (2014). *Recommendations for Action: Getting the Most out of Healthcare Teams*. The Conference Board of Canada. Retrieved from http://www.conferenceboard.ca/e-library/abstract.aspx?did=5988

Disler, R., Rochester, S., Kelly, M. A., White, H., & Forber, J. (2013). Delivering a large cohort simulation-beginning nursing students' experience: A pre-post survey. *Journal of Nursing Education and Practice, 3*(12), 133–142. doi:10.5430/jnep.v3n12p133

Dismukes, R. K., Gaba, D. M., & Howard, S. K. (2006). So many roads: Facilitated debriefing in healthcare. *Simulation in Healthcare, 1*(1), 23–25.

Dixon, G., Mercado, A., & Knowles, B. (2013). Followers and generations in the workplace. *Engineering Management Journal, 25*(4), 62–72. Retrieved from http://www.scimagojr.com/journalsearch.php?q=29088&tip=sid

Do, H. (2000). *EthnoMed: Chinese cultural profile*. Retrieved from https://ethnomed.org/culture/chinese/chinese-cultural-profile#section-2

Doane, G. H., & Varcoe, C. (2015). *How to nurse: Relational inquiry with individuals and families in changing health and health care contexts* (pp. 421–488). Philadelphia, PA: Wolters Kluwer.

Dolan, S., & Garcia, S. (2002). Managing by values: Cultural redesign for strategic organizational change at the dawn of the twenty-first century. *Journal of Management Development, 21*(2), 101–117. doi:10.1108/02621710210417411

Dolan, S. L., Garcia, S., & Auerbach, A. (2003). Understanding and managing chaos in organisations. *International Journal of Management, 20*(1), 23–35. Retrieved from http://www.journals.elsevier.com/journal-of-international-management/

Dongilli, T. A. (2016). Professional development for the next generation of simulation operations specialists. In L. Gantt & H. M. Young (Eds.), *Healthcare simulation: A guide for operations specialists*. Hoboken, NJ: Wiley and Sons, Inc.

Dongilli, T. A., Shekhter, I., & Gavilanes, J. S. (2015). Policies and procedures. In Palaganas, J. C., Maxworthy, J. C., Epps, C. A. & M. E. Mancini (Eds.), *Defining excellence in simulation programs*. Philadelphia, PA: Wolters Kluwer.

Doolen, J. (2015). Psychometric properties of the simulation thinking rubric to measure higher order thinking in undergraduate nursing students. *Clinical Simulation in Nursing, 11*(1), 35–43. doi:10.1016/j.ecns.2014.10.007

Doolen, J., Giddings, M., Johnson, M., de Nathan, G. G., & Badia, L. O. (2014). An evaluation of mental health simulation with standardized patients. *International Journal of Nursing Education Scholarship, 11*(1), 1–8. doi:10.1515/ijnes-2013-0075

Doolen, J., Mariani, B., Atz, T., Horsley, T. L., O'Rourke, J., McAfee, K., & Cross, C. (2016). High-fidelity simulation in nursing education: A review of reviews. *Clinical Simulation in Nursing, 12*(7), 290–302. doi:http://dx.doi.org/10.1016/j.ecns.2016.01.009

Doran, G. T. (1981). There's a S.M.A.R.T. way to write management's goals and objectives. *Management Review, 70*(11), 35.

Dorney, B., Walston, C., & Decker, S. (2014). Developing and building a simulation center. In B. Ulrich & B. Mancini (Eds.), *Mastering simulation: A handbook for success*. Indianapolis, IN: Sigma Theta Tau International.

Dorrenbos, A. Z., Schim, S. M., Benkert, R., & Borse, N. N. (2005). Psychometric evaluation of the cultural competence assessment instrument among healthcare providers. *Nursing Research, 54*(5), 324–331.

Douglas, M. K., Pierce, J. U., Rosenkoetter, M, Callister, L. C., Hattar-Pollara, M., Lauderdale, J., …, Pacquiao, D. (2009). Standards of practice for culturally competent nursing care: A request for comments. *Journal of Transcultural Nursing, 20*(3), 257–269. doi:10.1177/1043659609334678

Dowie, I., & Phillips, C. (2011). Supporting the lecturer to deliver high-fidelity simulation. *Nursing Standard, 25*(49), 35–40.

Dreifuerst, K. (2009). The essentials of debriefing in simulation learning: A concept analysis. *Nursing Education Perspectives, 30*(2), 109–114.

Dreifuerst, K. T. (2011). Debriefing for Meaningful Learning©: A reflective strategy to foster clinical reasoning. *Clinical Simulation in Nursing, 7*(6), e250. doi:10.1016/j.ecns.2011.09.023

Dreifuerst, K. T. (2015). Getting started with debriefing for meaningful learning. *Clinical Simulation in Nursing, 11*(5), 268–275. doi:10.1016/j.ecns.2015.01.005

Dreifuerst, K. T., & Decker, S. I. (2012). Debriefing: An essential component for learning in simulation pedagogy. In P. R. Jeffries (Ed.) *Simulation in nursing education: From conceptualization to evaluation* (2nd ed., pp. 105–129). New York, NY: National League for Nursing.

Drobac, P., & Naughton, B. (2014). Health equity in Rwanda: The New Rwanda, twenty years later. *Harvard International Reviews, 35*(4). Available from http://hir.harvard.edu/archives/5732

Drucker, P. F. (2006). *The effective executive: The definitive guide to getting the right things done*. New York, NY: Harper-Collins.

Duchscher, J. (2009). Transition shock: The initial stage of role adaptation for newly graduated registered nurses. *Journal of Advanced Nursing, 65*(5), 1103–1113. doi:10.1111/j.1365-2648.2008.04898.x

Duchscher, J. B. (2008). A process of becoming: The stages of new nursing graduate professional role transition. *Journal of Continuing Education in Nursing, 39*(10), 441–450.

Duchscher, J. E. B., & Myrick, F. (2008). The prevailing winds of oppression: The new graduate experience in acute care. *Nursing Forum, 43*(4), 191–206.

Dudley, F. (2012). *The simulated patient handbook. A comprehensive guide for facilitators and simulated patients.* London, UK: Radcliffe Publishing Ltd.

Duffield, S., & Whitty, S. J. (2015). Developing a systemic lessons learned knowledge model for organizational learning through projects. *International Journal of Project Management, 33*(2), 311–324. doi:10.1016/j.ijproman.2014.07.004

Dumas, P., Hollerbach, A. D., Stuart, G., & Duffy, N. D. (2015). Expanding simulation capacity: Senior-level students as teachers. *Journal of Nursing Education, 54*(9), 516–519. doi:10.3928/01484834-20150814-06

Duncan, S. M. (2014). Looking back, moving forward: The promise of nursing in the 21st century. In M. McIntyre & C. MacDonald (Eds.), *Realities of Canadian nursing; Professional, practice, and power issues* (4th ed., pp. 451–466). Philadelphia, PA: Lippincott Williams & Wilkins.

Dunn, R. (1996). How learning styles differ among groups of students. *Learning Styles Network Newsletter, 17*(1), 2.

Dunn, R., & Dunn, K. (1978). *Teaching students through their individual learning styles: A practical approach.* Reston, VA: Reston Publishing.

Dunn, R., & Dunn, K. (1992). *Teaching elementary students through their individual learning styles: Practical approaches for grades 3–6.* Boston, MA: Allyn & Bacon.

Dunn, R., Honigsfeld, A., Doolan, L. S., Bostrom, L., Russo, K., Schiering, M. S. ... Tenedero, H. (2009). Impact of learning-style instructional strategies on students' achievement and attitudes: Perceptions of educators in diverse institutions. *The Clearing House, 82*(3), 135–140.

Dunn, W. F. (Ed.). (2004). *Simulators in critical care and beyond.* Des Plaines, IL: Society of Critical Care Medicine.

Durham, C. F., & Alden, K. R. (2008, April). Enhancing patient safety in nursing education through patient simulation. In R. G. Hughes (Ed.), *Patient safety and quality: An evidence-based handbook for nurses.* Rockville, MD: Agency for Healthcare Research and Quality (US), Chapter 51. Available from http://www.ncbi.nlm.nih.gov/books/NBK2628/

Durham, C. F., Cato, M. L., & Lasater, K. (2014). NLN/Jeffries simulation framework state of the science project: Participant construct. *Clinical Simulation in Nursing, 10*(7), 363–372. doi:http://dx.doi.org/10.1016/j.ecns.2014.04.002

Dyer, W. G., Dyer, J. H., & Dyer, W. G. (2013). *Team building: Proven strategies for improving team performance.* San Francisco, CA: Jossey-Bass, Wiley and Sons, Inc.

eCunha, M. P., & Rego, A. (2010). Complexity, simplicity, simplexity. *European Management Journal, 28,* 85–94. Retrieved from http://www.elsevier.com/locate/emj

Edberg, M. (2013a). *Essentials of health, culture, and diversity: Understanding people, reducing disparities.* Burlington, MA: Jones & Bartlett Learning, LCC.

Edberg, M. (2013b). *Health, culture, and diversity: Understanding people, reducing disparities.* Burlington, MA: Jones & Bartlett Learning, LCC.

Eddins, E., Hu, J., & Liu, H. (2011). Baccalaureate nursing education in China: Issues and challenges. *Nursing Education Perspectives, 32*(1), 30–33.

Eder-Van Hook, J. (2004). *Building a national agenda for simulation-based medical education.* Washington, DC: Center for Telemedicine Law and Telemedicine and Advanced Technology Research Center, U.S. Army Medical Research and Materiel Command.

Edler, A. A., & Fanning, R. M. (2007). "A rose by any other name?" Toward a common terminology in simulation education and assessment. *Critical Care Medicine, 35*(9), 2237–2238. doi:10.1097/01.CCM.0000281643.88046.DC

Edmundson, A. (1999). Psychological safety and learning behavior in work teams. *Administrative Science Quarterly, 44*(2), 350–383.

Education Advisory Board. (2013). *Considerations for online medical simulation technician training programs.* Retrieved from http://www.eab.com/research-and-insights/continuing-and-online-education-forum/custom/2013/12/considerations-for-online-medical-simulation-technician-training-programs

Educause Learning Initiative. (2009). *7 Things you should know about location-aware applications.* Retrieved from https://net.educause.edu/ir/library/pdf/ELI7047.pdf

Eggerth, D. E., & Flynn, M. A. (2012). Applying the theory of work adjustment to Latino immigrant workers: An exploratory study. *Journal of Career Development, 39*(1), 76–98. http://doi.org/10.1177/0894845311417129

Eisen, L. A., & Savel, R. H. (2009). What went right: Lessons for the intensivist from the crew of US Airways Flight 1549. *Chest, 136*(3), 910–917. http://doi.org/10.1378/chest.09-0377

Eisert, S., & Geers, J. (2016). Pilot-study exploring time for simulation in academic and hospital-based organizations. *Clinical Simulation in Nursing, 12*(9), 361–367. http://dx.doi.org/10.1016/j.ecns.2016.04.005

Elfrink, V., Kirkpatrick, B., Nininger, J., & Schubert, C. (2010). Using learning outcomes to inform teaching practices in human patient simulation. *Nursing Education Perspectives, 31,* 97–100.

Elfrink Cordi, V. L., Leighton, K., Ryan-Wenger, N., Doyle, T. J., & Ravert, P. (2012). History and development of the Simulation Effectiveness Tool (SET). *Clinical Simulation in Nursing, 8*(6), 199–210. doi:10.1016/j.ecns.2011.12.001

Ellis Fletcher, S. (2015). *Cultural sensibility in healthcare: A personal and professional guidebook.* Indianapolis, IN: Sigma Theta Tau International.

Elton, J., & O'Riordan, A. (2016). *Healthcare disrupted: Next generation business models and strategies.* Hoboken, NJ: John Wiley & Sons, Inc.

Emanuel, E. J., & Pearson, S. D. (2012). Physician autonomy and health care reform. *JAMA, 307*(4), 367–368. doi:10.1001/jama.2012.19

Emanuel, L., Berwick, D., Conway, J., Combes, J., Hatlie, M., Leape, L., et al. (2008). What exactly is patient safety? In K. Henriksen, J. B. Battles, M. A. Keyes, et al. (Eds.), *Advances in patient safety: New directions and alternative approaches* (Vol. 1: Assessment). Rockville (MD): Agency for Healthcare Research and Quality. Retrieved from https://www.ncbi.nlm.nih.gov/books/NBK43629/pdf/Bookshelf_NBK43629.pdf

Emanuel, L. L., Taylor, L., Hain, A., Combes, J. R., Hatlie, M. J., Karsh, B. ... Walton, M. (Eds.), (2011). *The patient safety education program—Canada (PSEP Canada) curriculum. PSEP—Canada, 2011.* Retrieved from http://www.patientsafetyinstitute.ca/en/education/PatientSafetyEducationProgram/Pages/default.aspx

Embassy of Qatar in Rome (2015). Embassy of Qatar in Rome, Italy. Retrieved from https://www.embassypages.com/missions/embassy9305/

Emergency Nurses Association (ENA). (2014). Initial assessment. In *Trauma nursing core course provider manual* (7th ed.). Des Plaines, IL: Emergency Nurses Association.

Endacott, R., Scholes, J., Buykx, P., Cooper, S., Kinsman, L., & McConnell-Henry, T. (2010). Final-year nursing students' ability to assess, detect and act on clinical cues of deterioration in a simulated environment. *Journal of Advanced Nursing, 66*(12), 2722–2731. doi:10.1111/j.1365-2648.2010.05417.x

Endacott, R., Scholes, J., Cooper, S., McConnell-Henry, T., Porter, J., Missen, K., ... Champion, R. (2012). Identifying patient deterioration: Using simulation and reflective interviewing to examine decision making skills in a rural hospital. *International Journal of Nursing Studies, 49*(6), 710–717. doi:10.1016/j.ijnurstu.2011.11.018

Engward, H., & Davis, G. (2015). Being reflexive in qualitative grounded theory: Discussion and application of a model of reflexivity. *Journal of Advanced Nursing, 71*(7), 1530–1538. Retrieved from http://doi.org/10.1111/jan.12653

E-patients.net. (2016). *About us. Society for Participatory Medicine.* Retrieved on from http://e-patients.net/about-e-patientsnet

Epitropaki, O., Sy, T., Martin, R., Tram-Quon, S., & Topakas, A. (2013). Implicit leadership and followership theories "in the wild": Taking stock of information-processing approaches to leadership and followership in organizational settings. *The Leadership Quarterly, 24*(2013), 858–881. doi:10.1016/j.leaqua.2013.10.005

Eppich, W., & Cheng, A. (2015). Promoting excellence and reflective learning in simulation (PEARLS). *Simulation in Healthcare, 10,* 106–115. doi:10.1097/SIH.0000000000000072

Eppich, W. J., O'Connor, L., & Adler, M. D. (2013). Providing effective simulation activities. In J. Forrest, K. McKimm & S. Edgar (Eds.), *Essential simulation in clinical education* (pp. 213–234). Chichester, UK: Wiley-Blackwell.

Epstein, R. M. (2006). Making communication research matter: What do patients notice, what do patients want, and what do patients need? *Patient Education and Counseling, 60,* 272–278.

Epstein, R. M. (2013). Whole mind and shared mind in clinical decision-making. *Patient Education and Counseling, 90,* 200–206. doi:10.1016/j.pec.2012.06.035

Ericsson, K. A. (2004). Deliberate practice and the acquisition and maintenance of expert performance in medicine and related domains. *Academic Medicine, 79*(10), S70–S81.

Ericsson, K. A. (2006). The influence of experience and deliberate practice on the development of superior expert performance. In K. A. Ericsson, N. Charness, P. J. Feltovich & R. R. Hoffman (Eds.). *Cambridge handbook of expertise and expert performance* (pp. 685–706). Cambridge, UK: Cambridge University Press.

Ericsson, K. A. (2007). An expert-performance perspective of research on medical expertise: The study of clinical performance. *Medical Education, 41,* 1124–1130. doi:10.1111/j.1365-2923.2007.02946.x

Ericsson, K. A. (2008). Deliberate practice and acquisition of expert performance: A general overview. *Academic Emergency Medicine, 15,* 988–994. doi:10.1111/j.1553-2712.2008.00227.x

Ericsson, K. A. (2015). Acquisition and maintenance of medical expertise: A perspective from the expert-performance approach with deliberate practice. *Academic Medicine, 90*(11), 1–15. doi:10.1097/ACM.0000000000000939

Ericsson, K. A., Ericcson, K., Charness, N., Feltovich, P. J., & Hoffman, R. R. (2006). The influence of experience and deliberate practice on the development of superior expert performance. In K. A. Ericsson, N. Charness, P. J. Feltovich & R. R. Hoffman, (Eds.). *The Cambridge handbook of expertise and expert performance.* New York, NY: Cambridge University Press.

Errichetti, A. (2015). Standardized patient debriefing and feedback. In L. Wilson & R. A. Wittmann-Price (Eds.). *Review Manual for the Certified Healthcare Simulation Educator^{TM} (CHSE^{TM}) Exam* (pp. 209–221). New York: Springer Publishing Company, LLC.

Ertan, A., Putterman, L., & Fiszbein, M. (2012, August). *Determinants and economic consequences of colonization: A global analysis.* SSRN http://dx.doi.org/10.2139/ssrn.2129786

Ettorchi-Tardy, A., Levif, M., & Michel, P. (2012). Benchmarking: A method for continuous quality improvement in health. *Healthcare Policy, 7*(4), e101–e119.

Special Eurobarometer (EU 386). (2012). Europeans and their languages. Retrieved from http://ec.europa.eu/public_opinion/archives/ebs/ebs_386_en.pdf

European Union. (2015). Official websit of the European Union. Retrieved from http://europa.eu/index_en.htm

Evans, C. J., & Harder, N. (2013). A formative approach to student remediation. *Nurse Educator, 38*(4), 147–151. doi:10.1097/NNE.0b013e318296dd0f

Everett, L. Q., & Sitterding, M. C. (2011). Transformational leadership required to design and sustain evidence-based practice: A system exemplar. *Western Journal of Nursing Research, 33*(3), 398–426. doi:10.1177/0193945910383056

Everson, N., Levett-Jones, T., Lapkin, S., Pitt, V., van der Riet, P., Rossiter, R., ... Courtney-Pratt, H. (2015). Measuring the impact of a 3D simulation experience on nursing students' cultural empathy using a modified version of the Kiersma-Chen Empathy Scale. *Journal of Clinical Nursing, 24*(19–20), 2849–2858. doi:10.1111/jocn.12893

Eyre, E. (2015). *Forming, norming, storming, and performing: Understanding the stages of team formation.* Retrieved from http://www.mindtools.com/pages/article/newLDR_86.htm

Fabella, D. (2016a). *5 Augmented-reality games you can play while waiting for Pokémon Go.* Retrieved from http://cnnphilippines.com/life/culture/tech/2016/07/12/augmented-reality-games.html

Fabella, E. (2016b). *How can the Oculus Rift be used in healthcare?* Retrieved from http://www.forbes.com/sites/quora/2014/06/18/how-can-the-oculus-rift-be-used-for-healthcare/#1bff31c67718

Facteau, J., Dobbins, G., Russell, J., Ladd, R., & Kudisch, J. (1995). The influence of general perceptions of training environment on motivation and perceived training transfer. *Journal of Management, 21*(1), 1–25. doi:10.1177/0149206395021

Failla, K. R., & Macauley, K. (2014, November). Interprofessional Simulation: A concept analysis. *Clinical Simulation in Nursing, 10*(11), 574–580. http://dx.doi.org/10.1016/j.ecns.2014.07.006

Fairbanks, T. (2012, May). *Was it really a miracle on the Hudson? Aviation meets healthcare safety (plenary session video)*. National Patient Safety Foundation 2012 Meeting. Retrieved from https://youtu.be/kaydVvH7S4E

Fanning, R. M., & Gaba, D. M. (2007). The role of debriefing in simulation-based learning. *Simulation in Healthcare, 2*(2), 115–125. doi:10.1097/SIH.0b013e3180315539

Fanning, R. M., & Gaba, D. M. (2015). Debriefing. In D. M. Gaba, K. J. Fish, S. K. Howard & A. R. Burden (Eds.), *Crisis management in anesthesiology* (2nd ed., pp. 65–78). Philadelphia, PA: Elsevier Saunders.

Faure, E., Herrera, F., Abdul-Razzak, K., Lopes, H., Petrovsky, A. V., Rahnema, M., & Champion War, F. (1972). *Learning to be: The world of education today and tomorrow*. Paris, France: United Nations Educational, Scientific and Cultural Organization.

Fearless Leaders Group. (2014). *Over-romanticized, overlooked, and scientifically ignored*. Retrieved from http://www.fearlessleadersgroup.com/the-science-of-courage

Fernandez, R., Wang, E., Vozenilek, J. A., Hayden, E., McLaughlin, S., Godwin, S. A., ... Gordon, J. A.; for the Simulation Accreditation and Consultation Work Group on behalf of the SAEM Technology in Medical Education Committee. (2010). Simulation center accreditation and programmatic benchmarks: A review for emergency medicine. *Academic Emergency Medicine, 17*, 1093–1103. doi:10.1111/j.1553-2712.2010.00815.x

Fey, M. (2014). *Debriefing practices in nursing education programs in the United States*. (Doctoral dissertation). ProQuest Database Publication (Number 3621880).

Fey, M. K. (2016). Leading the way in simulation research. *Clinical Simulation in Nursing, 12*(3), 85–86. http://doi.org/10.1016/j.ecns.2016.01.001

Fey, M., Scrandis, D., Daniels, A., & Haut, C. (2014). Learning through debriefing: Students' perspectives. *Clinical Simulation in Nursing, 10*(5), e249–e256. doi:10.1016/j.ecns.2013.12.009

Figueiro, M. G., Rea, M. S., Rea, A. C., & Stevens, R. G. (2002). Daylight and productivity—A field study. Conference Proceedings of the American Council for an Energy-efficient Economy (ACEEE) Summer Study. Asilomar, CA.

Fineout-Overholt, E., Gallagher-Ford, L., Melnyk, B. M., & Stillwell, S. B. (2011). Evidence-based practice: Step by step: Evaluating and dissemination the impact of an evidence-based intervention: Show and tell. *The American Journal of Nursing, 111*(7), 56–59. doi:10.1097/01.NAJ.0000399317.21279.47

Fineout-Overholt, E., & Melnyk, B. M. (Eds.) (2005). *Evidence-based practice in nursing & healthcare: A guide to best practice* (3rd ed.). Philadelphia, PA: Lippincott Williams & Wilkins.

Fineout-Overholt, E., Melnyk, B. M., Stillwell, S. B., & Williamson, K. M. (2010a). Evidence-based practice: Step by step: Critical appraisal of the evidence: Part 1. *The American Journal of Nursing, 110*(7), 47–52.

Fineout-Overholt, E., Melnyk, B. M., Stillwell, S. B., & Williamson, K. M. (2010b). Evidence-based practice: Step by step: Critical appraisal of the evidence: Part 2. *The American Journal of Nursing, 110*(9), 41–48.

Fineout-Overholt, E. & Stillwell, S. B. (2015). Asking compelling, clinical questions. In B. M. Melnyk & E. Fineout-Overholt (Eds.), *Evidence-based practice in nursing & healthcare* (pp. 24–39). Philadelphia, PA: Wolters Kluwer Health.

Fineout-Overholt, E., Stillwell, S. B., Williamson, K. M., Cox, J., & Robbins, R. (2015). Teaching evidence-based practice in academic settings. In B. M. Melnyk & E. Fineout-Overholt (Eds.), *Evidence-based practice in nursing and healthcare: A guide to best practice* (3rd ed., pp. 330–362). Philadelphia, PA: Wolters Kluwer.

Fineout-Overholt, E., Williamson, K. M., Gallagher-Ford, L., Melnyk, B. M., & Stillwell, S. B. (2011). Evidence-based practice: Step by step: Following the evidence: Planning for sustainable change. *The American Journal of Nursing, 111*(1), 54–60. doi:10.1097/01.NAJ.0000393062.83761.c0

Fink, M., Linnard-Palmer, L., Ganley, B., Catolico, O., & Phillips, W. (2014). Evaluating the use of standardized patients in teaching spiritual care at the end of life. *Clinical Simulation in Nursing, 10*(11), 559–566. doi:10.1016/j.ecns.2014.09.003

Fisher, D., & King, L. (2013). An integrative literature review on preparing nursing students through simulation to recognize and respond to the deteriorating patient. *Journal of Advanced Nursing, 69*(11), 2375–2388. doi:10.1111/jan.12174

Fisher-Borne, M., Montana Cain, J., & Martin, S. L. (2015). From mastery to accountability: Cultural humility as an alternative to cultural competence. *Social Work Education, 34*(2), 165–181. http://dx.doi.org/10.1080/02615479.2014.977244

Flanagan, B. (2008). Debriefing: Theory and techniques. In R. H. Riley (Ed.), *A manual of simulation in healthcare* (pp. 155–170). New York, NY: Oxford University Press.

Flanagan, B., Nestel, D., & Joseph, M. (2004). Making patient safety the focus: Crisis resource management in the undergraduate curriculum. *Medical Education, 38*, 56–66. doi:10.1111/j.1365-2923.2004.01701.x

Fleiss, J. L. (1986). *The design and analysis of clinical experiments*. New York, NY: Wiley.

Flexner, A. (1910a). *Medical education in the United States and Canada*. Boston, MA: The Merrymount Press.

Flexner, A. (1910b). *Medical education in the United States and Canada: A report to the Carnegie Foundation for the Advancement of Teaching*, Bulletin No. 4. (p. 346). New York, NY: The Carnegie Foundation for the Advancement of Teaching.

Florida State University. (2017). *Office of faculty development* (Web page). Retrieved from http://med.fsu.edu/?page=facultyDevelopment.home

Foisy-Doll, C. (2013). Developing cultural competency in life and simulation: A year in Qatar as an exemplar. *Clinical Simulation in Nursing, 9*(2), e63–e69. doi:10.1016/j.ecns.2011.08.001

Foisy-Doll, C. (2017). Managing simulation program operations and human capital. In C. Foisy-Doll & K. Leighton (Eds.). *Simulation champions: Fostering courage, caring, and connection* (pp. xx–xx). Philadelphia, PA: Wolters Kluwer, Inc.

Foisy-Doll, C., & Leighton, K. (2015). SCORS—Simulation Cultural Organizational Readiness Survey. In C. Foisy-Doll & K. Leighton (Eds.). *Simulation champions: Fostering courage, caring and connection*. Philadelphia, PA: Wolters Kluwer, Inc.

Foisy-Doll, C., & Leighton, K. (2017). *Master simulation design template and intake form©*. In C. Foisy-Doll & K. Leighton (Eds.). Simulation champions: Fostering courage, caring, and connection. Philadelphia, PA: Wolters Kluwer, Inc.

Foisy-Doll, C., & Wild, C. (2017). Leading and developing effective simulation teams. In C. Foisy-Doll & K. Leighton (Eds.).

Simulation champions: Fostering courage, caring, and connection (pp. xx-xx). Philadelphia, PA: Wolters Kluwer, Inc.

Folkman, J. R. (2015). *Nine vital leadership behaviors that boost employee productivity: The keys to increasing discretionary effort.* Retrieved from www.zengerfolkman.com

Forneris, S., Neal, D., Tiffany, J., Kuehn, M., Meyer, H., Blazovich, B., ..., Smerillo, M. (2015). Enhancing clinical reasoning through simulation debriefing: A multisite study. *Nursing Education Perspectives, 36*(5), 304–310.

Foronda, C. (2008). Cultural sensitivity: A concept analysis. *Journal of Transcultural Nursing, 19*(3), 207–212. doi:10.1177/1043659608317093

Foronda, C., Baptiste, D., Ousman, K., & Reinholdt, M. (2016). Cultural humility: A concept analysis. *Journal of Transcultural Nursing, 27*(3). 210–217. doi:10.1177/1043659615592677

Foronda, C., & Bauman, E. (2014). Strategies to incorporate virtual simulation in nurse education. *Clinical Simulation in Nursing, 10*(8), 412–418. http://dx.doi.org/10.1016/j.ecns.2014.03.005

Foronda, C., Liu, S., & Bauman, E. (2013). Evaluation of simulation in undergraduate nurse education: An integrative review. *Clinical Simulation in Nursing, 9*(10), e409–e416. doi:10.1016/j.ecns.2012.11.003

Foronda, C., & MacWilliams, B. R. (2015). Cultural humility in simulation: A missing standard? *Clinical Simulation in Nursing, 11*, 289–290. doi:10.1016/j.ecns.2015.04.002

Foronda, C. L., Shubeck, K., Swoboda, S. M., Hudson, K. W., Budhathoki, C., Sullivan, N., & Hu, X. (2016). Impact of virtual simulation to teach concepts of disaster triage. *Clinical Simulation in Nursing, 12*(4), 137–144. http://dx.doi.org/10.1016/j.ecns.2016.02.004

Foronda, C., Swoboda, S., Bahreman, N., & Foisy-Doll, C. (2017). Cultural competence, safety, and humility in simulation education. In C. Foisy-Doll & K. Leighton (Eds.). (2018). *Simulation champions: Fostering courage, caring, and connection* (pp. xx–xx). Philadelphia, PA: Wolters Kluwer, Inc.

Forrest, F. C. (2008). Mobile simulation. In R. Riley (Ed.). *Manual of simulation in healthcare* (pp. 26–33). New York, NY: Oxford University Press.

Foster, J. (2009). Cultural humility and the importance of long-term relationships in international partnerships. *Journal of Obstetric, Gynecologic & Neonatal Nursing, 38*, 100–107. doi:10.1111/j.1552-6909.2008.00313.x

Fountain, R. A., & Alfred, D. (2009). Student satisfaction with high-fidelity simulation: Does it correlate with learning styles? *Nursing Education Perspectives, 30*, 96–98. http://dx.doi.org/10.1043/1536–5026-030.002.0096

Francis R. (2013). *Publication of the final report: Press statement.* The Mid Staffordshire NHS Foundation Trust Public Inquiry.

Frank, J. R., & Brien, S., (Eds.); on behalf of The Safety Competencies Steering Committee. (2008). *The safety competencies: Enhancing patient safety across the health professions.* Ottawa, ON: Canadian Patient Safety Institute.

Franklin, A. E., Boese, T., Gloe, D., Lioce, L., Decker, S., Sando, C. R., ... Borum, J. C. (2013, June). Standards of best practice: Simulation Standard IV: Facilitation. *Clinical Simulation in Nursing, 9*(6S), S19–S21. doi:10.1016/j.ecns.2013.04.011

Franklin, A. E., Burns, P., & Lee, C. S. (2014). Psychometric testing on the NLN Student Satisfaction and Self-Confidence in Learning, Simulation Design Scale, and Educational Practices Questionnaire using a sample of pre-licensure novice nurses. *Nurse Education Today, 34*(10), 1298–1304. http://doi.org/10.1016/j.nedt.2014.06.011

Franklin, A. E., & Lee, C. S. (2014). Effectiveness of simulation for improvement in self-efficacy among novice nurses: A meta-analysis. *Journal of Nursing Education, 53*(11), 607–614. doi:10.3928/01484834-20141023-03

Franklin, A. E., Leighton, K., Cantrell, M. A., & Rutherford-Hemming, T. (2015). Simulation research for academics: Novice level. *Clinical Simulation in Nursing, 11*(4), 214–221. doi:http://dx.doi.org/10.1016/j.ecns.2015.01.007

Fransen, J., Weinberger, A., & Kirschner, P. A. (2013). Team effectiveness and team development in CSCL. *Educational Psychologist, 48*(1), 9–24. doi:10.1080/00461520.2012.747947

Fraser, K., Huffman, J., Ma, I., Sobczak, M., McIlwrick, J., Wright, B., & McLaughlin, K. (2014). The emotional and cognitive impact of unexpected simulated patient death: A randomized controlled trial. *Chest, 145*(5), 958. http://doi.org/10.1378/chest.13-0987

Freire, P. (1972). *The pedagogy of the oppressed.* Harmondsworth, UK: Penguin.

Freire, P. (2000). *Pedagogy of the oppressed* (30th anniversary ed., M. B. Ramos, Trans.). New York, NY: Continuum International Publishing Group. (Original work published 1970).

Frenk, J., Chen, L., Bhutta, Z., Cohen, J., Crisp, N., Evans, T., ..., Zurayk, H. (2010). Health professionals for a new century: Transforming education to strengthen health systems in an interdependent world. *Lancet, 376*(9756), 1873–1958. doi:10.1016/S0140-6736(10)61854-5

Frey, B. B., Lohmeier, J. H., Lee, S. W., & Tollefson, N. (2006). Measuring collaboration among grant partners. *American Journal of Evaluation, 27*(3), 383–392.

Frost, R. (1914). *North of Boston.* New York: Henry Holt and Company.

Fu, C., & Bergeon, R. (2012). A Tao complexity tool: Leading from being. In J. D. Barbour, G. J. Burgess, L. L. Falkman & R. M. McManus (Eds.), *Leading in complex worlds* (pp. 227–251). San Francisco, CA: Jossey-Bass.

Fundación Garrahan (Garrahan Foundation), Argentina. (2015). *Home page.* Retrieved from http://www.fundaciongarrahan.org.ar/

Fung, L., Boet, S., Bould, M. D., Qosa, H., Perrier, L., Tricco, A., ... Reeves, S. (2015). Impact of crisis resource management simulation-based training for interprofessional and interdisciplinary teams: A systematic review. *Journal of Interprofessional Care, 29*(5), 433–444. http://doi.org/10.3109/13561820.2015.1017555

Fuselier, J., Baldwin, D., & Townsend-Chambers, C. (2015, June). *The effectiveness of the use of simulation: Mannequins of color in the nursing labs on enhancing the undergraduate nursing students' clinical experience and diversity awareness.* Poster presented at the 14th Annual International Nursing Association for Clinical Simulation Conference. Atlanta, GA.

Gaba, D. M. (1992). Improving anesthesiologists' performance by simulating reality. *Anesthesiology, 76*(4), 491–494.

Gaba, D. M. (1997). Simulators in anesthesiology. *Advanced Anesthesia, 14*, 55–94.

Gaba, D. M. (2004). The future vision of simulation in health care. *Quality & Safety in Health Care, 13*(Suppl 1), i2–i10. doi:10.1136/qshc.2004.009878

Gaba, D. M. (2010). Crisis resource management and teamwork training in anaesthesia. *British Journal of Anaesthesia, 105*(1), 3–6. http://doi.org/10.1093/bja/aeq124

Gaba, D. (2013). Simulations that are challenging to the psyche of participants: How much should we worry and about what? *Simulation in Healthcare, 8*(1), 4–7. doi:10.1097/SIH.0b013e3182845a6f

Gaba, D. M. (2014). Simulation as a critical resource in the response to Ebola virus disease. *Simulation in Healthcare, 9*(6), 337–338. http://doi.org/10.1097/SIH.0000000000000068

Gaba, D. M., & DeAnda, A. (1988). A comprehensive anesthesia simulation environment: Recreating the operating room for research and training. *Anesthesiology, 69,* 387–394.

Gaba, D. M., & DeAnda, A. (1989). The response of anesthesia trainees to simulated critical incidents. *Anesthesia and Analgesia, 68*(4), 444.

Gaba, D. M., Howard, S. K., Fish, K. J., Smith, B. E., & Sowb, Y. A. (2001). Simulation-based training in anesthesia crisis resource management (ACRM): A decade of experience. *Simulation and Gaming, 32,* 175–193. doi:10.1177/104687810103200206

Gaberson, K. B., & Oermann, M. H. (2010). *Clinical teaching strategies in nursing* (3rd ed.). New York, NY: Springer Publishing Company, LLC.

Galbraith, A., Harder, N., Macomer, C. A., Roe, E., & Roethlisberger, K. S. (2014). Design and implementation of an interprofessional death notification simulation. *Clinical Simulation in Nursing, 10*(2), e95–e102. http://dx.doi/org/10.1016/j.ecns.2013.08.003

Gallagher, C. J., & Issenberg, S. B. (2007). *Simulation in anesthesia.* Philadelphia, PA: Saunders Elsevier.

Galloway, S. J. (2009). Simulation techniques to bridge the gap between novice and competent healthcare professionals. *OJIN: The Online Journal of Issues in Nursing, 14*(2), Manuscript 3. doi:10.3912/OJIN.Vol14No02Man03

Gamble, A., Bearman, M., & Nestel, D. (2016). A systematic review: Children & adolescents as simulated patients in health professional education. *Advances in Simulation, 1*(1), 1–16. doi:10.1186/s41077-015-0003-9

Ganley, B. J., & Linnard-Palmer, L. (2012). Academic safety during nursing simulation: Perceptions of nursing students and faculty. *Clinical Simulation in Nursing, 8*(2), e49–e57. doi:10.1016/j.encs.2010.06.004

Gantt, L. (2013). The effect of preparation on anxiety and performance in summative simulations. *Clinical Simulation in Nursing, 9*(1), e25–e33. doi:10.1016/j.ecns.2011.07.004

Gantt, L. & Young, H. M. (2016). *Healthcare simulation: A guide for operations specialists.* Hoboken, NJ: John Wiley & Sons, Inc.

Gao, L.-L., Chan, S. W.-C., & Cheng, B.-S. (2011). The past, present and future of nursing education in the People's Republic of China: A discussion paper. *Journal of Advanced Nursing, 68*(6), 1429–1438. http://doi.org/10.1111/j.1365-2648.2011.05828.x

García, T. C., & Guisado, Y. M. (2013). *Simbase: Implementation handbook for simulation and ICT-based learning in training and healthcare centres.* http://www.simbase.co/

Gardiner, J. J. Z. (2009). Featured article: Transcendent leadership: Pathway to global sustainability. *Integral Leadership Review.* Retrieved from http://integralleadershipreview.com/1928-transcendent-leadership-pathway-to-global-sustainability

Garg, A., Haley, H., & Hatem, D. (2010). Modern moulage: Evaluating the use of 3-dimensional prosthetic mimics in a dermatology teaching program for second-year medical students. *Archives of Dermatology, 146*(2), 143–146.

Garrido, M. (M.), Dlugasch, L., & Graber, P. M. (2014). Integration of interprofessional education and culture into advanced practice simulations. *Clinical Simulation in Nursing, 10*(9), 461–469. http://dx.doi.org/10.1016/j.ecns.2014.06.001

Gates, B., & Gates, M. (2015). *2015 Gates Annual Letter.* Retrieved from http://www.gatesnotes.com/2015-Annual-Letter?page=0&lang=en

Gates, M. G., Parr, M. B., & Hugen, J. E. (2012). Enhancing nursing knowledge using high fidelity simulation. *Journal of Nursing Education, 51*(1), 9–15. doi:10.3928/014834-20111116-01

Gawande, A. (2009). *The checklist manifesto: How to get right.* New York, NY: Metropolitan Books.

Gazarian, P. K. (2010). Digital stories: Incorporating narrative pedagogy. *Journal of Nursing Education, 49*(5). doi:10.3928/01484834-20100115-07

George, M. L. (2005). *The lean six sigma pocket toolbook: A quick reference guide to nearly 100 tools for improving process quality, speed, and complexity.* New York, NY: McGraw-Hill.

George, N. M., Drahnak, D. M., Schroeder, D. L., & Katrancha, E. D. (2016). Enhancing prelicensure nursing students' use of an electronic health record. *Clinical Simulation in Nursing, 12*(5), 152–158. http://dx.doi.org/10.1016/j.ecns.2015.11.006

Gerlach, A. J. (2012). A critical reflection on the concept of cultural safety. *Canadian Journal of Occupational Therapy, 79*(3), 151–158. Retrieved from http://doi.org/10.2182/cjot.2012.79.3.4

Giger, J., Davidhizar, R., Purnell, L., Harden, J., Phillips, J., & Strickland, O. (2007). American Academy of Nursing expert panel report: Developing cultural competence to eliminate health disparities in ethnic minorities and other vulnerable populations. *Journal of Transcultural Nursing, 18*(2), 95–102.

Gilbert, J. H. V. (2005). Interprofessional learning and higher education structural barriers. *Journal of Interprofessional Care, 19*(S1), 87–106.

Gitembagara, A., Relf, M., & Pyburn, R. (2015). Optimizing nursing and midwifery practice in Rwanda. *Rwanda Journal Series F: Medicine and Health Sciences, 2*(2), 26–30.

Gladwell, M. (2002). *The tipping point: How little things can make a big difference.* New York, NY: First Back Bay Books.

Glaseroff, A. (2015). Editorial on "feasibility of 'standardized clinician' methodology for patient training on hospital-to-home transitions." *Simulation in Healthcare, 10*(1), 1–3. http://doi.org/10.1097/SIH

Glavin, R. (2008). A national simulation program influences teaching at a national level: Scotland. In W. Kyle & R. Murray (Eds.), *Clinical simulation operations, engineering, and management* (pp. 365–370). San Diego, CA: Academic Press.

Gloe, D., Sando, C. R., Franklin, A. E., Boese, T., Decker, S., Lioce, L., …, Borum. J. C. (2013, June). Standards of best practice: Simulation Standard II: Professional integrity of participant(s). *Clinical Simulation in Nursing, 9*(6S), S12–S14. doi:10.1016/j.ecns.2013.04.004

Glossary of Education Reform. (2014, May). *The competency based education.* Retrieved from http://edglossary.org/competency-based-learning/

Gobbi, M., Monger, E., Weal, M. J., McDonald, J. W., Michaelides, D., & De Roure, D. (2012). The challenges of developing and evaluating complex care scenarios using simulation in nursing education. *Journal of Research in Nursing, 17*(4), 329–345. doi.org/10.1177/1744987112449969

Godkin, M., & Savageau, J. (2003). The effect of a global multiculturalism track on cultural competence of preclinical medical students. *Family Medicine, 33,* 178–186.

Goldschmidt, A. (2009). *The evolution of Chinese medicine: Song dynasty, 960–1200.* http://dx.doi.org/SBN 0-203-94643-XMaster e-book ISBN

Goldsworthy, S. (2015). *The mechanisms by which professional development may contribute to critical care nurses' intent to stay* (Unpublished doctoral dissertation). The University of British Columbia, Vancouver, BC.

Goldsworthy, S., & Graham, L. (2012). *Simulation simplified: A practical guide for critical care nurse educators.* Philadelphia, PA: Lippincott Williams & Wolters.

Goleman, D. (1995). *Emotional intelligence.* New York, NY: Bantam.

Goleman, D. (1998). *Working with emotional intelligence.* New York, NY: Bantam: Doubleday Dell.

Goleman, D. (2006). *Emotional intelligence: Why it can matter more than IQ* (10th ed.). New York, NY: Bantam Books.

Goleman, D., Boyatzis, R., & McKee, A. (2002). *Primal leadership: Learning to lead with emotional intelligence.* Boston, MA: Harvard Business School Press.

Gonzalez, L., & Sole, M. L. (2014). Urinary catheterization skills: One simulated checkoff is not enough. *Clinical Simulation in Nursing, 10*(9), 455–460. doi:10.1016/j.ecns.2014.07.002

Goode T. (2013). *Applying cultural and linguistic competence to a framework for creating learning spaces for the enhancement of experiential learning.* Washington, DC: National Center for Cultural Competence, Georgetown University Center for Child and Human Development.

Goode, T., & Jones, W. (2009). *Research—Cultural and linguistic competence checklist for MCH training programs.* Washington, DC: National Center for Cultural Competence, Georgetown University Center for Child and Human Development.

Goode, T., & Bronheim, S. (2012). *Experiential learning: Cultural and linguistic competence checklist for MCH training programs.* Washington, DC: National Center for Cultural Competence, Georgetown University Center for Child and Human Development. Retrieved from http://nccc.georgetown.edu/resources/publicationstitle.html

Goode, T. D. (2004). *The cultural competence continuum.* National Center for Cultural Competence Georgetown University Center for Child and Human Development, University Center for Excellence in Developmental Disabilities. Retrieved from http://ncccurricula.info/documents/TheContinuumRevised.doc

Goode & Jones (2009). Definition of Linguistic Competence. National Center for Cultural Competence, Georgetown University Center for Child & Human Development. Retrieved 03/16/2017 from https://nccc.georgetown.edu/foundations/frameworks.html#lcdefinition

Goodson, P. (2010). *Theory in health promotion research and practice.* Sudbury, MA: Jones and Bartlett.

Gore, T. Hunt, C. W., Parker, F., & Raines, K. H. (2011). The effects of simulated clinical experience on anxiety: Nursing students' perspectives. *Clinical Simulation in Nursing, 7*(5), e175–e180. doi:10.1016/j.ecns.2010.02.001

Graham, C. L., & Atz, T. (2015). Baccalaureate minority nursing students' perception of high-fidelity simulation. *Clinical Simulation in Nursing, 11*(11), 482–488. http://dx.doi.org/10.1016/j.ecns.2015.10.003

Great Schools Partnership. (2014). *The glossary of education reform.* Retrieved from http://edglossary.org/competency-based-lesnowarning/

Green, M. L., Aagaard, E. M., Caverzagie, K. J., Chick, D. A., Holmboe, E., Kane, G., ... Iobst, W. (2009). Charting the road to competence: Developmental milestones for internal medicine residency training. *Journal of Graduate Medical Education, 1,* 5–20. doi:10.4300/01.01.0003

Greenawalt, J. A. (2014). Documentation in contemporary times: Challenges and successes in teaching. *Clinical Simulation in Nursing, 10*(4), e199–e204. http://dx.doi.org/10.1016/j.ecns.2013.11.008

Greenstock, L., Brooks, P., & Bingham, A. (2011). *Interprofessional learning (IPL) opportunities in simulation. Report prepared by the Australia Health Workforce Institute.* Available at www.hwa.gov.au/sites/uploads/sle-report-interprofessional-learning-201110.pdf

Greenwood, J. (1997). The role of reflection in single and double loop learning. *Journal of Advanced Nursing, 27,* 1048–1053.

Greenwood, M., de Leeuw, S., Lindsay, M. M., & Reading, C. (2015). *Determinants of Indigenous Peoples' heat in Canada: Beyond the social.* Toronto, ON: Canadian Scholar's Press.

Greidanus, E., King, S., LoVerso, T., & Ansell, L. D. (2013). Interprofessional learning objectives for health team simulations. *Journal of Nursing Education, 52*(6), 311–316. doi:10.3928/01484834-20130509-02

Griffin, M. (2004). Teaching cognitive rehearsal as a shield for lateral violence: An intervention for newly licensed nurses. *Journal of Continuing Education in Nursing, 35*(6), 257–263.

Griffin-Sobel, J. P., Acee, A., Sharoff, L., Cobus-Kuo, L., Woodstock-Wallace, A., & Dornbaum, M. (2010). A transdisciplinary approach to faculty development in nursing education technology. *Nursing Education Perspectives, 31*(1), 41–43. http://dx.doi.org/10.1043/1536-5026-31.1.41

Griswold-Theodorson, S., Ponnuru, S., Dong, C., Szyld, D., Reed, T., & McGaghie, W. C. (2015). Beyond the sim lab: A realist synthesis review of clinical outcomes of sim- based mastery learning. *Academic Medicine, 90*(11), 15513–1560. doi:10.1097/ACM.0000000000000938

Groom, J. A., Henderson, D., & Sittner, B. J. (2014). NLN/Jeffries simulation framework state of the science project: Simulation design characteristics. *Clinical Simulation in Nursing, 10*(7), 337–344. doi:http://dx.doi.org/10.1016/j.ecns.2013.02.004

Gropper, R., Harnett, N., Parker, K., Pearce, S., MacIver, D., Murray, L., ..., Zychla, L. (2010). The path to simulated learning: Developing a valid and reliable tool to evaluate performance of radiological technology students in patient interactions. *Journal of Allied Health, 39*(1), 28–33.

Grossman, S. C., & Valiga, T. M. (2013). *The new leadership challenge: Creating the future of nursing* (4th ed.). Philadelphia, PA: FA Davis.

Grove, S. K., Gray, J. R., & Burns, N. (2015). *Understanding nursing research: Building an evidence-based practice.* St. Louis, MO: Elsevier.

Gruppen, L. D., Mangrulkar, R. S., & Kolars, J. C. (2012). The promise of competency-based education in the health professions for improving global health. *Human Resources for Health, 10*(43), 1–7. doi:10.1186/1478-4491-10-43

Gutek, G. (2004). *Educational philosophy and changes* (3rd ed.). Boston, MA: Allyn & Bacon.

Hackett, M. (2013). *Medical holography for basic anatomy training.* Presented at the Interservice/Industry Training, Simulation, and Education Conference (I/ITSEC), Orlando, FL. Paper No. 13207.

Hacking Health. (2016). About us (web page). Retrieved from http://hackinghealth.ca/about-us/

Hackman, J. R. (2011). *Collaborative intelligence: Using teams to solve hard problems.* Oakland, CA: Berrett-Koehler Publishers

Hafferty, F. W., & Franks, R. (1994). The hidden curriculum, ethics teaching, and the structure of medical education. *Academic Medicine, 69*(11), 861–871.

Haines, T., Isles, R., Jones, A., & Jull, G. (2011). Economic consequences in clinical education. *Focus on Health Professional Education: A Multi-disciplinary Journal, 12*(3), 53–63.

Haines, T. P., Kent, F., & Keating, J. L. (2014). Interprofessional student clinics: An economic evaluation of collaborative clinical placement education. *Journal of Interprofessional Care, 28*(4), 292–298. doi:10.3109/13561820.2013.874983

Hallmark, B. (2015). Faculty development in simulation education. *Nursing Clinics of North America, 50,* 389–397. doi:http://dx.doi.org/10.1016/j.cnur.2015.03.002

Hallmark, B. F., Thomas, C. M., & Gantt, L. (2014). The educational practices construct of the NLN/Jeffries simulation framework: State of the science. *Clinical Simulation in Nursing, 10*(7), 345–352. doi:http://dx.doi.org/10.1016/j.ecns.2013.04.006

Halsall, P. H. (1998). *Modern history sourcebook: John Stuart Mill—On colonies and colonization, 1848.* Retrieved from http://sourcebooks.fordham.edu/mod/1849jsmill-colonies.asp

Hamilton, A. (2011). Europe's continental boundaries. *North American New Right.* Retrieved from http://www.countercurrents.com/2011/08/europes-continental-boundaries/

Hamilton, C., & Morris, A. H. (2012). Transformative learning in simulated environments. In A. G. Morris & D. R. Faulk, (Eds.), *Transformative learning in nursing: A guide for nurse educators* (pp. 107–118). New York, NY: Springer.

Hammick, M., Freeth, D., Koppel, I., Reeves, S., & Barr, H. (2007). A best evidence systematic review of interprofessional education. *Medical Teacher, 29*(8), 735–751. doi:10.1080/01421590701682576

Hamstra, S. J. (2012). Keynote Address: The focus on competencies and individual learner assessment as emerging themes in medical education research. *Academic Emergency Medicine, 19,* 1336–1343. doi:10.1111/acem.12021

Hamstra, S. J., Brydges, R., Hatala, R., Zendejas, B., & Cook, D. A. (2014). Reconsidering fidelity in simulation-based training. *Academic Medicine, 89*(3), 387–392. doi:10.1097/ACM.0000000000000130

Hanberg, A. D., & Madden, C. (2011). Tech-know-logy: Using multimodal simulation strategies to bring data management and patient care technologies to life. *Clinical Simulation in Nursing, 7*(4), e133–e139. doi:10.1016/j.ecns.2010.01.002

Hansen, J. J. (2008). A strategic plan template for dummies. *Woodhill Park Retreat.* Retrieved from http://www.edmonton.ca/programs_services/documents/PDF/StrategicPlanningForDummies.pdf

Hansen, K., & Davies, J. (2015). Designing a content management system to support the development of a multi-modality curriculum in an all-digital facility. *Weill Cornell College Professional Development Series.* Retrieved from https://qatar-weill.cornell.edu/cpd/designing-content-management-system.html

Harder, N. (2009). Use of simulation in teaching and learning in health sciences: A systematic review. *Journal of Nursing Education, 49*(1), 23–28. doi:10.3928/01484834-20090828-08

Harder, N. (2015). Replace is not a four-letter word. *Clinical Simulation in Nursing, 11,* 435–436. doi:http://dx.doi.org/10.1016/j.ecns.2015.07.001

Harding, T. (2013). Cultural safety: A vital element for nursing ethics. *Nursing Praxis in New Zealand, 29*(1), 4–11.

Hargraves, R. (2012). Standardized patient training. In L. Wilson & L. Rockstraw (Eds.), *Human simulation for nursing and health professions.* New York, NY: Springer Publishing Company.

Harper, M., & Markham, C. (2011). Clinical simulation: Exploring its history and evolution. *Technic: The Journal of Operating Department Practice, 2*(2), 11–14.

Harris, A. (2013). The times they are-a-changin': Are we? *Nursing Leadership, 26*(3), 15–18. Retrieved from http://www.longwoods.com/publications/nursing-leadership

Harrison, K. (n.d.). *Why employee recognition is so important.* Retrieved from http://www.cuttingedgepr.com/articles/emprecog_so_important.asp

Hart, J. A., & Chilcote, D. R. (2016). "Won't you be my patient?": Preparing theater students as standardized patients. *Journal of Nursing Education, 55*(3), 168–171. http://doi.org/10.3928/01484834-20160216-09

Hartigan-Rogers, J. A., Cobbett, S. L., Amirault, M. A., & Muise-Davis, M. E. (2007). Nursing graduates' perceptions of their undergraduate clinical placement. *International Journal of Nursing Education Scholarship, 4*(1), 1–12. doi:10.2202/1548-923X.1276

Hartrick Doane, G. (2002). Beyond behavioral skills to human-involved processes: Relational nursing practice and interpretive pedagogy. *Journal of Nursing Education, 41(9),* 400–404.

Hartrick Doane, G., & Varcoe, C. (2015). *How to nurse: Relational inquiry with individuals and families in changing health and health care contexts* (pp. 421–488). Philadelphia, PA: Wolters Kluwer.

Harvard Center for Medical Simulation (CMS). (2016). *Feedback for Assessment in Clinical Education (FACES).* Retrieved from https://harvardmedsim.org/feedback-assessment-clinical-education.php

Harvard Kennedy School. (2013). *Meta-leadership.* Retrieved from http://npli.sph.harvard.edu/meta-leadership/

Harvard Medical Simulation (2009). *Debriefing Assessment for Simulation in Healthcare* (DASH). Retrieved from https://goo.gl/N4jbUx

Haskvitz, L. M., & Koop, E. C. (2004). Students struggling in clinical? A new role for the patient simulator. *Journal of Nursing Education, 43*(4), 181–184. doi:10.3928/01484834-20040401-06

Hatchett, P., Haun, C., & Goldenhar, L. (2004). *Training standardized patients to give feedback to medical trainees: The state of the art*. Retrieved from http://www.aspeducators.org/files/project_awards/1280872305.pdf

Hatherly, A. (2011). *Leadership and management: Core education. ECE online*. Retrieved from http://eceonline.core-ed.org/groupcms/view/13898/leadership-and-management

Hawkins, S. F., & Morse, J. (2014). The praxis of courage as a foundation for care. *Journal of Nursing Scholarship, 46*(4), 263–270. doi:10.1111/jnu.12077

Hayden, J., Keegan, M., Kardong-Edgren, S., & Smiley, A. (2014). Reliability and validity testing of the Creighton Competency Evaluation Instrument for use in the NCSBN National simulation study. *Nursing Education Perspectives, 35*(4), 244–252. doi:10.5480/13-1130.1

Hayden, J. K., Smiley, R. A., Alexander, M., Kardong-Edgren, S., & Jeffries, P. R. (2014). The NCSBN national simulation study: A longitudinal, randomized, controlled study replacing clinical hours with simulation in prelicensure nursing education. *Journal of Nursing Regulation, 5*(2), S1–S41. http://dx.doi.org/10.1016/S2155-8256(15)30783-3

Hayden, J. K., Smiley, R. A., & Gross, L. (2014). Simulation in nursing education: Current regulations and practices. *Journal of Nursing Regulation, 5*(2), 25–27. doi:http://dx.doi.org/10.1016/S2155-8256(15)30084-3

Hayes, H. (2010, April). *Integrated data management: Managing data across its lifecycle*. Retrieved from https://www.ibm.com/developerworks/data/library/techarticle/dm-0807hayes/

Hays, J. M. (2010). High-performance teams and communities of practice. *Oxford Journal, 5*(1), 101–112. Retrieved from http://ojbe.org/

Health Workforce Australia. (2013). *Australia's health workforce series—Nurses in focus*. Adelaide, Australia: Author.

Health Workforce Australia. (2014). *Simulated learning environments*. Retrieved from http://www.hwa.gov.au/work-programs/clinical-training-reform/simulated-learning-environments-sles

Healthcare Insurance Reciprocal of Canada (HIROC). (2014). *Integrated risk management for healthcare organizations: Resource guide*. Toronto, Canada: Author.

Healthysimulation.com. (2016). *Building a medical simulation program website*. Retrieved from http://healthysimulation.com/2960/building-a-medical-simulation-program-website/

Heine, N., & Ferguson, D. (2015). Management of standardized patient program. In J. C. Palaganas, J. C. Maxworthy, C. A. Epps & M. E. Mancini (Eds.), *Defining excellence in simulation programs*. Philadelphia, PA: Wolters Kluwer.

Heinrichs, W. M., Bauman, E., & Dev, P. (2012). SBAR 'flattens the hierarchy' among caregivers. *Studies in Health Technology and Informatics, 173*, 175–182. Retrieved from http://www.iospress.nl/

Helmreich, R. L., & Foushee, H. C. (1993). Why crew resource management? Empirical and theoretical bases of human factors training in aviation. In B. Kanki, J. Anca & R. Helmreich (Eds.). *Cockpit Resource Management* (pp. 3–45). Philadelphia, PA: Elsevier. Retrieved from booksite.elsevier.com/samplechapters/9780123749468/9780123749468.pdf

Helping Babies Breathe. (2015). *Helping babies survive* Retrieved from http://www.helpingbabiesbreathe.org/about.html

Henderson, A., Cooke, M., Creedy, D. K., & Walker, R. (2012). Nursing students' perceptions of learning in practice environments: A review. *Nurse Education Today, 32*(3), 299–302. doi:10.1016/j.nedt.2011.03.010

Henneman, E., & Cunningham, H. (2005). Using clinical simulation to teach patient safety in an acute/critical care nursing course. *Nurse Educator, 30*(4), 172–177.

Henneman, E. A., Roche, J. P., Fisher, D. L., Cunningham, H., Reilly, C. A., Nathanson, B. H., & Henneman, P. L. (2010). Error identification and recovery by student nurses using human patient simulation: Opportunity to improve patient safety. *Applied Nursing Research, 23*(1), 11–21. doi:10.1016/j-apnr.2008.02.004

Herberg, P. (2012). Perspectives on international nursing. In M. M. Andrews & J. S. Boyle (Eds.), *Transcultural concepts in nursing care* (6th ed.). Philadelphia, PA: Wolters Kluwer, Lippincott Williams & Wilkins.

Herrmann, E. (1981). Mrs. Chase: A noble and enduring figure. *American Journal of Nursing, 81*(10), 1836.

Herrmann, E. K. (2008). Remembering Mrs. Chase. *NSNA Imprint, 55*, 52–55.

Heschong, L., Wright, R., & Okura, S. (2001). Daylighting impacts on human performance in schools. Journal of the Illuminating Engineering Society, Summer, 101–114.

Hetzel Campbell, S., & Daley, K. (2008). *Simulation scenarios for nurse educators: Making it REAL* (2nd ed.). New York, NY: Springer Publishing Company LLC.

Hetzel Campbell, S., Pagano, M. P., O'Shea, E. R., Connery, C., & Caron, C. (2013). Development of the Health Communication Assessment Tool: Enhancing relationships, empowerment, and power-sharing skills. *Clinical Simulation in Nursing, 9*(11), e543–e550. Retrieved from http://dx.doi.org/10.1016/j.ecns.2013.04.016

Hewson, M. G., & Little, M. L. (1998). Giving feedback in medical education: Verification of recommended techniques. *Journal of General Internal Medicine, 13*(2), 111–116.

Hibberd, J. M., Smith, D. L., & Wylie, D. M. (2006). Leadership and leaders. In J. M. Hibberd & D. L. Smith (Eds.), *Nursing leadership and management in Canada* (3rd ed., pp. 369–394). Toronto, ON: Elsevier.

Hickey, M. T. (2010). Baccalaureate nursing graduates' perceptions of their clinical instructional experiences and preparation for practice. *Journal of Professional Nursing, 26*(1), 35–41. doi:http://dx.doi.org/10.1016/j.profnurs.2009.03.001

Hidi, S. (1990). Interest and its contribution as a mental resource for learning. *Review of Educational Research, 60*, 549–571.

Hidi, S., & Baird, W. (1986). Interestingness—A neglected variable in discourse processing. *Cognitive Science, 10*, 179–194.

Hill, G., & Zinsmeister, D. (2012). Becoming an ethical teacher. In W. F. Buskist & V. Benassi (Eds.), *Effective college and university teaching* (pp. 125–133). Los Angeles, CA: Sage Publishing.

Himes, H., & Schulenberg, J. (2013). Theoretical reflections: Theory and philosophy should always inform practice. *Academic Advising Today, 36*(3). Retrieved from http://www.nacada.ksu.edu/Resources/Academic-Advising-Today/View-Articles/Theoretical-Reflections-Theory-and-Philosophy-Should-Always-Inform-Practice.aspx

Hirschfeld, M. J. (2008). Globalisation: good or bad, for whom? In V. Tschudin & A. J. Davis (Eds.), *The globalization of nursing*. Oxford, UK: Radcliffe Publishing Ltd.

Hober, C., & Bonnel, W. (2014). Student perceptions of the observer role in high fidelity simulation. *Clinical Simulation in Nursing, 10*(10), 1–27. http://doi.org/10.1016/j.ecns.2014.07.008

Hober, C., Manry, J., & Connelly, L. (2009, September). Simulation development: The Simmons family. *Clinical Simulation in Nursing, 5*, e173–e179. doi:10.1016/j.ecns.2009.05.001

Holden, L. M. (2005). Complex adaptive systems: Concept analysis. *Journal of Advanced Nursing, 52*(6), 651–657. doi:10.1111/j.1365-2648.2005.03638.x

Hong-Zhou, W. (2013). *Fundamentals of traditional Chinese medicine.* Retrieved from http://site.ebrary.com.proxy.cc.uic.edu/lib/uic/detail.action?docID=10775245

Hooper, B., Shaw, L., & Zamzam, R. (2015). Implementing high-fidelity simulations with large groups of nursing students. *Nurse Educator, 40*(2), 87–90. doi:10.1097/NNE.0000000000000101

Hope, A., Garside, J., & Prescott, S. (2011). Rethinking theory and practice: Pre-registration student nurses experiences of simulation teaching and learning in the acquisition of clinical skills in preparation for practice. *Nurse Education Today, 31*(7), 711–715. doi:10.1016/j.nedt.2010.12.011

Hopwood, N., Rooney, D., Boud, D., & Kelly, M. A. (2014). *Theorising simulation pedagogy differently: (virtual) realities, materialities, and simulacra.* Paper presented at the 2nd International ProPEL conference—'Professional Matters: Materialities and Virtualities of Professional Learning', Stirling, UK.

Hopwood, N., Rooney, D., Boud, D., & Kelly, M. A. (2016). Simulation in higher education: A sociomaterial view. *Educational Philosophy and Theory, 48*(2), 165–178. doi:10.1080/00131857.2014.971403

Horley, R. (2008). Simulation and skill centre design. In R. Riley (Ed.), *Manual of simulation in healthcare* (pp. 3–10). New York, NY: Oxford University Press.

Horsley, T. L., & Wambach, K. (2015). Effect of nursing faculty presence on students' anxiety, self-confidence, and clinical performance during a clinical simulation experience. *Clinical Simulation in Nursing, 11*(1), 4–10. http://dx.doi.org/10.1016/j.ecns.2014.09.012

Horton-Deutsch, S., & Sherwood, G. (2008). Reflection: An educational strategy to develop emotionally-competent nurse leaders. *Journal of Nursing Management, 16*, 946–954. doi:10.1111/j.1365-2834.2008.00957.x

Hou, J., Michaud, C., Li, Z., Dong, Z., Sun, B., Zhang, J. … Chen, L. (2014). Transformation of the education of health professionals in China: Progress and challenges. *The Lancet, 384*(9945), 819–827. http://doi.org/10.1016/S0140-6736(14)61307-6

Howley, L., & Martindale, J. (2004). The efficacy of standardized patient feedback in clinical teaching: A mixed methods analysis. *Medical Education Online, 9*, 18. http://dx.doi.org/10.3402/meo.v9i.4356

Huang, Y. M., & Dongilli, T. (2008). Simulation centre operations and administration. In R. H. Riley (Ed.), *Manual of simulation in healthcare.* New York, NY: Oxford University Press.

Huang, Y. M., Rice, J., Spain, A., & Palaganas, J. C. (2015). Terms of reference. In J. C. Palaganas, J. C. Maxworthy, C. A. Epps & M. E. Mancini (Eds.), *Defining excellence in simulation programs* (pp. xxi–xxxiv). Philadelphia, PA: Wolters Kluwer.

Huang, G. C., Sacks, H., DeVita, M., Reynolds, R., Gammon, W., Saleh, M., …, Passiment, M. (2012). Characteristics of simulation activities at North American medical schools and teaching hospitals: An AAMC-SSH-ASPE-AACN collaboration. *Simulation in Healthcare, 7*, 329–333. doi:10.1097/SIH.0b013e318262007e

Hubbard, E. (1899). *A message to Garcia.* Retrieved from http://www.govleaders.org/

Huitt, W. (2011). Motivation to learn: An overview. In *Educational Psychology Interactive.* Valdosta, GA: Valdosta State University. Retrieved from http://www.edpsycinteractive.org/topics/motivation/motivate.html

Hunt, C. W., Curtis, A. M., & Gore, T. (2015). Using simulation to promote professional development of clinical instructors. *Journal of Nursing Education, 54*(8), 468–471. doi:10.3928/01484834-20150717-09

Hunter, L. A. (2008). Stories as integrated patterns of knowing in nursing education. *International Journal of Nursing Education Scholarship, 5*(1), Article 38. doi:10.2202/1548-923X.1630

Hurwitz, M., & Hurwitz, S. (2015). *Leadership is half the story: A fresh look at followership, leadership, and collaboration.* Toronto, ON: University of Toronto Press.

Husebø, S. E., Friberg, F. Soreide, E., Rystedt, H. S., & Nestel, D. (2012). Instructional problems in briefings: How to prepare nursing students for simulation-based cardiopulmonary resuscitation training. *Clinical Simulation in Nursing, 8*(7), e307–e318. http://dx.doi.org/10.1016/j.ecns.2010.12.002

Husebø, S. E., O'Regan, S., & Nestel, D. (2015). Reflective practice and its role in simulation. *Clinical Simulation in Nursing, 11*(8), 368–375. http://dx.doi.org/10.1016/j.ecns.2015.04.005

Husson, N., & Zulkosky, K. D. (2014). Recruiting and training volunteer standardized patients in the NCSBN national simulation study. *Clinical Simulation in Nursing, 10*(9), 487–489. doi:10.1016/j.ecns.2014.05.01

IMI Association Executives. (2016). *What is an AMC?* Retrieved from http://www.imiae.com/about-imi/what-is-an-amc/

Imperial College London. (n.d.). *The London handbook for debriefing: Enhancing performance debriefing in clinical and simulated settings.* Retrieved from https://www1.imperial.ac.uk/resources/B4F0E6A4-0A0B-4AF1-A39F-23B615EF7922/lw2222ic_debrief_book_a5.pdf

Institute for Medical Simulation (IMS)—Center for Medical Simulation. (n.d.). *Simulation instructor training.* Retrieved from https://harvardmedsim.org/center-for-medical-simulation-ims.php

Institute for Patient-, and Family-Centered Care. (n.d.). *Patient- and family-centered care.* Retrieved from http://www.ipfcc.org/about/pfcc.html

Institute of Medicine (IOM). (1999). *To err is human: Building a safer healthcare system.* Washington, DC: National Academies Press.

Institute of Medicine (IOM). (2001). *Crossing the quality chasm: A new health system for the 21st century.* Washington, DC: National Academies Press.

Institute of Medicine (IOM). (2003). *Health professions education: A bridge to quality.* Washington, DC: Committee on the Health Professions Education Summit Board on Health Care Services.

Institute of Medicine (IOM). (2009). Committee on conflict of interest in medical research, education, and practice. In B. Lo & M. J. Field (Eds.), *Conflict of interest in medical research, education, and practice.* Washington, DC: National Academies Press.

Institute of Medicine (IOM). (2010a). *A summary of the February 2010 forum on the future of nursing: Education.* Washington, DC: The National Academies Press.

Institute of Medicine (IOM). (2010b). *The future of nursing: Leading change, advancing health.* Washington, DC: National Academies Press.

Institute of Medicine of the National Academies. (2015). *Measuring the impact of interprofessional education on collaborative practice and patient outcomes.* Washington, DC: The National Academies Press.

Instituto Nacional de Estadística Chile (National Institute of Statistics of Chile), INE. (2012). *Censo.* Retrieved from http://www.ine.cl/

Instituto Nacional de Estadística Chile (National Institute of Statistics of Chile). (2015). *INE, Población 2015.* http://www.ine.cl/

Interdisciplinary Health Education Partnership (IHEP). (2012). access to the future fund: Increasing programming capacity for interdisciplinary health sciences education: Simulated learning environments. Retrieved from http://iae.alberta.ca/media/119218/2007-2008_annual_report.pdf

International Alliance of Patients' Organizations (IAPO). (2006). *Declaration on patient-centered healthcare.* Retrieved from http://iapo.org.uk/sites/default/files/files/IAPO_declaration_English.pdf

International Civil Aviation Organization (ICAO). (2013). *Safety management systems* (ICAO - Doc 9859 AN/474). Retrieved from http://www.skybrary.aero/bookshelf/books/644.pdf

International Council of Nurses (ICN). (2006). *The ICN code of ethics for nurses.* Geneva, Switzerland: Author. Retrieved from http://www.icn.ch/icncode.pdf

International Council of Nurses (ICN). (2007). *Cultural and linguistic competence.* Retrieved from http://www.icn.ch/images/stories/documents/publications/position_statements/B03_Cultural_Linguistic_Competence.pdf

International Council of Nurses (ICN). (2013). *Position statement on cultural and linguistic competence* Retrieved from http://www.icn.ch/images/stories/documents/publications/position_statements/B03_Cultural_Linguistic_Competence.pdf

International Council of Nurses (ICN). (2014a). *Biennial report 2012–2013: Improving access impacting health.* Geneva, Switzerland: Author.

International Council of Nurses (ICN). (2014b). *Nursing education network bulletin, 4,* 1–5. Retrieved from http://www.icn.ch/images/stories/documents/networks/NursingEducation/Nursing_Education_Network_Bulletin_December_2014.pdf

International Data Corporation (IDC). (2016, August). *Press release: Worldwide revenues for augmented and virtual reality forecast to reach $162 billion in 2020, according to IDC.* Retrieved from http://www.idc.com/getdoc.jsp?containerId=prUS41676216

International Nursing Association of Clinical Simulation and Learning (INACSL). (2011). Standards of best practice: Simulation. *Clinical Simulation in Nursing, 7*(4S), Si–S19.

International Nursing Association of Clinical Simulation and Learning (INACSL). (2013). Standards of best practice: Simulation. *Clinical Simulation in Nursing, 9*(6S), S1–S32.

International Nursing Association of Clinical Simulation and Learning (INACSL) Board of Directors. (2011a). Standard III: Participant objectives. *Clinical Simulation in Nursing, 7*(4S), s10–s11. http://dx.doi.org/10.1016/j.ecns.2013.04.005

International Nursing Association of Clinical Simulation and Learning (INACSL) Board of Directors. (2011b). Standards of best practice: Simulation. *Clinical Simulation in Nursing, 7*(4S), s1–s20.

International Nursing Association of Clinical Simulation and Learning (INACSL) Board of Directors. (2013a). Standard I: Terminology. *Clinical Simulation in Nursing, 9,* S3–S11.

International Nursing Association of Clinical Simulation and Learning (INACSL) Board of Directors. (2013b). Standard II: Professional integrity of participant. *Clinical Simulation in Nursing, 9,* S12–S14.

International Nursing Association of Clinical Simulation and Learning (INACSL) Board of Directors. (2013c). Standard III: Participant objectives. *Clinical Simulation in Nursing, 9,* S15–S18.

International Nursing Association of Clinical Simulation and Learning (INACSL) Board of Directors. (2013d). Standard IV: Facilitation. *Clinical Simulation in Nursing, 9,* S19–S21.

International Nursing Association of Clinical Simulation and Learning (INACSL) Board of Directors. (2013e). Standard V: Simulation facilitator. *Clinical Simulation in Nursing, 9,* S22–S25.

International Nursing Association of Clinical Simulation and Learning (INACSL) Board of Directors. (2013f). Standard VI: The debriefing process. *Clinical Simulation in Nursing, 9,* S26–S29.

International Nursing Association of Clinical Simulation and Learning (INACSL) Board of Directors. (2013g). Standard VII: Participant assessment and evaluation. *Clinical Simulation in Nursing, 9,* S30–S32.

International Nursing Association of Clinical Simulation in Nursing (INACSL) Standards Committee. (2016). Standards of best practice: Simulation^SM. *Clinical Simulation in Nursing, 12*(S), S1–S50.

International Organization for Standardization (ISO). (2015). ISO 9001:2015 quality management systems—Requirements. Retrieved from https://www.iso.org/obp/ui/#iso:std:62085:en

Interprofessional Education Collaborative Expert Panel (IPECEP). (2011). *Core competencies for interprofessional collaborative practice: Report of an expert panel.* Washington, DC: Interprofessional Education Collaborative.

Ironside, P. M. (2013). Narrative pedagogy: Transforming nursing education through 15 years of research in nursing education. *Nursing Education Perspectives, 36*(2). doi:10.5480/13-1102

Ironside, P. M. (2014). Enabling narrative pedagogy: Inviting, waiting and letting be. *Nursing Education Perspectives, 35*(4), 212–218. doi:10.5480/13-1125.1

Ironside, P. M., & McNelis, A. M. (2010). *Clinical education in prelicensure nursing programs: Results from an NLN National Survey 2009.* New York, NY: National League for Nursing.

Irving, D. K. (2010). *Fundamentals of film directing* (pp. 2). Jefferson, NC: McFarland & Company, Inc.

Issenberg, S., McGaghie, W., Petrusa, E., Lee Gordon, D., & Scalese, R. (2005). Features and uses of high-fidelity medical simulations that lead to effective learning: A BEME systematic review. *Medical Teacher, 27*(1), 10–28.

Issenberg, S. B., Ringsted, C., Ostergaard, D., & Dieckmann, P. (2011). Setting a research agenda for simulation-based healthcare education: A synthesis of the outcome from an Utstein style meeting. *Simulation in Healthcare, 6*(3), 155–167. doi:10.1097/SIH.0b013e3182207c24

Iwasiw, C., & Goldenberg, D. (2014). *Curriculum development in nursing education* (3rd ed.). Burlington, MA: Jones and Bartlett Learning.

Iwasiw, C., Goldenberg, D., & Andrusyszyn, M. (2009). *Curriculum development in nursing* (2nd ed.). Burlington, MA: Jones and Bartlett Learning.

Jackson, B. H. (2015). Attentional leadership theory: A framework for the 2050 leader. In M. Sowcik, A. C. Andenoro, M. McNutt & S. E. Murphy (Eds.), *Leadership 2050: Critical challenges, key contexts, and emerging trends* (pp. 241–262). Bingley, UK: Emerald Group.

Jamal, A., Walling, K. D., & Arnold, J. L. (2015). Creating a fee structure. In J. C. Palaganas, J. C. Maxworthy, C. A. Epps & M. E. Mancini (Eds.), *Defining excellence in simulation programs* (p. 293). Philadelphia, PA: Wolters Kluwer.

James, K. M. G. (2010). Incorporating complexity science theory into nursing curricula. *Creative Nursing, 16*(3), 137–142. doi:10.1891/1078-4535.16.3.137

Jansen, D. A., Johnson, N., Larson, G., Berry, C., & Brenner, G. H. (2009). Nursing faculty perceptions of obstacles to utilizing manikin-based simulations and proposed solutions. *Clinical Simulation in Nursing, 5*(1), e9–e16. doi:10.1016/j.ecns.2008.09.004

Janzen, K. J., Jeske, S., MacLean, H., Harvey, G., Nickle, P., Norenna, L., ..., McLellan, H. (2016). Handling strong emotions before, during, and after simulated clinical experiences. *Clinical Simulation in Nursing, 12*(2), 37–43. http://dx.doi.org/10.1016/j.ecns.2015.12.004

Jeffreys, M. (2010). Cultural competence and nursing student retention. *Questionnaires and assessment tools.* Retrieved from http://www.mariannejeffreys.com/culturalcompetence/questionnaire.php

Jeffries, P. R. (2005). A framework for designing, implementing, and evaluating simulations used as teaching strategies in nursing. *Nursing Education Perspectives, 26*(2), 97–103.

Jeffries, P. R. (2007). *Simulation in nursing education: From conceptualization to evaluation.* New York, NY: National League for Nursing.

Jeffries, P. R. (2012a, May). *Clinical versus simulation: Outcomes, the evidence, and current research (symposium presentation).* Retrieved from http://www.wiser.pitt.edu/sites/wiser/ns12/pdfs/Clinical%20versus%20simulation_Jeffries.pdf

Jeffries, P. R. (2012b). *Simulation in nursing education: From conceptualization to evaluation* (2nd ed.). New York, NY: National League for Nursing.

Jeffries, P. R. (Ed.). (2014). *Clinical simulations in nursing education.* New York, NY: National League for Nursing/Wolters Kluwer.

Jeffries, P. R. (2015). *The NLN Jeffries simulation theory.* Philadelphia, PA: NLN and Wolters Kluwer.

Jeffries, P., & Battin, J. (2011). *Developing successful health care education simulation centers: The consortium model.* New York, NY: Springer Publishing Company.

Jeffries, P. R., Battin, J., Franklin, M., Savage, R., Yowler, H., Sims, C., ... Dorsey, L. (2013). Creating a professional development plan for a simulation consortium. *Clinical Simulation in Nursing, 9*(6), e183–e190. doi:10.1016/j.ecns.2012.02.003

Jeffries, P. R., Bauman, E. B., & Shaefer, J. J. (2014). The future of simulation in healthcare. In B. T. Ulrich & M. E. Mancini (Eds.), *Mastering simulation: A handbook for success.* Indianapolis, IN: Sigma Theta Tau International.

Jeffries, P. R., & Clochesy, J. M. (2012). Clinical simulations: An experiential, student-centered pedagogical approach. In D. M. Billings & J. A. Halstead (Eds.), *Teaching in nursing: A guide for faculty* (4th ed., pp. 352–368). St. Louis, MO: Elsevier Health Sciences.

Jeffries, P. R., & Rizzolo, M. A. (2007). Designing and implementing models for the innovative use of simulation to teach nursing care of ill adults and children: A national, multi-site, multi-method study. In P. R. Jeffries (Ed.), *Simulation in nursing education: From conceptualization to evaluation* (pp. 147–159). New York, NY: National League for Nursing.

Jeffries, P. R., & Rogers, K. J. (2012). Theoretical framework for simulation design. In P. R. Jeffries (Ed.), *Simulation in nursing education: From conceptualization to evaluation* (2nd ed., pp. 25–42). New York, NY: National League for Nursing.

Jeffries, P. R., Rogers, B., & Adamson, K. (2015). NLN Jeffries simulation theory: Brief narrative description. *Nursing Education Perspectives, 36*(5), 292–293.

Jeffries, P. R., Thomas-Dreifuerst, K., Kardong-Edgren, S., & Hayden, J. (2015). Faculty development when initiating simulation programs: Lessons learned from the national simulation study. *Journal of Nursing Regulation, 5*(4), 17–23. doi:http://dx.doi.org/10.1016/S2155-8256(15)30037-5

Johns, C. (2013). *Becoming a reflective practitioner* (4th ed.). Chichester, UK: Wiley-Blackwell.

Johnson, L., Adams Becker, S., Cummins, M., Estrada, V., Freeman, A., & Hall, C. (2016). *NMC horizon report: 2016 higher education edition.* Austin, TX: New Media Consortium. Retrieved from https://www.nmc.org/publication/nmc-horizon-report-2016-higher-education-edition/

Johnson, S. (n.d.). *Escaping conflict and the Karpman drama triangle.* Retrieved from http://bpdfamily.com/content/karpman-drama-triangle

Jones, A. L., Reese, C. E., & Shelton, D. P. (2014). NLN/Jeffries simulation framework state of the science project: The teacher construct. *Clinical Simulation in Nursing, 10*(7), 353–362. doi:http://dx.doi.org/10.1016/j.ecns.2013.10.008

Jones, E. R., Hennessey, R. T., & Deutsch, S. (1985). *Human factors aspects of simulation.* Washington, DC: National Academy Press.

Joseph, S., & Juwah, C. (2011). Using constructive alignment theory to develop nursing skills curricula. *Nurse Education in Practice, 12*(1), 52–59. doi:10.1016/j.nepr.2011.05.007

Josephsen, J. (2015) Cognitive load theory and nursing simulation: An integrative review. *Clinical Simulation in Nursing, 11,* 259–267. doi:http://dx.doi.org/10.1016/j.ecns.2015.02.004

Joshi, R., D'Costa, G., & Kura, M. (2010). Moulages of J.J. Hospital. *Indian Journal of Dermatology, Venereology & Leprology, 76*(5), 583–588. doi:10.4103/0378-6323.69088

Kable, A. K., Arthur, C., Levett-Jones, T., & Reid-Searl, K. (2013). Student evaluation of simulation in undergraduate nursing programs in Australia using quality indicators. *Nursing and Health Sciences, 15*(2), 235–243. doi:10.1111/nhs.12025

Kahrs, K., & Harmer, W. H. (2013). *Business plans handbook* (13th ed.). Boston, MA: Gale Cengage Learning Publishers.

Kaiser Permanente. (2016). *Electronic medical records.* Retrieved from http://www.kaiserpermanentejobs.org/electronicmedical-record.aspx

Kaiser, R. B., & Overfield, D. V. (2010). Assessing flexible leadership as a mastery of opposites. *Consulting Psychology Journal Practice and Research, 62*(2), 105–118. doi:10.1037/a0019987

Kalaniti, K. (2014). *In situ* simulation: Let's work, practice and learn together. *Acta Paediatrica, 103*, 1219–1220. doi:10.1111/apa.12802

Kalra, J. (2011). *Medical errors and patient safety: Strategies to reduce and disclose medical errors and improve patient safety.* New York, NY: Deutsche Nationalbibliothek.

Kameg, K. M., Szpak, J. L., Clinle, T. W., & Mcdermott, D. S. (2014). Utilization of standardized patients to decrease nursing student anxiety. *Clinical Simulation in Nursing, 10*(11), 567–573. doi:10.1016/j.ecns.2014.09.006

Kaminsky, J. (2011). Diffusion of innovation theory. *Canadian Journal of Nursing Informatics, 6*(2).

Kaplan, B. G., Abraham, C., & Gary, R. (2012). Effects of participation vs observation of a simulation experience on testing outcomes: Implications for logistical planning for a school of nursing. *International Journal of Nursing Education Scholarship, 29*(9), Article 14. doi:10.1515/1548-923X.2398

Kapralos, B., Hogan, M., Pribetic, A. I., & Dubrowski, A. (2011). Virtual simulations and seriousgames in a laptop-based university. *Interactive Technology and Smart Education, 8*(2), 106–120. http://dx.doi.org/10.1108/17415651111141821

Kardong-Edgren, S., Adamson, K. A., & Fitzgerald, C. (2010). A review of currently published evaluation instruments for human patient simulation. *Clinical Simulation in Nursing, 6*(1), e25–e35. doi:http://dx.doi.org/10.1016/j.ecns.2009.08.004

Kardong-Edgren, S., Dieckmann, P., & Phero, J. C. (2015). Simulation research considerations. In J. Palaganas, J. C. Maxworthy, C. A. Epps & M. E. Mancini (Eds.), *Defining excellence in simulation programs* (pp. 615–623). Philadelphia, PA: Wolters Kluwer, Inc.

Kardong-Edgren, S., Hanberg, A. D., Keenan, C., Ackerman, A., & Chambers, C. (2012). A discussion of high stakes testing: An extension of a 2009 INACSL round table. *Clinical Simulation in Nursing, 7*(1), e19–e24. doi:10.1016/j.ecns.2010.02.002

Kardong-Edgren, S., & Oermann, M. (2009). A letter to nursing program administrators about simulation. *Clinical Simulation in Nursing, 5*, e161–e162. doi:http://dx.doi.org/10.1016/j.ecns.2009.04.094

Kardong-Edgren, S., Willhaus, J., Bennett, D., & Hayden, J. (2012). Results of the National Council of State Boards of Nursing national simulation survey: Part II. *Clinical Simulation in Nursing, 8*, e117–e123. doi:10.1016/j.ecns.2012.01.003

Karpman, S. B. (2011, August). *The new drama triangles USATAA/ITAA conference lecture.* Retrieved from www.karpmandramatriangle.com

Karpman, S. B. (2014). *A game free life.* San Francisco, CA: Drama Triangle Publications.

Katz, G. B., Peifer, K. L., & Armstrong, G. (2010). Assessment of patient simulation use in selected baccalaureate nursing programs in the United States. *Simulation in Healthcare, 5*(1), 46–51. doi:10.1097/SIH.0b013e3181balf46

Kellerman, B. (2008). *Followership: How followers are creating change and changing leaders.* Boston, MA: Harvard Business Press.

Kellerman, B. (2014, July/August). Limits on leadership. *Capitol Ideas, 57*(4), 18–19. Retrieved from http://www.csg.org/pubs/capitolideas/index.aspx

Kelly, J., & Ahern, K. (2007). Preparing nurses for practice: A phenomenological study of new graduates in Australia. *Journal of Clinical Nursing, 18*(6), 910–918. doi:10.111/j.1365-2702.2008.02308.x

Kelly, M. (2009). International collaboration to advance simulation in nursing. *Clinical Simulation in Nursing, 5*(6), e201–e202. doi:10.1016/j.ecns.2009.05.063

Kelly, M. A. (2014). *Investigating the use of simulations in enhancing clinical judgement of nursing students to practice as registered nurses.* Dissertation University of Technology Sydney.

Kelly, M. A., Forber, J., Conlon, L., Roche, M., & Stasa, H. (2014). Empowering the registered nurses of tomorrow: Students' perspectives of a simulation experience for recognising and managing a deteriorating patient. *Nurse Education Today, 34*(5), 724–729. doi:10.1016/j.nedt.2013.08.014

Kelly, M. A., & Hager, P. (2015). Informal learning: Relevance and application to health care simulation. *Clinical Simulation in Nursing, 11*(8), 376–382. http://dx.doi.org/10.1016/j.ecns.2015.05.006

Kelly, M. A., Hager, P., & Gallagher, R. (2014). What matters most? Students' rankings of simulation components which contribute to clinical judgement. *Journal of Nursing Education, 53*(2), 97–101. doi:10.3928/01484834-20140122-08

Kelly, R. E. (2008). Rethinking followership. In R. E. Riggio, I. Chaleff & J. Lipman-Blumen (Eds.), *The art of followership: How great followers create great leaders and organizations* (pp. 5–15). San Francisco, CA: Jossey-Bass.

Kenaszchuk, C. MacMillan, K., van Soeren M., & Reeves, S. (2011). Interprofessional simulated learning: Short-term associations between simulation and interprofessional collaborations. *BMC Medicine, 9*, 29. doi:10.1186/1741-7015-9-29

Kennedy, P. (2002). Learning cultures and learning styles: Myth-understandings about adult (Hong Kong) Chinese learners. *International Journal of Lifelong Education, 21*(5), 430–445. http://dx.doi.org/10.1080/02601370210156745

Kerchner, C. T. (2011). A new culture of learning: John Dewey meets the Internet. *Learning 2.0 Series.* Retrieved from http://www.mindworkers.com/

Kessler, D. O., Artega, G., Ching, K., Haubner, L., Kamdar, G., Krantz, A., … Auerbach, M. (2013). Interns' success with clinical procedures in infants after simulation training. *Pediatrics, 131*(3), e811–e820. doi:10.1542/peds_2012-0607

Khatri, N., Brown, G. D., Hicks, L. L. (2009). From a blame culture to a just culture in health care. *Health Care Management Review, 34*(4), 312–322. doi:10.1097/HMR.0b013e3181a3b709

Kidder, R. M. (2005). *Moral courage.* New York, NY: Harper Collins.

Kiili, K. (2005). Digital game-based learning: Towards an experiential gaming model. *The Internet and higher education, 8*(1), 13–24. http://dx.doi.org/10.1016/j.iheduc.2004.12.001

Kilty, H. (2005). *Nursing leadership development in Canada.* Retrieved from http://www.cna-aiic.ca/sitecore%20modules/web/~/media/cna/page%20content/pdf%20fr/2013/09/05/19/21/nursing_leadership_development_canada_e.pdf

Kim, J., Neilipovitz, D., Cardinal, P., Chiu, M., & Clinch, J. (2006). A pilot study using high-fidelity simulation to formally evaluate performance in the resuscitation of critically ill patients: The University of Ottawa Critical Care Medicine, high-fidelity simulation, and crisis resource management I study. *Critical Care Medicine, 34*(8), 2167–2174.

Kim-Godwin, Y. S., Livsey, K. R., Ezzell, D., Highsmith, C., Winslow, H., & Aikman, A. N. (2013, November). Students like peer evaluation during home visit simulation experiences. *Clinical Simulation in Nursing, 9*(11), e535–e542. doi:http://dx.doi.org/10.1016/j.ecns.2012.06.002

Kimmel, P. J., Weygandt, J. J., Kieso, D. E., Trenholm, B., & Irvine, W. (2012). *Financial accounting: Tools for business decision-making* (6th Canadian ed.). Toronto, ON: John Wiley & Sons Canada, Ltd.

King, S., Carbonaro, M., Greidanus, E., Ansell, D., Foisy-Doll, C., & Magus, S. (2014). Dynamic and routine interprofessional simulations: Expanding the use of simulation to enhance interprofessional competencies. *Journal of Allied Health, 43*(3), 169–175.

King, S., Drummond, J., Hughes, E., Bookhalter, S., Huffman, D., & Ansell, D. (2013). An inter-institutional collaboration: Transforming education through interprofessional simulations. *Journal of Interprofessional Care, 27*(5), 429–431. doi:10.3109/13561820.2013.791260

King, S., Greidanus, E., Major, R., Loverso, T., Knowles, A., Carbonaro, M., & Bahry, L. (2012). A cross-institutional examination of readiness for interprofessional learning. *Journal of Interprofessional Care, 26*(2), 108–114. doi:10.3109/13561820.2011.640758

Kingma, M. (2006). *Nurses on the move: Migration and the global health care economy.* Ithaca, NY: Cornell University Press.

Kirkham, S., Van Hofwegen, L., & Pankratz, D. (2009). Keeping the vision: Sustaining social consciousness with nursing students following international learning experiences. *International Journal of Nursing Education Scholarship, 6*(1), 1–16. doi:10.2202/1548-923X.1635

Kirkman, T. (2013). High fidelity simulation effectiveness in nursing students' transfer of learning. *International Journal of Nursing Education Scholarship, 10*(1), 1–6. doi:10.1515/ijnes-2012-0009

Kirkpatrick, D. L. (1994). *Evaluating training programs: The four levels.* San Francisco, CA: Berrett-Koehler Publishers.

Kirkpatrick, J. D., & Kirkpatrick, W. K. (2010). ROEs rising star. *Association for Talent Development.* Retrieved from http://www.astd.org/TD/Archives/2010/Aug/Free/1008_ROEs_Rising_Star.htm

Kirkpatrick Partners, LCC. (2016). *Return on expectations.* Retrieved from http://www.kirkpatrickpartners.com/Our Philosophy/ReturnonExpectations/tabid/317/Default.aspx

Kirkwood, L. (2005). Enough but not too much: Nursing education in English language Canada (1874–2000). In C. Bates, D. Dodd & N. Rousseau (Eds.), *On all frontiers four centuries of Canadian nursing* (pp. 183–195). Ottawa, ON: University of Ottawa Press and the Canadian Museum of Civilization.

Kleinman, A. (1981). *Patients and healers in the context of culture: An exploration of the borderland between anthropology, medicine, and psychiatry.* Berkeley, CA: University of California Press.

Klipfel, J. M., Carolan, B. J., Brytowski, N., Mitchell, C. A., Gettman, M. T., & Jacobson, T. M. (2015). Patient safety improvement through in situ simulation interdisciplinary team training. *Urologic Nursing, 34*(1), 39–46. doi:10.7257/1053-816X.2014.34.1.39

Klokkerud, M. (2008). *Migration of health workers. Oslo University College.* Retrieved from http://eresearch.qmu.ac.uk/759/

Klopper, H. C., & Uys, L. (2013). *The state of nursing and nursing education in Africa: A country-by-country review.* Retrieved from http://d1wu7jj76b18bg.cloudfront.net/publications/Africa_Sample.pdf

Kneebone, R. (2003). Simulation in surgical training: Educational issues and practical training. *Medical Education, 37*, 267–277.

Knights, D., & O'Leary, M. (2006). Leadership, ethics and responsibility to the other. *Journal of Business Ethics, 67*(2), 125–137.

Knowles, M. (1990) *The adult learner: A neglected species* (4th ed.). Houston, TX: Gulf Publishing.

Knowles, M. S. (1968). Andragogy, not pedagogy. *Adult Leadership, 16*(10), 350–352, 386.

Knowles, M. S. (1980). *The modern practice of adult education: From pedagogy to andragogy* (2nd ed.). New York, NY: Cambridge Books.

Knowles, M. S. (1984). *The adult learner: A neglected species* (3rd ed.). Houston, TX: Gulf.

Kobayashi, L., Shapiro, M. J., Suner, S., & Williams, K. A. (2003). Disaster medicine: The potential role of high fidelity medical simulation for mass casualty incident training. *Medicine and Health Rhode Island, 86*(7), 196–200. Retrieved from http://search.proquest.com/openview/02542d5eb2a2f565850aca25084f2776/1?pq-origsite=gscholar

Koenig, A., Iseli, M., Wainess, R., & Lee, J. J. (2013). Assessment methodology for computer-based instructional simulations. *Military Medicine, 178*(10), 47–54. doi:10.7205/MILMED-D-13-00217

Koh, H. K., Garcia, N., & Alvarez, M. E. (2014). Culturally and linguistically appropriate services: Advancing health with CLAS. *New England Journal of Medicine, 371*(3), 198–201. doi:10.1056/NEJMp1404321

Kohn, L. T., Corrigan, J. M., & Donaldson, M. S. (Eds.) (2000). *To err is human: Building safer healthcare system.* Institute of Medicine (IOM). Washington, DC: National Academy Press.

Kolb, D. A. (1984). *Experiential learning: Experience as the source of learning and development.* Englewood Cliffs, NJ: Prentice-Hall.

Koltko-Rivera, M. E. (2006). Rediscovering the later version of Maslow's hierarchy of needs: Self-transcendence and opportunities for theory, research, and unification. *Review of General Psychology 10*(4), 302–317. Retrieved from http://academic.udayton.edu/jackbauer/Readings%20595/Koltko-Rivera%2006%20trans%20self-act%20copy.pdf

Kommers, P. (2012). Future developments in E-simulations for learning soft skills in the health professions. In D. Holt, S. Segrave & J. Cybulski (Eds.), *Professional education using e-simulations: Benefits of blended learning design* (pp. 370–393). Hershey, PA: Business Science Reference. doi:10.4018/978-1-61350-189-4.ch020

Konstantinos, N., & Ouzouni, C. (2008). Factors influencing stress and job satisfaction of nurses working in psychiatric units: A research review. *Health Science Journal, 2*, 183–195.

Koontz, H., & O'Donnell, C. (1972). *Principles of management: An analysis of managerial functions.* New York, NY: McGraw-Hill.

Koplan, J. P., Bond, T. C., Merson, M. H., Reddy, K. S., Rodriguez, M. H., Sewankambo, N. K., et al. (2009). Towards a common definition of global health. *The Lancet, 373*(9679), 1993–1995. http://doi.org/10.1016/S0140-6736(09)60332-9

Kotal, E. R., Sivertson, R. M., Wolfe, S. P., Lammers, R. L., & Overton, D. T. (2015). A survey of simulation fellowship programs. *The Journal of Emergency Medicine, 48*(3), 351–355. http://doi.org/10.1016/j.jemermed.2014.10.004

Kotter, J. P. (1996). *Leading change.* Boston, MA: Harvard Business School Press.

Kotter, J. P. (2008). *A sense of urgency.* Boston, MA: Harvard Business School Press.

Kotter, J. P. (2014). *XLR8: Accelerate.* Boston, MA: Harvard Business School Press.

Kotter, J. P., & Cohen, D. S. (2002). *The heart of change: Real life stories of how people change their organizations.* Boston, MA: Harvard Business School Press.

Kotter International. (2015a). *8 Steps to accelerate change in 2015.* Retrieved from http://www.kotterinternational.com/resources/landing-page/8-steps-to-accelerate-change-in-2015/

Kotter International. (2015b). *The heart of change.* Retrieved from https://www.kotterinternational.com/book/the-heart-of-change/

Kotter International. (2015c). *The 8-steps process for leading change.* Retrieved from http://www.kotterinternational.com/the-8-step-process-for-leading-change/

Koutonin, M. R. (2015, March). *Why are white people expats and the rest of us are immigrants?* Retrieved from http://www.theguardian.com/global-development-professionals-network/2015/mar/13/white-people-expats-immigrants-migration

Kouzes, J. M., & Posner, B. Z. (2007). *Leadership challenge* (4th ed.). San Francisco, CA: Wiley.

Kouzes, J. M., & Posner, B. Z. (2012). *The leadership challenge: How to make extraordinary things happen in organizations.* San Francisco, CA: Jossey-Bass.

Kouzes, J. M., & Posner, B. Z. (2014). *The student leadership challenge: Five practices for becoming an exemplary leader* (2nd ed.). San Francisco, CA: Wiley.

Kowch, E. G. (2013). Whither thee, educational technology? Suggesting a critical expansion of our epistemology for emerging leaders. *TechTrends, 57*(5), 25–34. doi:10.1007/s11528-013-0688-3

Kramer, M., Schmalenberg, C., & Maquire, P. (2010). Nine structures and leadership practices essential for a magnetic (healthy) work environment. *Nursing Administration Quarterly, 34*(11), 4–17. doi:10.1097/NAQ.0b013e3181c95ef4

Krathwohl, D. R. (2002). A revision of Bloom's taxonomy: An overview. *Theory Into Practice, 41*(4), 212–218.

Krishna, S. K. (2011). Modern moulage. *Indian Journal of Dermatology, Venereology & Leprology, 77*(1), 64. doi:10.4103/0378-6323.74987

Kruse, S. D., & Louis, K. S. (2009). *Building strong school cultures.* Thousand Oaks, CA: Corwin Press.

Kuiper, R. A., & Zabriskie, A. (2012). Developing a new state of the art simulation learning center. *Clinical Simulation in Nursing, 8*(9), e437–e442. doi:10.1016/j.ecns.2011.04.003

Kumashiro, K. K. (2000). Toward a theory of anti-oppressive education. *Review of Educational Research, 70*(1), 25–53.

Kutzin, J. M. (2016). Simulation design considerations 2.0: Optimizing space and operations. *Clinical Simulation in Nursing, 12*(6), 187–196. http://dx.doi.org/10.1016/j.ecns.2016.01.012

Kvarnström, S. (2008). Difficulties in collaboration: A critical incident study of interprofessional healthcare teamwork. *Journal of Interprofessional Care, 22,* 191–203. doi:10.1080/13561820701760600

Kyaw Tun, J., Alinier, G., Tang, J., & Kneebone, R. L. (2015). Redefining simulation fidelity for healthcare education. *Simulation and Gaming, 46*(2), 159–174. doi:10.1177/1046878115576103

Kyle, R. R., & Murray, W. B. (Eds.), (2008). *Clinical simulation: Operations, engineering and management.* Philadelphia, PA: Elsevier.

Laerdal. (n.d.). *Clinical skills managed educational network (CS MEN).* Retrieved from http://laerdalcdn.blob.core.windows.net/downloads/f1143/ACWLTXJW/5233_CSMEN_US.pdf

LaGrandeur, K. (2014, July). What is the difference between posthumanism and transhumanism? *Institute for Ethics and Emerging Technologies.* Retrieved from http://ieet.org/index.php/IEET/more/lagrandeur20140729

Lam, T., Wan, X., & Sau-Man, M. (2006). Current perspectives on medical education in China. *Medical Education, 40,* 940–949. http://dx.doi.org/10.1111/j.1365-2929.2006.02552.x

Landrigan, C. P., Parry, G. J., Bones, C. B., Hackbarth, A. D., Goldmann, D. A., & Sharek, P. J. (2010). Temporal trends in rates of patient harm resulting from medical care. *New England Journal of Medicine, 363*(22), 2124–2134. Retrieved from http://doi.org/10.1056/NEJMsa1004404

Lane, J. L., Ziv, A., & Boulet, J. (1999). A pediatric clinical skills assessment using children as standardized patients. *Archives of Pediatrics & Adolescent Medicine, 153*(6), 637–644. doi:10.1001/archpedi.153.6.637

Lange, E. (2004). Transformative and restorative learning: A vital dialectic for sustainable societies. *Adult Education Quarterly, 54*(2), 121–139. http://dx.doi.org/10.1177/0741713603260276

Lapkin, S., Levett-Jones, T., Bellchambers, H., & Fernandez, R. (2010). Effectiveness of patient simulation manikins in teaching clinical reasoning skills to undergraduate nursing students: A systematic review. *Clinical Simulation in Nursing, 6*(6), e207–e222. doi:http://dx.doi.org/10.1016/j.ecns.2010.05.005

Lasater, K. (2007a). Clinical judgment development: Using simulation to create an assessment rubric. *Journal of Nursing Education, 46*(11), 496–503.

Lasater, K. (2007b). High-fidelity simulation and the development of clinical judgment: Students' experiences. *Journal of Nursing Education, 46*(6), 269–276.

Lasater, K., & Nielsen, A. (2009). Reflective journaling for clinical judgment development and evaluation. *Journal of Nursing Education, 48*(1), 40–44.

Laszlo, A., Laszlo, K., & Johnsen, C. S. (2009). From high-performance teams to evolutionary learning communities: New pathways in organizational development. *Journal of Organizational Transformation & Social Change, 6*(1), 29–48. doi:10.1386/jots.6.1.29_1

Lateef, F. (2010). Simulation-based learning: Just like the real thing. *Journal of Emergencies, Trauma, and Shock, 3*(4), 348–352. doi:10.4103/0974-2700.70743

Launchship.com. (2016, October). *Why the university of the future will have no classrooms, no lectures, and lots of tech.* Retrieved from https://www.launchship.com/blog/why-the-university-of-the-future-will-have-no-classrooms-no-lectures-and-lots-of-tech

Lave, J., & Wenger, E. (1991). *Situated learning: Legitimate peripheral participation.* Cambridge, UK: Cambridge University Press.

Lazzara, D., Benishek, L. E., Dietz, A. S., Salas, E., & Adriansen, D. J. (2014, January). Eight critical factors in creating and implementing a successful simulation program. *The Joint Commission Journal on Quality and Patient Safety, 40*(1), 21–29. doi:http://dx.doi.org/10.1016/S1553-7250(14)40003-5

Leape, L. L. (1994). Error in medicine. *JAMA, 272*(23), 1851–1857. doi:10.1001/jama.1994.03520230061039

Learning Theories. (2016). *Learning paradigms and theories.* Retrieved from http://www.learning-theories.org/doku.php

Lederman, L. C. (1992). Debriefing: Toward a systematic assessment of theory and practice. *Simulation & Gaming, 23*, 145–160.

Lee, J., & Oh, P. J. (2015). Effects of the use of high-fidelity human simulation in nursing education: A meta-analysis. *Journal of Nursing Education, 54*(9), 501–507. doi:10.3928/01484834-20150814-04

LeFlore, J. L., & Anderson, M. (2009). Alternative educational models for interdisciplinary student teams. *Simulation in Healthcare, 4*(3), 135–142. doi:10.1097/SIH.0b013e318196f839

Lehr, S. T., & Kaplan, B. (2013). A mental health simulation experience for baccalaureate student nurses. *Clinical Simulation in Nursing, 9*, e425–e431. doi:10.1016/j.ecns.2012.12.003

Leigh, G. T. (2008). High-fidelity patient simulation and nursing students' self-efficacy: A review of the literature. *International Journal of Nursing Education Scholarship, 5*(1), 1–17. doi:10.2202/1548-923X.1613

Leigh, K., Whitted, K., & Hamilton, B. (2015). Integration of andragogy into preceptorship. *Journal of Adult Education, 44*(1), 9–17.

Leighton, K. (2015). Development of the clinical learning environment comparison survey. *Clinical Simulation in Nursing, 11*(1), 44–51. doi:10.1016/j.ecns.2014.11.002

Leighton, K. (2016). Innovations in facilitating learning using simulation. In M. Bradshaw & A. Lowenstein (Eds.), *Innovative teaching strategies in nursing and related health professions* (6th ed). Boston, MA: Jones & Bartlett, Inc.

Leighton, K., Ravert, P., Mudra, V., & Macintosh, C. (2015). Updating the simulation effectiveness tool: Item modifications and reevaluation of psychometric properties. *Nursing Education Perspectives, 36*(5), 317–323. doi:10.5480/15–1671

Leighton, K., & Scholl, K. (2009). Simulated codes: Understanding the response of undergraduate nursing students. *Clinical Simulation in Nursing, 5*(5), e187–e194. doi:10.1016/j.ecns.2009.05.058

Leininger, M. M. (1978). *Transcultural nursing concepts, theories and practices.* New York, NY: Wiley.

Leininger, M. M. (1988). Leininger's theory of nursing: Cultural care diversity and universality. *Nursing Science Quarterly, 1*(4), 152–160.

Leininger, M. M. (2007, January). Theoretical questions and concerns: Response from the theory of culture care diversity and universality perspective. *Nursing Science Quarterly, 20*(1), 9–15. doi:10.1177/0894318406296784

Leitch, R. A., Moses, G. R., & Magee, H. (2002). Simulation and the future of military medicine. *Military Medicine, 167*(4), 350–354. Retrieved from http://www.ncbi.nlm.nih.gov/pubmed/11977889

Leslie, R. (2003). Capturing the daylight dividend in buildings: Why and how? *Building and Environment, 38*(2), 381–385. doi:10.1016/s0360-1327(02)00118-x

Lett, M. (2001). A case for chaos theory in nursing. *Australian Journal of Advanced Nursing, 18*(3), 14–19. Retrieved from http://www.ajan.com.au/Vol18/Vol18.3-2.pdf

Levett-Jones, T. (Ed.). (2013). *Clinical reasoning: Learning to think like a nurse.* Sydney: Pearson.

Levett-Jones, T., Hoffman, K., Dempsey, J., Jeong, S., Noble, D., Norton, C., … Hickey, N. (2010). The 'five rights' of clinical reasoning: An educational model to enhance nursing students' ability to identify and manage clinically 'at risk' patients. *Nurse Education Today, 30*(6), 515–520. doi:10.1016/j.nedt.2009.10.020

Levine, A. I., DeMaria, S. Jr., Schwartz, A. D., & Sim, A. J. (2014). *The comprehensive textbook of healthcare simulation.* New York, NY: Springer Science + Business Media.

Levine, A. I., & Swartz, M. H. (2008). Standardized patients: The "other" simulation. *Journal of Critical Care, 23*, 179–184. doi:10.1016/j.jcrc.2007.12.001

Levinson, D. R. (2010). *Adverse events in hospitals: National incidence among Medicare beneficiaries.* Washington, DC: National Department of Health and Human Services, Office of the Inspector General.

Levintova, E., Johnson, T., Scheberle, D., & Vonck, K. (2011). Global citizens are made, not born: Multiclass role-playing simulation of global decision making. *Journal of Political Science Education, 7*(3), 245–274. doi:10.1080/15512169.2011.590075

Lewin, K. (1944). The dynamics of group action. *Educational Leadership, 1*(4), 195.

Lewin, K. (1947). Frontiers in group dynamics: Concept, method and reality in social science; social equilibria and social change. *Human Relations, 1*(1), 5–41. doi:10.1177/001872674700100103

Leymann, H. (1996). The content and development of mobbing at work. *European Journal of Work and Organizational Psychology, 5*(2), 165–184. doi:10.1080/13594329608414853

Li, J., Tang, Q., Di, J., Feng, J., Fu, J., Yu, Y., & Yand, C. (2012). The application of simulation teaching methods in clinical teaching of surgery of Chinese medicine. *Global Journal of Medical Research, 12*(8), 1–4. Retrieved from https://globaljournals.org/GJMR_Volume12/1-The-Application-of-Simulation.pdf

Libby, T., & Reeves, S. (2011). Using the sociological imagination in the interprofessional field. *Journal of Interprofessional Care, 25*(5), 317–318. doi:10.3109/13561820.2015.1035179

Lichtenstein, R., Alexander, J. A., McCarthy, J. F., & Wells, R. (2004). Status differences in cross-functional teams: Effects on individual member participation, job satisfaction and intent to quit. *Journal of Health and Social Behavior, 45*(3), 322–335.

Lindqvist, S., & Reeves, S. (2007). Faciliators' perceptions of delivering interprofessional education: A qualitative study. *Medical Teacher, 29*(4), 403–405. http://www.ncbi.nlm.nih.gov/pubmed/17786761

Lioce, L. (2015). *Faculty simulation evaluation self-assessment form.* Huntsville, AL: The University of Alabama.

Lioce L., Meakim C. H., Fey M. K., Chmil J. V., Mariani B., & Alinier G. (2015). Standards of best practice: Simulation standard IX: Simulation design. *Clinical Simulation in Nursing, 11*(6), 309–315. http://dx.doi.org/10.1016/j.ecns.2015.03.005

Lioce, L., Reed, C. C., Lemon, D., King, M. A., Martinez, P. A., Franklin, A. E., …, Borum, J. C. (2013). Standards of best practice: Simulation standard III: Participant objectives. *Clinical Simulation in Nursing, 9*(6S), S15–S18. http://dx.doi.org/10.1016/j.ecns.2013.04.005

Lipman-Blumen, J. (2005). The allure of toxic leaders: Why followers rarely escape their clutches. *IVEY Business Journal, 69*(3), 1–8. Retrieved from http://www.iveybusinessjournal.com

Lisko, S. A., & O'Dell, V. (2010). Integration of theory and practice: Experiential learning theory and nursing education. *Nursing Education Perspectives, 31*, 106–108.

Locsin, R. C. (2005). *Technological competency as caring in nursing: A model for practice.* Indianapolis, IN: Sigma Theta Tau International.

Lois, F. J., Pospiech, A. L., Van Dyck, M. J., Kahn, D. A., & DeKock, M. F. (2014). Is the "in situ" simulation for teaching anesthesia residents a lower cost, feasible and satisfying alternative to simulation centre? A 24 month prospective observational study in a university hospital. *Acta Anaesthesiologica Belgica, 65*(2), 61–71.

Lopreiato, J. O. (Ed.), Downing, D., Gammon, W., Lioce, L., Sittner, B., Slot, V., Spain, A. E. (Associate Eds.); and the Terminology & Concepts Working Group. (2016). *Healthcare Simulation Dictionary™*. Retrieved from http://www.ssih.org/dictionary

Loyd, G. E., Lake, C. L., & Greenberg, R. B. (Eds.), (2004). *Practical health care simulations.* Philadelphia, PA: Elsevier.

Lucas, C. V., Holmes, S. K., Cohen, A. B., Restuccia, J., Cramer, I. E., Shwartz, M., & Charns, M. P. (2007). Transformational change in healthcare systems: An organizational model. *Health Care Management Review, 32*(4), 309–320. doi:10.1097/01.HMR.0000296785.29718.5d

Luctkar-Flude, M., Baker, C., Hopkins-Rosseel, D., Pulling, C, McGraw, R., Medves, J., …, Brown, C. (2014). Development and evaluation of an interprofessional simulation-based learning module on infection control skills for prelicensure health professional students. *Clinical Simulation in Nursing, 10*(8), 395–405. doi:http://dx.doi.org/10.1016/j.ecns.2014.03.003

Luctkar-Flude, M., Baker, C., Medves, J., Tsai, E., Rivard, L., Goyer, M-C., & Krause, A. (2013). Evaluating an interprofessional pediatrics educational module using simulation. *Clinical Simulation in Nursing, 9*(5), e163–e169. doi:10.1016/j.ecns.2011.11.008

Lunger, K. (2017). Why you need more than a dashboard to manage your strategy. *Business Intelligence Journal, 11*(4), 8–17.

Lynn, M. C., & Twigg, R. D. (2011). A new approach to clinical remediation. *Journal of Nursing Education, 50*(3), 172–175. doi:10.3928/01484834-20101230-12

MacEwan University Figures. (2010). *MacEwan creed.* Retrieved from https://issuu.com/macewan.webmaster/docs/figures2010_web/31

MacLean, P. D. (1990). *The triune brain in evolution: Role in paleocerebral functions.* New York, NY: Plenum Press.

MacLellan, D. (2015). Evidence-based education in nutrition and dietetics. In T. Brown & B. Williams (Eds.), *Evidence-based education in the health professions: Promoting best practice in the learning and teaching of students* (pp. 486–501). London, UK: Radcliffe Publishing Ltd.

MacMillan, K. (2014). Guest editorial. *Nursing Leadership, 27*(4), 1–4. doi:10.12927/cjnl.2015.24146

Macy, R., & Schrader, V. (2008, October). Pediophobia: A new challenge facing nursing faculty in clinical teaching by simulation. *Clinical Simulation in Nursing, 4*(3), e89–e91. doi:10.1016/j.ecns.2008.07.001

Madhok, R. (2002). Crossing the quality chasm: Lessons from health care quality improvement efforts in England. *Proceedings (Baylor University Medical Center), 15*(1), 77–83.

Maguire, M. (2001). Methods to support human-centered design. *International Journal of Human-Computer Studies, 55*(4), 587–634. doi:10.1006/ijhc.2001.0503

Mahoney, A., Hancock, L., Iorianni-Cimbak, A., & Curley, M. (2013). Using high fidelity simulation to bridge clinical and classroom learning in undergraduate pediatric nursing. *Nurse Education Today, 33*(6), 648–654. doi:10.1016/j.nedt.2012.01.005

Makary, M. A., & Daniel, M. (2016). Medical error: The third leading cause of death in the US. *BMJ, 353*, i2139. doi:10.1136/bmj.i2139

Malekzadeh, S., Malloy, K., Chu, E., Tompkins, J., Battista, A., & Deutsch, E. (2011). ORL emergencies boot camp: Using simulation to onboard residents. *The Laryngoscope, 121*(10), 2114–2121. doi:10.1002/lary.22146

Maloney, S., & Haines, T. (2016). Issues of cost-benefit and cost-effectiveness for simulation in health professions education. *Advances in Simulation, 1*, 1–6. http://doi.org/10.1186/s41077-016-0020-3

Manser, T. (2009). Teamwork and patient safety in dynamic domains of healthcare: A review of the literature. *Acta Anaesthesiologica Scandinavica, 53*(2), 143–151. doi:10.1111/j.1399-6576.2008.01717.x

Maran, N. J., & Glavin, R. J. (2003). Low- to high-fidelity simulation across continuum of medical education? *Medical Education, 37*(Suppl 1), 22–28.

Marcelino-Sadaba, S., Gonzalez-Jaen, L. F., & Perez-Ezcurdia, A. (2015). Using projects management as a way to sustainability: From a comprehensive review to a framework definition. *Journal of Cleaner Production, 99*, 1–16. doi:10.1016/j.jclepro.2015.03.020

Marcus, L. (1979). Learning style and ability grouping among seventh grade students. *The Clearing House, 52*, 377–380.

Marquis, B. L., & Huston, C. J. (2012). *Leadership and management tools for the new nurse.* Philadelphia, PA: Wolters Kluwer Health.

Marshall, E. S. (2011). *Transformational leadership in nursing: From expert clinician to influential leader.* New York, NY: Springer.

Martin, A. (2007). The future of leadership: Where do we go from here? *Journal of Industrial and Commercial Training, 39*(1), 3–8. http://dx.doi.org/10.1108/00197850710721345

Martin, D. R., O'Brien, J. L., Heyworth, J. A., & Meyer, N. R. (2005). The collaborative healthcare team: Tensive issues warranting ongoing consideration. *Journal of the American Academy of Nurse Practitioners, 17*(8), 235–330. http://dx.doi.org/10.1111/j.1745-7599.2005.0054.x

Mashable Explains. (2014, April). *What is virtual reality and how does it work?*. Retrieved from https://youtu.be/HBNH8tzsfVM

Maslow, A. H. (1943). A theory of human motivation. *Psychological Review, 50*(4), 370–396. doi:10.1037/h0054346

Maxworthy, J., & Waxman, K. T. (2014). Simulation alliances, networks, and collaboratives. In J. Palaganas, J. Maxworthy, C. Epps & M. E. Mancini (Eds.), *Defining excellence in simulation programs* (pp. 423–432). Philadelphia, PA: Wolters Kluwer.

May, W., Park, J. H., & Lee, J. P. (2009). A ten-year review of the literature on the use of standardized patients in teaching and learning: 1996–2005. *Medical Teacher, 31*(6), 487–492. http://doi.org/10.1080/01421590802530898

Mayer, J. D. (2009, September). What emotional intelligence is and is not. *Psychology Today*. Retrieved from https://www.psychologytoday.com/blog/the-personality-analyst/200909/what-emotional-intelligence-is-and-is-not

McAllister, S. (2015). Best practice assessment in health professional education. In T. Brown & B. Williams (Eds.), *Evidence-based education in the health professions: Promoting best practice in the learning and teaching of students* (pp. 168–185). London, UK: Radcliffe Publishing Ltd.

McAllister, M., Levett-Jones, T., Downer, T., Harrison, P., Harvey, T., Reid-Searl, K., … Calleja, P. (2013). Snapshots of simulation: Creative strategies used by Australian educators to enhance simulation learning experiences for nursing students. *Nurse Education in Practice, 13*(6), 567–572. http://dx.doi.org/10.1016/j.nepr.2013.04.010

McAllister, M., Searl, K. R., & Davis, S. (2013). Who is that masked educator? Deconstructing the teaching and learning processes of an innovative humanistic simulation technique. *Nurse Education Today, 33*(12), 1453–1458. http://dx.doi.org/10.1016/j.nedt.2013.06.015

McClusky, H. Y. (1963). The course of the adult life span. In W. C. Hallenbeck (Ed.), *Psychology of adults* (pp. 10–19). Washington, DC: Adult Education Association.

McClusky, H. Y. (1970). An approach to a differential psychology of the adult potential. In S. M. Grabowski (Ed.), *Adult learning and instruction* (pp. 80–95). Syracuse, NY: ERIC Clearinghouse on Adult Education (ERIC Document Reproduction Service No. ED045867).

McClusky, H. Y. (1974). The coming of age of lifelong learning. *Journal of Research and Development in Education, 7*(4), 97–107.

McDavid, J. C., Huse, I., & Hawthorne, L. R. L. (2013). *Program evaluation and performance measurement: An introduction to practice* (2nd ed.). Thousand Oaks, CA: Sage Publications.

McDonald, M. E. (2013). *The nurse educator's guide to assessing learning* (3rd ed.). Burlington, MA: Jones & Bartlett.

McFadyen, A., Webster, V., Strachan, K., Figgins, E., Brown, H., & McKechnie, J. (2005). The readiness for Interprofessional Learning Scale: A possible more stable sub-scale model for the original version of RIPLS. *Journal of Interprofessional Care, 19*(6), 595–603.

McGaghie, W. C. (2008). Research opportunities in simulation-based medical education using deliberate practice. *Academic Emergency Medicine, 15*(11), 995–1001. doi:10.1111/j.1553-2712.2008.00246.x

McGaghie, W. C., Draycott, T. J., Dunn, W. F., Lopez, C. M., & Stefanidis, D. (2011). Evaluating the impact of simulation on translational patient outcomes. *Simulation in Healthcare, 6*(Suppl), S42–S47. http://doi.org/10.1097/SIH.0b013e318222fde9

McGaghie, W. C., Issenberg, S. B., Barsuk, J. H., & Wayne, D. B. (2014). A critical review of simulation-based mastery learning with translational outcome. *Medical Education, 48*(4), 375–385. doi:10.1111/medu.12391

McGahie, W. C., Issenberg, S. B., Petrussa, E. R., & Scalese, R. J. (2006). Effect of practice on standardized learning outcomes in simulation-based medical education. *Medical Educator, 40*(8), 792–797. doi:10.1111/j.1365-2929.2006.02528.x

McGaghie, W. C., Issenberg, S. B., Petrusa, E. R., & Scalese, R. J. (2010). A critical review of simulation-based medical education research: 2003–2009. *Medical Education, 44*(1), 50–63. doi:10.1111/j.1365-2923.2009.03547.x

McGibbon, E., Mulaudzi, R. M., Didham, P., Barton, S., & Sochan, A. (2014). Toward decolonizing nursing: The colonization of nursing and strategies for increasing the counter-narrative. *Nursing Inquiry, 21*(3), 179–191. doi:10.1111/nin.12042

McIntosh, C. E., Thomas, C. M., Allen, R. A., & Edwards, J. A. (2015). Using a combination of teaching and learning strategies and standardized patient for a successful autism simulation. *Clinical Simulation in Nursing, 11*(3), 143–152. doi:10.1016/j.ecns.2014.11.008

McKay, K. A. C., Buen, J. E., Bohan, K. J., & Maye, J. P. (2010). Determining the relationships of acute stress, anxiety, and salivary a-amylase level with student performance of student nurse anesthetists during human-based anesthesia simulator training. *American Academy of Nurse Anesthetists Journal, 78*(4), 301–309.

McKenna, K. D., Carhart, E., Bercher, D., Spain, A., Todaro, J., & Freel, J. (2015). Simulation use in paramedic education research (SUPER): A descriptive study. *Prehospital Emergency Care, 19*(3), 432–440. doi:10.3109/10903127.2014.995845

McKenna, L., Missen, K., Cooper, S., Bogossian, F., Bucknall, T., & Cant, R. (2014). Situation awareness in undergraduate nursing students managing simulated patient deterioration. *Nurse Education Today, 34*(6), e27–e31. doi:10.1016/j.nedt.2013.12.013

McLeod, R., & Schell, G. (2006). *Management information systems* (10th ed.). Upper Saddle River, NJ: Prentice-Hall, Inc.

McMaster University. (2013). *Research: Crisis resource management in healthcare*. Retrieved from http://simulation.mcmaster.ca/crmproject.html

McMullin, J. A. (2010). *Understanding social inequality: Intersections of class, age, gender, ethnicity, and race in Canada* (2nd ed.). Don Mills, ON: Oxford University Press.

McNeill, J., Parker, R., Nadeau, J., Pelayo, L., Robert, J. J., & Kleberg, H. C. (2012). Developing nurse educator competency in the pedagogy of simulation. *Clinical Simulation in Nursing, 8*(8), e409–e410. doi:10.3928/01484834-20121030-01

Meakim, C. (2007). Creating an environment for simulation in a school of nursing. *Clinical Simulation in Nursing, 3*(1), e11–e13. doi:10.1016/j.ecns.2009.05.033

Meakim, C., Boese, T., Decker, S., Franklin, A. E., Gloe, D., Lioce, L. … Borum, J. C. (2013). Standards of best practice: Simulation standard I: Terminology. *Clinical Simulation in Nursing, 9*(6S), S3–S11. http://dx.doi.org/10.1016/j.ecns.2013.04.001

MedData Group. (2014). *Physician perspectives and predictions of connected health in 2015*. Retrieved from https://www.meddatagroup.com/infographic-connected-health-2015/

Medical Education Technologies, Inc. (2010). *PNCI: Program for nursing curriculum integration*. Sarasota, FL: Author.

MedSim. (2015). *Medical simulation center directory*. Retrieved from http://halldale.com/files/halldale/attachments/MEdSim%20Simulation%20Center%20Directory%20web%20January%2023,%202015.pdf

Meichenbaum, D. H., & Deffenbacher, J. L. (1988). Stress inoculation training. *The Counseling Psychologist*, 16(1), 60–90. doi:10.1177/0011000088161005

Melnyk, B. M. & Fineout-Overholt, E. (Eds.). (2011). *Evidence-based practice in nursing & healthcare: A guide to best practice*. Philadelphia, PA: Lippincott, Williams & Wilkins.

Melnyk, B. M., & Fineout-Overholt, E. (2015a). Creating a vision and motivating a change to evidence-based practice in individuals, teams and organizations. In B. M. Melnyk & E. Fineout-Overholt (Eds.), *Evidence-based practice in nursing & healthcare* (3rd ed., pp. 316–329). Philadelphia, PA: Wolters Kluwer Health.

Melnyk, B. M., & Fineout-Overholt, E. (2015b). Making the case for evidence-based practice and cultivating a spirit of inquiry. In B. M. Melnyk & E. Fineout-Overholt (Eds.), *Evidence-based practice in nursing & healthcare* (3rd ed., pp. 3–23). Philadelphia, PA: Wolters Kluwer Health.

Melnyk, B. M., & Fineout-Overholt, E. (2015c). Organizational culture & readiness for system-wide integration of evidence-based practice survey. In B. M. Melnyk & E. Fineout-Overholt (Eds.), *Evidence-based practice in nursing & healthcare: A guide to best practice* (3rd ed.). Philadelphia, PA: Lippincott Williams & Wilkins.

Melnyk, B. M., & Fineout-Overholt, E. (Eds.). (2015d). *Evidence-based practice in nursing & healthcare: A guide to best practice* (3rd ed.). *Philadelphia, PA*: Wolters Kluwer Health.

Melnyk, B. M., Fineout-Overholt, E., Gallagher-Ford, L., & Kaplan, L. (2012). The state of evidence-based practice in US nurses: Critical implications for nurse leaders and educators. *Journal of Nursing Administration*, 42(9), 410–417.

Melnyk, B. M., Fineout-Overholt, E., Stillwell, S. B., & Williamson, K. M. (2009). Evidence-based practice: Step by step: Igniting a spirit of inquiry: An essential foundation for evidence-based practice. *The American Journal of Nursing*, 109(11), 49–52. doi:10.1097/01.NAJ.0000363354.53883.58

Melnyk, B., Gallagher-Ford, L., Long, L., & Fineout-Overholt, E. (2014). The establishment of evidence-based practice competencies for practicing registered nurses and advanced practice nurses in real-world clinical settings: Proficiencies to improve healthcare quality, reliability, patient outcomes, and costs. *Worldviews on Evidence Based Nursing*, 11(1), 5–15. doi:10.1111/wvn.12021

MENA Simulation User Network. (n.d.). Retrieved from https://www.linkedin.com/grp/post/6948474-5978389295516368900

Merriam-Webster Dictionary. (2016a). *Anxiety*. Retrieved from https://www.merriam-webster.com/dictionary/anxiety

Merriam-Webster Dictionary. (2016b). *Hologram*. Retrieved from https://www.merriam-webster.com/dictionary/hologram

Merriam-Webster Dictionary. (2016c). *Online dictionary*. Retrieved from http://www.merriam-webster.com/dictionary

Meskó, B. (2014, August). *The guide to the future of medicine: Technology and the human touch*. USA: Webcina Kft.

Meticulous Research. (2015). *Global medical simulation market outlook: 2013–2020—BT-990*. Retrieved from http://www.meticulousresearch.com/

Meurling, L., Hedman, L. Lidefelt, K., Escher, C., Felländer-Tsai, L., & Wallin, C. (2014). Comparison of high- and low equipment fidelity during paediatric simulation team training: A case control study. *BMC Medical Education*, 14, 221–229. doi:10.1186/1472-6920-14-221

Meyer, M. N., Connors, H., Hou, Q., & Gajewski, B. (2011). The effect of simulation on clinical performance: A junior nursing student clinical comparison study. *Simulation in Healthcare*, 6, 269–277. doi:10.1097/SIH.0b013e318223a048

Meyer, S. (Ed.). (2009). The imperative for interprofessional education. *American Journal of Pharmacy Education*, 73(4), 58.

Mezirow, J. (1991). *Transformative dimensions of adult learning*. San Francisco, CA: Jossey-Bass.

Mikasa, A. W., Cicero, T. F., & Adamson, K. A. (2013, September). Outcome-based evaluation tool to evaluate student performance in high-fidelity simulation. *Clinical Simulation in Nursing*, 9(9), e361–e367. http://dx.doi.org/10.1016/j.ecns.2012.06.001

Mileder, L., Urlesberger, B., Szyld, E., Roehr, C., & Schmölzer, G. (2014). Simulation-based neonatal and infant resuscitation teaching: a systematic review of randomized controlled trials. *Klinische Pädiatrie*, 226(5), 259–267. http://doi.org/10.1055/s-0034-1372621

Milesky, J., Baptiste, D., Foronda, C., Dupler, A., & Belcher, A. E. (2015). Promoting a culture of civility in nursing education. *Journal of Nursing Education and Practice*, 5(8), 90–94. doi:10.5430/jnep.v5n8p90

Mill, J., Astle, B.J., Ogilvie, L., & Gastaldo, D. (2010). Linking global citizenship, undergraduate nursing education and professional nursing. Curricular innovation in the 21st century. *Advances in Nursing Science*, 33(3), e1–e11.

Miller, G. E. (1990). The assessment of clinical skills/ competence/ performance. *Academic Medicine*, 6, s63–s67.

Miller, J. E., Leininger, M., Leuning, C., Pacquiao, D. F., Andrews, M., & Ludwig-Beyer, P. (2008). Transcultural nursing society position statement on human rights. *Journal of Transcultural Nursing*, 19(1), 5–8. doi:10.1177/1043659607309147

Miller, K. K., Riley, W., Davis, S., & Hansen, H. E. (2008). In situ simulation: A method of experiential learning to promote safety and team behavior. *The Journal of Perinatal & Neonatal Nursing*, 22(2), 105–113. http://doi.org/10.1097/01.JPN.0000319096.97790.f7

Minister of Public Works and Government Services Canada (PWGSC). (2011). Recent alcohol and drug workplace policies in Canada: Considerations for the nuclear industry. Retrieved from http://publications.gc.ca/pub?id=9.695657&sl=0

Ministry of Health and Human Resources for Health Program, Rwanda. Retrieved from http://www.hrhconsortium.moh.gov.rw/about-rwanda/health-system/

Ministry of Information and Communications Technology, Qatar. (2015). Ministry of transport and communications. Retrieved from http://www.ictqatar.qa/en

Missildine Martin, C., & Calabrese, M. (2011). *Performance appraisals managers will love*. Human Capital Institute. Retrieved from http://www.hci.org/lib/performance-appraisals-managers-will-love

Monachino, A., & Tuttle, S. (2015). Just-in-time training programs. In J. Palaganas, J. Maxworthy, C. Epps & M. Mancini (Eds.), *Defining excellence in simulation programs* (pp.127–134). Philadelphia, PA: Wolters Kluwer.

Montenery, S. M., Jones, A., Perry, N., Ross, D., & Zoucha, R. (2013). Cultural competence in nursing faculty: A journey, not a destination. *Journal of Professional Nursing, 29*(6), e51–e57. http://dx.doi.org/10.1016/j.profnurs.2013.09.003

Montessori, M. (1949). *The absorbent mind.* Madras, India: Theosophical Publishing House.

Moody, R. C., Horton-Deutsch, S., & Pesut, D. J. (2007). Appreciative inquiry for leading in complex systems: Supporting the transformation of academic nursing culture. *Journal of Nursing Education, 46*(7), 319–323. Retrieved from http://www.healio.com/nursing/journals/jne

Moran, C. M. W. (1967). *The anatomy of courage.* Boston, MA: Houghton Mifflin.

Moreno, R., & Mayer, R. E. (2000). A learner-centered approach to multimedia explanations: Deriving instructional design principles from cognitive theory. *Interactive Multimedia Electronic Journal of Computer-Enhanced Learning, 2*(2). Retrieved from http://imej.wfu.edu/articles/2000/2/05/index.asp

Morrison, J., & Deckers, C. (2015). Common theories in healthcare simulation. In J. Palaganas, J. Maxworthy, C. Epps & M. Mancini (Eds.), *Defining excellence in simulation programs.* (pp. 496–508) Philadelphia, PA: Wolters Kluwer.

Morrow, K. J. (2015). Leadership curricula in nursing education: A critical literature review and gap analysis. *Journal of Nursing Education, 54*(7), 367–371. doi:10.3928/01484834-20150617-02

Mortensen, J. (2005). *See-feel-change.* Retrieved from http://www.managementsite.com/483/see-feel-change.aspx

Mould, J., White, H., & Gallagher, R. (2011). Evaluation of a critical care simulation series for undergraduate nursing students. *Contemporary Nurse, 38*(1–2), 180–190. doi:10.5172/conu.2011.38.1-2.180

Moule, P., Wilford, A., Sales, R., Haycock, L., & Lockyer, L. (2006). *Can the use of simulation support pre-registration nursing students in familiarizing themselves with clinical skills before consolidating them in practice.* Bristol, UK: Centre for Learning and Workforce Research.

Mowry, M. J., & Crump, M. D. (2013). Immersion scenarios bridge the education-practice gap for new graduate registered nurses. *The Journal of Continuing Education in Nursing, 44*(7), 319–325. doi:10.3928/00220124-20130515-67

Mueller, G. (1997). A typology of simulators for medical education. *Journal of Digital Imaging, 10*(3 Suppl. 1), 194–196.

Mullan, P. C., Wuestner, E., Kerr, T. D., Christopher, D. P., & Patel, B. (2013). Implementation of an in situ qualitative debriefing tool for resuscitations. *Resuscitation, 84*(7), 946–951. http://doi.org/10.1016/j.resuscitation.2012.12.005

Munshi, F., Lababidi, H., & Alyousef, S. (2015). Low- versus high-fidelity simulations in teaching and assessing clinical skills. *Journal of Taibah University Medical Sciences, 10*(1), 12–15. http://dx.doi.org/10.1016/j.jtumed.2015.01.008

Murdoch, D., Bushell, C., & Johnson, S. (2012). Designing simulations for professional skill development in distance education: A holistic approach for blended learning. In D. Holt, S. Seagrave & J. Cybulski (Eds.), *Professional education using e-simulations: Benefits of blended learning design* (pp. 121–140). Hershey, PA: Business Science Reference.

Murphy, J. I. (2015). The role of research in simulation. In L. Wilson & R. A. Wittman-Price (Eds.), *Review manual for the Certified Healthcare Simulation Educator (CHSE) exam* (pp. 313–424). New York, NY: Springer Publishing Company, LLC.

Murray, S. (2016, August). *EDTECH: augmented reality and cloud computing are powering online learning.* Retrieved from http://www.businessbecause.com/news/mba-distance-learning/4118/ar-cloud-computing-power-online-learning

Myers Briggs Foundation (MBF). (2015). *MBTI basics.* Retrieved from http://www.myersbriggs.org/my-mbti-personality-type/mbti-basics/

Nagle, L. (2014a). An interview with Dr. Judith Shamian. *Nursing Leadership, 27*(1), 26–30. doi:10.12927/cjnl.2014.23761

Nagle, L. M. (2014b). Creativity core to the revolution of education. *Canadian Journal of Nursing Leadership, 27*(2), 1–3.

Nairn, S., Chambers, D., Thompson, S., McGarry, J., & Chambers, K. (2012). Reflexivity and habitus: Opportunities and constraints on transformative learning. *Nursing Philosophy, 13*(3), 189–201. http://dx.doi.org/10.1111/j.1466-769X.2011.00530.x

Najjar, R. H., Lyman, B., & Miehl, N. (2015). Nursing students' experiences with high fidelity simulation. *International Journal of Nursing Education Scholarship, 12*(1), 1–9. doi:10.1515/ijnes-2015-0010

Nance, J. (2008). *Why hospitals should fly: The ultimate flight plan to patient safety and quality care.* Bozeman, MT: Second River Healthcare Press.

Nanji, K. C., Baca, K., & Raemer, D. B. (2013). The effect of an olfactory and visual cue on realism and engagement in a health care simulation experience. *Simulation in Healthcare, 8*(3), 143–147. doi:10.1097/SIH.0b013e31827d27f9

National Academies of Practice. (2015). *Measuring the impact of interprofessional education on collaborative practice and patient outcomes.* Washington, DC: National Academies Press. Retrieved from http://www.nap.edu/catalog.php?record_id=21726

National Health Education and Training in Simulation Program. (2012). *Background.* Retrieved from http://www.nhet-sim.edu.au/nhet-sim-program-3/background/

National League for Nursing (NLN). (2005). *Core competencies of nurse educators with task statements.* Retrieved from http://www.nln.org/profdev/corecompetencies.pdf.

National League for Nursing (NLN). (2005). *Student satisfaction and self-confidence in learning scale.* Retrieved from http://www.nln.org/professional-development-programs/research/tools-and-instruments/descriptions-of-available-instruments

National League for Nursing (NLN). (2015b, April). A vision for teaching with simulation. *NLN Vision Series.* Retrieved from http://www.nln.org/docs/default-source/about/nln-vision-series-(position-statements)/vision-statement-a-vision-for-teaching-with-simulation.pdf?sfvrsn=2

National League for Nursing (NLN). (2015c, September). *Advancing care excellence for veterans (ACE/V) unfolding cases.* Retrieved from http://www.nln.org/professional-development-programs/teaching-resources/veterans-ace-v

National League for Nursing (NLN). (2015d). Debriefing across the curriculum. *NLN Vision Series.* Retrieved from National League for Nursing http://www.nln.org/docs/default-source/about/nln-vision-series-(position-statements)/nln-vision-debriefing-across-the-curriculum.pdf?sfvrsn=0

National League for Nursing (NLN). (2015e). *Leadership development program for simulation educators*. Retrieved from http://www.nln.org/professional-development-programs/leadership-programs/leadership-development-program-for-simulation-educators

National League for Nursing (NLN). (2015f). *vSim for Nursing*. Retrieved from http://www.nln.org/centers-for-nursing-education/nln-center-for-innovation-in-simulation-and-technology/vsim-for-nursing-medical-surgical

National League for Nursing (NLN), Board of Governors. (2005). Position statement: Transforming nursing education. *Nursing Education Perspectives, 26*(3), 195–197.

National League for Nursing Simulation Innovation Resource Center (NLN-SIRC). (2013). *SIRC glossary*. Retrieved from http://sirc.nln.org/mod/glossary/view.php?id=183

National League for Nursing Simulation Innovation Resource Center (SIRC). (2016). *SIRC courses*. Retrieved from http://sirc.nln.org/mod/page/view.php?id=842

Ndiwane, A., Koul, O., & Theroux, R. (2014). Implementing standardized patients to teach cultural competency to graduate nursing students. *Clinical Simulation in Nursing, 10*, e87–e94. doi:http://dx.doi.org/10.1016/j.ecns.2013.07.002

Nehring, W. M. (2008). U.S. Boards of Nursing and the use of high-fidelity patient simulators in nursing education. *Journal of Professional Nursing, 24*, 109–117. doi:10.1016/j.profnurs.2007.06.027

Nehring, W. M. (2010). History of simulation in nursing. In W. M. Nehring & F. R. Lashley (Eds.), *High fidelity patient simulation in nursing education* (pp. 3–26). Sudbury, MA: Jones & Bartlett Publishers.

Nehring, W. M., Ellis, W. E., & Lashley, F. R. (2001). Human patient simulators in nursing education: An overview. *Simulation & Gaming, 32*, 194–204.

Nehring, W. M., & Lashley, F. R. (2004). Current use and opinions regarding human patient simulators in nursing education: An international survey. *Nursing Education Perspectives, 25*, 244–248.

Nehring, W. M., & Lashley, F. R. (2009). Nursing simulation: A review of the past 40 years. *Simulation and Gaming, 40*, 528–552. doi:10.1177/10468781093332282

Nehring, W. M., & Lashley, F. R. (Eds.), (2010). *High-fidelity patient simulation in nursing education*. Boston, MA: Jones and Bartlett.

Nehring, W. M., Wexler, T., Hughes, F., & Greenwell, A. (2013). Faculty development for the use of high-fidelity patient simulation: A systematic review. *International Journal of Health Sciences Education, 1*(1), 4. Retrieved from http://dc.etsu.edu/ijhse/vol1/iss1/4

Neilipovitz, D. (2005). *Acute critical events simulation (ACES): Course syllabus*. Ottawa, CA University of Ottawa Press. Available at https://books.google.com/books?id=W32U3z50IHQC&pgis=1

Neill, M. A., & Wotton, K. (2011). High-fidelity simulation debriefing in nursing education: A literature review. *Clinical Simulation in Nursing, 7*(5), e161–e168. doi:10.1016/j.ecns.2011.02.001

Nelson, R. (2013). *The design and planning of multidisciplinary simulation centers*. Minneapolis, MN: HGA Architects and Engineers.

Nelson, S. (2012). The lost path to emancipatory practice: Towards a history of reflective practice in nursing. *Nursing Philosophy, 13*, 202–221. doi:10.1111/j.1466-769X.2011.00535.x

Nestel, D., & Bearman, M. (2014a). Introduction to simulated patient methodology. In D. Nestel & M. Bearman (Eds.), *Simulated patient methodology: Theory, evidence, and practice* (pp. 1–5). Malden, MA: Wiley Blackwell.

Nestel, D., & Bearman, M. (Eds.), (2014b). *Simulated patient methodology: Theory, evidence and practice*. Wiley-Blackwell.

Nestel, D., & Kelly, M. (2017). Strategies for research in healthcare simulation. In D. Nestel, M. Kelly, B. Jolly & M. Watson (Eds.), *Healthcare simulation education: Evidence, theory and practice* (Chapter 6). West Sussex, UK: John Wiley & Sons.

Nestel, D., Mobley, B. L., Hunt, E. A., & Eppich, W. J. (2014). Confederates in health care simulations: Not as simple as it seems. *Clinical Simulation in Nursing, 10*(12), 611–616. doi:http://dx.doi.org/10.1016/j.ecns.2014.09.007

Nestel, D., Watson, M., Marshall, S. D., & Bearman, M. (2014). *A national research agenda for healthcare simulation: Preliminary report*. Paper presented at SimHealth, Adelaide, Australia.

New Zealand Ministry of Health. (2015). *Health workforce*. Retrieved from http://www.health.govt.nz/our-work/health-workforce

Newman, O. (1972). *Defensible space: Crime prevention through urban design*. New York, NY: Macmillan.

Ng, C. (2015). Evidence-based education in radiography. In T. Brown & B. Williams (Eds.), *Evidence-based education in the health professions: Promoting best practice in the learning and teaching of students* (pp. 448–468). London, UK: Radcliffe Publishing Ltd.

Nguyen, D. N., Zierler, B., & Nguyen, H. (2011). A survey of nursing faculty needs for training in use of new technologies for education and practice. *Journal of Nursing Education, 50*(4), 181–189. doi:10.3928/01484834-20101130-06

Nicely, S., & Farra, S. (2015). Fostering learning through interprofessional virtual reality simulation development. *Nursing Education Perspectives, 36*(5), 335–336. doi:10.5480/13-1240

Nickel, S., Gesse, T., & MacLaren, A. (1992). Ernestine Wiedenbach: Her professional legacy. *Journal of Nurse-Midwifery, 37*(3), 161–167.

Nightingale, F. (1860). *Notes on nursing; what is, and what it is not*. New York, NY: Appleton & Company.

Nishisaki, A., Hales, R., Biagas, K., Cheifetz, I., Corriveau, C., Garber, N., … Morrison, W. (2009). A multi-institutional high-fidelity simulation "boot camp" orientation and training program for first year pediatric critical care fellows. *Pediatric Critical Care Medicine, 10*(2), 157–162. doi:10.1097/PCC.0b013e3181956d29

Norman, G., Dore, K., & Grierson, L. (2012). The minimal relationship between simulation fidelity and transfer of learning. *Medical Education, 46*(7), 636–647. doi:10.1111/j.1365-2923.2012.04243.x

Norman, J., Thompson, S., & Missildine, K. (2013). The 2-minute drills: Incorporating simulation into a large lecture format. *Clinical Simulation in Nursing, 9*(10), e433–e436. doi:10.1016/j.ecns.2012.08.004

Norman, L., Buerhaus, P., Donelan, K., McCloskey, B., & Dittus, R. (2005). Nursing students assess nursing education. *Journal of Professional Nursing, 21*(3), 150–158. http://dx.doi.org/10.1016/j.profnurs.2005.04.003

Nursing and Midwifery Board of Australia. (2017). *Registration standards*. Retrieved from http://www.nursingmidwifery-board.gov.au/Registration-Standards.aspx

Nursing and Midwifery Council (NMC). (2005). *NMC Circular 31/2005*. London: Author.

Nursing and Midwifery Council (NMC). (2006a, July). *NMC announce simulation and practice learning project*. London: Author 2006.

Nursing and Midwifery Council (NMC). (2006b). *NMC letter 17/03/2006*. London: Author.

Nursing and Midwifery Council (NMC). (2007). *Supporting direct care through simulated practice learning in the pre-registration nursing programmes*. NMC Circular 36/2007. London: NMC.

Nursing and Midwifery Council (NMC). (2008). *A review of pre-registration nursing education: Focus group report*. London: Author.

Nursing Council of New Zealand. (2005). *Guidelines for cultural safety, the Treaty of Waitanga and Maori health in nursing, midwifery, education and practice. Whanau Kawa Whakaruruhau*. Wellington, New Zealand: Author.

Nursing Council of New Zealand. (2008). *Code of conduct for nurses*. Wellington, New Zealand. Retrieved from http://www.nursingcouncil.org.nz/code%20of%20conduct%20March%202008.pdf

Nursing Management. (2011). *Delegation as a management function*. Retrieved from http://currentnursing.com/nursing_management/delegation.html

Nuzhat, A., Salem, R. O., Al Shehri, F. N., & Al Hamdan, N. (2014). Role and challenges of simulation in undergraduate curriculum. *Medical Teacher, 36*, S69–S73. doi:10.3109/0142159X.2014.886017

O'Donnell, J. F. (2014). The hidden curriculum—A focus on learning and closing the gap. In F. E. Hafferty & J. F. O'Donnell (Eds.), *The hidden curriculum in health professional education* (pp. 1–20). Hanover, NH: Dartmouth College Press.

O'Donnell, J. M., Decker, S., Howard, V., Levett-Jones, T., & Miller, C. W. (2014). NLN/Jeffries simulation framework state of the science project: Simulation learning outcomes. *Clinical Simulation in Nursing, 10*(7), 373–382. doi:10.1016/j.ecns.2014.06.004

O'Donnell, J. M., Goode, J. S., Jr., Henker, R., Kelsey, S. L., Bircher, N. G., Peele, P., ... Sutton-Tyrell, K. (2011). Effect of a simulation educational intervention on knowledge, attitude, and patient transfer skills: From the simulation laboratory to the clinical setting. *Simulation in Healthcare, 6*(2), 84–93. doi:10.1097/SIH.0b013e318212f1ef

Oermann, M. H. (Ed.). (2017). *A systematic approach to assessment and evaluation of nursing programs*. The National League for Nursing. Philadelphia, PA: Wolters Kluwer, Inc.

Oermann, M. H., Kardong-Edgren, S. E., & Odom-Maryon, T. (2011). Effects of monthly practice on nursing students' CPR psychomotor skill performance. *Resuscitation, 82*(4), 447–453. doi:10.1016/j.resuscitation.2010.11.022

Oermann, M. H., Yarbrough, S. S., Saewert, K. J., Ard, N., & Charasika, M. (2009). Clinical evaluation and grading practices in schools of nursing: National survey findings. Part II. *Nursing Education Perspectives, 30*, 352–357.

O'Grady, P. (2014). Leading the revolution in nursing practice: Advancing healthcare in the digital age. *Canadian Journal of Nursing Leadership, 27*(2), 14–19.

Oh, P. -J., Jeon, K. D., & Koh, M. S. (2015). The effects of simulation-based learning using standardized patients in nursing students: A meta-analysis. *Nurse Education Today*, 1–10. http://doi.org/10.1016/j.nedt.2015.01.019

Okuda, Y., Bryson, E. O., DeMaria, S., Jr., Jacobson, L., Quinones, J., Shen, B., & Levine, A. I. (2009). The utility of simulation in medical education: What is the evidence? *Mount Sinai Journal of Medicine: A Journal of Translational and Personalized Medicine, 76*(4), 330–343. http://doi.org/10.1002/msj.20127

O'Leary K, Ritter C, Wheeler H, Szekendi M, Brinton T, & Williams M. (2010). Teamwork on inpatient medical units: Assessing attitudes and barriers. *BMJ Quality & Safety, 19*(2), 117–121. doi:10.1136/qshc.2008.028795

Oldenburg, N. L., Maney, C., & Plonczynski, D. J. (2013). Traditional clinical versus simulation in 1st semester clinical students: Students perceptions after a 2nd semester clinical rotation. *Clinical Simulation in Nursing, 9*, 235–241. http://dx.doi.org/10.1016/j.ecns.2012.03.006

Onda, E. L. (2012, September). Situated cognition: Its relationship to simulation in nursing education. *Clinical Simulation in Nursing, 8*(7), e273–e280. doi:http://dx.doi.org/10.1016/j.ecns.2010.11.004

Onello, R., & Regan, M. (2013). Challenges in high fidelity simulation: Risk sensitization and outcome measurement. *OJIN: The Online Journal of Issues in Nursing, 19*(3), 1–8. doi:10.3012/OJIN.Vol18No03PPT01

Onello, R., Rudolph, J. W., & Simon, R. (2015). *Feedback for Clinical Education (FACE)—Rater Version*. Boston, MA: Center for Medical Simulation. https://harvardmedsim.org/_media/FACE.RV.RatingForm.pdf

Orchard, C., Curran, V., & Kabene, S. (2005). Creating a culture for interdisciplinary collaborative professional practice. *Medical Education Online, 10*(11), 1–13. http://dx.doi.org/10.3402/meo.v10i.4387

Oren, T., Elzas, M., Smit, I., & Birta, L. (2002). Code of professional ethics for simulationists. Proceedings of the Summer Computer Simulation Conference. San Diego, CA.

Orr, F., Kellehear, K., Armari, E., Pearson, A., & Holmers, D. (2013). The distress of voice-hearing: The use of simulation for awareness, understanding and communication skill development in undergraduate nursing education. *Nurse Education in Practice, 13*(6), 529–535. doi:10.1016/j.nepr.2013.03.023

Orriss, M. (2004). *The Karpman Drama Triangle*. Coaching Supervision Academy. Retrieved from http://coachingsupervisionacademy.com/thought-leadership/the-karpman-drama-triangle/

Orsini, M. (2015, April 9). What is the difference between expatriates and immigrants? Blog response. Retrieved from https://www.quora.com/What-is-the-difference-between-expatriates-and-immigrants

Ossowski, Y. (2015, March). The difference between expats and immigrants? It's passports, not race. *The PanAm Post: News and analysis of the Americas*. Retrieved from https://panampost.com/yael-ossowski/2015/03/26/the-difference-between-expats-and-immigrants-its-passports-not-race

Owens, R., & Taekman, J. M. (2013). Virtual reality, haptic simulators, and virtual environments. In A. I. Levine, S. DeMaria Jr., A. D. Schwartz & A. J. Sim (Eds.), *The comprehensive textbook of healthcare simulation* (pp. 223–253). New York, NY: Spring Science + Business.

Owens, T. L., & Gilva-McCovey, G. (2015). Standardized patients. In J. C. Palaganas, J.C. Maxworthy, C.A. Epps & M.E. Mancini (Eds.), *Defining excellence in simulation programs*, (pp. 199–212). Philadelphia, PA: Wolters Kluwer.

Ozkara San, E. (2015). Using clinical simulation to enhance culturally competent nursing care: A review of the literature. *Clinical Simulation in Nursing*, 11(4), 228–243. http://dx.doi.org/10.1016/j.ecns.2015.01.004

Page, D. (2010). IT's return on investments is tricky to pin down. *Hospital and Health Networks*, 84(6), 38.

Paige, J. B., & Daley, B. J. (2009). Situated cognition: A learning framework to support and guide high-fidelity simulation. *Clinical Simulation in Nursing*, 5(3). http://dx.doi.org/10.1016/j.ecns.2009.03.120

Palaganas, J. C., Epps, C., & Raemer, D. B. (2014). A history of simulation-enhanced interprofessional education. *Journal of Interprofessional Care*, 28(2), 110–115. doi:10.3109/13561820.2013.869198

Palaganas, J. C., Maxworthy, J. C., Epps, C. A., & Mancini, M. E. (Eds.), (2015). *Defining excellence in simulation programs*. Philadelphia, PA: Wolters Kluwer.

Palethorpe, R. J., & Wilson, J. P. (2011). Learning in the panic zone: Strategies for managing learner anxiety. *Journal of European Industrial Training*, 35(5), 420–438. doi 10.1108/03090591111138008

Paley, J. (2007). Complex adaptive systems and nursing. *Nursing Inquiry*, 14(3), 233–242. doi:10.1111/j.1440-1800.2007.00359.x

Palmer, P. J. (2007). A new professional: The aims of education revisited. *Change*, 39, 6–12. http://dx.doi.org/10.3200/CHNG.39.6.6-13

Palmer, R. (2014). *The TeleOSCE: Providing simulated telemedicine training for medical students*. Retrieved from http://www.ortelehealth.org/content/teleosce-providing-simulated-telemedicine-training-medical-students

Parker, B., & Myrick, F. (2010). Transformative learning as a context for human patient simulation. *Journal of Nursing Education*, 49(6), 326–332. doi:10.3928/01484834-20100224-02

Parker, B. C., & Myrick, F. (2009). A critical examination of high-fidelity human patient simulation within the context of nursing pedagogy. *Nurse Education Today*, 29(3), 322–329. doi:10.1016/j.nedt.2008.10.012

Parker, B. C., & Myrick, F. (2012). The pedagogical ebb and flow of human patient simulation: Empowering through a process of fading support. *Journal of Nursing Education*, 51(7), 365–372. doi:10.3928/01484834-20120509-01

Parsh, B. (2010). Characteristics of effective simulation clinical experience instructors: Interviews with undergraduate nursing students. *Journal of Nursing Education*, 49(10), 569–572. doi:10.3928/01484834-20100730-04

Paskins, Z., & Peile, E. (2010). Final year medical students' views on simulation based teaching: A comparison with the best evidence medical education systematic review. *Medical Teacher*, 32(7), 569–577. doi:10.3109/01421590903544710

Pastor, D. K., Cunningham, R. P., & Kuiper, R. A. (2015, February). Gray matters: Teaching geriatric assessment for family nurse practitioners using standardized patients. *Clinical Simulation in Nursing*, 11(2), 120–125. doi:http://dx.doi.org/10.1016/j.ecns.2014.09.002

Patankar, M. S., Brown, J. P., Sabin, E. J., & Bigda-Peyton, T. G. (2012). *Safety culture: Building and sustaining a cultural change in aviation and healthcare*. Aldershot, UK: Ashgate Publishing.

Patel, A. (2016). Finding the fit: What the simulation operations specialist has to offer and what the employer needs. In L. T. Gantt & H. M. Young (Eds.), *Healthcare simulation: A guide for operations specialists* (1st ed., pp. 78–90). Hoboken, NJ: Wiley.

Patterson, M. D., Blike, G. T., & Nadkarni, V. M. (2008). In situ simulation: Challenges and results. In K. Henriksen, J. B. Battles, M. A. Keyes & M. L. Grady (Eds.), *Advances in patient safety: New directions and alternative approaches* (Vol. 3: Performance and Tools). Rockville, MD: Agency for Healthcare Research and Quality (US). Retrieved from http://www.ncbi.nlm.nih.gov/books/NBK43682

Patterson, M. D., Geis, G. L., Falcone, R. A., LeMaster, T., & Wears, R. L. (2012). In situ simulation: Detection of safety threats and teamwork training in a high risk emergency department. *BMJ Quality & Safety*, 22(6), 468–477. doi:10.1136/bmjqs-2012-000942

Patterson, N., & Hulton, L. J. (2012). Enhancing nursing students' understanding of poverty through simulation. *Public Health Nursing*, 29(special edition), 143–151. doi:10.1111/j.1525-1446.2011.00999.x

Pattillo, R. E., Hewett, B., McCarthy, M. D., & Molinari, D. (2010). Capacity building for simulation sustainability. *Clinical Simulation in Nursing*, 6(5), e185–e191. doi:10.1016/j.ecns.2009.08.008

Paul, R., & Elder, L. (1997). *Foundation for critical thinking*. Retrieved from www.criticalthinking.org

Pelletier, K. L. (2011). Leader toxicity: An empirical investigation of toxic behaviour and rhetoric. *Leadership*, 6(4), 373–389. doi:10.1177/1742715010379308

Penn, H. (2014). Recognizing cultural safety issues for indigenous students in a baccalaureate nursing programme: Two unique programmes. *Whitireia Nursing and Health Journal*, 21, 29–33.

Perera, J., Perera, J., Abdullah, J., & Lee, N. (2009). Training simulated patients: Evaluation of a training approach using self-assessment and peer/tutor feedback to improve performance. *BMC Medical Education*, 9(37). doi:10.1186/1472-6920-9-37

Piaget, J. (1953). *To understand is to invent*. New York, NY: Grossman [French: Ou va l'education?, 1948].

Piaget, J. (1962). *Play, dreams and imitation*. New York, NY: Norton.

Piaget, J. (1972). Intellectual evolution from adolescence to adulthood. *Human Development*, 15, 1–12. doi:10.1159/000271225.

Plane Crash Information. (2015). *Accident history*. Retrieved from http://www.planecrashinfo.com/accidents.htm

Pocnet, C., Antonietti, J-P, Massoudi, K., Györkös, C., Becker, J., de Bruin, G. P., & Rossier, J. (2015). Influence of individual characteristics on work engagement and job stress in a sample of national and foreign workers in Switzerland. *Swiss Journal of Psychology*, 74(1), 17–27. http://dx.doi.org/10.1024/1421-0185/a000146

Polifroni, E. C., Packard, S. A., Shah, H. S., & MacAvoy, S. (1995). Activities and interactions of baccalaureate nursing students in clinical practica. *Journal of Professional Nursing*, 11(3), 161–169.

Polit, D. F., & Beck, C. T. (2012). *Nursing research: Generating and assessing evidence for nursing practice* (9th ed.). Philadelphia, PA: Wolters Kluwer Health/Lippincott Williams & Wilkins.

Pollard, C. L., & Wild, C. (2014). Nursing leadership competencies: Low fidelity simulation as a teaching strategy. *Nursing Education in Practice, 14*(6), 620–626. http://dx.doi.org/10.1016/j.nepr.2014.06.006

Pollard, K. C., Miers, M. E., & Gilchrist, M. (2004). Collaborative learning for collaborative working? Initial findings from a longitudinal study of health and social care students. *Health and Social Care in the Community, 12*(4), 346–358. doi:10.1111/j.1365-2524.2004.00504.x

Porter-O'Grady, T., & Malloch, K. (2003). *Quantum leadership: A textbook of new leadership.* Mississauga, ON: Jones and Bartlett.

Potter, J. Gatward, J. Kelly, M. McKay, L. McCann, E. Elliott, R. Perry, L. (2017). Simulation-based communication skills training for experienced clinicians to improve family conversations about organ and tissue donation. Unpublished manuscript.

Poulakou-Rebelakou, E., Karamanou, M., Rempelakos, A., & Androutsos, G. (2012). Depiction of venereal diseases on wax models in the Moulage museums of Paris and Athens. *European Urology Supplements, 11*(1), e829. doi:10.1016/S1569-9056(12)60826-4

Powell, D. L., Gilliss, C. L., Hewitt, H. H., & Flint, E. P. (2010). Application of a partnership model for transformative and sustainable international development. *Public Health Nursing, 27*(1), 54–70. doi:10.1111/j.1525-1446.2009.00827.x

Powers, B. A., & Knapp, T. R. (2011). *Dictionary of nursing theory and research* (4th ed.). New York, NY: Springer Publishing Company, LLC.

Prensky, M. (2001). Digital natives, digital immigrants. *On the Horizon, 9*(5), 1–6. http://dx.doi.org/10.1108/10748120110424816

Prensky, M. (2005a, September/October). Engage me or enrage me. *EDUCAUSE review.* Retrieved from http://net.educause.edu/ir/library/pdf/erm0553.pdf

Prensky, M. (2005b). Listen to the natives. *Educational Leadership, 63*(4), 8–13.

Prensky, M. (2007). Changing paradigms: From "being taught" to "learning on your own with guidance". *Educational Technology.* Retrieved from http://www.marcprensky.com/writing/Prensky-ChangingParadigms-01-EdTech.pdf

Prensky, M. (2011, November–December). A huge leap for the classroom true peer-to-peer learning, enhanced by technology. *Educational Technology.* Retrieved from http://marcprensky.com/writing/Prensky-EDTECHLearning Catalytics-Nov-Dec-2011-FINAL.pdf

Prensky, M. (2013a). Future-oriented education: A new way to describe our goal. *Educational Technology.* Retrieved from http://marcprensky.com/wp-content/uploads/2013/05/Prensky-3-Futureoriented_Education.pdf

Prensky, M. (2013b). Our brains extended. *Technology-Rich Learning, 70*(6), 22–27.

Prensky, M. (2013c). Time-travel as punishment: What our kids REALLY hate. *Educational Technology.* Retrieved from http://marcprensky.com/writing/Prensky-Time_Travel_as_Punishment-EDTECH-Jan-Feb%202013-FINAL.pdf

Prensky, M. (2014). *Accomplishment-based education not content or skills. Not artificial problem-solving. Education should be about students improving the real-world—NOW.* Retrieved from http://marcprensky.com/wp-content/uploads/2013/05/Prensky-4-Accomplishment-Based-_Education.pdf

Prensky, M. (2015, January–February). Innovating with future technologies keeping our kids ahead of the tech curve. *Educational Technology.* Retrieved from http://marcprensky.com/wp-content/uploads/2016/12/Prensky-Innovating_with_Future_Technologies-EDTEC-Jan-Feb-15.pdf

Prensky, M. R. (2010). *Teaching digital natives: Partnering for real learning.* Thousand Oaks, CA: Corwin Press.

Prion, S., & Adamson, K. (2012). Making sense of methods and measurement: The need for rigor in simulation research. *Clinical Simulation in Nursing, 8*(5), e193. doi:http://dx.doi.org/10.1016/j.ecns.2013.05.003

Pronovost, P. & Vohr, E. (2010). *Safe patients, smart hospitals.* New York, NY: Hudson Street Press.

Prosci Solutions, Inc. (2016). *Executive sponsor's importance and role.* Retrieved from https://www.prosci.com/change-management/thought-leadership-library/importance-and-role-of-executive-sponsor

Prus, J. S., & Strein, W. (2011). Issues and trends in the accreditation of school psychology programs in the United States. *Psychology in the Schools, 48*(9), 887–900. doi:10.1002/pits.20600

Purnell, L. (2005). The Purnell model for cultural competence. *Journal of Multicultural Nursing and Health, 11*(2). Retrieved from https://www.researchgate.net/profile/Larry_Purnell/publication/11265758_The_Purnell_Model_for_Cultural_Competence/links/00b495330173a7096d000000.pdf

Pyburn, R., & Bauman, E. (2013). Striving for cultural competency by leveraging virtual reality and game-based learning. In E. Bauman (Ed.), *Game-based teaching and simulation in nursing and healthcare* (pp. 147–176). New York, NY: Springer Publishing Company.

Qatar Culture and Traditions. (2015). Retrieved from http://qatarcultureandtraditions.blogspot.com/

Qatar Foundation. (2015). *Qatarization.* Retrieved from http://www.qf.org.qa/content/about/jobs/qatarization

Qatar National Health Strategy. (2015). Retrieved from http://www.nhsq.info

Qayumi, A. K. (2010). Centre of excellence for simulation and innovation (CESEI). *Journal of Surgical Education, 67*(4), 265–269. doi:10.1016/m.jsurg.2010.05.015

Qayumi, K., Donn, S., Zheng, B., Young, L., Dutton, J., Adamack, M., ... Cheng, A. (2012). British Columbia interprofessional model for simulation-based education in health care. *Simulation in Healthcare, 7*(5), 295–307. http://doi.org/10.1097/SIH.0b013e31825e8daa

Quality and Safety Education for Nurses (QSEN). (2014). *Competencies.* Retrieved from http://qsen.org/competencies/

Racine, L. (2014). The enduring challenge of cultural safety. *Canadian Journal of Nursing Research, 46*(2), 6–9. Retrieved from http://cjnr.archive.mcgill.ca/article/view/2445

Raemer, D. (2008). Society for simulation in healthcare. In R. Riley (Ed.), *A manual of simulation in healthcare* (pp. 529–532). Oxford, NY: Oxford University Press.

Raemer, D., Anderson, M., Cheng, A., Fanning, R., Nadkarni, V., & Savoldelli, G. (2011). Research regarding debriefing as part of the learning process. *Simulation in Healthcare, 6*(Suppl.), S52–S57. doi:10.1097/SIH.0b013e31822724d0

Raffo, D. M. (2014). Reflection and authentic leadership. In K. G. Schuyler, J. E. Baugher, K. Jironet & L. Lid-Falkman (Eds.), *Leading with spirit, presence, and authenticity* (pp. 179–195). San Francisco, CA: Jossey-Bass.

Rall, M., & Dieckmann, P. (2005). Crisis resource management to improve patient safety. *European Society of Anaesthesiology*. Retrieved from https://www.guysandstthomas.nhs.uk/resources/education-training/sail/reading/crisis-mgt-pt-safety.pdf

Ramazani, J., & Jergeas, G. (2015). Project managers and the journey from good to great: The benefits of investment in project management training and education. *International Journal of Project Management, 33*(1), 41–52. doi:10.1016/j.ijproman.2014.03.012

Rampersad, H. K., & El-Homsi, A. (2007). *TPS-lean six sigma: Linking human capital to lean six sigma: A new blueprint for creating high performance companies* (eBook). Charlotte, NC: Information Age Publishing.

Ramponi, D. R., & Ross, C. A. (2015). Preparing nurse practitioner students for international experiences using skills acquisition. *Clinical Simulation in Nursing, 11*(10), 458–461. doi:10.1016/j.ecns.2015.08.005

Raurell-Toredà, M., Olivet-Pujol, J., Romero-Collado, À., Malagon-Aquilera, M. C., Patino-Masó, J., & Baltasar-Bagué, A. (2015). Case-based learning and simulation: Useful tools to enhance nurses' education? Nonrandomized controlled trail. *Journal of Nursing Scholarship, 47*(1), 34–42. doi:10.1111/jnu.12113

Ravert, P., & McAfooes, J. (2014). NLN/Jeffries simulation framework: State of the science summary. *Clinical Simulation in Nursing, 10*(7), 335–336. doi:10.1016/j.ecns.2013.06.002

Reason, J. T. (1990). *Human error.* Cambridge, UK: Cambridge University Press.

Reason, J. T. (2000). Human error: Models and management. *British Medical Journal, 320*(7237), 768–770.

Reed, S. J. (2012). Debriefing experience scale: Development of a tool to evaluate the student learning experience in debriefing. *Clinical Simulation in Nursing, 8*(6), e211–e217. doi:10.1016/j.ecns.2011.11.002

Reedy, G. B. (2015). Using cognitive load theory to inform simulation design and practice. *Clinical Simulation in Nursing, 11*(8), 355–360. http://dx.doi.org/10.1016/j.ecns.2015.05.004

Reeves, S. (2016). Why we need interprofessional education to improve the delivery of safe and effective care. *Interface—Comunicação, Saúde, Educação, 20*(56), 185–197. http://doi.org/10.1590/1807-57622014.0092

Reeves, S., Boet, S., Zierler, B., & Kitto, S. (2015). Interprofessional education and practice guide no. 3: Evaluating interprofessional education. *Journal of Interprofessional Care, 29*(4), 305–312. doi:10.3109/13561820.2014

Reeves, S., Kitto, S., Alexanian, J., & Grant, R. (2016). *EIC-ICU toolkit. Enhancing interprofessional collaboration in the intensive care unit.* Gordon and Betty Moore Foundation. doi:10.13140/RG.2.1.1682.2800

Reeves, S., Lewin, S. Espin, S., & Zwarenstein, M. (2010). *Interprofessional teamwork for health and social care.* Oxford, UK: Wiley-Blackwell: Blackwell Publishing.

Reeves, S., & Pryce, A. (1998, October). Emerging themes: An exploratory research project of an interprofessional education module for medical, dental and nursing students. *Nurse Education Today, 18*(7), 534–541. doi:http://dx.doi.org/10.1016/S0260-6917(98)80003-8

Reeves, S., Tassone, M., Parker, K., Wagner, S., & Simmons, B. (2012). Interprofessional education: An overview of key developments in the past three decades. *Work, 41*(3), 233–245. doi:10.3233/WOR-2012-1298

Reeves, S., Zwarenstein, M., & Goldman, J. (2009). Interprofessional collaboration: Effects of practice-based interventions on professional practice and healthcare outcomes. *Cochrane Database of Systematic Reviews,* (3), CD000072. Retrieved from http://ipls.dk/pdf-filer/ip_collaboration_cochrane.pdf

Registered Nurses' Association of Ontario (RNAO). (2007). *Embracing cultural diversity in health care: Developing cultural competence.* Toronto, ON: Registered Nurses' Association of Ontario.

Registered Nurses' Association of Ontario (RNAO). (2012). *Managing and mitigating conflict in health-care teams.* Toronto, ON: Registered Nurses' Association of Ontario.

Registered Nurses' Association of Ontario (RNAO). (2013). *Developing and sustaining nursing leadership best practice guideline* (2nd ed.). Retrieved from http://rnao.ca/sites/rnao-ca/files/LeadershipBPG_Booklet_Web_1.pdf

Reid-Searl, K., Levett-Jones, T., Cooper, S., & Happell, B. (2014). The implementation of Mask-Ed: Reflections of academic participants. *Nurse Education in Practice, 14*(5), 485–490. doi:10.1016/j.nepr.2014.05.008

Reimer-Kirkham, S., & Brown, A. (2006). Toward a critical theoretical interpretation of social justice discourses in nursing. *Advances in Nursing Science, 29*, 324–339.

Rew, L., Becker, H., Cookston, J., Khosropour, S., & Martinez, S. (2003). Measuring cultural awareness in nursing students. *Journal of Nursing Education, 42*(6), 249–257.

Richardson, H., Goldsamt, L. A., Simmons, J., Gilmartin, M., & Jeffries, P. R. (2014). Increasing faculty capacity: Findings from an evaluation of simulation clinical teaching. *Nursing Education Perspectives, 35*(5), 308–314.

Richerson, P. J., & Christiansen, M. H. (Eds.), (2013). *Cultural evolution: Society, technology, language, and religion. Strüngmann Forum Reports, 12.* Cambridge, MA: MIT Press.

Ridenour, N., & Trautman, D. (2009). A primer for nurses on advancing health reform policy. *Journal of Professional Nursing, 25*(6), 358–362. doi:10.1016/j.profnurs.2009.10.003

Rideout, E. (2001). *Transforming nursing education through problem-based learning.* Sudbury, MA: Jones and Bartlett Publishers.

Ridley, B. (2013, April). *Virtual imaging for the medical industry.* Retrieved from https://www.mdtmag.com/article/2013/04/virtual-imaging-medical-industry

Ried, J. (1996). *A telemedicine primer: Understanding the issues.* Billings, MT: Innovative Medical Communication.

Rieteg, V., & Squires, A. (2015). *Building skills in North and Central America: Barriers and policy options toward harmonizing qualifications in nursing.* Washington, DC: Migration Policy Institute.

Riggio R. E., Chaleff, I., & Lipman-Blumen, J. (Eds.), (2008). *The art of followership: How great followers create great leaders and organizations.* San Francisco, CA: Jossey-Bass.

Riley, R., Grauze, A., Trewhella, N., Chinnery, C., & Horley, R. (2003). Three years of "CASMS": The world's busiest medical simulation centre. *Medical Journal of Australia, 179*(11), 626–630.

Ritala, P., & Huizingh, E. (2014). Business and network models for innovation: Strategic logic and the role of network position. *International Journal of Technology Management, 66*(2–3), 109–119. doi:10.1504/IJTM.2014.064608

Rizzolo, M. A., Durham, C., Ravert, P., & Jeffries, P. R. (2016). History and evolution of the NLN Jeffries theory. In P. R. Jeffries (Ed.), *The NLN Jeffries simulation theory*. Washington, DC: National League for Nursing.

Rizzolo, M. A., Kardong-Edgren, S. E., Oermann, M. H., & Jeffries, P. R. (2015). The National League for Nursing project to explore the use of simulation for high-stakes assessment: Process, outcomes, and recommendations. *Nursing Education Perspectives*, 36(5), 299–303. doi:10.5480/15-1639

Robert, H. M., Honemann, D. H., & Balch, T. J. (2011). *Robert's rules of order newly revised* (11th ed., p. 489). Philadelphia, PA: Da Capo Press.

Robert Wood Johnson Foundation. (2010, January 20). *Nursing leadership from bedside to boardroom: Opinion leaders' perception. Top line report.* Retrieved from http://www.gallup.com/poll/112264/Nurses-Shine-While-Bankers-Slump-Ethics-Ratings.aspx

Roberts, S. G., Warda, M., Garbutt, S., & Curry, K. (2014). The use of high-fidelity simulation to teach cultural competence in the nursing curriculum. *Journal of Professional Nursing*, 30(3), 259–265. doi:10.1016/j.profnurs.2013.09.012

Robinson, R., Molenda, M., & Rezabek, L. (2008). Facilitating learning. In A. Januszewski & M. Molenda (Eds.), *Educational technology: A definition with commentary*. New York, NY: Lawrence Erlbaum Associates.

Robinson, Sir K. (2011). *Out of our minds: Learning to be creative*. West Sussex, UK: Capstone Publishing.

Rochester, S., Kelly, M. A., Disler, R., White, H., Forber, J., & Matiuk, S. (2012). Providing simulation experiences for large cohorts of 1st year nursing students: Evaluating quality and impact. *Collegian*, 19(3), 117–124. doi:10.1016/j.colegn.2012.05.004

Rockstrom, J., Steffen, W., Noone, K., Persson, A., Chapin, F. S., Lambin, E. F., ..., Foley, J. A. (2009). *A safe operating space for humanity. Nature*, 461(7263), 472–475. http://doi.org/10.1038/461472a

Rogers, D. A., Peterson, D. T., Ponce, B. A., White, M. L., & Porterfield Jr J. R. (2015). Simulation and faculty development. *Surgical Clinics of North America*, 95(4), 729–737. http://dx.doi.org/10.1016/j.suc.2015.03.004

Rogers, E. M. (2003). *Diffusion of innovations* (5th ed.). New York, NY: Simon & Shuster.

Rogers, L., Miller, C., & Firmin, S. (2012). Evaluating the impact of a virtual emergency room simulation for learning. In D. Holt, S. Segrave & J. Cybulski (Eds.), *Professional education using E-simulations: Benefits of blended learning design* (pp. 100–120). Hershey, PA: Business Science Reference. doi:10.4018/978-1-61350-189-4.ch007

Roman, J. (2009). *Bigger than blockbusters: Movies that defined America*. Santa Barbara, CA: Greenwood Publisher.

Rooney, D., Hopwood, N., Boud, D., & Kelly, M. (2015). The role of simulation in pedagogies of higher education for the health professions: Through a practice-based lens. *Vocations and Learning*, 8(3), 269–285. doi:10.1007/s12186-015-9138-z

Rooney, D. M., Covington, B. J., Dionise, P. L., Nykamp, M. T., Pederson, M., Sahloul, J. M., . . . Cooke, J. (2017). What simulator is best? The creation and evaluation of the Simulator Value Index Tool. Unpublished manuscript.

Rosen, K. (2008). The history of medical simulation. *Journal of Critical Care*, 23, 157–166. doi:http://dx.doi.org/10.1016/j.jcrc.2007.12.004

Rosen, K. (2013a). Pioneers and profiles. In A. I. Levine, S. DeMaria Jr., A. D. Schwartz & A. J. Sim (Eds.), *The comprehensive textbook of healthcare simulation*. New York, NY: Springer Science + Business Media.

Rosen, K. R. (2013b). The history of simulation. In A. Levine, S. DeMaria, A. Schwartz & A. Sim (Eds.), *The comprehensive textbook of healthcare simulation* (pp. 1–49). New York, NY: Springer.

Rosen, M., Salas, E., Silvestri, S., Wu, T., & Lazzara, E. (2008). A measurement tool for simulation-based training in emergency medicine: The simulation module for assessment of resident targeted event responses (SMARTER) approach. *Simulation in Healthcare*, 3(3), 170–179. doi:10.1097/SIH.0b013e318173038d

Rosen, M. A., Hunt, E. A., Pronovost, P. J., Federowicz, M. A., & Weaver, S. J. (2012). In situ simulation in continuing education for the health care professions: A systematic review. *Journal of Continuing Education in the Health Professions*, 32(4), 243–254. doi:10.1002/chp.21152

Ross, J. G. (2012). Simulation and psychomotor skill acquisition: A review of the literature. *Clinical Simulation in Nursing*, 8(9), e429–e435. doi:10.1016/j.ecns.2011.04.004

Rothgeb, M. K. (2008). Creating a nursing simulation laboratory: A literature review. *The Journal of Nursing Education*, 47(11), 489–494.

Rourke, L., Schmidt, M., & Garga, N. (2010). Theory-based research of high fidelity simulation use in nursing education: A review of literature. *International Journal of Nursing Education Scholarship*, 7(1), 1–14. doi:10.2202/1548-923X.1965

Royal College of Nursing. (2012). *Quality with compassion: The future of nursing education*. Royal College of Nursing (on behalf of the independent Willis Commission on Nursing Education). Retrieved from www.rcn.org.uk/williscommission

Royal College of Physicians and Surgeons of Canada. (2016). *Accreditation of simulation programs*. Retrieved from http://www.royalcollege.ca/rcsite/cpd/accreditation-simulation-programs-e

Rudolph, J., Simon, R., Dufresne, R., & Raemer, D. (2015). Establishing a safe container for simulation learning. *Simulation in Healthcare* 9, 339–349.

Rudolph, J. W., Foldy, E., Robinson, T., Kendall, S., Taylor, S., & Simon, R. (2013). Helping without harming. The instructor's feedback dilemma in debriefing—A case study. *Journal of the Society for Simulation in Healthcare*, 8(5), 304–316. doi:10.1097/SIH.0b013e318294854e

Rudolph, J. W., McIntosh, C., Simon, R., & Raemer, D. B. (2015). Helping learners "buy in" to simulation. In J. C. Palaganas, J. C. Maxworthy, C. A. Epps & M. E. Mancini (Eds.), *Defining excellence in simulation programs* (pp. 579–580). Philadelphia, PA: Wolters Kluwer.

Rudolph, J. W., Raemer, D. B., & Simon, R. (2014). Establishing a safe container for learning in simulation: The role of a presimulation briefing. *Simulation in Healthcare*, 9(6), 339–349. doi:10.1097/SIH.0000000000000047

Rudolph, J. W., Simon, R., Dufresne, R. L., & Raemer, D. B. (2006). There's no such thing as "nonjudgmental" debriefing: A theory and method for debriefing with good judgment. *Simulation in Healthcare*, 1(1), 49–55.

Rudolph, J. W., Simon, R., & Raemer, D. B. (2007). Which reality matters? Questions on the path to high engagement in healthcare simulation. *Simulation in Healthcare, 2*(3), 161–163. http://doi.org/10.1097/SIH.0b013e31813d1035

Rudolph, J. W., Simon, R., Raemer, D. B., & Eppich, W. J. (2008). Debriefing as formative assessment: Closing performance gaps in medical education. *Academic Emergency Medicine, 15*(11), 1010–1016. doi:10.1111/j.1553-2712.2008.00248.x

Rudolph, J. W., Simon, R., Rivard, P., Dufresne, R. L., & Raemer, D. B. (2007). Debriefing with good judgment: Combining rigorous feedback with genuine inquiry. *Anesthesiology Clinics, 25*(2), 361–376. http://doi.org/10.1016/j.anclin.2007.03.007

Rundio. (2016). *The nurses manager's guide to budgeting and finance.* Indianapolis, IN: Sigma Theta Tau International.

Rutherford-Hemming, T., Kardong-Edgren, S., Gore, T., Ravert, P., & Rizzolo, M. A. (2014). High-stakes evaluation: Five years later. *Clinical Simulation in Nursing, 10*(12), e605–e610. doi:http://dx.doi.org/10.1016/j.ecns.2014.09.009

Rutherford-Hemming, T., Lioce, L., & Durham, C. (2015). Implementing the standards of best practice for simulation. *Nurse Educator, 40*(2), 96–100. doi:10.1097/NNE.0000000000000115

Rutherford-Hemming, T., Lioce, L., Kardong-Edgren, S. Jeffries, P. R., & Sittner, B. (2016). After the National Council of State Boards of Nursing simulation study—Recommendations and next steps. *Clinical Simulation in Nursing, 12*(1), 2–7. http://doi.org/10.1016/j.ecns.2015.10.010

Sachs, J. (2016). The age of sustainable development. *Coursera.* [Class notes, Lesson One]. Retrieved from https://www.coursera.org/learn/sustainable-development#syllabus

Saglyk Info. (2015). Retrieved from http://www.saglyk.info/english/about-us.html

Salas, E., Burke, C. S., & Cannon-Bowers, J. A. (2000). Teamwork: Emerging principles. *International Journal of Management Reviews, 2,* 339–356. doi:10.1111/1468-2370.00046

Salem-Schatz, S., Ordin, D., & Mittman, B. (2010). *Guide to the after action review.* Retrieved from http://www.cebma.org/wp-content/uploads/Guide-to-the-after_action_review.pdf

Salie, S., & Schlechter, A. (2012). A formative evaluation of a staff reward and recognition programme. *SA Journal of Human Resource Management, 10*(3), 1–11. doi:http://dx.doi.org/10.4102/sajhrm.v10i3.422

Salovey, P., & Mayer, J. D. (1990). Emotional intelligence. *Imagination, Cognition, and Personality, 9,* 185–211.

Saly, J. (2010). *Functional programming.* Retrieved from http://www.exac.ca/fileadmin/documents/pdf/en/ARE-Functional_Programming-2010_ENG.pdf

Samner, C. E., Lykens, K., Singh, K. P., Mains, D. A., & Lachan, N. A. (2010). What is patient safety culture? A review of the literature. *Journal of Nursing Scholarship, 42*(2), 156–165. doi:10.1111/j.1547-5069.2009.0130.x

San Miguel, C., & Rogan, F. (2009). A good beginning: The long-term effects of a clinical communication programme. *Contemporary Nurse, 33*(2), 179–190.

Sanders, A. E., & Lushington, K. (2002). Effect of perceived stress on student performance in dental school. *Journal of Dental Education, 66*(1), 5222–5228.

Sando, C. R., Coggins, R. M., Meakim, C., Franklin, A. E., Gloe, D., Boese, T., … Borum, J. C. (2013). Standards of best practice: Simulation: Standard VII: Participant assessment and evaluation. *Clinical Simulation in Nursing, 9*(6S), S30–S32. doi:10.1016/j.ecns.2013.04.007

Sando, C. R., Coggins, R. M., & Romanow, R. J. (2002). *Building on values: The future of health care in Canada* (Cat. No. CP32 85/2002E-IN). Retrieved from http://publications.gc.ca/site/eng/237274/publication.html

Sanko, J. S., Shekhter, I., Kyle, R. R., & Birnbach, D. J. (2015). Using embedded simulated persons (a.k.a "confederates"). In J. C. Palaganas, J. C. Maxworthy, C. A. Epps & M. E. Mancini (Eds.), *Defining excellence in simulation programs* (pp. 213–226). Philadelphia, PA: Wolters Kluwer.

Sanko, J. S., Shekhter, I., Kyle Jr, R. R., Di Benedetto, S., & Birnbach, D. J. (2013). Establishing a convention for acting in healthcare simulation: Merging art and science. *Simulation in Healthcare, 8*(4), 215–220. doi:10.1097/SIH.0b013e318293b814

Saravia, N. G., & Miranda, J. F. (2004, August). Plumbing the brain drain. *Bulletin of the World Health Organization, 82*(8), 608–615.

Sardari Nia, P., Heuts, S., Daemen, J., Luyten, P., Vainer, J., Hoorntje, J., …, Maessen, J. (2016). Preoperative planning with three-dimensional reconstruction of patient's anatomy, rapid prototyping and simulation for endoscopic mitral valve repair. *Interactive CardioVascular and Thoracic Surgery, 24*(2), 163–168. ivw308–6. doi:10.1093/icvts/ivw308

Saylor, J., Vemoony, S., Selekman, J., & Cowperthwait, A. (2016). Interprofessional education using a palliative care simulation. *Nurse Educator, 41*(3), 125–129. doi:10.1097/NNE.0000000000000228

Schaefer, J. J., Vanderbilt, A. A., Cason, C. L., Bauman, E. B., Glavin, R. J., Lee, F. W., & Navedo, D. D. (2011). Literature review: Instructional design and pedagogy science in healthcare simulation. *Simulation in Healthcare, 6*(Suppl), S30–S41. doi:10.1097/SIH.0b013e31822237b4

Schegel, C., Bonvin, R., Rethan, J., & Van der Vleuten, C. (2016). Standardized patient's perspectives on workplace satisfaction and work-related relationships: A multicenter study. *Simulation in Healthcare, 11*(4), 278–285. doi:10.1097/SIH.0000000000000160

Schein, E. H. (2009). *The corporate culture survival guide* (2nd ed.). San Francisco, CA: Jossey-Bass.

Schein, E. H. (2010). *Organizational culture and leadership* (4th ed.). San Francisco, CA: Jossey-Bass.

Scher, D. L. (2016). *5 Ways that virtual reality will transform healthcare.* Retrieved from https://insights.samsung.com/2016/06/24/five-ways-virtual-reality-will-transform-healthcare/

Schlairet, M. C., & Pollock, J. W. (2010). Equivalence testing of traditional and simulated clinical experiences: Undergraduate nursing students' knowledge acquisition. *Journal of Nursing Education, 49*(1), 43–47. doi:10.3928/01484834-20090918-08

Schleicher, J. (2014, January). *UNMC History 101: Medicine in wax.* Omaha, NE: University of Nebraska Medical Center. Retrieved from http://www.unmc.edu/news.cfm?match=12171

Schneider, B., & Barbera, K. M. (2014). *The Oxford handbook of organizational climate and culture.* New York, NY: Oxford University Press.

Schön, D. (1983). *The reflective practitioner. How professionals think in action.* London, UK: Temple Smith.

Schön, D. (1987). *Educating the reflective practitioner.* San Francisco, CA: Jossey-Bass.

Schram, A. P., & Mudd, S. (2015). Implementing standardized patients within simulation in a nurse practitioner program. *Clinical Simulation in Nursing, 11*(4), 208–213. doi:10.1016.j.ecns.2015.02.002

Schroeder, R., Linderman, K., Liedtke, C, & Choo, A.S. (2008). Six Sigma: Definition and underlying theory. *Journal of Operations Management, 26,* 536–554. doi:10.1016/j.jom.2007.06.007

Schultis, L., Domenech, M., Fritz, B., Starry, M., & Winton, E. (2006, November). *Contractual limitations of liability, warrantees, and remedies.* Pillsbury Global Sourcing. Retrieved from http://www.pillsburylaw.com/siteFiles/Publications/0C62DFD605F0471619ADF0E2E5576E98.pdf

Schwarz, M., Wojtczak, A., & Zhou, T. (2004). Medical education in China's leading medical schools. *Medical Teacher, 26,* 215–222. http://dx.doi.org/10.1080/01421590310001642939

Seely Brown, J. (2008). Forward. In T. Iiyoshi & M. S. Vijay Kumar (Eds.), *Opening up education: The collective advancement of education through open technology, open content, and open knowledge.* Cambridge, MA: The MIT Press.

Seely-Brown, J. (2012). Cultivating the entrepreneurial learner in the 21st century (keynote address). *2012 Digital Media and Learning Conference,* San Francisco, CA.

Seely Brown, J., & Adler, R. P. (2008). Minds on fire: Open education, the long tail, and learning 2.0. *EDUCAUSE Review, 43*(1), 16–32. Retrieved from http://creativecommons.org/licenses/by/3.0/

Sendjaya, S., & Sarros, J. (2002). Servant leadership: Its origin, development, and application in organizations. *Journal of Leadership and Organizational Studies, 9*(2), 57–64. doi:10.1177/107179190200900205

Senge, P. M. (2006). *The fifth discipline: The art and practice of the learning organization.* New York, NY: Doubleday.

Senger, B., Stapleton, L., & Gorski, M. S. (2012, November). A hospital and university partnership model for simulation education. *Clinical Simulation in Nursing, 8*(9), e477–e482. doi:10.1016/j.ecns.2011.09.002

Seropian, M. A., Alinier, G., Hussain, H., Driggers, B., Brost, B. C., Dongilli, T. A., & Lauber, M. C. (2015). Building a simulation centre: Key design considerations. In J. C. Palaganas, J. C. Maxworthy, C. A. Epps & M. E. Mancini (Eds.), *Defining excellence in simulation programs* (pp. 434–454). Philadelphia, PA: Wolters Kluwer.

Seropian, M. A., Brown, K., Gavilanes, J. S., & Driggers, B. (2004a). An approach to simulation program development. *Journal of Nursing Education, 43,* 170–174.

Seropian, M. A., Brown, K., Gavilanes, J. S., & Driggers, B. (2004b). Simulation: Not just a manikin. *Journal of Nursing Education, 43,* 164–169.

Seropian, M., Driggers, B., Taylor, J., Gubrud-Howe, J., & Brady, G. (2006). The Oregon simulation experience: A statewide simulation network and alliance. *Simulation in Healthcare, 1*(2), 56–61.

Seropian, M., & Lavey, R. (2010). Design considerations for healthcare simulation facilities. *Simulation in Healthcare, 5*(6), 338–345. doi:10.1097/SIH.0b013e3181ec8f60

Servicio de Información de Educación Superior (Information Service of Superior Education) (SIES). (2014). *Panorama de la Educación Superior en Chile, 2014.*

Seymour, N. E., Cooper, J. B., Farley, D. R., Feaster, S. J., Ross, B. K., Pellegrini, C. A., & Sachdeva, A. K. (2013). Best practices in interprofessional education and training in surgery: Experiences from American College of Surgeons-Accredited Education Institutes. *Surgery, 154,* 1–12. doi:10.1016/j.surg.2013.04.05

Sharma S., Boet, S., Kitto, S., & Reeves, S. (2011). Interprofessional simulated learning: The need for 'sociological fidelity'. *Journal of Interprofessional Care, 25*(2), 81–83. doi:10.3109/13561820.2011.556514

Sharpnack, P. A., Goliat, L., & Rogers, K. (2011). Using standardized patients to teach leadership competencies. *Clinical Simulation in Nursing, 9*(3), e95–e102. doi:10.1016/j.ecns.2011.10.001

Shearer, J. E. (2013). High-fidelity simulation and safety: An integrative review. *Journal of Nursing Education, 52*(1), 39–46. doi:10.3928/01484834-20121121-01

Sheehan, D., Robertson, L., & Ormond, T. (2007). Comparison of language used and patterns of communication in interprofessional and multidisciplinary teams. *Journal of Interprofessional Care, 21*(1), 17–30.

Shelton, D., & Pierce, S. T. (2011). Cyber innovation center: Building a virtual presence to enrich the educational experience. *Clinical Simulation in Nursing, 7*(6), e262–e263. http://doi.org/10.1016/j.ecns.2011.09.066

Shen, W., & Liu, Z. (2011). Bureaucratic regulation and interdisciplinary: The challenges in disciplinary management toward knowledge development. *Peking University Education Review, 2,* 25–36. Retrieved from http://en.cnki.com.cn/Article_en/CJFDTOTAL-BJPL201102007.htm

Sherwood, G. D., & Horton-Deutsch, S. (2012). *Reflective practice: Transforming education and improving outcomes.* Indianapolis, IN: Sigma Theta Tau International.

Sherwood, G. D., & Horton-Deutsch, S. (2015). *Reflective organizations: On the front lines of QSEN and reflective practice implementation.* Indianapolis, IN: Sigma Theta Tau.

Shin, S., Park, J. H., & Kim, J. H. (2015). Effectiveness of patient simulation in nursing education: Meta-analysis. *Nurse Education Today, 35*(1), 176–182. doi:10.1016/j.nedt.2014.09.009

Shinnick, M. A., Woo, M., Horwich, T. B., & Steadman, R. (2011). Debriefing: The most important component of simulation? *Clinical Simulation in Nursing, 7*(3), e105–e111. http://dx.doi.org/10.1016/j.ecns.2010.11.005

Shinnick, M. A., Woo, M. A., & Mentes, J. C. (2010). Human patient simulation: State of the science in prelicensure nursing education. *Journal of Nursing Education, 50*(2), 65–72. doi:10.3928/01484834-20101230-01

Silver, S., Wachowski, A., & Wachowski, L. (1999). *The matrix* [Motion picture]. United States: Warner Brothers.

Simington, M. (2011). Welcome to the future: Simulation training. Cutting-edge technology helps strengthen patient care. *Healthcare Executive, 26*(5), 60.

Simon, R., Raemer, D., & Rudolph, J. (2010). *Debriefing Assessment for Simulation in Healthcare (DASH)® rater's handbook.* Boston, MA: Center for Medical Simulation. Retrieved from https://harvardmedsim.org/_media/DASH.handbook.2010.Final.Rev.2.pdf

Simon Sinek, Inc. (2015). *The golden circle.* Retrieved from https://www.startwithwhy.com/default.aspx

Simpson, B., Skelton-Green, J., & Scott, J. (2011). Promising practices in leadership development. *Canadian Journal of*

Nursing Leadership, 24(3), 26–38. Retrieved from http://www.longwoods.com/publications/nursing-leadership/all

Sims, S., Hewitt, G., & Harris, R. (2015). Evidence of a shared purpose, critical reflection, innovation and leadership in interprofessional healthcare teams: A realist synthesis. *Journal of Interprofessional Care, 29*(3), 209–215. http://doi.org/10.3109/13561820.2014.941459

Simulation Australasia and the Australian Society for Simulation in Healthcare. (2012). *SimNET—connecting the health simulation community*. Retrieved from http://www.simnet.net.au/

Simulation Innovation Resource Center. (n.d.). *SIRC glossary*. Retrieved from http://sirc.nln.org/mod/glossary/view.php?id=183&mode=letter&hook=S&sortkey=&sortorder=&fullsearch=0&page=-1

Sinz, E. (2007). 2006 Simulation summit. *Simulation in Healthcare, 2*, 33–38. doi:10.1097/SIH.0b013e31803251cc

Sirimanna, P. V., & Aggarwal, R. (2013). Patient safety. In A. I. Levine, S. DeMaria Jr, A. D. Schwartz & A. J. Sim (Eds.), *The comprehensive textbook of healthcare simulation* (pp. 111–120). New York, NY: Spring Science + Business.

Sittner, B., Hertzog, M., & Ofe Fleck, M. (2013, November). Enhancing labor and delivery learning experiences through simulation. *Clinical Simulation in Nursing, 9*(11), e521–e530. http://dx.doi.org/10.1016/j.ecns.2013.04.012

Sitzman, K. L., & Eichelberger, L. W. (2011). *Understanding the work of nurse theorists: A creative beginning*. Sudbury, MA: Jones and Bartlett Publishers.

Skelton-Green, J., Simpson, B., & Scott, J. (2007). An integrated approach to change leadership. *Canadian Journal of Nursing Leadership, 20*(3), 1–15. doi:10.1297/cjnl.2007.19277

Skiba, D. (2016). Emerging technologies centre. On the horizon: Trends, challenges, and educational technologies in higher education. *Nursing Education Perspectives, 37*(3), 1–3. doi:10.1097/01.NEP.0000000000000019

Skiles, J. (2012, May). *Was it really a miracle on the Hudson? Aviation meets healthcare safety (Plenary session video)*. National Patient Safety Foundation 2012 Meeting. Retrieved from https://youtu.be/kaydVvH7S4E

Slater, L. Z., Bryant, K. D., & Ng, V. (2016, September). Nursing student perceptions of standardized patient use in health assessment. *Clinical Simulation in Nursing, 12*(9), 368–376. http://dx.doi.org/10.1016/j.ecns.2016.04.007

Slone, F. L., & Lampotang, S. (2015). A history of modern-day mannequins. In J. C. Palaganas, J. C. Maxworthy, C. A. Epps & M. E. Mancini (Eds.), *Defining excellence in simulation programs* (pp. 172–182). Philadelphia, PA: Wolters Kluwer.

Small, S. D., Wuerz, R. C., Simon, R., Shapiro, N., Conn, A., & Setnik, G. (1999). Demonstration of high-fidelity simulation team training for emergency medicine. *Academic Emergency Medicine, 6*(4), 312–323. Retrieved from http://www.ncbi.nlm.nih.gov/pubmed/10230983

Smith, B., & Gaba, D. (2001). Simulators. In C. Lake (Ed.), *Clinical monitoring: Practical application for anesthesia and critical care* (pp. 26–44). Philadelphia, PA: W.B. Saunders.

Smith, C. M., Gephardt, E. G., & Nestel, D. (2015). Applying the theory of Stanislavski to simulation: Stepping into role. *Clinical Simulation in Nursing, 11*(8), 361–367. http://dx.doi.org/10.1016/j.ecns.2015.04.001

Smith, S., & Clouder, L. (2010). Interprofessional and interdisciplinary learning: An exploration of similarities and dif-ferences. In A. Bromage, L. Clouder, J. Thistlethwaite & F. Gordon (Eds.), *Interprofessional e-learning and collaborative work* (pp. 1–13). Hershey, PA: Information Science Reference.

Smith-Stoner, M. (2011). Using moulage to enhance educational instruction. *Nurse Educator, 36*(1), 21–24. doi:10.1097/NNE.0b013e3182001e98

Snowden, D. (2015). *Summary article on origins of Cynefin*. Retrieved from http://cognitive-edge.com/articles/summary-article-on-cynefin-origins/

Snowdon, D. J., & Boone, M. E. (2007). A leader's framework for decision making. *Harvard Business Review, 85*, 66–76. Retrieved from http://www.HBR.org

Society for Simulation in Healthcare (SSH). (2012a). *Council for accreditation of healthcare simulation programs: Accreditation standards and measurement criteria*. Retrieved from http://ssih.org/search/search&keywords=accreditation%20standards&x=0&y=0

Society for Simulation in Healthcare (SSH). (2012b). *Policy and procedure manual*. Society for Simulation in Healthcare.

Society for Simulation in Healthcare (SSH). (2014a). *Core standards companion* (pdf). Retrieved from www.ssh.orgRidder

Society for Simulation in Healthcare (SSH). (2014b). *SSH accreditation process: Informational guide for the accreditation process from the SSH council for accreditation of healthcare simulation programs* (pdf). Retrieved from www.ssh.org

Society for Simulation in Healthcare (SSH). (2015a). *Core standards companion document*. Retrieved from www.ssh.org

Society for Simulation in Healthcare (SSH). (2015b). *SSH accreditation of healthcare simulation programs*. Retrieved from http://www.ssih.org/Accreditation

Society for Simulation in Healthcare (SSH). (2015c). *SSH certification programs*. Retrieved from http://www.ssih.org/Certification

Society for Simulation in Healthcare (SSH). (2015d). *The Standards fit any healthcare simulation programs*. Retrieved on November 2015 from http://www.ssih.org/Accreditation

Society for Simulation in Healthcare (SSH). (2016a). *About simulation*. Retrieved from http://www.ssih.org/About-Simulation

Society for Simulation in Healthcare (SSH). (2016b). *SSH certification programs*. Retrieved from http://www.ssih.org/Certification

Society for Simulation in Healthcare (SSH). (2016c). *Core standards companion document*. Retrieved from www.ssh.org

Society for Simulation in Healthcare (SSH). (2016d). *Council for Accreditation of Healthcare Simulation Programs Accreditation Standards*. Retrieved from http://www.ssih.org/Portals/48/Accreditation/14_A_Standards.pdf

Society for Simulation in Healthcare (SSH). (2016e). *SSH home page*. Retrieved from www.ssih.org

Society for Simulation in Healthcare (SSH) Accreditation. (2014a). *SSH accreditation informational guide*. Retrieved from http://www.ssih.org/Accreditation/Full-Accreditation

Society for Simulation in Healthcare Committee for Certification. (2014). *CHSOS handbook for the certification process from the SSH Committee for Certification*. Retrieved from http://www.ssih.org/Portals/48/Certification/CHSOS_Docs/CHSOS%20Handbook.pdf

Society for Simulation in Healthcare Council for Accreditation (SSH). (2014b). *SSH certified healthcare simulation operations specialist handbook*. Retrieved from http://www.ssih.org/Portals/48/Certification/CHSOS_Docs/CHSOS%20Handbook.pdf

Society in Europe for Simulation Applied to Medicine (SESAM). (2016). *SESAM Accreditation*. Retrieved from https://www.sesam-web.org/accreditation/

Solar, O., & Irwin, A. (2010). A conceptual framework for action on the social determinants of health. *Social Determinants of Health Discussion, Paper 2* (Policy and Practice). Geneva, Switzerland: World Health Organization.

Sole, M. L., Guimond, M. E., & Amedei, C. (2013). An analysis of simulation resources, needs, and plans in Florida. *Clinical Simulation in Nursing, 9*(7), e265–e271. doi:10.1016/j.ecns.2012.03.003

Sonnadara, R. R., Mui, C., McQueen, S., Mironova, P., Nousiainen, M., Safir, O., ... Reznick, R. (2014). Reflections on competency-based education and training for surgical residents. *Journal of Surgical Education, 71*(1), 151–158. doi:10.1016/j.jsurg.2013.06.020

Sorenson Marshall, E. (2011). *Transformational leadership in nursing: From expert clinician to influential leader*. New York, NY: Springer.

Southwick, F., Lewis, M., Treloar, D., Cherabuddi, K., Radhakrishnan, N., Leverence, R., ..., Cottler, L. (2014). Applying athletic principles to medical rounds to improve teaching and patient care. *Academic Medicine, 89*(7), 1018–1023. http://doi.org/10.1097/ACM.0000000000000278

Southwick, F. S. (2014). *Critically ill: A five-point plan to cure health care delivery*. Gainesville, FL: Southwick Press.

Sox, H. C., & Woloshin, S. (2000, November–December). How many deaths are due to medical error? Getting the number right. *Effective Clinical Practice, 3*(6), 277–283. Retrieved from http://ecp.acponline.org/novdec00/sox.htm

Spear, S., & Bowen, H. K. (1999). Decoding the DNA of the Toyota production system. *Harvard Business Review 77*(5), 97–106.

Spence, J. (2001). *The search for modern China*. Retrieved from http://iis-db.stanford.edu/docs/115/CRintro.pdf

Spielberger, C. D., Gorsuch, R. L., Lushene, R. E., Vagg, P. R., & Jacobs, G. A. (1983). *State-trait anxiety inventory for adults*. Menlo Park, CA: Mind Garden.

Sprehe, J., & Haley, J. A. (2012). Build it so they want to come: Establishing and developing a hospital simulation center. *Clinical Simulation in Nursing, 8*(8), e403–e404. http://doi.org/10.1016/j.ecns.2012.07.052

Squire, K. (2006). From content to context: Videogames as designed experience. *Educational Researcher, 35*(8), 19–29. doi:10.3102/0013189X035008019

St. Pierre, M., Hofinger, G., Buerschaper, C., & Simon, R. (2011). *Crisis management in acute care settings: Human factors, team psychology, and patient safety in a high-stakes environment*. Berlin/Heidelberg: Springer-Verlag.

Stanford University. (2015). *The MedSim eagle patient simulator*. Retrieved from http://med.stanford.edu/VAsimulator/medsim.html

Stavros, J. (2013). The generative nature of SOAR: Applications, results and the new SOAR profile. *AI Practitioner, 15*(3), 7–30. dx.doi.org/10.12781/978-1-907549-16-8-2

Stavros, J., & Hinrichs, G. (2007). SOARing to new heights of strategic planning to execution. *AI Practitioner*, 4–9.

Stefaniak, J. E., & Turkelson, C. L. (2014). Does the sequence of instruction matter during simulation? *Simulation in Healthcare, 9*(1), 15–20. doi:10.1097/SIH.0b013e3182a8336f

Steinemann, S., Berg, B., Skinner, A., DiTulio, A., Anzelon, K., Terada, K., ... , Speck, C. (2011). In situ, multidisciplinary, simulation-based teamwork training improves early trauma care. *Journal of Surgical Education, 68*(6), 472–477. doi:10.1016/j.jsurg.2011.05.009

Steiner, I. D. (1972). *Group process and productivity*. New York, NY: Academic Press.

Steinwachs, B. (1992). How to facilitate a debriefing. *Simulation & Gaming, 23*(2), 186–195.

Stewart, M., Brown, J. B., Donner, A., McWhinney, I. R., Oates, J., Weston, W., & Jordan, J. (2000). The impact of patient-centered care on outcomes. *Journal of Family Practice, 49*, 796–804.

Stillwell, S. B., Fineout-Overholt, E., Melnyk, B. M., & Williamson, K. M. (2010). Evidence-based practice: Step by step: Searching the evidence. *The American Journal of Nursing, 110*(5), 41–47. doi:10.1097/01.NAJ.0000372071.24134.7e

Storch, J. L., Starzomski, R., & Rodney, R. (2013). To boldly go forward: Epilogue and future horizons. In J. L. Storch, R. Rodney & R. Starzomski (Eds.), *Toward a moral horizon: Nursing ethics for leadership and practice* (2nd ed., pp. 527–536). Toronto, ON: Pearson.

Stroup, C. (2014). Simulation usage in nursing fundamentals: Integrative literature review. *Clinical Simulation in Nursing, 10*(3), e155–e164. http://dx.doi.org/10.1016/j.ecns.2013.10.004

Sui, H., Spence-Laschinger, H. K., & Finegan, J. (2008). Nursing professional practice environments: Setting the stage for constructive conflict resolution and work effectiveness. *Journal of Nursing Administration, 38*(5), 250–257. doi:10.1097/01.NNA.0000312772.04234.1f

Sullivan, N. (2015). An integrative review: Instructional strategies to improve nurses' retention of cardiopulmonary resuscitation priorities. *International Journal of Nursing Education Scholarship, 12*(1), 1–7. doi:10.1515/ijnes-2014-0012

Sunguya, B. F., Hinthong, W., Jimba, M., & Yasuoka, J. (2014). Interprofessional education for whom? Challenges and lessons learned from its implementation in developed countries and their application to developing countries: A systematic review. *PLoS One, 9*(5), e96724. doi:10.1371/journal.pone.0096724

Sweller, J. (1988). Cognitive load during problem solving: Effects on learning. *Cognitive Science, 12*(2), 257–285. doi:10.1016/0364-0213(88)90023-7

Sweller, J., Ayres, P., & Kalyuga, S. (2011). *Cognitive load theory*. New York, NY: Springer.

Swing, S. R. (2002). Assessing the ACGME general competencies: General considerations and assessment methods. *Academic Emergency Medicine, 9*(11), 1278–1288. doi:10.1197/aemj.9.11.1278

Sy, T. (2010). What do you think of followers? Examining the content, structure, and consequences of implicit followership theories. *Organizational Behavior and Human Decision Processes, 113*(2010), 73–84. doi:10.1016/j.obhdp.2010.06.001

SynDaver™ Labs. (2016). *SynDaver patient*. Retrieved from http://syndaver.com/shop/syndaver/synthetic-humans/syndaver-patient/

Szabo, L. (2015, January). 40 Patients mistakenly given unsterile intravenous fluid. *USA Today*. Retrieved from http://www.usatoday.com

Tagliareni, M. E., Cline, D. D., Mengel, A., McLaughlin, B., & King, E. (2012). Quality care for older adults: The NLN Advancing Care Excellence for Seniors (ACES) project. *Nursing Education Perspectives*, *33*(3), 144–149. doi:http://dx.doi.org/10.5480/1536-5026-33.3.144

Taibi, D. & Kardong-Edgren, S. (2014). Health care educator training in simulation: A survey and website development. *Clinical Simulation in Nursing*, *10*(1), e47–e52. doi:10.1016/j.ecns.2013.05.013

Talbot, T. B. (2013). Balancing physiology, anatomy, and immersion: How much biological fidelity is necessary in a medical simulation? *Military Medicine*, *178*(10), 28–36. doi:10.7205/MILMED-D-13-00212

Tan, S. B., Pena, G., Altree, M., & Maddern, G. J. (2014). Multidisciplinary team simulation for the operating theatre: A review of the literature. *ANZ Journal of Surgery*, *84*(7–8), 515–522. doi:10.1111/ans.12478

Tang, J. J., Kyaw Tun, J., & Kneebone, R. (2013). Distributed simulation. In K. Forrest, J. McKimm & S. Edgar (Eds.), *Essential simulation in clinical education* (pp. 196–210). Oxford, UK: John Wiley & Sons, Ltd.

Tanner, C. (2006). Thinking like a nurse: A research-based model of clinical judgment in nursing. *Journal of Nursing Education*, *45*(6), 204–211.

Taplay, K., Jack, S. M., Baxter, P., Eva, K., & Martin, L. (2014). Organizational culture shapes the adoption and incorporation of simulation into nursing curricula: A grounded theory study. *Nursing Research and Practice*, *2014*, 1–12. doi:10.1155/2014/197591

Tariq, U., Sood, M., & Goodsman, D. (2015). The facilitator's role in London's air ambulance's simulation "moulage" training. *Air Medical Journal*, *34*(2), 92–97. doi:10.1016/j.amj.2014.12.012

Tasmanian Government. (2014). *Tasmanian clinical education network. Simulated learning environment: Strategic plan.* Retrieved from http://www.tcen.com.au/sites/newtcen/files/documents/final_signed_sle_strategic_plan_march_2014.pdf

Taylor, E. (2009). Fostering transformative learning. In J. Mezirow & E. Taylor (Eds.), *Transformative learning in practice: Insights from community, workplace, and higher education* (pp. 3–17). San Francisco, CA: Jossey-Bass.

Technavio.com. (2016, January). *Global e-learning market 2016–2020.* Retrieved from http://www.technavio.com/report/global-education-technology-e-learning-market

Teo, G. (2016, September). *Healthcare is getting into VR—Here's why that matters.* Retrieved from https://www.linkedin.com/pulse/healthcare-getting-vr-heres-why-matters-gavin-teo

Tervalon, M., & Murray-Garcia, J. (1998). Cultural humility versus cultural competence: A critical distinction in defining physician training outcomes in multicultural education. *Journal of Health Care for the Poor and Underserved*, *9*(2), 117–125.

Texas Department of Health, National Maternal and Child Health Resource Center on Cultural Competency. (1997). *Journey towards cultural competency: Lessons learned.* Vienna, VA: Maternal and Children's Health Bureau Clearinghouse.

Thannhauser, J., Russell-Mayhew, S., & Scott, C. (2010). Measures of interprofessional education and collaboration. *Journal of Interprofessional Care*, *24*(4), 336–349. doi:10.3109/13561820903442903

The Human Body Exhibit. (2016). *Plastination.* Retrieved from http://thbexhibition.com/plastination.asp

The Joint Commission. (2008, July). Behaviors that undermine a culture of quality and safety. *Sentinel Even Alert*, *40*. Retrieved on from http://www.jointcommission.org/sentinel_event_alert_issue_40_behaviors_that_undermine_a_culture_of_safety/

The Joint Commission. (2012). *Sentinel event data: Root causes by event type 2004–2011.* Retrieved from http://www.joint-commission.org/

The Medical Futurist. (2016). *Grand challenges: Embrace disruptive medical technologies.* Retrieved from http://medicalfu-turist.com/grand-challenges/disruptive-medical-technology/

The Northern Territory Regional Training Network. (2013). *Northern Territory Government, Flinders University.* Retrieved from http://www.flinders.edu.au/medicine/courses/medical-course/nt-medical-program/nt-sim-lab/

The Royal College of Physicians and Surgeons of Canada. (2014, May). 3D printers, innovating medical education. *Dialogue: Newsletter For the Royal College of Physicians and Surgeons of Canada*, *14*(5). Retrieved from http://www.royalcollege.ca/portal/page/portal/rc/resources/publications/dialogue/vol14_5/3d_printers

The Royal College of Physicians and Surgeons of Canada. (2015). *Accreditation of simulation programs.* Retrieved on from http://www.royalcollege.ca/portal/page/portal/rc/members/cpd/cpd_providers_resources/simulation

The Royal College of Physicians and Surgeons of Canada. (n.d.). *Simulation educator training course.* Retrieved from http://www.royalcollege.ca/portal/page/portal/rc/resources/ppi/simulation_education_training_course

The Royal Society. (2014). *Climate change: Evidence and causes. An overview from the Royal Society and the US National Academy of Sciences.* Retrieved from https://royalsociety.org/~/media/Royal_Society_Content/policy/projects/climate-evidence-causes/climate-change-evidence-causes.pdf

The Secretary's Advisory Committee on National Health Promotion and Disease Prevention. (2008, October). *Objectives for 2020 phase i report recommendations for the framework and format of healthy people 2020.* Retrieved from http://www.healthypeople.gov/2010/hp2020/advisory/phasei/PhaseI.pdf

The World Bank. The World Bank Rwanda. Retrieved from http://www.worldbank.org/en/country/rwanda

The World Bank. (2015). *World Bank country and lending groups.* Retrieved from https://datahelpdesk.worldbank.org/knowledgebase/articles/906519

The World Bank. (2017). *Historical classification by income.* Retrieved from https://datahelpdesk.worldbank.org/knowledgebase/articles/906519-world-bank-country-and-lending-groups

Theilen, U., Leonard, P., & Jones, P. (2013). Regular in situ simulation training of paediatric medical emergency team improves hospital response to deteriorating patients. *Resuscitation*, *84*(2), 218–222. doi:10.1016/j.resuscitation.2012.06.027

Thibault, G. E. (2011). Interprofessional education: An essential strategy to accomplish the future of nursing goals. *Journal of Nursing Education*, *50*, 313–317. doi:10.3928/01484834-20110519-03

Thomas, C., Bertram, E., & Johnson, D. (2009). The SBAR communication technique: Teaching nursing students professional communication skills. *Nurse Educator*, *34*(4), 176–180. doi:10.1097/NNE.0b013e3181aaba54

Thomas, K. (2009, November/December). The four intrinsic rewards that drive employee engagement. *Ivey Business Journal.* Retrieved from http://iveybusinessjournal.com/publication/the-four-intrinsic-rewards-that-drive-employee-engagement/

Thorkelson, B. (2015). Mobile simulation. In J. C. Palaganas, J. C. Maxworthy, C. A. Epps & M. E. Mancini (Eds.), *Defining excellence in simulation programs* (pp. 99–104). Philadelphia, PA: Wolters Kluwer Inc.

Thorndike, E. L. (1923). The influence of first-year Latin upon the ability to read English. *School Sociology, 17,* 165–168.

Thorndike, E. L. (1924a). Mental discipline in high school studies. *Journal of Educational Psychology, 15*(1), 1–22. http://dx.doi.org/10.1037/h0075386

Thorndike, E. L. (1928). *Adult learning.* New York, NY: Macmillan.

Thorndike, E. L. (1932). *The fundamentals of learning.* New York, NY: Teachers College Press.

Todaro-Franchesci, V. (2012). *Compassion fatigue and burnout in nursing: Enhancing professional quality of life.* New York, NY: Springer Publishing.

Todd, M., Manz, J. A., Hawkins, K. S., Parsons, M. E., & Hercinger, M. (2008). The development of a quantitative evaluation tool for simulations in nursing education. *International Journal of Nursing Education Scholarship, 5*(1). doi:http://dx.doi.org/10.2202/1548-923X.1705

Toman, C. (2005). Body work. Medical technology, and hospital nursing practice. In C. Bates, D. Dodd & N. Rousseau (Eds.), *On all frontiers four centuries of Canadian nursing* (pp. 89–106). Ottawa, ON: University of Ottawa Press and the Canadian Museum of Civilization.

Torre, D. M., Aagaard, E., Elnicki, D. M., Durning, S. J., & Papp, K. K. (2013). Simulation in the internal medicine clerkship: A national survey of internal medicine clerkship directors. *Teaching and Learning in Medicine, 23,* 215–222. doi:10.1080/10401334.2011.586912

Tosterud, R., Hedlin, B., & Hall-Lord, M. (2013). Nursing students' perceptions of high and low-fidelity simulation used as learning methods. *Nursing Education Practice, 13*(4), 262–279. doi:10.1016/j.nepr.2013.02.002

Trotter, F., & Uhlman, D. (2013). *Hacking healthcare.* Sebastopol, CA: O'Reilly Media, Inc.

Truth and Reconciliation Commission of Canada (TRC). (2015). *Honouring the truth, reconciling for the future: Summary of the final report of the Truth and Reconciliation Commission of Canada.* Toronto, ON: James Lorimer & Company Ltd. Retrieved from www.trc.ca/websites/trcinstitution/File/.../Exec_Summary_2015_05_31_web_o.pdf

Tuckman, B. W. (1965). Developmental sequence in small groups. *Psychological Bulletin, 63*(6), 384–399. http://dx.doi.org/10.1037/h0022100

Tuckman, B. W., & Jensen M. A. (1977). Stages in small-group development revisited. *Group and Organizational Studies, 2*(4), 419–427.

Tutu Foundation. (2015). *Ubuntu.* Retrieved from http://www.tutufoundationuk.org/ubuntu/

Ultanir, E. (2012). An epistemological glance at the constructivist approach: Constructivist learning in Dewey, Piaget, and Montessori. *International Journal of Instruction, 5*(2), 195–212.

United Nations. (2008). *Universal declaration of human rights: Dignity and justice for all of us.* Retrieved from http://www.un.org/en/events/humanrightsday/2008/theme.shtml

United Nations. (2015). *Transforming our world: The 2030 agenda for sustainable development.* Retrieved from https://sustainabledevelopment.un.org/post2015/transformingourworld/publication

United Nations Educational Scientific and Cultural Organization (UNESCO). (2010). *Report of the International Bioethics Committee of UNESCO (IBC) On Social Responsibility and Health.* Paris, France: Author. Retrieved from unesdoc.unesco.org/images/0018/001878/187899E.pdf

United Nations Educational Scientific and Cultural Organization (UNESCO). (2013). *Rethinking education in a changing world: Meeting of the senior experts' group.* Paris, France: Author. Retrieved from http://unesdoc.unesco.org/images/0022/002247/224743e.pdf

United Nations General Assembly. (2012). *The future we want.* Resolution adopted by the General Assembly. Retrieved from www.un.org/disabilities/documents/rio20_outcome_document_complete.pdf

United Nations International Children's Emergency Fund (UNICEF). (2015). *Countries at a glance: Qatar.* Retrieved from http://www.unicef.org/infobycountry/qatar_statistics.html

United Nations Population Fund (UNPF). (2013). *International migration 2013* (wall chart). Retrieved from http://www.unfpa.org/resources/international-migration-2013-wall-chart

Universidad Finis Terrae (University of Finis Tarrae). (2008). *Archivos vicerrectoría académica. estudio de factibilidad y creación del curriculum de la carrera de enfermería, 2008.*

Universidad Finis Terrae. (2016). *Escuela de Enfermería.* Retrieved from http://facultadmedicina.finisterrae.cl/escuelas/enfermeria

University of Washington. (2016). *Course and syllabus design.* Retrieved from http://www.washington.edu/teaching/teaching-resources/preparing-to-teach/designing-your-course-and-syllabus/#Syllabus

Usman, T., Sood, M., & Goodsman, D. (2015). The facilitator's role in London's air ambulance simulation "moulage" training. *Air Medical Journal, 34,* 92–97. doi:10.1016/j.amj.2014.12.012

Utley-Smith, Q. (2004). 5 competencies needed by new baccalaureate graduates. *Nursing Education Perspectives, 25*(4), 166–170.

Valler-Jones, T. (2014). The impact of peer-led simulations on student nurses. *British Journal of Nursing, 23*(6), 321–326.

Van de Ridder, J. M., Stoking, K. M., McGaghie, W. C., & Ten Cate, O. T. J. (2008). What is feedback in clinical education? *Medical Education, 42*(2), 189–197 doi:10.1111/j.1365-2923.2007.02973.x

Van Soeren M., Cop, S., MacMillan, K., Baker L, Egan-Lee R., & Reeves, S. (2011). Interprofessional simulated education: An analysis of learning and teaching processes. *Journal of Interprofessional Care, 25*(6), 334–340. doi:10.3109/13561820.2011.592229

Van Der Vleuten, C. P. M., Schuwirth, L. W. T., Driessen, E. W., Govaerts, M. J. B., & Heeneman, S. (2015). Twelve tips for programmatic assessment. *Medical Teacher, 37*(7), 641–646. http://doi.org/10.3109/0142159X.2014.973388

Van Vugt, M., Hogan, R., & Kaiser, R. B. (2008). Leadership, followership, and evolution: Some lessons from the past. *American Psychologist, 63*(3), 182–196. doi:10.1037/0003-066X.63.182

Vertovec, S. (2010). Towards post-multiculturalism? Changing communities, conditions and contexts of diversity. *International*

Social Science Journal, 61(199), 83–95. doi:10.1111/j.1468-2451. 2010.01749.x

Victorian Department of Health and Human Resources (2014). *Sustainability blueprint, tools and templates.* Retrieved from https://vicknowledgebank.net.au/resource-library/project/sustainability-blueprint-tools-and-templates

Vollmer, J., Mönk, S., & Heinrichs, W. (2008). Staff education for simulation: Train-the-trainer concepts. In R. R. Kyle, Jr. & W. B. Murray (Eds.), *Clinical simulation: Operations, engineering and management* (pp. 625–642). London, UK: Elsevier.

Von Hagens Plastination. (2016). *True anatomy for new ways of teaching.* Retrieved from http://www.vonhagens-plastination.com/

Von Wyl, T., Zuercher, M., Amsler, F., Walter, B., & Ummenhoffer, W. (2008). Technical and non-technical skills can be reliably assessed during paramedic simulation training. *Acta Anaesthesiologica Scandinavica, 53,* 121–127. doi:10.1111/j.1399-6576.2008.01797.x

Vygotsky, L. S. (1978). *Mind in society: The development of higher psychological processes.* Cambridge, MA: Harvard University Press.

Wageman, R. Hackman, J. R., & Lehman. (2005). Team diagnostic survey: Development of an instrument. *Journal of Applied Behavioral Science, 41,* 4.

Waite, R., & McKinney, N. S. (2016). Capital we must develop: Emotional competence educating pre-licensure nursing students [Research Brief]. *Nursing Education Perspectives, 37*(2), 101–103. http://doi.org/10.5480/14-1343

Waldner, M. H., & Olson, J. K. (2007). Taking the patient to the classroom: Applying theoretical frameworks to simulation in nursing education. *International Journal of Nursing Education Scholarship, 4*(1), 1–14.

Walker, D., & Bauser, J. (2012, April). So you need (to improve) a governance committee? *Guide Star.* Retrieved from https://www.guidestar.org/Articles.aspx?path=/rxa/news/articles/2012/need-to-improve-a-governance-committee.aspx

Walker, R. A. (2013). Holograms as teaching agents. *Journal of Physics: Conference Series 415*(1), 1–5. doi:10.1088/1742-6596/415/1/012076

Wallace, P. (2007). *Coaching standardized patients for use in the assessment of clinical competence.* New York, NY: Springer Publishing Co.

Walsh, K., Reeves, S., & Maloney, S. (2014). Exploring issues of cost and value in professional and interprofessional education. *Journal of Interprofessional Care, 28*(6), 493–494. doi:10.3109/13561820.2014.941212

Walton, J., Chute, E., & Ball, L. (2011). Negotiating the role of the professional nurse: The pedagogy of simulation: A grounded theory study. *Journal of Professional Nursing, 27,* 299–310. doi:10.1016/j.profnurs.2011.04.005

Wang, A. L., Fitzpatrick, J., & Petrini, M. (2013). Use of simulation among Chinese nursing students. *Clinical Simulation in Nursing, 9,* e311–e317. http://dx.doi.org/10.1016/j.ecns.2012.03.004

Wang, W., Tat Keh, H., & Bolton, L. (2007). *Health remedies: From perceptions to preference to a healthy lifestyle.* Retrieved from http://knowledge.wharton.upenn.edu/wp-content/uploads/2013/09/1343.pdf

Wang, Z., Liu, Q., & Wang, H. (2012). Medical simulation-based education improves medicos clinical skills. *Journal of*

Biomedical Research, 27(2), 81–84. http://dx.doi.org/10.7555/JBR.27.20120131

Watcher, R. M. (2015). *The digital doctor: Hope, hype, and harm at the dawn of medicine's computer age.* New York: McGraw Hill.

Watson, K., Wright, A., Morris, N., McMeeken, J., Rivett, D., Blackstock, F., … Jull, G. (2012). Can simulation replace part of clinical time? Two parallel randomised controlled trials. *Medical Education, 46*(7), 657–667. doi:10.1111/j.1365-2923.2012.04295.x

Watson, R. (2014). Commentary: Nursing must learn to adapt. *Canadian Journal of Nursing Leadership, 27*(2), 21–23.

Watterson, L., Flanagan, B., Donovan, B., & Robinson, B. (2000). Anaesthetic simulators: Training for the broader health-care profession. *Australian & New Zealand Journal of Surgery, 70*(10), 735–737. doi:10.1046/j.1440-1622.2000.01942.x

Waxman, K. T. (2010). The development of evidence-based clinical simulation scenarios: Guidelines for nurse educators. *Journal of Nursing Education, 49*(1), 29–35. http://doi.org/10.3928/01484834-20090916-07

Waxman, K. T., & Miller, M. (2014). Faculty development to implement simulations: Strategies and possibilities. In P. Jeffries (Ed.), *Clinical simulations in nursing education: Advanced concepts, trends and opportunities* (pp. 9–21). Philadelphia, PA: Wolters Kluwer.

Waxman, K. T., Nichols, A. A., O'Leary-Kelley, C., & Miller, M. (2011). The evolution of a statewide network: The Bay area simulation collaborative. *Simulation in Healthcare, 6*(6), 345–351. doi:10.1097/SIH.0b013e31822eaccc

Wear, D. (2008). On outcomes and humility. *Academic Medicine, 83*(7), 625–626. doi:10.1097/ACM.0b013e318178379f

WeatherSpark. (2015). *Average weather for Kigali, Rwanda.* Retrieved from https://weatherspark.com/averages/29294/Kigali-Rwanda

Weaver, A. (2011). High-fidelity patient simulation in nursing education: An integrative review. *Nursing Education Perspectives, 32*(1), 37–40.

Weaver, S. J., Lyons, R., Diazgranados, D., Rosen, M. A., Salas, E., Oglesby, J., … King, H. (2012). The anatomy of health care team training and the state of practice: A critical review. *Academic Emergency Medicine, 85*(11), 1746–1760. doi:10.1097/ACM.0b013e3181f2e907

Weaver, S. J., Newman-Toker, D. E., & Rosen, M. A. (2012). Reducing cognitive skill decay and diagnostic error: Theory-based practices for continuing education in health care. *Journal of Continuing Education in the Health Professions, 32*(4), 269–278. http://doi.org/10.1002/chp.21155

Wei, C. N. (2013). Barefoot doctors: The legacy of Chairman Mao's health care. In C. N. Wei & D. E. Brock (Eds.), *Mr. Science and Chairman Mao's cultural revolution: Science and technology in modern China* (pp. 251–280). Retrieved from http://www.researchgate.net/publication/260248644_Barefoot_Doctors_The_Legacy_of_Chairman_Maos_Health_Care

Weller, J. M., Nestel, D., Marshall, S. D., Books, P. M., & Conn, J. J. (2012). Simulation in clinical teaching and learning. *Medical Journal of Australia, 196*(9), 594–598. doi:10.5694/mja.10.11474

Wenger, A. F. (1995). Cultural context, health and health care decision making. *Journal of Transcultural Nursing, 7*(1), 3–14.

Whatis.com. (2016). *Photovoltaic glass.* Retrieved from http://whatis.techtarget.com/definition/photovoltaic-glass-PV-glass

Wheatley, M. (2009). *Turning to one another*. San Francisco, CA: Berrett-Koehler Publishers, Inc.

Wheatley, M. (2011). *Walk out walk on: A learning journey into communities daring to live the future now*. San Francisco, CA: Berrett-Koehler Publishers, Inc.

Wheatley, M. (2012). *So far from home: Lost and found in our brave new world*. San Francisco, CA: Berrett-Koehler Publishers, Inc.

Wheatley, M. J. (2006). *Leadership and the new science: Discovering order in a chaotic world* (3rd ed.). San Francisco, CA: Berrett-Koehler.

Wheatley, M. J. (2010). *Perseverance*. San Francisco, CA: Berrett-Koehler.

Whitmarsh, T., & Thompson, S. (2015). *The romance between Greece and the east*. Oxford, UK: Cambridge University Press.

Whitmire, R. (2010). *Why boys fail: Saving our sons from an educational system that's leaving them behind*. New York, NY: AMACOM Books.

Wiedenbach, E. (1964). *Clinical nursing: A helping art*. New York, NY: Springer.

Wild, C., & Foisy-Doll, C. (2017). Simulation champions as leaders, followers, & managers: Advocating, dreaming, influencing, challenging, and executing! In C. Foisy-Doll & K. Leighton (Eds.), *Simulation champions: Fostering courage, caring, and connection* (pp. xx–xx). Philadelphia, PA: Wolters Kluwer, Inc.

Wilford, A., & Doyle, T. (2006). Integrating simulation training into the nursing curriculum. *British Journal of Nursing, 15*(11), 607–610. http://dx.doi.org/10.12968/bjon.2006.15.17.21907

Wilkinson, T. J., & Harris, P. (2002). The transition out of medical school—A qualitative study of descriptions of borderline trainee interns. *Medical Education, 36*, 466–471. doi:10.1046/j.1365-2923.2002.01209.x

Willems, A., Waxman, B., Bacon, A. K., Smith, J., & Kitto, S. (2013). Interprofessional non-technical skills for surgeons in disaster response: A literature review. *Journal of Interprofessional Care, 27*(5), 380–386. http://doi.org/10.3109/13561820.2013.791670

Willhaus, J. (2009). Using simulations to promote clinical decision making. In P. R. Jeffries (Ed.), *Clinical simulations in nursing education: Advanced concepts, trends, and opportunities* (pp. 219–227). Philadelphia, PA: Wolters Kluwer Health.

Willhaus, J. (2013). *Measures of physiological and psychological stress in novice health professions students during a simulated patient emergency*. (Doctoral dissertation). ProQuest database (UMI 3587191).

Williams, B., & Edwards, D. (2015). Evidence-based education in paramedics. In T. Brown & B. Williams (Eds.), *Evidence-based education in the health professions: Promoting best practice in the learning and teaching of students* (pp. 437–447). London, UK: Radcliffe Publishing Ltd.

Williams, B. R., & Dunn, S. E. (2002, 2008). *Brain-compatible learning for the block*. Thousand Oaks, CA: Corwin Press.

Williams, J. (2016). The basics of branding. Retrieved from https://www.entrepreneur.com/article/77408

Williamson, M., & Harrison, L. (2010). Providing culturally appropriate care: A literature review. *International Journal of Nursing Studies, 47*, 761–769. doi:10.1016/j.ijnurstu.2009.12.012

Winters, C. A., & Echeverri, R. (2012). Teaching strategies to support evidence-based practice. *Critical Care Nurse, 32*(3), 49–54. doi:10.4037/ccn2012159

Wiseman, A., Haynes, C., & Hodge, S. (2013). Implementing professional integrity and simulation-based learning in health and social care: An ethical and legal maze or a professional requirement for high-quality simulated practice learning? *Clinical Simulation in Nursing, 9*(10), e437–e443. doi.org/10.1016/j.ecns.2012.12.004

Womack, J. P., Jones, D. T., & Roos, D. (1990). *The machine that changed the world*. New York, NY: Free Press.

Wong, C., & Cummings, G. (2009). Authentic leadership: A new theory for nursing or back to basics? *Journal of Health Organization and Management, 23*(5), 522–538. doi:10.1108/14777260910984014

Woods, C. (2015). *Can higher education innovators help transform teaching and learning?* Retrieved from http://www.centerdigitaled.com/higher-ed/Can-Higher-Education-Innovators-Help-Transform-Teaching-and-Learning.html

Woodward, C., & Gliva-McConvey, G. (1995). Children as standardized patients: Initial assessment of effects. *Teaching and Learning in Medicine, 7*(3), 188–191. http://dx.doi.org/10.1080/10401339509539739

World Atlas. (2015). The richest countries in the world. Retrieved from http://www.worldatlas.com/articles/100008-the-richest-nations-in-the-world-the-ten-richest-countries-on-the-planet

World Health Organization (WHO). (1978). *Declaration of Alma-Ata*. Retrieved from http://www.who.int/publications/almaata_declaration_en.pdf

World Health Organization (WHO). (1997). *Health promotion: The Jakarta Declaration on leading health promotion into the 21st century*. Retrieved from http://www.who.int/healthpromotion/conferences/previous/jakarta/declaration/en/index2.html

World Health Organization (WHO). (2009a). *European Union standards for nursing and midwifery* (2nd ed.). Denmark: Author.

World Health Organization (WHO). (2009b). *Global standards for the initial education of professional nurses and midwives*. Geneva, Switzerland: WHO Press. Retrieved from http://www.who.int/hrh/resources/standards/en/

World Health Organization (WHO). (2010). *Framework for action on interprofessional education and collaborative practice*. Retrieved from http://www.who.int/hrh/resources/framework_action/en/

World Health Organization (WHO). (2011). *Multi-professional patient safety curriculum guide*. Retrieved from http://www.who.int/patientsafety/education/curriculum/tools-download/en/

World Health Organization (WHO). (2013). *Transforming and scaling up health professionals' education and training: World health organization guidelines 2013*. Retrieved from http://www.who.int/hrh/resources/transf_scaling_hpet/en/

World Health Organization (WHO). (2015a). *European strategic directions for strengthening nursing and midwifery towards Health 2020 goals*. Retrieved from http://www.euro.who.int/en/health-topics/Health-systems/nursing-and-midwifery/publications/2015/european-strategic-directions-for-strengthening-nursing-and-midwifery-towards-health-2020-goals

World Health Organization (WHO). (2015b). *Health systems/equity*. Retrieved from http://www.who.int/healthsystems/topics/equity/en/

World Health Organization. (2015c). *Healthcare waste fact sheet*. Retrieved from http://www.who.int/mediacentre/factsheets/fs253/en/

World Health Organization (WHO). (2015d). *Patient safety*. Retrieved from http://www.who.int/patientsafety/implementation/taxonomy/en/

Worm, A. M., Hadjivassilious, M., & Katsambas, A. (2007). The Greek moulages: A picture of skin diseases in former times. *Journal of European Academy of Dermatology and Venereology*, 21(4), 515–519. doi:10.1111/j.1468-3083.2006.02018.x

Wright, A. S., Kim, S., Ross, B., & Pellegrini, C. (2011). ISIS: The Institute for Simulation and Interprofessional Studies at the University of Washington. *Journal of Surgical Education*, 68(1), 94–96. doi:10.1016/j.jsurg.2010.05.030

Wu, H.-K., Lee, S. W.-Y., Change, H.-Y., & Liang, J.-C. (2013). Current status, opportunities and challenges of augmented reality in education. *Computers & Education*, 62, 41–49. doi:10.1016/j.compedu.2012.10.024

Wu, L., Wang, Y., Peng, X., Song, M., Guo, X., Nelson, H., & Wang, W. (2014). Development of a medical academic degree system in China. *Medical Education Online*, 19. doi:10.3402/meo.v19.23141

Wucherer, P., Stefan, P., Weidert, S., Fallavollita, P., & Navab, N. (2013). Development and procedural evaluation of immersive medical simulations. In D. Barratt. S. Cotin, G. Fichtinger, P. Jannin & N. Navab. (Eds.), *Information processing in computer-assisted interventions* (Vol. 7915, pp. 1–10). Berlin/Heidelberg: Springer. doi:10.1007/978-3-642-38568-1

Wulf, C. (2010). Education as transcultural education: A global challenge. *Educational Studies in Japan: International Yearbook*, (5), 33–47. Retrieved from http://www.eric.ed.gov/ERICWebPortal/recordDetail?accno=EJ916673

Wyatt Knowlton, L., & Phillips, C. C. (2013). *The logic model guidebook: Better strategies for results*. Los Angeles, CA: Sage Publications, Inc.

Wyrostok, L. J., Hoffart, J., Kelly, I., & Ryba, K. (2014, April). Situated cognition as a learning framework for international end-of-life simulation. *Clinical Simulation in Nursing*, 10(4), e217–e222. http://dx.doi.org/10.1016/j.ecns.2013.11.005

Xu, Y. (2006, August). Clinical differences in nursing between east and west: Implications for Asian nurses. *Home Health Care Management and Practice*, 18(5), 420–423. http://dx.doi.org/10.1177/1084822306288438

Yajamanyam, P. K., & Sohi, D. (2015). In situ simulation as a quality improvement initiative. *Archives of Disease in Childhood – Education & Practice Edition*, 100(3), 162–163. doi:10.1136/archdischild-2014-306939

Yao, C. (2015). Workplace stress in a foreign environment: Chinese migrants in New Zealand. *Equality Diversity and Inclusion: An International Journal*, 34(7), 608–621. http://dx.doi.org/10.1108/EDI-08-2014-0065

Yerkes, R. M., & Dodson, J. M. (1908). The relation of strength of stimulus to rapidity of habit formation. *Journal of Comparative Neurology and Psychology*, 18, 459–482. doi:10.1002/cne.920180503

Young, H. M. (2016). Healthcare simulation operations: Bridging the gaps. In L. T. Gantt & H. M. Young (Eds.), *Healthcare simulation: A guide for operations specialists* (pp. 5–14). Hoboken, NJ: Wiley and Sons, Inc.

Young, H. M., & Scherwitz, M. A. (2015). Transitioning to a new center. In J. C. Palaganas, J. C. Maxworthy, C. A. Epps & M. E. Mancini (Eds.), *Defining excellence in simulation programs* (pp. 479–486). Philadelphia, PA: Wolters Kluwer.

Youngblood, A. Q., Zinkan, J. L., Tofil, N. M., & White, M. L. (2012). Multi-disciplinary simulation in pediatric critical care: The death of a child. *Critical Care Nurse*, 32, 55–61. doi:10.4037/ccn2012499

Yuan, H. B., Williams, B. A., & Fang, J. B. (2012). A systematic review of selected evidence on improving knowledge and skills through high-fidelity simulation. *Nurse Education Today*, 32(3), 294–298. http://dx.doi.org/10.1016/j.nedt.2011.07.010

Yule, S., Flin, R., Paterson-Brown, S., & Maran, N. (2006). Non-technical skills for surgeons in the operating room: A review of the literature. *Surgery*, 139(2), 140–149. http://doi.org/10.1016/j.surg.2005.06.017

Zaleznik, A. (1977). Managers and leaders: Are they different? *Harvard Business Review*, 55(3), 67–78.

Zenger Folkman (2009). *Developing others checklist*. Retrieved from http://zengerfolkman.com/wp-content/uploads/2013/05/ZF-Developing-Others-Checklist.pdf

Zenger, J. H., & Folkman, J. R. (2014). *Key insights from the extraordinary leader: 20 new ideas about leadership development*. Retrieved from www.zengerfolkman.com

Zenger, J. H., Folkman, J. R., & Edinger, S. K. (2010). *Emotions at work*. Retrieved from www.zengerfolkman.com

Zenger, J., Sandholtz, K., & Folkman, J. (2014). *Leadership under the microscope: The science behind developing extraordinary leaders*. Retrieved from http://zengerfolkman.com/white-papers/

Zerdejas, B., Brydges, R., Wang, A. T., & Cook, D. A. (2013). Patient outcomes in simulation-based medical education: A systematic review. *Journal of General Internal Medicine*, 28(8), 1078–1089. doi:10.1007/s11606-012-2264-5

Zhenhui, R. (2001). *Matching teaching styles with learning styles in East Asian contexts*. Retrieved from http://iteslj.org/Techniques/Zhenhui-TeachingStyles.html

Zhou, Y. (2014). The experience of China-educated nurses working in Australia: A symbolic interactionist perspective. *PLoS One*, 9(9), 1–10. http://dx.doi.org/doi:10.1371/journal.pone.0108143

Zigmont, J. J., Kappus, L. J., & Sudikoff, S. N. (2011). The 3D model of debriefing: Defusing, discovering, and deepening. *Seminars in Perinatology*, 35(2), 52–58. doi:10.1053/j.semperi.2011.01.003

Ziv, A., Erez, D., & Berkenstadt, H. (2008). Clinical simulation on a national level: Israel. In W. Kyle & R. Murray (Eds.), *Clinical simulation operations, engineering, and management* (pp. 371–378). San Diego, CA: Academic Press.

Ziv, A., Erez, D., Munz, Y., & Vardi, A. (2006). The Israel Center for Medical Simulation: A paradigm for cultural change in medical education. *International Medical Education*, 81(12), 1091–1097. doi:10.1097/01.ACM.0000246756.55626.1b

Zulkosky, K. D. (2012). Simulation use in the classroom: Impact on knowledge acquisition, satisfaction, and self-confidence. *Clinical Simulation in Nursing*, 8(1), e25–e33. doi:10.1016/j.ecns.2010.06.003

Zwarenstein, M., & Reeves, S. (2006). Knowledge translation and interprofessional collaboration: Where the rubber of evidence-based care hits the road of teamwork. *Journal of Continuing Education in the Health Professions*, 26(1), 46–54. doi:10.1002/chp.50

Index

(Note: Page numbers followed by *"f"* and *"t"* denote figures and tables, respectively.)